THE ENCYCLOPEDIA OF

GENETIC DISORDERS AND BIRTH DEFECTS

THIRD EDITION

James Wynbrandt
and
Mark D. Ludman, M.D., F.R.C.P.C

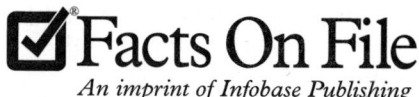

☑️ Facts On File

An imprint of Infobase Publishing

The information presented in this book is provided for research purposes only and is not intended to replace consultation with or diagnosis and treatment by medical doctors or other qualified experts. Readers who may be experiencing or witnessing a condition or disease described herein should seek medical attention and not rely on the information found here as medical advice.

The Encyclopedia of Genetic Disorders and Birth Defects, Third Edition

Copyright © 1991, 2000, 2008 by James Wynbrandt

Facts On File, Inc.
An imprint of Infobase Publishing
132 West 31st Street
New York NY 10001

Library of Congress Cataloging-in-Publication Data
Wynbrandt, James
The encyclopedia of genetic disorders and birth defects / James Wynbrandt and Mark D. Ludman.—3rd ed.
p. ; cm.
Includes bibliographical references and index.
ISBN 978-0-8160-6396-3 (hc : alk. paper) 1. Genetic disorders—Encyclopedias. 2. Abnormalities, Human—Encyclopedias. I. Ludman, Mark D. II. Title.
[DNLM: 1. Abnormalities—Encyclopedias—English. 2. Genetic Diseases, Inborn—Encyclopedias—English. 3. Genetics, Medical—Encyclopedias—English. QS 13 W985e 2007]

RB155.5.W96 2007
616'.04203—dc22   2006100640

Text and cover design by Cathy Rincon

Printed in the United States of America

VB Hermitage 10 9 8 7 6 5 4 3 2 1

This book is printed on acid-free paper and contains 30% post-consumer recycled content.

CONTENTS

PREFACE

Genetic disorders and birth defects comprise a vast galaxy of anomalous conditions and exert an extraordinary impact on the human population. Attempting even a partial catalog of them is daunting, indeed. More than 4,300 "single gene" disorders have been reported and are estimated to affect 1% of the population. The number of "multifactorial" disorders, those resulting from a combination of genes, is considered much greater. If late onset disorders are included, 60% of the population is thought to have a genetically influenced disease. Additionally, significant congenital anomalies, apparently unrelated to genetic influence, number in the thousands and are seen in approximately 2% to 3% of all live births.

We have included a little more than 1,000 entries in this encyclopedia, selected on the basis of the disorders' incidence and clinical and historical importance. We describe the condition, its prognosis, prevalence, mode of inheritance and the availability of carrier screening and prenatal diagnosis. For whom the condition is named and additional historical and anecdotal data are included where applicable and available. When known, the biochemical and molecular basis of the disorder is also given.

Entries for subjects and terminology important to genetic disorders and congenital anomalies are also included. Entry titles used within the text of other entries are in small capital letters the first time they appear, providing readers with numerous cross-references. However, we've attempted to make each entry stand alone, so that one can achieve a general understanding of a given topic without investigating additional entries. Resources to assist those seeking more information are listed in the appendixes. These are mostly private organizations. Addresses, phone numbers, Web site URLs and other contact information are found in the directory in the appendix. The appendix also contains an extensive listing of state, regional and federal government information resources. We urge readers to take advantage of these resources. Though entries were revised and updated through the final galley stage of this encyclopedia, rapid developments in the field of genetic and congenital anomalies add new knowledge to our understanding of this subject on an almost daily basis.

James Wynbrandt
Mark D. Ludman, M.D.

ACKNOWLEDGMENTS

We could not have created this encyclopedia without the help of many people and organizations. We wish to express our gratitude to them all, citing a few by name.

For their dedicated and tireless administrative assistance, we are deeply grateful to Emily Alexander, Gina Caimi, Deborah Hayes and Elizabeth Smith. For research and editorial assistance, heartfelt thanks to Leslie Brennan, Serena Chin, Betsy Hanson, Michael Herring, Gunnar Mengers, Rachel Pettman, Elizabeth Prata, Jed Russell, Linda Smith, M.D., Don Sontup, Dina Stein, Diann Peterson Trolle, Gayle Turim and Brian Wade. For encouragement and guidance, Allan Schanske, M.D., Rena Petrella, M.D., Ram Verma, M.D., and Anita Lustenberger. We would also like to thank Kurt Hirschhorn, M.D., who first interested Dr. Ludman in genetics and is responsible for the authors' collaboration on this encyclopedia. For their review and many helpful comments on the introductory essay, "A History of Human Genetics," very special thanks to Victor A. McKusick, M.D., and John M. Opitz, M.D.

Among the private and government organizations and their staffs that provided unfailing assistance, our gratitude to the March of Dimes Birth Defects Foundation, the Children's Defense Fund, the American College of Obstetricians and Gynecologists, the Centers for Disease Control, the American Academy of Pediatrics, the library and rare book collection of the New York Academy of Medicine, Johns Hopkins University, Mount Sinai School of Medicine, the DuPont Institute, the National Institute of Health, the National Center for Health Statistics, the National Center for Education in Maternal and Child Health, the National Institute of Child Health and Human Development, the Administration on Developmental Disabilities, the Clearinghouse on the Handicapped and, of course, the many support groups, associations and other organizations and individuals that were so generous with their time, resources and expertise.

We also wish to acknowledge all those physicians and scientists who have contributed to the knowledge that we have endeavored to summarize and catalog here, as well as the individuals and their families who have been touched by a genetic disorder or birth defect.

Dr. Ludman would also like to thank all those who taught him what he knows about genetics: instructors throughout his training; students, who constantly challenge him to learn more; and colleagues at the Mount Sinai School of Medicine in New York City and at the IWK Grace Health Centre, Atlantic Research Centre and Dalhousie University in Halifax, Nova Scotia.

Dr. Ludman expresses his appreciation to the Department of Human Genetics at Hadassah Medical Center in Jerusalem and the Department of Applied Human Nutrition at Mount Saint Vincent University in Halifax for providing research facilities during his sabbatical. It was at these institutions that much of the work for the encyclopedia's second edition was done. To his parents: Thanks for instilling the love of knowledge. And especially to his family for all the support they have given him throughout this project. He dedicates this book to his wife, Batya, and to his children, Benjamin Samuel, Aaron Joshua and Shayna Miriam. Dr. Ludman's wife now understands all too well why books are often dedicated to authors' spouses!

INTRODUCTION
A HISTORY OF HUMAN GENETICS

Little more than a century ago, in 1906, English zoologist William Bateson suggested to the scientific community that the study of heredity be named "genetics." Millennia of misconception preceded this christening, and the explosion of knowledge that has occurred since continues at a remarkable pace. It is a science with a singular ability to influence life, both in the general and individual sense, at its most profound level, a field with a promising future and a rich history.

Interest in the subject is as old as humankind and began with the realization that living things beget other living things in their own image and the observation of unique differences among individuals. Conditions arising from genetic aberrations have also been observed throughout human history. For example, archaeologists have found remains of dwarfs dating to prehistoric times. No doubt various legends and myths were created to explain these variations, both normal and abnormal, explanations probably no more fanciful than many that existed, even in scientific circles, from the beginning of recorded history until the dawn of the 20th century.

In a void without scientific understanding, the public historically has grappled with the causes and consequences of these conditions and variations on its own, resulting in a long tradition of fables and fallacies.

Babylonians regarded the birth of deformed infants or stillborn fetuses as portents from the gods. Astrological records from Babylon and Nineveh dating to 2800 B.C. indicate a great familiarity with anomalous congenital conditions in humans. Specific deformities were linked to specific prophesies, heralding events from war to natural disasters such as an earthquake, as well as peace or the favorable reign of a monarch. The Greeks had their tales of cyclopes and stories of hermaphrodites. In England in the Middle Ages, those who could not hear, and hence had not learned to speak, were thought to be stupid and labeled "dumb." And in the relatively recent past, the curious have flocked to see "prodigies" (such as Tom Thumb and Chang and Eng, the "Siamese" twins), individuals whose physical abnormalities formed the basis of performing careers that often brought them great fortune and renown.

The Roots of Genetics

What we now know as genetics has its roots in early history, with the development of agriculture. Animal and plant breeding were employed in Egyptian times; farmers crossed their best stock, surmising the offspring would also be superior. Babylonians are thought to have artificially cross-fertilized date palms. Stone carvings at least 4,000 years old from Chaldea (near the Persian Gulf) describe different pedigrees, showing the inheritance of specific traits of a horse's mane. Jews recognized a familial link in some diseases; according to the Tosafot, the commentary on the law of the Talmud, a boy need not undergo circumcision if his mother had previously given birth to two male infants who had bled to death at circumcision. This is obviously an allusion to hemophilia, a hereditary disorder seen almost exclusively in males, but whose pedigree pattern was not recognized by the scientific community until the 1800s.

It was likewise recognized that children often appeared to resemble their parents and that certain traits ran in families. Around 500 B.C., Pythagoras, the philosopher and mathematician, theorized that human life originated from a blend of male and female fluids, or semens, that came from within the body. Two centuries later, Aristotle, who believed males were primarily responsible for passing on hereditary characteristics, proposed that the semens were purified elements of blood, a belief that lingers today in phrases such as "blood relative" and "royal blood." Hippocrates, the father of medicine (ca. 460–377 B.C.), had his own ideas about these fluids: "The semen is produced by the whole body, healthy by healthy parts, sick by sick parts. Hence, when as a rule, baldheaded beget baldheaded, blue eyed beget blue eyed, and squinting, squinting." He had the mode of transmission wrong, but he clearly recognized the genetic nature of certain traits and disorders, as is further noted in his comments about epilepsy, the "divine" affliction (so called because those afflicted were said to have been blessed by the gods): "But this disease seems to me to be no more divine than others . . . Its origin is hereditary like that of other diseases . . . What is to hinder it from happening that where the father and mother were subject to this disease, certain of their offspring should be affected also?"

The Institutes of Manu in India during the first centuries of the Common Era proposed an agricultural model of heredity: Males provided the seed, while females provided the field in which the seed was planted and grew.

Despite these pioneering efforts, the nature of the connection between the parent and offspring, its method of transmission, how deformities arose, how hereditary patterns emerged or how they could remain hidden through generations was completely unknown. For centuries it remained a riddle, referred to as "the mysterious force." Erroneous assumptions based on classical Greek concepts persisted through the Middle Ages. Among them: The sex of a child is determined by the dominator of the sexual act; characteristics of offspring arise from the heat of the womb or which testis the sperm came from; sperm is secreted from all parts of the body during intercourse and responsible for reproducing that part of the body from which it was secreted. In the 1600s, the concept of the "manikin" was popular: Each sperm contained a small but complete "manikin," which would simply grow larger in the womb, rather than develop as a plant from a seed. In the 1700s, a theory of heredity popularized by French naturalist George-Louis Leclerc, comte de Buffon postulated that the male determined bodily extremities (head, tail, limbs) while the female was responsible for internal constituents and overall size and shape. A belief that persisted beyond that century was that the "essence" from each vital organ of the parents' bodies somehow blended to create a new individual. However, foreshadowings of modern concepts of heredity began to appear. In the mid-1600s, Dutch scientist Regnier de Graaf advanced the idea of a new being arising from the union of sperm and egg. (The question of whether the primary component of heredity transmission was the sperm or the egg led to a lively dispute between the so-called "ovists" and "spermatists.")

During the 1700s, pedigrees, the patterns whereby traits are transmitted from generation to generation, were recognized for the first time. (Members of the Hapsburgs, the ruling family of the Austrian Empire, were known in the Middle Ages for a characteristic "Hapsburg nose" and jutting chin seen in portraits extending over several centuries.) In 1751, French naturalist Pierre-Louis Moreau de Maupertuis invoked "elementary particles" as a transmission agent to explain a family in which several generations exhibited the trait of polydactyly (having more than the normal number of fingers and/or toes). In Système de la Nature, he also suggested that mutations might account for the diversity of life.

Botanists became interested in plant breeding, leading to horticultural experiments that laid the groundwork for modern genetics. When new species of plants appeared, as they did periodically, efforts were made to explain their occurrence. In 1760, Joseph Gottlieb Kolreuter created the first experimentally produced plant hybrid (the offspring of two different species), by mixing two species of the tobacco plant. This in turn helped generate extensive studies of the function of pollen. He also proposed, as had Maupertuis, that both parents contributed an equal hereditary element to their offspring. Yet, other than botanical studies, the scientific community showed little interest in questions of genetics and heredity, an attitude that changed markedly in the 19th century, as a spirit of inquiry and innovative technologies spread.

In 1814, Joseph Adams published "A Treatise on the Supposed Hereditary Property of Disease," a remarkably prescient work in which he indicated an appreciation for many of the hallmarks of hereditary theory. He distinguished between recessive and dominant conditions, noted hereditary predisposition in some disorders and the role of environmental influence in their development, and surmised that higher rates of familial diseases found in isolated populations could be due to inbreeding. He even invoked the concept of new mutations, by stating that the reproductive ability of many patients with hereditary conditions would eventually disappear were it not for their spontaneous appearance in healthy families.

Darwin and Mendel

During the mid-19th century, attention shifted from different species to variations within a given species (population groups) and the question of why various populations of a species were not all alike. The major catalyst for the shift was Charles Darwin's (1809–82) monumental *On the Origin of Species by Means of Natural Selection* (1859), which created an intense interest in the mechanics of evolution. Darwin was already well respected for his first book, *The Zoology of the Voyage of the Beagle* (1840), an account of his five-year voyage on H.M.S. *Beagle*, on which he sailed as an unpaid naturalist. At one stop, the Galápagos Islands, 15 small rocky outcroppings straddling the equator some 700 miles west of South America, Darwin noted that species of birds that had migrated to different islands had evolved slight differences. He

concluded the changes were the result of random variations. If the variation was beneficial, those possessing it were more likely to survive and multiply, a theory he called "natural selection." Darwin published his interpretation of these observations after his attention was brought to a manuscript by Alfred Russell Wallace, who was about to publish a paper with similar conclusions based on observations in the Malaysian islands. Darwin's theories, further delineated in *The Descent of Man* (1871), also addressed common ancestry among species, a concept often misinterpreted as man's having descended from apes. To this day, in the Western world, Darwin's theories of evolution are not universally accepted, primarily by those who find them incompatible with biblical accounts of the origin of life.

As science became more sophisticated in its outlook on genetics and heredity, so did the public. The hereditary nature of some disorders was now accepted. One of the characters in Nathaniel Hawthorne's *The House of the Seven Gables*, published in 1851, suffered from a disease (now speculated as being hereditary angioedema) that Hawthorne described as a fatal condition whose "mode of death has been an idiosyncrasy with this family, for generations past." Hemophilia was also known in New England to have a hereditary component. A familial link in color blindness had been recognized by the end of the 18th century.

It was also during this time that Gregor Johann Mendel (1822–84) was conducting experiments with garden peas. Mendel, an Austrian, was a monk in Brünn (now Brno), Moravia (now a part of the Czech Republic). Beginning his experiments in 1856, he noticed that pea plants had varying traits; some unripe pods were yellow, others green; some varieties were tall, while others were dwarfed. The position of the flowers, whether clustered at the top or distributed along the stem, also varied, as did the physical appearance of the peas themselves, being either smooth or wrinkled.

Using hybrid garden pea plants, Mendel's goal was to study the transmission of characteristics to their offspring, and the statistical relation of their subsequently appearing traits. Mendel had studied physics and mathematics, and he carefully recorded and attempted to explain his observations. During this time, he was also in written communication with Karl von Naegeli, one of the most respected botanists of his day.

Prevailing theory of the time held that heredity was a blending process. According to this theory, if two pea plants, one producing wrinkled peas and one producing smooth peas, were crossed, the first generation of their offspring should produce peas halfway between smooth and wrinkled: a blending of the parental traits. This wasn't what Mendel found when he crossed two true breeding strains (one always producing smooth, the other always producing wrinkled peas). The first (F1, or first filial) generation produced plants that yielded only smooth peas. Crossbreeding these F1 plants, he produced a second generation (F2). Three-quarters of the F1 plants produced peas that were smooth, and one-quarter produced wrinkled peas. Thus, the traits transmitted from parents didn't blend, but remained distinct, segregated, and had the ability to reappear in subsequent generations. This became the basis of his first law, the law of segregation. His hypothesis that the essence of heredity is particulate, that each trait is represented by only two alternate forms, one contributed by the male and one by the female, was a completely new idea, one that would eventually revolutionize genetics. (These alternative forms of traits are now known to reflect alternative forms of a gene, and are called "alleles.") He further proposed that these factors were either dominant or recessive: A dominant trait would override the influence of its complementary factor; the influence of recessive traits would recede when paired with a dominant complement.

Mendel presented his findings to the Natural History Society of Brünn in 1865, and they were published the following year in the society's proceedings, in a monograph entitled "Experiments in Plant Hybridization." No one appreciated their importance. Naegeli was unimpressed and suggested Mendel continue his experiments with another plant, the hawkweed. Mendel followed his advice, but the experiments proved frustrating, totally at odds with the results that would have been expected based on his experience with garden peas. This is not surprising, as it was later discovered that hawkweed reproduces asexually and therefore inherits the genetic endowment of only one parent. Eventually, Mendel was promoted to abbot of the monastery and no longer had the time to devote to his careful breeding experiments. He published only one other botanical paper, reporting his unsuccessful experience with hawkweed. However, he continued carefully to monitor and keep detailed records of meteorology. Upon his death, the succeeding abbot burned most of his papers.

New Theories and Discoveries

In the absence of a unifying theory that Mendel's work would have provided, others struggled to explain hereditary transmission. Most theories incorporated the now-accepted notion that heredity was based on a system of self-replicating, living units, which had variously been called "physiological units," "gemmules," "idioplasm," "micellae" and "pangenes." These theories included Darwin's "provisional hypothesis on pangenesis," offered in *Variation of Animals and Plants Under Domestication* (1868), and English philosopher and naturalist Herbert Spencer's (1820–1903) "theory of physiological units," proposed in *The Principles of Biology* (1864), which somewhat approximated Mendel's much more refined theories. Dutch botanist Hugo De Vries weighed in with "intracellular pangenesis." Other plant geneticists came close to Mendel's idea of discrete hereditary units, hinting at ideas of dominance and segregation without managing to articulate an overall interpretation. Among the stumbling blocks was the still-accepted view that heredity was a blending of traits. There was also the insistence that theories explain the inheritance of acquired traits, a theory initially proposed by French naturalist Jean-Baptiste de Lamarck (1744–1829) in 1809, and taken as an article of faith by many geneticists. According to this concept, a physical change in an individual can be passed on to offspring; for example, if enough mice in subsequent generations have their tails cut off, sooner or later, their offspring will be born without tails. (Despite his erroneous assumption, de Lamarck was perhaps the first to propose that species adapted to cope with changes in their environment, which would become a cornerstone in the theory of evolution.)

Francis Galton (1822–1911) contributed the idea of examining identical twins to study aspects of heredity. He deduced that twins must be genetically identical, and therefore were ideal to study the comparative influence of heredity and environment, which he referred to as "nature versus nurture." A proponent of the blending theory of genetics, he developed a method of statistical analysis he called "biometrics" that used complex mathematics to explain transmission of hereditary characteristics. In 1883 he formalized another idea that was to have a profound impact; he called it "eugenics," the improvement of a population by selective breeding of its best specimens. Though long practiced by farmers in plants and animals, Galton's concept of applying it to the human population was enthusiastically championed by many, initiating a eugenics movement that would hold sway for the next half century, until Nazi policies and atrocities committed in its name, as well as its ethical implications and practical problems, discredited it. In the United States and Canada, the movement was responsible for the passage of laws forbidding mentally deficient individuals from having children—statutes that were enforced through compulsory sterilization, and which remained on the books in some states and provinces until after World War II. The Cold Spring Harbor Laboratory, in Long Island, New York, one of the most respected genetics research centers in the world, began as the Eugenics Records Office, and became a center for the promulgation of many of these policies in North America.

Despite the prevalence of well-argued misconceptions, the 1800s was a century of scientific ferment, both literally and figuratively. Studies of the cell were well under way in the first half of the 19th century, with microscopy sufficiently advanced to be an invaluable research tool. (In the late 1600s, using a primitive microscope, Robert Hooke had seen structures in tissue he named "cells," giving birth to cytology, the science and study of cells.) In 1865, Louis Pasteur (1822–95) proposed his "germ theory of disease," hypothesizing that disease could be spread by invisible microbes, or germs. Pasteur also described the concepts of inoculation, pasteurization and fermentation, the last of which led to the discovery of enzymes, organic catalysts involved in life-sustaining chemical reactions within the cells. (When first discovered, they were called "ferments.") Advances in chemistry also aided research into the secrets of heredity; by 1810 the distinction between organic and inorganic compounds had been established, and scientists set about trying to re-create the compounds in laboratories. In the mid-1850s, these efforts led to another discovery—synthetic dyes. The aniline dyes developed in England created several fortunes for the chemists involved in their discovery, and also proved to be invaluable genetic research tools. It was soon noted that various structures in the cell absorbed dyes in varying amounts, making them easier to view under a microscope. Soon, Scottish botanist Robert Brown identified a central area of the cell, which he named the "nucleus."

Further studies revealed that cells contained carbohydrates, lipids and proteins. In 1871, Swiss chemist Friedrich Miescher reported isolating a new substance from the nucleus of the cell, and named it "nuclein." When it was later discovered to have the properties of an acid, it was renamed "nucleic acid." However, the importance of his discovery would remain unrecognized for three-quarters of a century. Also in this decade, German biologist Walther Flemming discovered a staining technique that revealed tiny thread-like bodies within the nucleus. Due to their ready absorption of dye, they became known as "chromosomes," colored bodies. In 1882 Flemming published drawings of these structures based on his observations, showing them in a cycle of positions in which they regularly aligned themselves. He was observing, for the first time, the splitting and replication of genetic material during cell division. This process was soon formally dubbed "mitosis," from the Greek "formation of threads."

Pondering the doubling of genetic material that accompanied mitosis, German physician August Weismann theorized that there must be a mechanism for reducing the genetic material in sex cells, the sperm and egg that united to create one new being. Otherwise, the joining of cells with two complete complements of chromosomes would create offspring with double the normal number of chromosomes in the first generation and, if they continued doubling, an astronomical number of chromosomes several generations in the future. In the mid-1880s, the existence of this reduction mechanism, to be called "meiosis," was confirmed in observations made by Eduard von Beneden.

By the beginning of the new century, it was known that nucleic acid and histone proteins were the basic components of chromosomes, and cytologists accepted chromosomes as the vehicle for hereditary transmission. But while some believed nucleic acid was the most important constituent of the chromosomes, many, particularly biologists, thought the proteins were more important. Nucleic acids were much simpler than the proteins. Far too simple, it was thought, to contain the information required to propagate a species, a view that persisted in some scientific quarters until the 1950s. But whatever the agents for hereditary transmission might be, as the 20th century dawned, the principles that governed their actions remained unknown.

Mendelism

While working on papers attempting to explain the heredity riddle, and in the course of investigating previous work in the field, three botanists—Hugo De Vries, Carl Correns from the University of Tubingen and Erich von Tschermak Seysenegg, an agricultural assistant who worked near Vienna—independently and within months of each other came upon the work of Gregor Mendel. They immediately recognized its importance and incorporated his findings in their own published work, all in 1900. (The question has been raised whether all of them had at first planned to credit Mendel in their papers; but prior to publication, all became aware of their mutual knowledge of his theories, voiding any possibility of denying Mendel his due.) Once his work was rediscovered, "Mendelism," as it came to be called, was an overnight sensation. The major champion of Mendelism before the scientific community was English zoologist William Bateson (1861–1926). He had Mendel's paper translated into English and published in the *Journal of the Royal Horticultural Society* in 1900. Botanists and scientists across the Continent hurriedly duplicated Mendel's results and hailed his theories' power and simplicity, which

explained the results of many of their own experiments. Bateson also introduced the term "genetics" in 1906, formally proposing to the scientific community that the term be used for the study of heredity and variation. (It first appears in a 1905 letter of his; however, the term "cytogenetics" has been dated to 1903, used by American Walter S. Sutton in a paper, "The Chromosomes in Heredity," published in the *Biological Bulletin*.)

With Mendel's theories providing the framework, genetic research advanced quickly in the first decade of the 20th century. Physician and biochemist Archibald E. Garrod, conducting research aided by Bateson, established the idea of an "inborn error of metabolism," a block at some point in a metabolic reaction sequence that he postulated was due to the congenital deficiency of a specific enzyme. In 1902, he identified alkaptonuria (an essentially benign disorder whose most noticeable feature is that the urine of affected individuals turns black when left standing in light) as such an inborn error of metabolism. This is considered the first proof of Mendelian inheritance in man. Brachydactyly (having unusually short fingers or toes) and the human ABO blood groups were also held to be examples of Mendelian inheritance by 1910. Garrod's work is considered the beginning of both modern biochemical genetics and medical genetics. In the same year that Garrod identified alkaptonuria as an inborn error of metabolism, American W. E. Castle began a systematic study of heredity with laboratory rodents and, beginning in 1905, with the fly *Drosophila melanogaster,* studies that had large impacts on genetic research. The term "gene" was introduced in 1909 by Wilhelm Ludwig Johannsen (1857–1927), a pharmacist's apprentice from Copenhagen who had gone on to become a respected geneticist and botanist, despite his lack of a university degree. He defined a gene as an accounting or calculating unit of heredity. He also introduced the term "genotype" (an individual's genetic makeup) and "phenotype" (an individual's physical appearance, which may or may not reflect his or her genotype).

By the middle of this decade, assaults on Mendel's law of segregation of traits had proved futile, and it was now the foundation of hereditary theory. Variations that could not be explained according to his theories were now accepted as being caused by spontaneous changes. The Hardy-Weinberg equation of 1908 also helped bolster the case for Mendel. The equation demonstrated gene distribution in randomly mating populations and explained the unanswered question of why dominant characteristics do not increase at the expense of recessive characteristics, thereby eventually replacing them. Independently postulated by English mathematician G. H. Hardy and German physician W. Weinberg, it formed a cornerstone of population genetics, the study of factors involved in human evolution.

By the end of the decade, Mendel's laws were accepted as applying to humans and animals as well as plants. The concept of genes was also now accepted, as was their role in controlling the production of enzymes. However, rearguard actions against Mendel's theories continued to be fought by Galton's disciples, the "biometricians," most notably Karl Pearson (1857–1936), who argued that Mendel's stark dominant and recessive approach failed to account for quantitative traits such as height, intelligence and body size. In an interesting coda to the battle, in 1918, English statistician and geneticist Sir Ronald Fisher (1890–1962) pointed out that there is no fundamental inconsistency between Mendelism and the blending concept of heredity; these quantitative traits involved the action of many genes, each behaving individually while blending with the action of others.

In 1910, American zoologist and geneticist Thomas Hunt Morgan (1866–1945) published his paper "Chromosomes and Heredity," ushering in the era of the "chromosome theory" of heredity. The foundations for this era had been laid in the previous decade. Sutton and Theodor Boveri of Germany independently suggested in 1903 that chromosomes were the carriers of genetic information and occurred in pairs, one inherited from the male and one from the female. Studies published in 1904 by A. B. Darbishire of two coat-color genes in the house mouse established the important concept of "linkage"; some individual traits tended to be inherited together. This was later demonstrated to be due to the genes for these traits being located on the same chromosome. (Mendel had been very fortunate; the genes for traits he chose to study were all located on different chromosomes of the pea plants and thus were not linked. Had they been, it would have been virtually impossible to interpret the results of his experiments correctly.) Inheritance of sex-linked traits was demonstrated in plumage patterns on Plymouth Rock fowls in 1909. (Sex chromosomes had been observed almost 20 years previously, by H. Henking in 1891, and their function identified soon after the rediscovery of Mendel's laws.)

At Columbia University, Morgan established what became known as the "fly group." When he began his work, Morgan was not a committed Mendelist, but his work with *Drosophila melanogaster* soon changed his mind about Mendel, and made *Drosophila* the subject of choice for geneticists. Often called the fruit fly, but actually the pomace or vinegar fly, *Drosophila* could quickly and easily be cultivated for study of transmission of traits; one female could provide several hundred offspring in less than two weeks, and simple breeding methods allowed easy analysis of specific traits. (Years later, it would be discovered that *Drosophila* also has "giant" chromosomes in its salivary glands, greatly easing visual examination of this material.) In 1910, Morgan noted a variation in one of his flies: The eyes were white instead of red. Breeding it produced more white-eyed flies, and further experiments revealed they were always males and eventually established the chromosomal basis of sex-linked inheritance. (In 1933, Morgan became the first geneticist to win the Nobel Prize.)

In 1911, E. B. Wilson identified the X chromosome as the location of the gene for color blindness, the first time a gene had been assigned to a specific chromosome, a pioneering demonstration of gene mapping. Hemophilia was recognized as an X-linked disorder during this same period. Later in the decade, sickle-cell anemia, a blood disorder found primarily in blacks, and whose characteristic "sickled," collapsed red blood cells had been first described in 1910, was identified as a recessive disorder.

During the period from 1910 to 1930, genetics slowly narrowed its focus from the chromosome to the gene. Research primarily involved experimental breeding, cytological observations and direct chemical and physical study of chromosomes and the proteins and nucleic acids from which they were built. With the basic laws and principles elucidated, the dramatic breakthroughs of the first decade gave way to exploring the territory that had so recently been claimed. The discovery of the mutagenic properties of X-rays was a major advance of this period. Previously, researchers had to wait for variations, which are useful for study and experimentation, to occur naturally, which rarely happened; genetic material appeared remarkably stable and impervious to alteration. But in 1927, Hermann J. Muller, who'd been a student of Morgan's, published "Artificial Transmutation of the Gene," a paper reporting that male flies exposed to heavy doses of X-rays exhibited new variation rates 15,000 times above normal. He called these changes "mutations." (He received the Nobel Prize for his work in 1946.) The following year, Lewis Stadler reported similar findings using maize, a corn plant, and barley.

Also during this period, unnoticed by most, an English microbiologist Frederick Griffith isolated a material from the cells that could influence heredity. Mixing the material with other cells, he found he could change hereditary characteristics of the bacterium he used in his research. His report of a "transformation" principle in 1928, overlooked at the time, represented the first isolation of DNA.

As improved health care conquered more infectious and nutritional diseases, the impact of genetically influenced disorders became more apparent. Antibiotics prolonged the lives of those affected with some of these conditions, revealing their previously unrecognized hereditary nature. Cystic fibrosis, among the most widely distributed hereditary disorders in white populations, was first definitively described in 1937. In 1934, Ivar Asbjørn Følling, a Norwegian physician, identified phenylketonuria, a common metabolic disorder that had previously resulted in mental retardation, but was ultimately found (in 1954) to be relatively easy to treat. This would lead in the 1960s to the first large-scale screening program for early detection of an inherited disorder.

However, it was also during these years that the study of genetics was subjected to political and ideological assault, particularly in the Soviet Union and Germany. Nazi eugenic breeding experiments and Soviet "geneticist" Trofim Denisovich Lysenko (1898–1976) dealt devastating blows to the science. Nazi physician Josef Mengele conducted experiments using 1,500 pairs of twins. Lysenko, whose ideas held sway in the Soviet Union for a quarter of a century, preached a socialist brand of Lamarckism, the theory of inheritance of acquired characteristics. He refused to acknowledge any hereditary property of chromosomes or genes, leading to the suppression of research and teaching of modern genetics in the Soviet Union from 1938 to 1963.

The Building Blocks of Heredity

The 1940s marked the dawn of molecular genetics. The seminal development was Dr. Linus Pauling's work with the sickle-cell trait, in which he identified the flaw in the hemoglobin molecule that results in sickle-cell anemia. This change altered the molecule's electrical charge. Thus, it behaved differently in an electrical field, a fact Pauling used to detect the abnormal molecules themselves. (He won the 1954 Nobel Prize in chemistry for his work.) This was also the era in which biochemical genetics flowered. George Beadle and Edward L. Tatum at California's Stanford University demonstrated the one-one correlation between genes and proteins. They began their experiments in the late 1930s with the mold *Neurospora crassa*. After inducing gene mutations with X-rays, they proved that a subsequent nutritional deficiency in the mold resulted from the lack of an enzyme the mutated gene was responsible for producing. This confirmed and explained the "inborn errors of metabolism" whose existence had been hypothesized at the turn of the century by Garrod. (Beadle and Tatum shared the Nobel Prize for their discovery in 1958.) By the end of the 1950s, a handful of the more than 250 recessive disorders then reported had been identified as enzyme deficiency diseases.

During this same period, DNA was established as the vehicle of hereditary transmission. In 1944, Dr. Oswald Avery at Rockefeller University in New York, building upon the earlier work of Griffith, demonstrated the transmission of characteristics from one strain of bacteria to another through DNA. By the end of the decade, the composition of nucleic acid was known, but its structure was not, setting the stage for one of genetics' major discoveries.

Drs. James D. Watson and Francis H. C. Crick of the Medical Research Council Laboratories in Cambridge, England, were among those trying to deduce the structure of DNA, basing their ideas on its behavior. They consulted extensively with Maurice Wilkins, a physicist who was attempting to make X-ray photographs of a DNA molecule. In 1953, Watson and Crick published their groundbreaking "Structural Implications of Deoxyribonucleic Acid," in which they proposed the double-helix model for DNA. Simultaneously, Wilkins published his X-ray photographs of the molecule, revealing a helical structure. (The three shared the Nobel Prize in 1962 for their work.)

As described by Watson and Crick, DNA consists of two long, linked strands, resembling a tightly coiled spiral staircase. It is composed of smaller units called nucleotides, which in turn are made of a sugar molecule, a phosphate and any one of four nitrogen bases: adenine, thymine, guanine or cystosine. These nitrogen bases link up with complementary bases on the other strand, forming "base pairs." Adenine always joins with thymine, and guanine is always paired with cytosine. The model explained both how DNA was built and how it functioned. It outlined how DNA replicated itself during mitosis and how it orchestrated the production of enzymes and proteins. In effect, the two strands would "unzip," separating at the base pairs, and each strand would then form a template, attracting new bases to construct a mirror image, exactly like the other strand, which was now also building its complement. When mitosis was complete, there would be two sets of the DNA, both exactly like the original. For the production of proteins, only a portion of the DNA would unzip, attracting ribonucleic acid (RNA) to re-create portions of the DNA, which held the code to building proteins from amino acids. The RNA would then leave the cell nucleus and itself become a template on which the proteins would be assembled. Watson and Crick's hypothesis was as simple and important in its own way as Mendel's postulations, providing a framework for all subsequent research in genetics.

There were other significant advances in the 1950s. After years of having to content themselves examining chromosomes from *Drosophila*, new techniques began to bring human chromosomes into better focus. In 1952, Dr. T. C. Hsu, at the University of Texas at Galveston, found that chromosomes exposed to a hypotonic solution, that is, one in which the concentration of sodium and chloride is less than in the cells, absorbed water and became more visible. By the middle of the decade the field of clinical genetics, the medical application of knowledge of genetics, was established, and a score of medical centers in the United States had medical genetics facilities. In 1956, Drs. Joe Hin Tjio and Albert Levan, using improved staining techniques they'd developed, demonstrated that humans have 23 pairs of chromosomes, or a total of 46. (It had been thought since 1923 that humans had 48 chromosomes.) The technique led to the identification of conditions caused by chromosome abnormalities. In 1958, French pediatrician Jerome Lejeune announced at a conference at McGill University the finding of a chromosomal abnormality in Down syndrome, and his findings were published the following year. By the end of the decade, the chromosomal basis of Turner syndrome, Klinefelter syndrome and other chromosomal abnormalities had been identified. (Down syndrome had been identified by English physician J. L. H. Langdon-Down in 1866, and Dutch physician P. J. Waardenburg suggested as early as 1932 that it could be caused by a chromosomal abnormality.)

New methods to halt various stages of mitosis, using chemicals, such as colchicine, as well as hypotonic solutions, made study of the chromosomes easier by suspending them in more advantageous viewing positions. Another chemical, phytohemaglutinin, was found to stimulate the division of lymphocytes, white blood cells. This led the way to genetic testing using blood, rather than tissue samples, greatly easing investigation of human genetic anomalies.

With these growing chromosome visualization abilities, scientists were now making microphotographs of human chromosomes to allow for their study. They would cut the pictures apart and arrange the individual chromosome pairs according to their size and the position of their centromere, the point at which the two chromosomes in a pair are joined. These blownup microphotos were called "karyotypes," and at a meeting of cytogeneticists in Denver in 1960, a standard method of arranging the human chromosomes in karyotypes was adopted, known as the Denver classification. Though since amended, the Denver classification remains the accepted method of karyotype display.

During the 1960s, modern medical-scientific study of genetic and congenital anomalies came into its own, as did clinical genetics and genetic counseling. The first catalog of genetic disorders, composed of a survey of X-linked traits, was published in 1962, assembled by Dr. Victor McKusick of Johns Hopkins University. (McKusick's survey grew into "Mendelian Inheritance in Man," a catalog of known or suspected single gene disorders that, by the end of the 1990s, contained some 4,300 autosomal dominant, autosomal recessive and X-linked conditions. By the end of 2007, the online version included more than 18,000 single gene disorders.) Prenatal diagnosis became a reality with the development of amniocentesis. First used for an intrauterine transfusion in 1963, in 1966 M. W. Steele and W. R. Breg demonstrated how the procedure could be used to collect and cultivate fetal cells whose chromosomes could then be examined and tested for any number of genetic disorders. By the end of the 1960s, the procedure was perfected.

This was also the decade in which the actual "genetic code," the chemical instructions contained in the DNA, was cracked: The code consists of a triplet of adjacent nucleotides, on a strand of DNA, that form a single message. Each nucleotide triplet is called a codon, and a gene was now defined as a series of codons that give the instructions for building a specific protein. Each codon may represent either a single one of the 20 amino acids found in humans, which make a protein, or it may be an instruction to stop or start production of a chain of amino acids.

But the size and complexity of DNA molecules continued to perplex researchers wishing to study individual genes and slowed progress in determining their secrets.

The early 1970s brought developments that helped isolate segments of DNA, greatly assisting the study of individual genes and groups of genes. Swiss microbiologist Werner Arber, working with *Escherichia coli* (*E. coli*), common intestinal bacteria, and Drs. Hamilton O. Smith and Daniel Nathans of Johns Hopkins University, using the bacteria *Hemophilus influenzae*, announced the discovery of enzymes produced by the bacteria that could cut the DNA of some viruses and bacteria at specific points. These became the first "restriction enzymes," which would become a key tool for genetic researchers. Ultimately, it enabled the isolation of short segments of DNA, assisting the search for specific genes. All three shared the Nobel Prize in 1979. (By the beginning of the 1990s, over 200 restriction enzymes had been isolated from bacteria, each of which can cut a DNA molecule at separate and specific points, based on the sequence of nucleotides on the DNA chain. By 2008, more than 3,800 restriction enzymes had been identified.) Once isolated, the function of some genes on these segments could be identified, or at least their location "mapped" to specific points on the chromosomes. Modern gene mapping had its genesis in the 1960s with the creation of human-mouse "hybrid cells." Human cells were fused together with cultured tumor cells from mice, combining the genetic material of the two species. After several cell divisions, only a portion of the human DNA, identifiable fragments of human chromosomes, would remain. By examining the human protein products of the hybrid cells, the location of the gene that controlled its production could now be placed on the human chromosome. But the difficulty of obtaining specific chromosome fragments had hindered progress. Once restriction enzymes were discovered, the ability to slice up DNA quickly and easily led to techniques to "recombine" the resulting fragments of DNA. This allowed investigators to take specific fragments of DNA from one cell and graft them into the DNA of another. "Recombinant DNA," as the reconstituted genetic material was called, could be placed into the nucleus of bacteria to study the influence of the human genes or to manufacture the enzyme the gene is responsible for producing. Using a combination of these techniques, by the early 1980s, human insulin and human growth hormone were being manufactured by genetically engineered *E. coli.*

Chromosome fragments created with restriction enzymes also proved vitally important in linkage studies, allowing the prenatal diagnosis of some genetic disorders even though the gene responsible had not been identified. This linkage was first used in 1978, to predict those at risk for developing sickle-cell anemia, demonstrated by Drs. Yuet Wai Kan and Andrees M. Dozy of the University of California at San Francisco. They found that some people have a benign variation in the DNA near the site of the gene for the production of hemoglobin. This was the first DNA polymorphism, an inherited variation in DNA sequence, ever found. These variations alter the points at which restriction enzymes would normally slice the DNA, creating DNA fragments of lengths not normally seen, called "restriction fragment length polymorphisms" (RFLP). By studying the DNA of many families of African Americans, the researchers linked this natural variation to the mutant gene for hemoglobin production, which causes sickle-cell anemia. They found individuals exhibiting this DNA variation were much more likely to have sickle-cell anemia than those without it. Thus, using fetal cells collected via amniocentesis, linkage studies could indicate pregnancies at risk for sickle-cell infants and pregnancies with greatly reduced risk. (Direct detection of the sickle-cell gene mutation became possible in 1981.)

DNA probes are another example of modern use of DNA fragments for diagnostic purposes. These are short, single-strand sections of DNA known to contain a specific group of genes and irradiated so they can be radioactively tracked. The probe is exposed to selected fragments of DNA from an individual being tested for a specific genetic anomaly. If the probe binds with the DNA fragment from the individual, the two contain a complementary gene sequence. Thus, if a probe containing a mutation is used and binds with the individual's DNA fragment, then the individual's DNA must likewise be flawed.

New banding techniques allowing better visualization of chromosomes were another significant development of the 1970s. These bands are the individual chromosome's "fingerprints"; every section of each chromosome has a distinctive banding pattern when exposed to specific dyes. By 1976, high resolution banding techniques, which examined stretched-out chromosomes, allowed the visualization of as many as 5,000 bands on the 23 pairs of human chromosomes. This enabled cytogeneticists to detect small chromosomal deletions in patients with a variety of disorders, ultimately assisting in the hunt for the genes that cause some of these genetic conditions. Concurrently, university centers and satellite clinics for study and treatment of genetic conditions proliferated. In 1979, the American Board of Medical Genetics was established. Also by the end of the decade, over 200 of the more than 700 recessive disorders then reported had been identified as enzyme deficiency diseases.

As the gene came closer into view, understanding of what exactly constituted a gene underwent further refinement. It was found that, rather than simply coding for an amino acid sequence of a polypeptide chain, almost every human and vertebrate gene analyzed has coding sequences, known as "exons," interspersed among intervening noncoding sequences, known as "introns," as well as "flanking regions," which are believed important in regulation of the gene's action. By the end of the 1980s, even Mendel's laws were undergoing modification, as research found that, at least among mammals, a mother and father's genes were not always equal in their hereditary power and differed in their ability to affect the development of some disorders in offspring through "imprinting."

During the 1980s, the number of identified genetic markers, normal genes often inherited along with or linked to an aberrant gene for a specific disorder, grew. Markers for cystic fibrosis, a number of cancers and Huntington's disease were identified. (However, in an example of certain limits of clinical genetics, only a small percentage of those at risk for developing Huntington's disease [that is, children and siblings of those with the disorder] indicated a desire to be tested; apparently a significant number of those at risk do not want to know if they will develop the disorder or are fearful of learning that indeed they will.)

In what were probably the most important discoveries of the 1980s, by the end of the decade the genes for Duchenne muscular dystrophy, cystic fibrosis and chronic granulomatous disease, among others, were isolated and identified solely on the basis of their chromosomal location, without prior knowledge of these genes' products or an understanding of the basic biochemical mechanism of the diseases. This process has been termed "reverse genetics," as opposed to the more usual method of genetic research, whereby identification of a gene product and its function precedes its molecular characterization.

Efforts also began in earnest to create a complete map of human genes. The Human Genome Project, a $3 billion, federally supported project, was established to identify every gene contained in the human genetic complement, or genome, by the year 2005. (By the late 1990s, a private commercial venture between Perkin-Elmer, a manufacturer of gene-sequencing machinery, and Dr. J. Craig Venter of the Institute for Genomic Research of Rockville, Maryland, began a parallel effort, turning the quest to map the human genome into something of a competition.)

The discovery of oncogenes, another major advance of the 1980s, held the promise of one day revolutionizing the diagnosis and treatment of cancer. These genes, involved in regulating cell growth, are thought to trigger abnormal growth after exposure to viral or other environmental assaults causes a mutation. Drs. J. Michael Bishop and Harold E. Varmus of the University of California shared a 1989 Nobel Prize for their pioneering work in developing the oncogene hypothesis. Anti-oncogenes, or tumor-suppressor genes, were subsequently found also to play a role in the process, by inhibiting the development of cancer. It appears that several oncogenes need to be "activated" and several anti-oncogenes "deactivated" in order for the uncontrolled cell growth that characterizes cancer to occur. If specific genes could be identified as promoting cancer, and the products they produce identified, it would be possible to identify at-risk individuals and eventually develop methods to block the genes' destructive action.

Treating disorders at this molecular level is the goal of gene therapy, and its first successful use, to correct adenosine deaminase deficiency (ADA), was reported in 1990. An affected four-year-old girl's lymphocytes were incubated with retroviral vector carrying a normal gene encoding for the missing enzyme, and after the healthy cells were reintroduced to her body, they multiplied.

The theories of Mendel underwent further revision in the 1990s with the discovery of mitochondrial inheritance and trinucleotide repeat disorders, methods of genetic transmission that explained patterns that had defied known laws of heredity. Mitochondria are organelles inside the cell with their own distinct genetic material, all of it inherited from the mother. It was discovered that aberrations in mitochondrial genetic material can cause inherited disorders, just as genetic material in the nucleus does. Yet mitochondrial disorders, like the genetic material responsible, can only be transmitted by females; even an affected male can't transmit the disorder. Trinucleotide repeat disorders involve a sequence of genetic material within a gene that becomes unstable and expands to abnormal lengths during replication, in some cases ultimately interfering with the gene's function and resulting in a genetic disorder. This explained the phenomenon of anticipation noted in some genetic disorders, whereby successive generations exhibited increasing severity and decreasing age of onset. This, it is now known, occurs as the repeat sequence becomes longer, and thus its effects become more pronounced with successive generations. Fragile X, in 1991, was the first identified trinucleotide repeat disorder, a roster that has grown to include Huntington disease, myotonic dystrophy, Friedreich ataxia and Machado-Joseph disease.

Important strides in the search for the genetic roots of cancer were highlighted by the 1994 discovery of the BRAC1 tumor-suppressor gene, and of BRAC2 the following year. These genes, when mutated, were found to confer susceptibility to breast and ovarian cancer. Their identification also enabled the possibility of screening women for the gene, particularly helpful for those with a family history of breast or ovarian cancer.

Also during this decade, definitive studies found folic acid, taken during pregnancy, significantly reduces the risk of neural tube defects (NTDs). This led to the addition of folic acid as a dietary supplement to all enriched foods in the United States, as well as efforts to educate women of child-bearing years on the need for folic acid, resulting in reduction in NTDs.

For parents to be, new prenatal screening methods offered more accurate and comprehensive prenatal diagnostic options. FISH (Fluorescence in situ hybridization) is able to reveal missing, duplicated and malpositioned chromosomal material that escapes routine cytogenetic tests. Maternal Serum Screening (MSS) provides a simple, more definitive prenatal test for estimating the probability of Down syndrome or open NTDs. And preimplanatation diagnosis enabled prospective parents with some known genetic defects to use in vitro fertilization to conceive and have the embryos tested for the genetic aberrations prior to being implanted in the womb.

Advances have continued in the new century. In 2000, by executive order, genetic discrimination was declared illegal in the federal workplace, prohibiting the government from demanding genetic tests of employees or making personnel decisions based on genetic considerations. In 2003, the first map of the entire human genome was completed. Meanwhile, the genetic roots and molecular basis of a growing number of disorders continue to be identified.

But despite great strides, human genetics can still be maddeningly imprecise, particularly when applied clinically. Diagnosis of genetic disorders in a given case may be impossible. Exciting breakthroughs have not eliminated the heartbreak many families endure. The answers medical geneticists can provide are often far outnumbered by the questions they are asked. Advances that may one day reduce this impotence and uncertainty have brought us to the threshold of ethical, moral and legal dilemmas that are as challenging and imperative to address as are the technical and theoretical ones. These are issues that society as a whole, not just geneticists, will face in coming years.

Yet, given even its current limitations, genetics has improved the lives of many, and its benefits are certain to increase, providing help, hope and even life where before there was none.

ENTRIES A to Z

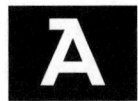

Aarskog syndrome (faciogenital syndrome) First described by Dr. Dagfinn A. Aarskog, professor of pediatrics at the University of Bergen, Norway, in 1970, this is a form of DWARFISM characterized by abnormalities of the hands, face and genitals. Inherited as an X-LINKED disorder, its full expression is seen only in males. However, females who carry a single GENE for the disorder tend to be below average height and may have minor facial or digital abnormalities.

Infants appear normal at birth, and the slowing of growth generally does not become apparent until two to four years of age. Thereafter, height remains below the third percentile for age.

Facially, the forehead is prominent, with wide-set eyes (HYPERTELORISM), often mildly slanted downward and away from the nose (antimongoloid obliquity), with drooping eyelids (PTOSIS). Vision problems are frequent. The nose is short, stubby and upturned (anteverted nares). The ears are low-set and cupped. Mild mental retardation is common.

Hands are short and broad, and fingers may appear "double-jointed" (HYPERMOBILITY of joints). Other digital abnormalities may include short (BRACHYDAC-TYLY), incurving (CLINODACTYLY), permanently flexed (CAMPTODACTYLY) or webbed (SYNDACTYLY) fingers. The feet may exhibit a stubby appearance.

The penis exhibits characteristic folds of skin of the scrotum that surround it, in a manner that has been likened to a shawl worn around the neck, an abnormality that is called "shawl scrotum." The testis may be undescended (CRYPTORCHISM).

Puberty is often delayed, although life span is normal. Adult height is usually below 5 feet 3 inches (157.6 cm).

The gene defect that causes Aarskog syndrome, discovered in 1994, appears to involve a TRANSCRIP-TION FACTOR. Considered relatively rare, approxi-mately 50 cases have been reported worldwide, though the frequency may be higher than this figure suggests. Prenatal diagnosis is not currently possible. Diagnosis in individuals suspected of having the disorder is based on the presence of the characteristic symptoms.

Aase syndrome See ANEMIA.

abetalipoproteinemia (Bassen-Kornzweig syndrome) First described in an 18-year-old Jewish female at New York's Mt. Sinai Hospital by Drs. F. A. Bassen and A. L. Kornzweig in 1950, this rare disease features intestinal fat malabsorption characterized by diarrhea and malnutrition. It may resemble celiac disease or CYSTIC FIBROSIS. Deterioration of the retina (pigmentary degeneration of the retina) leads to progressive loss of vision. Progressive loss of motor control with abnormalities of balance and gait (ataxic neuropathy), mental retardation (in one-third of cases) and abnormalities of the blood are also hallmarks.

Under microscopic examination, about 80% of red blood cells appear to have an abnormal shape, and are termed acanthocytes. These abnormal "burr-cells" are characteristic and appear to be covered by thorns. Other manifestations in the blood are very low levels of serum cholesterol and the absence of serum beta lipoprotein (which gives the disorder its name).

The disease usually begins prior to age one and the manifestations are progressive. While there is no cure, many of the manifestations of this disorder are the consequence of vitamin E deficiency, and treatment with vitamin E may alleviate some symptoms.

Inherited as an AUTOSOMAL RECESSIVE trait, of the approximately 40 published cases, 25% have been Ashkenazi Jews. The basic defect appears to be in the gene for microsomal triglyceride transfer protein (MTP), which is required for the normal assembly of beta-lipoprotein.

ablepharia   See CRYPTOPHTHALMOS.

abortion   The termination of a pregnancy before fetal viability, that is, before the FETUS can survive outside the womb (usually considered to be between the 20th and the 28th week of pregnancy). Abortion may occur spontaneously, often referred to as a miscarriage. Alternatively, it may result from an induced procedure for terminating a pregnancy and thus preventing childbirth. Induced abortion is among the reproductive options available in conjunction with GENETIC COUNSELING.

Miscarriage
Miscarriages, spontaneous abortions, may be the result of many influences, though it is possible to determine the exact cause in only about half of the cases, often only after comprehensive examination of fetal remains. Among the causes are chromosomal or genetic abnormalities, maternal infections, exposure to toxins, substance abuse, nutrition and immunologic, endocrine and reproductive system abnormalities.

The rate of miscarriage is estimated to be approximately 10% to 20% of all recognized pregnancies among women who have never previously miscarried. However, due to the potential number of unrecognized pregnancies, the true rate may be significantly higher, with estimates ranging as high as 31% of all implanted embryos.

Approximately 85% of all miscarriages occur during the first trimester, or three months, of pregnancy, and half of these fetuses are estimated to be chromosomally abnormal. Half of these are thought to be the result of trisomies, the triplication of individual chromosomes (see CHROMOSOME ABNORMALITIES). Genetic factors may play a role in some of the remainder as well.

The rate of miscarriage increases with maternal age. Women who have had one previous miscarriage have a 25% risk of recurrence, rising to between 25% and 30% for those who've had two previous spontaneous abortions. Approximately one woman in 300 has had three or more miscarriages, referred to as habitual abortions. These women have a 30% to 40% chance of a miscarriage in any subsequent pregnancy. Their miscarriages are more apt to be the result of maternal factors, such as reproductive system abnormalities, rather than chromosomal abnormalities. However, there is a possibility that they or their spouses carry a chromosomal rearrangement.

Reproductive system abnormalities include abnormalities of the uterus, deficiencies of the ovaries' ability to produce the hormone progesterone, and deficiencies of the immune system.

Women with underactive immune systems appear to lack an antibody that normally blocks rejection of foreign tissue during pregnancy, possibly causing the rejection of the fetus. In perhaps half of the estimated two million American women who have repeated miscarriages of normal fetuses, this is thought to be the cause.

Women who miscarry are prone to the same hormonal imbalance that leads to postpartum depression following normal childbirth.

Induced Abortion
When induced abortion is performed for genetic concerns, it usually follows prenatal diagnosis of a specific condition, and is generally performed by the 20th week of pregnancy. Abortions may be induced with drugs (e.g. methotrexate and misoprostol), performed by suction or surgical scraping of the embryo(s) from the uterus, or by injection of sterile hypertonic solutions into the womb. With more sensitive tests to determine pregnancy and improved ultrasound to locate the gestational sac, abortions may be performed as early as eight to 10 days after conception using a hand-held suction syringe.

A self-administered abortion-inducing pill, RU486 (mifepristone), manufactured and approved for use in France, can usually induce abortion when taken before the seventh week of pregnancy. It is used in conjunction with prostaglandin, a synthetic hormone that causes uterine contractions. Opposition by religious groups kept it from being used widely in the United States.

Abortions may also be performed selectively in cases of multiple embryos, where continued development of all the fetuses threatens their collective health and that of their mother. A small percentage of birth defects in infants born to young, unwed mothers may result from failed, self-induced abortions.

Partial-Birth Abortion
(intact dilation and extraction)

A procedure used for aborting a fetus in late term, usually in the third trimester, or after the 24th week of pregnancy. It involves vaginally delivering all but the head of the living fetus from the womb, then inserting scissors into the fetal brain to cause death. When a serious birth defect or threat to maternal life warrants consideration of terminating the pregnancy at this late date, this is often the only method of induced abortion possible.

Because of the nature of the procedure and the late stage at which it is carried out, partial birth abortions have become a lightning rod for opposition by groups opposed to abortion. In 2003, Congress passed the Partial-Birth Abortion Ban Act, which President George W. Bush signed into law in November of that year. The ban faced legal challenges in the courts of California, Nebraska and New York. District courts in all three jurisdictions subsequently found the law unconstitutional, rulings upheld by a U.S. Court of Appeals. The U.S. Justice Department appealed the decision to the U.S. Supreme Court. In April, 2007, the Supreme Court reversed the Court of Appeals decision and ruled the ban on partial-birth abortion was constitutional, in that it did not impose an undue burden on the due process right of women to obtain an abortion.

Selective Termination

The selective aborting of some of the fetuses in a multiple pregnancy. Increased use of fertility drugs, taken by an estimated 20,000 women in the United States in 1990, has led to an increase in the number of multiple pregnancies, those in which more than one embryo develops; in some cases as many as nine embryos may develop. Continued growth of all the fetuses in some multiple pregnancies is incompatible with the survival of any of the offspring, and may endanger maternal health as well. Selective termination may be employed in these cases. It is accomplished by the administration of a toxic solution directly into the embryos that are to be aborted, guided by the use of fetal imaging equipment. This procedure has also been done to selectively abort one TWIN affected with a genetic disorder or BIRTH DEFECT, which has been prenatally diagnosed, while allowing the continued pregnancy of the unaffected twin.

See also GRIEF; MULTIPLE BIRTHS; QUININE.

absent nails   See HEREDITARY ANONYCHIA.

absent testes (anorchia)   The absence of testes (anorchia) in individuals having otherwise well-differentiated male genitalia. It is not to be confused with agonadia, a more common condition in which not only are the testes absent, but the genital differentiation is abnormal as well. (See AMBIGUOUS GENITALIA.)

Anorchia occurs in unilateral and bilateral forms, that is, either one or both testes may be absent. Unilateral is more common but at least 100 cases of bilateral anorchia have been reported.

Diagnosis cannot be made until puberty and should involve surgical verification that the testes are absent and not merely undescended.

The cause of this condition is uncertain, although familial tendencies exist. Cases have been observed in which only one of a pair of identical (monozygotic) twins was affected. It is theorized that the testicular tissue is present in all affected fetuses until about 14 to 20 weeks into embryonic development, after which they seem to atrophy for an unexplained reason.

Absent testes usually occurs as an isolated ANOMALY, but can be seen with other abnormalities as part of SYNDROMES such as SIRENOMELIA. Treatment with male hormones can compensate for those hormones normally produced in the testes, but patients with bilateral anorchia remain infertile for life.

acanthocytosis   See ABETALIPOPROTEINEMIA.

acanthosis nigricans A hereditary skin disorder characterized by patches of gray or black, rough or velvety skin with a burned appearance, found around skin folds, most often about the armpits. The lesions tend to be symmetrical (that is, a lesion on one side of the body will have a corresponding lesion on the other side), and may also appear on the neck, face, backs of hands, forearms, between the breasts, groin, genitals, inner thighs, buttocks and around the anus. These darkened areas are caused by the excessive accumulation of melanin in the skin. Small warts, freckles and other skin abnormalities may be associated with the lesions. Affected areas may become hairless, and fingernails may deteriorate.

Acanthosis nigricans is more common in individuals with darker skin pigmentation. While its frequency in Caucasians is less than 1%, in Hispanics, it is 5.5%, and in African Americans, the frequency is 13.3%. The condition may be present at birth, but usually appears during childhood or early adolescence. It generally progresses during adolescence and regresses after puberty. In adults it is often associated with internal cancer.

Endocrine abnormalities are seen in approximately one-third of affected children. Those without hormonal abnormalities are often obese. It is frequently seen in individuals with diabetes. Insulin resistance is the most common association of acanthosis nigricans in the young. Overall, acanthosis nigricans associated with obesity is the most common form of the disorder. Among those so affected, the skin lesions generally are weight dependent and may improve, and even completely disappear, with weight loss. Many, but not all, of the obese patients have insulin resistance.

A benign form known as Miescher's syndrome is believed to be inherited as an AUTOSOMAL DOMINANT TRAIT. A form that appears mostly in young adult females, Gougerot-Carteaud syndrome, may also be hereditary, though the mode of transmission has not been established. It can also be seen in genetic disorders such as ALSTROM SYNDROME and LEPRECHAUNISM and can be induced by drugs such as oral contraceptives, insulin, human growth hormone and glucocorticoids.

acatalasemia See ACATALASIA.

acatalasia (acatalasemia; Takahara's disease) First discovered in Japan, this very rare disease of the oral tissue is most often seen in Asians. The gum (gingival) and oral tissues are very susceptible to bacterial infection, and the condition may result in oral ulcerations, gangrene and destruction of the bones around the tooth sockets.

Inherited as an AUTOSOMAL RECESSIVE disorder, it is caused by the absence of the ENZYME catalase, due to a defect in the gene encoding this enzyme, found on chromosome 11.

Accutane The trade name for an acne medication (generic name isotretinoin) marketed since 1982 for the treatment of severe cystic (nodular) acne that does not respond to other therapies. It is considered to present an extremely high risk of causing fetal malformations if used by a woman at the time of conception or during pregnancy, regardless of the level or length of exposure. Although only slightly more than 50 infants affected by Accutane had been reported to the Food and Drug Administration (FDA) by 1987, actual incidence was believed to be much greater. In one memorandum, the FDA estimated that from 900 to 1,300 infants were born with severe birth defects caused by maternal use of Accutane between 1982 and 1986. (Approximately 270,000 to 390,000 women between the ages of 15 and 44 took the medication during these years). The FDA also estimated that from 700 to 1,000 spontaneous ABORTIONS could be attributed to the drug, and that 5,000 to 7,000 women had induced abortions due to concern of fetal exposure to Accutane. Officials compared the drug to THALIDOMIDE in its potential for causing fetal damage.

Major fetal ANOMALIES related to Accutane that have been documented include brain anomalies, HYDROCEPHALUS, small head (MICROCEPHALY), small eyes (microphthalmia), abnormalities of the external ear, and cardiovascular anomalies. No dose, no matter how small, nor any exposure, no matter how short, can be considered safe; potentially all exposed fetuses could be affected.

Among those using it as an acne medication, Accutane has been associated with depression, psychosis and suicide. Women using Accutane are advised to use a contraceptive, and, if planning to become pregnant, to discontinue use of the medication from one month before conception to one month after delivery. Nursing mothers should also refrain from its use.

acetylator phenotype A genetic trait found in normal individuals that can help determine the likely outcome of some medical treatments and the impact of various doses of some commonly prescribed drugs. It refers to the speed with which the body breaks down the anti-tuberculosis drug, isoniazid. Those with a slow rate have an increased rate of adverse reactions to some drugs, such as isoniazid, hydralazine (a blood pressure medication) and some sulfa drugs. An individual is either a slow or fast acetylator. "Fast," is dominant to slow, thus an individual who is a "fast" acetylator has either one or two "fast" GENES while a "slow" acetylator has two "slow" genes.

achondrogenesis A rare, lethal form of DWARFISM characterized by abnormal development of the skeleton, a large head (possibly exceeding 40% of body length) and severe shortening of the limbs and trunk. Total body length at birth is rarely more than one foot. Most affected infants are stillborn or survive only a few days after birth. More than 100 cases have been reported worldwide.

While the head size is actually normal, due to the dwarfing of the rest of the body it appears disproportionately large. The forehead is broad and the face and scalp are swollen (hydropic), with an extremely flattened nose and nasal bridge. The mouth is small, and the ears are low-set and blunted. The head appears attached directly to the trunk, as the neck is hidden by skin folds. The chest is extremely shortened, and the abdomen is disproportionately large. The limbs are extremely short, and are sometimes referred to as "flipper-like." There is almost a total absence of ossification (formation of bones) in the vertebral column. Heart defects and malformation of the respiratory system are also common.

Several types have been described and their nomenclature can be confusing and has changed over the years. The types are differentiated on the basis of clinical and X-ray features, as well as by microscopic examination of cartilage and by biochemical and molecular studies. For example, in type I the ribs are generally thin and multiple fractures may be seen. Type I is divided into two forms, types IA and IB. IA is now referred to as the Houston Harris form and type IB, the Fraccaro form. The defect in type IA is not known, but the inheritance is probably AUTOSOMAL RECESSIVE. The defect in type IB is known: It is a different MUTATION in the same GENE as that for DIASTROPHIC DYSPLASIA, the diastrophic dysplasia sulfate transporter [*DTDST*] gene, located on the long arm of chromosome 5. In addition to diastrophic dysplasia and achondrogenesis type IB, two other autosomal recessive phenotypes are seen with mutations in the *DTDST* gene: atelosteogenesis type II and recessive multiple epiphyseal dysplasia. This gene is also known as *SLC26A2*. Mutations in the type II collagen gene (*COL2A1*), in addition to producing achondrogenesis type II, can also cause hypochondrogenesis, spondyloepimetaphyseal dysplasia, spondyloepiphyseal dysplasia, Kniest dysplasia and Stickler syndrome. Thus, achondrogenesis and diastrophic dysplasia are allelic disorders see ALLELE). Type II, Langer Saldino type, is caused by mutations in the type II collagen gene found on the long arm of chromosome 12. Previously incorrectly thought to be autosomal recessive as well, it is now known that it is an AUTOSOMAL DOMINANT trait, with most cases representing new mutations.

(A disorder called Grebe disease has been referred to as "Brazilian achondrogenesis," but it is not actually a form of this condition.)

PRENATAL DIAGNOSIS is possible via ULTRASOUND and X-rays, which can detect the gross abnormalities of fetal development that characterize this condition. Type IB can be diagnosed prenatally by molecular studies on CVS. Heterozygous carriers can also be identified by molecular studies. If an individual (such as the partner of a known HETEROZYGOTE) is tested for the five most common mutations in the *SLC26A2* gene and these five mutations are excluded, the risk of carrying a *SLC26A2* mutation is reduced from the general population risk of 1:100 to about 1:300.

achondroplasia The most common and best-known form of short-limbed DWARFISM, characterized by relatively normal trunk size, disproportionately short arms and legs and disproportionately large head.

Achondroplasts have been noted throughout history. Skeletal remains of prehistoric achondroplasts have been unearthed by archaeologists. In Egypt, they appear to have occupied favored positions in royal courts of the pharaohs, and the deity Bes was depicted with achondroplastic features. A Roman statue of a gladiator with achondroplasia dates to the Emperor Domitian (A.D. 51–96). Don Sebastian de Morro, an achondroplast nobleman in the court of Philip V of Spain, can be seen in a portrait by Velasquez. There have even been suggestions that Attila the Hun had achondroplasia. (However, not all those so labeled have had true achondroplasia; many other forms of short-limbed dwarfism have similar features.)

A disorder of bone growth, achondroplasia is a form of "rhizomelic dwarfism," so called because the limbs are shortened in a rhizomelic fashion: The bones closest (proximal) to the trunk display the greatest shortening. Thus, it is most pronounced in the thighs and upper arms. It is one of a group of congenital conditions called "chondrodystrophies," disorders affecting the development of bone from cartilage. Special growth curves and infant developmental charts have been created to help pediatricians monitor the growth and development of children with achondroplasia.

Facially, affected individuals have prominent foreheads, depressed nasal bridge and protruding jaw. The teeth are crowded, and upper and lower teeth often are poorly aligned (malocclusion). The skull may be somewhat squat (brachycephaly).

The upper spine tends to be straight, and the lower spine presents an exaggerated curve, giving a swayback appearance (lumbar lordosis). The legs are often bowed (genu varum). The feet may point inward (talipes varus). Additional limb abnormalities include inability to extend elbows fully, and hands with short, stubby fingers. The fingers are often abnormally positioned so that they appear to present three groups of digits (trident hand).

Achondroplasia is caused by MUTATIONS in the GENE encoding the fibroblast growth factor receptor 3 [FGFR3]. This gene is located on the short arm of chromosome 4 (4p16.3). More than 99% of affected individuals have one of two specific mutations in this gene, both causing the same amino acid substitution, which likely accounts for the consistent characteristic features of the disorder in affected individuals. (This also makes PRENATAL DIAGNOSIS by molecular means on CVS tissue feasible.) A different distinct mutation in the FGFR3 gene causes THANATOPHORIC DYSPLASIA, a lethal neonatal form of dwarfism. Yet another extremely rare mutation in this gene results in a disorder termed severe achondroplasia with developmental delay and acanthosis nigricans (SADDAN). The stature in SADDAN is extremely short and the developmental delay profound.

Achondroplasia is inherited as an AUTOSOMAL DOMINANT trait, though at least 80% of cases are believed to be the result of new mutations, often associated with increased paternal age. It is estimated to occur in one in 40,000 births, and accounts for approximately half of all cases of dwarfism. The total population of achondroplasts is thought to be approximately 5,000 in the United States and 65,000 worldwide. Yet while it is the most common form of short-limbed dwarfism, it is not as widespread as once believed; previously, virtually all infants with short-limbed dwarfism were routinely classified as achondroplastic.

While it can be diagnosed at birth, the disorder becomes more pronounced with age. Intelligence is normal, though developmental milestones may be retarded in infancy due to the physical problems associated with short limbs. Affected individuals are prone to middle ear infections in childhood, which, if not properly treated, can lead to significant hearing loss. Mean adult height for males is 52 inches (132 cm), for females 48 inches (123 cm). There is a tendency toward OBESITY and 50% of those under medical care exhibit some neurologic and spinal complications. The most serious complications include hydrocephalus, compression of the spinal cord or brain stem and upper airway obstruction.

Prenatal diagnosis of achondroplasia is possible via ultrasonographic examination (see ULTRASOUND) of the fetal bones of the limbs. Pregnancies of achondroplastic females must be carefully monitored, and delivery is always via cesarean section (See CESAREAN DELIVERY). Should two achondroplastic parents each transmit the dominant GENE for this condition to an offspring (that is, have a child who is HOMOZYGOUS for the trait), the result is a lethal form of achondroplasia.

ACHOO syndrome (autosomal dominant compelling heliophthalmic outburst syndrome) Benign hereditary condition characterized by nearly uncontrollable paroxysms of sneezing caused by exposure to intensely bright light, usually sunlight, after an individual's eyes have adjusted to a darkened environment. The number of successive sneezes is typically two or three, but has been reported as high as 43. It is also known as photic or solar sneeze reflex and Peroutka sneeze.

First described in medical literature in 1964, it was named by Dr. William R. Collie of Seattle, Washington, and three colleagues in 1978, all of whom described the condition in their own families. Limited surveys have found that the condition exists in as many as 23% to 33% of individuals, though many are unaware of possessing this reflex reaction. It is transmitted as an AUTOSOMAL DOMINANT trait.

The "stomach sneeze reflex" or "gastric sneezing" is a similar curiosity. First described in 1989 in a single family, this autosomal dominant trait involves paroxysms of uncontrollable sneezing after the stomach has become full following a meal.

achromatopsia A rare congenital hereditary disorder that results in total or near-total colorblindness and poor visual acuity. It is caused by defective development of the cones, the photoreceptors in the retina responsible for vision in daylight and other high-illumination conditions. Cones come in three forms: red, blue and green, each stimulated by the wavelength of light associated with that color. The mixing of the pigments produced by this stimulation is what results in color vision. An achromate, as affected individuals are known, must rely on the rods, the photoreceptors responsible for vision at night and in low-light situations, for vision at all times. Rods, which surround the periphery of the retina, are poor at perceiving color and discerning detail. As illumination levels increase, visual acuity declines.

Rod monochromacy, the most common form of achromatopsia, is an autosomal recessive disorder. In complete achromatopsia, or rod monochromacy, the most severe form, all the cones are affected. Incomplete rod monochromats are affected to lesser degrees. A rare form, blue cone monochromacy, an X-lined recessive trait, is seen almost exclusively in males. In blue cone monochromacy, the cones form normally, but the retina is unable to provide the red and green pigment, leaving only blue to be perceived. Mutations in more than one gene can cause achromatopsia. Studies have linked genes on chomrosome 2 and chromosome 8 to the disorder. Expressiveness is highly variable. Incidence is estimated at one per 33,000 births in the United States and most of the world, though incidence is higher in some areas with isolated populations.

Historically, the nomenclature used to classify and identify individuals with achromatopsia has been inconsistent. It has frequently been identified as cone dystrophy. Unlike that condition, achromatopsia is not progressive and does not result in blindness. Nystagmus (crossed eyes), one of the symptoms, is most noticeable during infancy and childhood. Dr. Oliver Sacks wrote of the condition in *The Island of the Colorblind,* about Pohnpie, an island with a cluster of people from the atoll of Pingelap. A relatively high proportion of these people carry the recessive gene and thus exhibit a high incidence of the disorder. Sacks referred to the condition as "achromatopia" and those affected as "achromatopes."

acne (acne vulgaris) Common acne (an inflammation of the sebaceous glands most often seen on the face, with onset at puberty), has demonstrated a familial tendency, though the exact genetics are unclear. So-called neonatal acne occurs in nearly half of all newborns. Termed *milia* it results from overly active sebaceous, or oil, glands in the baby's skin. It can also be a feature of several genetic disorders, for example, later onset forms of some of the adrenogenital syndromes. Acne has been said to affect 85% to 100% of people at some time during their lives. Medications taken to alleviate acne by pregnant or childbearing-age women can have an adverse impact on fetal development. These medications include tetracycline and retinoic acids (see ACCUTANE). It is recommended that tetracycline not be used from the fourth month of pregnancy, nor administered to children under the age of 12, because of its effects on tooth and bone development.

acquired immunodeficiency syndrome   See AIDS.

acrocentric   Any of the five CHROMOSOME pairs (chromosome 13, 14, 15, 21 and 22) whose two chromatids, or strands, are joined at an off-center point.

The chromatids of most chromosomes are joined somewhere near their midpoint. This intersection is the centromere. However, the centromeres in the acrocentric chromosomes are located near one end. These chromosomes are frequently involved in a form of translocation known as Robertsonian translocations, in which two chromosomes (e.g., a chromosome 14 and a chromosome 21) fuse at the centromere. This can have important genetic consequences. (See CHROMOSOME ABNORMALITIES.)

acrocephalosyndactyly   See APERT SYNDROME; CARPENTER SYNDROME; PFEIFFER SYNDROME.

acrocephaly   See CRANIOSYNOSTOSIS.

acro-osteolysis   A FAMILIAL DISEASE with onset in childhood, in which the bones at the tips of the extremities (the most distal bones of the fingers and toes) with no history of trauma, dissolve in a severe osteoporosis-like process. Pain, swelling and deformity result. The cause is unknown, and most cases are autosomal dominantly inherited, although other inheritance patterns have been described. About 30 cases have been reported worldwide. The term "acro-osteolysis" has been used in a variety of syndromes in which the bones of the extremities of the limbs dissolve. These include PYCNODYSOSTOSIS, RHEUMATOID ARTHRITIS, hyperparathryoidism and polyvinylchloride poisoning. When accompanied by changes in the skull and lower jaw bone (mandible), as well as other features, the disorder is known as the autosomal dominant Hajdu-Cheney syndrome.

Neurogenic acroosteolysis is another name for hereditary sensory and autonomic neuropathy (HSAN) type II. This is an autosomal recessive disorder that has as its features impairment of pain, temperature and touch sensation due to a decreased number of or absence of peripheral sensory nerves. The condition begins in early childhood and results in extensive tissue damage to the limbs in a "glove and stocking" distribution, including spontaneous amputation. The causative gene is found on chromosome 12p.

acute intermittent porphyria   See PORPHYRIA.

Adam and Eve   Evidence indicates all humans share a portion of their genetic endowment, which can be traced to a single set of ancestral parents. This male and female have been dubbed Adam and Eve in popular accounts of the research pointing to their existence, though this "couple" didn't necessarily live in the same time, nor were they the first humans.

Examination of genetic material found in the mitochondria, which is only passed on by the mother, evidences a common female ancestor, thought to have lived in Africa some 200,000 years ago. Examination of segments of the Y CHROMOSOME, passed on from fathers to sons, likewise indicates a common male ancestor dating to that same era. They are thought to have been members of a small group of early humans, a group whose other members failed to pass on their genetic endowment.

The first convincing evidence for a common male ancestor came from research at the University of Arizona that examined the DNA of eight Africans, two Australian Aborigines, two Europeans and three Japanese. Results were published in 1995.

ADAM complex   See AMNIOTIC BAND SYNDROME.

adenosine deaminase deficiency, ADA   See SCID, under IMMUNE DEFICIENCY DISEASES.

adrenogenital syndromes (congenital adrenal hyperplasia, CAH) A group of disorders characterized by genital abnormalities due to deficiencies of the enzymes of the adrenal glands, which result in disruptions at specific stages of the synthesis of the steroid hormone cortisol. Located above the kidneys, the adrenal glands produce hormones involved in the metabolism of sodium and potassium, and androgens, estrogens, and progestins, which are important in the development and functioning of the reproductive system. The pituitary gland senses the cortisol deficiency and in response secretes massive amounts of the adrenal stimulating hormone, ACTH, or corticotropin, in an attempt to raise the cortisol levels to normal. The ACTH overproduction in turn causes the adrenal glands to overproduce certain other hormones (adrenal hyperplasia). Many of these have androgenlike effects on the fetus and child, leading to changes in the genitalia.

In addition to cortisol, in certain forms, the other major adrenal steroid hormone, aldosterone, is also deficient. This hormone is involved in sodium, potassium and water balance.

Because of the failure to metabolize sodium properly, affected individuals also exhibit excessive sodium loss, which can be life-threatening, and, in some forms of adrenogenital syndrome, the individuals may be prone to hypertension. In the sodium-losing form, newborns develop symptoms shortly after birth, including dehydration, shock and cardiac arrhythmias, which can be fatal within the first few weeks of life.

The most common form (over 90% of cases brought to medical attention) is 21-hydroxylase deficiency. In females, this disorder causes the female genitalia to appear "masculinized." It is thus a cause of AMBIGUOUS GENITALIA. The degree of masculinization of the genitals is variable, ranging from slight enlargement of the clitoris to development of a male phallus, and may lead the infant to be raised as a male. (Internally, there is development of the uterus and ovaries.) The nipples and genitals may exhibit excessive pigmentation. In the absence of treatment with hormones, no pubertal changes will occur.

Males appear normal at birth, but later may exhibit premature enlargement of the penis and precocious development of secondary sex characteristics.

In both males and females with 21-hydroxylase deficiency, bones develop at an accelerated rate. Though there is accelerated early growth, closure of the growing portion of bone prematurely results in ultimate short stature. Other associated features include excessive salt loss and dehydration.

Treatment is required and involves replacement of steroid hormones. Genital abnormalities may require corrective cosmetic surgery.

An AUTOSOMAL RECESSIVE disorder, 21-hydroxylase deficiency is estimated to occur in one in 12,000 live births in the United States, though incidence is increased among the Inuit or Eskimo Native Americans living in Alaska. The incidence among the Yupik Eskimos has been found to be as high as 1:282. Newborn screening for the disorder is done in some places. The diagnosis of 21-hydroxylase deficiency is made by measuring levels of the steroid precursor 17-hydroxy progesterone in the blood. The causative gene is called *CYP21A2* and is found on chromosome 6p. Molecular genetic testing of the *CYP21A2* gene for a panel of nine common mutations and gene deletions detects about 90% to 95% of disease-causing alleles in affected individuals and carriers.

PRENATAL DIAGNOSIS is possible, using analysis of tissue obtained by CHORIONIC VILLUS SAMPLING or AMNIOCENTESIS. In females, treatment with steroids in utero may minimize the virilizing effects of the syndromes.

Another relatively common form of CAH is 11-hydroxylase deficiency (5% to 8% of cases of CAM), occurring in one in 100,000 births and appearing very much like 21-hydroxylase deficiency. Sodium wasting is not a feature but hypertension is.

Another form, 3-beta hydroxysteroid dehydrogenase deficiency, results in genital ambiguity and incomplete virilization in males, characterized by a penis with a malplaced urethral opening, and defective development of the scrotum with undescended testes. Affected children also lose excessive salt in the urine. Infants with complete deficiency of this enzyme usually don't survive more than a few hours unless promptly diagnosed and treated.

Other rare forms are deficiencies of 12-hydroxylase, cholesterol desmolase, 17,20-lyase and corticosterone methyl oxidase, which together account for less than 1% of all cases of adrenogenital syndrome.

A final syndrome is nonclassic adrenal hyperplasia. This late onset disorder results from a deficiency of 21-hydroxylase and leads to excessive hair growth and infertility. Symptoms also include severe acne, and often short stature in males or premature sexual development. These features all result from excess androgens. Nonclassic 21-hydroxylase deficiency may be present at any birth. Many affected individuals are asymptomatic throughout their lives, or symptoms may develop during or after puberty or after a pregnancy and delivery. It occurs in approximately three in 1,000 individuals in the general white population and about one in 30 Ashkenazi Jews and may be an important cause of infertility in this ethnic group. Mild forms of CAH may be found in about one in 40 Hispanics, one in 50 Yugoslavians and one in 300 Italians.

Most CAHs are autosomal recessive disorders and in most forms a gene mutation has been found.

adrenoleukodystrophy (ALD) Lipid storage disease and form of LEUKODYSTROPHY. Storage diseases take their name from the abnormal accumulation, or storage, of substances within cells. In this disorder, the accumulation of very-long-chain fatty acids (VLCFA) in the white matter of the brain and in the adrenal gland interferes with the ability of cells to function. The disease results from deficient activity of the enzyme that normally breaks down VLCFA. ALD was first recognized in 1923, and was named by Dr. Michael Thaw in 1971. Several hundred cases have been reported around the world.

Inherited as an X-LINKED trait, adrenoleukodystrophy affects only males. Several forms of the disease exist: they exhibit X-linked and AR (AUTOSOMAL RECESSIVE) inheritance patterns and various ages of onset (childhood, adult and neonatal).

In its classic and most severe form, affected children develop normally until four to 10 years of age. Initial symptoms include attention deficit, memory lapses, vision problems and difficulty with walking and coordination; the afflicted are often described as walking into walls. The dysfunction of the adrenal gland may cause increased skin pigmentation, or "bronzing," as well as nausea, vomiting and

weakness. Symptoms become progressively more pronounced (though the rate of deterioration varies considerably), leading to inability to communicate (aphasia) or control motor functions (apraxia), dementia and blindness. Death usually occurs within one to 10 years of diagnosis. Childhood ALD was the subject of the 1992 movie *Lorenzo's Oil*, adapted from a true story of a family's search for treatment for their afflicted son.

A milder, adolescent or adult onset form, adrenomyeloneuropathy (AMN), affects the spinal cord and results in stiffness and clumsiness in the legs, accompanied by general fatigue, weight loss, pigmentation and bouts of nausea and vomiting. The progression of this form is slower, but dementia and other deterioration in function of the brain can also occur. Motor control of the legs deteriorates progressively over a period of five to 15 years, requiring the use of cane or wheelchair. Life expectancy is only moderately diminished.

Childhood ALD and adult onset AMN can both occur in different individuals in the same family pedigree, and result from the same MUTATION within the family. The basis for this is unknown, however, other factors must be involved in the expression of the disease. It has been suggested that immunological factors contribute to the pathogenesis of the central nervous system involvement in ALD.

The underlying defect appears to be a mutation in the GENE encoding for the adrenoleukodystrophy protein, one of what appears to be a group of proteins that bind ATP and act as transporters. The mutation leads to a deficiency of the enzyme lignoceroyl-CoA synthetase. The gene involved, *ABCD1*, is the only gene associated with X-ALD. More than 400 different mutations have been identified in *ABCD1*; these mutations are usually unique to an individual family.

Treatment includes adrenal steroid replacement for the adrenal deficiency symptoms, and symptomatic therapies, such as the use of anticonvulsant drugs and physical therapy, for the neuorologic features. Investigational treatments include dietary restrictions of VLCFAs, administration of oils such as glycerol trioleate or erucic acid (Lorenzo's Oil). The efficacy of these potentially toxic therapies has yet to be demonstrated despite the apparent success suggested by the film of this name. Bone marrow or cord blood stem cell transplants can provide long-term benefits for boys who have both early symptoms and changes on MRI, but the procedure carries a high risk of serious complications or death. Thus it is not recommended for those whose symptoms are already severe, who are without symptoms or who have the adult-onset or neonatal forms.

Diagnosis of ALD is made on the basis of high levels of very-long-chain fatty acids in plasma and/or cultured skin fibroblasts, and testing appears to be highly (close to 100%) accurate. Female CARRIERS can be detected with approximately 90% accuracy by plasma and cultured skin fibroblast analysis. About 20% of heterozygous carrier females can also have some mild to moderate, progressive or nonprogressive spinal cord involvement. This neurologic involvement resembles adrenomyeloneuropathy, but the symptoms in manifesting females have a later onset (35 years or later) and milder expression than in affected males. PRENATAL DIAGNOSIS in at-risk pregnancies is also possible by examination of very-long-chain fatty acid levels in fetal cells obtained by AMNIOCENTESIS or CVS. Molecular analysis of the *ABCD1* gene may be used for determination of carrier status in at-risk female relatives and for prenatal diagnosis, when the mutation has been previously identified in the family.

There is also an AUTOSOMAL RECESSIVE neonatal form with features common to both X-linked ALD and ZELLWEGER SYNDROME. These children are neurologically abnormal at birth and die generally within the first five years of life. It shares the common features of leukodystrophy and adrenal dysfunction with X-linked ALD but has additional features of Zellweger syndrome, including characteristic dysmorphic facial appearance. This disorder is caused by more generalized abnormalities of the peroxisome, a subcellular organelle, a structure that is a component of the cell.

The distinct autosomal recessive neonatal form is a peroxisomal biogenesis disorder. These disorders involve abnormal development of peroxisomes, organelles in the cell that control a variety of metabolic functions. Mutations in twelve different genes encoding peroxins, the proteins required for normal peroxisome assembly, termed *PEX* genes, have been identified in the spectrum of peroxisomal biogenesis disorders. Mutations in *PEX1* are most commonly observed, accounting for about 65% of cases.

adrenomyeloneuropathy   See ADRENOLEUKO DYSTROPHY.

affective disorders   See MANIC-DEPRESSION.

agammaglobulinemia   See IMMUNE DEFICIENCY DISORDERS.

agenesis   The failure of a part of the body or an organ to develop.

Agent Orange   A chemical defoliant used extensively in the Vietnam War, which many American servicemen were exposed to.

There has been considerable controversy concerning the impact of direct and indirect exposure to Agent Orange, including reports of increased incidence of CANCER and other health problems in those directly exposed, and increased incidence of BIRTH DEFECTS in their offspring, particularly NEURAL TUBE DEFECTS. A study by the National Academy of Sciences released in 1996 found a tentative link between exposure and an increased risk of SPINA BIFIDA and recommended further research. However, no conclusive link between paternal exposure to Agent Orange and birth defects in their offspring has been established. (See also TERATOGEN.)

age-related macular degeneration   A progressive condition resulting in declining visual acuity. Age-related macular degeneration (AMD) typically refers to cases with onset after the age of 55.

The macula is the center of the retina, where central vision is focused. As the condition progresses, the light-sensitive photoreceptor cells, rods and cones begin to fail. The sharpness of vision declines, ultimately leaving a dark hole at the center of the visual field, with vision restricted to blurry peripheral images. AMD rarely causes complete blindness, but it is the leading cause of vision loss and legal blindness in adults over 60 in the United States. Affected individuals may lose the ability to read, drive, recognize individuals, cook, use computers or accomplish other leisure and essential tasks of living.

AMD occurs in two forms, distinguished primarily by the amount of retinal damage: dry form and wet form. The dry form is more common and less severe. In a significant proportion of cases, the condition has a hereditary basis. In its hereditary form, AMD is thought to be multifactorial, caused by a combination of genes in concert with environmental factors. In studies published in 2005, a mutation of a gene on chromosome 1 was identified as raising the risk of developing AMD from two to seven times. The gene produces a protein, complement factor H, which limits immune response and inflammation. The mutation renders the protein less effective, and it is suspected this allows the development of a chronic inflammation that may be at the root of the condition. However, not all individuals with the defective genes have been found to show signs of AMD, and some who did exhibit the condition did not have this mutation. Individuals with two copies of the defective gene are most at risk of developing AMD.

Earlier studies linked a mutation in the *ABCR* gene, which creates a protein for the rod cells, with 16% of affected individuals. The same mutation is associated with Stargardt's disase, a form of hereditary macular degeneration with onset in early adulthood. Genetic testing for these mutations is not recommended, as the results cannot be definitively interpreted.

More than 10 million Americans are thought to have macular degeneration, and AMD is the fastest growing type. It may account for 20% to 50% of all cases and affects an estimated 14% to 24% of the U.S. population aged 65 to 74, and 35% of those aged 75 and older. AMD appears to be more prevalent among whites than among other ethnic groups. The number of those affected is expected to grow as baby boomers age.

Cigarette smoke is believed to contribute to its onset by reducing the blood flow to the photoreceptors in the macula, which have high oxygen requirements. Obesity and fatty diets that can lead to plaque buildups in the blood vessels supplying these cells are also possible causative factors. Diets rich in leafy green vegetables, certain vitamins and zinc are associated with lower risk.

Because of the brain's ability to compensate for defects in vision, the disorder may initially go unrecognized. By the time those affected usually seek medical attention, the disorder is relatively advanced. Medication can slow the development of AMD, but cannot stop or reverse its progress. Low Vision Rehabilitation, which incorporates special visual devices and training, allows greater independence and range of activities for those affected.

Aicardi syndrome   Seen only in females, this severe developmental defect is named for French physician Jean Aicardi, who first observed it in 1965. Aicardi syndrome is considered extremely rare. It involves AGENESIS (lack of development) of the corpus callosum of the brain along with lesions in the retina called lacunae.

The corpus callosum is the large bundle of nerve fibers normally found between and connected to the two cerebral hemispheres. The nerve bundle fails to form, or form completely, in this disorder. The characteristic features include mental retardation and seizures, typically of the infantile spasm type. Symptoms typically develop between the ages of three and five months.

Skeletal abnormalities include severe vertebral and rib abnormalities.

The underlying cause for this disorder is unknown. It may be inherited as an X-LINKED dominant trait, with male fetuses dying IN UTERO. Each case would represent a new MUTATION. However, no clear MENDELIAN inheritance pattern has been demonstrated.

It should also be noted that agenesis of the corpus callosum can occur as an isolated defect or as a part of a number of other syndromes. It can be seen in CHROMOSOME ABNORMALITIES (trisomy 13 or 18, for example). When found in isolation, with no other associated brain ANOMALIES, corpus callosum agenesis can be completely asymptomatic.

AIDS (acquired immunodeficiency syndrome)   Disorder characterized by a breakdown in the immune system, rendering affected individuals vulnerable to multiple infections (see IMMUNE DEFICIENCY DISEASE). It is caused by a virus termed "human immunodeficiency virus," or HIV. Definitive diagnosis of the condition is made by blood tests that reveal the presence of antibodies produced by the immune system in response to the virus. Those who have these antibodies are said to be HIV positive. Due to an incubation period that may range from several months to several years, not all HIV-positive individuals exhibit symptoms of AIDS.

While initially associated primarily with homosexual men and intravenous drug users and their sexual partners, the rate of HIV infection has been rising most rapidly among heterosexual women. AIDS can be passed from infected women to their offspring during pregnancy or delivery, resulting in infants who are born with AIDS. Additionally, the virus can be transmitted from infected women to infants by breast feeding. The first report of an infant with congenital AIDS was published in 1983. The mode of transmission is poorly understood.

The incubation period is shorter in infants than in adults, and symptoms may appear within three or four months of birth. Recurrent infections and fluid in the ears may be the first signs. Growth failure and craniofacial abnormalities may also be evident. Affected infants are prone to brain damage due to the effect of the disorder on the developing nervous system; as many of 75% exhibit some neurologic damage. Brain development may cease, and developmental abilities may regress. Infants become weak and apathetic.

In addition to brain damage, there are three other hallmarks of pediatric AIDS. One is susceptibility to bacterial infections (rather than the viral and fungal infections more commonly seen in adult patients) similar to typical childhood bacterial diseases, only much more severe and resistant to treatment. The two other hallmarks are susceptibility (as in adults) to pneumocystis carinii pneumonia (PCP), which causes pneumonia, and, unlike adults, to lymphocytic interstitial pneumonitis (LIP), a poorly understood abnormality of the lung's immune response. Both cause severe breathing problems. Other symptoms include FAILURE TO THRIVE, warts on the hands, swollen lymph nodes and a yeast infection known as "thrush" in the mouth. There is no cure.

Prognosis is poor, though it has been noted that infants born with AIDs may remain asymptomatic for several years.

For adults with AIDS, though the disease was formerly invariably fatal, improved drug therapies, such as protease inhibitors, have dramatically altered the outlook for many, changing it from a fatal disease to a controllable chronic condition. By 1997, about 150,000 people were taking protease inhibitors. It appears to be successful for about 70% to 75% of those taking them. However, protease inhibitors are not approved for children under two and rarely used among older children because of uncertainties about side effects.

The antiviral drug zidovudine (AZT), administered either to pregnant women with AIDS, or to their babies within two days of birth, reduces the chances of maternal transmission of AIDS. On average, without treatment about 25% of infected women pass along the virus to their offspring. In 1994 the U.S. Public Health Service issued guidelines recommending use of the drug by pregnant HIV-infected women, and subsequently, increased testing of expectant mothers in combination with the drug therapy has reduced AIDS cases in newborns. Between 1992 and 1995 the number of newborns with AIDS declined 27%, according to the Centers for Disease Control. Use of the AZT rose from 17% of HIV-infected pregnant women to 80%. An estimated 500 infants are born with AIDS each year, and the Centers for Disease Control estimated in 1997 there were 3,200 children under 13 living with AIDS in the U.S. and thousands more who are HIV positive.

Even as AZT has reduced the toll of congenital AIDS, the success of the therapy has raised the issue of mandatory testing and provoked debates about privacy vs. public health and the rights of a mother vs. that of her unborn child. Of the approximately four million women who give birth annually in the United States, an estimated 6,000 to 7,000 are HIV infected.

While exact statistics are difficult to ascertain, a disproportionate number of congenital cases occur in urban minority communities. Of approximately 1,200 infants born with AIDS and identified by the federal Centers for Disease Control (CDC) from 1983 to 1989, more than 80% were black or Hispanic (824 infant deaths had been attributed to the disorder by 1989).

Nevarapine, a cornerstone of antiretroviral AIDS treatment in developing countries, has been found effective in preventing transmission of AIDS during childbirth without compromising a woman's subsequent ability to undergo antiretroviral treatments with the drug.

Among the experimental treatments that have been tried are intravenous transfusions of gamma globulin, antibodies isolated from blood that help fight a variety of bacterial and viral agents. Treatment of infants with AIDS dysmorphic syndrome with AZT may prevent developmental delay.

In a curious reversal of the often tragic consequences of noteworthy genetic anomalies, mutations have been found that inhibit the transmission of the disease and slow its progression in infected individuals. The mutations are in the *CKR2* and *CKR5* GENES, which produce chemokine receptors, a group of proteins found on the surface of immune system blood cells. The mutations render the genes unable to produce the proteins, which HIV needs to invade a cell. Individuals without normal copies of both *CKR5* genes do not become infected despite repeated exposure to AIDS. Those with one missing copy can become infected, though the progression of the disease is much slower than in people with two normal copies of the gene. (Patients with mutated *CKR2* gene develop AIDS up to four years later than those with normal *CKR2* gene.) Thus, immunity to AIDS can be said to be a recessive trait, with strong expression for the characteristic in HOMOZYGOTES. Individuals with one mutated *CKR5* gene account for about 30% of long-term survivors. Among some populations, almost 14% have one copy of *CKR5* and 1% have two. These are very high percentages for a genetic MUTATION. Researchers at the National Cancer Institute have asserted the *CKR5* mutation arose in Europe when the Black Death swept the Continent in the 14th century. This has led to speculation that its relative ubiquity may result from protection against bubonic plague it perhaps afforded.

A disproportionate number of hemophiliacs (see HEMOPHILIA) in the United States also harbor the AIDS virus, resulting from transfusions containing blood products from AIDS-infected blood donors.

Prior to 1984, screening procedures for donated blood did not detect the presence of the virus. In 1997, the CDC reported just over 2,500 hemophiliacs taking part in federal health care programs were HIV positive. (About 17,000 males in the United States have hemophilia A or B, the most common forms.) Yet hemophiliacs who test positive for the virus seem to develop symptoms less frequently than affected members of other risk groups. Hemophiliacs with AIDS do not pose a greater threat of transmitting the disorder than do other affected individuals, despite their prolonged bleeding; the primary bleeding problem in hemophilia is an inability to staunch internal bleeding. Thus, fears of their spreading the disease by bouts of excessive bleeding are greatly exaggerated.

AIP   See PORPHYRIA.

Alagille syndrome (arteriohepatic dysplasia; Watson-Alagille syndrome)   A hereditary liver disease of infants and young children. It has many of the features of other childhood liver diseases (see ALPHA-1-ANTITRYPSIN DEFICIENCY, BILARY ATRESIA, GALACTOSEMIA), such as jaundice, FAILURE TO THRIVE within the first three months, itching, fatty deposits under the skin, and stunted growth and development during early childhood. However, this disorder also involves the cardiovascular system, spinal column, eyes, nervous system, kidneys and other organs.

Abnormalities in the cardiovascular system (peripheral pulmonary artery stenosis) and spinal column are usually benign and can help in diagnosing the condition. Abnormalities in the eyes and kidneys may lead to minor degenerative changes.

Though the first cases of this disorder were described by G. H. Watson and V. Miller in 1973, the eponymic designation of this disorder is for French pediatrician Daniel Alagille, who delineated more features of the disorder in 1975 in the *Journal of Pediatrics*. This disorder is now recognized more frequently among children with chronic liver diseases. There are well over 100 described cases. Prevalence is estimated to be 1/100,000 live births. At birth, there is an insufficiency of bile ducts, causing bile to back up within the liver and damage liver cells. Scarring of the liver (fibrosis or cirrhosis) occurs in 30% to 50% of affected infants. A small number of patients (about 15%) develop severe liver disease and require liver transplantation.

It has been suggested that individuals with this syndrome also present a typical facial appearance, with a prominent, broad forehead, deep-set eyes, bulbous nose and small, pointed chin.

While many adults with the syndrome are leading normal lives, overall life expectancy is unknown. Infant mortality rate is approximately 10–20%. The severity of liver damage and complications caused by abnormalities in other organ systems is a factor in the long-term outlook. However, prognosis is generally better than for infants with other forms of childhood liver disease.

Alagille syndrome is transmitted as an AUTO-SOMAL DOMINANT trait. It appears to be caused by MUTATIONS of the *JAG1* gene located on chromosome 20, a GENE which appears to be involved in cell differentiation in embryonic development. At one time thought to be a CONTIGUOUS GENE DISOR-DER, all of the features of this syndrome have been seen to result from mutations of the *JAG1* gene.

Prenatal testing of fetal cells obtained by chorionic villus sampling (CVS) or amniocentesis is available for affected families in which previous genetic testing has found a mutation in the *JAG1* gene. Testing available early in the 21st century could identify abnormalities (mutations or gene deletions) involving *JAG1* in about three-fourths of clinically diagnosed cases.

albinism One of the most widely recognized and striking of all genetic conditions, this describes a group of inherited metabolic disorders characterized by a reduction or absence of a pigment called melanin in the skin, hair and eyes. In addition to a lack of pigment, common features in all are visual abnormalities, including decreased visual acuity, rapid, involuntary back and forth darting of the eyes (nystagmus), increased sensitivity to light (photophobia), and crossed eyes, caused by a muscle imbalance of the eyes (STRABISMUS). Affected individuals may be far-sighted (hyperopia)

or near-sighted (myopia), and often have astigmatism, a condition wherein light focuses poorly on the retina due to abnormal curvature of the cornea. Some forms may be associated with other problems such as difficulties with blood clotting (see below) or hearing impairment. (Albinism should be differentiated from hypopigmentation, in which there is a reduction of the normal amount of pigment, but vision is unaffected. Many forms of hypopigmentation are associated with deafness. (See WAARDEN-BURG SYNDROME.)

Albinism occurs in plants, insects, fish, reptiles, amphibians, birds, marsupials and mammals. The Greeks referred to it as "leukoethiopes," from *leuko*, the word for white. Pliny and Aulus Gellius described the condition in the first century. Historically, people with albinism have been singled out and occupied social positions ranging from outcasts to semigods.

Noah is thought to have been an albino, due to Midrashic accounts (interpretive texts of Hebrew scripture), which state "his hair was white as snow, and his eyes like the rays of the sun." However, there is a similar description of Christ, who has not historically been regarded as an albino, in Revelations 1:14: "His head and his hair were white like wool, as white as snow; and his eyes were like a flame of fire." The term "albino" was first used in about 1660 by a Portuguese explorer in describing white Negroes he had observed in Africa, and comes from the Latin "albus," meaning white. Early explorers to the New World found a high frequency of albinism in several Indian tribes. The English Rev. Dr. Spooner, a brilliant classicist whose amusing errors of speech became known as "spoonerisms," was an albino. His errors of speech are thought to be related to his nystagmus, which caused a jumbling of information from the printed page, leading to a verbal jumbling of speech.

Albinos are popularly thought to have red eyes, but actually most have blue or grayish eyes. In some types, the iris appears to have a violet or reddish hue, because light is reflected back from the reddish retina, similar to the effect seen in some flash photos where eyes appear red.

Visual problems are caused by pigmentary deficiency. The eye needs pigment to develop normal vision, though the reason for this requirement is unknown. The retina develops improperly during fetal life, and vision cannot be totally corrected, even with corrective lenses. Nerve signals from the retina to the brain do not travel along the proper nerve routes. Normally light enters the eye only through the pupil—the dark opening at the center of the iris. But in albinism, the iris doesn't have enough pigment to screen out excess light, and it passes through the iris, as well.

Treatment generally consists of attempts to alleviate ocular deficiencies. Surgery, though sometimes helpful for cosmetic reasons, does not seem to improve vision. Corrective and tinted lenses and specialized magnifiers and small telescopes may be of help in addressing vision problems. Albinism generally does not affect life span, though there is an increased incidence of skin cancer due to the lack of pigmentation, which serves to protect the skin from damage caused by ultraviolet radiation. Sunscreens are recommended for reducing exposure to the harmful ultraviolet rays.

There are two major forms of albinism: oculocutaneous albinism, in which pigment is reduced in the hair, skin and eyes; and ocular albinism, in which pigment is reduced only in the eyes. Overall, some type of albinism occurs in approximately one in 17,000 live births. Prevalence in African Americans in the United States is about 1/10,000; in Hopi Amerindians 1/227, and 1/240 among Zuni Amerindians.

Oculocutaneous Albinism

Researchers have described 10 types of oculocutaneous albinism. The most common types are termed either OCA1 and OCA2. These were formerly referred to as "ty-negative" and "ty-positive" respectively, based on whether or not the enzyme tyrosinase is present. This is an ENZYME that converts tyrosine, an AMINO ACID, into melanin in the production of pigment.

Differentiation between OCA1 and OCA2 on the basis of physical examination is not always possible as there is a considerable overlap between the phenotypes, or characteristics of the two. The most helpful feature is that most individuals with OCA1 (ty-neg) have white hair, "milky white skin," and blue eyes at birth. The determination is made by plucking a few hairs from the scalp of a person with

albinism, and incubating the roots, or "bulbs," in a chemical solution of tyrosine. Hair bulbs that don't turn dark in this test are termed "ty-neg,"—that is, they don't produce melanin from tyrosine. If the hair bulbs turn dark, they are termed "ty-pos"—melanin is present. A tyrosinase assay measures the rate at which tyrosine in hair bulbs is converted to dopa, which is then made into pigment.

The hair bulb incubation and tyrosinase assays that have been used to differentiate between OCA1 and OCA2 are not precise, and overlap exists in their results. The GENES that cause OCA1 and OCA2 have been identified, and molecular testing of the involved genes provides the most accurate means of diagnosis.

OCA1 (formerly Tyrosine-negative oculocutaneous albinism) Without tyrosinase activity, the skin and hair stay white throughout life. There is a greater susceptibility to developing skin cancer than in ty-pos albinism. The genetic abnormality in OCA1 is in the tyrosinase gene found on the long arm of chromosome 11. Many different mutations have been found. Classical OCA1 individuals have mutations which result in complete absence of enzyme activity. Some individuals have mutations which reduce but do not eliminate enzyme activity. While generally they have white skin and hair at birth, some hair pigment may develop in the first years of life and their appearance may be that of so-called yellow albinism with blond hair. Yellow albinism has been particularly described in the Amish.

CARRIERS can be identified through hair bulb analysis, measuring the rate at which they produce pigment, and prenatal diagnosis is possible through testing fetal hair bulbs obtained by FETOSCOPY. Visual problems are severe. OCA1 albinism occurs in about one in 28,000 blacks and one in 39,000 whites in the United States.

OCA2 (formerly Tyrosine-positive oculocutaneous albinism) At early ages, this form closely resembles ty-neg albinism. However, there is partial activity of tyrosinase, leading to the gradual accumulation of pigment with age. The hair becomes yellow or reddish and the skin may become freckled or have pigmented nevi. Ocular problems are less severe than in ty-neg, and tend to improve with age. This form is estimated to occur in one in 15,000 blacks and one in 37,000 whites in the United States. It is particularly common in some Indian tribes.

Individuals with OCA2 have mutations in a gene found on the long arm of chromosome 15, known as the *P* gene. Like tyrosinase, many different mutations have been found. The gene appears to encode a transporter protein integral to the membrane of the melanosome, the intracellular organelle that contains the pigment cell's melanin.

CHEDIAK-HIGASHI SYNDROME is a rare form of OCA2 (formerly ty-pos albinism). While oculocutaneous symptoms are moderate, it is usually fatal in childhood due to leukocyte abnormalities that lead to repeated infections and a condition that mimics leukemia. The gene involved in Chediak-Higashi syndrome is the lysosomal trafficking regulator gene found on chromosome 19.

Hermansky-Pudlak-type albinism exhibits a progressive and potentially life-threatening bleeding tendency. Most affected individuals are of Puerto Rican descent, but it has been found rarely in other populations. The frequency in Puerto Rico is about 1/2000, making it the most frequent single gene disorder in Puerto Rico. Lung disease and intestinal problems (colitis) are also features of this disorder. The gene involved was discovered in 1996; it is found on chromosome 10 and appears to encode an important protein component of multiple organelles found in the cell.

Ocular Albinism

In these forms of albinism pigment is reduced only in the eyes. There are several recognized types. The most prevalent forms are X-LINKED and therefore affect primarily males. The gene for X-linked OA, named *OA1*, has been identified on the short arm of the X CHROMOSOME. Female CARRIERS can generally be identified through subtle abnormalities in the eye that are detectable through ophthalmologic examination.

An AUTOSOMAL RECESSIVE form previously thought to be a type of ocular albinism affects males and females equally. In this form, mutations have been found in either the tyrosinase or P genes. Thus, this is actually a form of OCA with minimal cutaneous features and primarily ocular involvement.

Albright hereditary osteodystrophy (pseudo-hypoparathyroidism)   Syndrome marked by short stature, obesity and, in most cases, MENTAL RETARDATION. Named for Dr. Fuller Albright, it is not to be confused with polyostotic fibrous dysplasia, also known as MCCUNE-ALBRIGHT SYNDROME. It is caused by errors of mineral metabolism, which frequently result in skeletal and dental abnormalities, including poorly formed teeth with delayed eruption and a proneness to develop cavities. Hand ANOMALIES are common. Cataracts are also a feature. The severity of expression of the disorder is variable. Life span is normal.

Affected individuals have elevated levels of serum parathyroid hormone (PTH), low levels of calcium and exhibit symptoms of hypoparathyroidism. Pseudohypoparathyroidism was the first endocrine syndrome in humans to be recognized as a failure of end-organ response to a hormone.

Affected infants frequently have seizures due to decreased concentration of calcium in the blood (hypocalcemia), muscle cramps and intermittent muscle spasms (tetany). These individuals don't respond normally to parathyroid hormone.

At birth, infants have prominent foreheads and a round face. The nasal bridge is low, and the neck is short. The most striking characteristic is shortening and malformation of fingers and toes (especially the fourth and fifth) due to shortening of the metacarpal and metatarsal bones, which gives the appearance of an "absent" fourth and fifth knuckle.

This is an inherited condition, though its genetics are not entirely clear. It appears to be an AUTOSOMAL DOMINANT trait, yet the ratio of female to male reported cases is 2:1. This discrepancy, in what should be a 1:1 ratio, awaits explanation. Both sex-limited autosomal dominant and X-LINKED dominant inheritance have been suggested. The possibility of other inheritance patterns exists, but most cases have been found to have MUTATIONS in the GNAS1 GENE on chromosome 20q. Various mutations have been found in this gene, which provides the blueprint for the alpha subunit of the membrane-bound G_s protein. This protein is involved in stimulation of the enzyme adenyl cyclase, which triggers the formation of cAMP in the cell. A cellular messenger, cAMP plays a crucial role in the action of a number of hormones. PTH normally works by stimulating this cAMP production, and thus, in this disorder the response to PTH is deficient or absent. Treatment consists of cautious dietary supplementation with vitamin D and calcium.

alcoholism   A chronic and progressive disorder characterized by the inability to control the consumption of alcohol. It may lead to death due to the internal consequences of long-term alcohol abuse, which include cirrhosis of the liver, cardiac arrest and cancers of the liver, pancreas, lung, colon and rectum.

Alcoholism is most likely a MULTIFACTORIAL disorder caused by the action of several GENES in concert with environmental influence. Inherited tendencies that may play a role include how an individual metabolizes alcohol, an individual's hormonal and behavioral response to alcohol, and his or her tolerance for levels of alcohol in the blood. Biochemically, those prone to alcoholism may experience more pleasurable effects than others. (A preference for alcohol can be selectively bred into experimental animals.)

A familial link has been recognized in alcoholism since ancient times, and numerous studies have found increased risks for the disorder among relatives of those affected. Estimates on the percentage of the general population that will develop alcoholism generally range from 3% to 10% of males and 1% to 3% of females. (Estimates of the number of alcoholics in the United States are generally put at approximately 10 million.) Sons and brothers of alcoholic males may have three to five times this risk, and daughters of female alcoholics three times. In identical (monozygotic) TWINS there is a concordance (both display the trait) of more than 50%, while the concordance is less than 30% for fraternal (dizygotic) twins of the same sex. Familial alcoholism tends to develop early in life.

Studies of adoptees indicate that heredity plays a stronger role than environment in producing alcoholics, with the rates among adopted children of male alcoholics more reflective of the risks associated with their biological than their adoptive fathers. Also, sons of alcoholics who are themselves not alcoholics have a higher tolerance for alcohol than sons of non-alcoholics.

Some ethnic groups show an increased incidence of alcoholism and some a markedly decreased tolerance for alcohol. Native Americans and individuals of Irish descent are among the former group, while Asians are among the latter. Many Asians lack an enzyme responsible for breaking down acetaldehyde, a toxic stimulant that is a byproduct of alcohol metabolism. Individuals with this enzyme deficiency become flushed, dizzy and experience headaches and nausea after ingestion of small amounts of alcohol. An estimated two-thirds of Asians exhibit ill effects from alcohol, while only about 5% of whites are similarly affected.

A small molecule, alcohol is easily absorbed throughout the body, and, in pregnant women, can enter the fetal blood via the placenta. The developmental ANOMALIES that may occur as a result are termed FETAL ALCOHOL SYNDROME.

Alexander disease   One of the rarest forms of LEUKODYSTROPHY, this progressive and fatal infant-onset disorder is seen mostly in males. Named for New Zealand pathologist W. S. Alexander, who described it in 1949, it is characterized by progressive enlargement of the head, spasticity and dementia. It results from defective formation or destruction of myelin, the protective sheath that covers nerve tissue. Seizures may also be a feature. Characteristic microscopic Rosenthal fibers are seen in the brain. Treatment is limited to symptomatic and supportive therapies. Death usually occurs one to two years after onset of symptoms. It is caused by mutations in the gene for glial fibrillary acidic protein (GFAP), located on the long arm of chromosome 17. Most cases are sporadic, and hereditary forms are transmitted in an autosomal dominant manner. Rare cases of multiple affected siblings with unaffected parents seem to be due to gonadal mosaicism. The risk to the siblings is generally felt to be less than 1/200. No more than 300 cases have been reported.

alkaptonuria   Inherited as an AUTOSOMAL RECESSIVE trait, this rare disorder results from a lack of the ENZYME hepatic homogentisic acid oxidase. Although this enzyme defect can be detected from birth by a urine test, affected infants and young adults are usually asymptomatic and fail to notice its most characteristic manifestation: Their urine, if left to stand, turns brown or black. The gene causing Alkaptonuria, mapped to 3q, was identified in 1996. A number of MUTATIONS underlying the disorder have been found.

This condition occupies an important place in the history of genetics. It is one of the first disorders in humans shown to be caused by MENDELIAN inheritance; it was identified as a recessive disorder by English physician Archibald E. Garrod in 1902. It is also one of the four disorders Garrod hypothesized were due to an "inborn error of metabolism" (the title of his 1909 monograph), an important concept in human genetics whose value was not appreciated until the 1940s. (The other three of these metabolic disorders were ALBINISM, CYSTINURIA and pentosuria.)

With age, dark spots may develop on the whites (sclerae) of the eyes. Pigmentation also develops in the cartilage, nails and skin, particularly on the cheeks, forehead, armpits (axillae) and genitals. Ear wax (cerumen) is often black or brown. A later symptom is arthritis, especially in the spine. Joints often stiffen completely (ankylosis).

At least 1,000 cases of alkaptonuria have been described; this is likely an underestimate. The incidence of alkaptonuria in the United States is estimated to be one in 250,000 to 1,000,000 live births. Incidence is reportedly unusually high in the Dominican Republic and the Czech Republic. Affected individuals have normal intelligence and life span, although arthritis may limit their mobility.

allele One of two or more alternative forms of any particular gene located on a GENE pair. Gene pairs, found at corresponding positions (loci) on CHROMOSOME pairs, represent two alleles.

Many genes have more than one allele, such as those for blood type, with the alleles for types A, B and O all found at the same gene locus. Additionally, advances in molecular genetics have demonstrated that what were previously considered as simply either dominant or recessive traits, or genes, may actually be produced by a variety of different versions, or alleles of a given gene.

In some circumstances different mutant alleles in the same gene may lead to the same disorder (although the exact clinical picture may vary somewhat), while in other cases different mutant alleles in the same gene may lead to very different disorders. In this latter category, for example, alternate MUTATIONS in the fibroblast growth factor receptor genes result in various forms of craniosynostosis, and thus all have a common cause.

allergy An acquired hypersensitivity to a normally benign substance. The term is taken from the Greek *altos,* meaning "altered," and *ergia,* "reactivity." Any substance that provokes an allergic reaction is known as an allergen.

Allergic reactions are a unique form of autoimmune disease, possibly evolved from a genetic mechanism that protected the body against worms and parasites. The allergens may in some way mimic these invading organisms. It appears that individuals inherit a genetic predisposition to develop a particular allergy, though the mode of transmission is unclear. It is likely to be POLYGENIC and/or MULTIFACTORIAL, though single GENES may be involved as well in some allergies, inherited in an AUTOSOMAL DOMINANT manner.

Common allergens include pollen, dust, hair, fur, feathers, scales, wool, chemicals, drugs, insect bites, and such foods as eggs, chocolate, milk, wheat, tomatoes, nuts, citrus fruits, shellfish, oatmeal, sulfite preservatives and potatoes. Evidence also indicates deer can make some hunters sneeze, cockroaches can prompt asthma attacks in asthmatics, physicians can develop an allergy to latex and some individuals are literally allergic to exercise. Concern over peanut allergies has provoked efforts to ban peanut butter in schools.

The prevalence of allergies is unknown, though it is thought potentially to represent the largest population of chronically diseased individuals in the United States. Common allergic conditions include hay fever (vasomotor or allergic rhinitis), bronchial asthma, eczema (a skin condition) and hives (urticaria). An estimated 40 million Americans have hay fever, 9 million asthma, from 10 million to 20 million have had occasional hives and an untold number have food allergies. Because of the prevalence of these disorders and their morbidity and economic impact (consider absenteeism in schools and workplace related to asthma alone) much effort has been made to identify the genes involved, which may eventually allow for a pharmacogenetic approach to treatment.

Symptoms of the reaction commonly involve the respiratory tract or the skin. In the respiratory tract this usually takes the form of congestion, runny nose, watery eyes, sneezing and breathing difficulty caused by swelling and constriction of the bronchial tubes. Cutaneous involvement includes itching, rashes and lesions.

Allergies usually develop following a number of exposures to a given substance, after enough antibodies are produced to trigger the response to the allergen. The antibodies are a class of immunoglobulins, IgE, with a specific form for each allergen. When allergens are present, the IgE antibodies attach themselves to cells in the lining of the nose and bronchial passages, where they bind to the allergens. This triggers the cells to eject histamine or histamine-like substances, causing an irritation accompanied by sneezing, itching and watery eyes. Severe reactions can cause death by blockage of air passages or a precipitous drop in blood pressure.

Genes have been found that may increase susceptibility to allergies that result in asthma and hay fever attacks. Individuals with one such gene often have high levels of IgE in their blood, an indicator of allergic overreaction. Another implicated gene codes for production of interleukin 4, a protein that regulates the body's production of IgE. Individuals with a mutated copy of this gene are 10 times likelier than the general population to have an allergy.

Atopic eczema, which is often associated with asthma and other allergic phenomena, is extremely common, affecting 0.7% of the population. Some believe that it may even be determined by an autosomal dominant gene with highly variable expression. The risk of developing some allergic problem where one parent is affected approaches 50% and is slightly higher when both parents are affected.

ized by the loss of hair in distinct round or oval patches about the head, though hairless patches may appear anywhere. Onset is usually between the ages of 20 and 50, with the average about 30 years of age. In most cases, hair regrows after several months, though episodes may recur. Alopecia areata may progress, particularly in childhood cases, to alopecia totalis, resulting in total loss of hair of the head, or alopecia universalis, in which all body hair is lost, usually without regrowing. Between 5% and 30% of those with alopecia areata develop alopecia totalis.

About 2.5 million people in the United States have alopecia areata. It is estimated that 10% of alopecia areata cases and 20% of alopecia totalis demonstrate a familial aggregation. For those with a relative under medical treatment for alopecia, the chance of developing the condition is estimated at 100 times the general population's.

Familial forms of alopecia are thought to involve an abnormality of the immune system. Many cases go into spontaneous remission. Treatments with the steroid cortisone and other drugs have been effective in some cases. Steroid injections in the scalp can restore hair loss in alopecia areata, but its effects may be temporary. Absence of hair can also be a component of many syndromes, in particular the ECTODERMAL DYSPLASIAS. When genetic, it is probably most often MULTIFACTORIAL, but cases with AUTOSOMAL DOMINANT, AUTOSOMAL RECESSIVE and X-LINKED recessive inheritance have all been described.

The first human GENE linked to hair loss was found in 1997 by studying members of an extended Pakistani family who exhibited alopecia totalis from birth. Located on chromosome 8, this gene (autosomal recessive) codes for a transcription factor, a protein that regulates other genes and thus is believed to play a role in the hair growth cycle. This transcription factor is absent in those with alopecia totalis, though this particular gene mutation has been seen only in this Pakistani kindred.

(See also MALE PATTERN BALDNESS.)

alopecia   A general term for any type of hair loss. Several forms of alopecia exist, with the most common being alopecia areata, a condition character-

alpha-fetoprotein (AFP)   A protein excreted by the FETUS into the AMNIOTIC FLUID and from there into the mother's bloodstream through the placenta. During the second trimester of pregnancy, usually the 16th week, a blood test to measure the level of maternal AFP can aid in assessing the presence of certain defects in the developing fetus.

Elevated levels of AFP are an indication of possible neural tube defects, which occur in about one to two of every 1,000 births. High levels can also indicate the possibility of multiple births, underestimation of the age of the fetus, other ANOMALIES, LOW BIRTH WEIGHT and fetal death. Low levels of AFP can indicate an overestimation of the age of the fetus or the more ominous possibility of genetic chromosomal disorders, such as DOWN SYNDROME.

The maternal blood test presents no risk to the fetus or to the mother, but it is not a positive indication of either NEURAL TUBE DEFECTS or other disorders. However, an abnormal test result will allow the physician and patient to determine if further testing is necessary. Usually, a second AFP blood test will be performed as a confirmation of the first result. If the second test result is the same, a decision can be made to try ultrasonography (see ULTRASOUND), followed, if necessary, by a determination of the level of AFP in the amniotic fluid. Assaying the concentration of AFP in the amniotic fluid can be a more positive confirmation of abnormalities, especially neural tube defects. Chromosome analysis can also be done on cells in the fluid to look for Down syndrome. However, this test requires AMNIOCENTESIS, which involves a small (less than 1%) risk of miscarriage, infection or fetal death.

alpha-1-antitrypsin deficiency (AAT deficiency)

An inherited disorder that can lead to hepatitis in infants and emphysema in adults. Progressive emphysema is the most common manifestation. Initial symptoms of the lung disease may be seen in homozygous individuals (see HOMOZYGOTE) as early as the teens or 20s, with clinical disease developing by the 30s or 40s. In patients with intermediate levels (such as HETEROZYGOTES), the onset of symptoms is generally during the 40s with full clinical disease by the late 50s. The earliest symptom may be progressive shortness of breath, especially with exertion, generally accompanied by chronic cough. Recurrent respiratory infections may be seen.

AAT deficiency is a relatively common inborn error of metabolism, caused by mutations in the SERPINA1 gene, located on the long arm of chromosome 14. Transmitted as an AUTOSOMAL RECESSIVE trait, its incidence is estimated at between one in 700 and one in 2,500 live births. The disorder is most common in individuals of northern and central European descent. About 5% of people in Sweden are CARRIERS of the deficiency GENE, and one in 1,700 has two deficiency genes. AAT deficiency should be suspected when emphysema occurs in a woman, a relatively young man, a nonsmoker, or in someone with a family history of emphysema.

The disorder gained attention in the medical community in 1963 when its link to the development of emphysema was demonstrated. Its association with juvenile cirrhosis was established a few years later.

The primary role of AAT is unclear, though it is known to be an enzyme-inhibitor that limits the action of ENZYMES active in the breakdown of protein. It may facilitate "safe handling" of these caustic enzymes, which are otherwise capable of digesting and destroying cells and proteins of the body.

There are over 75 genetic variants involved in the synthesis of AAT that may differ substantially in the levels of alpha-1 antitrypsin found in the body, leading to a wide variation in the manifestations and severity of this disorder. But what is inherited is the deficiency of AAT, not the disease. For unknown reasons, only 10% to 20% of babies born with the deficiency will develop liver disease. Individuals will either be asymptomatic, will develop a liver disease in the first weeks or months of life or will develop emphysema in middle age.

Symptoms of the disorder often appear in the newborn period. They include jaundice, swelling of the abdomen and poor feeding. If the onset is during childhood or adolescent years, symptoms include fatigue, poor appetite, swelling of the abdomen and legs or enlargement of the liver (hepatomegaly).

If they develop cirrhosis (scarring of the liver), the change in blood flow that results can cause significant complications. There may be nosebleeds, bruising, excess body fluid and enlarged veins in the inside of the stomach and esophagus (varices). Increases in pressure in these veins may make them leak, resulting in internal bleeding. Later complications include sleepiness after eating protein (due to increased blood ammonia levels) and increased risk of infection. Approximately 15% of those who come to medical attention develop cirrhosis.

Cirrhosis may be caused by abnormal forms of AAT, which are retained by the liver cells, where it may lead to liver damage. The alpha-1-AT deficiency's association with the development of emphysema may be due to the unchecked action of enzymes it is responsible for blocking. Released at the site of lung inflammation or irritation, the caustic action of the protein-digesting enzymes may eventually reduce elasticity in the underlying tissue, resulting in greatly reduced lung capacity.

It is estimated that 20,000 to 40,000 individuals in the United States have this disease. Two percent to 3% of the white population of the United States is thought to have a variety of alpha-1-trypsin deficiency that puts them at risk for developing emphysema, particularly if they smoke. This is because heterozygotes (carriers) of this variation are at risk of developing emphysema in later life.

Carrier screening is available. PRENATAL DIAGNOSIS using RECOMBINANT DNA techniques is possible in a select number of laboratories. The gene is known to be on chromosome 14.

Research is currently under way on the treatment of this disorder by replacement therapy. AAT is given intravenously. Early results appear promising. Importantly, "treatment" includes avoidance of both cigarette smoke and environmental exposure to respiratory irritants.

Alpha-Thalassemia X-Linked Mental Retardation syndrome   A form of mental retardation affecting only males, characterized by major developmental delays, dysmorphic craniofacial features and genital anomalies. Developmental delays are evident from infancy, though the degree of retardation can vary from mild to severe. Some affected individuals never become ambulatory or capable of significant speech.

At birth, muscle tone is weak (hypotonia) and a variety of finger and toe and skeletal abnormalities may be present. The head is small (microcephaly), and dysmorphic features of the mid-face can include telecanthus (widely separated eyes) and epicanthus (folds of skin over the inner corners of the eyelids). Nostrils are small and upturned (anteverted nares). Teeth are widely spaced and the tongue protrudes. The features coarsen over time. Genital abnormalities are usually minor and include hypospadias, undescended testicles and ambiguous genitalia. Genital anomalies are typically similar among affected individuals within a family. In isolated cases, males have what appear to be normal female genitalia.

Alpha thalassemia, with which this form of retardation is associated, is a chronic anemia. However, many patients with this syndrome have normal red cell function and normal hemoglobin. The causative gene (the *ATRX* gene, mapped to Xq13) apparently also acts as a brake on the expression of the alpha thalassemia. The mutation may be inherited from the mother (as in most X-linked disorders, females carriers remain asymptomatic) or may result from a de novo mutation.

Diagnosis is made on the basis of characteristic features and family history. Molecular testing for the defective gene is available and can identify the mutation in about 90% of affected individuals and female carriers and be used for prenatal testing. Females who carry the defective gene exhibit skewed X-chromosome inactivation. This can help identify carriers either preliminarily or in the absence of definitive results from molecular testing. Linkage analysis to find a marker for the defective gene can be performed in cases where an ATRX mutation has not been found and can also be used for carrier testing and prenatal diagnosis. This requires acquiring samples from several family members.

Prevalence is unknown. At least 100 individuals have been definitely diagnosed by genetic testing laboratories. The condition is believed to be underreported.

Alport syndrome   See FAMILIAL NEPHRITIS.

ALS   See AMYOTROPHIC LATERAL SCLEROSIS.

Alstrom syndrome   An endocrine disorder first described by C. H. Alstrom in 1959, characterized by early onset vision and hearing impairment. Loss of central vision, due to RETINITIS PIGMENTOSA, begins before one year of age, progressing to functional blindness by adolescence. Hearing loss due to nerve DEAFNESS begins in childhood and progresses to clinical deafness by adolescence. Other ocular manifestations reported include nystagmus, CATARACTS and glaucoma. Heart disease characterized by enlarged and weakened cardiac muscles (dilated cardiomyopathy) with onset in infancy or adolescence occurs in over 60% of affected individuals.

OBESITY is common in affected children, and in early adulthood non-insulin dependent (type II) DIABETES MELLITUS or glucose intolerance is sometimes seen. ACANTHOSIS NIGRICANS, ALOPECIA of the scalp, hyperuricemia and hyperlipidemia have also been reported in Alstrom patients. Chronic nephropathy may be present, possibly leading to renal failure. Hypogonadism, or failure of the sex organs to develop, resulting in delayed puberty, has also been reported in males. Secondary sexual characteristics may develop normally.

Inherited as an AUTOSOMAL RECESSIVE trait, Alstrom syndrome is caused by mutations in the *ALMS1* gene on chromosome 2p. The locus of the gene was initially identified based on linkage data from a large Acadian kindred. About 300 cases have been reported worldwide, the majority of them males.

Alzheimer's disease (AD)   An adult onset degenerative brain disorder characterized by memory loss, deterioration of mental function and disturbances of speech and movement. AD is the most common cause of dementia. It was first described in 1906 by German neurologist and psychiatrist Alois Alzheimer (1864–1915), who noted the "neurofibrillary tangles," damaged brain cells that are a hallmark of this disorder. (These distorted brain cells can only be seen upon autopsy; thus, definitive diagnosis of Alzheimer's disease cannot be made until after death.)

The disease was originally thought to be rare, but as knowledge of the disorder has grown, the extent of its impact on the population has been revised upward. By the latter 1980s the total number of those affected in the United States was thought to be 2.5 million. That number was revised upward

again in 1989 when a major, federally financed study by Brigham and Women's Hospital in Boston found 10.3% of individuals over age 65 and 47.2% over age 85 had mental impairments most likely caused by Alzheimer's disease. A 2007 survey of data by the Alzheimer's Association concluded more than 5 million Americans were afflicted with the disorder. The survey also found that 13% of those over 65 years of age and 42% of those older than 85 are affected. A 1986 study by Dr. D. Morrison Smith for the Alzheimer's Society of Canada estimated that 300,000 Canadians had Alzheimer's, and that by 2020, 700,000 Canadians will have it. The number of affected individuals in the United States is expected to triple by 2050.

Onset may occur anywhere from the 30s to the 80s, though it rarely occurs before the age of 45; most cases occur after age 70. Early signs are forgetfulness and minor mood swings, progressing to loss of memory, the ability for rational thinking and the ability to care for oneself. There is no cure, and affected individuals invariably succumb to infections, malnutrition or other complications within 10 years of onset.

This disorder is thought to involve the accumulation of large concentrations of amyloid, a protein, in abnormal brain structures of amyloid plaques and neurofibrillary tangles, as well as in the walls of the cerebral blood vessels. In 1989, researchers found the abnormal amyloid beta protein outside the brain for the first time, a development which may lead to a practical diagnostic test for the disease. Aluminum is present in increased concentrations in the brains of those affected as well, but this is thought to be a result rather than a cause of the disorder.

Most cases are sporadic, but familial forms of Alzheimer's disease are thought to account for 10% to 30% of those under medical attention. Most SPORADIC cases are thought to be MULTIFACTORIAL, precipitated by the action of several GENES in concert with environmental factors. But between 6% and 10%, by some estimates, of all those affected with Alzheimer's have inherited it as an AUTOSOMAL DOMINANT trait.

A number of GENES have been found to be related to the development of AD and there are at least three different etiologies for early onset (before age 60) forms. The first gene identified is the *beta-amyloid precursor protein* gene, found on chromosome 21. This appears to be associated with a small number (less than 3%) of families with early onset AD. A gene believed to be responsible for a buildup of amyloid has been identified on the long arm of chromosome 21. Interestingly, this is the same chromosome that, when an extra copy is present, results in DOWN SYNDROME; individuals affected with Down syndrome frequently develop amyloid plaques and succumb to an Alzheimer-like dementia in their forties. A more frequent gene in familial early onset AD (80% of early onset families) is the *presenilin-1* gene found on chromosome 14. A third gene involved is the *presenilin-2* gene found on chromosome 1. A MUTATION in this gene is found in individuals of Volga German descent with early onset AD. The Volga German families are a group of individuals that descended from a colony of ethnic Germans who moved to the Volga valley of Russia in the 1760s. The gene may cause AD in non-Volga Germans as well.

The genetics of late onset (variously defined as after ages 60 to 70) AD, the most frequent form of the disease, is even more complex. The presence of a specific defective gene on the long arm of chromosome 19 (19q13) is the most significant risk factor for familial and sporadic cases of late onset AD identified to date. The gene involved is the apolipoprotein (apo) E locus. There are three common ALLELES at this locus: E2, E3, and E4, the frequencies of which in the United States are 7%, 78% and 15% respectively. An increased risk and lower age of onset of AD was shown to be related to the "dose" of the apoE4 allele inherited. An individual with one copy of the E4 allele has double the risk that a person with no E4 has of developing AD. An individual with two copies has eight times the risk. The apoE2 allele is, furthermore, protective: It is associated with a decreased risk and with a later age of onset of AD when it does occur. It is important to note that most E4 carriers do not develop dementia, and about one-half of AD is not associated with the E4 allele. Thus the apoE4 allele is neither necessary nor sufficient for the development of AD. It is a susceptibility gene, and other genetic and environmental factors clearly must exist for the development of AD. Other factors identified include variations in mitochondrial energy metabolism genes and head injury, which interact with apoE4 to increase the risk of developing AD.

Indeed, apoE4 produces a genetic susceptibility to the effects of head injuries. In a study of boxers conducted at New York Hospital–Cornell Medical Center, among the 30 pugilists examined, those who had one copy of the allele and had competed in 12 or more bouts had a significant increase in brain injury compared to boxers of equivalent experience without the allele. Another study found the effects of head injuries worked synergistically with apoE4, increasing the risk of developing AD tenfold. Those with this allele are said to have the ApoE genotype.

A link to defects in two mitochondrial genes that code for cytochromec oxidase, a key enzyme in the metabolism of oxygen, has also been reported.

A variant of the *SORL1* gene, which has been mapped to the long arm of chromosome 11 (11q23.2-24.2) has been implicated in AD as well. The variant was isolated from Dominicans in Manhattan whose families exhibited three times the usual incidence of AD. Researchers believe individuals with a variant form of this gene produce less *SORL1*, a protein used in nerve cells. This is thought to disrupt the movement of proteins in nerve cells and allow the amyloid precursor protein to be converted into a toxic form.

High doses of vitamin E have been found to slow the progression of AD, as has selegiline, a drug usually prescribed for Parkinson's disease. Both appear to shield brain cells from the damaging effects of oxygen. At least five drugs that slow onset of the disease's symptoms for six to 12 months in half the individuals who take them have been approved by the Food and Drug Administration.

Predisposition testing for estimating the risk to develop AD is fraught with many ethical and psychosocial concerns. Moreover, the link between the apo E4 gene and AD is of limited predictive value even in members of families with clusters of AD. The apoE4 gene is also associated with heart disease, increasing the risk 30–50%. Many people with dangerously high cholesterol levels are tested for the gene to target them for preventive treatment for heart disease. Physicians conducting the tests rarely mention the link to Alzheimer's.

Blacks and Hispanic Americans have been found to have an elevated risk of developing Alzheimer's disease independent of the APOE4 gene. Blacks without the gene were found to be four times more likely than whites to develop AD, and Hispanic Americans two times.

ambiguous genitalia   A general term for maldevelopment of the genitals. These conditions have their genesis in the eighth week of fetal development, when the sexual organs begin to develop. At this time, in the female embryo, müllerian ducts develop into fallopian tubes and uterus, and in the male embryo, wolffian ducts develop into the epididymis, vas deferens and seminal vesicle. If there are errors in this process, the female reproductive organs may become overly masculinized, or the male organs may be inadequately masculinized. In some such cases, it may be difficult to determine the gender of the baby at birth; an enlarged clitoris appears similar to a penis with undescended testes in newborn infants.

A GENE that disrupts normal genital development in males has been found and mapped to the X CHROMOSOME. Named DDS, the gene can overcome or mitigate the influence of the gene for maleness, SRY, found on the Y CHROMOSOME. If, through a genetic error, a duplicated, rather than a single DDS gene is inherited by a male, external sex organs are somewhat feminized. However, if through a genetic error no copy of the DDS gene is inherited by a male, about half such infants will be born with undescended testes while the rest appear unaffected.

Approximately one in 1,000 babies is born with some degree of gender ambiguity. Medical texts have described ambiguous genitalia as "a true genetic emergency." Reconstructive surgery and hormonal therapy are often prescribed in cases of indeterminate gender, with physicians deciding whether to mold the infant as male or female, regardless of their true sex as determined by their chromosomes. In the majority of cases the female gender is chosen as it is easier to surgically construct a vagina than a penis. Some individuals who've undergone such therapy as infants have later criticized this approach, arguing against surgical and hormonal remedies in favor of a less crisis-oriented view of ambiguous genitalia.

Among the disorders characterized by ambiguous genitalia are ADRENOGENITAL SYNDROMES, HERMAPHRODITISM and PSEUDOHERMAPHRODITISM.

amelogenesis imperfecta   Defective formation of the enamel of a child's teeth without any apparent accompanying disease or external cause characterizes this hereditary disorder. It may be seen alone or in conjunction with other problems (e.g., retinal dystrophy, spine dysplasia, seizures). It occurs in AUTOSOMAL DOMINANT, AUTOSOMAL RECESSIVE, and X-LINKED dominant and recessive forms. The most widely accepted classification system for amelogenesis imperfecta subdivides the disorder into four main types based on the enamel defects and further delineates these forms into 14 distinct subtypes based on clinical appearance (phenotype) and mode of inheritance.

Enamel is the outermost covering of the teeth and the hardest tissue in the body. It contains two important proteins: enamelin and amelogenin. The defective protein in amelogenesis imperfecta is amelogenin. The GENE for this protein is located on the distal portion of Xp. There may be a corresponding locus on the Y CHROMOSOME. These chromosomal assignments are consistent with the hypothesis that the amelogenin gene is involved in X-linked types of amelogenesis imperfecta and that the Y-chromosomal location may participate in regulating tooth size and shape. Another gene maps to chromosome 4q where the ameloblastin gene is located. This may be involved in some of the autosomal forms of the disorder.

Defects vary considerably with the genetic type. Dental abnormalities include thin, incompletely developed (hypoplastic) enamel; pitted, grooved and discolored enamel; lack of contact between adjacent teeth (malocclusion); teeth that do not grow through the gum (unerupted) due to partial absorption in their sockets; teeth sensitive to temperature changes; easily broken or pulverized (friable) enamel; enamel that is deficient in hardening (hypocalcification) or incompletely grown (hypomaturation) and soft enough to allow a metal probe to be pushed through; and teeth that turn brown or black from food stains.

Defects are apparent at the time of tooth eruption by visual examination and by X-ray examination, which may disclose a lack of contrast between the enamel and the basic bony tissue (dentin) of the teeth.

The prevalence of the disorder has been studied in only a few populations and has been reported to range from one in 700 to one in 15,000 or fewer. It occurs in about one in 16,000 births among North American white children. Amelogenesis imperfecta can lead to early loss of teeth, periodontal disease and psychosocial problems because of unsightly teeth. Orthodontics and special dental restoration procedures can be effective in correcting the problems. Identification of carriers is possible in the case of the X-linked recessive type. Currently, there is no method for PRENATAL DIAGNOSIS.

amino acid   The building blocks of proteins, and members of a large group of organic compounds. While more than 80 amino acids are found in nature, only 20 are required for human life. Eight of these are only available from food, and these are called essential amino acids: isoleucine, leucine, lysine, methionine, phenylalanine, threonine, tryptophan and valine. During infancy, arginine and histidine are also essential; these amino acids are the end product of digestion.

A variety of inborn errors of metabolism in synthesis or breakdown of amino acids lead to inherited disorders of amino acid metabolism. These include HOMOCYSTINURIA, PHENYLKETONURIA (PKU), and the UREA CYCLE DEFECTS. (See also AMINOACIDEMIA and MAPLE SYRUP URINE DISEASE.)

aminoacidemia (aminoaciduria; aminoacidopathies)   Any one of almost 100 inborn errors of AMINO ACID metabolism. They include ALKAPTONURIA, CYSTINURIA, HOMOCYSTINURIA, PHENYLKETONURIA (PKU) and MAPLE SYRUP URINE DISEASE.

aminoaciduria   See AMINOACIDEMIA.

Amish   A religious isolate population living primarily in Lancaster County, Pennsylvania. Intermarriage within the community has contributed to the documentation of a number of rare hereditary disorders in higher incidence than would be expected in a random population. The disorders include cartilage-hair hypoplasia (METAPHYSEAL CHONDRODYSPLASIA), CRIGLER-NAJAR SYNDROME, ELLIS-VAN CREVELD SYNDROME, GLUTRAIC ACIDURIA and MAPLE SYRUP URINE DISEASE.

Some 250,000 Amish live in the United States, all descendants of about 200 families that immigrated from the lower Rhine Valley in the 18th century. A Mennonite population in the Lancaster County area also exhibits an increased incidence of rare hereditary conditions. As groups, members of these religious communities, which eschew the use of electric- and gas-powered equipment, are known as the Plain People. The Clinic for Special Children was established in Strasburg, Pennsylvania, in 1989 to identify and treat the rare syndromes seen in the population, as was the DDC Clinic for Special Needs Children in Middlefield, Ohio, in 2002.

amniocentesis   The most widely used invasive diagnostic procedure for prenatal detection of hereditary disorders and CONGENITAL defects.

During pregnancy, the fetus is surrounded by a sac of AMNIOTIC FLUID, which protects and cushions the developing embryo and into which fetal cells are released. In amniocentesis, these cells are collected, examined and analyzed, along with amniotic fluid itself, to provide information regarding the condition of the fetus and to detect possible genetic or metabolic defects. Normally, this procedure is performed at the 15th to 17th week of pregnancy to ensure that sufficient amniotic fluid is present to provide the amount of fluid required for proper analysis. It can take two to five weeks to culture and prepare the fetal cells in the laboratory for analysis, so the matter of the timing of this procedure is important in the event that amniocentesis discloses a defect or disorder that may indicate considering the option of terminating the pregnancy.

Often the first step is injection of local anesthetic. A needle is then inserted through the mother's abdominal wall and the wall of the uterus, and into the amniotic sac. A syringe is used to withdraw a sample of the amniotic fluid.

ULTRASOUND is used in conjunction with amniocentesis to present an image of the fetus and its position in the uterus, and to aid the physician in guiding the needle into the amniotic sac. With the use of ultrasound and the image of the fetus projected on the screen, a skilled physician can guide the needle into and through a space as small as a quarter-inch in diameter.

A report published in 1963 described the technique, which was used in this account to give a blood transfusion to a fetus with maternal Rh blood factor incompatibility (see HEMOLYTIC DISEASE OF THE NEWBORN). In 1966, M. W. Steele and W. R. Bregg described how the technique could be used to collect and culture fetal cells for chromosomal analysis from the amniotic fluid. The technique was perfected for use in PRENATAL DIAGNOSIS by 1969.

Disorders that can be detected through amniocentesis include TAY-SACHS DISEASE, SICKLE-CELL ANEMIA, SPINA BIFIDA, NEURAL TUBE DEFECTS (NTD), ENZYME deficiencies, CHROMOSOME ABNORMALITIES and blood disorders. Using molecular diagnostic studies with linked GENETIC MARKERS, many other diseases, such as CYSTIC FIBROSIS and Duchenne MUSCULAR DYSTROPHY can now be diagnosed as well. Amniocentesis can also disclose the sex of the unborn child, although the procedure is not performed solely for this purpose.

Amniocentesis is an invasive procedure and involves risks, both to the mother and the fetus. Strict antiseptic procedures must be followed to prevent infection and extreme care must be taken to keep the needle from puncturing the fetus. Other potential adverse effects include hemorrhage of either the mother or the fetus, leakage of amniotic fluid, and spontaneous ABORTION. There is a one in 200 risk of miscarriage in addition to the normal risk of miscarriage at this point in pregnancy. The other potential complications are much less often encountered. Some studies have suggested that the risk of early amniocentesis is more comparable to CVS than to routine midtrimester amniocentesis.

The use of amniocentesis earlier in pregnancy (11th or 12th week) has also been investigated. A large Canadian study found a link between early amniocentesis and increased foot deformities and stillbirth. Infants exposed to standard amniocentesis exhibited a foot deformity rate of 0.1%. Among those tested via early amniocentesis, the rate was 1.3%, or a 13-fold increase. This is thought to result from loss of amniotic fluid, leading to compression of the fetus. Rates of STILLBIRTH were about 1% higher.

Despite its widespread use as a prenatal diagnostic procedure, the decision to use amniocentesis should be carefully considered by the physician and parents in consultation, with the risks weighed against potential benefits. However, it is commonly recommended for pregnancies of women over 35 years of age due to increased risk of DOWN SYNDROME and other chromosomal abnormalities, after maternal serum screening indicates an elevated risk of having a fetus with a CHROMOSOME ABNORMALITY, as well as in pregnancies involving a known and detectable risk of birth defects or GENETIC DISORDERS.

amniotic band syndrome (ADAM complex) Term referring to a variety of anomalies associated with fibrous bands that entangle the fetus in the womb, interfering with fetal development. The fibrous bands are thought to result from ruptures of the amniotic membranes within the womb. The earlier and more severe the intrauterine damage, the greater the impact on the infant. It may simply constrict a portion of the fetus or cause more widespread problems by cutting off blood supply to a region of the body of the fetus.

In its most common form, only the limbs are involved, ranging from constriction rings that appear around digits or limbs to amputation of digits or limbs. There may be fusion of the ends of digits (distal pseudosyndactyly). The most severe form involves both limb malformations and crainiofacial anomalies, and has been referred to by the acronym ADAM, (Amniotic Deformity, Adhesions, Mutilations) Complex.

The craniofacial malformations may include CLEFT LIP and palate, an increase in cerebral fluid causing enlargement of the head (HYDROCEPHALUS), gross clefts of the midface and protrusion of the brain through fissures in the skull (ENCEPHALOCELE). A number of ocular and nasal abnormalities may also be present.

Part of the intestine may protrude through the abdominal wall, covered only by a thin membrane.

The failure of the abdominal wall to close is referred to as "gastroschisis."

This nonhereditary congenital condition is estimated to occur in one in 5,000 to one in 10,000 live births, with at least 600 cases reported. While some genetic conditions may cause similar malformations, they tend to be symmetrical, that is, the limb defects are mirror images of each other.

PRENATAL DIAGNOSIS may be possible in severe cases, due to the association of elevated alpha-fetoprotein levels with ADAM complex, as well as by ultrasound examination. Simple cases may cause only cosmetic problems. Congenital limb amputations require prosthetic limbs, and MENTAL RETARDATION may be associated with cases involving craniofacial defects. Many cases of the ADAM complex may result in STILLBIRTH or death soon after birth.

amniotic fluid The colorless, almost transparent fluid that surrounds the developing FETUS in the womb. Amniotic fluid is composed of fluid from the mother as well as fetal urine and other body secretions. It contains cells, for example, shed from the fetus's skin as well as fetal bladder cells excreted in the urine.

This protective fluid is rapidly recirculated throughout the mother's body, with a complete replacement requiring approximately three hours. The fetus swallows some of the fluid, and if there is, for example, an obstruction in the fetus's intestinal tract or the fetus has a neurologic disorder that impairs swallowing, the fluid accumulates. This condition of excess fluid is termed polyhydramnios. If the fetal kidneys are not working properly and no fetal urine is produced, there is a deficiency of amniotic fluid. This is termed oligohydramnios.

In the genetic testing procedure of AMNIOCENTESIS, amniotic fluid is withdrawn from the womb via a surgical needle for later examination.

amyloidosis A rare metabolic disorder marked by deposition of amyloid, a starchlike protein, in organs and tissues, leading to slowly progressive deterioration of nerves (in adulthood) and ultimately death. AUTOSOMAL DOMINANT hereditary forms have been identified in isolated families and populations around the world, caused by a mutation in the *TTR* gene on the long arm of chromosome 18.

In the United States approximately 1:100,000 to 1:1,000,000 people are CARRIERS of the defective GENE that causes hereditary amyloidosis. It can affect many different organs in the body including the nervous system, heart, kidneys, liver and gastrointestinal tract. In addition to the autosomal dominant hereditary form it can be found secondary to another chronic inflammatory disease, FAMILIAL MEDITERRANEAN FEVER, an AUTOSOMAL RECESSIVE disorder.

amyotrophic lateral sclerosis (ALS) Known as "Lou Gehrig's disease" after perhaps the best-known patient, the New York Yankees' all-star of the 1920s and '30s, ALS is a progressive and fatal degenerative disease of the neuromuscular system. (Gehrig's life story was recounted in the 1942 movie *Pride of the Yankees*. Other famous affected individuals have included physicist Steven Hawking, Vice President Henry A. Wallace, boxing champion Ezzard Charles, jazz musician Charles Mingus, actor David Niven and U.S. senator Jacob Javits.)

ALS attacks the motor neurons, among the largest nerve cells, which reach from the brain to the spinal cord and from the spinal cord to muscles throughout the body. The destruction of these neurons leads to complete loss of voluntary muscle movement and total paralysis. It was first described by French neurologist Jean-Martin Charcot in 1869. The name is derived from Greek. *A* means "without" or "negative," *myo* refers to muscle, and *trophic* means "nourishment." When a muscle has no nourishment, it withers and wastes away. "Lateral" refers to the area of the spinal cord (the lateral columns) where portions of the affected neurons are located. The degenerative changes produce scarring, or hardening, referred to as "sclerosis" of the muscle and nerve tissue.

Onset usually occurs between the ages of 40 and 70, though it may begin as early as the teen years. Early symptoms include tripping, dropping objects, abnormal fatigue of the arms or legs, slurred speech, muscle cramps and twitching and involuntary bouts of laughing or crying.

The hands and feet are usually affected first, progressing to the muscles of the trunk. It eventually affects chewing, breathing and swallowing, and requires permanent mechanical breathing assistance to maintain life.

Mental functions, and senses of sight, touch, hearing, taste, smell and muscles of the eyes and bladder are generally unaffected.

Worldwide, ALS occurs in four to eight per 100,000 individuals. Some 5,000 people in the United States are newly diagnosed annually. An estimated 30,000 have the disease at any given time, with approximately 300,000 presently unaffected individuals expected to develop the disease in the future. Half live at least three years after diagnosis, 25% five years or more, and 10% survive for more than 10 years. Lifetime risks of ALS are one in 600 for men and one in 850 for women. More than 90% to 95% of amyotrophic lateral sclerosis cases are classified as sporadic. The remaining cases of ALS are familial, inherited in an autosomal dominant fashion. Inherited types of amyotrophic lateral sclerosis can be caused by mutations in the *SOD1*, *ALS2* or *KIAA0625* (also called *SETX*) genes. Mutations in the gene for Cu/Zn binding superoxide dismutase (*SOD1*) have been found to account for 15% to 20% of familial cases. How these mutations cause the disease is unclear, and conflicting hypotheses have been advanced, but it appears that toxicity of free radicals plays an important role. A number of other genes appear to be involved in rare hereditary forms.

A very rare recessive form of ALS, a juvenile form with the mean age of onset of symptoms being 12 years of age, has a relatively high prevalence in Tunisia. A gene for this form has been linked to chromosome 2q. Other rare forms of the disease include the AUTOSOMAL DOMINANT ALS with dementia, and the ALS-Parkinsonism-Demetia complex of Guam, which may be of polygenic or environmental etiology.

In 1995, the Food and Drug Administration approved the world's first drug to treat the disease, riluzole. Clinical studies had shown it could slightly prolong lives.

Currently, there is no method of PRENATAL DIAGNOSIS for ALS. Other inherited motor system diseases include SPINAL MUSCULAR ATROPHY, Werdnig-Hoffman disease and Kugelberg-Welander disease.

Andersen disease   See GLYCOGEN STORAGE DISEASE.

anemia   Not a disease, but a manifestation of a group of disorders of the red blood cells, which collect oxygen absorbed in the lungs and carry it throughout the body. Among the more prevalent causes: The blood cells themselves may be abnormal, as in spherocytosis (see below); the levels of HEMOGLOBIN, the pigment that carries the oxygen in the blood cell, may be abnormally low, as in THALASSEMIA; the hemoglobin itself may exhibit abnormalities, as is the case in SICKLE-CELL ANEMIA; if hemoglobin production is normal, the red blood cells may be broken down (hemolyzed) in the body faster than they can be replaced (this is called a "hemolytic" anemia). There can be decreased production of red cells as in the hypoplastic anemias or the cells can be trapped and destroyed in an enlarged spleen, as in GAUCHER DISEASE.

Several conditions causing anemia are inherited, and it is also a feature of numerous hereditary disorders. These include ABETALIPOPROTEINEMIA, Gaucher disease, FANCONI ANEMIA, DYSKERATOSIS CONGENITA, METHYLMALONIC ACIDEMIA, CYSTINOSIS, OSTEOPETROSIS (see INFANTILE OSTEOPETROSIS), Chediak-Higashi syndrome and thrombocytopenia-absent radius (TAR) syndrome. Anemia may also result from dietary or vitamin deficiencies (e.g., iron, folic acid), drugs or other disease processes such as blood loss. It tends to be highly variable in expression, ranging from mild to severe.

Regardless of the cause, the symptoms in all forms may include weakness, general malaise, headaches, drowsiness, sore tongue, loss of libido, slight fever, hunger for air and breathing difficulties (dyspnea), and heart palpitations. The skin, gums, eyes and nail beds may exhibit a pallor or paleness. In severe cases anemia may induce cardiac disease, resulting in chest pain or heart failure.

Although individuals with anemia exhibit a reduced number of functioning red blood cells within a given volume of blood, there is no precise definition for specific levels below which anemia is said to exist. The defined level must also take into account age and gender. If the onset is slow, the body may adjust so well that there is no functional impairment, despite extremely low

levels of hemoglobin. Diagnosis requires integration of information about patient history, physical examination, blood tests including blood counts, and red cell indices and appearance as well as other laboratory testing. (The red cells may exhibit characteristic deformities suggestive of, for example, sickle-cell disease, spherocytosis or elliptocytosis.)

Congenital Hemolytic Anemias

These inherited chronic diseases are characterized by hemolysis (breakdown) of red blood cells at an accelerated rate. While symptoms are the same as in other forms of anemia, there may be jaundice, or yellowing of the skin and eyes, as well. This results from an excess of bilirubin, a yellow pigment, which is released when red blood cells are hemolyzed. The spleen, which is where most hemolysis occurs, may become enlarged and is one of the signs of the disorder.

There is also a familial, non-congenital form of hemolytic anemia, as well as acquired forms. Hemolytic anemia is also a feature of numerous specific disorders, such as sickle-cell anemia and thalassemia, spherocytosis, elliptocytosis, glucose-6-phosphate dehydrogenase deficiency (G6PD) and other red cell enzyme deficiency disorders.

Spherocytosis

This is a hereditary form of hemolytic anemia that results from the red blood cells being abnormally small and round (that is, spherocytic; red cells are normally biconcave disks). It is caused by a defect in the red cell membrane and occurs as an AUTOSOMAL DOMINANT trait. This is the most common hereditary hemolytic anemia in whites (particularly of northern European extraction). Most cases are due to deficiency of one of the red blood cell membrane proteins, ankyrin or spectrin. Incidence has been estimated at 2.2 per 10,000 live births, with about one-quarter of the cases being SPORADIC. Symptoms are the same as for congenital hemolytic anemia. In most cases the anemia is mild. Diagnosis often requires red cell fragility tests.

The increased production of bilirubin leads to gallstone disease, a major complication of this disorder, which can be prevented by the removal of the spleen. In some cases, removal of the spleen may cure the accelerated destruction of red blood cells.

Elliptocytosis

This is characterized by abnormalities of the membrane imparting an oval or cigar shape to the red blood cells. Inherited as an autosomal dominant trait, incidence is estimated at approximately one in 2,500 live births. Most affected individuals are asymptomatic, though about 12% exhibit symptoms similar to spherocytosis. Several distinct forms exist, resulting from mutations in any one of several genes for different red blood cell membrane proteins.

Congenital Hypoplastic Anemia

A rare condition which seems to be due to impairment of red blood cell progenitor differentiation. Incidence is estimated to be about five per 1,000,000, and several hundred affected individuals have been reported in the medical literature. Both autosomal dominant and AUTOSOMAL RECESSIVE inheritance have been postulated but the genetics are unclear. Some families clearly show autosomal dominant patterns, though most cases have been sporadic. About 10% to 15% of cases occur in families with more than one affected individual. Symptoms, beginning with skin pallor, usually have onset within the first three months of life. The pulse becomes rapid as anemia increases, and cardiac enlargement and dilation may develop. Heart failure and pneumonia may ensue.

The disorder is sometimes known as the Blackfan-Diamond syndrome, for U.S. physicians K. D. Blackfan and L. K. Diamond, who first described it in 1938. About 25% of affected children also have physical abnormalities, most commonly short stature. Some affected infants have also had two thumbs on one hand, or thumbs with an extra joint (triphalangeal thumbs). About 25% of cases of Blackfan-Diamond anemia are caused by mutations in the gene encoding ribosomal protein S19 (*RPS19*), which maps to 19q. At least 10% of Blackfan-Diamond anemia, and possibly a larger proportion, result from mutations in genes other than the *RPS19* gene. There is considerable overlap between Blackfan-Diamond and Aase syndrome (named for physician J. M. Aase who published the first description in 1969) and they are probably the same disease. Other physical abnormalities described include short, webbed neck, cleft palate,

and structural abnormalities of the heart or kidney. Many of these same physical features are also seen in Fanconi anemia, from which this must be differentiated.

Anemia may also be associated with pregnancy. A 1987 survey of lower income women by the Centers for Disease Control found that in the first three months of pregnancy, 13% of black women and 4% of white women had hemoglobin levels indicating anemia. In the second trimester the rates rose to 18% and 6%, respectively, and in the last trimester, 38% and 19%. Anemia during pregnancy increases the risk of premature birth, LOW BIRTH WEIGHT and fetal death.

anencephaly   A severe NEURAL TUBE DEFECT (NTD) that results in absence of most of the brain and, in extreme cases, the spinal cord as well. Additionally, there are often multiple malformations of the skeleton and internal organs. The cranial vault, or top of the skull, is absent, and the brain tissue, if present, is exposed. Though the cerebral hemispheres are usually missing, the lower brain stem, which controls internal organs, is present. Almost all the bones in the skull are abnormal. Defects in skull formation cause characteristic facial anomalies. The eyes protrude, the nose is prominent and CLEFT LIP WITH OR WITHOUT CLEFT PALATE is often seen. Malformations of limbs, thoracic cage, the abdominal wall, gastrointestinal tract and genitourinary system are relatively common. The heart, lungs, kidneys and adrenal glands are also often malformed.

The disorder is thought to develop between the 23rd and 26th days following conception, due to a failure of part of the neural tube to close.

While there have been reports of cases believed to be transmitted in AUTOSOMAL RECESSIVE and X-LINKED patterns, anencephaly appears to be a MULTIFACTORIAL condition. Incidence in the United States is estimated at one in 1,000 live births, with 2,000 to 3,500 anencephalics born annually. However, prevalence varies with geography, racial and ethnic background and sex of the fetus, and socioeconomic conditions. In some areas of Ireland and Wales, incidence is as high as five to seven per 1,000 live births. (In South Wales, the disorder has been reported as high as one in 105 live births.) Neural tube defects as a whole have a low incidence among blacks, Ashkenazi Jews (those of Eastern European ancestry) and Asians. Affected females outnumber affected males by at least a 2:1 ratio. There is an approximately 3–5% risk of recurrence of a neural tube defect (either SPINA BIFIDA or anencephaly) in subsequent pregnancies, after the birth of a child with a neural tube defect. Recent evidence from studies with folic acid supplementation support the view that the majority of NTDs are caused by a combination of genetic and environmental factors.

Parents of infants with neural tube defects appear to have a higher than average incidence of defects of spinal cord development, including spine bifida occulata.

Taking folic acid (a B-complex VITAMIN) before conception and during early pregnancy can reduce the occurrence of NTDs, though the mechanism of this preventative effect is not understood. Women who had one or more pregnancies affected by an NTD and who subsequently used supplemental folic acid significantly reduced their risk to have another child with an NTD to about 1%. These findings led the FDA to approve fortification of food with folic acid in 1998, the first new fortification allowed since 1943. It has been recommended that all women of childbearing age who have had a pregnancy affected with a NTD should take 4–5 mg of folic acid per day and that all women of childbearing age (especially those planning a pregnancy) should take 0.4 mg of folic acid a day.

Prenatal screening for elevated maternal serum alphafetoprotein levels, in conjunction with ULTRASOUND (and AMNIOCENTESIS) is thought to be capable of diagnosing 90% of cases.

This condition is incompatible with life, and most anencephalic infants are either stillborn, or die within a few days of birth. Some anencephalic infants have been kept alive by artificial means in order to preserve their organs for transplant. Without life support, the organs deteriorate by the time these infants are legally dead. Typically, the organs sought are liver, heart, heart valves and corneas. It is estimated that 40% to 70% of children under two years old on waiting lists for organ transplants die before suitable organ donors are found.

In the 1980s, the Loma Linda University Medical Center, in Loma Linda, California, developed

the first guidelines in the United States for accepting anencephalic organ donors and keeping them alive. Though parents of anencephalic infants have requested that their infant's organs be donated in this manner, the practice raises troubling ethical and legal issues, and the program at Loma Linda was suspended soon after its inception and remains dormant. As in other states, organs are often unusable due to deterioration by the time the donor meets current California standards defining death.

In 1996, the American Medical Association took a position opposing the harvesting of organs from infants with anencephaly or other brain developmental disorders incompatible with life.

aneuploidy The state of having an abnormal number of CHROMOSOMES. Normally, humans have 23 pairs of chromosomes in each cell. A cell, or an individual, that has a number of chromosomes that is not an exact multiple of 23 (e.g., 47 instead of 46) is said to be aneuploid. Some CHROMOSOME ABNORMALITIES are characterized by aneuploidy. Conditions of aneuploidy include DOWN SYNDROME and TURNER SYNDROME.

Angelman syndrome (AS; happy puppet syndrome)
First described by Dr. Harry Angelman in 1965, this disorder is characterized by severe MENTAL RETARDATION, developmental delays and growth deficiency. It takes its name from an abnormal, puppet-like gait and frequent paroxysms of laughter unconnected to emotions of happiness; affected individuals seem constantly and inappropriately happy, smiling and laughing. These laughing fits are thought to result from a defect in the brain stem. Gait is wide-based with jerky limb movements and flapping hands. Characteristic facial appearance includes a small, squat skull, decreased ocular pigmentation resulting in pale blue eyes, a large mouth with a large, protruding tongue (macroglossia), and widely spaced teeth. Absent speech is a feature. Seizures are frequent.

More than 50% of cases result from chromosomal deletions in one copy of chromosome 15 involving a specific segment of the long arm of that chromosome. The deleted segment is lost from the chromosome 15 inherited from the mother. (Deletions of the same segment of the chromosome inherited from the father result in PRADER-WILLI SYNDROME.) In very rare cases, AS patients are found to have inherited two copies of chromosome 15, both from the father. This is called uniparental disomy. (See CHROMOSOME ABNORMALITIES.) These two situations have in common the lack of a maternal gene contribution from this region of the long arm of chromosome 15, an example of IMPRINTING. About 6% of patients with AS have a mutation in the chromosome 15 imprinting center that makes the maternal chromosome look like a paternal one (it fails to get the imprint of its maternal origin). The imprinting center is a gene on the chromosome that controls imprinting and therefore affects the function of those genes on the chromosome susceptible to imprinting's influence.

Recently a specific gene, *UBE3A*, was found to be involved in Angelman syndrome; mutations in the gene can cause the syndrome. Only the maternally imprinted copy of this gene is expressed in the brain.

This syndrome affects an estimated one in 10,000 to 20,000 people. The risk to siblings of an affected child who has a deletion or uniparental disomy is typically less than 1%. The risk can be as high as 50% to the siblings of a child with an imprinting defect or a mutation of the *UBE3A* gene. The vast majority (>85% at least) of cases are sporadic, and therefore recurrence risks are low.

angioneurotic edema, hereditary See HEREDITARY ANGIONEUROTIC EDEMA.

aniridia The absence of all or part of the iris, the pigmented circle that gives eyes their color. This condition affects both eyes (bilateral) and is usually detected at birth. Accompanying visual disturbances include CATARACTS, glaucoma and malformation of the cornea.

Affected individuals with isolated aniridia have acute visual problems but normal life expectancy and intelligence. However, it has been associated with disorders including partial or complete absence

of the kneecap (patella), speech disturbances, psychomotor malfunction, CHROMOSOME ABNORMALITIES (deletions of the short arm of chromosome 11), WILMS TUMOR of the kidney and varying degrees of MENTAL RETARDATION. Aniridia may also be seen as part of the WAGR syndrome. This SYNDROME consists of the occurrence together of two or more of the following: Wilms tumor (a kidney tumor), aniridia, genitourinary abnormalities and MENTAL RETARDATION. The genitorurinary abnormalities include AMBIGUOUS GENITALIA, gonadoblastoma, CRYPTORCHISM and hypospadias.

The WAGR syndrome is a contiguous GENE SYNDROME resulting from the deletion of contiguous genes located next to one another on 11p. In WAGR, the *PAX6* and *WT1* genes are disrupted to varying degrees along with other as yet unidentified genes (e.g., one causing mental retardation.) The genitourinary abnormalities seem to result from the *WT1* mutation. The size and nature of the deletion determines which features the affected child will have.

Aniridia occurs in all cases of WAGR, and Wilms tumor is seen in about 90% of those with WAGR. Isolated aniridia is transmitted as an AUTOSOMAL DOMINANT trait and results from mutations in the *PAX6* gene, located on the short arm of chromosome 11. This developmental gene seems to affect not only the development of the eye but also the migration and differentiation of neuronal progenitor cells in the developing brain. *PAX6* mutations have also been described in Peters anomaly, an opacity of the central cornea, though this mutation has not been detected in the majority of affected individuals. *PAX 6* mutations have also been seen in other ocular malformations, including Ectopia pupillae, the displacement of the pupil from the center of the iris, and juvenile cataracts. The *PAX6* mutation is seen in about one-third of cases of aniridia, and these are often found to have cytogenetically detectable deletions of the short arm of chromosome 11. If the deletion is extensive enough, the WAGR syndrome results.

As an isolated condition, aniridia occurs in approximately one in 50,000 live births. PRENATAL DIAGNOSIS is theoretically possible in cases where aniridia is associated with Wilms tumor or chromosomal anomalies.

ankyloglossia (tongue-tie) Movement of the tongue is severely restricted by this defect, also known as tongue-tie. It results from an abnormal shortness of the membrane that anchors the underside of the tongue to the floor of the mouth (frenulum linguae). An affected person cannot raise his or her tongue above the corners of the mouth when it is wide open. Efforts to stick the tongue out make the edges protrude while the anchored tip remains in place, giving it a grooved or forked appearance.

The cause is not known, but evidence suggests an AUTOSOMAL DOMINANT mode of inheritance in some cases. The defect occurs in about one in 330 live births. Male and female infants are affected equally. The defect can be identified at birth.

ankylosing spondylitis (AS) A chronic arthritis involving the joints of the spine, AS takes its name from the Greek terms for stiffening (ankylosing) and inflammation of the spinal joints (spondylitis). The disorder is variable in its expression, ranging from mild aches and pains to severe stooping posture caused by fusing of the joints, rendering them immobile. (In 20% of cases, joints of the pelvis, shoulders, hips and knees may also be involved.) It is the third most common form of chronic arthritis in the United States, affecting an estimated 500,000 individuals.

AS has been identified in 4,000-year-old Egyptian mummies, and, as with other diseases characterized by inflammation of the joints (arthritic diseases), a strong familial link has been established. Previously thought to affect only males, females are now known to be equally at risk, though they are usually less severely affected.

Onset is gradual, typically beginning between the ages of 18 and 30 years, with episodes of lower back pain that may be acute at night. Frequently, the back pain improves with exercise and grows worse with rest, making it distinguishable from common lower back pain.

The basic defect that causes the inflammation of the joints is unknown. However, a GENETIC MARKER for the condition, *HLA B27*, has been identified. This particular variation of HLA antigen (see HUMAN LEUKOCYTE ANTIGEN), the "tissue type" marker on cell surfaces, is found in almost everyone with AS,

and unaffected individuals with *HLA B27* have 300 times the susceptibility to develop the condition as those without it. Still, only 2%–8% of all *HLA B27* individuals develop AS. Whether this is due to other genetic differences in predisposition or due to environmental exposure is not known, but it is likely to be a combination of the two. Some of the difference is likely to be due to a variation with the *B27* GENE itself. There are nine subtypes of *B27* and some of these are more associated with AS than others, though it appears other genes are also involved in the development of this disorder.

While there is no cure, proper diagnosis and treatment (generally consisting of nonsteroid anti-inflammatory drugs, to alleviate inflammation, and daily exercise for the joints) can minimize the effects of the disorder.

annular pancreas   A malformation of the pancreas during fetal development leading to intestinal obstruction. The pancreas is a gland that, in addition to secreting the hormone insulin, releases ENZYMES for the proper digestion of fats, proteins and carbohydrates. The pancreas is situated behind the stomach and connects to the duodenum, the first portion of the small intestine through which food passes from the stomach. Pancreatic juices are released into the duodenum through an opening in the wall of the duodenum. This opening also acts as the point of release for bile, a liver secretion that emulsifies fats in food.

In this condition, during development of the embryo, portions of the pancreas form an abnormal collar or ring encircling the duodenum. This can lead to an intestinal obstruction in the duodenum, symptoms of which can include intermittent vomiting, bile-stained vomit, FAILURE TO THRIVE, and in rare cases later in life, inflammation of the pancreas (pancreatitis) and biliary tract disease.

Frequently (perhaps in 70% of cases), the malformation is associated with other ANOMALIES. Duodenal stenosis or atresia occurs most commonly. Occasionally annular pancreas only becomes symptomatic in adulthood where symptoms may mimic gallbladder disease. The syndrome it is most often associated with is DOWN SYNDROME. As many as 15–20% of infants who exhibit intestinal obstruction due to annular pancreas have Down syndrome, and one study found 6% of children with Down syndrome also suffered from the obstructive symptoms of annular pancreas.

Annular pancreas occurs in about one of every 10,000 live births and can be detected from birth on. Most cases are sporadic, though a few families in which it appears to be transmitted as an AUTOSOMAL DOMINANT trait have been reported. The intestinal obstruction can be corrected surgically. Life expectancy is normal, except in cases where pancreatitis or biliary tract disease occur.

anomaly   An IN UTERO developmental deviation from normal form or structure, such as a missing organ or limb, or an extra digit. Synonym: congenital anomaly.

Anomalies may be divided into two categories: malformations and deformations. A malformation occurs where the body part or organ, is different because of an intrinsically abnormal developmental process (e.g., a congenital HEART DEFECT or a CLEFT LIP). A deformation occurs when a previously normally formed body part is altered in shape or structure (e.g., a CLUBFOOT or CONGENITAL hip dislocation) by mechanical forces, such as compression against the wall of the womb due to deficient AMNIOTIC FLUID. (See also BIRTH DEFECTS.)

anonychia, hereditary   See HEREDITARY ANONYCHIA.

anophthalmia   The congenital absence of one or both eyes. It is associated with several syndromes involving mental retardation and congenital anomalies. Anophthalmia with anomalies of the hands and feet has been identified as a distinct hereditary condition, identified in at least 18 families. Consanguinity was noted in 90% of these families.

Anopthalmia is a rare condition. Autosomal recessive inheritance has been suggested. Exposure to a variety of teratogens in utero, including X-rays, chemicals, drugs, pesticides, radiation or viruses, increases the risk of anophthalmia. Prenatal diagnosis via ultrasound may be possible.

anorchia See ABSENT TESTES.

anosmia (congenital anosmia) The complete absence of the sense of smell (anosmia) and an abnormally decreased sense of smell (hyposmia) are, by themselves, quite rare among newborns. Risk, prevalence and the ratio of males to females are unknown for isolated cases. However, either condition may accompany certain congenital endocrine disorders, defects in head or facial shape, and hearing or visual disabilities. Failure to respond to parathyroid hormone (pseudohypoparathyroidism) and abnormally decreased activity of the gonads (hypogonadotropic hypogonadism) are two endocrine abnormalities often associated with anosmia. When no other abnormalities are present, anosmia and hyposmia are usually detected by clinical surveys during childhood. Neither condition, by itself, affects normal life span or intelligence.

While the cause of both conditions is unknown, it is believed that developmental abnormalities in the sense of smell (olfactory system) are to blame, particularly a lack of development of the olfactory bulb in the embryo. Other hypothesized causes are trauma to the fetus, inflammation and lack of vitamin A during gestation. There is no known treatment for either disorder, and therapy for associated endocrine imbalances does not restore olfactory function. Isolated anosmia has been described with X-LINKED recessive and AUTOSOMAL DOMINANT inheritance. The condition has also been described in REFSUM DISEASE, with frontal or temporal lobe brain tumors, and in cadmium poisoning.

The combination of anosmia and hypogonadotropic hypogonadism is known as KALLMAN SYNDROME, for Franz Josef Kallman, who described the disorder in 1944. It is most commonly inherited as an X-linked recessive disorder affecting males. Individuals with hypogonadotropic hypogonadism exhibit delayed puberty, abnormal development of secondary sexual characteristics and infertility as well as CRYPTORCHISM (undescended testes) and in some instances micropenis. Renal ANOMALIES can also be present. Transmitting females have hyposmia or anosmia. About one in 10,000 males is affected. The GENE responsible, KAL1, is found on the short arm of the X CHROMOSOME and is involved in neuronal migration. There are also autosomal dominant and autosomal recessive forms. The genetic basis for these are unknown.

antenatal diagnosis See PRENATAL DIAGNOSIS.

anticonvulsants Medications used to control seizures. Some have been linked to birth defects when taken during pregnancy. It is not clear whether the association of anticonvulsants and congenital defects is due to the drugs, the underlying disease itself, other genetic factors or a combination of all of the above. Clearly, there is some evidence pointing to the drugs as a causative factor. Overall risk of fetal abnormalities in women treated with anticonvulsants is about two to three times that of the general population.

Hydantoins, such as phenytoin, prescribed for epileptic seizures, may cause fetal hydantoin syndrome characterized by distinctive facial malformations, such as a short nose, bowed upper lip, broad nasal bridge, wide space between the eyes, and CLEFT LIP or CLEFT PALATE. Underdeveloped fingertips, with small or missing nails are also common. Slow growth both before and after birth, an abnormally small head (MICROCEPHALY), MENTAL RETARDATION and heart defects are additional symptoms of the syndrome.

About 10% of infants born to women taking hydantoins have the full-blown SYNDROME. An additional 30% show some of the abnormalities. Some facial deformities and heart defects may require surgical correction. The susceptibility of the fetus to the teratogenic effects of hydantoins depends on the fetal genotype, that is, an interaction between genetics and environment.

The anticonvulsants trimethadione, paramethadione and primidone are known to cause birth defects, but are rarely prescribed to women during their childbearing years. In 20% to 50% of exposed infants, trimethadione and paramethadione have been linked to a syndrome characterized by INTRAUTERINE GROWTH RETARDATION, small head circumference, delayed development, mental retardation, deformed ears and heart defects. Other features include V-shaped eyebrows, a short nose with a

broad, depressed bridge, a small jaw, and cleft lip or palate and hearing loss.

Children with primidone syndrome grow more slowly than normal and have an abnormally small head, jitteriness, a hairy forehead, deformed nostrils, a small jaw, underdeveloped fingernails and heart defects.

Valproic acid, another anticonvulsant, has been associated with an increase in SPINA BIFIDA. It occurs in the offspring of about 1–2% of the women who take it during pregnancy. A fetal valproate syndrome has also been described, consisting of a high forehead, epicanthic folds, small upturned nose with a low nasal bridge, small mouth, long philtrum and thin upper lip, long, thin fingers and toes, and congenital heart defects.

Several reports have linked carbamazepine to an increased risk of ANOMALIES, including a characteristic facial appearance and an increased risk of spina bifida. Insufficient information on other anticonvulsants exists to ascertain their safety or potential adverse effects.

All the major anticonvulsant drugs (carbamazepine, sodium valproate, phenytoin, phenobarbitone and mysoline) are teratogenic. The main risk to the developing fetus appears to be when the mother is on more than one drug, especially if one is valproate. The majority of the malformations seen are minor and include hypertelorism, an abnormal midface, epicanthic folds, microcephaly, transverse palmar creases and minor skeletal abnormalities. More serious malformations include spina bifida and congenital heart disease. These can be screened for in utero with ultrasound. The risk of an infant having congenital anomalies can be minimized by using only one drug in the lowest possible dose. Folic acid supplements before conception are advisable, and some recommend that women with epilepsy should receive high-dose folate supplements (4mg). It has been suggested that oral vitamin K should be given to a mother receiving enzyme-inducing antiepileptic drugs (phenytoin, carbamazepine or phenobarbitone) in the last month of pregnancy to protect the fetus against haemorrhagic disease of the newborn. Two newer anticonvulsant drugs (gabapentin and lamotrigine) do not appear to be teratogenic in animal studies, though there is little data on women taking these drugs in pregnancy.

Topiramate, a more recently licensed anticonvulsant, has been shown to cause limb abnormalities in animal studies. (See also TERATOGEN.)

antidepressants Many women of child-bearing age take antidepressants. The effects of these drugs on the developing fetus have been closely examined, but findings have been inconclusive or contradictory. Some studies have suggested selective serotonin reuptake inhibitors (SSRIs), the most commonly prescribed antidepressants, are relatively safe to take during pregnancy. These antidepressants include fluoxetine (Prozac), paroxetine (Paxil), citalopram (Celexa), and sertraline (Zoloft). Other research contradicts those findings.

An analysis of past research showed that babies whose mothers take SSRIs during pregnancy may be more likely to be born prematurely, have low birth weight, spend time in a neonatal intensive care unit and have trouble adapting to life outside the womb. This was particularly the case for babies of women who were also taking other drugs for mental conditions or who smoked or drank alcohol. However, no significant difference in the rates of miscarriages and stillbirth between women who take SSRIs and women who do not has been found.

Two large studies published in 2005 found babies of women who took Paxil and Prozac in the first trimester had a greater risk of birth defects. One study found that babies whose mothers took SSRIs in the second half of their pregnancy were six times more likely to be born with persistent pulmonary hypertension, a serious breathing problem that typically occurs in 1:1,000 live births. Other recent studies have noted withdrawal symptoms in nearly one-third of newborns whose mothers were treated with SSRIs near the end of their pregnancy. The symptoms, though relatively benign and short-lived, included tremors, convulsions, irritability and increased crying. Some physicians recommend pregnant patients taper to a lower dosage or stop taking antidepressants 10 to 14 days before their due date to prevent withdrawal symptoms in newborns. In 2005, the Food and Drug Administration ordered a new warning label for paroxetine (Paxil) after two studies linked it to heart defects in newborns.

The findings give pregnant women who have been prescribed antidepressants a difficult choice. Without the medication, some women may have difficulty sleeping, eating and gaining enough weight for a healthy pregnancy. Additionally, research has shown that infants of mothers suffering postpartum depression are more likely to have trouble with cognitive, social and psychological development.

Antidepressants known as monoamine oxidase inhibitors (MAOIs), such as phenelzine (Nardil) and tranylcypromine (Parnate), may cause birth defects and are not considered safe to use during pregnancy.

antiphospholipid syndrome (antiphospholipid antibody syndrome) An autoimmune disorder affecting blood coagulation that results in recurring thromboses, or the formation of blood clots within the heart or blood vessels, before the age of 45. It is also associated with repeated spontaneous abortions in young women. It is one of several forms of thrombophilia, clotting disorders in which the blood has a tendency to clot, or thrombose. Some thrombophilias are hereditary, but antiphospholipid syndrome is an acquired form. Abnormal bleeding and coagulation occur most frequently in the arms, legs and gastrointestinal tract, though it may occur in many organs or parts of the body. The characteristic blood clots often lead to strokes or transient ischemic attacks and, in women, repeated spontaneous ABORTIONS.

antitrypsin deficiency See ALPHA-1-ANTITRYPSIN DEFICIENCY.

Apert syndrome (acrocephalosyndaclyly) A form of CRANIOSYNOSTOSIS, a condition caused by the premature closure of the gaps, or sutures, of the skull bones, resulting in an abnormal shape of the head. This form is named for Eugene Apert (1868–1940), a senior pediatrician at the Hopital des Enfants Malades in Paris, who published the definitive description in 1906.

The most characteristic features are a peaked, pointed head (ACROCEPHALY; turribrachycephaly) and webbed fingers and toes (SYNDACTYLY).

The deformities of the hands and feet are symmetrical; that is, both appendages exhibit similar abnormalities. The first and fifth finger are often partially attached to the fused three middle fingers. The joints and fingers gradually become more stiff, and the bones of the hands, feet and spine progressively grow together (synostosis).

Most affected individuals are mentally retarded. Facial acne is common in adolescence. The eyes are wide-set (HYPERTELORISM), and the midface is often underdeveloped, with a depressed nasal bridge, making the jawbone appear large. One-third are reported to have cleft palate.

Many other abnormalities, including non-skeletal ones, have been described in affected individuals. Central nervous system abnormalities are common and may account for the mental retardation present in a significant number of patients, as early neurosurgical intervention does not prevent it.

The syndrome is caused by a mutation in the *fibroblast growth factor receptor 2* GENE (*FGFR2*), located on the long arm of chromosome 10. Different MUTATIONS in the same gene cause other CRANIOSYNOSTOSIS syndromes: CROUZON DISEASE, JACKSON-WEISS SYNDROME and PFEIFFER SYNDROME, as well as Beare-Stevenson cutis gyrata syndrome.

While this disorder is inherited as an AUTOSOMAL DOMINANT trait, most cases are SPORADIC. Increased paternal age has been noted, which may be a factor in the appearance of the new MUTATIONS that may cause these sporadic cases. The chance for recurrence for unaffected parents of a child with Apert syndrome, on the basis of a new mutation, is considered to be negligible, while that for an affected individual is 50%. More than 250 affected individuals have been reported, and the condition is estimated to occur in 15.5 per million live births. Due to the high neonatal mortality rate, prevalence in the general population is estimated at one in 2 million.

PRENATAL DIAGNOSIS has been successful using FETOSCOPY to detect malformations of the hands and feet. These should also be identifiable by prenatal ULTRASOUND. In familial cases, molecular testing could be used for prenatal diagnosis.

The exact trigger for the abnormal development (DYSPLASIA) of the skull, hands and feet is unknown. Facial surgery can correct some abnormalities, and digits of the hands are often separated surgically.

For other forms of craniosynostosis, see CAR-PENTER SYNDROME, CROUZON DISEASE, PFEIFFER SYNDROME and SAETHRECHOTZEN SYNDROME.

aplasia cutis congenita   Congenital absence of a portion of the skin due to an in utero disruption of skin development. Usually a benign, isolated defect, it is most frequently confined to a single area, such as the scalp (70–85% of cases), but may be widespread. The size of the lesions are also variable, from 0.5 cm–10 cm across, as is the shape, from ovoid and circular to linear or stellate. In some cases, the lesions are symmetrical, mirrored on opposites sides of the body. The depth of the missing skin can be superficial or deeply ulcerated and involve subcutaneous tissue. If on the scalp, the area will be hairless. In some newborns, lesions may have already healed, leaving signs of parchmentlike scarring. The condition usually resolves itself, with no treatment other than application of topical ointments. In more severe cases, corrective grafting surgery has been used.

Incidence is unknown. Though more than 500 cases have been reported, its benign nature makes it likely that most cases are unreported. It is believed to result from genetic factors, teratogens (methimazole), deficient blood supply to the fetal skin and trauma. Though it occurs most commonly as an isolated anomaly, it is also associated with a variety of syndromes and suspected causative agents. Triplet patches are often seen in infants with trisomy 13. It is also associated with fetus papyraceous.

arachnodactyly (spider fingers)   Abnormally long and slender fingers and toes. This is seen as several genetic conditions, MARFAN SYNDROME being perhaps the most well known.

argininemia   See UREA CYCLE DEFECTS.

argininosuccinic aciduria   See UREA CYCLE DEFECTS.

arteriohepatic dysplasia   See ALAGILLE SYNDROME.

arteriovenous malformation (AVM)   Defects of the circulatory system composed of snarled tangles of arteries and veins that are thought to arise during embryonic or fetal development or soon after birth. These defects can disrupt the cyclical flow of blood through the body, and though they can cause fatal complications, the majority of affected individuals are asymptomatic. Malformations are typically found incidentally, usually during autopsy or treatment for an unrelated disorder. AVMs can develop at a variety of sites, but those in the brain or spinal cord (neurological AVMs) are the most potentially dangerous. About 300,000 Americans are thought to have neurological AVMs.

In about 12% of those affected (approximately 36,000) the condition causes health problems, most commonly seizures and headaches of varying severity. Seizures can be partial or total, involving a loss of control over movement, convulsions, or a change in level of consciousness. Headaches can vary in frequency, duration, and intensity. AVMs also can cause a variety of neurological symptoms, including localized muscle weakness or paralysis, a loss of coordination (ataxia), dizziness, visual disturbances, memory problems, hallucinations or dementia. AVMs may also cause subtle learning or behavioral disorders during childhood or adolescence.

As symptoms tend to result from a slow buildup of neurological damage over time they are most often noticed when people are in their twenties, thirties, or forties. In some cases surgical repair or removal of an AVM is possible, and about 5,000 people per year in the U.S. undergo such procedures. About 1% of those with AVMs die, annually as a result of the condition.

AVM affects males and females of all racial and ethnic groups equally. Among women, pregnancy can cause a sudden onset or worsening of symptoms due to accompanying cardiovascular changes, especially increases in blood volume and blood pressure.

A severe form of AVM, vein of Galen defect, a lesion located deep in the brain, is associated with hydrocephalus, and symptoms include swollen veins visible on the scalp, seizures, failure to thrive, and congestive heart failure. Children born with this condition who survive past infancy often remain developmentally impaired.

arthritis See RHEUMATOID ARTHRITIS.

arthrogryposis (arthrogryposis multiplex congenita, AMC) The presence of multiple joint contractures at birth, representing a large group of congenital disorders. A contracture is a limitation in the range of motion of a joint. There is a wide variability in the expression of this problem. In some cases only a few joints may be affected, and the range of motion will be nearly normal. In classic cases, hands, wrists, elbows, shoulders, hips, feet and knees are affected, and in the most severe cases, almost every body joint may be involved, including the jaw and back. Frequently, muscle weakness accompanies joint contractures, further limiting movement.

AMC was first described in 1841 by A. G. Otto, who referred to it as "congenital myodystrophy." The term *arthrogryposis* was first applied to the condition in 1923.

AMC is estimated to occur in approximately one of every 3,000 to 4,000 live births. Many varieties of hereditary arthrogryposis have been identified, including an X-LINKED recessive form, which resolves spontaneously, and AUTOSOMAL DOMINANT and RECESSIVE forms; it can be a feature of many multiple ANOMALY SYNDROMES as well. The most common hereditary form, distal arthrogryposis (autosomal dominant), is characterized by overlapping fingers and clenched fist, which eventually opens with use, leaving a residual loss of movement in adults. There may also be foot deformities. The gene that causes autosomal dominant distal arthrogryposis has been mapped to chromosome 9. However, hereditary forms account for only 30% of all cases. The majority of cases are caused by non-genetic factors during fetal development. Overall recurrence rate is about 5%.

Non-genetic forms have their origin in several developmental aberrations. The most common of these forms is amyoplasia, characterized by flexed wrists and extended elbows, as well as involvement of the shoulders and feet. All cases have been sporadic.

Anything that prevents normal joint movement during fetal development can result in joint contractures, even if the joint itself is normal. This can occur if there is insufficient room in the uterus for normal movement, due to low levels of AMNIOTIC FLUID or abnormal shape of the uterus. If movement is restricted, extra connective tissue may grow around the joint, fixing it in position. Additionally, tendons may lose their ability to stretch or contract.

Muscles responsible for joint movement may also fail to develop properly, due to muscle diseases (such as congenital muscular dystrophies) or environmental exposures such as viruses which can damage cells responsible for transmitting nerve impulses to the muscles. In some cases, tendons, bones, joint linings or joints themselves may develop abnormally for unknown reasons.

Arthrogryposis can also result from malformations of the central nervous system and spinal cord, though in these cases the condition is usually accompanied by a wide range of other disorders.

PRENATAL DIAGNOSIS for hereditary forms has been attempted for at-risk pregnancies using ULTRASOUND to monitor prenatal movement.

Physical therapy is the primary recommended treatment. Surgery is sometimes performed as an adjunct, most commonly on the ankles to assist in supporting weight and walking. These measures can provide substantial improvement in functional ability.

arthrogryposis multiplex congenita, AMC See ARTHROGRYPOSIS.

aspartylglucosaminuria The most distinctive physical feature of this disorder is the thick, sagging skin observed on the cheeks of affected infants, though it also causes severe MENTAL RETARDATION and susceptibility to frequent infections. Affected infants resemble those with MUCOPOLYSACCHARIDOSIS. Though the first symptoms occur in infancy, the course is slowly progressive, with death by the fourth decade. In Finland, where most affected individuals have been identified, incidence is estimated at one in 26,000 births. It is extremely rare elsewhere. Inherited as an AUTOSOMAL RECESSIVE trait, the GENE responsible is located on the long arm of chromosome 4. It is a lysosomal storage disease, resulting from a specific ENZYME deficiency. CARRIER testing and PRENATAL DIAGNOSIS by measurement of this enzyme is possible.

asphyxiating thoracic dysplasia   See JEUNE SYN-DROME.

asplenia syndrome (Ivemark syndrome)   Affected individuals have no spleen and usually exhibit many internal abnormalities. A distinctive feature is a strong tendency for organs or pairs of organs that are normally asymmetric to develop symmetrically. This is a SYNDROME of bilateral "right-sidedness," i.e., left-sided organs or members of pairs of organs have the structural characteristics of their right-sided counterparts, but in mirror images. The alteration of the normal left-right arrangement of internal organs is termed *heterotaxy*.

In at least 90% of the cases, the left lung has three lobes, instead of the normal two. In 40% of the cases, the right and left lobes of the liver are equal in size. In about half the cases, the stomach is located on the right side instead of the midline. Usually the intestinal tract has failed to rotate normally, resulting in abnormalities of the position of the colon.

Infants with this anomaly also have complex cardiovascular defects. Partial or complete obstruction to pulmonary arterial blood flow is found in at least 70% of the cases.

Symptoms are usually evident within days or weeks of birth and include blue discoloration of the skin (CYANOSIS), breathing problems, feeding difficulties and congestive heart failure. Prognosis is poor, with most infants dying during the first year. Infants who survive for any length of time often fail to thrive and suffer from infections.

Asplenia is about twice as prevalent in males as in females. Though usually occurring sporadically, AUTOSOMAL RECESSIVE, AUTOSOMAL DOMINANT and X-LINKED recessive inheritance have all been described. The factors responsible for the left-right organ rearrangement are not understood. A number of genes that appear to be important in this process have been identified. One form of heterotaxy is caused by defects in the *Zic3* gene, located on the X chromosome.

In polysplenia, a condition of having two spleens, there is bilateral left-sidedness. Both bilateral right sidedness (asplenia) and bilateral left sidedness (polysplenia) have been seen in different members of the same family, suggesting two different presentations of an underlying primary genetic defect in body lateralization and symmetry. Asplenia/polysplenia are also known as isomerism sequence or laterality sequence. Taken together, they have a frequency of about one in 22,000. Recurrence risks for siblings of about 5–10% have been suggested.

asthma   See VITAMINS.

ataxia-telangiectasia (AT; Louis-Bar syndrome)   Ataxia is derived from the Greek word *ataxias*, meaning "without order" or "incoordination." Ataxia is a neurological disorder characterized by disturbances of muscular coordination and the inability to control muscular action and balance, caused by degeneration of the cells of the spinal cord and brain. There are several hereditary ataxias, such as Marie's ataxia (hereditary cerebellar ataxia), striatonigral degeneration (Joseph's or AZOREAN DISEASE) and FRIEDREICH'S ATAXIA, with AT being one of the more prevalent.

AT is a chromosomal fragility SYNDROME, inherited as an AUTOSOMAL RECESSIVE disorder. An inability to properly repair DNA damaged by ionizing radiation (such as found in X-rays) is thought to be responsible for chromosomal breakage and rearrangement, which results in characteristics of the disorder.

Along with progressive cerebellar ataxia and inability to control movement (apraxia) of the eyes, a striking characteristic is the development of "telangiectasias," vascular lesions formed by the dilation of small blood vessels that appear on the eyes, ears, face, chest, hands, feet and folds of the elbows and knees.

The telangiectasias usually become apparent by the age of five, appearing on parts of the body most exposed to the sun. Graying of the scalp hair is common, even in children. With continued exposure to the sun, the skin becomes hardened and mottled with hyperpigmented and depigmented areas.

Growth is greatly diminished in more than 65% of affected individuals. They tend to have thin faces, with a relaxed, dull or sad expression. The head is often held to one side, and individuals often present a stooped posture with drooping shoulders.

The loss of motor control is progressive, with speech becoming difficult due to loss of control over vocal cords and mouth. Drooling is frequent. Additionally, there is often endocrine malfunction, intellectual decline and development of immune deficiency disorders.

Over the past 20 years, the life expectancy of individuals with AT has increased considerably; most now live past 25 years of age and some have survived into their 40s and 50s. Death typically results from infection or, less frequently, the development of malignant growths. Homozygotes have an increased risk for malignancies of about 38%. Leukemias and lymphomas account for about 85% of these malignancies.

The condition can be diagnosed by chromosomal analysis, which can detect characteristic changes in the chromosomes of affected individuals. A 7:14 chromosomal translocation is identified in 5–15% of cells in routine chromosomal studies on peripheral blood of individuals with AT.

Incidence of the disorder is thought to be between two and three per 100,000 live births. One percent of the population is thought to be CARRIERS. Carriers can be identified by deficiencies in DNA repair ability and have a fivefold increase in tumors of all types. Heterozygous carriers have a risk of developing cancer four times that of the general population, primarily from breast cancer. Exposure to X-irradiation may trigger the development of cancer, according to some authorities, though this assertion is somewhat controversial. Mutations in the *ATM* gene (*AT* mutated) on the long arm of chromosome 11 underlie the disorder. Sequencing the *ATM* gene can discover about 90% of the mutations underlying *AT*. When the mutation in a family is known, carrier detection and prenatal diagnosis by molecular techniques are possible. PRENATAL DIAGNOSIS may also be possible by evaluating the sensitivity of cultured fetal cells, obtained via AMNIOCENTESIS, to ionizing radiation.

attention deficit hyperactivity disorder (ADHD)

A heritable consistent inability to focus the attention required to complete tasks and/or activities. First diagnosed by a pediatrician in 1902, ADHD is the most common childhood-onset behavioral disorder. For many years ADHD was considered only a childhood disorder, but it is now recognized as affecting all ages, and current studies estimate it affects from 6 million to 9.5 million adults.

Affected individuals are typically inattentive, hyperactive and impulsive. The American Psychiatric Association bases its diagnosis on the presence of any of six of the following symptoms for a period of six months: failure to pay attention to details or making careless mistakes; difficulty sustaining attention to work or play activities; seeming failure to listen when spoken to; failure to complete assignments or chores; difficulty organizing tasks and activities; avoidance of tasks requiring sustained mental effort; repeated loss of implements required for tasks or activities; forgetfulness. With therapy, affected individuals show high adaptability, often using notes to overcome organizational deficits. The drug Ritalin is prescribed in many cases. It increases the level of dopamine, believed to be at low levels in ADHD, and helps affected individuals concentrate.

ADHD affects approximately 5% to 10% of children and adolescents. Boys are affected about eight times more frequently than girls. Though the cause is unknown, there is evidence of involvement of multiple different genes. Familial aggregation has been noted. Studies have also linked ADHD to fetal exposure to teratogens such as cigarettes, alcohol and lead.

Children diagnosed with the disorder are twice as likely to have a 7-repeat form of the *dopamine D4 receptor* gene as those without it. This same GENE, on 11p, was proposed as being the gene for thrill-seeking behavior in a 1996 study, but subsequent research failed to confirm that finding.

atypical cholinesterase (pseudocholinesterase deficiency) See CHOLINESTERASE.

auditory canal atresia   Absence (atresia) of the auditory canal. It may take the form of a visible

block where the canal would normally begin at the outer ear, or it may resemble a funnel leading down to a block farther within the canal. The outer ear may appear normal, or it may be set lower than normal on the side of the head with minor variations in shape. Persons with atresia of both auditory canals suffer complete hearing loss and impairment of speech development. The defect may be detected by careful examination at birth, or it may escape detection until the hearing loss becomes apparent.

It is not known how the defect develops, but it is hypothesized that early in fetal development the primitive auditory canal fails to form properly.

Associated defects and malformations seen in some cases include excessive distance between paired organs, such as the eyes (HYPERTELORISM), skin folds covering the inner corner of the eyes (EPICANTHUS), small nose, flattened midface, CLEFT PALATE, webbing or fusion of fingers or toes (SYNDACTYLY) and CLUBFOOT. This ANOMALY has also been seen as a component of a number of SYNDROMES, most important in the deletion of the long arm of chromosome 18 (18q-), a CHROMOSOME ABNORMALITY.

The condition is rare. Cause and the risk of occurrence are unknown. The life span of an affected person is generally normal if no serious associated defects exist.

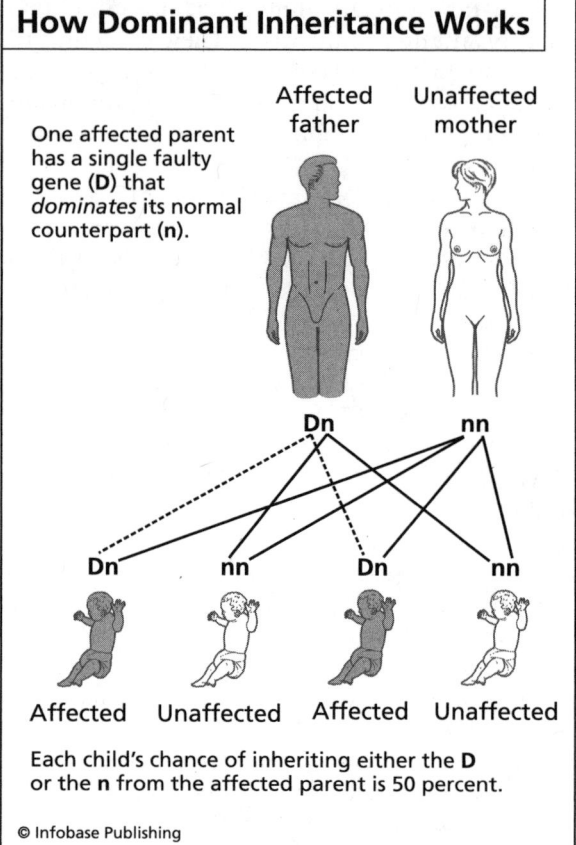

How Dominant Inheritance Works

One affected parent has a single faulty gene (**D**) that *dominates* its normal counterpart (**n**).

Affected father   Unaffected mother

Dn   nn

Dn   nn   Dn   nn

Affected   Unaffected   Affected   Unaffected

Each child's chance of inheriting either the **D** or the **n** from the affected parent is 50 percent.

© Infobase Publishing

autism, infantile   See INFANTILE AUTISM.

autosomal dominant (dominant)   A method of transmission of a hereditary trait. It is the confirmed or suspected mode of transmission of more than 2,100 GENETIC DISORDERS or conditions. While popularly referred to as "dominant" traits, they are more properly termed "autosomal dominant," reflecting the location on the autosomes, any of the 22 non–sex chromosome pairs, of the aberrant GENES responsible for the disorders. (Genetic disorders involving the sex chromosomes, the 23rd chromosome pair, are termed X-LINKED; they may also be dominant traits, although most X-linked disorders are recessive.)

Autosomal dominant disorders have their origins in MUTATIONS or defects in a single gene or a gene pair. They are called dominant due to their ability to override, or dominate, their normal gene counterpart. Hence, an individual who inherits a single copy of the gene for a dominant disorder will usually exhibit that disorder.

In general, autosomal dominant disorders show a wide variability of severity, and not all who inherit the defective gene will exhibit its associated disorder. The ratio of those who exhibit the disorder to those who inherit the gene for the disorder is referred to as PENETRANCE, and is expressed as a percentage. (For example, if half of those who possess the gene exhibit the disorder, penetrance is 50%.) For an individual to have a dominant disorder, one parent is generally affected; unlike AUTOSOMAL RECESSIVE disorders, dominant conditions generally do not skip generations. The exceptions:

(1) an individual may have unaffected parents, if that individual has the disorder as the result of a new mutation that has occurred in the sperm, egg or fertilized zygote that has gone on to produce that individual; and (2) as a result of lack of penetrance, an individual who has inherited the gene for a disorder may not display the manifestations of the disorder and appear unaffected.

Among couples in which one individual has a dominant disorder, each child has a 50% chance of inheriting the gene, and therefore the disorder, from the affected parent, and a 50% chance of being unaffected. Affected individuals are said to be "HETEROZYGOTES," that is, the two genes in the gene pair are dissimila—one is faulty and one is normal. "HOMOZYGOTES," those who have two identical faulty genes, are extremely rare in dominant disorders (both parents would have to have the disorder), and homozygosity usually results in severe, lethal forms of dominant conditions. If both parents are affected, each child has a 25% chance of being homozygous for the condition and a 25% chance of being unaffected. (See Table I.)

TABLE I
FREQUENCIES OF THE MOST COMMON DOMINANT DISORDERS FOUND IN A SURVEY CONDUCTED IN BRITISH COLUMBIA*, CANADA

Dominant Condition	1952–63		1964–73		1974–83		Total	
	N	Rate[1]	N	Rate[1]	N	Rate[1]	N	Rate[1]
Retina, malignant neoplasm	6	13.7	14	40.6	16	41.3	36	30.8
Neurofibromatosis	34	77.7	33	95.7	32	82.5	99	84. 6
Other disorders of metabolism	1	2.3	7	20.3	11	28.4	19	16.2
Hereditary spherocytosis	12	27.4	18	52.2	20	51.6	50	42.7
Von Willebrand disease	5	11.4	7	20.3	8	20.6	20	17.1
Myotonic disorders	14	32.0	8	23.2	6	15.5	28	23.9
Hereditary retinal dystrophies	13	29.7	0	0.0	0	0.0	13	11.1
Nystagmus and other irregular eye movements	14	32.0	2	5.8	3	7.7	19	16.2
Sensorineural deafness	3	6.9	15	43.5	4	10.3	22	18.8
Congenital cataract and lens anomalies	21	48.0	10	29.0	5	12.9	36	30.8
Polydactyly	6	13.7	16	46.4	14	36.1	36.1	30.8
Other anomalies of upper limbs, including shoulder girdle	3	6.9	2	5.8	9	23.2	14	12.0
Anomalies of skull and face bones	9	20.6	11	31.9	14	36.1	34	29.1
Chondrodystrophy	48	109.7	21	60.9	20	51.6	89	76.1
Osteodystrophies	24	54.9	31	89.9	29	74.8	84	71.8
Other specified anomalies of muscle, tendon, fascia, etc.	13	29.7	14	40.6	7	18.1	34	29.1
Unspecified anomalies of musculoskeletal system	2	4.6	8	23.2	0	0.0	10	8.5
Other specified congenital anomalies of skin	11	25.1	5	14.5	6	15.5	22	18.8
Tuberous sclerosis	13	29.7	23	66.7	22	56.7	58	49.6
Other specified congenital anomalies	17	38.9	16	46.4	9	23.2	42	35.9
All other dominant conditions[2]	110	251.4	85	246.6	81	208.9	276	235.9
Total	379	866.3	346	1,003.9	316	815.1	1,041	889.8
Sum of highest individual rates								1,395.4

*Statistics reflect local population bias.
N = Number of patients.
[1]Per 1 million live births.
[2]Each individual rate was used to determine the sum of the highest individual rates for these conditions.
Source: Patricia A. Baird, "A Population Study of Genetic Disorders in Children and Young Adults," *American Journal of Human Genetics* 42 (1988): 677–693.

autosomal recessive (recessive) A method of transmission of a hereditary trait. It is the confirmed or suspected mode of transmission of more than 1,950 GENETIC DISORDERS or conditions. While popularly referred to as "recessive" traits, they are more properly termed "autosomal recessive," reflecting the location on the autosomes, any of the 22 non–sex chromosome pairs, of the aberrant GENES responsible for the disorders. (Genetic disorders involving the sex chromosome, the 23rd chromosome pair, are termed X-LINKED; most X-linked traits are recessive, though there are X-linked dominant disorders, as well.)

Autosomal recessive disorders have their origins in MUTATIONS, or defects in both genes in a gene pair. They are called recessive because the influence of the faulty gene remains recessed, or suppressed, if paired with a normal gene. Hence, individuals must inherit a faulty gene from both the mother and father for the associated condition to manifest itself.

Individuals who possess one recessive gene may pass the gene on to their offspring, but will rarely exhibit any symptoms of the disorder itself. (These individuals, who remain asymptomatic, are termed CARRIERS.) As a result, recessive disorders can skip one or more generations, and will appear only when two individuals, both possessing the faulty gene, have offspring. Even in those circumstances, the offspring will not necessarily (that is, 100% of the time) inherit the condition unless both parents are actually affected by the disorder.

Carrier testing, when possible, can establish whether an individual possesses the recessive gene.

Among couples where only one member has a single recessive gene for a disorder, each offspring has a 50% chance of inheriting the gene and being a carrier, and a 50% chance of not inheriting the gene. If one parent has a recessive disorder (two faulty genes) and the other parent has no recessive genes for the disorder, all offspring will be carriers.

Among couples where both members have a single recessive gene, each child has a 25% chance of inheriting two recessive genes and therefore inheriting the disorder, a 50% chance of inheriting one faulty gene and being a carrier, and a 25% chance of inheriting no recessive genes.

If one parent has a recessive disorder and the other a single recessive gene for it, each child will either be a carrier or have the disorder, with the chances for either being 50%.

If both parents have a recessive disorder, all their offspring will inherit the disorder.

Affected individuals are said to be "HOMOZYGOTES," that is, the two genes in the gene pair are identical—both faulty. Carriers, those capable of transmitting the faulty gene without having the condition themselves, are said to be "HETEROZYGOTES"—the genes are dissimilar, one faulty, one normal. The unaffected parents or offspring of an individual with a recessive disorder are termed obligate heterozygotes, since they must have one copy of the recessive gene.

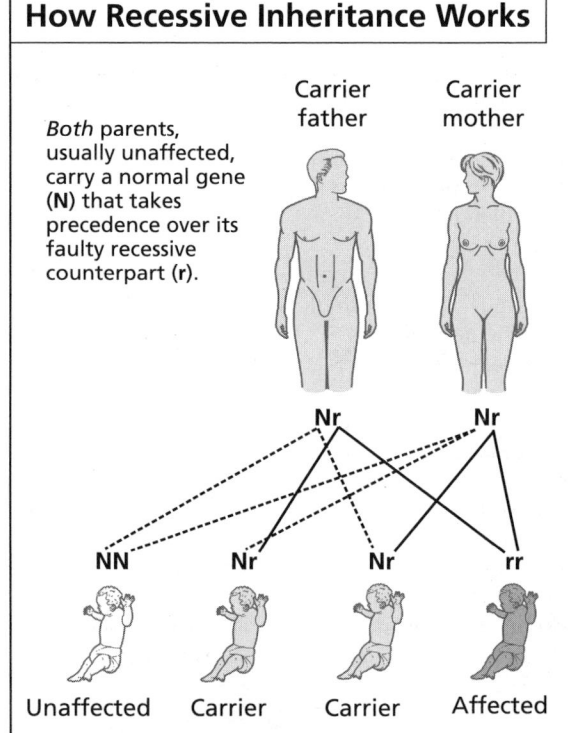

How Recessive Inheritance Works

Both parents, usually unaffected, carry a normal gene (**N**) that takes precedence over its faulty recessive counterpart (**r**).

Carrier father
Carrier mother

Nr   Nr

NN   Nr   Nr   rr

Unaffected   Carrier   Carrier   Affected

The odds for each child are:
1. a 25 percent risk of inheriting a "double dose" of **r** genes, which may cause a serious birth defect
2. a 25 percent chance of inheriting two **N**s, thus being unaffected
3. a 50 percent chance of being a carrier as both parents are

© Infobase Publishing

TABLE II
FREQUENCIES OF THE MOST COMMON RECESSIVE DISORDERS FOUND IN A SURVEY
CONDUCTED IN BRITISH COLUMBIA*, CANADA

Recessive Condition	1952–63		1964–73		1974–83		Total	
	N	Rate[1]	N	Rate[1]	N	Rate[1]	N	Rate[1]
Hyperaldosteronism	13	29.7	7	20.3	1	2.6	21	18.0
Adrenogenital disorders	5	11.4	8	23.2	12	31.0	25	21.4
Phenylketonuria	26	59.4	18	52.2	31	80.0	75	64.1
Other disturbances of aromatic amino acid metabolism	22	50.3	19	55.1	16	41.3	57	48.7
Glycogenosis	3	6.9	12	34.8	8	20.6	23	19.7
Lipidoses	4	9.1	10	29.0	4	10.3	18	15.4
Cystic fibrosis	80	182.9	105	304.6	87	224.4	272	232.5
Mucopolysaccharidosis	8	18.3	11	31.9	2	5.2	21	18.0
Deficiency of humoral immunity	4	9.1	12	34.8	4	10.3	20	17.1
Thalassemias	15	34.3	7	20.3	16	41.3	38	32.5
Cerebral lipidoses	5	11.4	10	29.0	3	7.7	18	15.4
Werdnig-Hoffman disease	6	13.7	19	55.1	15	38.7	40	34.2
Other myoneural disorders	18	41.1	4	11.6	0	0.0	22	18.8
Hereditary progressive muscular dystrophy	19	43.4	3	8.7	0	0.0	22	18.8
Hereditary retinal dystrophies	21	48.0	10	29.0	0	0.0	22	18.8
Sensorineural deafness	9	20.6	12	34.8	8	20.6	29	24.8
Unspecified deafness	1	2.3	8	23.2	7	18.1	16	13.7
Cystic kidney disease	11	25.1	10	29.0	7	18.1	28	23.9
Osteodystrophies	1	2.3	8	23.2	7	18.1	16	13.7
Other specified congenital anomalies	7	16.0	18	52.2	21	54.2	46	39.3
All other recessive conditions[2]	104	237.7	91	264.0	126	325.0	321	274.4
Total	401	916.6	406	1,178.0	372	959.5	1,179	1,007.8
Sum of highest individual rates								1,655.3

*Statistics reflect local population bias.
N = Number of patients.
[1]Per 1 million live births.
[2]Each individual rate was used to get the sum of the highest individual rates for these conditions.
Source: Patricia A. Baird, "A Population Study of Genetic Disorders in Children and Young Adults," *American Journal of Human Genetics* 42 (1988): 677–693.

In general, autosomal recessive disorders tend to be less variable in expression and more uniformly severe than AUTOSOMAL DOMINANT disorders. (See Table II.)

Azorean disease (Machado-Joseph disease; Joseph disease; spinopontine atrophy) A fatal disorder of the central nervous system that predominantly affects individuals of Portuguese ancestry, and is characterized by progressive weakening and spasticity of the extremities. Onset is usually between the ages of 15 and 35 years, though it may appear earlier or much later. The rate of progression is variable. Symptoms include awkward body movements and a staggering, lurching gait that is easily mistaken for drunkenness. Affected individuals have difficulty speaking and swallowing. Bulging eyes and involuntary facial movements are characteristic. Life expectancy following onset is generally between 10 and 30 years.

First documented in the 1970s, two separate individuals have been identified as the "original" case: William Machado, a native of the Azores, a group of islands off the coast of Spain, and Antone Joseph, a Portuguese sailor, also from the Azores, who jumped ship in California in 1845. In fact, they may both have had a common ancestor, three generations back, who was the original case. However, this AUTOSOMAL DOMINANT disorder has been reported in many non-Azorean families in many countries and has come to be regarded as one of the most common autosomal dominant spinocerebellar degenerations. Also known as SCA3, the designations Azorean neurologic disease or Machado-Joseph disease (MJD) are used as well.

The responsible GENE has been mapped to the long arm of chromosome 14 (14q). MJD and type 3 spinocerebellar ataxia are produced by an expansion of a CAG repeat in the MJD gene. The gene normally has a series of 3 DNA base pairs (CAG) that are repeated a number of times in a row. In normal individuals the gene contains between 13 and 36 of these CAG repeats. Most patients with clinically diagnosed MJD show expansion of the repeat number in the range of 61 to 84 repeats. This is an example of a trinucleotide repeat amplification (see TRINUCLEOTIDE REPEAT DISORDER), a type of MUTATION capable of causing genetic diseases. Other genetic disorders found to have trinucleotide repeat amplification as the underlying causative mutation include MYOTONIC DYSTROPHY, HUNTINGTON DISEASE, FRAGILE X, SCA1, KENNEDY DISEASE and FRIEDRICH'S ATAXIA.

Presymptomatic and PRENATAL DIAGNOSIS are possible using molecular techniques.

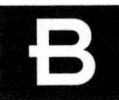

Baby Doe Name used to identify anonymous infants in several court cases involving the withholding of treatment from newborns who require medical intervention for survival.

Parents and doctors have allowed some infants with severe congenital defects to expire from complications of their conditions, a practice termed "passive euthanasia," rather than intervene medically to attempt to sustain their lives. In some situations, third parties have mounted legal efforts to compel the provision of medical treatment. One of the seminal cases involved an infant with DOWN SYNDROME and esophageal atresia who was allowed to die of starvation in Indiana in 1982. Controversy following the death led the federal government to define non treatment of newborns with congenital anomalies as discrimination against the handicapped, making institutions involved at risk for losing federal funds. This federal policy was subsequently invalidated by the Supreme Court. Withholding treatment in these situations is not currently illegal under federal statutes, but courts continue to be asked to rule on individual cases, with the affected infants usually designated as Baby Doe.

baldness See ALOPECIA.

baldness, male pattern See MALE PATTERN BALDNESS.

Bardet-Biedl syndrome (Laurence-Moon-Biedl syndrome) Syndrome characterized by obesity, abnormally small genitals (hypogenitalism), extra fingers and toes (polydactyly), degenerative disease of the retina (pigmentary retinopathy) and psychological and neurological disorders.

It bears the name of George Louis Bardet (b. 1885), a French physician, and Arthur Biedl (1869–1933), a professor of experimental pathology at the University of Prague. It has also been identified with the names of John Zachariah Laurence (1829–70), an English ophthalmologist, and Richard Charles Moon (1845–1914), his assistant.

Birth weight is usually above average, and by the age of one year nearly one-third of affected children are obese, with the extra weight typically found disproportionately within the trunk of the body. Tending toward shortness of stature, most exhibit infantile, unstable personalities (labile) and are mentally retarded.

They may experience kidney problems and nearly 35% of those afflicted with this syndrome die from kidney failure. Other problems include mild spasticity of the extremities, abnormalities in brain structures affecting body movements (extrapyramidal disorders), deafness, lack of eye coordination (nystagmus) and glucose intolerance. Urine shows decreased levels of gonad-stimulating hormones (gonadotropin).

Inherited as an AUTOSOMAL RECESSIVE trait, over 600 cases have been reported. The incidence is greatest among Bedouin Arabs, where it occurs in at least one in 13,500. Genes in at least 12 different locations (*BBS1-12*) have been associated with this syndrome, and these 12 have been identified. One particular mutation in the *BBS1* gene (located on the long arm of chromosome 11) appears to be a common cause of this syndrome. In rare cases, the presence of three mutations (that is mutations in both alleles of one *BBS* gene and another mutation in one allele of another *BBS* gene) is required in order for the disease to express itself. This is known as triallelic inheritance. Hypogenitalism also implies immature functioning of genitals—delayed puberty, absence of secondary sexual characteristics, lack of menstruation in females or male sterility. Prenatal diagnosis is possible only if extra digits are observed by ultrasonic scanning (see ULTRASOUND), for example. In some families who have been carefully studied, prenatal diagnosis might be possible with molecular testing.

Though sometimes referred to as Laurence-Moon-Biedl syndrome, many authors prefer to use the Bardet-Biedl syndrome after the two authors who described this disorder in the 1930s. Laurence and Moon described a similar disorder in 1865, but those patients did not have polydactyly or obesity.

basal cell carcinoma (skin cancer)   A heritable, and the most common and easily treatable, form of cancer. Affected individuals are predisposed to develop cancerous lesions on the skin as a result of cumulative exposure to sunlight.

About 750,000 individuals in the United States develop basal cell carcinoma annually, according to the National Cancer Institute. Most are fair-skinned and of Northern European extraction. (The skin of all people chronically exposed to sunlight has been found to have up to 10 times more genetic mutations capable of causing skin cancer than protected skin.) When treated promptly, skin cancer is easily curable by excising cancerous lesions. However, left untreated, lesions may become malignant and spread to other parts of the body.

Sunlight causes a mutation of the gene *p53,* one of the genes linked to the disorder. Another gene that plays a role in the disorder, *PTC,* or "patched," is a tumor suppressor gene on chromosome 9. The *PTC* gene is absent, damaged or defective in affected individuals, allowing cell growth to go unchecked. The region of chromosome 9 where the defective gene is located has previously been linked to nevoid basal cell carcinoma syndrome (basal cell nevus syndrome (BCNS)), a rare hereditary disorder affecting about one in every 200 basal cell carcinoma patients.

The *PTC* gene was first identified in a fruit fly. When mutated forms were observed to cause developmental problems in the insects' offspring, researchers were able to focus on corresponding development problems wrought by the human counterpart gene. Knowledge of the gene may yield new treatment and screening methods.

See also NEVOID BASEL CELL CARCINOMA SYNDROME.

basal cell nevus syndrome   See NEVOID BASAL CELL CARCINOMA SYNDROME.

Bassen-Kornzweig syndrome   See ABETALIPOPROTEINEMIA.

Batten disease   See NEURONAL CEROID LIPOFUSCINOSIS.

Beare-Stevenson cutis gyrata syndrome   An autosomal dominant disorder characterized by congenital skin abnormalities in combination with craniosyntosis, the premature fusing of bones of the skull, which results in a malformed head and mental deficiency. It bears the names of J. M. Beare and R. E. Stevenson, who described it in 1969 and 1972, respectively.

Affected individuals have prominent, bulging eyes and a poorly developed mid-face that appears flat. Ears are low set and rotated backwards. The most distinctive of the characteristic skin abnormalities is the ridged, corrugated appearance of the skin (cutis gyrata). Thick, dark, velvety patches of skin (acanthosis nigricans) may appear on the hands and feet. Genital abnormalities may also be present.

An autosomal dominant disorder, it is caused by a mutation in the *FGFR2* gene, located on 10q, which produces fibroblast growth factor receptor 2, a protein that helps control cell growth during and after embryonic development. The mutation reduces the effectiveness of the protein, which is believed to hinder skeletal and skin development. All reported cases have been the result of new mutations, as there was no history of the disorder in families of affected individuals. However, some individuals with the disorder do not have this mutation.

Affected individuals typically die in infancy or early childhood. Incidence is unknown, but the condition is very rare, with only some 10 cases reported.

Becker's muscular dystrophy   See MUSCULAR DYSTROPHY.

Beckwith-Wiedemann syndrome   A condition encompassing a vast and varied constellation of congenital symptoms, most notably an enlarged tongue (macroglossia) that pushes out of the mouth, protrusion of a portion of the intestine through a defect in the abdominal wall (OMPHALOCELE), severe low blood sugar (hypoglycemia) that disappears within a year of birth and large size. Other frequently seen characteristics include facial birthmarks, and grooves and pits on the ears and earlobes. Umbilical and INGUINAL HERNIA are common, as is intestinal malrotation. Mild to moderate MENTAL RETARDATION is frequent.

It bears the names of J. B. Beckwith and H. R. Wiedemann, who independently described it in 1964.

In general, gigantism is a feature of Beckwith-Wiedemann syndrome. Mean weight at birth is generally high (3,900 g or 8.6 lb.), even though approximately 25% of births are premature. Stature and weight eventually are above the 90th percentile, with advanced bone age. One half of the body may be noticeably larger than the other (HEMIHYPERTROPHY). Hemihypertrophy occurs in about 25% of cases. The visceral organs are commonly enlarged, as is the clitoris in females. Cells of the adrenal cortex are large (cytomegaly), and the kidneys often develop abnormally.

Prognosis is fair. Most deaths in infancy occur due to complications of the syndrome, but later malignant tumors of the kidneys or adrenal cortex occur in approximately 5–10% of cases. When deaths occur in infancy (21% of cases) they are generally due to complications of the syndrome due to the abdominal defects, difficulty with breathing or swallowing due to the large tongue or due to seizures because of the low blood sugar. Surgery can correct omphalocele, intestinal rotation and macroglossia. As children grow older, characteristics become less noticeable.

The genetics of this disorder are complex. Most cases arise sporadically, but inheritance in familial cases appears to be autosomal dominant with incomplete penetrance and great variability. The mechanisms underlying this syndrome involve abnormalities in the expression of a number of genes located in what has been termed the BWS critical region located at 11p15. Most of these genes are normally modified by a process known as IMPRINTING whereby the maternally and paternally derived copies (ALLELES) of the gene are uniquely chemically modified leading to different expression of the gene depending on which parent it came from. The chemical modification is called methylation, and, in BWS, certain genes that are normally methylated may not be or certain genes that are not usually methylated are.

Many different chromosomal and molecular abnormalities involving chromosome 11 and specifically 11p15 have been described in different individuals affected with BWS. UNIPARENTAL DISOMY, whereby only paternal copies of 11p15 are seen (and the maternally imprinted copy of genes in the region are absent), may be found. Chromosome abnormalities resulting in paternal 11p15 duplication or maternal deletion may also be seen. There may be mutations in the gene *CDKN1C*, which codes for a protein known as cyclin dependent kinase inhibitor 1C. This gene is normally expressed almost exclusively from the maternal chromosome 11. Mutations in this gene have been found in 5–10% of sporadic cases of BWS and about 40% of families where the syndrome has been inherited in an AUTOSOMAL DOMINANT manner. In other BWS cases, certain genes that are normally methylated, such as *KCNQ1OT1*, are found not to be methylated, and in other cases, genes not usually methylated, such as *H19*, are methylated. It appears that in general the cause of the condition is too much expression of paternally expressed growth-promoting genes or too little expression of maternally derived genes that usually suppress growth (such as *CDKN1C*). Hemihypertrophy seems to be associated with cases with paternal UPD, and Wilms tumor risk seems higher with cases of *H19* methylation. Recurrence risks within a family will depend on the underlying genetic mechanism and can range from virtually zero to 50%.

Affected children should be checked for low blood sugar in the newborn period (first three days) and should be screened with abdominal ultrasound every three months until the age of three, and then every six months to the age of seven to monitor the development of tumors.

Prenatal diagnosis has been accomplished by ULTRASOUND; ALPHA-FETOPROTEIN levels may also be elevated in the presence of an abdominal wall defect. The condition affects both sexes equally and is estimated to occur in one in 15,000 live births. Approximately 15% of infants with omphalocele have this syndrome.

behavior Personality traits and complex human behaviors have become the subject of research of the sort usually reserved for genetic disorders. The traits for which genetic links have been sought and/or reportedly found include anxiety, violence, hyperactivity, happiness, sociability and sexual orientation. Some of these behaviors have been studied in mice, whose genes can be manipulated to produce strains that are excessively violent or asocial. However, it is generally believed that behaviors in humans are most likely controlled by the action of several genes working in combination.

Human personality traits that can be reliably measured by standard psychological tests have shown a considerable degree of heritability. Studies dating to the early 1950s, for example, have suggested panic disorder, or anxiety neurosis, exhibits autosomal dominant inheritance. A 1996 study linked a polymorphism in the serotonin transporter gene (SLC6A4) to some cases of anxiety. Novelty- or thrill-seeking has been linked to genetic variability in dopamine transmission. In 1996, this behavior was linked to a polymorphism, a 7-repeat ALLELE at the site of the *dopamine receptor D4 gene (DRD4)*, which family studies indicate results from genetic transmission. In 1993, researchers at the National Cancer Institute reported a gene or genes on a section of the X chromosome may have a role in homosexuality.

The genetic basis of cognitive ability, or intelligence, is also being probed. In 1998, a variant of the *IGF2 (insulin growth factor 2) receptor* gene on the long arm of chromosome 6 was associated with superior intelligence, though it is thought that 50 or more genes affect mental development.

The 1998 book *Living With Our Genes* examined this subject and explored the social implications of evidence that genetics plays a role in behavior.

benign familial hematuria (thin basement membrane nephropathy) This benign disorder, inherited as an AUTOSOMAL DOMINANT trait, is characterized by the presence of blood in the urine. It is nonprogressive and not associated with kidney failure, nor is it associated with conditions such as deafness, which is seen in other syndromes involving hereditary kidney malfunction like ALPORT SYNDROME. However, a link between the two disorders appears to exist. At least some cases have had mutations in the gene for the alpha 3 or alpha 4 chain of type 4 collagen (COL4A4). This is a protein found in the basement membrane of the glomerulus of the kidney. Mutations in these genes have been identified in cases of autosomal recessive Alport syndrome. Other cases of benign familial hematuria are not linked to these two genes, and thus mutations in other genes must also be able to cause this disorder.

bent stick syndrome See PEYRONIE DISEASE.

bifid uvula (split uvula; cleft uvula) The uvula is the small, soft tissue that hangs from the roof of the mouth over the root of the tongue. In approximately 1% of whites and 10% of American Indians and Japanese, the uvula is split by a central fissure. The frequency in SIBLINGS, parents and children (first degree relatives) of affected persons is reported to be about 18%. This defect can be considered a minor form of cleft palate, and, as in that anomaly, MULTIFACTORIAL inheritance is thought to be the cause of this benign condition. It may also be seen in CRI DU CHAT SYNDROME, Opitz syndrome, female CARRIERS of type II oto-palatodigital syndrome or in other syndromes where cleft palate may be a component.

In persons with cleft uvula, the complete removal of the adenoids may produce hypernasal speech.

biliary atresia This rare disease, seen in very young infants, is caused by inflammation and obstruction of the bile ducts, which carry bile from the liver into the small intestine. Due to the blockage, bile backs up into the liver, resulting in destruction of healthy liver cells and scarring of the liver (cirrhosis). The scarring interferes with blood flow through the liver, resulting in further damage.

The symptoms, which usually appear between two days and six weeks after birth, are a yellowing of the skin (jaundice), frequently accompanied by the enlargement and hardening of the liver, and a swelling of the abdomen. Stools are usually pale or grayish, resembling the color of clay. The urine appears dark. Some babies may develop intense itching (pruritus), which makes them extremely uncomfortable and irritable. As the disease progresses, it results in ANEMIA, malnutrition and growth retardation.

Biliary atresia mimics the symptoms of other liver diseases, especially neonatal HEPATITIS, requiring several tests before the diagnosis can be made conclusively. These tests may include blood and urine tests, liver function tests, blood counts and clotting function tests, liver biopsy, liver scans using radioisotopes, and ULTRASOUND to determine the size of liver and bile ducts.

In the past, this condition was always fatal. Now some cases can be successfully treated with the surgical creation of a new bile duct fashioned from a piece of the small intestine. However, it must be performed in the first three months of life. Called the Kasai procedure, after Dr. Morio Kasai, a Japanese surgeon who developed it, the operation is successful in one-third to one-half of cases. An additional one-third continue to manifest signs of liver disease, but can lead relatively normal lives. Affected infants who do not respond to this treatment generally face increasing complications from cirrhosis, and may succumb by age two. Liver transplants are sometimes attempted if the Kasai procedure is ineffective. The Kasai operation may also be considered a temporizing measure to support patients and allow them to grow until a liver transplant is more easily done. Transplantation has improved the outlook for children affected with biliary atresia; nearly 75% of recipients treated for this condition are alive and in good health five years later.

Biliary atresia is not a HEREDITARY DISEASE. Although the exact cause is not known, a viral infection near the time of birth may be responsible for the inflammation and obstruction of the bile ducts. The condition occurs in an estimated one in 10,000 to 15,000 live births. Males and females are equally affected. In Europe, approximately 700 infants are born with bilary atresia annually. A European Biliary Atresia Registry (EBAR) was founded in 2001 to raise awareness of the disease and promote international and interdisciplinary cooperation in research and treatment. There is an increased incidence in Japanese and Hawaiians of Chinese ancestry. Abnormalities of the heart, kidney and spleen may also be observed.

biochemical assays   A laboratory test for ENZYME activity that may be used for diagnosis of some HEREDITARY DISEASES. An enzyme is a protein involved in chemical reactions in living matter. Hundreds of genetic disorders are caused by lack of a certain enzyme or its reduced activity, which produces a biochemical imbalance. These include a form of ANEMIA, ALBINISM and TAY-SACHS DISEASE. (In the diagnosis of other genetic disorders the amount of non-enzyme biochemicals in body fluids may also be assayed or measured. These substances include amino acids and mucopolysaccharides.)

The deficiency or absence of an enzyme or other substance can often be determined either through biochemical assay of the individual's blood or prenatally, through analysis of cultured amniotic fluid cells gathered via AMNIOCENTESIS or CHORIONIC VILLUS SAMPLING.

bird-headed dwarfism   See SECKEL SYNDROME.

birth, premature   See PREMATURITY; LOW BIRTH WEIGHT.

birth control   See CONTRACEPTIVE.

birth defect   A CONGENITAL abnormality. Literally thousands of types of birth defects have been reported and identified, ranging from mild conditions with only minor cosmetic significance, to lethal conditions, which may result in STILLBIRTH. About 2% to 3% of infants are born with a significant birth defect or defects, though not all are detected at birth or even soon after. For example, some congenital HEART DEFECTS may be identified only during autopsy following a death they have precipitated. Conversely, some defects visible at birth may in some cases spontaneously correct themselves. For example, some BIRTHMARKS called HEMANGIOMAS, red-colored marks that are composed of dilated blood vessels, may spontaneously fade during infancy. Due to reductions in the mortality rates associated with PREMATURITY, infection and injuries, birth defects are now the leading cause of infant deaths in the developed world.

Birth defects have been noted throughout recorded history. Official records of ancient astrologers of Nineveh and Babylon, dating to 2800 B.C., mention the birth of "monsters," severely deformed infants or aborted fetuses. These births were given great weight, and various deformities of specific limbs or other body parts were considered portents with highly specific meanings, heralding war, peace, natural disasters or the success or failure of a monarch's reign. Based on the specific nature of these prophesies, numerous congenital malformations must have been known to the Babylonians. Aristotle was also familiar with birth defects and wrote, in *On the Generation of Animals*, that "In man the male is more often born with deformity than the female," which appears to be the case for a number of congenital ANOMALIES.

TABLE III
CONGENITAL ANOMALIES FOUND IN A SURVEY CONDUCTED IN BRITISH COLUMBIA*, CANADA

Congenital Anomaly	1952–63		1964–73		1974–83		Total	
	N	Rate[1]	N	Rate[1]	N	Rate[1]	N	Rate[1]
Anencephaly	74	169.1	60	174.1	89	229.6	223	190.6
Spina bifida	377	861.7	267	774.7	261	673.2	905	773.6
Encephalocele	12	27.4	26	75.4	46	118.6	84	71.8
Congenital hydrocephalus	182	416.0	273	792.1	347	895.0	802	685.5
Other nervous system disorders	158	361.1	268	777.6	372	959.5	798	682.1
Eye	382	873.1	507	1,471.0	603	1,555.3	1,492	1,275.4
Ear, face, neck	158	361.1	606	1,816.3	858	2,213.0	1,642	1,403.6
Heart and circulation	1,981	4,528.0	3,628	10,526.2	5,073	13,084.7	10,682	9,130.9
Respiratory	38	86.9	748	2,170.2	748	1,929.3	1,5 34	1,311.3
Cleft palate and cleft lip	812	1,856.0	757	2,196.3	809	2,086.6	2,378	2,032.7
Pyloric stenosis	38	86.9	900	2,611.2	1,063	2,741.8	2,001	1,710.4
Hirschsprung disease, etc.	16	36.6	81	235.0	89	229.6	186	159.0
Other digestive system disorder	212	484.6	667	1,935.2	1,277	3,293.7	2,156	1,842.9
Hypospadias and epispadias	174	397.7	788	2,286.3	990	2,553.5	1,952	1,668.6
Other genito-urinary disorder	421	962.3	2,866	8,315.3	3,369	8,689.6	6,656	5,689.5
Clubfoot	1,065	2,434.3	1,896	5,501.0	2,694	6,948.6	5,6 55	4,833.9
Congenital dislocation of hip	313	715.4	1,109	3,217.6	1,713	4,418.3	3,135	2,679.8
Congenital dislocatable hip	4	9.1	23	66.7	779	2,009.3	806	689.0
Other musculoskeletal disorders	1,255	2,868.6	2,256	6,545.5	3,261	8,411.0	6,772	5,788.7
Integument disorders	227	518.9	678	1,967.1	1,165	3,004.9	2,070	1,769.4
Chromosomal anomalies	665	1,520.0	574	1,665.4	630	1,624.9	1,869	1,597.6
Other	137	313.1	248	719.5	424	1,093.6	809	691.5
Total diagnoses	8,701	19,887.8	18,671	54,171.4	26,660	68,763.6	54,032	46,186.2
Total cases	7,065	16,148.4	14,707	42,670.4	20,474	52,808.2	42,246	36,111.6

*Statistics reflect local population bias.
N = Number of patients.
[1]Per 1 million live births.
Source: Patricia A. Baird, "A Population Study of Genetic Disorders in Children and Young Adults," *American Journal of Human Genetics* 42 (1988): 677–693.

TABLE IV
CONGENITAL ANOMALIES WITH SPECIFIC GENETIC ETIOLOGY FOUND IN A SURVEY
CONDUCTED IN BRITISH COLUMBIA*, CANADA

Congential Anomaly	1952–63		1964–73		1974–83		Total		Sum % of Highest Individual Rates[1]	
	N	Rate[1]	N	Rate[1]	N	Rate[1]	N	Rate[1]		
Dominant conditions	202	461.7	198	574.5	181	466.8	581	496.6	741.5	2.8
Recessive conditions	52	118.9	71	206.0	74	190.91	197	168.4	290.3	1.1
X-linked conditions	10	22.9	13	37.7	20	51.6	43	36.8	66.4	0.2
Autosomal chromosome conditions	586	1,339.4	524	1,520.3	533	1,374.8	1,643	1,404.4	1,693.1	6.4
Sex-chromosome conditions	64	146.3	39	113.2	33	85.1	136	116 .3	152.3	0.6
Multifactorial conditions	. . .	. . .	. . .	. . .	. . .	. . .	. . .	. . .	23,076.0	86.8
Genetic unknown	247	564.6	176	510.6	116	299.2	539	460.7	564.62	2.1
Total	. . .	. . .	. . .	. . .	. . .	. . .	. . .	. . .	26,584.2	100.0

*Statistics reflect local population bias.
N = Number of patients.
[1]Per 1 million live births.
[2]Sum for the decade (1952–63) showing the highest rate.
Source: Patricia A. Baird, "A Population Study of Genetic Disorders in Children and Young Adults," *American Journal of Human Genetics* 42 (1988): 677–693.

Such has been the ubiquity of these conditions throughout history that laws have been passed and policies established dating at least to Roman times to deal with questions of inheritance, culpability for criminal acts and baptism among those born with significant deformities. (For example, while it is unclear if it was necessary to invoke these statutes, according to Roman law one member of a set of CONJOINED TWINS could not be put to death for a capital offense since it would require killing the innocent twin as well. Additionally, in the eyes of the church each individual head required a baptism; if a malformation resulted in two heads joined to a single trunk, two baptisms would be performed.) These canons have been referred to as "monster laws."

However, despite the recognition of various anomalous conditions, little effort was made by the medical community to study them until the 19th century. Among the first to apply scientific standards to the investigation of birth defects was zoologist Isidore Geoffroy Saint-Hilaire (1805–61), who gave the name "teratology" from the Greek *teras,* for "monster," to their study and classification.

It has only been recently, perhaps since the 1960s, that classification and causes of birth defects have received extensive research attention, coinciding with the development of diagnostic procedures that can identify the chromosomal, molecular or chemical basis of some disorders. Prior to this time, medical authorities tended to lump birth defects together in broad categories such as DWARFISM or MENTAL RETARDATION, without concern for the subtle differences between many anomalies or the tremendous diversity of developmental defects that often exhibit almost identical characteristics. Additionally, little attention was given to the unexplained causes of death in early infancy following FAILURE TO THRIVE, which can now often be attributed to specific conditions. Thus there is a paucity of historical data on many GENETIC and congenital conditions.

Generally, defects that occur in one or more per 1,000 live births are considered common. However, there is no consensus for what constitutes a rare condition. While there is ample documentation on conditions that have been seen in far fewer than 100 individuals worldwide, or in just one family, there is no way of knowing the true incidence of many of these or other rarely reported disorders.

Birth defects are the leading cause of infant mortality, and can be caused in several ways. Genetically, they may result from the action of a single mutant GENE or gene pair, or may be due to abnormalities involving entire chromosomes or sections of them (see CHROMOSOME ABNORMALITIES). They may also be caused by the action of several genes in concert with an environmental trigger (MULTIFACTORIAL traits) or by the action of several genes alone (POLYGENIC).

Non-genetic causes include fetal exposure to TERATOGENS, substances that can have a harmful impact on fetal development. Birth defects may also result from mechanical forces within the womb. CLUBFOOT, for example, is the result of uterine crowding of a normally developed foot. Due to their diversity in origin and expression, congenital anomalies are classified a number of ways. Birth defects caused by defective or abnormal development of an organ or body part are referred to as malformations. These include CONGENITAL HEART DEFECTS, SPINA BIFIDA and biochemical disorders that may manifest after birth, such as CYSTIC FIBROSIS, MUSCULAR DYSTROPHY and SICKLE-CELL ANEMIA. "Deformation" refers to a congenital anomaly caused by damage that occurs in the womb to a normally developed part, such as clubfoot. DYSPLASIA refers to abnormal tissue development, and may involve skin, bones, nerves, organs or other tissue. Some ANOMALIES, which may occur in isolation, are frequently seen together in a recognizable pattern. This group of defects is termed a SYNDROME.

More than 250 birth defects can now be detected prenatally. While the incidence of major birth defects has remained remarkably constant, improvements in prenatal detection and treatment, as well as societal attitudes about these conditions, continue to offer more options and opportunities for affected individuals and their families. (See also DATING; EDUCATION; GENETIC DISORDERS; HANDICAP and the Introduction.)

birth injury   An injury to a newborn that occurs during the birth process. It may result from forces due to maternal factors, such as an abnormal position of the newborn during birth, or as a result of medical intervention, such as the use of forceps to assist a prolonged labor.

Injuries include hemorrhaging, damage to organs and nerves, trauma that causes fluid buildup in the tissues (edema), and fractures. The most common fractures are of the collarbone (clavicle), and are most prone to occur during delivery of large infants. Hemorrhaging of the retina is the most common birth injury involving the eye, and may occur in as many as 35% of all live births, though typically there is no lasting damage.

Injuries to abdominal organs and nerves (most commonly facial nerves) are other noted birth injuries. Facial nerve paralysis is estimated to occur in one in 400 live births, though it is usually a self-correcting condition.

The majority of serious birth injuries are thought to result from trauma associated with breech delivery, in which an infant emerges from the womb feet, instead of head, first. Spinal cord injuries are the most common complication in these deliveries and may result in death. (Spinal cord injuries are extremely rare is deliveries where the infant emerges head first.)

Kaiser Wilhelm II of Germany was delivered in a breech birth, and as a result of ensuing nerve damage his left arm was atrophied. It has been suggested that this birth trauma may have contributed to World War I; the psychological effects of his permanent injury were said to have enhanced his aggressive militaristic tendencies.

Statistics on birth injuries appear to be somewhat unreliable, and while they indicate a declining trend over the past several decades, trauma associated with delivery may be underreported, particularly in the case of minor injuries.

birthmark   Well-defined areas of colored skin present at birth to some degree on most people.

In whites, birthmarks are usually dark brown, the result of hyperpigmentation, and may lighten and become slightly raised in time. They may also be strawberry-colored, the result of vascular lesions consisting of masses of small blood vessels (capillaries) just below the surface of the skin. These lesions are called HEMANGIOMAS.

Birthmarks are generally benign, though in rare cases they may become cancerous. Additionally, large strawberry-colored birthmarks may be associated with some hereditary disorders, such as STURGE-WEBER SYNDROME. (See also NEVUS; PORT

WINE STAIN.) Coffee-colored birthmarks, known as café au lait spots, are seen in NEUROFIBROMATOSIS.

birth palsy   Paraplegia or hemiplegia caused by a birth injury. (See PARAPLEGIA.)

Blackfan-Diamond syndrome   See ANEMIA.

bladder, exstrophy of   See EXSTROPHY OF BLADDER.

bleeder's disease   See HEMOPHILIA.

blepharophimosis syndrome (BPES; blepharophimosis, ptosis, and epicanthus inversus)   Blepharophimosis, a vertical fold of skin covering the outer portion of the eyelid, is the most distinguishing of the four anomalies of the eyelid that characterize this hereditary syndrome. The other signature features are ptosis (drooping upper eyelid), epicanthus inversus (a fold of skin extending from the nose to the eyebrow that covers the inner portion of the eyelid) and telecanthus (increased distance between the inner corners of the eyelids). Additional ophthalmic malformations may be present, including strabismus (crossed eyes) and defects in the tear ducts. A broad nasal bridge and low-set ears are observed in some affected individuals.

BPES, an autosomal dominant disorder, occurs in two forms. Type I, affecting only women, consists of the eyelid anomalies and infertility resulting from premature ovarian failure. BPES type II consists of eyelid and associated anomalies alone. The gene FOXL2, mapped to 3q23, has been linked to both forms of BPES. About 70% of those affected have a mutation in this gene. Some 135 mutations and variants of this gene have been identified. About half of all BPES cases are thought to result from de novo mutations (occurring during embryonic development). It has been suggested BPES type 1 is caused by the inability of a normal gene's protein production to compensate for deficiencies of the mutated gene (haploinsufficiency), while Type II results from the defective gene's production

of elongated defective proteins. Lifespan and intelligence are unaffected.

Diagnosis is possible by molecular genetic testing using sequence analysis of the single coding exon of FOXL2, and by FISH, which can identify microdeletions at the 3q23 locus. Prenatal testing may be available for women in families in which the FOXL2 mutation has been identified. The prevalence of BPES has not been established.

blindness   The eye is particularly sensitive to genetic influences. A vast array of hereditary ocular disorders have been identified, some affecting the eyes alone and many others existing as part of more complex SYNDROMES that effect other body systems as well. These disorders may be inherited as AUTOSOMAL DOMINANT, AUTOSOMAL RECESSIVE, X-LINKED, POLYGENIC or MULTIFACTORIAL conditions.

About 124,000 individuals in the United States under 45 years old are legally blind, and genetic aberrations account for almost half such cases. In addition, severe visual impairment or blindness in childhood affects about one of every 2,000 children in developed countries, and it is estimated that well over half such vision loss is attributable to genetic causes.

Some of the many eye findings that may indicate the presence of a hereditary disorder are CATARACTS (any opacities in the lens that result in blurred vision); CHERRY-RED SPOT; corneal clouding (opacity); nystagmus (rapid involuntary movement of the eyes from side to side, up and down, or in circular fashion); pain; pale or absent iris; photophobia (abnormal intolerance to light, causing intense eye discomfort accompanied by tight contractions of the eyelids or other attempts to avoid the light); PTOSIS (drooping of the upper eyelid); retinal detachment (frequently associated with severe myopia); small or malformed eye; STRABISMUS (any abnormal alignment of the two eyes accompanied by double vision).

Hereditary visual disorders include CONGENITAL GLAUCOMA, LEBER'S OPTIC ATROPHY and RETINOBLASTOMA.

GENETIC DISORDERS associated with visual defects include ALBINISM, ALSTROM SYNDROME ANIRIDIA, BARDET-BIEDL SYNDROME, CROUZON DISEASE, DOWN

SYNDROME, FABRY DISEASE, GALACTOSEMIA, HOMO-CYSTINURIA, KNIEST DYSPLASIA, Lenz syndrome, LOWE SYNDROME, MARFAN SYNDROME, MUCOLIPIDOSIS, MUCO-POLY-SACCHARIDOSIS, MYOTONIC DYSTROPHY, NEURO-FIBROMATOSIS, OSTEOGENISIS IMPERFECTA, REFSUM DISEASE, RETINITIS PIG-MENTOSA, RIEGER SYNDROME, SPHINGOLIPIDOSIS, USHER SYNDROME, WAARDENBURG SYNDROME, WERNER SYNDROME, WILMS TUMOR, WIL-SON DISEASE and XERODERMA PIGMENTOSUM.

Bloom syndrome   Condition characterized by low birth weight and short stature, a characteristic facial appearance, development of skin rashes on the face during the first year of life, sun-sensitivity and a predisposition to develop CANCER. An immune defect is usually associated with Bloom syndrome, and frequently there are infections of the ear and respiratory tract as well. Physical growth remains stunted. Mild mental deficiency, though not a typical feature, has also been seen in a few individuals with this syndrome. A tendency to develop diabetes in the teens or twenties is also characteristic.

Since it was first described in 1954 by Dr. David Bloom, a New York City dermatologist with an interest in GENETICS, more than 300 affected individuals have been identified, almost half of them Ashkenazi Jews (those of eastern European ancestry). The genetic basis (AUTOSOMAL RECESSIVE inheritance) was identified in 1963. Approximately one in 120 Ashkenazim are estimated to be CARRIERS of the defective gene.

Males average under five pounds (2.5 kg) at birth and females approximately four pounds (1.8 kg). The skin appears normal, but late in infancy or early childhood, reddish rashes (telangiectasias) appear, caused by dilated capillaries near the surface of the skin. These lesions most often appear on the face, primarily around the nose, lips and cheeks. In approximately half, the lesions appear on the forearms, backs of the hands, ears and neck as well. Exposure to the sun exacerbates the skin eruptions. At puberty, these areas of the skin scar, atrophy and become depigmented. Café au lait spots (irregularly shaped, coffee-colored splotches) frequently appear.

Body proportions, though normal, have a slender and delicate appearance. Affected individuals show a striking resemblance to each other. They have small, narrow faces. The nose is prominent, and the distance between the nose and the back of the head is greater than average. (This skull shape is referred to as dolichocephalic.) The ears protrude, and the voice tends to be high-pitched. Though they appear to be dwarfed in childhood, adolescent growth generally removes them from the category of true dwarfs, though height rarely reaches five feet. INFERTILITY appears to be the rule in males. Life span is shortened due to the development of malignant cancers at an early age. About one in four has developed a malignancy, most commonly leukemia or digestive tract cancers.

MUTATIONS in a GENE for an ENZYME involved in DNA replication and repair are the cause of this disease. The gene is found toward the end of the long arm of chromosome 15, and is a member of a family of genes known as RecQ helicases, involved in maintaining the proficiency of recombination. The genes had previously been characterized in the bacteria *E. coli*. A specific mutation has been found in affected Ahkenazi Jews, confirming that all affected individuals are descended from a common "founder" ancestor who carried this mutation. Different mutations in this gene underlie the disorder in other populations. Identification of the gene and mutations involved permits carrier detection and PRENATAL DIAGNOSIS, and allows confirmation of diagnosis in individuals suspected of being affected on the basis of clinical and cytogenetic manifestations.

Confirmation of the diagnosis based on physical characteristics is accomplished by findings of diminished immunoglobulin levels and cultured blood and skin cells showing chromosomal "instability," that is, the tendency of the chromosomes to break and rearrange themselves, which is a characteristic of this disorder. An increase is seen in sister chromatic exchange (exchange of DNA segments between the two parallel strands of a CHROMO-SOME, each of which becomes a chromosome in the daughter cell during mitosis or cell division).

blue baby (congenital cyanosis)   Any infant with a cyanotic form of congenital HEART DEFECT causing poor oxygenation of the blood shortly after birth, and resulting in a blue tint of the skin. Poor oxygenation (cyanosis) can also be a manifestation of respiratory disease in a newborn or result from a defect in the oxygen carrying molecule of the blood, hemoglobin, as is seen in methemoglobinemia. (See also PATENT DUCTUS ARTERIOSUS; CONGENITAL CYANOSIS.)

blue diaper syndrome   A very rare metabolic disorder that takes its name from the blue urine stain of an infant's diaper that is often the first sign of the syndrome's presence. Affected infants typically exhibit irritability, FAILURE TO THRIVE, constipation, poor appetite, vomiting, and frequent infections and fevers. Vision is often poor due to ocular abnormalities.

Inherited as an AUTOSOMAL RECESSIVE trait, the cause is thought to relate to defective intestinal absorption of tryptophan (see AMINO ACID). Intestinal bacteria convert the excess tryptophan into indican and related substances that turn the urine blue. Antibiotics may help control intestinal bacteria.

bottled water   A series of studies by the California Department of Health Services conducted in the Silicon Valley area found that women who reported drinking only bottled water while pregnant had a lower rate of miscarriage and birth defects in their children than did women who reported drinking tap water.

Over the course of four surveys involving 5,000 women, bottled water drinkers had miscarriage rates ranging from zero to 7.7%, while tap water drinkers had miscarriage rates within the normal range of 8% to 14%. Birth defects in children of the former group ranged from zero to 1.6%, and in children of the latter group, 2.6% to 6.2%, higher than the 2% to 3% national average.

Other factors such as smoking, alcohol consumption and exercise were taken into account in comparing the two groups. Researchers were unable to explain the findings and the results were noted mainly as a curiosity. It should not be taken as an advertisement for bottled water nor as evidence that tap water is dangerous. However, it does point out how difficult it can be to prove whether a drug or environmental exposure is safe or dangerous.

bowleg   A skeletal deformity in which the lower limbs bow outward. Synonyms: genu varum; bandy leg.

Brachmann–de Lange syndrome   See CORNELIA DE LANGE SYNDROME.

brachy   Taken from the Greek *brachys*, meaning "short," this is a prefix used with a variety of terms to describe, among other conditions, abnormalities often associated with CONGENITAL anomalies and inherited conditions. Common terms using this prefix include

bachycephaly—Abnormally short head
brachychelia—Abnormally short lips
brachydactyly—Abnormally short fingers or toes
brachygnathia—Abnormally short lower jaw

brachycephaly   See CRANIOSYNOSTOSIS.

brachydactyly   Shortness of the fingers due to malformation of bones in the hand (metacarpals) or fingers (phalanges), from Greek *brachys*, meaning "short," and *dactyl*, meaning "digit." There are seven distinct genetic variations of the disorder, some of which cause shortness of the toes as well as fingers.

In Type A1, the middle phalanges (the middle of the three bones in each finger) are rudimentary and sometimes fused to the bones at the tips of the fingers (terminal phalanges). In the thumbs, the bones nearest the hand (proximal phalanges) are also short, as are the corresponding phalanges on the big toes. Type A1 brachydactyly was the first malformation attributed to single gene inheritance, earning the distinction in 1905.

In Type A2, all the fingers are normal except the middle phalanges of the index fingers and second toes.

Type A3 is characterized by shortened middle phalanges of the little fingers.

In Type B, not only are the middle phalanges short, but the terminal phalanges are also rudimentary or absent altogether. Both fingers and toes are involved.

Type C is marked by shortened middle and proximal phalanges of the index and middle fingers. The middle phalanx of the fifth finger is also short. The index finger characteristically deviates away from the thumb. MUTATIONS in a GENE known as CDMP1 have been found to cause AUTOSOMAL DOMINANT type C brachydactyl.

In Type D, the terminal phalanges of the thumbs and big toes are short and broad. It has also been known as "Potter's thumb" and "Murderer's thumb."

In Type E, the bones of the hands and feet (metacarpals and metatarsals) are shortened. Short stature and a round face are also characteristic of this variation. This type is also seen ALBRIGHT'S HEREDITARY OSTEODYSTROPHY.

Types A3 and D are the most common variations. Brachydactyly may occur as an isolated malformation (unaccompanied by malformations of other parts of the body) or may occur as a part of a SYNDROME. For example, type A3 brachydactyly is seen in DOWN SYNDROME, type D in RUBINSTEIN-TAYBI SYNDROME and type E in TURNER SYNDROME. Isolated type D brachydactyly (stub thumbs) is common among Jews.

Isolated brachydactyly is generally inherited as an autosomal dominant trait. It may be detected at birth but often remains undiagnosed until late in childhood. Life span is not affected by the condition, and it is sometimes surgically correctable. Routine PRENATAL DIAGNOSIS is not currently available, but in severe cases Brachydactyly may be detectable by prenatal ULTRASOUND.

brain malformations   Improper formation of the brain during embryonic development. The most common brain malformations include agenesis of the corpus callosum, anencephaly, Arnold-Chiari malformation (also called Chiari II malformation), Dandy-Walker malformation, encephalocele, holoprosencephaly, hydrocephalus, lissencephaly, neuronal migration disorders, intracranial cysts and lipomas and schizencephaly.

Congenital brain defects may be caused by inherited genetic defects, spontaneous mutations within the developing embryo or the effects of maternal infection, trauma or drug use. Several brain mal-

formations result from trisomy, the inclusion of a third copy of a chromosome, which normally exist in pairs. Trisomy of chromosome 9 can cause some cases of Dandy-Walker and Arnold-Chiari malformation. Some cases of holoprosencephaly are caused by trisomy of chromosome 13, while abnormalities in chromosomes 7 or 18 are responsible for others. Mutations in individual genes can also cause congenital brain malformations. Drugs that can cause these malformations include anticonvulsants, retinoic acid and tretinoin, anticoagulants and alcohol.

Diagnosis is made from physical examination or imaging studies including magnetic resonance imaging (MRI) and computerized tomography (CT) scans. Prenatal diagnosis of some brain malformations is possible through ultrasound or MRI and via amniocentesis, which reveals chromosomal abnormalities.

branchial cleft cysts or sinuses   A painless cyst on the neck, which may be present at birth. It slowly enlarges, and may grow larger during infections, and subside afterward. Males are affected three times as frequently as females. The cause is unknown, but it is thought to result from a fetal developmental defect. The cyst can be removed surgically. Life span is normal, except in rare cases where the cyst becomes malignant. Most cases are SPORADIC but AUTOSOMAL DOMINANT inheritance has been described. It is also a feature of syndromes such as branchio-oto-renal syndrome where it is associated with ear malformations, hearing loss and kidney anomalies.

breast cancer   This is the most common form of CANCER among women. Each year, more than 210,000 cases of invasive breast cancer are diagnosed in women in the United States. The average American woman has a lifetime risk of approximately 11% for developing breast cancer. Factors involved in its development include GENETICS, hormones, viruses and chemical agents.

After rising precipitously at the end of the 20th century (from 1980 to 1987, incidence of breast cancer rose almost 4% per year; and from 1987 to 2002, incidence rose about 0.3% annually), cases of the most common form of breast cancer, estrogen-positive tumors, dropped 15% from mid-2002 to the end of 2003 to a rate that has held steady in the following years. The decline is believed to have resulted from women's large scale abandonment of hormone replacement therapy used to alleviate symptoms of menopause. In 2002, such treatments were identified as causing an increased risk of breast cancer.

Between 15% and 30% of all breast cancers are thought to be genetically determined and heterogeneous, that is, they represent various GENETIC DISORDERS with a common symptomatic expression. A familial link was noted by the Romans as early as 100 A.D. Familial breast cancer may also be associated with other forms of cancer, particularly ovarian, uterine, prostate and colon cancer, and acute leukemias.

Among the indications that a given case is familial are a family history of breast cancer, an earlier-than-average age of onset and the appearance of the cancer in both breasts (bilateral). If a woman's mother or sister had breast cancer, her risks are two to three times above average; if both mother and sister were affected, the risk rises to six times above average. If her mother had breast cancer and a sister had bilateral breast cancer prior to menopause, her risk is increased 40 times. It is suggested that women with increased risk undergo careful periodic examinations.

An estimated 5 to 10 percent of all breast cancers are caused by inherited specific gene mutations, primarily in the *BRCA1* or *BRCA2* genes. In the general population, about one in 500 people have a mutation in a *BRCA* gene that increases their risk of developing cancer. *BRCA1*, on chromosome 17, plays a role in suppressing malignant changes. Discovered in 1994, a variety of mutations have been identified in the gene, each inactivating it in a different way.

As many as 1% of Ashkenazi Jews (those whose ancestors lived in Eastern and Central Europe) may have a particular mutation, *185delAG*, associated with the disorder, a high percentage for a genetic disorder. The mutation is thought to be present in about one in 800 non-Jews.

Women with the mutation and a family history of breast cancer appear to have up to an 80–90% chance of developing breast cancer in their life time and up to a 40–50% chance of developing ovarian cancer.

BRCA2, located on chromosome 13, was identified in 1995. Women with a defective copy face more than an 85% risk of developing breast cancer. A *BRCA2* mutation, *6174delT* (deletion of the letter "T" at position *6174*) occurs in about 2% of Ashkenazi women, so that about one in 50 can have a gene predisposing them to breast or ovarian cancer. These two genes account for about 4% of all breast cancers.

The mutations involve deletions of sections of the gene. The function of the genes is to repair double strand breaks in the DNA.

These genes have also been linked to ovarian cancer. Women with a mutated *BRCA1* gene have up to a 60% chance of developing ovarian cancer, while women with *BRCA2* mutations face a 25% chance of developing ovarian cancer.

Males can be affected as well. Men who inherit the abnormal *BRCA2* gene have an increased risk for male breast cancer. This risk is approximately 6% to 7% over a man's lifetime, which is about 80 times greater than the lifetime risk of men without a *BRCA2* abnormality. In 2005, about 1,700 men in the United States developed breast cancer, making it some 125 times more rare in men that women. About 460 men died from breast cancer that same year. Men with a *BRCA1* mutation do not appear to face a significantly increased risk for breast cancer, but can transmit the mutation to their daughters. Men with either an altered *BRCA1* or *BRCA2* gene have an increased risk of prostate cancer. Mutations in the *BRCA2* gene have also been associated with an increased risk of lymphoma and melanoma, as well as cancers of the pancreas, gallbladder, bile duct and stomach in both men and women.

Mutations in the *BRCA1* and *2* genes are transmitted in an AUTOSOMAL DOMINANT manner. There is a 50% chance that an individual who carries a mutated gene will transmit it to his or her child. Clinical testing is available for changes in the *BRCA1* and *BRCA2* genes. In addition to the three mutations seen in Ashkenazi Jewish individuals, other *BRCA1* or *BRCA2* mutations are more common among people of Norwegian, Icelandic and Dutch ancestry. Mutations in other genes have also been found to increase the risk of developing breast cancer. These genes include *p53*, *CHEK2*, *STK11*, *PTEN* and *ATM*.

The National Cancer Institute (NCI) recommends that women in their 40s have a mammogram every one to two years. The NCI estimates screening of women at risk could reduce mortality rates by 17%. However, scientific evidence for the benefits is not as convincing as it is for screening for women in their 50s. Several studies have demonstrated that magnetic resonance imaging (MRI) may be more accurate at detecting breast cancer in *BRCA1* and *BRCA2* mutation carriers than mammography. In 2007, the American Cancer Society recommended women who have had breast cancer or are at high risk undergo annual breast MRI scans starting at age 30.

Self-examinations and mammography are useful methods of early detection. (However, a widely used computerized system for examining mammograms, computer-aided detection, or CAD, has been associated with significantly higher false positive rates and biopsy rates with significantly lower overall accuracy.) Treatment generally consists of surgery to remove the growth, in conjunction with chemo-, hormonal or radiation therapy.

Some women who test positive for a *BRCA1* or *BRCA2* mutation may choose to undergo a bilateral prophylactic mastectomy, the surgical removal of the breasts, in order to reduce the risk of getting breast cancer. Studies suggest that prophylactic mastectomy can reduce breast cancer risk by at least 90% in women who carry *BRCA1* or *BRCA2* mutations. Women who test positive for a *BRCA1* or *BRCA2* mutation also may choose to have a bilateral prophylactic oophorectomy, the surgical removal of both ovaries. The available data suggest that bilateral prophylactic oophorectomy reduces the risk of ovarian cancer by at least 95%. Several studies suggest that this surgery also can reduce the risk of breast cancer by about 50%. These two operations do not remove all breast or ovarian tissue, and a woman may still get breast cancer and/or ovarian cancer in the remaining tissue. Both operations have significant emotional and physical risks that must be carefully considered along with the potential benefits.

In 1998, the Food and Drug Administration determined tamoxifen, a drug long used to treat breast cancer, could prevent breast cancer, after a large study found it reduced the incidence of the disease 45% among women using it. However, the drug is associated with a slightly increased risk of endometrial cancer (cancer of the uterine lining) and potentially fatal blood clots, particularly for women over age 50. The drug's effect on reducing breast cancer among women with predisposing genetic mutations awaits further study.

brittle bone disease   See OSTEOGENESIS IMPERFECTA.

Bubble Boy   The popular designation given to a child named David in Houston, Texas, with severe combined immunodeficiency disease or SCID (see IMMUNE DEFICIENCY DISEASE); his story was dramatized in a made-for-television movie starring John Travolta, *The Boy in the Plastic Bubble*, first aired in 1976. The extremely rare disorder made his body unable to defend itself against viral, bacterial or parasitic agents, and his survival required a sterile environment completely sealed from the outside world. Hence, he lived in a plastic, room-sized "bubble" in a hospital.

An older sister was immunodeficient, and an infant brother died of a similar disorder before David's birth. Upon birth, David was placed in isolation, tested, found to be immunodeficient and remained in isolation throughout his life. Efforts were made to find a suitable donor for a bone marrow transplant, which can sometimes enable recipients to produce components of the immune system that their own body is unable to manufacture. David died on February 22, 1984, at age 12, shortly after an unsuccessful bone marrow transplant procedure.

Burkitt lymphoma   A lymph CANCER most commonly found in Central Africa, named for D. O. Burkitt, a contemporary physician posted in Uganda. Although the Epstein-Barr virus plays a role in its development, a specific translocation (see CHROMOSOME ABNORMALITIES) involving the myconcogene and the immunoglobulin genes found on chromosomes 8 and either 14, 2 or 22 appears to work as a genetic trigger of the disease.

Burton's agammaglobulinemia   See IMMUNE DEFICIENCY DISEASES.

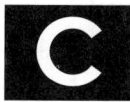

CADASIL (cerebral autosomal dominant arteriopathy with subcortical infarcts and leukoencephalopathy) A hereditary degenerative disorder of the small blood vessels, primarily in the brain. It can cause strokes (the most common feature), migraine headaches and increased risk of heart attack, as well as emotional and mental disorders and ultimately dementia (the second most common feature). It is the first known genetic form of vascular dementia whose causative gene has been identified. (Vascular dementias are the second most common type of dementia after Alzheimer's disease.)

A connection between mental disorders and cerebral vascular disease has been noted for more than a century. Researchers first described the hereditary syndrome now identified as CADASIL in 1977.

Symptoms begin from the mid-20s to about 45 years of age. Progression is slow and expression is highly variable. Some individuals may experience migraines alone, others exhibit strokes, which may be recurring. It can progress to dementia 20 years after onset. Patients typically die by age 65.

An autosomal dominant trait, CADASIL is caused by mutations in the *NOTCH3* gene on 19q, which makes the Notch3 receptor protein. This protein is involved in the development and functioning of the vascular smooth muscle cells that surround the blood vessels. As a result of the mutation, an abnormal version of the protein is produced and accumulates in the vascular smooth muscle cells. This is thought to lead to their degeneration. A few rare cases have resulted from sporadic mutations.

CADASIL affects both males and females. Prevalence is unknown. No treatment protocol currently exists. Some 400 families with the disorder have been described. One study estimated incidence at two in 100,000 adults. It is thought to be underdiagnosed.

Magnetic Resonance Imaging (MRI) scans of the brain of affected patients reveal unusual signals in the "white matter" area, but these anomalies are nonspecific. Diagnosis is made on the basis of an MRI scan in conjunction with a skin biopsy to detect a characteristic abnormality in the small arteries of the skin, or by DNA analysis to identify the mutation. Prenatal testing is available.

caffeine In laboratory studies, rats fed large quantities of caffeine—the equivalent of 80 cups of coffee daily—gave birth to offspring with below average birth weights and a higher incidence of bone abnormalities. Recent studies have also suggested a link between caffeine intake and infertility. However, there is lack of agreement on whether or at what level ingesting caffeine during pregnancy increases the risk of miscarriage (see ABORTION), STILLBIRTH or premature birth (see PREMATURITY) in humans. It has not been directly linked to BIRTH DEFECTS, however studies indicate consumption of greater than 300 mg/d (milligrams per day) during pregnancy, the equivalent of three cups of coffee, is potentially harmful. It has been associated with LOW BIRTH WEIGHT and fetal loss, though its safety in pregnancy is considered unresolved.

In view of the uncertainties, in 1980, the U.S. Food and Drug Administration advised women to avoid coffee, tea, chocolate, cocoa, soft drinks and other foods that contain caffeine, as well as cold medicines, painkillers and weight control drugs that list caffeine among their ingredients during pregnancy. (See also TERATOGEN.)

Cammurati-Engelmann's disease (progressive diaphyseal dysplasia) A rare hereditary form of osteochondrodysplasia, or maldevelopment of the bones, primarily affecting the long bones, those of the arms and legs. "Diaphyseal" in the disorder's secondary name refers to the *diaphysis,* the shaft of a long bone. A symmetrical accretion of excess osseous, or bony material, occurs on the shafts of the long bones. Affected individuals walk with a waddling gait and also frequently experience muscular weakness, fatigue and limb pain. In severe cases, the skull and spinal cord may be involved. Muscle mass may be below normal.

Neurological manifestations include cranial nerve dysfunction and complications arising from increased intracranial pressure from skull malformation. Therapy frequently involves mitigation of bone pain. In cases of excessive intracranial pressure, surgery has been used to relieve the pressure.

At its root, Cammurati-Engelmann's disease appears to be a metabolic disorder that involves the defective regulation of calcium in the body. It is inherited as an autosomal dominant disorder. The gene responsible, *TGFbeta1,* has been mapped to 19q13.1. The gene codes for a growth factor that affects bone development, as well as the ongoing breakdown and rebuilding of bones. A variety of mutations of the gene have been associated with Cammurati-Engelmann's disease. X-rays play an important role in the diagnosis of the disorder. More than 200 cases have been identified worldwide.

Onset typically occurs by age 10, but can appear as early as 20 months or as late as adulthood. In at least one affected family, the disorder exhibited anticipation, that is, onset occurred at younger ages in succeeding generations. In other families, individuals who have inherited the mutated gene have been unaffected, though the disorder has occurred in the offspring of some such individuals. Intelligence and lifespan are unaffected in many affected individuals.

camptodactyly   A permanent flexing of finger(s) or toe(s). It is most common in the little finger, though any finger or toe may be affected. Also, though any joint may be affected, it is most commonly seen in the middle joints.

As an isolated ANOMALY, it is inherited as an AUTOSOMAL DOMINANT trait with variable PENETRANCE. It is a feature of many GENETIC DISORDERS, including SYNDROMES with multiple contractures. (See also ARTHROGRYPOSIS.)

camptomelic dysplasia (CMD; camptomelic dwarfism)   A rare form of neonatal DWARFISM characterized by CONGENITAL bowing of the bones of the legs (campomelia is the bending of the limbs) along with defects of the ribs and pelvis and facial anomalies. The bones of the arms are rarely bowed, but may be mildly short. The skull is large with a disproportionately small, flat face, low-set ears, small jaw (micrognathia) and wide-set eyes (HYPERTELORISM). Disarray of the hair (unruly hair) and CLEFT PALATE are sometimes present. There is generally a decreased number of ribs, which are slender in appearance, producing a small chest.

Death usually occurs soon after birth, generally due to respiratory distress caused by the decreased size of the rib cage.

Twice as many female as male cases have been reported. This may be due to the external sex reversal that sometimes occurs in this condition (i.e., genetic males fail to develop masculine characteristics and thus have female external genitalia combined with XY chromosomal constitution). Previously thought to be an AUTOSOMAL RECESSIVE disorder, now that the molecular defect is known, it is clear that this is an AUTOSOMAL DOMINANT trait; only one of the two GENES is mutated in affected individuals. Most cases are new MUTATIONS. Familial cases may be due to gonadal MOSAICISM or some other disorder resembling CMD. The gene involved is SOX9, a sex determining gene found on the long arm of chromosome 17. Mutations account for both the sex reversal seen and the skeletal malformations. Approximately 100 cases have been reported.

PRENATAL DIAGNOSIS has been accomplished using ULTRASOUND to measure fetal long bone length.

Canavan disease (spongy degeneration of the brain)   A form of LEUKODYSTROPHY, a group of progressive, degenerative disorders of the nervous system. In Canavan disease, white matter in the brain is replaced by microscopic, fluid-filled spaces, hence its "spongy degeneration" appellation. It is named for M. M. Canavan (1879–1953), who reported her patient in 1931.

Onset is in early infancy, beginning with feeding difficulties, poor muscle tone (hypotonia), progressive MENTAL RETARDATION, apathy and weakness, especially in the muscles supporting the head. As the disorder progresses, the head becomes enlarged as the brain enlarges, and the bones of the skull fail to fuse properly. Spasticity and paralysis develop. Vision, and sometimes hearing, deteriorate. Death usually occurs by 18 months to four years of age. There is no cure.

The basic defect that causes this disorder has been identified as a deficiency of the ENZYME aspartoacylase. Although computerized axial tomography (CAT scan) can reveal severe changes in the white matter of the brain, previously the only way to confirm the disease was upon autopsy, with the finding of spongy degeneration of the gray and white matter of the brain. Now it has been demonstrated that affected individuals have deficient aspartoacylase and excrete excessive amounts of N-acetyl aspartic acid in their urine.

Inherited as an AUTOSOMAL RECESSIVE trait, Canavan disease is a rare disorder, though it has increased frequency in Ashkenazi Jews (those of Eastern European ancestry), where incidence is 1:6400 (one in 40 is a CARRIER). Symptoms resemble TAY-SACHS DISEASE, another HEREDITARY DISEASE exhibiting increased incidence in this ethnic group. (The latter stages of Canavan disease also resemble KRABBE DISEASE, another form of leukodystrophy.) Enlargement of the head is also seen in ALEXANDER DISEASE.

The GENE for aspartoacylase, on the short arm of chromosome 17, has been identified. Three MUTATIONS account for about 99% of the mutations that cause Canavan disease in Ashkenazi Jews; one of these accounts for over 60% of the causative mutations. This has allowed for development of carrier screening (by DNA methods) among Ashkenazi Jews, even in the absence of family history. One mutation accounts for 40–60% of the mutations in non-Jewish cases. DNA testing is the preferred method of PRENATAL DIAGNOSIS as the enzyme is expressed at only very low levels in chorionic villus tissue and amniocytes. Research is ongoing into treatment—gene therapy is being investigated. With the identification of a biochemical defect, carrier detection and prenatal diagnosis are now possible.

cancer Term describing more than 100 distinct disorders characterized by uncontrolled cell growth.

Taken from the Latin for crab, cancer refers to the extension, like legs of a crab, of the neoplasm, or new growth, into adjoining tissue (though not all cancers exhibit this characteristic). If a neoplasm is not self-limiting and resists efforts to contain it, it is said to be malignant.

More than a score of hereditary cancer SYNDROMES have been identified, resulting in about 1.0% of cancer patients. However, it is not cancer that is inherited, but the predisposition to develop the disease (see FAMILIAL DISEASE).

Cancers may be associated with CHROMOSOME ABNORMALITIES, single mutant GENES or exposure to viral or environmental agents. Additionally, there are approximately 200 inherited disorders in which cancer has been reported as a regular or occasional feature, and the existence of some "cancer families" with a demonstrated predisposition to develop malignancies has long been recognized. Though the causes of cancer, either in general or in specific cases, are poorly understood, most are thought to result from a combination of genetic and environmental factors.

Assessing a genetic link in a given case may be difficult, though there are several characteristics associated with hereditary cancers: They tend to appear at an earlier age than would generally be expected for a given form of cancer, and in approximately 50% of the cases the cancer develops simultaneously in more than one area, whereas this only occurs in 3% to 5% of SPORADIC cases of cancer. Medical histories of family members may be useful in making a determination.

Genes that play a role in the development of cancer are divided into two major groups, ONCOGENES and tumor-suppressor genes. Oncogenes trigger aberrant cell growth. More than 50 have been identified, and many are located at the sites of the chromosome rearrangements seen in various cancers, such as the Philadelphia chromosome observed in many leukemia patients. Tumor-suppressor genes are involved in diverse functions regulating cellular growth, differentiation and death, and appear to inhibit the formation of cancer. A MUTATION that inactivates a tumor-suppressor can result in neoplasia, though it is thought a number of cumulative errors must occur before cell growth becomes uncontrolled. Genes involved with DNA maintenance and repair may also play a large, though more indirect role in the development of cancer. When inactivated, these genes appear to facilitate mutations of oncogenes and tumor-suppressor genes, which affect cellular proliferation. It is likely that the actions of oncogenes and tumor-suppressor genes underlie most if not all cancers, and it is only how the cancers are triggered that differs from situation to situation.

In some cancers, exposure to toxic substances may trigger the development of neoplasms by transforming a normal gene into one that orchestrates uncontrolled cell growth.

Currently, cancers caused by single gene mutations account for 5% to 10% of all cases, with most of these inherited as AUTOSOMAL DOMINANT traits. About 25% of cancers are familial; though family members exhibit a greatly increased risk for developing cancer, affected individuals demonstrate no known pattern of inheritance. Typically, the risk of developing a cancer in these families is greater than within high-risk groups in the general population, such as heavy smokers or workers exposed to cancer-causing environmental agents.

Genetic syndromes associated with cancer include LIFRAUMENI SYNDROME, NEUROFIBROMATOSIS, BECK-WITH-WIEDEMANN SYNDROME, VON HIPPEL–LINDAU SYNDROME, MULTIPLE ENDOCRINE NEOPLASIA, MULTIPLE EXOSTOSES, ATAXIA TELANGIECTASIA, BLOOM'S SYNDROME and FANCONI ANEMIA. The genetics involved in some of the more common forms of cancer is less clear. They include:

Leukemia. This cancer of the white blood cells is the most common childhood malignancy, though numerically it is much more common in adults. About 27,000 new cases are reported annually in the United States, with children accounting for an estimated about 16–20% of them. More than half of all cases occur after age 60. The disorder is characterized by the production of abnormal white blood cells. Onset and progression may be rapid, as in acute leukemia, or may progress slowly, as in chronic leukemia.

Families with successive generations with leukemia (where affected individuals have had no contact) have been well documented, establishing a strong genetic link in at least some cases.

Additionally, many chronic leukemia patients exhibit a chromosome translocation, with a rearrangement involving chromosomes 9 and 22. This chromosome abnormality is referred to as "Philadelphia chromosome." Children with DOWN SYNDROME are also at increased risk for developing leukemia. Previously a uniformly fatal disease, many affected individuals now survive.

Lung cancer. Lung cancer accounts for about 15% of all cancer cases, and is the greatest cause of cancer death in the United States and Canada, accounting for approximately 135,000 American and 16,800 Canadian deaths a year. While smoking is considered the major cause, genetic predisposition is also involved. The risk of developing lung cancer is thought to be 14 times above average for smokers with a close relative with lung cancer. A deletion of genetic material from chromosome 3 has been linked to small-cell lung cancer, a form that causes 35,000 to 40,000 fatalities annually in the United States.

Melanoma. A rapidly progressive and lethal form of skin cancer. Though it accounts for only about 4% of all skin cancers, it accounts for the great majority of skin cancer deaths. The disorder was first noted by Hippocrates. Most cases are sporadic, but 3% to 15% of all melanomas that result in malignancies appear in familial clusters. An inherited mutation, a shared environmental exposure or both are involved in these cases.

The familial form may have been described as early as 1820 by an English surgeon, W. Norris, who observed multiple skin moles and melanoma in three generations of one family.

The primary initial indication of melanoma is a change in the size, shape, color or feel of a mole. Moles are nothing more than clusters of melanocytes (the epithelial, or skin cells that produce melanin, the pigment that colors the skin) amalgamated with surrounding tissue. Physicians refer to a mole as a nevus (pl. nevi).

If diagnosed early in its development, melanoma is highly curable. But melanoma can metastasize (the process by which a cancer spreads) rapidly and can quickly involve other organ systems and cause death within weeks.

The incidence of melanoma varies around the world, but is greatest in areas with light-skinned populations, strong sun and an emphasis on out-door activities. Exposure to ultraviolet radiation from the Sun plays a large role in its onset. It most often occurs between the ages of 45 to 55, but one-quarter of all cases have their onset before age 40. Melanoma is rare among blacks and oth-ers with dark skins. In these groups, melanoma most often occurs in areas with little pigmenta-tion: under finger- or toenails or on the palms or soles. In the United States, where people have spent growing leisure hours in outdoor activi-ties, the incidence of melanoma has increased. Between 1973 and 2002, the number of new cases diagnosed rose from 5.7 to 14.3 per 100,000 people, one of the fastest rates of increase of any cancer. Despite its relative rarity, it is one of the leading causes of cancer in young adults. In 2004, about 55,000 new cases were diagnosed, and about 7,900 succumbed to melanoma.

Two types of familial melanomas have been identified, though they can be difficult to dif-ferentiate: Familial Atypical Mole Melanoma (FAMM) and Familial Predisposition to Cutane-ous Melanoma. Familial melanomas can alter-natively be grouped in three categories: sporadic melanomas in familial clusters, familial melano-mas triggered by low-risk mutations and mela-nomas caused by high-risk mutations.

In members of families with a history of mela-noma, the risk of developing the cancer is estimated to be 30 to 70 times higher than in the general population. Several different genetic mutations associated with an increased risk of developing melanoma have been identified. In some families, the propensity to develop malignant melanomas follows autosomal dominant inheritance patterns. In other families, the lack of clear Mendelian inheritance patterns (that is, either dominant or recessive) suggests multifactorial polygenic inheri-tance, involving several defective genes in combi-nation with environmental factors.

The most common form of hereditary mela-noma results from a mutation in a single gene, *CDKN2A*. This accounts for about 20–40% of hereditary melanoma and about 0.2–2.0% of all cases of melanoma. Harmful mutations in *CDKN2A* are estimated to increase the lifetime risk of developing melanoma to as high as 76%.

In other words, more than three out of four peo-ple with the mutation will develop melanoma. One group of studies found that individuals with this mutation have a lifetime risk of developing melanoma more than 50 times greater than the general population's. In families with members known to possess the mutation, individuals free of the genetic aberration nonetheless have an 80% higher risk of developing melanoma. A mutation in this gene is also associated with an increased risk of pancreatic cancer in some families.

Some cases of hereditary melanoma are caused by a mutation in the *P14ARF* gene and the *CDK4* gene. These two forms are much more rare. Other genes involved in susceptibility to melanoma likely await discovery. (See *nevoid basal cell carcinoma; xeroderma pigmentosa*.)

Skin cancer. Skin cancer is the most common form of cancer in the United States, and the most eas-ily treatable. The primary cause is thought to be exposure to ultraviolet radiation from sunlight, though genetic predisposition is a factor.

Prostate cancer. Prostate cancer is the most common cancer in males, with rates comparable to breast cancer in women. The test for prostate specific antigen, or PSA, developed in the 1980s, enabled greatly enhanced detection of prostate cancer. Taken via blood test, elevated levels of PSA (above 4.0 ng/ml) are associated with an increased chance of the presence of prostate cancer.

(For other forms of hereditary cancer, see BREAST CANCER; FAMILIAL ADENOMATOUS POLYPOSIS; HEREDI-TARY NONPOLYPOSIS COLORECTAL CANCER and PEUTZ-JEGHERS SYNDROME under COLORECTAL CANCER. See also RETINOBLASTOMA; WILMS TUMOR; BURKITT'S LYM-PHOMA.)

cannabis   See MARIJUANA.

carbamyl phosphate synthetase deficiency, CPS-I See UREA CYCLE DEFECTS.

cardioauditory syndrome   See JERVELL AND LANGE-NIELSEN SYNDROME.

cardiomyopathy Cardiomyopathy, a deterioration of the heart muscle, primarily affects middle-aged individuals. However, hereditary forms occur in children and are one of the leading causes of juvenile cardiac-related deaths. Cardiomyopathy occurs in three major types: dilated congestive, hypertrophic and restrictive. Dilated congestive, the most common, is the form seen in children and occurs in autosomal dominant, X-linked and sporadic forms.

Dilated cardiomyopathy is characterized by an enlarged and weakened heart, often exhibiting arrhythmias (abnormal rhythms). About 30% of cases of dilated cardiomyopathy are transmitted in an X-linked autosomal disorder (familial X-linked dilated cardiomyopathy). It is caused by a mutation of the *dystrophin* gene. The gene produces dystrophin, a protein, found in muscle fibers. Mutations of this gene have also been associated with certain types of muscular dystrophy. The chromosomal locations of several other genes believed involved in an autosomal dominant form have been identified. Several cases studied appeared to be sporadic, that is, arising from a new mutation, as no other family members had ever been affected. Researchers suspect mutations in mitochondrial DNA may also be responsible for some cases. Mitochondria are organelles within every cell that provide energy, and the DNA within them is transmitted only maternally, that is the genetic endowment is passed on from the mother, and it remains unchanged from generation to generation.

Congestive heart failure occurs in the majority of affected individuals. Little treatment is available. In some cases a heart transplant may be required for survival.

This condition is also associated with Barth syndrome, a rare genetically linked cardiac disease that affects male infants, typically in the first year of life. Affected infants also often exhibit short stature, a predisposition to infections and neutropenia, a decrease in the white blood cell count.

Carney Complex (CNC) An autosomal dominant syndrome consisting of cardiac tumors (myxomas), pigmented skin lesions, endocrine tumors and tumors involving nerve sheaths (schwannoma). It was first described by J. A. Carney in 1985. The myxomas, containing connective tissue, can appear in any or all chambers of the heart. They may interfere with proper functioning of the heart, resulting in pulmonary congestion or mitral valve insufficiencies. Should these benign tumors become life threatening, treatment typically consists of surgical removal of the myxomas.

Myxomas without the association of these other anomalies may occur sporadically in both infancy and adulthood and are among the most common forms of all tumors, and the most common form of primary cardiac tumor. Isolated cardiac myxomas occur in about seven out of 10,000 individuals. Carney Complex is estimated to account for 7% of cardiac myxomas.

Myxomas typically develop at a young age, and median age of diagnosis is 20 years. The tumors can mimic other cardiac conditions, and echocardiograms are used in diagnosis. Lifespan is unaffected in most cases, but some patients die at an early age, lowering the average life expectancy for those affected to 50 years.

Mutations responsible for the syndrome have been linked to the short arm of chromosome 2 (2p16) and the long arm of chromosome 17 (17q22-24). This latter site is associated with a tumor suppressor gene (*PRKAR1A*) that is mutated in about half the members of families with a history of Carney Complex. This is the first human disease known to be caused by mutations of the PKA holoenzyme, a critical component of cellular signaling. There is no clinical differentiation in the disorder between affected individuals whose genetic anomaly has been mapped to chromosome 17 and those in whom is has been linked to chromosome 2. About 30% of cases have been linked to the anomaly in chromosome 2. It is possible that an unidentified mutation site is involved in some cases.

The presence of the *PRKAR1A* mutation can be identified through sequence analysis of the gene's coding region in about 50% of cases in which it exists. Prenatal testing for at-risk pregnancies is possible.

The Carney Complex is considered to include cases of what were previously designated as LAMB (lentigines, atrial myxomas, mucocutaneous myxomas and blue nevi) syndrome and NAME (nevi, atrial myxoma, myxoid neurofibroma, and ephelides) syndrome. More than 400 cases have been reported. About 30% are the result of de novo, or new, mutations that occur early in gestation.

carnitine deficiency   Carnitine helps to regulate the cellular rate of long-chain fatty acid oxidation. Deficiency of the carnitine protein can result in impaired oxidation of fat with episodes of coma or a muscle disorder related to increased lipid storage. Some patients may have MENTAL RETARDATION. Although the basic cause is often unknown, carnitine deficiency in the muscle may be due to defective absorption of carnitine by the muscle fiber, to defective carnitine synthesis in the liver, or to depletion of the body's stores of this compound. The diagnosis is based on finding decreased levels of carnitine in the blood.

The first carnitine deficiency disorder was identified by Dr. W. Engle in 1970, who published a description in the journal *Science*. Symptoms generally appear during the 20s or 30s or earlier, and include muscle cramping following exercise. Affected individuals may have had prolonged fasts or may indulge in high-fat diets.

The long-term prognosis is uncertain. However, progressive muscle and liver damage may occur. Primary treatment may target avoidance of such exacerbating factors as strenuous exercise, severe dietary restriction and high-fat diets.

The mode of transmission of this very rare disorder is generally AUTOSOMAL RECESSIVE.

People with primary carnitine deficiency have defective proteins called carnitine transporters, which bring carnitine into cells and prevent its escape from the body. Primary carnitine deficiency affects one in every 40,000 live births in Japan and one in every 37,000 to 100,000 newborns in Australia. Primary carnitine deficiency can be caused by mutations in the *SLC22A5* gene, mapped to the long arm of chromosome 5.

Most carnitine deficiency is not primary, but rather occurs secondary to other diseases, mainly the organic acidurias, including propionic acidemia or the more recently described acyl-coA dehydrogenase deficiencies, primary disorders of fatty acid breakdown. In secondary carnitine deficiency it is not the deficiency of carnitine that is the fundamental problem, but rather that deficiency occurs

as a result of a primary defect of another ENZYME involved in fatty acid utilization. Nevertheless, the carnitine deficiency in those circumstances causes problems in addition to those caused by the underlying metabolic disorder. Carnitine deficiency can also accompany treatment with the anticonvulsant drug valproic acid, antiretrovial therapy in AIDS, use of a ketogenic diet, and with chronic hemodialysis.

Carpenter syndrome (acrocephalopolysyndactyly type II)   A form of CRANIOSYNOSTOSIS, skull malformations caused by premature closure of the gaps (sutures) between one or more skull bones. Head growth is thus directed in aberrant directions. Two sisters with this form were first described in 1901 by English pediatrician George Alfred Carpenter (1859–1910).

Carpenter's syndrome is distinguished by the presence of extra toes, which may be webbed. Cardiac abnormalities, OBESITY, poorly developed genitalia and MENTAL RETARDATION are sometimes present. Early surgical treatment may reduce incidence of mental retardation by relieving cranial pressure.

Inherited as an AUTOSOMAL RECESSIVE trait, about 35 affected individuals have been reported. For other forms of craniosynostosis, see APERT SYNDROME; CROUZON DISEASE; PFEIFFER SYNDROME and SAETHRE-CHOTZEN SYNDROME.

carrier   An individual who is heterozygous for a particular GENE. Generally used for an individual with a single recessive gene for a particular disorder; a HETEROZYGOTE for a recessive disease. The term is also often applied to a female who possesses a gene for an X-LINKED disorder. The carrier will usually not exhibit any signs of the disorder, but is capable of passing the gene to his or her offspring, or of having an infant with the disorder if he or she mates with another carrier. (See also AUTOSOMAL RECESSIVE.) The term is also sometimes used for an individual who is heterozygous for an AUTOSOMAL DOMINANT gene but does not (yet) express any features related to the mutant ALLELE he or she carries. An example would be someone who "carries" an autosomal dominant gene that predisposes to the development of cancer, but who has not yet developed a tumor, or an individual carrying a MUTATION that causes ALZHEIMER'S DISEASE or HUNTINGTON CHOREA but does not yet manifest any symptoms.

cartilage-hair hypoplasia   See METAPHYSEAL CHONDRODYSPLASIA.

cataracts   Opacities or clouding of the lens of the eye that can result in decreased vision and, in some cases, BLINDNESS. The severity of CONGENITAL cataracts varies greatly, ranging from functionally insignificant to blindness caused by a totally opacified lens.

An estimated one in 250 infants is born with a cataract, as a result of either GENETICS or other prenatal influence. Their formation is poorly understood. They account for 11.5% of blindness in preschool children. About 25% of congenital cataracts are believed to be genetically induced, most often the result of AUTOSOMAL DOMINANT inheritance. AUTOSOMAL RECESSIVE and X-LINKED inheritance is rare.

Additional ocular defects are seen in approximately 50% of all affected individuals. Congenital cataracts are also an associated feature of a number of GENETIC DISORDERS as well as of other systemic diseases or SYNDROMES. These include GALACTOSEMIA, cerebral cholesterinosis, congenital ICHTHYSOSIS, CHONDRODYSPLASIA PUNCTATA, WERNER SYNDROME, LOWE SYNDROME, MYOTONIC DYSTROPHY, ZELLWEGER SYNDROME, SMITH-LEMLI-OPITZ SYNDROME, CEREBRO-OCULO-FACIAL SKELETAL SYNDROME and STICKLER SYNDROME, in addition to disorders such as congenital rubella, diabetes and chromosomal aberrations.

Total congenital cataracts, possibly with X-linked inheritance, have been observed in the We-Sorts, a biracial group of southern Maryland.

Management depends on the severity of the opacities, whether they are unilateral or bilateral and their association with other ocular defects or systemic problems. Early surgery is needed in bilateral, complete cataracts. This is followed by contact lens fitting, even in the infant.

CATCH 22 (deletion 22q11.2 syndrome)   An acronym given to a constellation of overlapping SYN-DROMES all resulting from a deletion of a portion of chromosome 22 (22q11). This is the most common autosomal deletion known. The acronym stands for cardiac anomaly/abnormal facies, T cell defect due to thymic hypoplasias, CLEFT PALATE, and hypocalcemia due to hypoparathyroidism. The syndromes include the DI GEORGE SYNDROME, velocardiofacial syndrome (Shprintzen syndrome), conotruncal anomaly face syndrome (Takao syndrome) and isolated defects of the outflow tract of the heart (TETRALOGY OF FALLOT, truncus arteriosis and interrupted aortic arch). The current view is that all of these are one syndrome, though a name for it remains undecided. Deletion 22q11.2 syndrome appears to be one of the favored designations.

Recognition of the deletion's role in the development of cardiac malformations represents a major advance in the understanding of these abnormalities. Family members of affected individuals have exhibited deletions along with cardiac abnormalities and characteristic facial features. The palpebral fissures are short, narrow and upslanting. Because of its association with cardiac defects, physicians may recommend genetic analysis for the deletion among family members when a child is affected with a cardiac condition. The presence of the deletion constitutes the CATCH 22 genotype.

The deletion has an estimated frequency of one in 4,000 live births. It is detectable by fluorescence in situ hybridization (FISH). Over 90% of affected individuals have a de novo, or new, mutation, and between 5–10% have inherited the deletion from a parent. In some of these latter cases, the parent's manifestations are so mild or absent that the parent is an apparently asymptomatic carrier. The spectrum of involvement is great, and variation even within affected members of the same family can be wide. Prenatal diagnosis is available. Affected individuals may also show immune dysfunction causing recurrent infections, feeding problems and learning difficulties. Adults show an increased risk of developing mental illnesses such as schizophrenia and bipolar disorder.

cat eye syndrome   Condition named for the vertical appearance of the pupil of those affected, caused by a fissure or cleft of the iris (coloboma). The two major features of the SYNDROME are this "cat eye" and an anus that has failed to open during fetal development (IMPERFORATE ANUS). Several other conditions are commonly seen in those with the syndrome. MENTAL RETARDATION of varying severity is present in between 55% and 80% of cases. Forty percent have abnormally small heads (MICROCEPHALY), and cardiovascular ANOMALIES occur in about 55%. CLEFT LIP or CLEFT PALATE occur in about 25% and genital and kidney malformations in about 20%.

Additional eye anomalies often associated include wide-set eyes (HYPERTELORISM), seen in about 40% and small eye(s) (microophthalmia), in 25%.

It results from a CHROMOSOME ABNORMALITY in which there are extra copies of portions of chromosome 22. Usually an extra chromosome is present, derived from two identical pieces of chromosome 22, including duplication of the entire short arm and the first portion of the long arm. Thus an individual carrying this extra chromosome fragment has four copies of a segment of chromosome 22. Other cases, previously thought to have no extra chromosome 22 material, have been found to have a chromosome 22 in which there is a duplication of the proximal portion of its long arm. Other chromosome abnormalities, e.g., trisomy 22, may have similar features. FISH studies can document the duplications of chromosome 22 segments. Prenatal diagnosis is possible using chromosome analysis, perhaps accompanied by FISH studies, on fetal tissue derived from amniocentesis or CVS.

PRENATAL DIAGNOSIS of a baby with cat eye syndrome is theoretically possible by finding the chromosome fragment in fetal cells collected via AMNIOCENTESIS or CHORIONIC VILLUS SAMPLING.

Surgery can correct the imperforate anus and other associated anomalies. Life span may be shortened in those individuals with cardiac and renal malformations associated with the syndrome.

cats   Cats are believed to be a vector for transmitting the microorganism that causes toxoplasmosis, a disease that, if contracted during pregnancy, can cause fetal development anomalies that may result in MENTAL RETARDATION or death.

Evidence indicates that the feces of infected cats may harbor the microorganisms, thereby contaminating soil or litter boxes, which may remain infectious for weeks or months. It has been advised that all individuals wash their hands after handling or disposing of cat litter, and that pregnant women avoid contact with used cat litter.

CBAVD (congenital bilateral absence of the vas deferens)   The maldevelopment of the vas deferens, the tube which carries sperm from the testes to the penis. Sperm is viable, but there is no way for it to travel to the penis for insemination. The condition is closely associated with cystic fibrosis (CF).

CBAVD accounts for 1 to 2% of male infertility. The condition is present at birth, but most affected males remain unaware of it until they experience fertility difficulties and seek medical counsel. Most cases are caused by an allele, or variation in the cystic fibrosis transmembrane conductance regulator (CFTR) gene on chromosome 7, which causes CF. Almost all men with cystic fibrosis (CF) have CBAVD. Those with CBAVD without CF may exhibit some CF symptoms. Now that its genetic basis is known, CBAVD is considered a mild form of CF. Between 64 and 84% of men with CBVAD without CF have at least one variation in the CF gene. Individuals with CBVAD should be examined to assure that they don't have lung or digestive problems seen in CF. Those with the *R117H* mutation and the 5T allele are most likely to exhibit these symptoms. (There are more than 30 common mutations in the CF gene.)

Affected males have assisted reproductive options that enable them to conceive, such as ICSI (intracytoplasmic sperm injection) using sperm collected via Microsurgical Epididymal Sperm Aspiration (MESA).

cebocephaly   See HOLOPROSENCEPHALY.

celiac disease   See GLUTEN-INDUCED ENTEROPATHY.

cell bank   A repository for collecting, storing and distributing CELL CULTURES for scientific research. The Human Genetic Mutant Cell Repository, at the Coriell Institute for Medical Research in Camden,

New Jersey, for example, maintains, a collection of human cells preserved for the study of GENETIC DISORDERS. With some 8,500 cell lines and 2,000 DNA samples donated from individuals affected with various HEREDITARY DISEASES and disorders associated with aging, it is the largest facility of its kind in the world.

About 500 to 600 new samples are received annually. In many cases, samples are donated by several family members exhibiting a hereditary disorder whose exact genetic cause has yet to be determined. Cells from donated tissue samples are cultured and then stored at minus 316 degrees Fahrenheit. Portions of the repository's cell samples are thawed and sent to researchers around the world. Studies of these cells may help unravel the genetic secrets of hundreds of inherited disorders. Other institutions also maintain similar, often more specialized, collections.

cell culture   The growth of cells in vitro, that is, in glass, such as a test tube, for experimental purposes. The cells proliferate but do not organize into tissue. Cells taken from AMNIOTIC FLUID or fetal tissue for use in prenatal diagnostic procedures are cultured prior to their analysis. Other types of cells (for example from skin) can be maintained in culture (see CELL BANK) for experimental studies. (See also AMNIOCENTESIS.)

central core disease   Characterized by weak muscles and lack of muscle tone (hypotonia), this rare AUTOSOMAL DOMINANT trait is a form of benign familial polymyopathy (disorders that affect skeletal muscles). Described in 1956, though not named until later, it was the first example of a stationary muscle disorder. (Stationary muscle disorders are nonprogressive, as opposed to the MUSCULAR DYSTROPHIES.) It produces a FLOPPY INFANT and is usually observed in early infancy. In initial stages it resembles Duchenne muscular dystrophy, except for its nonprogressive nature. Walking and muscular development are delayed.

In most if not all cases this disorder is caused by mutations in the ryanodine receptor-1 GENE found on the long arm of chromosome 19. Other MUTATIONS in this gene have been found to cause malignant hyperthermia. The gene codes for an ion channel component of the skeletal muscle fiber. The name is derived from the fact that when affected muscle fibers are stained and examined microscopically, there is a central "core" of fibers that do not stain the same way as the fibers at the margins.

cerebral gigantism   See SOTOS SYNDROME.

cerebral palsy (CP; congenital cerebral palsy)   A group of disabling conditions resulting from damage to the central nervous system; "cerebral" refers to the brain, and "palsy" refers to a lack of muscle control that is a frequent feature of the disorders. Characteristics of CP may include spasms, involuntary movements and disturbances of gait and mobility, which may be accompanied by abnormal sensation and perception.

The early-onset disorders of movement and posture that characterize CP are chronic and nonprogressive. That is, they persist throughout life but do not get worse with time. Though primarily disturbances of movement, they may have associated abnormalities of vision or hearing, seizures or MENTAL RETARDATION. It was formerly named "Little's disease," for British physician William John Little (1810–94), who was among the first to study this disorder.

There are four major types of CP: spastic, characterized by stiff and difficult movement; athetoid, characterized by uncontrolled, abnormal movement; and ataxic, characterized by a disturbed sense of balance and depth perception; and mixed, in which individuals exhibit characteristics of any combination of the three other types. (There are other, rarer types of movement disorders that are not really CP; for example, LESCH-NYHAN SYNDROME has been considered a severe form of cerebral palsy, but it is really an inherited metabolic disease that affects only males and is progressive in nature.)

There is great variability in the expression of CP, ranging from severe cases that result in total inability to control body movements and mental retardation, to mild cases that may result only in slight speech impairment. The severity of the condition is dependent on the part of the brain affected and the extent to which it has been damaged.

The cause of CP is not clearly or fully understood. Cerebral palsy is thought to be caused by damage to the brain before, during or shortly after birth. There are numerous possible ways for this damage to occur. For example, it is clear that maternal viral infections during pregnancy (such as German measles; see TORCH SYNDROME) can seriously affect fetal development. A blood type incompatibility conflict between the mother and the fetus can also cause damage to the fetus and result in CP, if Rh factor is absent from the mother's blood and present in the father's (see HEMOLYTIC DISEASE OF THE NEWBORN). Head injuries, infections such as meningitis and other insults to the brain in the first few months of life are also thought capable of causing CP.

Lack of oxygen reaching the fetal or newborn brain may also be a cause of CP, and may result from infant breathing problems associated with premature birth, or complications in pregnancy and labor. While in the past it was thought that most cases of CP were caused by oxygen deprivation related to the birthing process, such as awkward birth position, extended labor or interference with the umbilical cord, recent data is making it clear that this is not the case. Large studies in the United States and Australia have shown that most newborns with lack of oxygen at birth do not suffer from CP, and most children with CP were not deprived of oxygen at birth. Clearly, other poorly understood factors must occur before birth that play a role in causing CP. Because of this link to delivery, a growing number of lawsuits have been brought by parents of affected individuals, claiming obstetrical malpractice caused the condition in their child, though this is generally not the case.

An estimated 500,000 to 700,000 children and adults in the United States manifest one or more CP symptoms. The United Cerebral Palsy Association has estimated that between one in 1,000 and three in 1,000 infants develop CP each year, resulting in about 9,000 new cases annually.

Improvements in treatments for affected individuals in recent years have lessened their isolation. Medication for controlling seizures, surgery for correcting some physical problems, counseling to assist emotional adjustment, and mechanical aids such as communication equipment, specially equipped cars and page turners, have helped increase opportunities for affected individuals. New muscle relaxants are also being tried to relieve the muscle spasticity. Additionally, an increase in available programs offering physical therapy, occupational therapy and speech therapy have assisted in helping these individuals become more integrated into society. Yet controversy over the murder conviction of a Canadian farmer, Robert Latimer, who killed his severely affected daughter in 1993 to relieve her of pain and suffering, focused attention on treatments and their limits.

cerebro-hepato-renal syndrome See ZELLWEGER SYNDROME.

cerebro-oculo-facio skeletal syndrome (COFS) Rare AUTOSOMAL RECESSIVE disorder that typically leads to death from emaciation and respiratory failure, or from repeated respiratory infections within the first three to five years of life.

Affected infants are usually small; though typically born at term with normal birth weights, there is virtually no growth. Other features include a small head, often with a sloping forehead, CATARACTS or small eyes, high nasal bridge, large ears, overhanging upper lip and small jaw. There are also skeletal abnormalities, such as narrow pelvis, prominent heels, "rocker bottom feet" and, importantly, flexion contractures of the limbs and fingers. These congenital contractures (see ARTHROGRYPOSIS) are due to an apparent neurologic degeneration occurring before birth.

PRENATAL DIAGNOSIS may be possible using ULTRASOUND. The disorder appears to be etiologically heterogeneous, that is, it can be caused by any one of several mutations. The first described cases, from a native family in Manitoba, were found to have changes in the *ERCC6* gene, a DNA repair gene located at 19q13.2. This gene also causes Cockayne syndrome, type B or type II. Individuals diagnosed with COFS syndrome who have this mutation are considered to have Cockayne syndrome type II, and COFS syndrome is now considered part of the spectrum of Cockayne syndrome disorders. A child of Ashkenazi Jewish descent with COFS was found to carry a unique mutation in another DNA-repair gene, *ERCC2*, mapped to 19q13.3. Mutations in this gene also cause a form of xeroderma pigmentosum.

cesarean delivery (cesarean section; C section) A method of childbirth in which the baby is surgically removed from the uterus through an incision made in the abdomen. Cesarean deliveries were practiced as early as 3000 B.C. in Egypt, and the name of the procedure is taken from a set of Roman laws, the Lex Caesare, dating to 715 B.C., which mandated the surgical removal of a FETUS following maternal death. (Julius Caesar was also said to have been delivered this way, as was Macduff in Shakespeare's *Macbeth*.)

Historically, cesarean deliveries have been a high risk to both mother and infant, due to the likelihood of infection and the primitive surgical techniques employed. However, as these risks have dropped, the rates of cesarean childbirth have climbed dramatically. From 5.5% of births in 1970, the percentage of cesarean to vaginal deliveries grew to 24.5% in 1988, and, in 2005, reached 27.5% of the more than 4 million births in the United States, making C sections the most common major surgery performed in the country. Nineteen percent of women giving birth for the first time have their babies delivered via C section. (The rate of vaginal deliveries among women who have previously had C sections is 11 per 100 births.) The Centers for Disease Control advocates a rate of no more than 15%.

Despite improved medical techniques, C sections are still associated with increased risks to both maternal and infant health. Maternal mortality is approximately one in 2,500 for cesarean deliveries, as compared with one in 10,000 for vaginal deliveries. A 2006 study of almost six million births found the neonatal mortality rate for cesarean delivery among low-risk women was 1.77 deaths per 1,000 live births, while the rate for vaginal delivery among this group was 0.62 deaths. Infants delivered by cesarean section are at increased risk for respiratory ailments and fetal distress caused by the anesthesia administered to the mother. Moreover, labor releases hormones in babies that are beneficial to healthy breathing, and the physical compression of vaginal deliveries helps remove fluid from the neonatal's lungs.

The continued high rates of cesarean deliveries are due to several factors: Since the procedure is safer than it once was, many infants who would be difficult to deliver vaginally due to complications of labor, termed dystocia, are instead delivered via C section. (Dystocia refers to a broad range of labor complications, including a mismatch between the size of the baby and that of the mother's pelvis or the position of the fetus.) The accepted notion that once a woman has had a cesarean she will always deliver by that method has also made it more common. (More than 98% of U.S. women who have had a cesarean delivery continue to deliver this way in subsequent childbirths.) Cesarean deliveries also allow more control over when an infant will be delivered.

The current consensus among maternal and childcare authorities is that the rates of cesarean deliveries should be reduced and that, where possible, vaginal delivery should be the method of choice. The American College of Obstetricians and Gynecologists, noting both the additional risks and costs of surgical delivery, has recommended that most women who have had a cesarean delivery try to have vaginal deliveries in subsequent births.

cesarean section   See CESAREAN DELIVERY.

CF   See CYSTIC FIBROSIS.

CGH (comparative genomic hybridization) A molecular cytogenetic technique for identifying mutations and aberrant chromosomal regions and genes in the DNA of cancerous tissue. This technique has been used to find genetic anomalies in a variety of malignancies. It is much faster than earlier methods in that it allows screening of the entire genome in a single test. The tumor DNA and normal DNA are first labeled with different fluorescent marker chemicals. Images taken during hybridization are analyzed by computer. Differences in the binding of the two labeled DNAs indicate regions of the genome that are gained or lost in the DNA of the tumor. The genetic alterations are denoted as DNA losses and gains, and these chromosomal and subchromosomal mutations exhibit a characteristic pattern.

CGH detects only unbalanced chromosome changes. Structural chromosome aberrations such as balanced reciprocal translocations and inversions cannot be detected.

Charcot-Marie-Tooth disease, CMT (peroneal muscular atrophy; hereditary motor and sensory neuropathy) A group of GENETIC DISORDERS characterized by degeneration of the motor and sensory nerves that control movement and feeling in the arm below the elbow and in the leg below the knee. There is progressive muscle atrophy and wasting, resulting in severe weakness in the wrists, hands and fingers, as well as in the feet, ankles and lower legs. Simple tasks requiring manual dexterity, such as buttoning buttons, picking up small objects and writing, may become difficult. In the legs, degenerative changes may limit mobility. Reflexes slow considerably.

It is named for French neurologists Jean M. Charcot and Pierre Marie and British neurologist Howard Tooth, who simultaneously described the disorder in 1866.

The severity of the disorder is highly variable, even among members of the same family. Some researchers believe a large number of mildly affected individuals are never diagnosed. Symptoms most frequently appear in adolescence. Typically it begins with weakness in muscles of the feet, progressing to the calf muscles and muscles of the lower arms. Due to atrophy of muscles in the foot, the toes become cocked and the foot becomes foreshortened and may develop a very high arch (pes cavus) or become uncommonly flat. Affected individuals develop a high-stepping drop-foot gait, with the foot raised well above the ground (stork leg), in order to prevent the forefeet from dragging on the ground and tripping them. The foot slaps as it hits the ground. Affected individuals cannot run very fast, and due to weakness in the ankles, they often have frequent sprains. Changes in the shape of the foot may lead to blistering of the toes and other problems due to the unaccommodating shape of normal shoes. Loss of feeling occurs to a variable degree.

The disorder is slowly progressive, may stabilize for long periods of time, and may stop progressing entirely at any time. Therefore, affected individuals can never be sure about the extent of the ultimate severity of their condition. Life span is unaffected. The majority of therapy is focused on care of feet and lower legs to ease mobility and to reduce problems caused by weakening and degenerative changes in the feet. Surgery can sometimes reduce hand, foot ankle and toe problems.

CMT in its various forms adds up to be the most common inherited peripheral neuropathy, with an incidence of about 1:2500. It is estimated that about 125,000 individuals in the United States have CMT. Affected individuals show an enhanced likelihood of neurotoxicity when treated with the cancer chemotherapy drug vincristine.

An inherited disorder, CMT is transmitted in AUTOSOMAL DOMINANT, AUTOSOMAL RECESSIVE and X-LINKED forms. Some cases appear to be the result of new MUTATION. The majority of cases are autosomal dominant, followed by the X-linked form. One study in western Norway found the prevalence of autosomal dominant forms to be 36 in 100,000 people, of X-linked to be 3.6 in 100,000 and autosomal recessive, 1.4 in 100,000.

About 15% of cases are apparently SPORADIC: They are more likely to be autosomal dominant rather than autosomal recessive; GENETIC COUNSELING can be complex in these circumstance. Understanding the molecular basis for this group of disorders allows molecular testing which can clarify the genetic basis of the disorder in an individual family.

The most common form of CMT is the autosomal dominant form with slow nerve conduction. (Nerve conduction velocities are determined by electrophysiologic studies of the patient.) This is known as type 1, which is further delineated into subtypes A–F.

Most CMT patients have type 1A CMT. And approximately 70% of all individuals presenting to neuromuscular clinics with a chronic peripheral neuropathy have CMT1A (*PMP22* duplication) as its cause. The average age of onset is 12 and the disease is almost 100% penetrant by adulthood (see PENETRANCE). This type has been found to be due to mutations in the GENE for a protein known as peripheral myelin protein 22. The gene (*PMP22*) is found on the short arm of chromosome 17, and the major cause of CMT is its duplication. Molecular testing can reveal this mutation and allow for prenatal and presymptomatic diagnosis. Another gene, the *MPZ* gene, which codes for the major structural protein of myelin, myelin protein zero, and is found on the long arm of chromosome 1, causes type 1B CMT. Although this is an autosomal dominant form, males with type 1B are generally more severely affected than females, who may be asymptomatic.

Some cases of autosomal dominant CMT type 1 are caused by mutations in genes other than *PMP22* or *MPZ*; these rare types are currently classified as types C–F.

In type 2 the onset of the disease is somewhat later, the disorder progresses more slowly, and nerve conduction velocities are more normal. This is also an autosomal dominant form, and at least 10 genetic loci on a number of different chromosomes may be involved, including 1p and 3. The autosomal recessive forms are known as CMT4. At least 7 different genes may be involved. Some autosomal recessive cases have involved the *PMP22* locus. There appear to be at least three different gene loci involved in X-linked CMT. The major one involves the gene for connexin-32; this codes for a protein involved in the structure of a channel between contacting adherent cells known as a gap junction, which allows the transport of materials between the connecting cells. This gene is found on the long arm of the X chromosome, and this form of CMT shows X-linked dominant inheritance or perhaps more appropriately an intermediate X-linked inheritance, as affected females are generally more mildly affected.

Other mutations in the *PMP22* and *MPZ* genes lead to a different and more severe neuropathy known as Dejerine Sottas disease. Still other mutations in the *PMP22* gene lead to yet another neuropathy known as "hereditary neuropathy with liability to pressure palsies." Finally there are yet rarer forms of CMT which may be associated with deafness, and/or optic atrophy which may be either autosomal dominant, autosomal recessive, or X-linked. Another rare X-linked form is also associated with a scalp defect. A form of the disorder linked with DEAFNESS has been reported to be unusually frequent in the hill country of western North Carolina.

CHARGE association This rare SYNDROME results from defects in embryonic development summarized by the acronym CHARGE: fissure of the eye (COLOBOMA); heart disease; a block in the nasal passages (atresia choanal); retarded growth and development; genital ANOMALIES and deformed ears or DEAFNESS. In addition, kidney anomalies, or abnormal connection between the windpipe and esophagus (TRACHEOESOPHAGEAL FISTULA), feeding difficulties, an abnormally small jaw (micrognathia), CLEFT LIP and CLEFT PALATE may occur. The abnormalities are believed to originate during the second month of gestation, when the differentiation of tissues and organs in the fetus takes place.

Most cases are SPORADIC, and prevalence is thought to be 1:12,000 births. The majority of affected individuals are mentally deficient. Facial palsy and swallowing difficulties are common. Visual or hearing handicaps may also influence their ability to function. If the defects are severe, death may occur soon after birth.

Most children with CHARGE have a mutation in the *CHD7* gene on chromosome 8.

Char syndrome A triad of anomalies comprised of characteristic dysmorphic facial features, patent ductus arteriosus (PDA) and malformations of the fifth finger. It is named for F. Char who first described it in 1978. The midface is flat, eyes are set wide, eyelids are droopy (ptosis), the palpebral fissures slant downward, the philtrum (the midline groove extending from the nose to the lip) is short, lips are "duck bill"-like and the mouth is triangular. Ears are set low. The middle phalanges of the fifth fingers exhibit aplasia or hypoplasia.

An autosomal dominant disorder, the gene responsible, *TFAP2B* on 6p, makes the protein transcription factor AP-2 beta. Several mutations have been identified in affected individuals. Individuals with isolated PDA do not have these mutations. Prevalence of this rare disorder is unknown. An undetermined percentage arise from de novo mutations. Prenatal testing may be available for families in which the mutation has been identified in an affected family member in a clinical or research laboratory. In pregnancies at increased risk, ultrasound examination may reveal the characteristic hand anomalies and the congenital heart defect (PDA).

Chediak-Higashi syndrome A lethal metabolic disorder, named after M. Chediak, a Cuban physician who described it in 1952, and O. Higashi, a Japanese pediatrician who published a description in 1954. A form of ALBINISM, it is characterized by decreased pigmentation of hair and eyes, sensitivity to light (photophobia), constant, involuntary movement of the eyes (nystagmus), abnormal susceptibility to infection and a peculiar malignant lymphoma. Nerve damage is also present. There is muscle weakness, foot drop (a peculiar gait) and decreased muscle stretch reflexes. Affected infants may have convulsions and MENTAL RETARDATION, and often have frequent recurring infections, especially of the gastrointestinal tract, skin and respiratory tract, and fevers of unknown origin. Inherited as an AUTOSOMAL RECESSIVE trait, it is very rare. Most cases have been of European ancestry, especially Spanish, and most have died in childhood due to infection, often before the age of seven. Those that survive beyond infancy generally die of a rapidly developing malignancy. Most patients require bone marrow transplantation. The GENE involved is the *lysomal trafficking regulator* gene found on chromosome 1.

CARRIER detection is possible in some cases by the presence of abnormally large granules in the blood cells. A similar or identical blood cell disorder has been found in Aleutian mink, Hereford cattle, Beige mice and a killer whale.

cherry-red spot An abnormal red circular area in the retina of the eye. One of the hallmarks of TAY-SACHS DISEASE, it results from swelling of the nerve cells around the macula of the retina (the central area of vision on the retina) which makes the macula stand out as a red circle. It can also be seen in other storage diseases, though Tay-Sachs is the most common causitive disorder.

chicken pox See VARICELLA.

chimera Taking its name from the mythological hybrid beast with a lion's head, goat's body and serpent's tail, this is an individual with, or the condition of having, genetic material from two different fertilized eggs (zygotes) or embryos. The two genetically different zygotes from which the cells of a chimera are derived may be from the same or different species. It is most common in the blood of fraternal twins due to the mixing of the fetal blood cells during embryonic development. True HERMAPHRODITES with an XX/XY chromosomal constitution also may be chimeras. Additionally, individuals who have had transplants, in particular, bone marrow transplants, are often referred to as chimeric, as their blood cells are thereafter derived from another individual, and therefore from a different embryo.

Chimerism can be produced experimentally as well, and is being used to make chimeras involving different species. In 2003, scientists at China's Shanghai Second Medical University successfully fused human skin cells with rabbit eggs. The embryos were reported to be the first human-animal chimeras successfully created. These chimeras were allowed to develop for several days in a laboratory petri dish before the investigators destroyed the embryos and harvested their stem cells. Researchers at the Mayo Clinic have created pigs with human blood by introducing human stem cells into gestating pig fetuses. At Stanford University, investigators have made mice that have brains that are 1% human.

Chinese restaurant syndrome (monosodium glutamate sensitivity) An estimated 25% of the general population may be sensitive to MSG (monosodium glutamate), a chemical used as a flavor enhancer. Its heavy use in some Chinese foods is the reason these individuals often experience a characteristic reaction following a meal in a Chinese restaurant. Symptoms include a tightening in the back of the neck, pressure around the eyes, headache, flushed face and nausea. So-called hot dog headache and migraine headaches triggered by diet may be similar sensitivities. (Individuals who think they are allergic to MSG actually have this inherited sensitivity [see ALLERGY].)

The sensitivity may be inherited as an AUTOSOMAL RECESSIVE trait, though this is not proven. The basic defect involved in the reaction is unknown, but may be due to an inborn error of metabolism.

choanal atresia   A life-threatening condition caused by the failure of the opening between the nasal passages and the airway to develop, which causes a blockage of the nasal passage. This creates a serious problem because newborns normally breathe through their noses, and must learn to breathe through their mouths. Since they have not learned mouth breathing, and the normal nasal passage is blocked, affected infants exhibit severe respiratory problems. Occurring in one in 7,000 live births, the male to female ratio is 1:2, and uni-lateral/bilateral relationship is 2:1. Unilateral cases rarely cause respiratory distress, but only a mucoid discharge. Mouth breathing is learned at about four to six weeks after birth. Associated ANOMALIES including CHARGE in 50% of cases. (Choanal atresia is itself a feature of the CHARGE ASSOCIATION.)

The genetics of this disorder are poorly understood. Like CLEFT LIP and CLEFT PALATE, it is most likely a MULTIFACTORIAL trait. It has been reported in both affected single and successive generations, with about 8% of the cases being familial.

choledochal cyst   A CONGENITAL cyst found in the bile duct, which manifests itself as a mass in the right upper quadrant of the abdomen, frequently accompanied by jaundice and pain due to blockage of the flow of bile. Affecting females four times as often as males, incidence is less than 1:200,000 in the general population, and it appears most commonly in the Japanese. The exact cause is unknown and appears to be non-genetic. It is usually not associated with other malformations of other organ systems, but may occur with other abnormalities of the pancreas or biliary system. It may remain asymptomatic for a long period of time and may be difficult to diagnose.

Without treatment, this defect is lethal due to inflammation of the bile ducts (cholangitis) and prolonged jaundice caused by chronic retention of bile (biliary cirrhosis). It can be treated by surgery, often biliary-intestinal drainage, or complete removal of the cyst.

It is detected in the first year of life in approximately 20% of cases, and between the ages of one and 10 years in an additional third. Eighty percent of all cases are identified in the first 30 years of life. Over 500 cases have been reported.

PRENATAL DIAGNOSIS may be possible by identifying the cyst via ULTRASOUND.

cholesterol ester storage disease (CESD)   An extremely rare hereditary condition, apparently caused by a deficit of acid lipase, an ENZYME that breaks down cholesterol esters (a particular form of fat). As a result, abnormally high levels of cholesterol esters and triglycerides accumulate in the liver, spleen and intestine. The liver is enlarged (hepatomegaly), and the spleen may be as well (splenomegaly). Lipid levels in blood, plasma and bone marrow are extremely high. There is also an indication that premature coronary vascular disease may be a part of this condition.

Transmitted as an AUTOSOMAL RECESSIVE trait, very few cases have been documented. Females may be more often affected than males. The disease can be detected at birth by measuring levels of the affected enzyme. There is no treatment. PRENATAL DIAGNOSIS has been accomplished. Life expectancy appears shortened, though the exact cause of death has not been fully established.

CESD and WOLMAN DISEASE both result from lysosomal acid lipase (LAL) deficiency. CESD has a later onset and much less fulminant course of the disease whereas Wolman disease causes more serious manifestations much earlier in life with death within a few months of birth. The two diseases result from different MUTATIONS in the same GENE, that for LAL, found on chromosome 10. The mutations that cause Wolman disease leave no residual enzyme activity.

cholinesterase   A hereditary defect in the ENZYME necessary to reverse the effects of the skeletal muscle relaxant succinylcholine, often administered with anesthesia during surgery. The result is a prolonged cessation of breathing (apnea) following administration of this relaxant.

Succinylcholine acts at the neuromuscular junction to block the effects of acetylcholine, which transmits neural impulses across the nerve junction. Under ordinary circumstances, succinylcholine is a shortacting drug (about 10 minutes); plasma levels fall rapidly due to the action of plasma cholinesterase. However, if plasma cholinesterase levels are low, the effects of succinylcholine are greatly prolonged, and the ability to breathe without respiratory assistance is delayed.

Theoretically, diagnosis is possible at any time with laboratory tests. However, the condition will not be discovered unless a specific history is taken or tests are run before surgery. Often, it is not evident until prolonged apnea occurs after succinylcholine administration. Prognosis is good, provided the apnea is recognized and respiratory assistance is given.

Inherited as an AUTOSOMAL RECESSIVE trait, the most common form of atypical cholinesterase (dibucaine-resistant) is estimated to occur in approximately one in 2,000 to one in 4,000 live births in various populations. The responsible GENE is located on the long arm of chromosome 3 (3q). Two variations (fluoride-resistant and silent gene variant) are much rarer.

Individuals with this disorder should alert their relatives to be tested before surgery, and people with relatives who died from an unexplained cause during surgery should also be tested before undergoing an operation. If the enzyme defect is detected, succinylcholine should not be used.

chondrodysplasia punctata

A group of dwarfing conditions characterized by multiple abnormalities in the development of the bones, especially the bones of the upper leg (long bones) and the bones in the fingers. "Chondro" refers to cartilage, "DYSPLASIA" to abnormal development and "punctata" refers to the characteristic pinpoint spots of calcification found by X-rays in cartilage of developing bones. In addition, affected individuals may have a characteristic facial appearance and other defects as well. Scalp hair tends to be sparse and coarse, and the skin tends to be dry and scaly.

There are several forms of chondrodysplasia punctata. They are clinically and etiologically heterogeneous and the differentiation and classification of them is confusing and changing. The majority are genetically determined. As a HEREDITARY DISEASE, it occurs in AUTOSOMAL DOMINANT, AUTOSOMAL RECESSIVE, and X-LINKED dominant and recessive forms. Maternal ingestion of certain drugs (e.g., anticoagulants such as warfarin) during pregnancy has also been associated with this disorder. The punctate calcifications have also been seen in other disorders, such as ZELLWEGER SYNDROME.

Detection by ULTRASOUND has been accomplished in several of the forms. Identification of a specific underlying biochemical abnormality has made PRENATAL DIAGNOSIS of the recessive form possible (see below).

Conradi-Hunermann type Bearing the name of E. Conradi and C. Hunermann, who published descriptions in 1914 and 1931, respectively, this skeletal dysplasia is marked by asymmetry of the limbs. The face appears flat, with a depressed nasal bridge. Other common characteristics include scoliosis (often developing in the first year of life) and contractures of the large joints. Dry scaly skin or loss of hair (alopecia) occur in about 25% of cases. cataracts occur in less than 20% of cases. Congenital heart defects are sometimes present. Previously thought to be autosomal dominant, this type is now generally considered to be X-linked dominant; it seems to affect only females. Hemizygous males ("hemizygous" means someone possessing only one copy or allele of a given gene pair see heterozygote; X-linked) are unaffected because it is lethal for them in utero. There is a wide variability in this form. Though severe cases may be stillborn, for those who survive beyond the first weeks of life, life expectancy and mental development are normal. The Conradi Hunermann type is caused by defects in sterol-Δ8-isomerase, which catalyzes an intermediate step in the conversion of lanosterol to cholesterol. The diagnosis may be confirmed by measuring the plasma concentration of sterols. Most cases are thought to be the result of new mutation.

Rhizomelic type Rhizomelic is a term denoting disproportionate shortening of those parts of the limbs closest (proximal) to the body (i.e., the upper arm and thigh). This is the autosomal recessive form of chondrodysplasia punctata. It is rare and usually fatal. Infants fail to thrive and die in the first weeks of life from respiratory difficulties. Those who survive the first year of life are severely retarded and usually die in early childhood.

In addition to the disproportionate shortening of the proximal portions of the limbs, other findings may include a small head (MICROCEPHALY) and CLEFT PALATE. Swelling of the cheeks due to blockage of the lymph glands (lymphedema) give the cheeks a "chipmunk" appearance. CATARACTS in both eyes (bilateral) are found in 70% to 80% of cases. In Australia, the depressed bridge of the nose (saddle nose) seen in many cases led to the designation "koala bear syndrome" for this disorder in 1970.

As in other rare recessive disorders, the frequency of CONSANGUINITY appears high in the parents of infants with this disorder.

Rhizomelic chondrodysplasia punctata has recently been found to be due to a defect in the function of the subcellular organelles called peroxisomes, which play an important role in many metabolic processes. The peroxisomal disorders are a newly recognized group of disorders caused by the dysfunction of this organelle. They include the Zellweger syndrome, ADRENOLEUKODYSTROPHY, Refsum disease and rhizomelic chondrodysplasia punctata. There are specific biochemical abnormalities identifiable now in rhizomelic chondrodysplasia punctata that not only shed light on the origin (pathogenesis) of this disorder but also permit precise prenatal (by CHORIONIC VILLUS SAMPLING or AMNIOCENTESIS) and postnatal diagnosis. There are several specific peroxisomal ENZYMES whose functions are impaired in this disorder. It has been found that the underlying defect lies in the receptor required for the proper targeting of these enzymes to the peroxisome. The GENE for this is known as *PEX7*.

X-linked   The X-linked recessive form has the skeletal manifestations of chondrodysplasia punctata, along with icthyosis-type skin lesion which may have linear or whorled appearance, short stature and MENTAL RETARDATION. The disorder results from MUTATIONS in the gene for arylsulfatase (ARSE), found on the short arm of the X chromosome. In many patients this mutation results from a chromosomal deletion or translocation and may affect contiguous genes resulting in other manifes-

tations of other GENETIC DISORDERS (such as KALLMAN SYNDROME and deficiency of other sulfatases such as arylsulfatase C) as well. Warfarin inhibits the activity of ARSE and it appears the fetal warfarin syndrome occurs because of this (see WARFARIN EMBRYOPATHY).

An X-linked recessive form has been described with mild physical symptoms and mental deficiency.

chondrodystrophy   See ACHONDROPLASIA.

chondroectodermal dysplasia   See ELLIS–VAN CREVELD SYNDROME.

chorea, hereditary benign   See HEREDITARY BENIGN CHOREA.

chorea, Huntington, chronic   See HUNTINGTON CHOREA.

chorion   One of the membranes surrounding the fetus and containing another membrane, the amnion, the sac that holds the fetus and the AMNIOTIC FLUID. The placenta develops from this membrane. In early gestation the chorion contains finger-like projections, the chorionic villi. Sampling of these pieces of tissue (CHORIONIC VILLUS SAMPLING, or CVS) allows for early PRENATAL DIAGNOSIS of some genetic conditions in the first trimester of pregnancy.

chorionic villus sampling (CVS)   An invasive prenatal diagnostic procedure. First introduced in the United States in 1983, an advantage over the older and more widely used AMNIOCENTESIS procedure is that CVS can be performed much earlier in a pregnancy—usually about the 10th–12th week—thus providing diagnostic information during the first trimester.

The CHORION is a membrane that forms early in pregnancy and later develops into the placenta, through which the fetus is nourished. At the edge of the chorion are villi, tiny frondlike projections containing blood vessels. The villi connect the chorion to the lining of the uterus and contain many fetal cells, which can be analyzed in the laboratory to aid in prenatal diagnosis of possible genetic defects and CHROMOSOME ABNORMALITIES.

In chorionic villus sampling, a small piece of villus tissue is removed by one of two methods. In the first, which was the original technique employed, a catheter is inserted into the mother's vagina and, with the aid of ultrasound imaging, the catheter is guided through the cervix and into the uterus to the chorionic villi. A syringe is then used to suction out the required tissue sample. In the second method, a needle is inserted through the mother's abdominal wall, as in amniocentesis, and the chorionic villus sample is obtained in this manner.

Once removed, the tissue sample can be analyzed quickly. Fetal cells from chorionic villi may not require extensive culturing in the laboratory, as do cells obtained from the amniotic fluid in amniocentesis, and test results can often be available in about a week. PRENATAL DIAGNOSIS becomes a more private issue as the woman is not yet "showing," and a termination of pregnancy, if such an option is chosen, is safer (see ABORTION). Chorionic villas sampling can aid in prenatal diagnosis of a range of GENETIC DISORDERS including DOWN SYNDROME and Duchenne MUSCULAR DYSTROPHY.

A major disadvantage of chorionic villas sampling is that risks of miscarriage and fetal death seem to be somewhat greater than with amniocentesis, on the order of 1/2–1%.

In 1991, a new risk was recognized: an increased frequency of limb defects in infants exposed to CVS. It is now acknowledged that there is the possible small increase in risk of limb reduction defects, primarily absence of parts of one or more fingers or toes, estimated at three to six times over the general population's risk but still quite small (1/1000–1/3000). Rate and severity seem to be associated with procedures done before 10 weeks and those that are difficult, involving more trauma to the placenta. Rare cases have had more severe limb defects, primarily in early procedures, which is why CVS is now done after 10 weeks. Thus, the decision whether to use chorionic villus sampling is made only after careful consideration of all factors involved.

choroideremia   A rare X-LINKED hereditary vision disorder. It affects the choroid, the dark brown vascular coat of the eye between the white of the eye (sclera) and the retina. Females are rarely affected.

Early symptoms are night blindness and a gradual constriction of the visual field. As the condition progresses, the choroid and the retina undergo complete atrophy, resulting in BLINDNESS.

Vision is usually normal in female CARRIERS, but they may exhibit striking changes in the pigmentation of the eye.

Choroideremia has an estimated prevalence of about one in 50,000. The gene responsible, *CHM*, encodes for the Rab escort protein-1 (REP1), which is involved in membrane trafficking. Its gene has been mapped to chromosome locus Xq21. In the Salla region of northeastern Finnish Lapland, there is an unusually high frequency of this disorder, and it affects one in 40 individuals. The cases in the pedigree account for one-fifth of the world's patients. The specific mutation found in the Salla pedigree is unique. DNA-based diagnosis is now available for carrier detection and prenatal diagnosis.

Christmas disease   Hemophilia B. It takes its name from the surname of the first patient with the disease who was studied. (See also HEMOPHILIA.)

chromosome   Strands of genetic material that contain our entire genetic heritage, and are responsible for the expression of hereditary traits that distinguish us as individuals and as members of a particular species. They are found in the nucleus of all cells, with the exception of red blood cells.

In the 1880s, German biologist Walther Flemming, using synthetic dyes, discovered a staining technique that revealed tiny threadlike bodies within the nucleus of the cell. In 1882, he published drawings of his observations, showing a cycle of positions in which these bodies regularly aligned themselves. He was observing, for the first time, the process of mitosis, whereby chromosomes replicate.

Due to their ability to absorb dye, these structures were called chromosomes, colored bodies. In 1903, American Walter S. Sutton and German Theodor Boveri independently suggested that chromosomes were the carriers of genetic information, and that they occurred in pairs, one from the mother and one from the father. Proof of their importance to heredity came in 1944 with the experiments of Oswald Avery at Rockefeller University in New York. He demonstrated that chromosomal material could, when transferred into the nucleus of a cell, transmit characteristics from one strain of bacteria to another.

Chromosomes are composed of a double helix of DEOXYRIBONUCLEIC ACID (DNA), a shape reminiscent of a twisted ladder, constructed of pairs of GENES, locked together rung by rung. (There are between 50,000 and 100,000 gene pairs in human chromosomes.) The chromosomes can be visualized as strings of individual genes—one after another. Chromosomes occur in pairs (except in sperm and egg cells), and humans have a normal complement (karyotype) of 23 chromosome pairs. Twenty-two of the chromosomes or chromosome pairs are referred to as "autosomes" or "somatic chromosomes." The 23rd chromosome or chromosome pair are the sex chromosomes, or X and Y chromosomes, and determine gender. (Males have an X and a Y chromosome, females have two X chromosomes.) It is estimated that if the chromosomal material found in a single human cell were uncoiled and stretched out, it would measure approximately six feet in length.

Aberrations in mitosis and meiosis, the process whereby chromosomes replicate themselves, are responsible for many GENETIC DISORDERS. (See also CHROMOSOME ABNORMALITIES; X CHROMOSOME; Y CHROMOSOME.)

chromosome abnormalities   Aberrations in the structure or composition of the CHROMOSOMES, which can result in a multitude of development difficulties, GENETIC DISORDERS and BIRTH DEFECTS. Many CONGENITAL disorders previously regarded as being of unknown origin have been identified as resulting from specific chromosomal abnormalities through high-resolution microscopy and cytogenetic techniques. Many of these abnormalities involve small deletions or rearrangements, the majority found at the ends, or telomeres, of chromosomes. These cytogenetic diagnostic techniques, which use molecular technologies, include Fluorescence In Situ Hybridization (FISH) and Comparative Genetic Hybridization (CGH) (often using microarrays or gene chips).

Normally, humans possess 46 chromosomes, divided into 23 pairs. Each parent provides one chromosome of each pair. (There are 23 chromosomes in the female ovum, or egg, and 23 in each of the male sperm. When sperm and egg unite at conception, the resulting fertilized egg has 23 pairs of chromosomes.) Twenty-two of these chromosome pairs are called autosomes. The 23rd is composed of what are called SEX CHROMOSOMES. At a particular point in cell division, each individual chromosome consists of a double strand that appears joined at an off-center point (the centromere), resembling a narrowed X with a misplaced intersection. Each autosome pair is numbered (1 through 22) and the individual sex chromosomes are identified as X or Y CHROMOSOMES. (Females have a pair of X sex chromosomes; males have one X sex chromosome and one Y sex chromosome; the presence of a Y determines "maleness.") The individual chromosomes are recognized in cytogenetic examination based on their size, exact position of the centromere and their staining characteristics of light or dark bands when stained with special microscope dyes (see CHROMOSOME BANDING) or with fluorescently labeled DNA PROBES. Any disruption of the normal arrangement or number of chromosomes is considered a chromosomal aberration. While some aberrations are benign, others can have severe consequences. (See Tables V and VI.)

The abnormality may be in the number of chromosomes, the loss of chromosomal material (deletion), duplication of chromosomal material, or the transfer of chromosomal material to another chromosome or to a different part of the same chromosome.

The general location of an abnormality is defined as being on either the long arm or the short arm of a chromosome, a position determined with reference to the centromere. The letter q designates a position on the long arm; the letter p (which stands for "petite"), on the short arm. Thus, 13q designates a position on the long arm of chromosome 13.

TABLE V
FREQUENCIES OF AUTOSOMAL CHROMOSOME CONDITIONS FOUND IN A SURVEY
CONDUCTED IN BRITISH COLUMBIA*, CANADA

Autosomal Chromosome	1952–63		1964–73		1974–83		Total	
	N	Rate[1]	N	Rate[1]	N	Rate[1]	N	Rate[1]
Down syndrome	571	1,305.1	460	1,334.6	394	1,016.2	1,425	1,218.1
Patau syndrome (trisomy 13)	3	6.9	15	43.5	22	56.7	40	34.2
Edward syndrome (trisomy 18)	1	2.3	31	89.9	57	147.0	89	76.1
Autosomal deletion syndromes	4	9.1	4	11.6	26	67.1	34	29.1
Other conditions due to autosomal anomalies	6	13.7	14	40.6	31	80.0	51	43.6
Anomaly of unspecified chromosome	1	2.3	0	0.0	3	7.7	4	3.4
Total	586	1,339.5	524	1,520.3	533	1,374.8	1,643	1,404.4
Sum of highest individual rates								1,693.2

*Statistics reflect local population bias.
N = Number of patients.
[1]Per 1 million live births.
Source: Patricia A. Baird, "A Population Study of Genetic Disorders in Children and Young Adults," *American Journal of Human Genetics* 42 (1988): 677–693.

Chromosomal abnormalities may be inherited, they may occur before conception, during the formation of the sperm or egg, or they may occur early in embryonic development. (In this last case, some cells will have the normal complement of chromosomes, and some will not, a condition referred to as MOSAICISM.) In some cases of infants with chromosomal abnormalities, the chromosomal change is found in one of the parents, as well. If both parents exhibit normal KARYOTYPES (chromosomal arrange-

ments), the abnormality in their offspring is said to have occurred "de novo" in the sperm or egg.

About one in every 200 liveborn infants has a detectable chromosomal abnormality. In about half of these cases, the abnormality is basically benign. In the other half, the aberrant condition causes congenital malformations, MENTAL RETARDATION or abnormalities that develop later in life. An estimated 12% of mentally retarded children have chromosomal abnormalities.

TABLE VI
FREQUENCIES OF SEX CHROMOSOME CONDITIONS FOUND IN A SURVEY
CONDUCTED IN BRITISH COLUMBIA*, CANADA

ICD9, Sex-chromosomal Condition	1952–63		1964–73		1974–83		Total	
	N	Rate[1]	N	Rate[1]	N	Rate[1]	N	Rate[1]
Gonadal dysgenesis	33	75.4	26	75.4	23	59.3	82	70.1
Klinefelter syndrome	28	64.0	11	31.9	5	12.9	44	37.6
Other sex-chromosome anomalies	3	6.9	2	5.8	5	12.9	10	8.5
Total	64	146.3	39	113.2	33	85.1	136	116.3
Sum of highest individual rates								152.3

*Statistics reflect local population bias.
N = Number of patients.
[1]Per 1 million live births.
Source: Patricia A. Baird, "A Population Study of Genetic Disorders in Children and Young Adults," *American Journal of Human Genetics* 42 (1988): 677–693.

Chromosomal abnormalities are also found in approximately half of all spontaneously aborted FETUSES, and in an estimated 7% of STILLBIRTHS and cases of prenatal death (see ABORTION). (Perinatal refers to the period from the 28th week of pregnancy to 28 days after birth.)

General Terms

Aneuploidy   A deviation in the number of chromosomes that is not an exact multiple of 23, the number of chromosomes present in a sex cell. (Thus TRIPLOIDY and tetraploidy, while they are numerical aberrations are not aneuploidy.) The most common forms of aneuploidy are MONOSOMY and trisomy. These most commonly result from nondisjunction, an abnormality in the normal process whereby the pair of chromosomes split to form sperm and egg, each of which contain only a single copy of each chromosome. In nondisjunction, both copies of the pair go into a single daughter cell.

Monosomy   The absence of one chromosome of a particular pair. The total number of chromosomes is thus 45 (22 pairs, plus one unpaired chromosome). It is usually caused by abnormalities during the formation of sperm or egg cells (meiosis). Turner syndrome is the only common condition that results from monosomy. All other forms of monosomy are extremely rare and generally lethal. Only monosomy X (Turner syndrome) usually survives to the stage of a recognizable pregnancy among non-mosaic monosomies.

Trisomy   The presence of an extra, third chromosome in what would normally be a pair. The total number of chromosomes is 47 (22 pairs, plus three chromosomes where there should be only two). This is the result of nondisjunction during meiosis. Down syndrome, for example, is also known as trisomy 21, indicating the presence of an entire extra chromosome 21.

While the origin of the extra chromosome may be either maternal or paternal, it is believed to be contributed by the mother in 75% of cases. The frequency of trisomy increases with maternal age.

Additional abnormalities occur in which entire extra sets of chromosomes are present, such as in the aforementioned triploidy and tetraploidy.

Triploidy   Having three, rather than the normal complement of two copies of each chromosome. Instead of a total of 46 chromosomes (2 x 23), individuals with triploidy have 69 (3 x 23). It generally results from either fertilization by 2 sperm cells or from a failure of a maturation division in either the egg or more frequently the sperm. Most triploid conceptions result in miscarriage but a few triploid infants have been liveborn and survive only briefly. They have severe growth retardation and many malformations. Older maternal age is generally not a factor.

Tetraploidy   Having four copies of each chromosome, instead of the normal two. Individuals have 92 chromosomes in all (4 x 23). This is caused by the abnormal cell division of a normal fertilized egg. This condition is extremely rare, and infants generally die within 19 weeks of birth.

Rearrangements   In addition to abnormalities involving entire chromosomes, many abnormalities involve only portions of a single chromosome, as a result of chromosomal breakage that does not properly repair itself. These are abnormalities not in chromosome number but in chromosome structure. These rearrangements can also have severe consequences. Their more common forms include the following:

Deletion   A section of one chromosome in a pair is absent. This is sometimes referred to as "partial monosomy." A "-" sign indicates a deletion. Thus, the syndrome "18q-" indicates a deletion of a section of the long arm of chromosome 18.

Duplication   An extra section of one chromosome in a pair is present. This is sometimes referred to as "partial trisomy." A "+" sign indicates a duplication. Thus, "+4p" is a syndrome associated with a duplication of a section of the short arm of chromosome 4.

Translocation   A section of one chromosome is interchanged with a section of another chromosome (reciprocal translocation) or with a section of the same chromosome. In balanced translocation, no genetic materials lost (deleted) or gained (duplicated) but is only rearranged; in an unbalanced translocation, material is deleted and/or duplicated.

Inversion   A broken section of a chromosome has reattached in the same place on the same chromosome but in reverse direction ("upside-down" or inverted).

High resolution microscopy techniques and FISH recently identified several well-known hereditary conditions as also exhibiting chromosomal rearrangements, generally small deletions. These conditions include PRADER-WILLI SYNDROME, RETINOBLASTOMA, ANIRIDIA-Wilm's tumor syndrome, DI GEORGE SYNDROME, LANGER-GIEDION SYNDROME and Miller-Diecker lissencephaly.

Even within recognized syndromes caused by duplication or deletion of portions of a chromosome, there may be a high degree of variability of expression, due to the variability of the length, or the exact position, of the section that is duplicated or deleted.

Syndromes

Listed below are some of the most documented chromosome syndromes; other common or important syndromes have separate entries. About 100 distinct chromosomal syndromes have been delineated. The vast majority are extremely rare.

+3q Birth weight is usually somewhat below average. Infants have poor muscle tone (hypotonia), presenting a "floppy infant" appearance. The head is small (microcephaly), and the face tends to be square-shaped. Abnormal head shape due to craniosynostosis is seen in 92% of cases. Characteristic facial features include wide-set eyes (hypertelorism), dense eyebrows that join above the nose (synophrys), upturned nose (anteverted nares), downturned corners of the mouth and low-set or malformed outer ears. Hirsutism (excessive hair) is common.

Nearly all exhibit a high-arched or CLEFT PALATE or BIFID UVULA. The neck is short and the chest is often deformed, with widely spaced nipples. The extremities are usually short, and some of the toes may be fused together (SYNDACTYLY). Over 75% of cases have congenital heart abnormalities, and malformations of the urogenital tract are common.

Infants often have a low-pitched, growling cry. Almost half die before one year of age. Those that survive exhibit severe mental and growth retardation. These children resemble those with CORNELIA DE LANGE SYNDROME; recurrent cases of this syndrome may be due to familial translocation leading to +3q.

4p- See WOLF-HIRSCHHORN SYNDROME.

+4p This condition results in mental and motor retardation and a characteristic facial appearance. Infants have small heads (MICROCEPHALY), serious ocular defects, a short, large nose with a rounded fleshy tip ("boxer nose") and prominent chin. The eyebrows are dense and may be joined above the nose (synophrys). The ears may be unusually large and rotated slightly backward. The neck is short and the hairline low.

More than 35 cases have been reported. Growth is retarded in about half of affected infants. About one-quarter to one-third have died by two years of age due to infections, respiratory complications or heart disease. Puberty appears to be delayed in those who survive. IQs are in the 20 to 65 range. Most cases have resulted from a familial translocation.

4q- This condition is marked by mild early growth retardation and moderate to severe mental retardation. Birthweight is normal. Facially, the eyes are wide-set (hypertelorism), the nasal bridge is depressed and the nose upturned (anteverted nares). The ears are low-set and rotated slightly backward. The chin is small (micrognathia), and cleft palate, with or without CLEFT LIP, is frequent. Malformations of the hands and feet and cardiac anomalies are seen in about one quarter of the cases. Mental retardation is moderate to severe. Over two-thirds of infants succumb within two years of birth to respiratory infections or congenital HEART DEFECTS.

+4q Severe mental and motor retardation, often accompanied by cardiac and genitourinary abnormalities, are hallmarks of this syndrome. IQ is generally below 50. It usually results from a translocation.

While the facial features are variable, they may include a small head (microcephaly) with sloping forehead, bushy eyebrows, mouth with downturned corners and a horizontal dimple below the lower lip, or a "pursed mouth." There may be anomalies of the hands and feet, as well.

The prognosis for survival for these infants is poor, due to the severe mental and motor retardation.

5p- See CRI DU CHAT SYNDROME.

+7q A few dozen cases of this syndrome have been reported. The skull is usually asymmetrical, with a bulging forehead. The scalp hair is fuzzy. The eye slits (palpebral fissures) are long and narrow, and have been described as "almond-shaped." The nose is small and becomes pointed as infants age. The tongue may be large (MACROGLOSSIA) and the upper lip may overhang the lower. The ears are low-set and rotated slightly backward. Abnormalities of the spine may be seen as well as with the limbs, especially hip dislocation, foot position deformities and stiffness of the fingers.

The prognosis for affected individuals is based on the section of the long arm of the chromosome that is duplicated. Duplications of larger segments may be associated with malformations of brain, heart and kidneys. Many have a shortened life span, especially when the trisomic segment is large. While some infants die by the age of one year, generally this condition is not incompatible with life.

Trisomy 8   One of the more common autosomal chromosomal abnormalities, at least 80 cases have been confirmed. At birth, the skull is long and narrow, the forehead is prominent, the nose bulbous and the lower lip is thick and turned outward. The eyes are deep set. The jaw is small (micrognathia), the ears are low-set, prominent and malformed. Individuals have been described as having a "what-me-worry?" face. Mental retardation ranges from mild to extreme.

Contractures of the fingers and toes, and restricted mobility of joints, are frequent, as are abnormalities of the spinal column. Undescended testes (CRYPT-ORCHISM) occur in about half of affected males. Obstruction of urinary outflow and kidney and ureter malformations are characteristic. One-quarter have congenital heart disease. Approximately 90% exhibit mild mental retardation.

This condition is compatible with a normal life span. However, language development may be severely affected. The joint contractures become more pronounced with age, and may require treatment. There is a very high frequency (approximately 85%) of MOSAICISM. The most common autosomal aneuploidy after trisomies 21, 13 and 18, incidence is estimated at between one in 25,000 and one in 50,000 live births. Males are affected three to five times as frequently as females.

9p-   All reported cases exhibit mental retardation and mild skull abnormalities. Facial features, while characteristic in childhood, become less so as individuals age. The head is triangular in shape from early suture closure (see craniosynostosis). The eye slits (palpebral fissures) are short and up-slanting away from the nose (mongoloid obliquity). The nasal bridge is flat and the nose is upturned (anteverted nares). The mouth appears small, with a narrow upper lip. The ears are low-set and may exhibit external and internal malformations. The neck is short, the hairline is low and the nipples are widely spaced. The fingernails are characteristically square-shaped, and the fingers long and thin (arachnodactyly).

Life span is generally normal, as is adult height, and rare affected individuals have IQs above 50. They tend to be friendly, affectionate and sociable. Adults tend toward obesity in their trunks, though the extremities remain thin.

+9p   This condition appears to be somewhat common, with twice as many affected females as males. Various sections of the short arm of chromosome 9 may be duplicated and the exact manifestations and clinical severity vary with the size and nature of the duplicated segment. Over 100 cases have been reported. It is characterized by variable mental retardation, typical facial appearance and short fingers and toes with small nails and poor development of the tips of the digits.

Facially, the forehead is high and broad. The skull is short. The eye slits (palpebral fissures) are slanted down away from the nose (antimongoloid obliquity). The nose is large and bulbous, as is the mouth, which angles downward, with a turned-out lower lip. The philtrum (the groove from the bottom of the nose to the top of the lip) is extremely short. The ears are large and low set. Affected individuals have an "unworried look."

The neck is short, and the hairline low. Shoulders may be underdeveloped, there may be anomalies of the spinal cord, and individuals may be knock-kneed (genu valgum). Other skeletal malformations are common. The nipples may be darkly pigmented.

Growth retardation is sometimes noted, as is delayed sexual development and severe speech delay. Mental retardation is generally in the IQ range of 30 to 65. Life span is normal.

Trisomy 9   Both mosaic and homogeneous trisomies of chromosome 9 have been seen. Characteristic features include small head (microcephaly) with sloping forehead. The eyes are deep-set and the palpebral fissures (eye slits) are short and upslanting. The nose has a bulbous tip, the ears are low set and malformed. The jaw is small (micrognatia) and the upper lip covers the receding lower lip. Joint anomalies are common and characteristic, including hip dislocation, dislocation of knees or elbows, and contractures. Congenital heart defects are found in about two-thirds of cases. Brain, kidney or digestive malformations may also be seen. Most die in the first few months of life. Those who survive exhibit severe failure to thrive and mental retardation.

+10p   This syndrome is characterized by severe mental and psychomotor retardation, growth retardation, seizures, poor muscle tone (hypotonic) and hyperextensibility of joints.

The skull tends to be long and narrow, with a high, prominent forehead and low hairline. The cheeks are prominent, the nose upturned (anteverted nares), with a long philtrum (the groove extending from the bottom of the nose to the top of the upper lip). The mouth has been described as triangular or as appearing like a "turtle's beak," with a protruding upper lip. Ears are large, low-set and rotated slightly backward. Cleft lip or cleft palate is present in about half the cases. Elbows, wrists, fingers and ankles may be permanently bent (flexion contractures). The feet may be clubbed (talipes equinovarus).

Approximately half die early in life, and those who survive are severely retarded (IQ is approximately 20).

+10q   This condition is marked by extreme mental retardation. Height, weight and head size are well below average (typically below the third percentile).

The face appears flattened and wide. The eye slits (palpebral fissures) are unusually small, the eyebrows are arched and fine. The nose is small and beaked, the cheeks are prominent and the mouth is bow-shaped with a protruding upper lip.

The eyelids have a tendency to droop (PTOSIS) in about half of the reported cases, and the same percentage have cleft palate. The hands and feet may be deformed, with digits abnormally flexed (CAMPTODACTYLY) or curving inward (CLINODACTYLY). The bottom of the foot may be convex (rock-

erbottom foot). About half of those under medical care exhibit congenital heart defects. Several kidney (renal) abnormalities have also been associated with this disorder. Kidney defects are seen in about 50% of cases.

Death usually occurs prior to four years of age in about half of the cases, due to cardiac, renal or respiratory complications. Individuals who survive are severely retarded, usually bedridden and without the ability to communicate.

11p-   See WILMS TUMOR. Associated with ANIRIDIA–Wilms tumor syndrome.

+12p   The severity of this syndrome is dependent on the amount of chromosomal material that is duplicated on the 12th chromosome. There may be severe congenital malformations of the brain, heart, intestinal tract and kidneys. Additionally, various abnormalities of skull development are frequent features. The majority of cases result from parental translocation.

In general, the head is broad, with a high forehead. The face tends to be rectangular and flat. Eyebrows are thick, high and arched, and slanted downward. The nasal root is broad, the nose short and upturned (anteverted nares). The upper lip is thin, the lower lip wide and turned outward. The ears may be low-set and rotated slightly backward. The neck is short and cloaked in folds of skin. The nipples may be misplaced, and there may be more than two of them. Hands and feet often show abnormalities, such as short, broad, overlapping and malformed digits.

Mental retardation is a constant feature. Those manifesting severe congenital abnormalities rarely survive the first six weeks of life (neonatal period). Those who survive have normal life expectancies, though there is severe delay of motor development, such as head control, sitting and standing, and poor speech development. Growth is also retarded, and most individuals are of short stature.

13q-   Well over 100 cases of this condition have been reported. Affected individuals exhibit psychomotor retardation, poor muscle tone (hypotonia) and small heads (microcephaly). Birthweight is usually low.

The characteristic facial features include a triangular shape of the forehead (trigoncephaly), large, low-set ears and several defects of the eye, such as drooping lids (ptosis), fissures of the iris (COLOBOMA and abnormal smallness of the eye (microphthalmia). The upper incisor teeth are large and protruding and described as "rabbit-like," the chin is small (micrognatia) and the neck is short and webbed. In some cases, the thumbs may be absent.

About one-third of those affected have congenital heart defects. Over half the males have genital abnormalities, including undescended testicles (cryptorchism), micropenis and an abnormal opening in the subsurface of the penis that connects with the urethra (HYPOSPADIASIS). Retinoblastoma, a malignant eye tumor, is seen with deletion of the band 13q14; a "retinoblastoma gene" has been found in this region.

Trisomy 13   See PATAU SYNDROME.

15q-   Associated with Prader-Willi syndrome and ANGELMAN SYNDROME.

18p- syndrome (short arm 18 deletion syndrome)   Unusual facial characteristics and mild to severe mental retardation caused by the deletion of the short arm of chromosome 18. Facial abnormalities are apparent at birth, though there is a large variability in expression of the phenotype. The abnormalities include hypertelorism (wide-set eyes), ptosis (drooping eyelids), epicanthal folds, low nasal bridge, micrognathia and downturned mouth. The face itself is rounded and ears are large and protruding.

Females are affected at twice the rate of males. IQs range from 25 to 75, with an average of 45–50. Most affected individuals cannot speak even simple sentences until the age of seven to nine years. However, some have no mental impairment. Mild-to-moderate growth deficiency is also characteristic, as is hypotonia, poor concentration, emotional lability, fear of strangers and restlessness. Life expectancy is not affected.

First noted by de Grouchy in 1963, more than 100 cases have been reported to date. Above average parental age may be a factor in its occurrence. The mean parental age of affected individuals is 32 for mothers and 38 for fathers.

18q-   The condition is marked by mental retardation and characteristic facial features, including a bulging forehead (bossing), deeply set eyes, poor development of the midface area, a "carp-shaped" mouth, prominent chin and short neck. There may be subcutaneous nodules in the cheeks at the usual site of dimples.

A number of defects of the eyes may also occur, and ear abnormalities are common. In particular, the external ear canal funneling sound to the middle ear is often narrow or even undeveloped. Thus, about half the affected individuals have impaired hearing. Additionally, there may be genital abnormalities, clubbed feet (talipes equinovarus) and minor anomalies of the fingers and toes. Congenital heart defects are frequent, and infants have poor muscle tone (hypotonic) and seizures. Life expectancy is greatly reduced. At least 65 cases have been reported.

Trisomy 18   See EDWARD SYNDROME.

Trisomy 21   See DOWN SYNDROME.

For other chromosome syndromes, see CAT EYE SYNDROME; FRAGILE X SYNDROME (X-linked mental retardation); KLINEFELTER SYNDROME (XXY); TRIPLOIDY; XXXXY SYNDROME; XXXXX SYNDROME and XYY SYNDROME.

chromosome banding   A laboratory technique for staining chromosomes with a chemical dye to delineate various regions or bands of the chromosomes so that they may be examined and analyzed. The word chromosome means "colored body," and it is so named due to its ability to darken dramatically when dyed. Each chromosome or chromosome fragment has a unique identifiable pattern of bands observable under a microscope after it has been stained, and these serve as reference points for identifying the different chromosomes (e.g., 13 vs. 14 vs. 15) as well as the positions of specific genes on individual chromosomes.

The development of improved banding techniques, which underwent significant advances in the 1970s, has had a major impact on genetic research, greatly assisting in the mapping of individual genes and linked genes to specific points on the chromosomes. Using high-resolution banding techniques, including FISH, it is possible to visualize as many as 5,000 bands on the 23 pairs of human chromosomes. (See Introduction. Also see FLUORESCENCE IN SITU HYBRIDIZATION).

chronic granulomatous disease   See IMMUNE DEFICIENCY DISEASE.

cigarettes While cigarettes can be branded as bad for a smoker's health, the effects of exposure IN UTERO are less clear. Smoking cigarettes during pregnancy has not been associated with an increase in MENTAL RETARDATION, but some studies have suggested that there is an increase in birth defects such as CLEFT LIP and CLEFT PALATE. However, the more a pregnant woman smokes, the lower the weight of her child at birth; LOW BIRTH WEIGHT infants are prone to numerous health problems. Also, smokers have twice as many premature deliveries as non-smokers, and an increased risk of miscarriage, STILLBIRTH and infant death. The cause of this association is unknown, but may be due to carbon monoxide in the smoke, which is absorbed through the placenta, reducing levels of oxygen in the FETUS and therefore interfering with proper development. Maternal smoking during pregnancy also contributes to childhood asthma. Beyond this, smoking has been implicated as a risk factor for a number of diseases which may have genetic components, such as CANCERS (e.g., lung, esophageal, bladder), cardiovascular disease, emphysema (see below) and CROHN DISEASE. It is suspected of being a factor in the development of manifestations in individuals carrying a MUTATION for LEBER OPTIC ATROPHY. Importantly it leads to an earlier onset and more severe emphysema in individuals with ALPHA-1- ANTITRYPSIN DEFICIENCY. Not only HOMOZYGOTES for that disease are at risk, but HETEROZYGOTES also have a greater predilection for emphysema.

A genetic component involved in tobacco addiction and cigarette smoking itself has also been suggested. In 1998, researchers at the University of Toronto identified a mutation in the gene CY P2A6 that seemingly reduces an affected individual's chances of becoming a cigarette smoker, and reduces the risk of cancer among those with the mutation who do smoke. The gene produces an ENZYME involved in the metabolism of nicotine. Those with a mutation to the gene can't metabolize nicotine, and are less likely to become smokers. Individuals with two copies of the defective gene, or homozygotes (estimated at 1% of the population) are least likely to smoke. Additionally, those with the mutation who do smoke are less likely to develop cancer, as their bodies are less efficient at transforming the ingredients of tobacco smoke into carcinogens.

cirrhosis, familial See FAMILIAL CIRRHOSIS.

citrullinemia See UREA CYCLE DEFECTS.

clawfoot A deformity of the foot in which the arch is abnormally high and the toes are long and permanently bent (flexion contracture). It may be present at birth or may occur as a result of nerve or muscle disease.

Synonyms: pes cavus; gampsodactyly; griffe des orteils; talipes caves.

cleft A split or fissure in a body part caused by improper union during fetal development. CLEFT LIP and CLEFT PALATE are the most common forms, though clefts may appear on many parts of the body. Among the more common sites of clefting besides the lip and palate are the hand, foot or cheek. (See also CLEFT LIP, CLEFT PALATE AND ASSOCIATED CLEFTING CONDITIONS.)

cleft lip, cleft palate and associated clefting conditions Cleft lip and cleft palate are the most common CONGENITAL clefting conditions, and may occur individually or together. However, cleft lip, which may be seen with or without cleft palate, is a separate and distinct condition from cleft palate alone. In about 25% of those affected, cleft lip alone occurs; cleft lip with cleft palate is seen in about 45%, and cleft palate alone in 30%.

Cleft lip is caused by the incomplete closure of the primary palate, which forms the lip and gum. Closure usually occurs by the 45th day of fetal development, and if it has not occurred by then, the infant will have a cleft lip. Cleft palate is caused by the incomplete closure of the secondary palate, which occurs by the ninth week of pregnancy. Where both cleft lip and cleft palate are present, the clefting of the primary palate is blamed for interfering with the closure of the secondary palate.

TABLE VII
ESTIMATED RISKS FOR ISOLATED CLEFTS

	CL With or Without CP (%)	Isolated CP (%)
General population	0.1	0.04
One affected sibling	4–7	2–5
One affected parent	2–4	7
One affected parent and one affected sibling	11–14	14–17
Two affected siblings	9–10	10

A careful check of other family members may reveal or rule out subtle signs, such as a sub-mucous cleft or a high arched palate, allowing more precise risk estimation.

Key: CL = cleft lip; CP = cleft palate

The first historical evidence of clefting was found in a mummified Egyptian dating from 2400–1300 B.C. A 2,000-year-old statue of a king from Colombia, South America, appears to depict a cleft lip, and an African mask with a cleft lip and palate has been described.

The causes of these conditions are unclear. The majority are thought to be MULTIFACTORIAL, that is, caused by the action of several GENES in concert with environmental factors. They may also be caused by single GENE (MENDELIAN disorders, CHROMOSOME ABNORMALITIES or environmental agents, and are seen in association with almost 400 genetic SYNDROMES. These include LIP PITS, EEC, STICKLER SYNDROME, SHPRINTZEN SYNDROME, SMITH LEMLI OPITZ SYNDROME, Kniest syndrome and SPONDYLO-EPIPHYSEAL DYPLASIA. Up to 13% of babies with oral/facial clefts have other birth defects. Studies suggest that taking multivitamins containing folic acid before conception and during the first two months of pregnancy may help prevent cleft lip with or without cleft palate and isolated cleft palate.

cleft lip with or without cleft palate (CL/P) The frequency of CL/P varies widely across population groups, and severity is highly variable as well. More than 70% of babies with cleft lip also have cleft palate. The lip may be cleft on one side (unilateral, 80%) or both (bilateral, 20%). If the cleft of the lip is bilateral, the cleft of the palate may be bilateral, as well.

An estimated 7% to 13% of those with cleft lip alone have additional CONGENITAL defects, a proportion that rises to between 11% and 14% for those with both cleft lip and cleft palate.

Various races exhibit substantially different frequencies of CL/P, frequencies that persist in differing geographical areas. Among Asians, it is estimated at one per 600 births. Whites have a frequency of one per 1,000 and blacks of one per 2,500. Among blacks, females are more often affected, while males are more commonly affected in whites.

Children and SIBLINGS of affected individuals have an approximately 4% risk of CL/P. If both a parent and child have CL/P, risk to a subsequent child is estimated at approximately 15% to 17%. If two children (but no parent) are affected, risk to a third is placed at 9%. Second-degree relatives (nieces, nephews, uncles and aunts) have a 0.7% risk and cousins a 0.4% risk. (See Table VIII, p. 82) The severity of the cleft also influences severity recurrence risk: There is a higher risk of occurrence in families when the affected individual has a bilateral cleft lip and palate, and a lower risk when there is only a unilateral cleft lip.

Midline or median cleft lip has a different embryologic basis and is considered to be separate genetically as well. It also has its own specific syndromic associations (e.g., ELLIS-VAN CREVELD SYNDROME). Lateral and oblique orofacial clefts are also distinct entities.

Affected infants may have feeding difficulties. Speech therapy, orthodontic treatments and psychosocial counseling may be helpful. CL/P can be repaired surgically. An interdisciplinary team of specialists is usually required for optimal care management.

cleft palate The palate is the structure that forms the roof of the mouth. Cleft palate is a rarer condition than CL/P, and is a separate and distinct condition. It appears to be associated with genetic syndromes more frequently than is cleft lip with or without cleft palate. Cleft palate may involve the hard palate (the tissue toward the front of the mouth), the soft palate (the tissue toward the back of the mouth) or both. There may be one cleft (unilateral) of the palate or it may appear on both sides (bilateral). The fissure may be complete, extending through the palate, or incomplete. (BIFID UVULA is a minor form of cleft palate, and cleft palate is also a cardinal feature of ROBIN ANOMALY.)

As with CL/P, frequency varies with race. It occurs in Native Americans as frequently as 80 per 1,000 live births. Asians have an incidence of one in 1,500 births. Among whites, frequency is one per 2,500 births, and in blacks, one per 5,000 births. Females appear to be affected slightly more often than males.

SIBLINGS of affected individuals have about a 2% recurrence risk, while individuals with an affected sibling and parent have approximately a 7% risk. Among whites, recurrence risk in an infant with an affected sibling and parent is close to 15%.

Babies with cleft palate often have difficulty in feeding, swallowing and respiration. Their heads are usually smaller than those of unaffected individuals. Approximately one third to one-half exhibit additional abnormalities, including CLUBFOOT, deformities of the limbs and ears, and umbilical hernia.

There is evidence that many cases go unreported and that the actual incidence may be more than 50% higher than present statistics indicate. Cleft palate can be treated surgically, and speech therapy, orthodontic treatments and psychosocial counseling can also be helpful.

ULTRASOUND has been used to detect clefts prenatally.

cleft uvula   See BIFID UVULA.

cleidocranial dysplasia   A hereditary disorder that affects the formation and development of cartilage and bone. The most obvious symptom, recognized early in infancy, is a missing or incompletely developed collarbone (clavicle). Affected individuals appear to have a long neck and narrow shoulders. They also have a wide range of motion of the shoulders; some can bring their shoulders together in front of the chest. The incidence of this disorder is 1:1,000,000, yet over 1,500 cases have been reported. The proband (first family member known to exhibit the disorder) of the most noted affected family was a Chinese Muslim in South Africa named Arnold, who had seven wives. A geneticist in the middle of the last century was able to trace 356 of his descendants, 70 of whom were affected by the disorder, called *Arnold head* locally. It is estimated that today more than 1,000 descendants of the first progenitor have had cleidocranial dysplasia.

Additional symptoms are a protruding forehead or top of the head (bossing), causing the face to appear small. The skull may appear to be short or broad (brachycephalic), and often the bones of the skull do not fuse together. This causes the "soft spot" of the skull, the fontanelle, to remain open or "soft" for an abnormally long time. The nasal bridge is broad, and the eyes are set far apart (HYPERTELORISM). Other skeletal malformations include fingers of asymmetric length, knock-knees (genum valgum), SCOLIOSIS and deformed teeth.

The severity of expression of the disorder varies widely. Affected individuals live a normal life span and have normal intelligence. Hearing and dental problems may occur. Because of a pelvic deformity, affected females may have to give birth by CESAREAN DELIVERY.

The basic defect in this rare disorder, transmitted as an AUTOSOMAL DOMINANT trait, is a mutation in the gene for the transcription factor *CBFA1*, also known as *RUNX2*, for *runt-related transcription factor 2*, found on the short arm of chromosome 6. Approximately one-third of cases represent new mutations.

clinodactyly   The permanent sideways curvature of one or more fingers or toes. It most commonly affects the fifth finger, and is often caused by lack of development of the middle of the three bones in the digit. It is associated with many CONGENITAL and genetic anomalies.

clomiphene citrate   A nonsteroidal drug used to stimulate ovulation in women who have had difficulty conceiving, though they have potentially functioning pituitary and ovarian systems. Women who become pregnant as a result of this treatment have an increased incidence of MULTIPLE BIRTHS.

cloning   The process of artificially creating a genetically identical organism from an individual's DNA, rather than by combining the DNA of two parents. In 1997 the possibility of cloned humans came a step closer to reality with the announcement of the successful creation of a cloned sheep, Dolly, in England. Society is now struggling with the ethical questions raised by the specter of human cloning, though most of the public and the scientific community appear opposed to its application.

Cloning can also be used to reproduce portions of genetic material, and this technique has been important in the identification of many GENETIC DISORDERS.

cloverleaf skull   See KLEEBLATTSCHADEL ANOMALY.

clubfoot   Misalignment of the bones in the front part of the foot resulting in an abnormal shape. The general medical term for this condition is talipes, and it is further delineated by direction of the misalignment. In the great majority of cases (approximately 95%) the front of the foot turns inward and downward (talipes equinovarus). In the remaining cases the front of the foot turns outward and upward (talipes calceneovalgus; talipes calceneovarus), deviates toward the midline (metatarsus adductus), or the inner side of the foot doesn't touch the ground when walking (metatarsus varus).

As an isolated malformation, the condition often results from crowding in the uterus. It may be corrected surgically, or with splints and casts during infancy. Left uncorrected, affected individuals will usually develop an awkward gait. Clubfoot is also associated with many genetic SYNDROMES.

George Gordon, Lord Byron (1788–1824), the English Romantic poet, had this condition.

Clubfoot is caused by MULTIFACTORIAL inheritance, the action of several GENES in concert with environmental influence, with both likely interfering with prenatal growth of foot structures. It occurs

in from one to three in 1,000 live births. Talipes equinovarus is the more severe form and occurs most often in males (two to one). The risk for SIBLINGS is around 3%, with the risk for siblings of a female patient being higher (5%) than for those of a male patient (2%).

CMT   See CHARCOT-MARIE-TOOTH DISEASE.

CMV   See TORCH SYNDROME.

cocaine   An alkaloid refined from the leaves of the coca plant, this stimulant is thought to be the illegal drug most widely abused by pregnant women. It is typically ingested by inhalation, either through the nostrils in powder form or by smoking derivatives such as crack, or by injection. Studies (conducted by urine screening and self-reporting) through the mid-1990s found cocaine use among pregnant women at rates varying from 1% to 2% to 7% to 15% of them. Contemporaneous newborn screening studies found exposure rates varying from 4% to 31%. Among newborns of women receiving no prenatal care, cocaine exposure has been reported at over 60%. In 1999, the Department of Health and Human Services put the number of babies born annually in the United States who are exposed to cocaine IN UTERO at between 50,000 and 375,000.

Maternally ingested cocaine flows through the placenta into the FETUS, causing a decrease in fetal blood supply and resulting in abnormalities of fetal development. Use during pregnancy increases the risk of miscarriage, premature birth and STILLBIRTH (see ABORTION, LOW BIRTH WEIGHT, PREMATURITY). Infants exposed before birth also tend to be smaller than average and exhibit higher-than-average incidence of central nervous system defects, abnormal development of the small intestine, and genital and urinary tract anomalies, including seriously malformed kidneys. A survey of 5,000 infants born with BIRTH DEFECTS in the Atlanta area, conducted by the federal Centers for Disease Control from 1968 to 1980, found the risk of urinary tract defects was 4.8 times higher in infants whose mothers reported using cocaine from one month prior to conception through the first trimester of pregnancy. (The normal risk for urinary tract defects is 1.5. per 1,000 live births; among the infants exposed to cocaine in utero, these defects occurred in 7.2 per 1,000 births.) Since some people do not admit cocaine use, these statistics may be conservative, and the true increased risks actually may be higher.

Because studies of cocaine use in pregnancy are hard to conduct for social and methodological reasons, it is difficult to reach conclusions regarding its effects. The major findings continue to indicate evidence of an increase in genitourinary abnormalities. Other research indicates SUDDEN INFANT DEATH SYNDROME occurs 10 times more frequently than the norm in these infants. (Given the growing recognition that some deaths labeled as SIDS may actually result from child abuse, a link between drug and child abuse underlying this last statistic cannot be discounted.)

As they grow, these infants are often hypersensitive and irritable, and have motor difficulties that make their limbs stiff and interfere with learning to crawl and walk. It has been suggested that as these children grow older their neurological problems will be manifested as learning disabilities, hyperactivity and attention deficits. Studies of infants exposed before birth to crack, a concentrated, smokable form of cocaine, have found they exhibit subnormal emotional development, though these infants are capable of achieving normal intelligence.

Cockayne syndrome A rare AUTOSOMAL RECESSIVE condition characterized by DWARFISM, precociously senile appearance, ocular abnormalities, and MENTAL RETARDATION, in addition to other common features. It bears the name of Edward A. Cockayne (1880–1956), a senior dermatologist at the Hospital for Sick Children in London, who described it in 1936.

At birth, weight is appropriate and affected infants appear normal. Symptoms begin in the second year of life. Growth slows, and mental and motor development become abnormal. Dwarfing and mental retardation become more pronounced with time.

As the condition progresses, there is retinal degeneration, optic atrophy and cataracts, leading to BLINDNESS. Hearing loss leads to DEAFNESS. The head is abnormally small (MICROCEPHALY and the face takes on a strikingly senile appearance due to the absence of a subcutaneous layer of fat. Hair is sparse, and the nose is thin and beaked. There may be absence of some permanent teeth. There is also sensitivity to sunlight, causing severe skin rashes (photosensitive skin rash), and deficient perspiration. Susceptibility to infections is increased.

Arms and legs appear disproportionately long, and hands and feet are large. Joints of the ankles, knees, hands and elbows may become permanently bent (flexion contractures), eventually leading to total immobility.

By the late teens affected individuals are unable to care for themselves, with death occurring from respiratory infection or from a debilitated condition due to lack of nutrition (inanition). No reported cases have survived beyond the age of 31. Despite the bleak outlook for all affected individuals, a wide variability of expression has been reported.

Among the fewer than 200 reported cases, males have outnumbered females by a ratio of three to one, though the reason for this preponderance is unknown. The prevalence of Cockayne syndrome is unknown, but it probably occurs in fewer than one in 100,000 individuals.

There are several forms of Cockayne syndrome though the differences among them may be more at the molecular level than the clinical one. However, the age of onset may differ. The basic defects are being elucidated and the GENES involved identified. The major forms involve genes on chromosomes 5 and 10 and result in defects in various proteins that play a role in the repair of the DNA of active or transcribed genes. Yet overall, DNA repair is normal, and there is no predisposition to malignancy or infectious complications seen in other DNA repair diseases like BLOOM SYNDROME or ATAXIA-TELANGIECTASIA. The difference in the type of DNA repair defect seems to account for this.

Type I is the classic form of the disease, while type II is more severe and presents at birth as CEREBRO-CULO-FACIO-SKELETAL SYNDROME (COFS). Type III is milder, with a later onset, and another form is found in individuals who have combined features of both Cockayne syndrome and XERODERMA PIGMENTOSUM. Mutations in the *CKN1* gene (also known as *CSA* or the *ERCC8* gene) located on the long arm of chromosome 5 account for about 25% of cases of Cockayne syndrome. Mutations in the *ERCC6* gene account for about 75% of cases. Mutations in the ERCC6 gene have been identified in patients with the cerebro-oculo-facial-skeletal syndrome (COFS), and those patients should be considered to have Cockayne syndrome type II. The *ERCC6* gene (also known as *CKN2* or *CSB*) is mapped to the long arm of chromosome 10. The full name of the gene is *excision repair cross-complementing rodent repair deficiency, complementation group 6,* and the gene is involved in both repair of damaged DNA and production of protein. *ERCC6* mutations have also been found in certain patients with xeroderma pigmentosum, particularly those with a subtype known as the de Sanctis-Cacchione form, which is a severe form that includes problems with the nervous system.

Fetal cells have shown a reduction in the ability to form colonies and decreased synthesis of DNA and RNA (see RIBONUCLEIC ACID) after exposure to ultraviolet light. PRENATAL DIAGNOSIS has been accomplished by exposing cultured cells from the amniotic fluid to ultraviolet light to test for reduction in their DNA and RNA synthesis or ability to grow. Now that the genes for Cockayne have been found and some of the MUTATIONS identified, CARRIER detection and prenatal diagnosis using molecular techniques may be possible. Thus far mutations are only known for specific individual patients, and testing is available primarily on a research basis.

codon A sequence of three nucleotides (the individual molecules making up nucleic acids) in the DNA or RNA (see RIBONUCLEIC ACID) chains that provides the code for a specific AMINO ACID or step required for the production of a protein. There are 64 of these nucleotide triplet sequences. Sixty-one codons "code" for the 20 amino acids found in proteins, and three are "termination" codons that signal a halt to the formation of the sequence of amino acids producing the protein.

If the codon is changed (a MUTATION) the result may be that the wrong amino acid is incorporated into the protein or the protein chain may be prematurely terminated. For example, a change in just one of the three nucleotides in just one codon of the hundreds encoding HEMOGLOBIN (the oxygen-carrying pigment in red blood cells) results in SICKLE-CELL ANEMIA.

Coffin-Lowry syndrome First identified by Grange S. Coffin, a pediatrician in San Francisco, in 1966, and R. Brian Lowry, professor of medical GENETICS at the University of Calgary, Canada, in 1971, Coffin-Lowry syndrome features a characteristic facial appearance, severe MENTAL RETARDATION, anomalies of the hand, and short stature. Males are much more severely affected than females.

In early childhood, males display a prominent square forehead, coarse, straight hair, wide-set eyes (HYPERTELORISM) that slant down and away from the nose (antimongoloid obliquity), an upturned nose (anteverted nares), prominent chin (PROGNATHISM), large, protruding ears, thick lips and open mouth. The fingers are short, thick, puffy and tapered. A variety of oral deformities, including malocclusion and absent permanent teeth are also characteristic. The facial features become more pronounced with age. Affected males have been described as having a "pugilistic nose."

The hands appear large and soft, with thick, tapering fingers. The skin is loose and easily stretched. Skeletal features include either a protruding "pigeon breast" (PECTUS carinatum) or a depressed chest (pectus excavatum) and curvature of the spinal column (kyphoscoliosis).

Affected individuals also have a characteristic clumsy gait. All males are severely retarded, with IQs below 50. Most females exhibit mild mental retardation and tend toward OBESITY.

The underlying genetic defect in the disorder has been identified: Various MUTATIONS in the *RSK2* GENE on the short arm of the X CHROMOSOME result in the SYNDROME. The *RSK2* gene is also known by its official gene symbol as the *RPS6KA3* gene, which stands for ribosomal protein S6 kinase, 90kDa, polypeptide 3 gene. The protein this gene encodes is involved in cell signaling and cell proliferation and differentiation. PRENATAL DIAGNOSIS and CARRIER detection by DNA analysis should be possible in families in which the mutation is characterized.

Coffin-Lowry syndrome is believed to be transmitted as an X-LINKED dominant trait. Life span is normal, though the condition may be lethal in severely affected males. The incidence is unknown, but it is thought to affect about one in 40,000 to 50,000 births. About 70–80% of affected individuals have no family history of the syndrome and about 20–30% have more than one affected family member.

This disorder should not be confused with the unrelated COFFIN-SIRIS SYNDROME (see below) also described first by Coffin.

Coffin-Siris syndrome (fifth digit syndrome) A CONGENITAL disorder characterized by MENTAL RETARDATION, short stature and malformations of the fifth digit, named for G. S. Coffin and E. Siris, who described three patients in 1970. Mild to moderate growth deficiency begins IN UTERO. The nail on the fifth finger or toe may be hypoplastic or absent. Joint laxity and mild-to-severe hypotonia may also be present. Feeding problems and frequent respiratory infections are common, and dental and motor development may be retarded.

The characteristic coarse facial features include a wide nose and/or mouth, low nasal bridge and thick lips. Body hair is generally excessive, though scalp hair may be sparse. Skin, skeletal, genital and cardiac defects have also been reported. Some patients also have DANDY-WALKER SYNDROME.

More than 30 cases have been reported. AUTOSOMAL RECESSIVE inheritance is suspected. Females are affected four times as often as males; it may possibly be lethal to males in utero.

Cohen syndrome (Pepper syndrome) Hypotonia, truncal obesity with mid-childhood onset, low white blood cell count, prominent incisors and MENTAL RETARDATION are the hallmarks of this rare GENETIC DISORDER.

Affected individuals have LOW BIRTH WEIGHT and postnatal growth deficiency. The head may be microcephalic, and characteristic facial features include a high nasal bridge, mild downward slant of palpebral fissures, short philtrum (the mid-face groove between the nose and upper lip) and open mouth. The prominent incisors manifest as the infant grows. The jaw may develop abnormally. Ocular abnormalities include RETINITIS PIGMENTOSA and decreased clarity of vision.

Though truncal obesity develops in childhood, the hands and toes are long and slender, and syndactyly of the fingers may be present. Deformities of the knees, elbows and spine, including SCOLIOSIS, are also characteristic. CRYPTORCHISM and delayed puberty may also be present. IQ's range from 30 to 70.

Inherited as an AUTOSOMAL RECESSIVE trait, it was first reported by M. M. Cohen in 1973, who described two affected siblings and one isolated case of the disorder. Since then over 80 cases have been reported. It is one of the disorders that are overrepresented in the FINNISH population, though it affects individuals of Eastern European Jewish descent as well. The syndrome is caused by mutations in the COH1 gene on the long arm of chromosome 8.

coloboma An ocular defect in which there is a fissure or cleft in the structures of the eye, usually in the iris or choroid, or in the eyelid. The retina and optic nerve can also be involved. It is associated with many CONGENITAL and genetic ANOMALIES. As an isolated defect it may be inherited as an AUTOSOMAL DOMINANT trait, with the fissure usually located in the lower part of the iris. (See CAT EYE SYNDROME.)

Individual families have also had other inheritance patterns. (See CHARGE ASSOCIATION.) Another SYNDROME in which this is a cardinal feature is that of optic nerve coloboma with renal anomalies. MUTATIONS have been found in the developmental GENE PAX2 in this last syndrome.

colon aganglionosis See HIRSCHSPRUNG DISEASE.

colon cancer See COLORECTAL CANCER.

color blindness A group of visual disorders more properly termed "color deficiencies" characterized by inability to distinguish various wavelengths of light. There are approximately one dozen of these CONGENITAL conditions. Most are inherited as X-LINKED traits, affecting males almost exclusively. These defects are less frequent among males of African (3–4%) or Asian (3%) origin. A familial link had been noted for several centuries before PEDIGREES of color-blind families, documented by Swiss ophthalmologist J. F. Homer (1831–86), established its hereditary nature for the scientific community. In 1876 he first demonstrated that a man with red-green color blindness transmitted the trait to his male grandchildren through his unaffected daughter. Color blindness was the first GENE to be assigned to a specific CHROMOSOME (on the X CHROMOSOME, as this is an X-linked trait) in a pioneering example of GENE MAPPING by E. B. Wilson in 1911.

Normal human vision is trichromatic, or three-colored; color is perceived by the response of red, green and blue visual pigments, or light absorbing proteins, to wavelengths of light falling on the retina, the interior surface of the back of the eyeball. The mixture of these three primary color pigments determines how color is seen. A defect or deficiency of any of the three pigments (or the cones from which they are produced) will result in abnormal color vision.

Daltonism The majority of color defects are in red/green vision, affecting approximately 8% of Caucasian males and 0.5% of females. These defects are popularly known as "color blindness," in which males are unable to distinguish various colors. The group of conditions has also been called "Daltonism," for John Dalton (1766–1844), the English chemist and physicist considered the father of atomic theory. In 1794, he published a paper, "Extraordinary Facts Relating to the Vision of Colours," in which he reported that he did not perceive colors as others do. Dalton discovered the fact when, as a Quaker, he embarrassed himself by wearing a scarlet garment instead of the somber black garb he thought he was donning. In school, affected individuals may have difficulty with color-coded diagrams in math books. They may also have problems distinguishing a red stop sign against a background of green foliage.

Clinical chart tests (such as Ishihara plates) are typically used to detect red-green color vision defects. The two genes associated with red-green color vision defects are the *OPN1LW* gene (which stands for *opsin 1 long wave*), which encodes the red pigment, and *OPN1MW* (for *opsin 1 middle wave*), which encodes the green pigment.

Protanopia (red blindness) Marked by the inability to distinguish certain pastel shades and by a reduced sensitivity to red light. Affected individuals may, when driving, have difficulty ascertaining whether traffic lights are operating, and may confuse red and green lights. (Partial red blindness is called protanomaly.)

Deuteranopia (green blindness) Often renders individuals unaware they have defective color vision. Visual acuity is normal, but they may exhibit atypical color combinations in their clothing. Red and green are perceived as varying shades of yellow. Once identified, experience and education can help them adjust to chromatic deficiencies, though they may be unsuitable for occupations requiring proper identification of colors within this spectrum, such as with colorcoded electronic wiring. (Partial green blindness is called deuteranomaly.)

Tritanopia (blue-yellow color confusion) Rare, inherited as an autosomal dominant trait, it occurs in one in 500 individuals or probably fewer. The gene for blue pigment is located on chromosome 7. As well as the red and green pigment genes, located on the long arm of the X chromosome, it has been identified and cloned.

Achromatopsia (total color blindness) Very rare, and inherited as an autosomal recessive condition, affecting males and females equally. Color is perceived as various shades of gray, as on a black and white TV. These individuals generally also have poor visual acuity and extreme sensitivity to light (photophobia), restricting their vision and requiring squinting in even ordinary light. It is also called "day blindness" because vision is better at night. They can learn to interpret color to some degree by differences in brightness. Achromatopsia is caused by mutations in the *CNGA3*, *CNGB3*, and *GNAT2* genes and its estimated incidence is one in 30,000 live births, though on Pingelap, a Caroline Island in the South Pacific, incidence may be as high as six per 100.

English physicist John William Strutt, Lord Rayleigh (1842–1909), developed the anomaloscope, a device that remains the primary tool for testing color vision. However, no single instrument or test is totally reliable in detecting visual color deficiencies, and standard color vision tests are only effective in screening vision that deviates from normal; they cannot properly classify specific abnormalities.

Other diseases affecting the retina also affect color vision.

In the 1996 presidential debates, a system had to be developed to let the candidates know when they were on camera. Both President Bill Clinton and Senator Bob Dole have inherited red/green color vision confusion and would have had difficulty with signals based on individual colored lights, so a system using three lights was used.

color deficient   A term sometimes preferred for COLOR BLINDNESS, the inability to identify one or more of the primary colors. It has been noted that affected children may become alarmed by hearing the word "blindness," and therefore the more technically correct "color deficient" is used.

colorectal cancer   Colorectal cancer—cancers of the colon and rectum—is the fourth most common form of cancer in the United States, following skin, prostate and lung cancer in men, and skin, lung and breast cancer in women. More than 145,000 new cases were diagnosed in 2005, and that same year it caused more than 56,000 deaths, according to the National Cancer Institute. In Canada, about 19,200 new cases were reported in 2004, and some 8,300 patients succumbed to the disease. (The great majority of cases are colon, rather than rectal cancers.) As in other forms of cancer, most are thought to be multifactorial, involving the action of several genes as well as environmental factors such as diet. Overall, first-degree relatives (parents, siblings or children) of individuals with a colorectal cancer have a two- to threefold increased risk of colorectal cancer. When the family history includes two or more relatives with colorectal cancer, the possibility of the presence of a genetic syndrome is increased.

A number of hereditary and familial forms have been identified. Among the most studied are various polyposis syndromes, so named due to the char-

acteristic polyps that develop throughout the colon and, sometimes, the gastrointestinal tract. Polyps are small growths that in many cases may become malignant. About 75% of patients with colorectal cancer have sporadic cases, with no apparent evidence of having inherited the disorder. Single gene mutations are estimated to account for only about 5% to 6% of cases of colorectal cancer.

Familial adenomatous polyposis (FAP)   Inherited as an autosomal dominant trait displaying high penetrance and highly variable expressivity, FAP is characterized by the development of from hundreds to thousands of polyps throughout the colon, often beginning in childhood or early adulthood. The polyps frequently become malignant and spread rapidly. Carcinoma may arise from late childhood to the sixties, with a mean age at diagnosis of 40 years.

Polyps also develop in the upper gastrointestinal tract and malignancies may occur in other sites including the brain and the thyroid. Associated ANOMALIES include pigmented retinal lesions known as CONGENITAL hypertrophy of the retinal pigment, jaw cysts, sebaceous cysts and osteomata.

Multiple polyposis of the colon, hereditary polyposis coli, familial multiple polyposis and familial polyposis of the colon (FPC) were early terms for this disorder. The designation familial adenomatous polyposis (FAP) is most often used today. Adenomatous refers to a cancerous growth.

In the United States, FAP affects about one in 30,000 people, with about 800 to 1,000 new cases detected each year. Approximately 75–80% of individuals with FAP have an affected parent. FAP is estimated to occur in one in 8,000 births and accounts for perhaps 1% of colon cancers. The gene for this disorder has been mapped to chromosome 5. A variant of FAP called attenuated familial adenomatous polyposis is seen in some individuals and families in which polyps are usually found later in life. Typically, fewer polyps are seen in this form.

Congenital hypertrophy of the retinal pigment epithelium is a frequent finding (at least 90%) and is a valuable diagnostic clue, as the lesions may precede the onset of other signs. The gene has been characterized, its protein identified, and a variety of MUTATIONS cataloged. The APC gene at 5q21 is mutant in FAP. Allelic deletion occurs in most colorectal tumors and desmoids (cysts) of patients with FAP. Some, but not other aspects of the PHE-NOTYPE may be related to the site of the mutation. For example, CHRPE lesions were almost always absent if the mutation occurred before, and present if after, exon 9. The prevalence of the mutant gene is estimated as at least 1/26,000, with 24% of carriers representing new mutations.

FAP accompanied by dental anomalies and jaw cysts, sebaceous cysts, fibromas, lipomas, or osteomas was formerly named GARDNER SYNDROME, for E. J. Gardner (b. 1909), who described it in 1950. However, this is now considered a form of FAP, with onset usually around age 20 and symptoms including mild diarrhea with mucous and blood. While some affected individuals remain asymptomatic, in the rest malignancies develop 15 to 20 years after symptoms first appear. Death from colon cancer usually occurs between the ages of 40 and 50. Incidence is estimated at one in 16,000 births.

A milder type of FAP, autosomal recessive familial adenomatous polyposis, or *MYH*-associated polyposis, has also been found. Individuals with the autosomal recessive type of FAP, like patients with attenuated FAP, have fewer polyps than those with the classic type, typically less than 100, rather than hundreds or thousands. The autosomal recessive type is caused by mutations in a different gene (the *MYH* gene, found on chromosome 1p) than classic and attenuated types of FAP. A change in the *APC* gene called *I1307K* has been described. This variation is found in about 6% of people of Ashkenazi Jewish descent and appears to be associated with an approximately twofold increase in the risk to develop colorectal cancer.

Peutz-Jeghers syndrome   This autosomal dominant disorder is characterized by benign polyps found throughout the gastrointestinal tract and abnormal patterns of pigmentation, particularly about the lips. It bears the names of Dutch physician J. L. A. Peutz, who described it in 1921, and U.S. physician H. Jeghers, who described it in 1949. The polyps typically develop in adolescence, while the characteristic "black freckles" are present from birth.

Symptoms include severe, recurrent bouts of abdominal pain. However, the polyps become malignant in only 2% to 3% of those under medical attention. If all polyps are removed surgically in adulthood, no new ones develop. Affected individuals are also at a higher risk for cancers of the intestine, breast, pancreas, testis and ovary.

In 1998, the causative gene was mapped to 19p (the short arm of chromosome 19) and several mutations have been identified. The gene produces a protein kinase ENZYME, the first time a protein kinase gene has been identified as a tumor suppressor. Protein kinase disorders are typically the result of the overproduction of the enzyme, but in the case of Peutz-Jeghers syndrome, the cause is its absence.

Hereditary   nonpolyposis   colorectal   cancer (HNPCC; Lynch syndrome; cancer family syndrome) Early onset colorectal cancer associated with an increased risk for other cancers, mostly of the uterus (endometrial), ovary, stomach, small bowel and urinary tract. Overall, there is an increase in proximal colon cancers, that is, those on the right side of the colon. HNPCC is thought to be responsible for about 2 to 7% of all diagnosed cases of colorectal cancer.

The majority of individuals with a family history of colon cancer do not exhibit the autosomal dominant inheritance pattern indicative of genetic predisposition. In 1991, researchers adopted minimum criterion for identifying HNPCC families, standards which include: at least three affected relatives, with one a first-degree relative of the other two; at least two successive generations affected; onset before age 50 in at least one, and familial adenomatous polyposis ruled out as a diagnosis. These criteria were later modified to include the other HNPCC-related cancers. However, many patients have been found to have HNPCC and not meet these criteria.

Inherited as an autosomal dominant trait, this is a genetically heterogeneous disorder; mutations in any one of several different genes can result in HNPCC. Genetic mutation analysis is typically done of *MSH2* or *MLH1*. Often an initial screening procedure is done in suspected HNPCC patients. This consists of an evaluation of the colorectal tumor DNA for the presence of what is termed "high level microsatellite instability" and/or for absence of expression of either the *MSH2* or *MLH1* proteins. At least four have been identified: *MLH1* (mapped to 3p), *MSH2* (mapped to 2p), *MSH6* (mapped to 2p), and *PMS2* (mapped to 7q). Mutations in *MLH1* and *MSH2* account for approximately 90% of detected mutations in families with HNPCC. *MSH6* mutations occur in approximately 7–10% of families with HNPCC while *PMS2* ones account for less than 5%. All these genes are involved in the repair of mismatched DNA. For those with mutations, the lifetime risk of developing colorectal cancer is estimated at 80%.

Genetic testing allows for the identification of the majority of individuals with HNPCC. However, careful interpretation of the results are required, since not all with the gene will develop a cancer. Average age of diagnosis is 45, but cancers may develop as early as the 20s. Those at risk are recommended to undergo colonoscopy every one to three years from ages 20 to 25 on. Some with extreme indications of risk or previous cancers may opt for preventive removal of portions of their colons. Excretory functions can still be performed normally following the procedure.

Endometrial cancer is the second most common form seen in HNPCC families, and on average exhibits earlier onset than SPORADIC cases. Lifetime risk of developing such cancer among female HNPCC mutation CARRIERS is estimated at 20–60%. Risk to first-degree relatives is 15%, compared to 3% in the general population. Ovarian cancers occur 3.5 times more frequently in HNPCC families than in the general population, though risk is still under 10% at age 70.

Juvenile polyposis A rare, childhood-onset, autosomal dominant disease. It is genetically heterogeneous and presents with a different type of polyposis from FAP, termed hamartomatous polyposis. These polyps may occur throughout the gastrointestinal tract and can present with diarrhea or GI tract hemorrhage. The majority of patients with juvenile polyposis appear to be sporadic. Juvenile polyposis syndrome is caused by germline mutations in the MADH4 gene (mapped to chromosome 18q) in about 15% to 20% of cases, and mutations in the BMPR1A gene (on chromosome 10q) in approximately 25% to 40% of cases.

Non-polyposis syndromes with predisposition to colorectal cancer The majority of genetically determined colon cancers appear to be familial, without a clear Mendelian hereditary pattern. Families have been identified that are predisposed to developing bowel cancer and ulcerative colitis, an inflammatory bowel disorder that may lead to colon cancer. In these families, other family members may exhibit a variety of malignancies.

combined hyperlipidemia See CORONARY ARTERY DISEASE.

common variable immunodeficiency See IMMUNE DEFICIENCY DISORDERS.

complete androgen insensitivity See TESTICULAR FEMINIZATION SYNDROME.

concordance The expression of a specific trait in both members of a pair of TWINS. (See also DISCORDANCE.)

congenital A condition or abnormality that is present at birth. See BIRTH DEFECTS; ANOSMIA; BLUE BABY; CONGENITAL GLAUCOMA; HEART DEFECTS; CONGENITAL DISLOCATION OF THE HIP; CONGENITAL HYPOTHYROIDISM; LACTIC ACIDOSIS; CONGENITAL NEPHROSIS.

congenital absence of the pituitary See PITUITARY DWARFISM SYNDROMES.

congenital adrenal hyperplasia See ADRENOGENITAL SYNDROMES.

congenital agammaglobulinemia See IMMUNE DEFICIENCY DISEASE.

congenital analgesis See INDIFFERENCE TO PAIN.

congenital anomaly See ANOMALY.

congenital bilateral absence of the vas deferens, CBAVD   See CYSTIC FIBROSIS.

congenital cerebral palsy   See CEREBRAL PALSY.

congenital cyanosis   See BLUE BABY.

congenital dislocation of the hip (congenital dysplasia of the hip)   A CONGENITAL defect of the hip joint most likely due to MULTIFACTORIAL inheritance (the action of several genes in concert with environmental influence), though it is often noted following breech delivery. It is approximately three to four times more common in females than in males. Joint laxity, which is normally greater than in males, probably accounts for some of the preponderance of affected females. Ethnic variation is also seen. The genetic component of its cause is likely due to the shape of the hip socket of the pelvis (the acetabulum) in addition to joint laxity.

Ultrasound or X-rays (particularly in older infants) of the hip are helpful in the diagnosis. Treatment involves positioning with a device or a cast to keep the legs in a frog leg position, and, in some cases, surgery may be necessary.

Incidence is estimated at between one and five per 1,000 live births. Risk of recurrence when a SIBLING is affected is estimated at 1% for males and 11% for females. If a parent is affected, risk of recurrence is 5% for males and 17% for females. If one parent and one child are affected, risk for recurrence in future births is estimated at 36%. Congenital hip dislocation is also associated with single GENE disorders of bone and connective tissue, including MARFAN SYNDROME, EHLERS-DANLOS SYNDROME and LARSEN SYNDROME. In addition to association with connective tissue disease it is also seen in neuromuscular diseases.

This condition occurs with high frequency in German shepherd dogs.

congenital erythropoietic porphyria   See PORPHYRIA.

congenital facial diplegia   See MOEBIUS SYNDROME.

congenital glaucoma   Elevated pressure in the eyes due to a blockage in the trabecular meshwork (supporting connective tissue in the eye), preventing the eye fluid (aqueous humor) from flowing normally. It results in clouding or enlargement of the cornea, tiny rips in the inner corneal lining (COLOBOMA), excessive tearing and hypersensitivity to light. In 75% of cases, both eyes are affected (bilateral). It is diagnosed within the first year of life in four out of five cases. MENTAL RETARDATION may be associated.

Glaucoma mostly affects adults, where it often remains asymptomatic until after it damages the optic nerve. It is one of the three most common causes of blindness in the world; in the United States it is the second most common form of irreversible blindness. CONGENITAL infantile glaucoma, unlike adult glaucoma, is rare.

If eye pressure is elevated at birth, there is less chance of cure than if the symptoms appear after the second month. Surgery (most often trabulectomy, the removal of the trabecular meshwork) successfully saves the eyes in 80% of the latter cases, though vision may remain poor. Rare spontaneous remissions have been reported.

More males than females develop congenital glaucoma. It may be inherited as an AUTOSOMAL RECESSIVE trait or, more commonly, it occurs in a seemingly SPORADIC fashion. At present, CARRIERS of the autosomal recessive trait cannot be identified. The defect occurs in approximately one of 10,000 births. Risk to SIBLINGS born after a single affected child is about 10%.

Congenital glaucoma may be associated with many other conditions including NEUROFIBROMATOSIS, ANIRIDIA, RETINOBLASTOMA, forms of GOINIODYSGENESIS, congenital RUBELLA, LOWE SYNDROME, STURGE-WEBER SYNDROME, STICKLER SYNDROME, FETAL ALCOHOL SYNDROME, COCKAYNE SYNDROME, HOMOCYSTINURIA and MARFAN SYNDROME.

congenital heart defects, CHD   See HEART DEFECTS.

congenital hemolytic anemism   See ANEMIA.

congenital hyperammonemia   See UREA CYCLE DEFECTS.

congenital hypothyroidism   In affected infants the thyroid gland is absent, malpositioned and poorly formed, or unable to properly synthesize thyroid hormones. The condition is asymptomatic at birth; however, unless detected and treated prior to one month of age, brain development and growth will be severely retarded. ("Cretinism" was the term previously used to describe the condition.) Screening involves a blood test to detect levels of thyroid hormones (blood thyroxine and/or thyroid stimulating hormone [TSH]) in newborns, a relatively simple procedure. Every state in the United States and every province in Canada mandates that all newborns be screened for this condition. Treatment is simple, and involves daily replacement with synthetic thyroid hormone medication. Hypothyroidism (both CONGENITAL and later onset) is more common in infants with DOWN SYNDROME.

Most cases occur sporadically. Overall, congenital hypothyroidism affects about one in 3,000 to 4,000 newborns. It affects more than twice as many females as males. Defects in thyroid hormone production occur in an estimated one in 30,000 births. Defects in the function of the hypothalamus and pituitary glands, which also cause congenital hypothyroidism, are estimated at about one in 20,000 births.

About 15 to 20% of cases are inherited. Most inherited cases are inherited in an AUTOSOMAL RECESSIVE manner. Defects in thyroid hormone production have found to be caused by mutations in the *SLC5A5, TG, TPO,* and *TSHB* genes. Dominant *PAX8* gene mutations may cause thyroid dysgenesis.

congenital infantile lactic acidosis   See LACTIC ACIDOSIS.

congenital myodystrophy   See ARTHROGRYPOSIS.

congenital myopathies   A group of disorders of the striated muscles (myopatahies) present at birth. (These exclude MUSCULAR DYSTROPHIES.) Distinctive features are observed in the muscles when sample tissue is examined microscopically. Low muscle tone (hypotonia) and weakness are the major features.

See CENTRAL CORE DISEASE; CENTRONUCLEAR MYOPATHY; NEMALINE MYOPATHY; MYOTONIA CONGENITA; PARAMYOTONIA CONGENITA.

congenital nephrosis (congenital nephrotic syndrome, Finnish type)   A fatal CONGENITAL kidney disease. Affected infants typically exhibit LOW BIRTH WEIGHT and size, as well as an abnormal pooling of fluid in the tissues (edema). Diagnostic tests usually reveal a decrease or abnormally low level of the amount of protein in the blood (hypoproteinemia), decreased albumin in the blood (hypoalbuminemia), excessive blood cholesterol (hypercholesterolemia) and large amounts of protein in the urine (proteinuria).

This disease in generally fatal, with most infants dying within one year of birth, usually as the result of infection or kidney failure. Recent advances in kidney dialysis and transplantation may alter the previously gloomy outlook for these infants.

About 200 cases have been reported, most in Finland or in areas of other countries where there is a large population of Finnish extraction. This is one of over 30 diseases that is seen in Finland but is rare or absent elsewhere. (See ETHNIC GROUPS.) Incidence in this population is estimated at 1:8000.

It is inherited as an AUTOSOMAL RECESSIVE TRAIT. Mothers at risk of bearing a child with this condition exhibit a high level of ALPHA-FETOPROTEIN after the 15th week of pregnancy. The causitive gene has been mapped to the long arm of chromosome 19. The involved gene encodes a protein named nephrin. This protein belongs to the immunoglobulin family of cell adhesion molecules and is specifically expressed in renal glomeruli. A high incidence of this disorder has also been found in the Old Order Mennonites in Lancaster County, Pennsylvania. In fact, the incidence is 20 times greater than that observed in Finland.

Other disorders may also cause nephrotic syndrome in newborns, such as neonatal SYPHILIS (as well as other TORCH infections), NAIL-PATELLA SYNDROME and kidney disease associated with brain malformations.

congenital nephrotic syndrome, Finnish type   See CONGENITAL NEPHROSIS.

conjoined twins (Siamese twins) TWINS physically united at birth as a result of the incomplete separation of a single ovum that has split in the process of twinning. (The splitting of the ovum that produces identical twins occurs on about the 20th day of gestation.) This condition is commonly referred to by the public as "Siamese twins" and has been seen throughout history. There is an illustration of conjoined twins IN UTERO in the first printed treatise on obstetrics, the Rosengarten, by Rosslin, printed in 1513; grown conjoined twins, united at the head (craniopagus), appear in a German woodcut dated 1510. Historical accounts of conjoined twins are rather common, and many of these united individuals achieved considerable notoriety. In addition, there are many reports of individuals to whom a partially formed body, or "parasitic" twin, was attached from birth, and who lived their lives in permanent union with this bodily encumbrance.

The popular contemporary appellation "Siamese twins," dates to Chang and Eng Bunker (1811–74), conjoined Chinese twins born in Siam and exhibited as a circus attraction by P. T. Barnum. He touted them with the following quatrain:

> The Twins of Siam
> Rarest of Dualities
> Two Ever Separate
> Ne'er Apart Realities

Joined by tissue at the trunk, an autopsy following their deaths (they died hours apart at age 63) revealed that they could most likely have been separated by surgical means. Chang and Eng married sisters and fathered at least 21 children between them. Two of their granddaughters produced two normal sets of twins. Other conjoined twins have also gained attention in modern times, exhibiting, for example, musical talents in addition to their anatomical abnormalities.

Conjoined twins may be united at various parts of the body. The suffix *pagus*, which is appended to several body parts, comes from the Greek word *pagos*, meaning "that which is fixed." Frequently these conditions are not compatible with life, and many conjoined twins die at birth or soon after.

Craniopagus. Two complete twins joined at the head. This accounts for approximately 2% of cases.
Dicephalus. A single body with two heads.
Dipygus. Twins joined at the hip with one head, thorax and abdomen with two pelves and four legs.
Omphalopagus. Two complete twins joined at the abdomen.
Pyopagus. Twins joined at the lower back. This accounts for about 19% of conjoined twins.
Rachiopagus. Twins joined at the upper back.
Syncephalus. A single head, with the body separated into twins at some point below.
Thoracopagus. Twins joined at the chest. This accounts for approximately 74% of cases.

Conjoined twins have lived far into adulthood without being separated. However, surgical separation is the treatment of choice whenever possible, though both individuals may not survive when certain organs are shared. Surgical separations now occur more frequently and with greater success than in previous years, though ethical debate about such procedures continue. Conjoined twins with one heart have never survived with or without surgery. In 1987, twins joined at the head who shared part of their cerebral blood supply and brain tissue were separated at Johns Hopkins University, the first time this surgery had been accomplished without causing severe brain damage or death.

Varying statistics on incidence have been reported, ranging from approximately one in 30,000 to one in 100,000 live births. Conjoined twins occur in six out of every 100,000 live births in India and Africa, and four of every 100,000 live births in Europe and the Americas. It affects seven females to every three males. No case of recurrence has ever been reported, either in parents of conjoined twins, or a child of a conjoined twin. PRENATAL DIAGNOSIS is possible by X-ray or ULTRASOUND techniques.

Conradi-Hunermann-type chondrodysplasia See CHONDRODYSPLASIA PUNCTATA.

consanguinity The mating of two individuals with recent common ancestors. Consanguinity is often associated with an increased risk of GENETIC DISORDERS or BIRTH DEFECTS in offspring, due to the potential for expression of aberrant recessive hereditary characteristics, and a slightly increased risk for MULTIFACTORIAL disorders requiring a combination of several GENES for expression.

It is estimated that the average individual has about five to seven mutant recessive genes. While any particular MUTATION, or combination of mutations, would be extremely rare in the general population, the chances that a close relative shares the same mutation are much greater. (First cousins share an average of one-eighth of their genes.) Thus the offspring of close relatives would be more likely to have two copies of the recessive gene and be affected with the disorder that this gene causes. Yet, unless there is a known aberrant genetic condition in the family, the risk for a genetic disorder in the offspring of first cousins is only approximately 3%, as compared to 2% in the general population. (See Table VIII.)

In families with a history of known recessive genetic disorders the risk of having an offspring with the condition rises dramatically. For example, an individual with a first degree relative (parent, child or sibling) with a rare AUTOSOMAL RECESSIVE disorder might have a one in 600 chance of having a child with the condition. However, in a marriage with a third-degree relative (e.g., first cousin), the risk of having an affected infant could be as high as one in 12.

Consanguinity is found with increased frequency in parents of individuals diagnosed as having genetic disorders, CONGENITAL anomalies and MENTAL RETARDATION. Infants resulting from incestuous matings clearly have a higher incidence of hereditary or congenital anomalies.

Consanguineous relationships are common in some cultures and isolated populations, and have historically been associated with royal families, where a desire to cement strategic relationships and assure alliances frequently resulted in intermarriage.

Acceptance of consanguineous relationships varies. For example, marriages of third-degree relatives (first cousins, half-uncle, half-aunt, etc.), relatively common in some cultures, are illegal in some states in the United States.

Consanguineous unions are also more likely to produce offspring affected with disorders associated with specific ethnic groups, such as TAY-SACHS DISEASE among Ashkenazi Jews and SICKLE-CELL ANEMIA among blacks.

constitutional disease Any disease that results from one's hereditary constitution. These can include not only single GENE disorders (i.e., disorders inherited in AUTOSOMAL DOMINANT, RECESSIVE or X-LINKED manner, like HUNTINGTON CHOREA, CYSTIC FIBROSIS or HEMOPHILIA) but also MULTIFACTORIAL diseases, such as MANIC-DEPRESSION or PYLORIC STENOSIS, and CHROMOSOME ABNORMALITIES such as DOWN SYNDROME.

contiguous gene syndrome (segmented aneusomy syndromes, SAS) Disorders caused by the deletion or duplication of adjacent GENES in a specific chromosomal region. Thus, these disorders involve more than one GENE. First described by R. D. Schmickel in 1986, among the disorders now included in this category are WILLIAMS SYNDROME and LANGER-GIEDION SYNDROME. Testing for these conditions involves the use of both conventional

TABLE VIII
PROPORTION OF GENES SHARED BY RELATIVES

Relationship	Genes (%)
First-degree relatives	
Sibs	50
Parent-child	50
Second-degree relatives	
Half-sibs	25
Grandparents	25
Uncle, aunt-niece, nephew	25
Third-degree relatives	
First cousins	12.5
Half uncle, half aunt-niece, nephew	12.5
Fourth-degree relatives	
First cousins once removed	6.25
Fifth-degree relatives	
Second cousins	3.12

chromosome analysis and FLUORESCENCE IN SITU HYBRIDIZATION (FISH).

contraceptive   Any method of preventing conception and pregnancy; birth control.

Some couples whose offspring are at risk of inheriting a GENETIC DISORDER (or those couples in which the female has a genetic or other condition that may be complicated by pregnancy) practice contraception. The decision to avoid pregnancy in these cases is usually made after consultation with a medical geneticist or other appropriate specialist and a thorough review of probability figures for infant abnormalities or health risks for the mother. Once they understand these figures, couples who choose to avoid having children may practice any of several methods of contraception. These methods include oral contraceptives, spermicides, condoms, diaphragms, cervical caps, intrauterine devices (IUDs), sponges, implants and injectable contraceptives, vasectomies, tubal ligation and natural methods.

Oral contraceptives are synthetic steroids that mimic natural hormones (estrogen or progesterone), thus preventing ovulation. These include what is commonly called "the pill," and "morning after" contraceptives.

A high dose of oral contraceptives has been found to prevent pregnancy when taken within 72 hours of unprotected sex by preventing the fertilized egg from attaching itself to the uterine wall. In 1997 the Food and Drug Administration pronounced this method safe and effective.

Depending on the type of oral contraceptive used, the failure rate is estimated to result in one to 10 pregnancies per 100 users over the course of a year.

Spermicides in the form of jellies, foams, creams and vaginal suppositories act by killing sperm. Inserted into the vagina prior to intercourse, they have a failure rate estimated to result in 10 to 25 pregnancies per 100 users over the course of a year.

Condoms are thin-skinned rubber or natural membrane tubes, closed at one end. Fit over the penis, the condom prevents sperm from entering the vagina. Over the course of a year, they are estimated to have a failure rate resulting in three to 15 pregnancies per 100 users.

The diaphragm is a circular, domed-shaped rubber cup. Inserted in the vagina prior to intercourse, it covers the cervix, the entrance to the uterus, preventing sperm from reaching the egg. It is used in conjunction with a spermicide. Failure rate is estimated to result in four to 25 pregnancies per 100 users over the course of a year.

The cervical cap is similar to the diaphragm but smaller. Although it can be difficult to learn to use, it can be left in place for several days. Its failure rate is similar to that of the diaphragm.

IUDs are small plastic or metal devices inserted into the uterus, where they may be left in place for several years. They are believed to work by preventing the fertilized egg from attaching itself to the uterine wall. Use of IUDs has declined significantly since some (particularly the Dalkon Shield) were found capable of causing uterine infections resulting in scarring, pain and INFERTILITY. In 1983 IUDs were the method of choice of an estimated 7% of women practicing birth control. By 1988 the percentage had declined to an estimated 3%. IUDs are thought to have a failure rate resulting in one to five pregnancies per 100 users over the course of a year.

The sponge acts as a barrier and releases a spermicide. Though convenient, its failure rate is high, resulting in 15 to 30 pregnancies per 100 users over the course of a year.

Implants and injectable contraceptives operate on the same principle as oral contraceptives, but over a much longer period of time and at lower doses, since they are absorbed directly into the body rather than being ingested. Capsules surgically implanted under the skin may be effective for as long as five years. The Norplant is one such implant. Failure rates for these forms of birth control are low, typically resulting in one or fewer pregnancies per 100 users over the course of a year.

Hormone shots of Depo-Provera every 12 weeks prevent the release of an egg, thicken the cervical mucus preventing penetration by the sperm, and prevent a fertilized egg from attaching to the wall of the uterus. Considered very effective, fewer than one pregnancy per 100 users over the course of a year.

Norplant, an implantable contraceptive, is comprised of small, matchsticklike rubber rods impregnated with the hormone progestin. They are placed under the skin of a woman's upper arm by a physician. Once implanted, the rods slowly release progestin. There are two types: a two-rod and a six-rod implant, which provide contraception for up to two and five years, respectively. The rods are also removed by a physician.

The Patch is a skin patch worn on the lower abdomen, buttocks, or upper body that releases the hormones progestin and estrogen into the bloodstream. A new patch is applied once a week for three weeks. The patch is not worn during the fourth week, and the menstrual period occurs. Approved by the FDA in 2001, the failure rate, or number of pregnancies expected per 100 women per year, is between one and two. The patch appears to be most effective in women weighing less than 198 pounds.

Emergency contraception (morning-after pill); Post-Coital Contraceptives (RU-486 [Mifeprex], Preven and Plan B) are pills containing either progestin alone or progestin plus estrogen. Taken within 72 hours of copulation, they prevent a fertilized egg from attaching to the uterine wall. The pills were approved by the FDA in 1998–1999, but in the United States their availability was initially curtailed by government policy. In 2006, the FDA approved over-the-counter sales of Plan B to women 18 years of age and older. Morning after pills reduce by 80% the risk of pregnancy for a single act of unprotected sex. By 2006, RU-486 had been used in more than 560,000 abortions, and the risk of death among women who used it was estimated at slightly greater than one in 100,000. The risk of death from surgical abortion is estimated at about one in one million. Pill-based abortions are five to 10 times as likely to fail as surgical ones, and those that do fail require a follow-up surgical procedure.

The vaginal ring is a doughnut-shaped device inserted like a diaphragm, though it remains in the vagina between periods. It releases a low level of hormones similar to those used in oral contraceptives.

Natural methods of birth control include avoiding intercourse during the female's monthly fertile period (the "rhythm" method) and withdrawal of the penis during intercourse prior to ejaculation. Neither of these natural methods is considered reliable.

Permanent birth control methods include vasectomies for men (which may be reversible), in which the ducts that bring sperm from the testicles to the penis are tied or severed, and tubal ligation for women, in which the fallopian tubes that bring the eggs from the ovaries to the uterus, are tied closed.

Cooley's anemia   See THALASSEMIA.

coproporphyria   See PORPHYRIA.

cordocentesis (percutaneous umbilical blood sampling, PUBS; fetal blood sampling)   A technique for fetal blood sampling, available since the mid-1980s. An outpatient procedure generally taking less than 10 minutes, it is usually performed after 18 weeks of pregnancy but can be performed any time after the 12th week. About 3 to 4 ml of blood generally can be taken from the FETUS. The procedure can be used for PRENATAL DIAGNOSIS in a variety of situations, including obtaining blood for CHROMOSOME analysis when results are needed more quickly than can be provided by AMNIOCENTESIS (in about three days rather than three weeks) or when there have been previously unclear chromosome results from either amniocentesis or CHORIONIC VILLUS SAMPLING. It is also used in the evaluation of potential fetal blood disorders (such as HEMOPHILIA), infection (such as TORCH SYNDROME) or other situations in which fetal blood must be tested. It has been used not only to take blood from the fetus but also for transfusions or to administer drugs directly into fetal circulation. The fetal loss rate is four to five times higher when the procedure is used for fetal transfusion than for blood sampling.

After administration of local anesthesia, a needle is placed through the mother's abdominal wall and uterus directly into a fetal blood vessel in the umbilical cord, guided by ULTRASOUND.

PUBS is not a replacement for amniocentesis; rather it is an alternative in specific, well-defined situations. The procedure is more difficult to perform and carries a higher risk to the fetus (about 1%) of inducing a miscarriage than amniocentesis.

Cori disease   See GLYCOGEN STORAGE DISEASE.

corneal dystrophy The cornea is the transparent membrane covering the eye. There are more than 20 corneal dystrophies that affect all parts of the cornea. Several hereditary forms have been documented. The degree of vision problems they create is variable as is their age of onset. Most are inherited as AUTOSOMAL DOMINANT traits, though AUTOSOMAL RECESSIVE forms also occur. Though they may be slowly progressive, most forms rarely cause severe vision problems.

Typically, opacities will form on the cornea, clouding the vision. These opacities can often be removed surgically. Corneal dystrophies may also be found as part of mucolipidoses (especially type IV) and other disorders, for example, the MUCOPOLYSACCHARIDOSES.

Cornelia de Lange syndrome (de Lange syndrome; Brachmann–de Lange syndrome) A SYNDROME consisting of growth deficiency, MENTAL RETARDATION, anomalies of the extremities and characteristic facial appearance. It is named for pediatrician Cornelia de Lange (1871–1950), professor of pediatrics at the University of Amsterdam, Holland, who described two girls with the syndrome in 1933. It is sometimes called Brachmann–de Lange syndrome, as Dr. W. Brachmann described a patient with similar features in 1916.

Infants have LOW BIRTH WEIGHT, typically under five pounds. Height and weight remain below the third percentile for their age. Other common features include recurrent respiratory infections and gastrointestinal problems, diminished sucking and swallowing ability, congenital HEART DEFECTS, CLEFT PALATE and bowel abnormalities. Permanent bending (flexion contractures) of the elbows are reported in 80% of cases. Hands are small and spadelike, with tapering fingers, a curved fifth finger and a single deep transverse crease across the palm (SIMIAN CREASE). There may be shortening of the limbs. In severe cases, there may be missing limbs or fingers. Hearing loss is also frequent (60%). Autistic and self-destructive behaviors are sometimes seen.

The characteristic facial appearance consists of a small head (MICROCEPHALY), excessive hair (hirsutism), thick, bushy eyebrows that meet above the nose (SYNOPHYRYS), unusually long eyelashes, small nose with upturned nostrils (anteverted nares), small, widely spaced teeth and low-set ears. The lips are thin and the mouth is turned down. There is a small "beak" in the middle of the upper lip and a corresponding notch in the lower lip. These features may not all be visible during the first year of life.

All cases exhibit moderate to severe MENTAL RETARDATION. The IQ is usually below 50. There is significant developmental delay, particularly in speech, even among those only mildly affected by the disorder. Life expectancy is diminished due to susceptibility to infections.

Diagnosis is made by a thorough medical evaluation, which includes X-rays and CHROMOSOME analysis. This is because duplication of a band on the long arm of chromosome 3 leads to a pattern of abnormalities similar to de Lange syndrome (see CHROMOSOME ABNORMALITIES).

Mutations in the *NIPBL* gene, mapped to the short arm of chromosome 5 and which makes a protein called delangin, cause Cornelia de Lange syndrome. Transmitted as an AUTOSOMAL DOMINANT TRAIT, most cases are sporadic, the result of new mutation. Less than 1% of individuals diagnosed with this condition have an affected parent. A few cases of multiple SIBLINGS of normal parents being affected with this disorder have been reported. When the parents of an affected child are apparently clinically unaffected, the risk to the siblings of a child with de Lange syndrome has been estimated to be about 1.5% because of the possibility of germ-line MOSAICISM.

The incidence is estimated at one in 20,000 live births. Currently, PRENATAL DIAGNOSIS of this condition by ULTRASOUND detection of the anomalies seen in the syndrome is theoretically possible.

coronary artery disease (CAD) Encircling the heart like a crown, the coronary arteries bring oxygenated blood to heart muscle. Disease of the coronary arteries is the consequence of atherosclerosis, the accumulation of fats, carbohydrates, components of blood, fibrous tissue and calcium into plaque on the artery's inside wall. According to one theory, the plaque develops at a site where the lining of the artery has been damaged or roughened by a mechanical, chemical or toxic factor or substance. As the plaque enlarges, it restricts or shuts off completely the flow of blood to an area of the heart, injuring or even killing heart muscle fibers. This event is called a myocardial infarction or, popularly, a "heart attack." It may also cause extreme pain (angina pectoris), loss of normal heart beat (fibrillation) and death. CAD is the leading cause of death in the United States for both men and women. In fact it results in more fatalities than all forms of cancer combined. At the beginning of the 21st century, about 500,000 people a year died of CAD, and some 13,000,000 were affected by the disorder. The chance of having coronary artery disease after age 40 is 49% for men and 32% for women. Atherosclerosis accounts for about 50% of death in industrialized populations.

Perhaps the first to recognize a familial link in coronary artery disease was English poet and essayist Matthew Arnold (1822–88). While visiting the United States in 1887, he experienced severe chest pains (angina pectoris), and wrote to a friend, "I began to think that my time was really coming to an end. I had so much pain in my chest, the sign of a malady which had suddenly struck down in middle life, long before they came to my present age, both my father and my grandfather." Arnold died less than a year later. The noted English physician Sir William Osler (1849–1919) cited the Arnold family in 1897 in proposing a genetic factor in the development of coronary disease.

People who smoke, have high blood pressure or high levels of fat-related substances in their blood, such as cholesterol and triglycerides (also termed lipids, or lipoproteins), are more likely than others to develop coronary artery disease. Some inherit a tendency to have high levels of these substances in the blood. These HEREDITARY DISEASES include familial HYPERCHOLESTEROLEMIA and familial HYPERTRIGLYCERIDEMIA, as well as other familial forms of hyperlipoproteinemia.

High levels of LDLs (low-density lipoproteins), a cholesterol-carrying particle, are critical to the development of atherosclerosis. Genetic variations exist in many lipoproteins, in addition to familial hypercholesterolemia, which are associated with increased susceptibilities to atherosclerosis and CAD. The presence of such lipoproteins is not predictive of an individual's risk, but as a group, those with some variations are at a higher risk for developing CAD. These include apo-AI and AII, apo-b, Lp(a) lipoprotein, and they may be important risk determinants in individual families. Higher levels of HDLs (high-density lipoproteins) are associated with lower risks of atherosclerosis. Other identified risk factors include hyperhomocystemia, OBESITY, high blood pressure and diabetes, each of which have genetic determinants. Clearly multiple genetic loci (see LOCUS) are involved along with environmental factors, like diet and smoking, in the onset of CAD. In addition there are rare GENETIC DISORDERS associated with premature vascular (blood vessel) disease, such as PSEUDOXANTHOMA ELASTICUM, HOMOCYSTINURIA, PROGERIA, COCKAYNE SYNDROME and WERNER SYNDROME. The classification of the hyperlipidemias is also evolving—many are now categorized based on their underlying genetic abnormality rather than the lipid profile.

Familial Hypercholesterolemia

A characteristic sign of familial hypercholesterolemia (FH) is development of yellowish fat-laden nodules (xanthomas), particularly on the Achilles tendon or tendons of the hand. It is the result of a dominant MUTATION in the GENE coding for a cell surface receptor for LDLs. As a result of the mutation LDLs continue circulating in the blood instead of being picked up and carried off for disposal. Low-density lipoproteins are about 75% lipid, and about two-thirds of the lipid is cholesterol. The accumulation of LDLs in arterial pathways leads to formation of plaque.

FH should be suspected if the blood level of cholesterol is higher than 350 mg/dl, but in some cases the blood level may be lower. The disorder does not account for all instances of elevated cholesterol, some of which are likely to be due to other POLYGENIC and environmental factors. The Nobel prize in medicine was shared in 1985 by molecular geneticists Joseph Goldstein (b. 1940) and Michael Brown (b. 1941) of the University of Texas for their discovery of the LDL receptor and its role in the regulation of cholesterol levels.

FH occurs in about one in every 500 persons. In men with FH, heart attacks typically occur in the 40s to 50s. About 85% of men with FH have had a heart attack by the age of 60. Treatment includes diet, exercise and drug therapy. A variety of cholesterol-reducing drugs are available for this condition. Certain populations have an increased incidence with a specific mutation due to a FOUNDER EFFECT. These include French Canadians, Afrikaners and Lebanese. A related disorder which also leads to high cholesterol levels is known as familial defective apo-B100. In this disorder the gene for the lipoprotein apo-B100 (which is a component of LDL) has a mutation that interferes with its (and therefore LDL's) binding to the LDL receptor. It also slightly raises cholesterol levels but not as much as FH, and xanthomas are not seen. Its incidence is slightly lower than FH (about 1/800). About one in 1 million people inherits two copies of a mutant LDL receptor gene. In these individuals with homozygous familial hypercholesterolemia, plasma levels of cholesterol are enormous and heart attacks occur in childhood and adolescence.

Familial Hypertriglyceridemia

Triglycerides are fatty substances that, like cholesterol, can contribute to the formation of atherosclerotic plaques. Low-density lipoproteins are rich in triglycerides. The concentration of very low-density lipoprotein (VLDL) and triglycerides are elevated in the plasma. There is an associated increased risk of coronary artery disease and pancreatitis. Genetic defects in lipoprotein lipase and in the gene for lipoprotein apoCII have been found. Familial cases appear to be AUTOSOMAL DOMINANT, and frequency is estimated at one in 300 individuals in the United States. Only 10% to 20% of carriers of the gene for familial hypertriglyceridemia show signs of the disorder before 20 years of age. It is the rare homozygotes and not heterozygotes that develop hyperlipidemia. Most affected persons exhibit OBESITY.

Combined Hyperlipidemia

Combined hyperlipidemia is frequently found in young to middle-aged adults recovering from heart attacks caused by clogged arteries (coronary atherosclerosis). It is diagnosed by elevated levels of plasma cholesterol and triglycerides—fatty substances associated with clogged arteries—in the blood. Many of these individuals exhibit impaired glucose tolerance and obesity, and may succumb to coronary heart disease between the ages of 30 and 60.

Some studies suggest this disorder may be inherited as an autosomal dominant trait. Risk of occurrence is from approximately one per 500 to one per 1,000 in the general population. The cause is uncertain, but dietary modification is a generally effective treatment. This is the most common familial lipid disorder among survivors of a premature heart attack (‹60%). The frequency appears to be about 1/200.

Type III Hyperlipoproteinemia

Hyperlipoproteinemia III rarely appears before 30 years of age. Cholesterol levels are high, ranging from 400 mg to 600 mg/dl and triglycerides range from 175 mg to 1,500 mg., though individuals have usually consumed a regular diet. LDLs have an increased ratio of cholesterol compared to triglycerides. The defect lies in the structure of a protein named apolipoprotein E. Lipoprotein deposits in skin creases of the palm (xanthomata) may appear after age 25. Coronary disease and peripheral vascular disease may appear in males over 45 years of age and in females over 55 years of age.

Glucose tolerance is abnormal in about 40% of those brought to medical attention. The mode of transmission of this inherited disorder is not completely understood, but the risk of occurrence is considered infrequent. Rarely appearing before 30 years of age, it is usually seen in individuals between 40 and 60 years old. It can be managed with dietary restriction and lipid lowering drugs.

This appears to be an AUTOSOMAL RECESSIVE trait. The frequency is about 1/5000, and among heart attack survivors about 1/100. (See also ABETALIPOPEOTEINEMIA; CHOLETERYL ESTER STORAGE DISEASE; TANGIER DISEASE.)

Cowden disease (multiple hamartoma syndrome)

A hereditary disorder characterized by hamartomatous neoplasms (benign tumors which develop from normal tissue) on the skin, mucous membranes, gastrointestinal tract, central nervous system, eyes and genitourinary tract and an increased risk of developing cancers. It is named for the family of Rachel Cowden, in which the autosomal dominant inheritance pattern of the disorder was first identified in 1963.

Onset can occur from birth to the mid-40s. Most affected individuals come to medical attention when they seek help for the skin lesions. One of more than 50 genodermatoses, or genetically influenced skin disorders, at least one of four types of skin lesions are seen in all cases: facial papules, which are flesh-colored, flat-topped dry or warty growths around the mouth, nostrils and eyes; oral lesions, smooth whitish spots on the gums and palate that join together to create a cobblestone appearance known as papillomatosis; acral keratoses, which are flesh-coloured or slightly pigmented smooth or warty papules on the upper surface of the hands and feet; and palmoplantar keratoses, scaly spots on the palms and soles.

Cowden disease is also associated with several types of malignancies, particularly breast cancer in females and thyroid cancer in males. At least 40% of patients have at least one cancer. Lifetime risk of breast cancer for affected women is 25–50%, and both breasts may be affected. Lifetime risk of thyroid cancer is 3–10%. Polyps of the colon and intestines may also occur. Development of malignant tumors is the primary risk to normal lifespan. Benign tumors can also lead to death in affected individuals. However, if detected early, the cure rate for the cancers is high with appropriate treatment. Central nervous system involvement occurs in about 40% of cases.

Cowden disease is caused by a mutation in the *PTEN* gene, a tumor suppressor gene on chromosome 10q. The gene makes a phosphatase protein that is believed to promote cell death. The mutated gene manufactures a nonfunctioning protein, which may lead to a proliferation of cells, resulting in growth of the characteristic tumors. However, other factors are also believed to be involved in the development of the neoplasms, as the same mutation occurs in another hereditary disorder, Bannayan-Zonana syndrome, which has a much lower predisposition to cancer.

A rare disorder, prevalence has been estimated at 1:200,000–250,000 in the Dutch population. More than 200 cases have been described, some involving families with several generations of affected members. Onset is typically at a young age. Affected individuals are advised to undergo annual medical and physical examinations and tests to check for internal malignancies. Relatives of affected individuals should undergo genetic counseling.

Coxsackie virus This virus takes its name from Coxsackie, New York, the home town of the patients in whom it was first isolated. Though the illness produced by the virus is mild, infection during first trimester of pregnancy has been associated with an increased incidence of CONGENITAL heart lesions in newborns. Some studies have also suggested a role for this virus in the etiology of insulin-dependent DIABETES MELLITUS. (See also HEART DEFECTS.)

craniocarpotarsal dysplasia See WHISTLING FACE SYNDROME.

craniodiaphyseal dysplasia A very rare disorder characterized by severe developmental defects of the skull and short stature. This is the condition that affected the youth who became the subject of the popular 1985 movie *Mask*. The skull bones thicken, resulting in severe facial deformities, which in turn cause nasal obstruction and cranial nerve compression that often leads to BLINDNESS, DEAFNESS, facial paralysis and seizures. Most affected individuals have exhibited MENTAL RETARDATION. Inherited generally as an AUTOSOMAL RECESSIVE trait, it is progressive, leading to death in the second or third decade of life.

craniometaphyseal dysplasia There are two genetic forms of this disorder: one transmitted by a recessive GENE and the other by a dominant gene. The dominant form is less severe and more common (see AUTOSOMAL DOMINANT and AUTOSOMAL RECESSIVE). Both forms can be recognized during the first year of life and display the same facial abnormalities, which include a long and narrow skull (scaphocephaly), thickening of the frontal and side skull bones, with wide-set eyes (HYPERTELORISM) that may bulge outward (proptosis), broadening of the root of the nose and a depressed nasal bridge, imperfect positioning and contact of the upper and lower teeth (dental malocclusion) and mouth breathing caused by narrowed nasal passages.

Other manifestations include facial paralysis, difficulties with eye movement and defective vision caused by wasting of the optic nerve (optic atrophy), as well as poor hearing caused by alterations in the bone structure around the eyes and ears. The latter may lead to sound distortion in the inner ear (sensorineural DEAFNESS), which occurs before puberty. The alterations in bone structure result in narrowing of the passage through which the nerves to the face, ears and eyes traverse, compressing them and disturbing their function.

X-ray examination discloses hardening and thickening (sclerosis) and abnormal growth (hyperostosis) of bone tissues of the front and back of the skull, increased bone growth in the skull spaces around the nose (paranasal sinuses) and below the ears, and a club-shaped thickening (flaring) to the tubular shafts of the long bones, especially in the upper extremities.

The basic defect causing this disorder is not known. It tends to be progressive, and some of the complications may require neurosurgery. Intelligence is not affected. The gene responsible for the recessive form maps to the long arm of chromosome 6. Currently, there is no method for PRENATAL DIAGNOSIS.

craniosynostosis Deformities of the skull resulting from premature closure of the gaps, or sutures, between the skull bones. Normally, the bones of the skull are not joined at birth, allowing the head to grow evenly. In individuals with craniosynostosis, the sutures where the skull bones meet have closed, or closed prematurely. "Synostosis" means a union of adjacent bones.) As a result, the expanding skull bones grow abnormally, and the abnormal skull shape becomes more pronounced as the infant grows. The shape is dependent on which sutures have closed, and various abnormalities have specific names.

Acrocephaly; oxycephaly; turricephaly. These denote a pointed (high) head, caused by the premature closure of all sutures.
Brachycephaly. This denotes an abnormally short, squat skull, caused by the premature closure of the two coronal sutures, which cross the top front portion of the skull, widthwise.
Dolichocephaly; scaphocephaly. These denote an abnormally long front-to-back distance of the skull, caused when the sagittal suture, which runs lengthwise along the top of the skull, is closed.
Plagiocephaly. This denotes a somewhat lopsided, asymmetric, pointed appearance, caused by premature closure of sutures that cross the top of the skull widthwise (coronal sutures in the front, lambdoidal sutures in back), on only one side (unilateral).
Trigonocephaly. This denotes a triangular shape at the top of the skull, caused by the closing of the metopic suture, which runs lengthwise along the top front of the skull, forward of the sagittal suture and anterior fontanelle (the "soft spot" at the top front portion of an infant's skull).

The sagittal sutures are involved in over 50% of craniosynostosis cases. The coronal sutures are involved in between 20% and 30%. Least frequently involved are the metopic suture and labdoidal sutures. MENTAL RETARDATION may occur in these disorders, and is more likely in cases where the closure of the sutures is greatest. The abnormal growth of the skull can have many effects on the brain and nervous system. Intracranial pressure may be raised and blood flow to the brain may be impaired. Vision and hearing impairments and airway obstruction may occur. Even in the absence of mental retardation, learning difficulties may be present, and despite improving surgical treatments these problems may remain.

Both genetic and environmental factors can contribute to craniosynostosis. Abnormal mechanical forces such as external pressure from uterine crowding or even postnatal positioning, or a deficiency of underlying brain growth, which can have numerous causes, may underlie many cases. The presence of associated anomalies or a family history is evidence of a genetically caused condition. Now over 100 SYNDROMES associated with craniosynostosis have been described, not including the many (more than 25) in which it is a secondary or occasional feature. Most common forms have an AUTOSOMAL DOMINANT inheritance pattern. Many of the craniosynostosis SYNDROMES also have limb abnormalities.

A number of GENES whose MUTATIONS cause craniosynostosis have been identified. These include the genes for the fibroblast growth factor receptors type 1, 2 and 3, as well as the MSX2, fibrillin 1, and TWIST genes. Among these the FGFR2 gene, located on the long arm of chromosome 10, is the most important. Many different mutations (›50) in this gene have been found, and specific ones result in one or more of the well-known syndromes. That is, the same mutation has been found to cause several possible disorders. (e.g., one mutation has been found to underlie either PFEIFFER SYNDROME, CROUZON DISEASE, or JACKSON-WEISS SYNDROME in different families. These disorders differ on the basis of the limb anomaly seen and in some cases may represent variable expressions of the same mutation.)

Most cases of isolated craniosynostosis are SPORADIC with MULTIFACTORIAL inheritance, but AUTOSOMAL DOMINANT and AUTOSOMAL RECESSIVE forms have been reported. About 10% of cases are familial (see FAMILIAL DISEASE). Craniosynostosis is estimated to occur in from one in 1,000 to one in 2,500 live births. PRENATAL DIAGNOSIS has been achieved by X-rays in late pregnancy, revealing closed sutures, and by ULTRASOUND, indicating the unusual shape of the head.

Among those who don't exhibit mental retardation, there are few complications caused by this disorder other than cosmetic and sociopsychological problems. The craniosynostoses are treated surgically by removing the affected suture(s). (See also APERT SYNDROME; SAETHRECHOTZEN SYNDROME; CARPENTER SYNDROME.)

cri du chat syndrome CHROMOSOME ABNORMALITY that takes its name from the distinctive, mewing cry of affected infants, which has been likened to a kitten in distress. Birthweight is low, and infants exhibit FAILURE TO THRIVE and short stature. The condition is also referred to as monosomy 5p, as the cause has been traced to the deletion of a small section of the short arm of chromosome 5. All affected individuals are severely retarded, though survival into adulthood is common.

While facial features do not show any signature abnormalities, the head is small (MICROCEPHALY), eyes wide set (HYPERTELORISM), chin receding and the face round, with a paradoxically alert expression. The hair may gray prematurely. About 20% have congenital HEART DEFECTS.

Incidence is estimated at approximately one in 50,000 in the general population. PRENATAL DIAGNOSIS is possible by analysis of fetal chromosomes obtained by AMNIOCENTESIS. In about 10% to 15% of cases the SYNDROME results from an inherited translocation and thus is associated with an increased recurrence risk.

Crigler-Najar syndrome A rare hereditary liver enzyme deficiency characterized by severe jaundice in early infancy. It is named for Drs. John Crigler and Victor Najar, who first identified the disorder in 1952. An autosomal recessive disorder, the syndrome is caused by a mutation in the UDP-*glycuronosyltransferase* gene (*UGT1A1*) located on 2q. The mutation results in a deficiency of the enzyme glucuronal transferase, resulting in accumulation of bilirubin in the blood. The jaundice may cause brain damage or death; some affected infants die in the first weeks or months of life. However, some affected infants suffer no long-term neurological damage. Treatment consists of phototherapy, exposure to hot, bright, blue-toned lights that break down the bilirubin, or liver transplantation, preferably performed at an early age before irreversible neurological effects occur. About 90 cases in the United States have been identified.

Crohn disease (regional ileitis) An inflammatory bowel disease characterized by abdominal distress, which slowly progresses to more severe bowel symptoms. Crohn disease and ulcerative colitis comprise the two inflammatory bowel diseases (IBD). It is named for U.S. physician B. B. Crohn (b. 1884), who first described it in 1932. Ashkenazi Jews have a higher risk of developing IBD than other ETHNIC GROUPS. Prevalence of Crohn is about 30–100/100,000. About 20% of cases have an affected first degree relative, usually a sibling. Recurrence risks of IBD to SIBLINGS is 2–5%; to parents 1–5%; to offspring 1–4%. (Some studies suggest it may be as high as 8–9% for siblings and offspring in Ashkenazi Jews.)

It appears to be MULTIFACTORIAL in its causation. Although the cause is unknown, one of the genes involved in susceptibility to Crohn disease has been mapped to chromosome 16.

Crouzon disease   A form of CRANIOSYNOSTOSIS, ANOMALIES of skull development characterized by oddly shaped heads. In this form, the head is pointed and there is defective development (hypoplasia) of the mid-face. It is named for French neurologist Octave Crouzon (1874–1938), a neurologist at the Salpêtrière Hospital in Paris, who noted the disorder's familial occurrence in 1912 when he first described the SYNDROME.

The pointed head is caused by premature closure of sutures of the skull, forcing the bones to grow abnormally. The eyes are large and wide-set (HYPERTELORISM), with shallow orbits, so that they appear somewhat bulging. Approximately half of affected individuals have vision problems, and progressive vision loss may require surgical intervention in some cases.

The mouth is small, the nose, beaklike. Deviated septum and obstruction of the nasal passages is common. The ears, depending on the degree of skull malformation, may be displaced downward. There are often defects of the middle and inner ear, as well. Defects in formation of the bones of the inner ear (ossicles) lead to conductive hearing loss in over half of those under medical treatment. Spine anomalies are present in almost one-third. Some affected individuals are mentally retarded.

The abnormal growth of the head begins during the first year of life and is usually complete by three years of age. It is inherited as an AUTOSOMAL DOMINANT trait, with new MUTATIONS responsible for perhaps 33% to 50% of cases. Increased paternal age has been associated with these SPORADIC cases. While there is currently little published data regarding PRENATAL DIAGNOSIS, it has been accomplished by ULTRASOUND and in previously characterized families by molecular based techniques identifying the mutation in the family in CVS material.

Incidence is estimated at about 16 per million newborns. Crouzon is the most common of the craniosynostosis syndromes, comprising about 3% to 7% of patients with such conditions.

Life expectancy is normal, and facial surgery can correct some of the cosmetic aspects of the disorder. However, effective treatment takes many years and requires a team of specialists.

The disorder can be highly variable, even among affected individuals within a single family, in terms of the degree of craniosynostosis, age of onset, and associated features. Frequency is said to be about 1/25,000.

Crouzon disease results from mutations in the *FGFR2* gene (see CRANIOSYNOSTOSIS). Most patients with APERT SYNDROME as well as PFEIFFER SYNDROME or JACKSON-WEISS SYNDROME also have mutations in this gene, and some patients with either Pfeiffer or Jackson-Weiss syndromes have had mutations identical to those seen in Crouzon. There is considerable overlap among these disorders, which differ primarily on the basis of the limb anomaly seen. Patients with Crouzon disease have not been considered to have limb anomalies, whereas in Pfeiffer syndrome, broad thumbs and great toes are seen, and in Jackson-Weiss, broad great toes and bony fusions in the feet are characteristic. Thus, some of these cases appear to be variable expressions of the same genetic defect, and previous clinical delineation used by geneticists may have to be revised.

cryptophthalmos (ablepharia)   The CONGENITAL absence or reduction in size of the eyelids. The most severe cases are bilateral, that is, involve both eyes, and there may be no recognizable differentiation of the lids (e.g., the lids are completely fused or absent). Eyelashes and eyebrows are also absent. Less severe forms may be unilateral or incomplete, with only the upper or lower lid lacking. Pliny the Elder in the first century A.D. described the Lepidus family in which three children were born with a membrane over the eye, typical of this rare ANOMALY. In mild cases fused eyelids can be separated surgically, allowing normal vision. However, in more severe cases there may be malformations of ocular structures as well, resulting in BLINDNESS.

Other multiple malformations may be associated. In 1962, G. R. Fraser described a distinctive "cryptophthalmos SYNDROME." This AUTOSOMAL RECESSIVE condition includes ear anomalies, genital abnormalities and SYNDACTYLY (webbed or fused digits). In fact, cryptophthalmos is not always a feature of the "cryptophthalmos syndrome," and thus, the eponymic FRASER SYNDROME is preferable for the condition. Fraser syndrome may be caused by mutations in the *FRAS1* gene (on the long arm of chromosome 4) (in about 50% of cases) or in the *FREM2* gene (on the long arm of chromosome 13).

cryptorchidism   See CRYPTORCHISM.

cryptorchism (cryptorchidism)   The condition of having undescended testicles, or the failure of the testicles to descend into the scrotum. It is seen in many GENETIC DISORDERS. Individuals with cryptorchism exhibit much higher rates of testicular malignancies than unaffected individuals.

About 2–3% of full-term and 15–30% of preterm male infants will have an undescended testis. One fourth of these will be bilateral. By age one year though, the incidence falls to 0.7% as the testes descend when testosterone levels rise over the first three months of life. An undescended testes has about a 20–40 times higher risk of cancer. Fertility appears to be unaffected in boys who have had a unilateral undescended testis repaired early, but those with bilateral cryptorchism may have decreased fertility, even with early surgery.

C section   See CESAREAN DELIVERY.

cutis laxa   A group of inherited conditions characterized by excess skin that hangs loosely in folds, about the face and body, often giving affected individuals a prematurely aged appearance. The Latin *cutis laxa* means "loose skin." The loose skin may be thickened and dark. If it affects the skin around the eyes symptoms such as burning, redness, light sensitivity and loss of eyebrows and lashes may occur. The skin is inelastic and, if pulled, does not spring back upon release. It is not fragile, and the joints are not loose and hypermobile. While it is usually evident at birth, there have been reports of a few late-onset cases. There is also an acquired form that doesn't manifest until puberty or later, which often

follows an inflammatory illness and appears to have an autoimmune basis. Affected individuals are said to have "hound dog faces" and are often described as appearing "mournful." They have a beaked nose and long upper lip. Frequently, other abnormalities are associated with cutis laxa, and cardiorespiratory complications and inguinal hernias may also be seen.

These disorders are very rare, with approximately 40 cases reported. Four types are recognized.

Type I. In this relatively benign form, the laxity of skin is the only abnormality exhibited. Though the excess of skin is mildest in this form, adolescent children may appear older than their unaffected parents. It is inherited as an AUTOSOMAL DOMINANT trait. This form can be caused by mutations in the elastin gene. (Mutations in the gene encoding fibulin-5 can cause either autosomal dominant or autosomal recessive cutis laxa.)

Type II. This, the most common form, is severe or lethal. Affected individuals also have emphysema, which interferes with their ability to breathe, as well as other cardiopulmonary problems. There may be mild malformations of the gastrointestinal and genitourinary tracts. Infants typically have hoarse, harsh, deep and resonant voices caused by the laxity of vocal cords. This form is inherited as an AUTOSOMAL RECESSIVE trait. Death usually occurs early in life due to complications from emphysema.

Type III. In addition to loose skin, individuals exhibit retarded physical development, with height typically below the 10th percentile for age. Mild MENTAL RETARDATION is also common. Joint laxity and CONGENITAL hip dislocation are seen. It is thought to be inherited as an autosomal recessive trait.

Type IV. Type IV cutis laxa is the only form in which the basic defect causing the disorder has been identified. A deficiency of lysyl oxidase interferes with the normal activity of collagen, an important component in the formation of skin. This form is inherited as an X-LINKED recessive trait. It is caused by mutation in the Cu(2+)-transporting ATPase, alpha polypeptide gene, the same one that causes Menkes syndrome.

Type IV is the same entity as EHLERS-DANLOS SYNDROME, Type IX. It is also known as occipital horn SYNDROME, because of the nubby protuberances at the back of the skull (occiput). These individuals have lax skin, hypermobile joints and other bony abnormalities. It appears as a result of a fundamental abnormality of copper metabolism, copper being necessary to lysyl oxidase activity.

CVS   See CHORIONIC VILLUS SAMPLING.

cyanosis, congenital   See CONGENITAL CYANOSIS.

cyclopia (cyclops)   The most extreme form of HOLOPROSENCEPHALY, a group of rare ANOMALIES caused by maldevelopment of the forebrain in the embryo resulting in various degrees of brain defects and fusion of the optic nerves. In cyclopia there is a single eye, and typically no nose, though there may be a proboscis-like structure above the eye.

Cyclops have been a staple of legend since antiquity. Perhaps the most well known is the giant Cyclops in Homer's epic poem *The Odyssey*. There was also a belief dating to early Western civilization that certain tribes in Scythia (the area north of the Black Sea), Ethiopia and India existed that had but one eye in the middle of their heads. According to Pliny, the Roman scholar of the first century A.D., there was a nation of these people called Arimaspi. The true condition of cyclopia, however, is incompatible with life. Most affected infants die at birth or within a few hours, although one was reported to have lived for 10 years. The cause of this extremely rare disorder is unknown, although it has been associated with various CHROMOSOME ABNORMALITIES (e.g., trisomy 13).

cyclops   See CYCLOPIA.

cystic fibrosis (CF)   Cystic fibrosis is among the most common GENETIC DISORDERS in white populations, and the most common fatal HEREDITARY DISEASE in this group. Inherited as an AUTOSOMAL RECESSIVE trait, CF is a disorder of the exocrine (outward-secreting) glands, which causes the body to produce an abnormal amount of excessively thick, sticky mucus that clogs the lungs and pancreas, interfering with breathing and digestion. In some people, the respiratory system is primarily affected, while in others the digestive system is more affected. Respiratory complications arise from the blockage of bronchial passages. Eventually, cilia, the small hairs lining the respiratory tract and responsible for clearing mucus, are destroyed. Additionally, CF mucus traps bacteria, which leads to lung infections and lung damage. In the digestive system, mucus may block ducts of the pancreas, which provides the ENZYMES necessary to help digest food. If the ducts become blocked, the enzymes are unavailable to assist in digestion, and nutrients cannot be absorbed.

Females may experience delayed puberty and infertility. More than 95% of males are sterile.

The underlying problem in CF involves the defective transport of chloride across membranes leading to dehydrated, thickened secretions. This leads to the thick, sticky mucus. Almost two-thirds of patients are diagnosed in the first year of life. Average age of survival as of 1995 is 30 years. In a 1995 study, 35% of young adults with CF worked full time and almost 90% completed a high school education. Severity of lung disease is the most important determinant of quality of and length of life. (CF patients may have an increased risk of developing GI tract cancers.)

Incidence in Caucasians is 1 in 3,300 and CARRIER frequency is 1/29. Hispanics also have a relatively high frequency, 1/9,500, giving a carrier frequency of 1/46. While it is rare in native Africans and native Asians, higher incidences are seen in American populations of these ETHNIC GROUPS (1/15,300 and 1/32,100 respectively, giving carrier frequencies of 1/60 and 1/90 respectively.) More than 25,000 Americans have CF, and about 850 new cases are diagnosed annually.

Identified as a specific disease in 1938, CF became, in 1989, the first disease whose genetic basis was elucidated entirely on the basis of its map location without the availability of CHROMOSOME ABNORMALITIES such as translocations or deletions, as had been available for example with Duchenne type MUSCULAR DYSTROPHY or chronic granulomatous disease.

The disorder usually appears in infancy, though rare, mild cases may not become apparent until adulthood. Symptoms include persistent coughing, recurrent wheezing, more than one bout of pneumonia, excessive appetite with poor weight gain, salty-tasting skin, and bulky, foul-smelling stools. However, the symptoms show a great variability, and often mimic other childhood diseases. Respiratory symptoms may initially be diagnosed as asthma, pneumonia or other respiratory conditions. Digestive symptoms of CF (malabsorption and malnutrition) may be confused with celiac disease or other digestive disorders. Ten percent of newborns with CF have obstruction of their small bowel because the meconium (the dark green intestinal contents that constitute the newborn's first bowel movement) that these infants produce is overly thick and sticky and "plugs up" their intestine (a process called "meconium ileus"). Liver disease is also seen in some individuals with CF.

Sweat glands of affected individuals produce perspiration with an abnormally high level of salt. A finding of excessive levels of salt in sweat is the primary method for diagnosing CF.

Physical therapy and medication can help alleviate respiratory and digestive problems associated with the disorder. Bronchial drainage (also called postural drainage), a form of physical therapy, helps break up mucus accumulations in small airways and move them into larger passages where they can be coughed up. Antibiotics are used to treat infections in the lungs. For digestive problems, regulated diet, pancreatic enzymes and nutritional supplements are usually prescribed. Heart-lung transplants have also been performed on a very limited basis. New treatments include the use of inhaled DNase which breaks down the DNA from white blood cells in the lung, and drug treatments that modify ion transport to aid in loosening mucus secretions. GENE therapy is currently under active investigation, but this potential cure is "not anticipated in the near future" to quote a 1997 National Institute of Health statement.

The gene that causes CF has been identified, located on the long arm of chromosome 7 (see CHROMOSOME). Known as the *CFTR* gene, it codes for a protein termed the CF transmembrane regulator. One MUTATION resulting in an abnormality in the *CFTR* protein accounts for almost 70% of the mutations causing CF. It is known as the delta F508 mutation. A single AMINO ACID is deleted from this protein in these mutations. As of 2006, more than 1,000 different mutations in the *CFTR* gene have been identified. About 15–20 of these are "common" and account for an additional 2–15% of mutant ALLELES. Most of the others are rare. In U.S. Caucasians, about 90% of CF CARRIERS can be identified by molecular-based carrier screening. In some populations 90–95% of carriers can be found, including Ashkenazi Jews, Celtic Britons, French Canadians from Quebec, and some Native Americans. There is some controversy about whether or not routine carrier testing and screening should be offered, how and to whom.

In families in which a previous pregnancy resulted in CF, both carrier and PRENATAL DIAGNOSIS are possible, through the use of DNA-based molecular testing. Pilot studies of neonatal screening are under way based on blood tests for immunoreactive trypsin. The trypsin is elevated in the newborn's blood because of pancreatic disease.

The finding of fetal echogenic bowel (one creating a strong reflective image) on routine prenatal ultrasound examination can be associated with a slightly increased risk for CF in a pregnancy that had otherwise not been known to be at increased risk for CF.

Routine newborn screening has been implemented in some states. PREIMPLANTATION DIAGNOSIS has been used to allow the birth of a healthy child to known carrier parents. Conception was by in vitro fertilization (IVF). The embryo was tested by removing one cell at the eight-cell stage. Testing was done for the mutation known to be in the family. Only embryos which did not have two copies of the CF mutation were transferred to the uterus for continued development and ultimate birth.

Virtually all males with classic CF have CONGENITAL bilateral absence of the vas deferens (CBAVD). It has now been discovered that there is a population of otherwise entirely healthy men (1/1,000) who have CBAVD and who have a high frequency of CF mutations. About one half of these men have a specific mutation (known as the 5T mutation).

Overall, more than half, and probably about 70% of men with CBAVD have at least one CFTR mutation with about 15–25% having two. Sweat chlorides may be elevated in these men. (Other patients with CBAVD (about 20%) also have renal malformations. These patients are unlikely to have CFTR mutations.)

CF is among the most common fatal inherited diseases. Yet the prognosis for CF has grown much more favorable than when it was first identified. In the early 1950s, children born with the disorder typically died before reaching elementary school age. Today, half live beyond the age of 21. For all ages, prognosis is poorer for females than for males. Repeated lung infections and blocked air passages eventually leading to respiratory failure are the major causes of death.

The fundamental defect is now known, and research is ongoing to use this knowledge to create improved therapies. A transgenic mouse model of CF has been developed. These mice have the same intestinal disease (from which they die in infancy) but no lung disease. Understanding this may give important information in the development of treatment strategies for CF.

The frequency of CF has led to speculation about possible benefits a single copy of the mutated gene may afford carriers. Research indicates such individuals may be more resistant to cholera's lethal ravages.

cystic hygroma   A tumor consisting of enlarged lymphatic vessels or channels that usually appear in various locations on the neck. These structures consist of intact and collapsed cysts held together by connective tissue (stroma) and containing a clear or cloudy fluid. In most of the cases, the cyst is present at birth; in the remainder, it nearly always becomes apparent by the age of two. The cysts vary in size from 2.5 to 15 cm. (1 to 6 inches), and may grow rapidly or slowly. They are not painful unless they become infected. Skin may be stretched thin over this underlying sac, and may have a bluish hue. Large cysts, especially those in CONGENITAL cases (present at birth), may also involve the armpit, structures within the chest, tongue or mouth. Respiratory obstruction is common because of dis-

placement of the windpipe (trachea). Cystic hygromas may be diagnosed before birth by ULTRASOUND.

While the cause of the condition is thought to be generally non-genetic, there have been reports of multiple affected sibs suggesting the possibility of AUTOSOMAL DOMINANT inheritance in some families. Cystic hygromas are also frequently found in association with CHROMOSOME ABNORMALITIES (particularly TURNER SYNDROME). Cystic hygromas IN UTERO, which later resolve (with the fluid being reabsorbed), lead to redundant skin and are the cause of the webbed neck in disorders such as Turner syndrome, NOONAN SYNDROME and FETAL ALCOHOL SYNDROME. Amniotic fluid AFP may be elevated in affected pregnancies.

cystine storage disease   See CYSTINOSIS.

cystinosis (cystine storage disease)   A genetic metabolic disorder, inherited as an AUTOSOMAL RECESSIVE trait and first described in 1903, that causes abnormal amounts of cystine, an AMINO ACID, to accumulate in various cells in the body. Primary sites of accumulation are the eyes, liver, white blood cells, muscles and the kidneys; most of the damage occurs in the kidneys, ultimately leading to kidney failure and death.

Cystine enters the cells normally and is stored in lysosomes, small digestive organelles found within each cell. However, it is unable to be transported out of the lysosomes, reaching from 10 to 1,000 times the normal level, disrupting cellular activity and eventually destroying the cell itself.

The disorder is estimated to occur in one in 150,000 live births in the United States. For unknown reasons, the incidence is on the order of one in 30,000 in Brittany, France. The gene defect is on the short arm of chromosome 17. Designated *CTNS*, the gene encodes, or directs, the production of a protein known as cystinosin. Affected individuals tend to look younger than their age, and most are fair-skinned and blond, even though their parents may have dark complexions and hair.

Although present at birth, there is a variability in age of onset and progression. Typically, it is diagnosed between nine and 18 months of age.

Symptoms are excessive thirst, excessive urination, fever, vomiting, FAILURE TO THRIVE, failure to walk or the development of rickets. Individuals are short statured and usually thin, with small pot bellies. Accumulation of cystine in the eye causes progressive sensitivity to light (photophobia), and ocular defects of the retina and cornea may cause BLINDNESS. Though patients have IQ scores within the normal range, they have been shown to have global intellectual defects. The finding of sugar in the urine leads to frequent misdiagnosis of diabetes (see DIABETES MELLITUS). Further testing reveals other hallmarks of cystinosis, such as excess waste products and acid in the body, ANEMIA and a loss of alkali in the urine. X-rays reveal bone disease. Cystine crystals in the eyes, or cystine in the white blood cells, provide confirmation of the presence of the disorder.

Ultimately, kidney (renal) failure results, generally between the ages of nine and 12 years, and the condition is usually fatal by age 16. Dialysis and kidney transplants are prolonging life among a growing number of affected individuals. However, complications, including possible nervous system disorders, result from the continued accumulation of cystine.

A milder benign or adult form of the disease also exists, with normal renal function but with cystine deposits in the cornea. An intermediate juvenile or adolescent form has renal manifestations occurring in the teens or twenties. The drug cysteamine has been approved for oral use in this condition by the FDA. It is a cystine depleting agent. Cornea transplantation has been used in the management of the corneal disease.

PRENATAL DIAGNOSIS in at-risk pregnancies is possible via CHORIONIC VILLUS SAMPLING. CARRIER detection is possible in families with an affected family member. However, this test is not widely available.

cystinuria An inherited inborn error of AMINO ACID metabolism leading to the formation of pebble-like deposits of the amino acid cystine in the kidney, ureter or bladder.

Symptoms of the kidney stones may include increased volume of urine excreted, pain to the back or flank from the kidney or ureter, blood in the urine and difficult or painful urination. Urinary tract infections are common. Because of poor kidney function, toxic wastes may accumulate in the blood. Onset of symptoms is generally between the ages of 10 and 30. Less than 3% of known urinary tract stones are cystine stones. They are most common in adults under age 40.

Diagnosis is made by finding increased cystine or cystine crystals in the urine. Some recommend that all patients with urinary "stones" be screened for this disorder. Occurring in about one in 10,000 live births, it is inherited as an AUTOSOMAL RECESSIVE trait. There are at least three variants due to MUTATIONS: Types I, II and III. About two-thirds of all CARRIERS are Type I HETEROZYGOTES (heterozygotes have only one of the two recessive genes required for expression of a recessive trait), whose condition can be detected only by studies of intestinal absorption or transport of cystine. Type II and Type III heterozygotes excrete increased amounts of cystine in urine.

Treatment includes a high fluid intake, ingestion of sodium bicarbonate to keep the urine alkaline, and drugs including D-penicillamine and alphamercaptopropionyglycine, which have been approved by the FDA for use in this disorder. Other new drugs are also being investigated. Without treatment kidney obstruction from the stone deposits can lead to kidney failure. Life span is shortened by more than 10 years in affected males and less than 10 years in females, with death due to kidney failure.

cytogenetics The visualization and study of CHROMOSOMES. Examining chromosomes for abnormalities in size, structure and other aspects provides the means for diagnosing many GENETIC DISORDERS in the fetus. This field of research has led, for example, to identification of the cause of DOWN SYNDROME (an extra chromosome 21) and other genetic conditions caused by CHROMOSOME ABNORMALITIES. Use of the term *cytogenetics* has been dated to "The Chromosomes in Heredity," a paper published in 1903 by Walter S. Sutton of the United States, predating by three years William Bateson's formal proposal to name the study of heredity "genetics."

Cytogenetic analysis for PRENATAL DIAGNOSIS begins with the extraction, primarily through

AMNIOCENTESIS, of sufficient fetal cells for study. The cells are cultured and prepared in the laboratory and stained by a variety of methods to allow effective visualization under a microscope. A photograph of the microscopic image (KARYOTYPE) of the chromosome complement of a cell allows the 23 chromosome pairs each human cell possesses to be arranged in descending order of size and studied for abnormalities that will indicate genetic defects.

An additional aspect of cytogenetic analysis is that the sex of the fetus can be determined by the X and Y chromosome makeup of the fetal cell being examined through the karyotype. A male child will have one X and one Y CHROMOSOME; a female will have two X CHROMOSOMES. Such information will be of value in diagnosing any sex-linked genetic defects.

Cytogenetic analysis may be performed for prenatal diagnosis of chromosome abnormalities primarily among pregnant women 35 years of age or older or among those who have had a previous child with a documented chromosome ANOMALY, or following maternal serum screening that suggests a higher risk for chromosomal abnormalities. Cytogenetic studies are also done on blood (or other tissues) for a variety of other indications. These include individuals who have manifestations suggesting a chromosome abnormality or have multiple malformations, especially when associated with disturbances of growth or MENTAL RETARDATION, newborns with AMBIGUOUS GENITALIA (that is, whose sex is unclear), certain individuals with INFERTILITY, couples who have had multiple miscarriages (see ABORTION) and individuals with leukemias (see CANCER) and certain other tumors where chromosome anomalies have been described and may help determine the prognosis of the disorder. (See also CONTIGUOUS GENE SYNDROME and the Introduction)

cytomegalovirus   See TORCH SYNDROME.

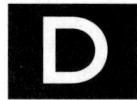

Daltonism   See COLOR BLINDNESS.

Dandy-Walker syndrome   A developmental mal-formation of the fourth ventricle of the brain that frequently results in CONGENITAL HYDROCEPHALUS. The ventricles are the cavities within the brain filled with cerebrospinal fluid. The malformation is char-acterized by hypoplasia or absence of a portion of the middle cerebellum called the vermis and the presence of a large, thin-walled cyst formed at the roof of the fourth ventricle, behind the cerebellum.

Macrocrania is common, as are signs of increased intracranial pressure, including hypotonia, leth-argy, nausea, vomiting and headaches, though indications of cranial nerve dysfunction are rare.

The majority of patients reportedly have addi-tional central nervous system abnormalities. Intel-lectual ability ranges from retarded to normal.

Most patients are diagnosed in the first year of life, though some may not be identified until adult-hood. Radiographs, ventriculography, PEG (pneumo encephalogram) and arteriography have been used for diagnosis, though CT, radionucleotide scanning and sonography are now preferred. Inherited as an AUTOSOMAL RECESSIVE trait, it is also associated with teratogenic and chromosomal SYNDROMES, and is a feature of several genetic and congenital disorders, including AICARDI SYNDROME, CRYPTOPHTHALMOS, cytomegalovirus (TORCH SYNDROME), CORNELIA DE LANGE SYNDROME, maternal diabetes, ELLIS-VAN CREVALD SYNDROME, RUBINSTEIN-TAYBI SYNDROME and prenatal exposure to WARFARIN.

PRENATAL DIAGNOSIS may be possible via sonogra-phy (ULTRASOUND). Karyotyping to look for deriva-tive CHROMOSOMES may be appropriate in high-risk cases. The syndrome is estimated to comprise 3% of cases of hydrocephalus. With hydrocephalus esti-mated to affect 1%–1.5% of the population, Dandy-Walker occurs in one in 2,500 to one in 3,500 live births. Control of the hydrocephalus is the primary treatment, and a variety of shunting methods have been used.

Studies in the mid 1980s found a 27% overall mortality rate, though more recent studies indicate a more positive outlook for affected individuals without serious associated disorders.

Darwin tubercle   A small, visible thickening or protuberance of the cartilage of the rim of the outer ear, common in many populations. Inherited as an AUTOSOMAL DOMINANT trait, it is a benign condition, of interest mainly as a genetic curiosity. It is esti-mated to occur in about 50% of the population in England and Finland, and about 20% in Germany.

dating   While conditions associated with many genetic anomalies and BIRTH DEFECTS have restricted social interactions for many affected individuals, the importance of developing social and sexual rela-tionships for their emotional well-being is increas-ingly recognized.

deafness   The complete or partial loss of hear-ing. Hearing loss is common, with at least 6 mil-lion individuals in the United States believed to be hearing impaired or deaf. Hearing impairment is most frequent among the elderly (thought to be a MULTIFACTORIAL trait, arising from both hereditary and environmental factors). In fact, the chance of developing hearing loss increases with age, and half of all people older than 80 years have impaired hearing. However, some 400,000 children are also affected: About 2/1,000 under the age of three, and 4/1,000 children under the age of 19, are hearing impaired.

About 70–80% of inherited deafness is not associated with any other problems beyond the hearing loss. Severe CONGENITAL deafness or early profound hearing loss occurs in approximately one in 1,000 infants in the United States, and an equal number become deaf or have severely impaired hearing by the age of 16. About half of these conditions of deafness are thought to be genetically caused. Over 400 hereditary SYNDROMES featuring or associated with serious hearing loss have been identified. As an isolated problem, congenital deafness may be inherited in AUTOSOMAL DOMINANT (20% to 30%), AUTOSOMAL RECESSIVE (40% to 60%), MULTIFACTORIAL (20% to 30%) or X-LINKED (2%) forms, though they may be indistinguishable. Mitochondrial inheritance accounts for a very small percentage of hearing loss problems (see MITOCHONDRIAL DISEASES). Even if the mode of inheritance is known, it may be impossible to specify the type of deafness in a given case.

More than 30 different genes have been identified, mutations in which can cause non-syndromic deafness. MUTATIONS in the *GJB2* gene (connexin 26), on chromosome 13q, account for 50% of autosomal recessive non-syndromic hearing loss. The CARRIER rate in the general population for a recessive deafness-causing connexin 26 mutation is about one in 33. A single common mutation, which is called either 30delG or 35delG, is found in over two-thirds of persons with autosomal recessive non-syndromic hearing loss. At least 21 other disease-causing mutations have been identified. The connexin 26 protein is a gap junction protein which functions in the cell-to-cell channels of adhering cells. Overall, the specific mutation 30delG is responsible for 10% of all childhood hearing loss and for 20% of all childhood hereditary hearing loss.

Deafness at birth may also be the result of BIRTH INJURIES, maternal infections or exposure to drugs. Rubella was a major cause of congenital hearing impairment until a vaccine for the virus was developed. Exposure to cytomegalovirus (TORCH SYNDROME) and herpes simplex type 2 virus can also result in congenital hearing loss.

Malformations of the ears may also cause deafness, and are reported in approximately 35 per 10,000 live births. These may accompany significant malformations of the middle or inner ear, and are thought to account for about 2% of conductive hearing loss.

Hearing disorders are classified as either conductive or sensorineural. Conductive hearing loss is caused by abnormalities in the hearing organs; sensorineural hearing loss involves defects in the nerves that transmit auditory impulses to the brain. However, even in these latter cases, some hearing, particularly of low tones, may be possible.

Severe congenital or early childhood deafness is most likely to be sensorineural and affect both ears (bilateral).

As an isolated disorder, affected infants may go undiagnosed for some time, especially since they make sounds until about nine months of age. It is important to detect hearing disorders as early as possible in order to begin and maximize the effectiveness of communication therapy. Congenital hearing loss can be identified through universal newborn screening, which has been advocated by the National Institutes of Health and others. This screening is available in most states.

More than 400 genetic syndromes that include hearing loss have been described.

Genetic conditions of deafness with onset after childhood are more likely to be inherited as autosomal dominant disorders, and more likely to be conductive. These are classified by the age of onset, rate of progression, frequencies involved and severity. Beyond this, it is often impossible to identify or attach a specific designation to them. Additionally, in familial cases there may be a wide variability of expression, such that members may be unaware of a common problem.

If parents with normal hearing have more than one deaf child, the condition is usually an autosomal recessive disorder. If two generations are affected, it is usually dominant. If only one child has congenital deafness and careful investigation has eliminated syndromic or environmental causes, the estimated risk for recurrence in a SIBLING is one in six. If only one parent is affected, the estimated risk is 5%.

If two congenitally deaf people marry, there is a 70% to 80% chance that all their offspring will have normal hearing. Even if the parents both have autosomal recessive hearing disorders, unless the disorders are identical, children will be carriers of the disorders, rather than affected by them. Only 5% to 14% of the offspring of two congenitally deaf individuals are deaf children.

Historically those with severe hearing disorders were often thought to have low intelligence, and the word dumb, from the Old English root meaning mute or unable to speak, a condition exhibited in many with congenital deafness, gradually came to mean unintelligent. However, efforts in the late 19th century to improve education and opportunities for those with hearing disorders have helped reverse this misconception.

Hearing-impaired individuals now have a cohesive and structured social system of their own, in addition to an increased integration into society at large, and many do not regard their condition as a deficit. It has been reported by genetic counselors that some deaf couples or individuals would prefer to have a hearing-impaired child than a child with normal hearing with whom they might not be able to cope.

For syndromes associated with deafness, see ALPORT SYNDROME; MIDDLE-EAR INFECTIONS; OTOSCLEROSIS; PENDRED SYNDROME; TREACHER-COLLINS SYNDROME; USHER SYNDROME and WAARDENBURG SYNDROME.

deafness and functional heart disease   See JERVELL AND LANGE-NIELSEN SYNDROME.

deformity   See ANOMALY.

de Lange syndrome   See CORNELIA DE LANGE SYNDROME.

deoxyribonucleic acid (DNA)   The supermolecule from which CHROMOSOMES are made, and which carries the GENETIC CODE. Nucleic acid was found in the nucleus of the cell by Swiss chemist Friedrich Miescher in 1871, and DNA, its major component, was isolated by English taxonomist Fred Griffith, which he reported in 1928. While many geneticists suspected it played an important part in heredity, this was not proved until 1944, when Oswald Avery of Rockefeller University in New York used DNA to transmit characteristics from one strain of bacteria to another.

Its structure remained a mystery until James D. Watson and Francis H. C. Crick, of the Medical Research Council Laboratories in Cambridge, England, working with physicist Maurice Wilkins, defined its structure. Wilkins had taken X-ray photographs of the molecule revealing a helical shape. In 1953, Watson and Crick published their paper, "Structural Implications of Deoxyribonucleic Acid," in which they proposed the double helix model of the molecule and its functioning, and Wilkins simultaneously published his X-ray photographs. (The three shared the Nobel Prize for their work in 1962.)

As described by Watson and Crick, DNA consists of two long, linked strands, resembling a tightly coiled spiral staircase. Each strand is composed of smaller units called nucleotides which, in turn, are made of a sugar molecule, a phosphate and any one of four nitrogen bases: adenine, thymine, guanine or cytosine. Nucleotides on each strand are linked with a nucleotide on the opposite strand by the nitrogen bases; each nitrogen base joins only with a complementary nitrogen base, and these are called "base pairs." Adenine always joins with thymine, and guanine always pairs with cytosine. A sequence of three nucleotides is called a CODON.

Each DNA strand is made up of millions of nucleotides. The makeup and order of the four different bases within each codon determines the specific AMINO ACIDS that assemble to make proteins. Thus the order of bases determines the specific sequence of a protein's amino acids, which in turn determines that protein's individual function. The DNA bases (ATGC) are like letters of the alphabet that combine to form words (amino acids), which join together to form sentences (proteins) that have specific meanings (functions in the cell).

When the DNA replicates during cell division, the two strands divide down the middle, with the base pairs unlocking, and each strand becomes a template, attracting mirror-image segments of nucleotides. When the entire new chain of nucleotides is complete, there is a new, identical double helix of DNA.

DNA controls protein synthesis in a similar fashion: DNA forms a template for RIBONUCLEIC ACID (RNA). The assembled RNA chain exits the nucleus, and itself becomes a template for the construction of the amino acid chains that form proteins and ENZYMES. Thus, genes may be considered a series of codons that give the instructions for assembling a specific protein. The complex process of copying information from DNA to RNA is known as transcription, and the process whereby the RNA instruction set is used by ribosomes in the cytoplasm to construct proteins is known as translation.

Changes or MUTATIONS of individual nucleotides, and changes in DNA, which provides the blueprint, may result in defective formation of proteins and enzymes, and are the basis of many GENETIC DISORDERS. (See also the Introduction.)

dermoid cyst (teratoma)   Rare condition marked by cysts, or sacs containing skin-type tissue (dermoids) or more complex benign tumors composed of tissue not usually found at that site (teratomas). Cysts of both kinds appear most commonly in infancy (dermoid cysts occur almost exclusively in infants and young children) but may not cause symptoms until adulthood.

Dermoid and teratomatous cysts most commonly occur on the lower portion of the spinal chord, accounting for about 2% of spinal tumors. Symptoms of compression of the spinal cord, which vary depending on the specific location, often bring these cases to medical attention. The cysts occur primarily in the lumbosacral region and often accompany occult spina bifida. The second most common sites of teratomas are the sex organs, the ovary or testis. They may also occur on the head and neck.

Teratomas are usually detected in the first two years of life. Malignant degeneration can occur within a teratoma wherever it is. Teratomas account for about 3% of childhood tumors. Most are SPORADIC but some families with an AUTOSOMAL DOMINANT predisposition to ovarian teratomas have been described. Genetic factors seem to play a role in their development and the tumors themselves appear to have two sets of maternal CHROMOSOMES rather than one maternal and one paternal. The size and location of the cyst, or tumor, typically determines its impact and treatment.

Nasal dermoids, which may appear as a small pit or depression on the bridge of the nose with a hair protruding from it, are usually detected shortly after birth. They are slightly more prevalent in males and may be associated with obstructed nasal passages and mucus in the nose.

Infants born with nasopharyngeal teratomas may also have respiratory problems. These tumors, located in the airway between the nose and throat, are six times more prevalent in females than males.

With a teratoma of the orbit (eye), the infant is usually born with a mass behind one eye. This may cause the eye to bulge and may decrease vision. The tumor may extend through defects in the orbit or skull into the brain or nasal cavity.

Tumors that occur in the neck region (cervical teratomas) are usually present at birth and are rare after age one. Symptoms may include noisy or temporary cessation of breathing, a bluish tinge to the skin and difficulty swallowing.

The cause of these tumors and cysts is uncertain. They contain bizarre mixes of malplaced tissues. For example, teratomas often contain skin, hair, bone, teeth and even liver or kidney tissue.

Surgical removal of all tumors is necessary to prevent recurrences and other complications, though tumors rarely become malignant. If the tumor is completely removed, a normal life span can be expected.

DES   See DIETHYLSTILBESTROL.

deuteranomaly   See COLOR BLINDNESS.

deuteranopia   See COLOR BLINDNESS.

developmental disability   Any condition resulting from a CONGENITAL abnormality, trauma, disease or deprivation that interrupts or delays normal growth and development. Children with developmental disabilities may have multiple handicaps with or without MENTAL RETARDATION.

diabetes mellitus   A group of disorders caused by the absence of, or the body's inability to use, insulin. Insulin is a hormone necessary for regulating the blood levels of glucose (blood sugar), which is the body's main source of energy.

The condition known as diabetes has been recognized for millennia. Described in the Egyptian Ebers Papyrus, written about 1500 B.C., it was named by early Greek physicians, who called it diabetes, Greek for "fountain" or "siphon," due to the copious urination that is one of the hallmarks of the disorder in its early, untreated state. They also noted that the urine had a sweet odor and taste, hence the term *mellitus,* which comes from the Latin word for honey. The familial nature of this disorder has been recognized for at least 300 years.

The primary symptoms are elevated blood sugar levels (hyperglycemia), frequent urination, excessive thirst, increase in appetite and weight loss. There can be emaciation, weakness, debility and a low resistance to infections as well as leg cramps, "pins and needles" sensations in the fingers and toes, and blurred vision. Sugar is excreted in the urine. Unsuspected cases of diabetes may first be recognized in a routine urine test. (Sugar in the urine is not always a sign of diabetes; it may merely indicate the kidneys are unable to process normal amounts of sugar. Conversely, sugar is not always present in the urine of diabetics. A glucose tolerance test, which measures the body's reaction to large amounts of sugar or glucose, is another diagnostic test, though individuals who display glucose intolerance do not always develop diabetes.)

If diabetes is undiagnosed and untreated, the body may accumulate incompletely metabolized fats, called ketones, leading to ketoacidosis. This condition is marked by fruity, sweetish breath odor, tremendous thirst and dryness of the tongue and skin, weakness and vomiting. If untreated, ketoacidosis can progress to diabetic coma and death.

Other complications of diabetes may affect the heart, kidneys, eyes, circulatory and nervous systems. Individuals are two to four times more likely to die of heart disease, and their incidence of strokes is two to six times higher than average. Kidney failure and kidney infections are common. Circulatory problems may lead to gangrene in the limbs, sometimes requiring amputation. Diabetes can damage any part of the eye, and is now the leading cause of new adult blindness in the United States, with 6,000 new cases a year developing. Over 90% of those who've had diabetes for 20 years or longer have damage to the blood vessels in the retina. In the nervous system, diabetes can slow reflexes, cause pain, impotence and loss of sensation.

The exact mechanism by which diabetes leads to complications in organ systems is unclear, but high blood glucose levels are thought to play a part. It is a major cause of death, with approximately 150,000 to 300,000 people in the United States dying from diabetes and its complications annually.

The disorder is centered in the islets of Langerhans, small clusters of hormone-producing tissue in the pancreas. The islets contain beta cells, which produce insulin.

There are two major types of diabetes: Type I, formerly referred to as juvenile, insulin-dependent (IDDM) diabetes mellitus; and Type II, formerly adult-onset, non-insulin-dependent (NIDDM) diabetes. Type I involves destruction of the pancreatic beta cells which normally produce insulin. This leads to an absolute insulin deficiency. Type II diabetes involves a combination of insulin resistance in the tissues (a failure to use insulin properly) along with a relative deficiency of insulin.

Type I diabetes (juvenile diabetes; insulin-dependent diabetes mellitus, IDDM)   This is the more severe form, as well as the more care of the two, comprising perhaps 10% of cases. Though most commonly diagnosed from infancy to the late 30s, it can appear at any age. Symptoms usually develop rapidly.

Juvenile diabetes is thought to be an autoimmune disorder (see IMMUNE DEFICIENCY DISEASES). Antibodies, proteins that destroy bacteria and other foreign tissue within the body, perhaps triggered by some infections, attack and destroy the beta cells that produce insulin. Individuals must take daily insulin injections to stay alive.

Familial aggregation in Type 1 has long been noted. However, the disease is not inherited; what is inherited is a susceptibility to develop the disease. Type I is clearly genetically heterogeneous (see HETEROGENEITY). Environmental factors are thought to play a role, and more than one gene may be involved in this predisposition. The environmental triggers in Type 1 diabetes include viral infections. It has also been proposed that dietary exposures, in particular cow's milk, may be a trigger, though this remains unresolved. The HLA genes appear to play a major role in determining the susceptibility to develop diabetes. In addition to HLA genes, other loci (see LOCUS) also play a role: Research is under way to identify these genes. Many (about 15) suspected loci have been mapped. Clearly it is a very complex process. The risk that a SIBLING of an individual with the disorder will develop it is estimated at between 10% and 15%. The risk that a child of an individual with the disorder will develop it is 2% to 5%.

Type II (adult-onset, non-insulin dependent [NIDDM]) diabetes This milder form primarily affects people over the age of 40. Far more common than Type I, it comprises 90% or more of all cases of diabetes. Insulin is produced in varying amounts by beta cells, but the body is unable to use it effectively. Maturity-onset diabetes has a greater genetic component than juvenile diabetes. Virtually 100% of identical twins show concordance for the disorder, that is, if one twin has it, so will the other. The risk that a first-degree relative (sibling or offspring) of an individual with the disorder will develop it is estimated at 10–15%. Thus, genetic susceptibility seems to be the primary determinant of type II. In 2006, a common variant of *Transcription Factor 7-Like 2 (TCF7L2)*, a gene mapped to chromosome locus 10q25.3, was identified as having a role in susceptibility to the disease. It regulates the activity of other genes and may control the levels of hormones that work with insulin to set blood sugar levels. Thirty-eight percent of Americans have inherited one copy of the variant gene, and they have a 45% greater risk of developing Type 2 diabetes than do those without the variant gene. About 7% of the population have two copies of the variant gene and are 141% more likely to develop the disease than those without the genetic anomaly. Nongenetic factors also play a strong role. Being overweight usually contributes to its onset.

Type II is usually treated with diet, weight control and exercise. Oral medication or insulin may be required by some individuals.

There is also a rare form of adult-onset diabetes, maturity-onset diabetes of the young (MODY),

which is transmitted as an AUTOSOMAL DOMINANT trait in some families, with onset usually in adolescence or young adulthood. Among the gene mutations that can cause MODY are those for glucokinase and the *hepatocyte nuclear favor-1 alpha* genes.

Types I and II serve as an exception to a general rule regarding genetic disorders: Usually, the most severe form of a disorder shows the clearest genetic basis. But in this disorder, the genetics of the more severe Type 1 juvenile form are less clear than that of the milder Type 1I adult-onset type.

Taken together, these are among the most common human disorders, estimated to affect 7–10% of the adult population of the Western world. The National Institutes of Health (NIH) estimated in 2005 that 20.8 million Americans had diabetes—6.2 million of the cases undiagnosed. The great majority—90–95%—are Type II diabetes. In Canada, an estimated 2,250,000 had diabetes in 2003, and in aboriginal communities rates of diabetes are two to five times higher than the national average. The World Health Organization estimates 177 million were affected worldwide in 2000, and the figure will reach 300 million by 2025. It causes about 4 million deaths a year, about 9% of the global total.

Black Americans are twice as likely as whites to develop diabetes, and black women are particularly vulnerable, with one in four over the age of 55 having the disorder. The reasons for the disparities in incidence are unclear.

Though it is impossible to calculate the suffering and toll exacted by any disorder, a study by the American Diabetes Foundation found the cost of diabetes in the United States, in medical expenditures and lost productivity, was an estimated $132 billion annually. Based on census bureau population statistics, an estimated 17.4 million Americans will be diagnosed with diabetes by 2020, with costs projected at $192 billion. This figure represents an increase from earlier estimates, as the prevalence of diabetes has increased. A 2003 study by the National Institutes of Health calculated the costs of diabetes in Latin America and the Caribbean at more than $65 billion. In addition to physical complications, diabetes takes a high emotional toll on individuals.

Diabetes and glucose intolerance are also features of many GENETIC DISORDERS and over 70

SYNDROMES, including CYSTIC FIBROSIS, HEMOCHRO-MATOSIS, PRADER-WILLI SYNDROME.

Diabetes—Pregnancy

Diabetes can have a profound impact on pregnancy. Control over the disorder may be complicated by pregnancy, which requires a normalization of blood sugar that may risk frequent hypoglycemia. The risk of a major CONGENITAL malformation in an infant of a diabetic mother is estimated at two to three times greater than the general population's. The overall incidence of BIRTH DEFECTS in offspring of insulin-dependent diabetic mothers is estimated to be 6% or higher. Among the malformations are the caudal regression sequence, an otherwise rare malformation combining failure of the bones of the lower spine and thighs to form properly. The kidneys and cardiovascular system may also be affected, and NEURAL TUBE DEFECTS or other ANOMA-LIES of the central nervous system may occur.

The cause of this teratogenic effect is not under-stood. However, poor control over the disorder seems to increase the risk of congenital malformations. It is imperative that pregnancies of diabetic women be carefully monitored. There is also a condition called gestational diabetes that most commonly appears in pregnancies of overweight women over the age of 35 who have had large babies, were large babies themselves and have a family history of diabetes. While symptoms are mild in the mother, it can pro-duce the same complications for the newborn as other forms of diabetes. Affected infants tend to be large babies with low blood sugar and exhibit respi-ratory distress, though gestational diabetes does not increase the risk of congenital malformations. PRENATAL DIAGNOSIS studies include ULTRASOUND, fetal echocardiography and maternal serum ALPHA-FETOPROTEIN screening, and are recommended as is preconceptional folic acid supplementation.

diaphragm, eventration of the   See EVENTRATION OF THE DIAPHRAGM; DIAPHRAGMATIC HERNIA.

diaphragmatic hernia   Difficulty in breathing is a hallmark of this disorder, an abnormality of the diaphragm, the muscular membrane separating the abdomen from the thoracic (chest) cavity. The lungs are in the thoracic cavity, and the motion of the diaphragm controls breathing.

There are two types of diaphragmatic her-nias. In posterolateral diaphragmatic hernias, the breathing difficulty is caused by the protrusion of an abdominal organ through the diaphragm into the chest cavity. (Posterolateral refers to the loca-tion of the hernia, in back and to the side of the breast bone [sternum].) Infants with this condi-tion may appear bluish at birth. Symptoms prog-ress with this condition as swallowed air distends hollow internal organs and tissues, pushing them into the chest and causing further heart/lung com-pression. The less developed the lungs are, the earlier the onset of symptoms and the higher the risk of death.

This condition occurs twice as often in males as in females. It is thought to be the result of an imbalance in timing in fetal development. As a result, the intestines may migrate into the chest (thoracic) cavity through an abnormal opening in the diaphragm and compress the undeveloped lung buds. Posterolateral hernias are also known as Bochdalek hernias. Fetal surgery has been employed in repair of diaphragmatic hernias. The role of this therapy in general treatment is not yet clear. Incidence of poserolateral hernia is 16–21 per 100,000 births.

The second type of diaphragmatic hernia, called a retrosternal hernia, may also affect newborns but usually isn't recognized until later in infancy and childhood. (Retrosternal refers to the location of the hernia, directly behind the sternum.) Incidence of retrosternal hernia is probably less than one in a million. In most cases these extremely rare her-nias occur on the right side of the body and seldom are they large enough to cause serious symptoms. It is theorized that this type of hernia occurs due to failure of muscular ingrowth during fetal develop-ment, or failure of the diaphragm to fuse properly.

Inheritance modes for either of these condi-tions have not yet been determined. Diaphragmatic defects may be identified prenatally by ULTRASOUND examinations. Individuals with diaphragmatic her-nias may enjoy a normal life span without disability if the repair is straightforward, lung development is normal and there are no other irregularities.

diastrophic dysplasia The name of this form of short-limbed DWARFISM was borrowed from the field of geology in 1960: Diastrophism is the process of the bending of the earth's crust that creates mountains, ocean basins and other features of the planet's surface. In this disorder it refers to the flexion contractures, or permanent bending of the knees, elbows and hips exhibited in some affected individuals. The disorder is variable in its expression.

Like many other forms of short stature caused by defective skeletal development, for many years this disorder was erroneously classified as a form of ACHONDROPLASIA. Many cases of "achondroplasia with CLUBFOOT" are actually diastrophic dwarfism. Additionally, it has been said that this disorder has frequently been erroneously labeled as ARTHROGRYPOSIS in hospital diagnostic files.

At birth, individuals exhibit severe clubfoot (talipes equinovarus) and malformations of the hands, particularly the so-called hitchhiker's thumb. Other joint limitations are also seen. Fingers are short and broad, and their mobility is reduced. About 25% have CLEFT PALATE. Mesomelic limb shortening (shortening of forearm and lower leg) is universal and CONGENITAL joint dislocations are common. In most cases, cysts of the cartilage of the ears swell soon after birth, resulting in a "cauliflower ear" deformity, though in most cases hearing remains unimpaired.

The trunk has an extreme swayback appearance (lumbar lordosis) beginning at an early age. As individuals grow, the face takes on a characteristic appearance, with a narrow nasal root, long, broad philtrum (the groove extending from the bottom of the nose to the upper lip), prominent mouth and square jaw. These features were referred to by the now outdated term "cherub dwarf." Individuals have a distorted gait, due to congenital joint dislocations, with a tendency to walk on their toes. The chest is barrel-shaped, and there may be lateral curvature of the spine (SCOLIOSIS) as well. These abnormalities of the spinal column may cause severe neurological complications. Defects of development of the larynx produce a characteristic soft, rasping or hoarse voice. Intelligence is normal. Average male height is approximately 125 cm (about 49 inches).

Diastrophic dysplasia is inherited as an AUTOSOMAL RECESSIVE trait. About one quarter of affected infants under medical care die due to respiratory difficulties. (A lethal variety of this disorder, also inherited as an autosomal recessive trait, has been reported.) The GENE defect in this disorder involves MUTATIONS in a novel sulfate transporter gene (*DTDST*) found on the long arm of chromosome 5. The gene is also known as the *SLC26A2* gene. More than 20 *SLC26A2* mutations have been identified in people with diastrophic dysplasia. Impaired function of this transporter gene leads to defective sulfate incorporation into important component molecules of cartilage, which now affects how cartilage turns into bone. Other mutations in this gene cause recessive multiple epiphyseal dysplasia, as well as achondrogenesis, type 1B and atelosteogenesis, type 2, which is particularly prevalent in Finland. Impaired function of this transporter gene leads to defective sulfate incorporation into important component molecules of cartilage, which affects how cartilage turns into bone.

PRENATAL DIAGNOSIS has been achieved using ULTRASOUND to detect skeletal abnormalities in the FETUS.

diethylstilbestrol, DES A synthetic estrogen, a female sex hormone, previously prescribed for women suspected of being at risk for developing complications (such as miscarriage) during pregnancy.

Between 1940 and 1971, approximately 2 to 3 million pregnant women were treated with DES, the majority between the years 1946 and 1960. In 1971 the drug was linked to cervical and vaginal CANCER in women (usually 19 to 25 years of age) whose mothers used the drug during pregnancy. These women have been called "DES daughters."

It is estimated that for every 10,000 women exposed during fetal development, approximately 1.4 to 14 develop cervical cancer. A significantly larger proportion (estimated at between 20% and 60%) exhibit other abnormalities of the reproductive system, including structural defects of the cervix, vagina and fallopian tubes. DES daughters are also prone to INFERTILITY, miscarriage and premature delivery. Most DES daughters are now entering middle age and little is known about how exposure will affect menopause. However, DES daughters 40 and older have been found to have nearly twice the risk of breast cancer as unexposed women, and the increased risk is even greater for DES daughters 50 and older. These findings support the hypothesis that one risk factor for breast cancer is prenatal exposure to higher than normal levels of estrogen. The use and safety of hormone replacement therapy in this group is now discouraged as it has been linked to increased risk of breast cancer. There appears to be no known increase in risk of health problems or infertility in DES sons, but some have had minor genetic abnormalities.

Di George syndrome (thymic alymphoplasia) CONGENITAL developmental ANOMALY characterized by abnormalities of the immune system and congenital HEART DEFECTS. The immune system deficiencies are caused by the failure of the thymus gland to develop (see IMMUNE DEFICIENCY DISEASE). In addition, the parathyroid glands, which regulate blood calcium, fail to develop. First described by U.S. pediatrician A. M. Di George (b. 1921) in 1965, it results from an abnormality in the development of the third and fourth pharyngeal pouches of the embryo, from which the aorta forms. Within days of birth, infants may exhibit the grayish or dark purple discoloration of the skin (cyanosis) caused by abnormal amounts of lowhemoglobin blood due to cardiac abnormalities. Seizures may occur as a result of low calcium. There is FAILURE TO THRIVE, and most die within a month of birth from severe cardiac abnormalities or infections.

In half of the cases, the thymus has completely failed to develop, and is underdeveloped in the other half. Once the immune deficiency is identified, infants must be isolated. Those that survive face increased susceptibility to respiratory infections.

More than half of affected infants share characteristic facial features. The placement of the eyes on the face is uneven; one may be slightly below the other or they may be wide-set (HYPERTELORISM). The eye slits (palpebral fissures) are slanted toward the nose. The nose itself is upturned (anteverted nares), and the groove below the nose that meets the lip (philtrum) is short. The upper and lower lip form a cupid-bow shape. The outer ears (pinnae) may be small, low-set or rotated slightly backward, and malformed.

In most cases a deletion in the upper portion of the long arm of chromosome 22 has been found. The deletion is usually only detectable with FISH studies. Cases with this deletion overlap with other presentations of deletion 22 syndrome, and the long-term problems of those affected and natural history of the disorder are the same as those seen in Shprintzen syndrome (see CATCH 22).

Other chromosome abnormalities have also been found in some cases of this etiologically heterogeneous SYNDROME (see HETEROGENEITY). The offspring of women taking Isotretinoin (ACCUTANE) once a day in the treatment of severe cystic acne, have features that resemble the Di George syndrome. Exposure to alcohol IN UTERO may also cause similar features.

The incidence is unknown, but it has been found in 3% of children who succumb to congenital heart disease.

disability, developmental See DEVELOPMENTAL DISABILITY.

discoid lupus erythematosus See LUPUS.

discordance The expression of a specific trait in only one member of a pair of TWINS. (See also CONCORDANCE.)

DNA See DEOXYRIBONUCLEIC ACID.

DNA banking The storage of DNA material for future testing. It is useful in situations where currently available tests cannot definitively identify the genetic basis of a disorder or anomaly exhibited by the donating individual. If a definitive test becomes available in the future, the banked DNA material could then be examined, and the results could prove useful either to the donor or his or her relatives. It is often used in situations when molecular genetic testing is available only on a research basis. The DNA material is typically extracted from white blood cells.

DNA fingerprinting (genetic fingerprinting, DNA profiling)   The use of DNA to identify an individual or their genetic heritage. It is used in clinical genetics to test for hereditary disorders, both prenatally and after birth. The disorders it can identify include cystic fibrosis, hemophilia, Huntington's disease, sickle cell anemia, thalassemia, familial Alzheimer's and many others. The process was introduced by Alec Jeffreys at the University of Leicester in 1985. DNA fingerprinting is also used to identify the remains of otherwise unidentifiable individuals, and in forensics to determine or eliminate suspects in criminal investigations and trials.

DNA probes   Short segments of DEOXYRIBONUCLEIC ACID (DNA) of a specific sequence that can be used to identify some genetic abnormalities. The DNA segments are typically synthesized in a laboratory using biotechnology processing methods to string together the appropriate nucleotides, after identifying the desired sequence. These segments will bind to and identify a specific target segment of DNA. Machines called oligonucleotide synthesizers have been developed specifically to create the probes.

A DNA probe is prepared from normal CHROMOSOMES with the normal complement of GENES. Each probe is specially labeled with either a radioactive or chemical tag that identifies the DNA gene sequence of the particular segment being used. The probe can then be used as a standard against which the DNA of an individual can be compared.

After obtaining a DNA sample from an individual, often a fetus, the DNA is cut into fragments by use of RESTRICTION ENZYMES and mixed in solution or on a filter with selected DNA probe fragments. Similar fragments from both sets of DNA will stick together, while the others wash away. Often, other individuals in the family will also have been tested and a study made of the family's normal genetic makeup. Thus, genetic deviations or abnormalities in the DNA of the individual being tested can be disclosed by a comparison of the family's DNA structure and the segments of the DNA probe that unite with the DNA of the tested person. Where no family study has been possible DNA probes can be used in some instances where previous research has established the presence or absence of a particular

genetic sequence at a specific location indicating a genetic defect, as in PRENATAL DIAGNOSIS using FISH studies.

dolichocephaly   See CRANIOSYNOSTOSIS.

dominant   See AUTOSOMAL DOMINANT.

Donahue syndrome   See LEPRECHAUNISM.

double cortex syndrome (Subcortical band heterotopia; X-linked lissencephaly)   An X-linked disorder characterized by mild to severe mental retardation, behavioral problems and epilepsy. The name of the disorder refers to an extra layer of neurons under the normal gray matter of the brain cortex seen in affected individuals. Double cortex syndrome primarily affects females, though males who inherit the disorder are much more severely affected. They exhibit lissencephaly, or smooth brain, which is associated with severe mental retardation. A mutation of the doublecortin gene has been identified in about half the cases studied, but not in other cases. Moreover, a significant number of cases appear to be sporadic, or resulting from new mutations, because the doublecortin mutation does not appear in other family members of some affected individuals.

Diagnosis is made on the basis of an MRI finding of the brain, which would reveal a characteristic bilateral band of heterotopic gray matter between the lateral ventricles and cortex, separated by normal-appearing white matter.

Down syndrome   Characterized by mental deficiency and typical facial features, Down syndrome is the most common identifiable form of MENTAL RETARDATION. It is named for J. Langdon Down (1828–96), a British physician and early champion of education for the retarded, who in 1866 described a condition he called MONGOLISM in a series of lectures entitled "On some of the mental afflictions of childhood and youth." "Mongolism" referred to the vertical folds of skin obscuring the juncture of the upper and lower eyelids on either side of the nose (epicanthal folds), which, along with the upslanting of the eyes, give individuals an Oriental appearance. However, use of the term *mongolism* is presently discouraged.

Down syndrome is a CHROMOSOME ABNORMALITY. Most cases (95%) result from the presence of a third copy of chromosome 21, a condition called trisomy 21. It is the first condition in humans that was found to be caused by a chromosomal abnormality, and was identified as such in 1959 by French pediatrician Jerome Lejeune. (However, in 1932, Dutch physician P. J. Waardenburg speculated that this could be the cause). The presence of the third chromosome is most often the result of a cell-division error during meiosis, when chromosome pairs normally split in the formation of sperm and egg cells. Thus, the sperm or egg has two chromosome 21s prior to conception, instead of the normal single copy. (In 95% of the cases, the extra chromosome is thought to be in the egg, and in 5% in the sperm.)

In approximately 4% of cases, Down syndrome may result from a translocation, in which extra chromosome 21 material, rather than an entire extra chromosome, is present. In translocation cases there is no association with advanced maternal age but there is a higher recurrence risk if one parent carries a balanced translocation, especially if it is the mother. (In a balanced translocation, no genetic material is lost or gained; it is only rearranged. The carrier parent with a balanced translocation for Down syndrome has material from chromosome 21 switched with another chromosome. An affected offspring of this parent would have two normal copies of chromosome 21, along with additional chromosome 21 material from the gene involved in the balanced translocation. Thus, they essentially have three copies of chromosome 21 material.) Perhaps another 1% of cases are the result of MOSAICISM, a condition in which the error in cell division occurs after the egg has been fertilized, so that some of the individual's cells exhibit the extra chromosome 21, while other cells have only the normal pair. These individuals are generally less severely affected.

Characteristic facial features, in addition to epicanthal folds, include eyes slanted upward away from the nose (mongoloid obliquity), possibly with a speckling at the periphery of the iris (Brushfield spots), and large tongue (MACROGLOSSIA) that often protrudes from an open mouth, making normal speech difficult. Cognitive development HANDICAPS further speech development. (Speech development in infancy is estimated to lag seven months behind unaffected infants.) Other oral abnormalities include fissured lip, delayed eruption or missing teeth and, rarely, CLEFT PALATE. The chin is usually small (micrognathia) and the neck short with extra skin. The outer ears (auricles) tend to be small, and hearing loss is common, with an estimated 75% exhibiting some degree of hearing impairment. Hands are typically short and broad, with a mild incurving (CLINODACTYLY) of the fifth finger. A single crease in the palm (SIMIAN CREASE) is present in about 30% of those with the syndrome. Muscle tone is frequently poor and newborns are often "floppy" (hypotonic).

CONGENITAL cardiac abnormalities are present in about 40% to 50% of affected individuals, and they may lead to death in infancy. An estimated 75% of Down syndrome conceptions are lost before birth most commonly as first trimester spontaneous ABORTIONS. They also have 20 times the risk of the general population of developing leukemia (see CANCER). Incidence of leukemia is about 1%. One fourth of those born with congenital HEART DEFECTS will die in first year of life. Survival rates are highest in those without heart disease. About 12% may have digestive tract problems such as esophageal or intestinal blockages. Ultimately, individuals with Down syndrome develop an Alzheimer's-like dementia, characterized by the development of amyloid plaques in the brain (see ALZHEIMER'S DISEASE) and many succumb to complications by the age of 35. About 1/2 survive beyond 50, and one in 7 is still alive at 68.

Overall incidence is about one in 800. About 7000 affected children are born in the United States each year. Risks of having an affected infant rise dramatically with maternal age (as they do for all chromosomal abnormalities). Under age 30, the chances of having an affected child are estimated at one in 1,000, while chances are put at one in 35 for women aged 44 and one in 10 at age 49. The reason for the increased risk is unknown but is thought to be due to the female's possessing all her oocytes, or egg cells, at birth. Thus, they may be exposed to environmental agents or deteriorate over time, so that they are more prone to errors when being transformed into eggs at advanced maternal age. There is also increased risk among women who have had a previous child with the SYNDROME, or those who themselves have Down syndrome (though pregnancy is rare in this condition).

There is a wide variation in the degree of retardation among affected individuals. Until the 1970s, the majority were institutionalized, but new attitudes and educational opportunities are enabling many of them to lead productive and meaningful lives. A little over half have IQs of 30 to 50, classified as moderate retardation, and are capable of achieving some degree of self-sufficiency. Children with Down syndrome tend to be very sociable and loving. A television series about a family with a teenager with Down syndrome, *Life Goes On*, appeared in 1989.

A number of controversial treatment therapies have been proposed for Down syndrome. Plastic surgery has been advocated to change their physical appearance with the view that it is easier to change the individual's appearance than to remove the misconceptions and prejudices in others that the appearance triggers. Treatments with vitamin and mineral supplements have also been advocated. There has been no convincing evidence that this costly endeavor is beneficial, and, in fact, high dose megavitamin supplements may have potentially harmful side effects.

PRENATAL DIAGNOSIS with AMNIOCENTESIS and CHORIONIC VILLUS SAMPLING is recommended for all pregnancies beyond the age of 35. As a result of the availability of less invasive prenatal screening techniques, using ULTRASOUND, such as NUCHAL TRANSLUCENCY SCREENING, in 2007, the American College of Obstetricians and Gynecologists recommended all pregnant women undergo screening for Down syndrome. While infants born to older women are at greater risk for the condition, the majority of those affected are born to younger women, simply because this segment of the population is responsible for more births. Prenatal screening is now available using maternal serum screening with ALPHA-FETOPROTEIN, hCG and other analytes. It enables calculation of risk that the pregnancy is affected with Down syndrome or certain other abnormalities, but it does not detect the abnormality itself. Like those pregnancies suspected to be affected on the basis of ULTRASOUND detected "markers," confirmation is by chromosome analysis of fetal cells obtained by a procedure such as amniocentesis.

drug abuse   A large number of infants are believed to be exposed to illegal drugs IN UTERO due to mater-

---

TABLE IX
EMPIRIC RISKS* FOR DOWN SYNDROME LIVE BIRTH

Source	Risk (%)
Young mother with previous trisomy 21 (or other trisomy) live birth, miscarriage or stillbirth	About 1
Occurrence of trisomy 21 in a 2nd- or 3rd-degree relative; maternal age below 35	Somewhat increased but still less than 1
Rare families with two or more cases of trisomy 21	Risk markedly increased for 1st- and 2nd-degree relatives
Mother with a 21/13, 21/14, or 21/15 translocation	About 15
Father with a 21/13, 21/14, or 21/15 translocation	About 5
Mother with a 21/22 translocation	About 10
Father with a 21/22 translocation	About 12
Either parent with a 21/21 translocation	100
Decreased levels of maternal serum alphafetoprotein	Studies indicate increased risk

*Maternal-age specific risks not included.
Reproduced with the permission of the National Genetics Foundation, Inc., from R. B. Berini and E. Kahn (eds.), *Clinical Genetics Handbook* (Orodell, N.J.: Medical Economics Co., Inc., 1987). All rights reserved.

nal drug abuse. Surveys of pregnant women in hospitals across the United States have found at least 11% of women use illegal drugs during pregnancy, exposing an estimated 430,000 newborns a year to potential damage, at the turn of the century. This estimate is considered conservative. The drugs include COCAINE, MARIJUANA, heroin, methadone, amphetamines and PCP, and their use appears to transcend social and economic boundaries.

These figures do not include maternal abuse of alcohol, which is considered to be a larger problem. (Abuse of prescription drugs can also interfere with pregnancy and fetal development.)

Infant damage associated with maternal drug abuse includes prenatal strokes, retarded fetal growth, premature birth (see PREMATURITY), LOW BIRTH WEIGHT, abnormalities of the development of genital, urinary and abdominal organs, and seizures after birth.

Additionally, pregnant drug abusers may have a difficult time receiving help for their dependency; due to liability concerns, some addiction treatment programs will not knowingly treat pregnant women. (See also FETAL ALCOHOL SYNDROME; TERATOGEN.)

Dubowitz syndrome Infants with this disorder, first described in 1965 by Victor Dubowitz, professor of pediatrics at the Royal Postgraduate Medical School in London, usually have LOW BIRTH WEIGHT, an unusually small head (MICROCEPHALY) and are slightly built. They also have a distinct facial appearance marked by sparse hair, a high sloping forehead, flattening of the ridges above the eyes, drooping upper eyelids (PTOSIS), folds of skin at the inner corners of the eyes (EPICANTHUS) and prominent or low-set ears. The features resemble those of FETAL ALCOHOL SYNDROME.

During the first year of life the infant usually develops a skin rash on the face and limbs (eczema) and may suffer from chronic diarrhea. Affected males may have undescended testes (CRYPTORCHISM) and may have a condition known as HYPOSPADIAS, where the opening of the urethra is located on the underside of the penis.

As they grow, affected individuals usually develop an uneven jaw, a high nasal bridge and general facial asymmetry. Some are retarded (generally mildly)

and most have a hoarse, high-pitched voice. Behavioral problems including hyperactivity are common, as are learning difficulties and speech deficits.

Inherited as an AUTOSOMAL RECESSIVE disorder, to date over 50 cases have been reported, most occurring within a few families. Overall prognosis for a normal life span is favorable.

Duchenne muscular dystrophy See MUSCULAR DYSTROPHY.

ductus arteriosus, patent, PDA See PATENT DUCTUS ARTERIOSUS.

duodenal atresia or stenosis The CONGENITAL blockage of the upper segment of the intestine, the duodenum. In those affected, usually the duodenum is constricted (stenosis), rather than completely unconnected (atresia) due to developmental failure. Generally, it is not diagnosed until a few days after birth. If not treated and repaired surgically, death will result, though more than 60% of affected infants survive.

Occurring in an estimated one of every 10,000 births, a little over half of those with this condition under medical care were LOW BIRTH WEIGHT infants. Most cases are SPORADIC. It is often associated with other ANOMALIES, and can be seen in other SYNDROMES, particularly DOWN SYNDROME; approximately 30% of individuals with the condition have this intestinal blockage as well, though the reason is unknown. Other associated syndromes include fetal hydantoin or THALIDOMIDE exposure, OPITZ G/BBB SYNDROME and TOWNES-BROCKS SYNDROME. Recurrence risks are low (‹5%).

Dupuytren contracture Disorder characterized by progressive flexion deformities of the fingers, particularly the fourth and fifth digits, resulting in permanent bending of the affected fingers. Onset may begin in infancy, though symptoms are most obvious after age 40. Eventually, the hand loses functional ability due to the inability to extend the fingers. The deformity results from abnormal growth of fibrous connective tissue bands within the palm of the hand. It primarily affects adult white males of Northern European origin. In the United States, an estimated 5–15% of males older than 50 years are affected. In studies, 27–68% of patients present a positive family history.

It is named for Guillaume Dupuytren (1775–1835), the preeminent French surgeon of the early 19th century, who first published a report of the disorder in 1833. A brilliant but ruthlessly ambitious, obsessive-compulsive perfectionist, contemporaries labeled Dupuytren "first among surgeons and last among men" and the "Napoleon of surgery." Dupuytren contracture exhibits familial aggregation (see FAMILIAL DISEASE) and is thought to be inherited as an AUTOSOMAL DOMINANT disorder with partial sex-limitation; the ratio of affected males to females is 6:1. It is often seen in association with PEYRONIE DISEASE.

dwarfism   A general term for conditions of short stature. Prior to 1900, classification of dwarfism was rather unrefined, leading to frequent misdiagnosis of various forms and leaving little reliable historical data on incidence or other aspects of the disorders. Classification has improved greatly in recent years due to advanced diagnostic techniques and increased research. The medical profession now recognizes some 200 conditions associated with dwarfism. About half are specific disorders; the remainder represent rare, unidentified conditions that have been seen in one family or individual. ACHONDROPLASIA accounts for approximately half of all cases of dwarfism.

There are more than 500,000 adults below 5 feet in height, and an estimated 500,000 children with growth deficiencies. (Individuals are generally considered dwarfed if their full-grown height is below 4 feet 10 inches [145.4 cm]. Approximately 3% of adult females are estimated to be under 4 feet 11 inches in height, and 3% of adult males under 5 feet 4 inches [160.2 cm].) However, the majority of infants seen by doctors—due to parental concern about growth deficiencies—merely exhibit delayed development and ultimately reach normal adult height.

In the majority of types of dwarfism, life span and intelligence are normal, though some forms are lethal or associated with severe mental impairment.

Dwarfs have been seen in the human population throughout history. They are believed to have been given magical significance in the prehistoric world, and they often occupied unique positions of importance in recorded history. Skeletal remains of achondroplastic dwarfs have been found by archaeologists at prehistoric sites, and figurines and amulets in their shape dating to these same periods have also been found. The pharaohs and their nobles are said to have delighted in having dwarfs in their households, and there are many statues, drawings and records attesting to their special status in Egypt. The Egyptian god Ptah was sometimes depicted as a dwarf, and mummified remains of dwarfs have been found in royal tombs as well as in tombs of dwarfs themselves. They were also invoked in spells involving childbirth and other rituals. Dwarfs continued as court favorites during the Roman Empire; many emperors kept dwarfs, sometimes as trusted advisers. Through the Middle Ages their popularity in royal households remained constant, and they were seen in nearly every court, often fulfilling the role of jester. This practice lingered in Russia and Sweden well into the 19th century, while in the United States of the era, the public appeal of the dwarf was personified by TOM THUMB.

The term *dwarf*, was formerly used to describe short-statured individuals with disproportionate physiques. MIDGET was used to describe a short-statured individual of normal body proportions. (This dwarfing is not actually proportionate, as upper/lower body segment ratios may not be in the normal range.) However, contemporary short-statured individuals regard the term midget as derogatory. The origins of the objection to this term are believed to derive from its circus sideshow associations as well as resentment from a time when proportionate short-statured individuals were perceived by those of abnormal proportions as having fewer social disadvantages. Preferred terminology today includes *dwarfs* and *small, little* or *short* people.

Proportionate dwarfing (physiologic dwarfing) is usually caused by one of several factors:

Chromosome abnormalities. Missing or abnormal (e.g., rearranged) CHROMOSOMES are responsible for some forms of short stature, for example, TURNER SYNDROME.

Hormone failure. There may be disturbances or deficiencies of the pituitary or thyroid glands, which are responsible for regulating normal growth.

Primary growth disturbances. Some infants do not respond to normal growth factors. This is often the case in certain malformation syndromes. (See PITUITARY DWARFISM SYNDROMES.)

Secondary growth failure. Growth may be stunted by disease, such as kidney failure, or as a result of fetal exposure to certain TERATOGENS.

Poor nutrition. Chronic malnutrition can result in short stature.

Inherited short stature. This is the most common form of short stature. If parents are short-statured, their offspring tend to be short-statured as well.

(For information on specific forms of proportionate dwarfing, see also SECKEL SYNDROME; HALLERMANN-STREIFF SYNDROME; PYGMIES; CORNELIA DE LANGE SYNDROME; LEPRECHAUNISM; NOONAN SYNDROME.)

Disproportionate dwarfing is usually the result of defective skeletal development (skeletal DYSPLASIA). There are over 100 recognized dysplasias that result in short stature, usually caused by an inherited single GENE, a metabolic disturbance or an unknown factor. The molecular basis of number of forms of skeletal dysplasia is being elucidated. The genes involved include those for the fibroblast growth factor receptors, collagen genes, and transporter proteins (e.g. the diastrophic dysplasia sulfate transporter).

Disproportionate forms of dwarfism are classified as either short-limb or short-trunk types, depending on whether the limbs or trunk show the most evidence of dwarfing. The short limb type is further classified by the section of the limb most affected. In rhizomelic dwarfing, the sections closest (proximal) to the trunk, the upper arms and thighs, are most shortened. Mesomelia indicates primary involvement of the middle portion of the limbs. Acromelia designates the distal portions, or the extremities of the limbs, the hands and feet. Most cases of disproportionate dwarfing are hereditary, but a significant number are the result of new MUTATIONS.

For information on specific forms of disproportionate dwarfism, see also ACHONDROGENESIS; CAMPTOMELIC DYSPLASIA; DIASTROPHIC DYSPLASIA; METAPHYSEAL CHONDRODYSPLASIA; HYPOCHODROPLASIA; KNIEST DYSPLASIA and PYCNODYSOSTOSIS.

Diagnosis may require multiple specialists, e.g., geneticist, endocrinologist, orthopedist and diagnostic procedures, including X-rays, hormone tests, chromosome analysis or other tests.

Treatment is usually multidisciplinary, involving orthodontist, endocrinologist, geneticist, neurologist, physical therapy, often dentist, psychologist and ophthalmologist. Psychosocial and GENETIC COUNSELING can help answer questions from affected individuals and relatives. Hormone replacement with growth hormones may be of use in cases of growth hormone deficiency (pituitary dwarfism syndrome) and perhaps in Turner syndrome.

PRENATAL DIAGNOSIS may be possible for some skeletal dysplasias using ULTRASOUND. Diagnosis is dependent on specific disorder.

Dyggve-Melchior-Clausen syndrome A rare inherited form of short trunk DWARFISM. Infants born with the SYNDROME have a short neck, protruding broad chest (PECTUS carinatum) and small head (MICROCEPHALY). Signs of MENTAL RETARDATION may develop in the first year of life. As the child learns to walk, a waddling gait becomes noticeable. Other characteristics include short, broad pelvic hip bones (ilia), short fingers, toes and wrists, and pronounced curvature of the lower back (lumbar lordosis). Restricted joint mobility and contractures are seen. X-rays reveal the spinal column is abnormally shifted toward the front of the body, which may result in damage to the spinal cord. Surgical procedures are available to correct bone abnormalities. The disorder resembles the MUCOPOLYSACCHARIDOSES but does not involve the same biochemical pathways.

First described by Danish physicians Holger V. Dyggve, Johannes C. Melchior and Jorgen Clausen in 1962, the original patients were three children from an uncle-niece marriage in Greenland. About 50 cases have been reported, with a disproportionate number of them of Lebanese background.

The illness is thought to be an AUTOSOMAL RECESSIVE syndrome. There is no test at present to diagnose the disorder prenatally. The life span of affected individuals is difficult to predict, but those with mental retardation generally live into their 20s, while those of normal intelligence live into their

40s. Some patients with the identical features but with no mental retardation have been described. This is sometimes differentiated as Smith-McCort dwarfism.

dysautonomia   See FAMILIAL DYSAUTONOMIA.

dyschondrosteosis   See MESOMELIC DYSPLASIA, LANGER TYPE.

dysgenesis   Defective or abnormal formation of an organ or portion of the body, particularly during embryonic development.

dyskeratosis congenita   A rare HEREDITARY DISEASE characterized by hyper- and/or hypopigmentation of the skin, progressive dystrophy (deterioration) of the nails and formation of hard, patches (leukoplakia), occasionally fissured, primarily on the neck, upper chest and arms. Hyperpigmentation may be present at birth, but most of the characteristic symptoms occur between the ages of five and 15 years of age.

Overgrowth of skin on the palms and soles (hyperkeratosis) may result in lack of fingerprints or footprints. The palms and feet are also prone to excessive sweating (hyperhidrosis), and chronic tearing may also be present due to the absence of the ducts (lacrimal puncta) at the corner of each eyelid that normally drain tears. The mucous membranes of the lips, mouth, eyes, uretha and/or anus may also exhibit the characteristic hard, fissured patches found on the upper trunk. MENTAL RETARDATION is an occasional feature. Reduction in the number of blood cells due to bone marrow failure (pancytopenia) is seen in about 50% of cases. Affected patients are predisposed to developing cancer, particularly those affecting the head and neck or gastrointestinal tract, as well as leukemias.

First reported by H. N. Cole in 1930, about 120 cases have been reported. Two genes have been identified as causing this disorder, but do not account for all cases. The *DKC1* gene, which encodes a protein known as dyskerin, accounts for the X-linked form, and a gene variously known as *DKC2* or *TERC* appears to account for the autosomal dominant form seen in some families. Male-to-male transmission has been documented. Sporadic cases represent a significant proportion of the reported total. About 75% of affected patients are male.

Invariably fatal, the average age of death is 24. Most patients succumb before the age of 30 from infections, pancytopenia or malignancies arising from the leukoplakia.

dyslexia   A defect in reading and writing unaccompanied by other impairment of intellectual function. The concept of a specific SYNDROME involving the inability to read evolved in the 19th century, and was articulated in German neurologist Adolf Kussmaul's description of "word blindness" in 1881. The term *dyslexia* was first used in 1887 by Rudolf Berlin, a physician and professor in Stuttgart, Germany who noted a loss of reading ability among some patients who suffered stroke or trauma.

Dyslexia is a biologic problem distinct from less specific reading difficulties. It is thought to be caused by a central nervous system inability to organize graphic symbols. One of the hallmarks of the disorder is the inversion and transposition of letters and numbers when writing or reading, but this is actually not present in the majority of cases. An alternative diagnostic indication is a reading level less than 80% of mathematical level.

While dyslexia likely has numerous origins, familial cases are well documented. One study of the immediate family of children with dyslexia found that 45% of 75 first-degree relatives examined were considered affected. A hereditary form, transmitted as an AUTOSOMAL DOMINANT trait, with reduced PENETRANCE in females, has been identified. Investigators have identified a biologic marker for dyslexia: a striking difference in brain activity and in the functional organization of the brain's visual system in adults with dyslexia. It is elicited by their viewing of moving dots, and the brain activity is studied using a technique called function magnetic resonance imaging.

A developmental gene that guides the axons, or nerve connections linking the brain's two hemispheres, *ROBO1* has been linked to dyslexia. It is located on the short arm of chromosome 3 (3p12). A second gene that appears to play a role in the disorder, *DCDC2,* is active in the reading centers in the human brain. It has been mapped to the short arm of chromosome 6 (6p22.1). Other genes associated with dyslexia have been mapped to a region of chromosome 6 associated with the immune system. Dyslexics are known to often have hay fever, asthma, rheumatoid arthritis, ulcerative colitis or other immune disorders, and this suggests there may be a link between autoimmune diseases and dyslexia.

dysostosis   A general term for defective bone formation, or ossification, a characteristic of many GENETIC DISORDERS affecting the skeletal system. However, it is more properly used to describe malformations of individual bones either singly or in combination. This is, as opposed to the osteochondrodysplasias, more generalized abnormalities of cartilage or bone growth and development. Examples of dysostoses are CRANIOSYNOSTOSIS, KLIPPEL-FEIL SYNDROME, SPONDYLOTHORACIC DYSPLASIA, TREACHER-COLLINS SYNDROME and POLYDACTYLY.

dysplasia   The abnormal organization of cells into tissues during embryonic development. It involves the process of histogenesis (the origin and development of tissue) and is rarely confined to single organs.

dysplasia of the nails with hypodontia   See TOOTH-AND-NAIL SYNDROME.

dysplastic nevus syndrome (malignant melanoma syndrome)   A disorder marked by the formation of potentially malignant nevi or moles during adolescence or young adulthood (see NEVUS). The nevi may vary in size, shape and color, and appear most frequently on the trunk. Some may exhibit excessive growth (hyperplasia) of melanin-forming cells, and may develop into malignant melanomas.

Multiple heritable forms, transmitted as autosomal dominant traits, exist, caused by mutations in

genes including *CDKN2A* on the short arm of chromosome 9, and *CDK4* on the long arm of 12. The disorder may occur sporadically, and many cases are likely multifactorial. Males and females are affected in an equal ratio. Affected individuals are advised to avoid excessive exposure to the Sun and undergo periodic dermatologic examination for changes to nevi. Even in those cases that involve changes in the *CDKN2A* gene, exposure to UV radiation from sun exposure plays a large role. Since 1960, mortality from melanoma in the United States has risen more than mortality from any other cancer except carcinoma of the lung. Mutations in the *CDKN2A* gene in patients with familial melanoma syndrome are also predisposed to other cancers including pancreatic cancer. (See CANCER: MELANOMA.)

dystonia (torsion dystonia; dystonia musculorum deformans)   Incapacitating neurologic (nerve) disorder whose major manifestation is sustained involuntary muscle contraction which can result in repeated and uninterrupted twisting and writhing movements. It may affect a single muscle, a group of muscles, such as those in the arms, legs or neck, or the muscles of the entire body. In children, the legs, back and arms are most frequently affected, while in adults, manifestations in the face and neck are most common. It is a disorder of movement that does not affect memory, intellect or physical senses.

Early symptoms may be very mild and noticeable only after long exertion, or during times of stress or fatigue. Handwriting may deteriorate after a few lines. There may be footcramps, or one foot may drag or tend to pull up after walking or running. The neck may turn involuntarily, especially when tired. There may be tremors and speech difficulties. Dystonic motions may lead to permanent physical deformities by causing tendons to shorten and connective tissue to build up in the muscle.

First described in 1907, the prevalence of the disorder is uncertain, with estimates of between 11 per million and 248 per million of the population, though these estimates may be low due to undiagnosed cases. There is no definitive test for the condition. Diagnosis is based on observation of symptoms and tests of muscles. The cause is unknown, though it is thought to involve the basal ganglia, which lie at the base of the brain and are responsible for controlling movement. Generalized dystonia is thought to be more common in Ashkenazi Jews (those of eastern European ancestry) and possibly individuals of northern Swedish extraction.

Dystonia is clearly etiologically heterogeneous (see HETEROGENEITY) and occurs in a number of different forms which differ on the basis of their clinical presentations as well as the underlying genetic basis. It also results from other causes, for example lesions of the basal ganglia caused by trauma (including BIRTH INJURY), or infection; certain neuroleptic drugs (as in neuroleptic induced tardive dyskinesia) or other exposures (e.g., carbon monoxide, heavy metals), or due to other identified neurologic disorders (e.g., WILSON DISEASE or type I GLUTARIC ACIDURIA). Other forms of torsion dystonia are also associated with other symptoms, often neurologic, such as Parkinsonian symptoms (tremor and rigidity) or deafness. Torsion dystonia has been found to have AUTOSOMAL DOMINANT, AUTOSOMAL RECESSIVE and X-LINKED variants. A number of different genes have been mapped.

Autosomal Dominant Dystonia

The classic form of torsion dystonia appears to be autosomal dominant with reduced PENETRANCE (only about 30–40% of those who carry the disease-causing MUTATION manifest symptoms). This is the type found to cause classic early-onset generalized dystonia, found at greatest prevalence in Ashkenazi Jews. It is the most severe and common form of hereditary dystonia.

The age of onset is between five and 16 years, usually beginning in the foot or, less often, the hand. Involuntary dystonic movements may progress rapidly to all limbs and torso. The progression slows considerably after adolescence.

A GENE for dominant dystonia, *DYT1*, has been mapped to the long arm of chromosome 9. (The gene is also known as the *TOR1A* gene and encodes the torsin A protein.) The mutations in the *DYT1* gene are thought to account for approximately 30–60% of early-onset dystonia in non-Jews and about 90% in Ashkenazi Jews. But because only a minority of all dystonia is the early onset type, the rate of *DYT1* as a percentage of all dystonia is low.

Almost all cases (in both Ashkenazi Jews and other populations) have an identical, unique mutation with a deletion of three base pairs from this gene. The mutation seems to have arisen independently in different ethnic populations. Identification of this mutation allows DNA-based diagnosis of the disorder, even in apparently sporadic cases.

Currently there is no treatment for the disorder, but symptoms can sometimes be controlled with muscle relaxants or by drugs that affect the metabolism of chemicals responsible for transmitting nerve impulses. Early diagnosis and counseling to help deal with the emotional adjustment to the illness are important. A number of surgical treatments have been used in an effort to interrupt the pathways causing the abnormal movements. Deep brain stimulation has been used with some success. A treatment for certain types of dystonia involves the use of injections of botulinum toxin into affected muscles.

In some patients with dominant dystonia, the symptoms emerge in late adolescence or early adulthood. In these cases, symptoms often begin in the torso, and a common feature is involuntary neck muscle movements (torticollis). Progression, while slow, is continual.

Another autosomal dominant form of dystonia is responsive to L-dopa, and displays marked variation over the course of the day. It has been found to result from point mutations in the *GTP cyclohydrolase I* gene found on chromosome 14q.

Autosomal Recessive Dystonia

An autosomal recessive form of dopa-responsive dystonia results from point mutations in the *tyrosine hydroxylase* gene on 11p. (A point mutation is a mutation in a single base pair of DNA; one single letter of the DNA code is altered, and one letter is substituted for another.) Other loci map to 1q, 2q, 8 and 18p as well as the long arm of the X chromosome (dystonia-Parkinsonism).

Focal Dystonia

Though often not hereditary, these localized dystonias represent some of the most interesting and perplexing movement disorders, and include writer's cramp, blepharospasm (characterized by uncontrolled blinking, which may eventually render an individual unable to see), and oromandibular dystonia, which causes the mouth to pull open or shut tight, creating difficulties of speech and swallowing. Meige's disease, a combination of blepharospasm and oromandibular dystonia, is also called Brueghel's syndrome, because the 16th-century Flemish artist, Peter Brueghel the Elder, painted individuals with this condition. Torticollis, also known as cervical dystonia, affects the neck muscles, causing the head to twist to one side, and often forward or backward. It can occur at any age, although most individuals first experience symptoms in middle age. About 10 to 20% of those with torticollis may experience a spontaneous remission, but it may not be lasting. This is the most common of the focal dystonias. (Blepharospasm is the second most common focal dystonia.) Overall, adult-onset focal dystonia is the most common form of dystonia.

dystonia musculorum deformans   See DYSTONIA.

dystrophin   The *dystrophin* gene, located on Xp, makes a protein of the same name. This protein is a vital part of a protein complex that connects a muscle fiber's cytoskeleton, or structure that maintains a cell's shape, to the surrounding connective tissue through the cell membrane. The mutation of this gene, and the resulting deficiency of this protein, is one of the causes of the muscular dystrophies. Its absence also can result in fibrosis, a condition characterized by the hardening of muscles. The protein was identified in 1987 by Louis M. Kunkel, the year after the discovery of the gene mutation responsible for Duchenne muscular dystrophy.

A different mutation of the same gene causes defective dystrophin, leading to Becker's muscular dystrophy (BMD). Dystrophin is the longest gene identified to date, measuring 2.4 megabases. It is so large it accounts for 0.1% of the human genome.

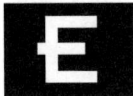

ear, hairy   See HAIRY EAR.

Ebstein anomaly   A congenital HEART DEFECT that manifests (as do many others) in heart murmurs, congestive heart failure and a bluish or grayish color of the skin (cyanosis) caused by insufficient oxygen. Named for Wilhelm Ebstein (1836–1912), a German physician who described it in 1866, the anomaly consists of the downward displacement of the tricuspid valve (which separates the right atrium and right ventricle), possibly interfering with nerve impulses that control the muscular contractions of the heart, increasing the risk of sudden cardiac arrest and death.

The extent of the defect is highly variable and may be severe enough to cause fetal or neonatal death. Among those who survive, symptoms include shortness of breath (dyspnea) following exertion, weakness and fatigue, and abnormally rapid heart beat (tachycardia). The heart may appear enlarged upon examination by X-ray.

Inheritance is believed to be MULTIFACTORIAL, though AUTOSOMAL RECESSIVE transmission has also been suggested in some cases. Maternal ingestion during pregnancy of lithium, a drug often used to treat MANIC-DEPRESSION has been implicated as a cause in some cases.

Incidence is estimated at one in 50,000 in the general population and one in 20,000 live births. It is thought to account for perhaps one in 200 cases of CONGENITAL heart disease.

ectodermal dysplasia (ED)   A group of rare disorders resulting from abnormal development of the ectoderm, the outer layer of fetal tissue that develops into skin, hair, teeth, nails, sweat glands, glands of the mouth, the nervous system, parts of the eye, the pineal gland and parts of the pituitary and adrenal glands. Any disorder that involves defective development of more than one ectodermal structure is considered to be a form of ED.

Historical data concerning this group of disorders dates back to an account by W. Wedderburn, whose description, in 1838, of the "toothless men of Scinde," members of a Hindu kindred in the vicinity of Hyderabad, India, was cited by Charles Darwin in *The Variations of Animals and Plants Under Domestication* in 1875.

> I may give an analogous case, communicated to me by Mr. Wedderburn, of a Hindoo family in Scinde, in which ten men, in the course of four generations, were furnished, in both jaws taken together, with only four small and weak incisor teeth and with eight posterior molars. The men thus affected have very little hair on the body, and become bald early in life. They also suffer much during hot weather from excessive dryness of the skin. It is remarkable that no instance has occurred of a daughter becoming affected . . . though the daughters in the above family are never affected, they transmit the tendency to their sons: and no case has occurred of a son transmitting it to his sons. The affection thus appears only in alternate generations, or after long intervals.

The condition was named ectodermal dysplasia by Dr. Ashley A. Weech in 1929, in a report in the *American Journal of Diseases of Children.* A dysplasia refers to any abnormal development. (German F. G. Danz, in 1792, had described two Jewish boys born with no hair and no teeth.)

As the teeth are so often affected, individuals need early and ongoing comprehensive dental care.

Any ectodermal structure may be involved. The skin may be lightly pigmented, thin, delicate and prone to infections or rashes. Scalp and body hair may be thin, sparse or lightly pigmented. Some or all of the teeth may be missing or malformed. Teeth that are present tend to erupt late and may be peg-shaped or pointed. Eyes may have CATARACTS, corneal clouding, nystagmus, STRABISMUS and other ocular defects. There may be a hearing disorder. Some individuals exhibit learning disabilities.

Though there is great variability among the forms of ED, and within individual cases of any given form, ED is often divided into two major types, based on whether or not the individual can sweat normally. In hidrotic EDs, the production of sweat is normal. In hypohidrotic EDs, which tend to be more severe, sweat is greatly reduced or absent.

The increased severity of hypohidrotic EDs is generally the result of the deficiencies of the sweat glands, which render the body unable to regulate internal temperature. Overheating, often to the point of heat exhaustion, may occur, especially in hot weather. Additionally, respiratory infections are common as the protective secretions of the mouth and nose are absent.

Characteristic facial features of this form include flat face around the cheekbones and nose, with a depressed nasal bridge. The forehead is broad, with prominent ridges above the eyes. The lips may protrude, and the eyes may be dry and prone to develop abrasions or cataracts.

Because the ectoderm forms so many structures, ectodermal dysplasias take many different forms. The primary features of some of the more recognized of the over 100 different syndromes are listed below.

Christ-Siemens-Touraine syndrome, CST; hypohidrotic ED (AUTOSOMAL RECESSIVE, X-LINKED recessive). This is the best known of EDs, characterized by decreased sweating, absent or undeveloped eyebrows and eyelashes, sparse hair, small and missing teeth, deficient tears and sensitivity to light (photophobia). Nails are unaffected. Beard and mustache hair are normal. The GENE for this form is named *ED1* and deletions and point MUTATIONS found. Classic CST is an X-linked recessive trait affecting only males, though HET-

EROZYGOTE females may be missing teeth or have patchy areas of decreased hair (hypotrichosis) or decreased sweating. These female CARRIERS may also have hypoplasia of breasts. In appropriate families, carrier testing and PRENATAL DIAGNOSIS may be possible using either detection of the mutation known in the family or linkage methods. An autosomal recessive form has a similar PHENOTYPE and is very rare. Mutations in the *EDAR* and *EDARADD* genes underlie both the autosomal recessive form (which is clinically indistinguishable from the X-linked form) and an autosomal dominant form, which is milder.

Clouston ED; hidrotic ED (AUTOSOMAL DOMINANT). Total baldness, severe nail dysplasia and thickening of skin on palms and toes characterize this disorder. Sweating is normal as are teeth, generally, though NATAL TEETH—present at birth—may be a feature, along with scanty eyebrows and lashes. The gene maps to long arm of chromosome 13. This form appears to be more common in French Canadians.

Ectrodactyly–ED–cleft lip–palate. See ECTRODACTYLY-ECTODERMAL DYSPLASIA CLEFTING SYNDROME.

Hay-Wells syndrome (autosomal dominant). Fused eyelids (ankyloblepharon), hair, nail and skin abnormalities, CLEFT LIP and CLEFT PALATE, and mildly diminished sweating and abnormal teeth are features of this very rare form of ED. It is caused by mutations in the *TP73L* gene, which encodes the p63 protein. Mutations in this gene, located on the long arm of chromosome 3, also underlie split-hand/foot malformation (ectrodactyly), the EEC SYNDROME, limb-mammary syndrome, acro-dermato-ungual-lacrimal-tooth (ADULT) syndrome, and Rapp-Hodgkin syndrome.

Hypertrichosis lanuginosa (autosomal dominant). Excessive hair, of extreme degree; affected individuals often appeared as "sideshow" performers. Descriptions have included "The Dog-Faced Boy" or "The Sacred Hairy Family."

Hypomelanosis of Ito (autosomal dominant). Characterized by asymmetric, bizarre hypopigmented areas of skin (whorls or lines), ocular defects, abnormal or missing teeth, hypohydrosis, MENTAL RETARDATION and seizures. Affected individuals may be found to have chromosomal or genetic MOSAICISM: In fact, it appears that hypomelanosis of Ito is a manifestation of an etiologically heterogeneous group of disorders (see HETEROGENEITY), the most common factor being the presence of two genetically distinct cell lines which differ in one of several ways: by a point mutation (a mutation in a single base pair of DNA) of a specific pigmentation gene, a chromosome translocation (frequently involving a translocation between an X chromosome and one of the autosomes), ANEUPLOIDY, deletion, or tetraploidy. Females are affected more often than males.

Incontinentia pigmenti (Bloch-Sulzberger syndrome) (X-linked dominant). Lethal in affected males IN UTERO. Among females, hair is either absent or abnormal. Skin involvement is the most consistent feature. The condition initially manifests as redness and areas of inflammation and progresses to blisters in first weeks of life. These heal, leaving thickened, rough warty growths which persist for six to 12 months. Between three to six months, hyperpigmented lesions, typically in streaks and whorls appear, leaving a marbled pattern to the skin. One-third will have mental retardation, MICROCEPHALY, spasticity and/or seizure. Over 600 cases have been reported. Mutations in the *IKK-gamma* gene, which is also called *NEMO* and *IKBKG*, and maps to Xq28, cause incontinentia pigmenti. A variety of malformations of the eye, teeth, skeleton, heart and other organs may been seen in this disorder. Carrier detection and prenatal diagnosis using molecular genetic testing are available if the disease-causing *IKBKG* gene mutation has been identified in an affected individual in the family.

ectopia cordis   Ectopia refers to the CONGENITAL displacement or malposition of an organ or body part. Cordis refers to the heart. In this condition, the infant is born with the heart outside of the thoracic cavity. It is generally incompatible with life. See congenital HEART DEFECTS.

ectopia lentis   Subluxation, or dislocation of the lens of the eye. The condition can lead to GLAUCOMA. In rare cases it may occur as an isolated defect. More commonly it is a manifestation of a number of multisystem diseases, including MARFAN SYNDROME, HOMOCYSTINURIA, Weil-Marchesani syndrome, to name a few. As an isolated defect, both AUTOSOMAL DOMINANT and AUTOSOMAL RECESSIVE inheritance have been seen.

ectrodactyly   A congenital absence or malformation of the fingers or toes, ranging from partial to complete absence of a finger or toe, which occurs sporadically, to CLEFT hand or foot deformity (lobster claw deformity) or to absence of all but the fifth finger or toe. Cleft hand and foot deformities are generally characterized by absence of the central finger or toe and clefting into the near portion of the hand or foot, with webbing of the remaining fingers or toes on each side of the cleft. It also includes cases known as split-hand/foot malformation. The more severe malformations usually occur in both hands (bilaterally), and foot involvement is frequent.

Several genetically distinct traits appear to be associated with the defect, generally showing AUTOSOMAL DOMINANT transmission with considerable variability in severity. GENES for a number of different forms of isolated or syndromic ectrodactyly have been mapped to various CHROMOSOMES. Some cases have been found to have mutations in the *TP73L* that maps to the long arm of chromosome 3 and encodes the p63 protein. Mutations in this gene also underlie Hay-Wells syndrome, the EEC SYNDROME, limb-mammary syndrome, acro-dermato-ungual-lacrimal-tooth (ADULT) syndrome, and Rapp-Hodgkin syndrome. Ectrodactyly (as manifested by cleft hand) occurs in approximately one in 55,000 to one in 70,000 newborns. Reconstructive surgery may be helpful in repairing the deformity. PRENATAL DIAGNOSIS has been accomplished by ULTRASOUND. (See also ECTRODACTYLY-ECTRODERMAL DYSPLASIA CLEFTING SYNDROME.)

ectrodactyly-ectrodermal   dysplasia   clefting syndrome (EEC syndrome)   The primary manifestations of this rare SYNDROME are lobster claw deformity of the hand (ECTRODACTYLY), abnormalities of skin and its appendages (ECTODERMAL DYS-

PLASIA) and CLEFT LIP and CLEFT PALATE. Other oral features of the syndrome include absence of teeth, usually the permanent incisors, decreased formation of enamel, deeply furrowed tongue and dryness of the mouth.

The absence of a tear duct opening may be associated with increased tearing and inflammation of the eyelids and the tear sac. There may also be simultaneous inflammation of the corneas and the mucous membrane covering the eyeball (which occurs due to dryness) and sensitivity to light (photophobia).

The scalp hair, eyelashes and eyebrows may be sparse, and nails may be underdeveloped and brittle. Skin biopsy may reveal absence of sweat glands or irregular clustering of sweat pores. A child with the syndrome may have difficulty regulating body temperature due to a decrease in sweating.

ULTRASOUND examination during pregnancy may detect many of these abnormalities. The majority of patients with hand or foot deformity and cleft lip/palate require surgical correction of the anomaly. Opening of the tear duct is essential to prevent chronic inflammation, which can lead to blindness. Intelligence and life span are rarely affected.

It is inherited as an AUTOSOMAL DOMINANT trait with a variable degree of severity of its manifestations among affected individuals, even within families. Some cases have been found to have mutations in the *TP73L* that maps to the long arm of chromosome 3 and encodes the p63 protein. Mutations in this gene also underlie Hay-Wells syndrome, some cases of isolated ectrodactyly (split-hand/foot malformation), limb-mammary syndrome, acro-dermato-ungual-lacrimal-tooth (ADULT) syndrome, and Rapp-Hodgkin syndrome. There appear to be at least two other loci (site of the GENES) for this syndrome, one on chromosome 7 and the other on 19. A large number of patients live in Denmark.

education Individuals affected with some genetic or CONGENITAL conditions associated with MENTAL RETARDATION (such as DOWN SYNDROME) were historically regarded as largely uneducable. However, new approaches and opportunities for their education reveal a higher degree of learning ability than previously thought possible.

In the United States, individuals handicapped by a GENETIC DISORDER, or congenital ANOMALY, or for any other reason, must, by law, have access to the same educational opportunities as non-handicapped individuals (see HANDICAP). The 1975 Education of the Handicapped Act provides federal financial assistance to states to ensure that each child with handicap(s) receives a free, appropriate public education.

Institutions receiving this financial assistance must provide educational services that meet handicapped children's individual needs as adequately as those services provided for non-handicapped children. Additionally, it is required that handicapped and non-handicapped children be educated together, to the extent possible. Parents and guardians may review education and placement decisions made on behalf of their child, and be given due process to challenge those decisions.

Children with handicap(s) must also have equal opportunity to participate in extracurricular activities such as counseling, physical education, recreational athletics and transportation.

These guidelines apply to primary, secondary and postsecondary education.

Edward syndrome (trisomy 18) A CHROMOSOME ABNORMALITY in which an extra chromosome 18 is present. Named for English medical geneticist J. H. Edward (b. 1928) who published a description in 1960, it occurs in an estimated one in 7,000 live births, with females being affected three times as often as males. It is characterized by a variety of developmental abnormalities of the chest, hands and feet, joints, skeletal muscles, heart, kidneys and genitals. Fingerprints are also abnormal. The hands, often clenched (with the index finger overlapping the third and the fifth over the fourth), are frequently held next to the head in what has been described as a "pleading" position.

The characteristic face includes an elongated, narrow skull (dolichocephaly; see CRANIOSYNOSTOSIS) with a prominent bulge at the back of the head (prominent occiput). Ocular abnormalities include small eyes (microphthalmia), eye slits (palpebral fissures) that are short, and clouding of the cornea. The mouth is small, as is the chin (micrognathia).

The ears are low set and poorly formed. The breast bone (sternum) is characteristically short. The "rocker-bottom" feet have prominent heels.

Infants have LOW BIRTH WEIGHT and FAILURE TO THRIVE. About one-third succumb within the first month of life, half within the first two months, and 90% within one year. Females tend to survive much longer than males (134 days mean survival time vs. 15 for males). Mental and developmental retardation is universal.

It is caused by nondisjunction, or improper distribution of chromosomes, in this case a third chromosome 18, most often resulting from a cell division error during meiosis, when chromosome pairs normally split in the formation of sperm and egg cells. Thus, the affected sperm or egg has two chromosome 18s prior to conception, instead of the normal single copy. Risk of having an affected child rises with maternal age. Incidence is estimated at one in 5,000 to one in 7,000

EEC syndrome See ECTRODACTYLY-ECTODERMAL DYSPLASIA CLEFTING SYNDROME.

Ehlers-Danlos syndrome (EDS) A group of disorders of the connective tissue, which includes tendons, ligaments, skin, bones, cartilage and the membranes surrounding blood vessels and nerves. These highly variable disorders can be characterized by easily bruised and highly elastic skin that is prone to tear, extreme joint laxity giving the appearance of double-jointedness, and multiple chronic dislocations and broken bones. Premature birth is common in some forms, due to early rupture of the fetal membranes (see PREMATURITY). At birth, there are often scars on the forehead and chin. The ears frequently stick outward. The skin is often described as "velvety," or like chamois. Bruised skin heals with peculiar, "cigarette paper" scars. Normal bumps and bruises can result in serious injury. In some patients most surgery can be undertaken only at great risk, due to fragile tissue and uncontrollable bleeding, and in some forms of the disorder major heart problems, rupture of major blood vessels, aortic aneurisms and internal bleeding can create lethal complications.

The SYNDROME is named for eminent Danish dermatologist Eduard Ehlers (1863–1937) and French dermatologist Henri A. Danlos (1844–1912), who described various forms of the condition in the early 1900s.

An inherited disorder, at least 10 varieties have been identified, transmitted in AUTOSOMAL DOMINANT, AUTOSOMAL RECESSIVE and X-LINKED forms. The forms vary in their severity. Some are associated with mild symptoms. Others can result in severe disability and death, as described above. Typically, there is little variability among affected family members. In 1997, researchers proposed a simpler classification that reduces the number of major types from the previously delineated 10 down to six.

The basic cause is not known for all types of the disorder. In some forms, defective biosynthesis of collagen appears to play a role. Tissue strength and limited elasticity are associated with normal collagen structures.

Type I (gravis) Severe "classic" features as described above of soft, fragile, hyperextensible skin, "cigarette paper" scars, easy bruisability, and large and small joint hypermobility. Hernias and varicose veins are frequent. An autosomal dominant disorder, at least some cases are caused by mutations in the gene for the alpha-1 chain of a type V collagen (*COL5A1*).

Type II (mitis) Classic features with milder expression. Scarring, bruising and joint hypermobility are less severe. Varicose veins and hernias are less common. This is the most common variant of EDS. An autosomal dominant disorder, some cases are allelic to the type I form caused by *COL5A1*; that is, mitis involves different mutations to the same gene. Types I and II are grouped together in the new classification as classical type. Less commonly, mutations in the *COL5A2*, *COL1A1* and *COL1A2* genes, or even more infrequently in another gene, *TNXB*, cause the classical type.

Type III (benign familial hypermobility) Minimal skin involvement, marked large and small joint hypermobility, recurrent joint dislocations and early osteoarthritis are the hallmarks of this autosomal dominant form. While in most cases the underlying molecular defect of this very common type of Ehlers-Danlos syndrome is unknown, mutations in one copy of the TNXB gene may be responsible for the condition in 5–10% of cases. This gene encodes a protein called tenascin-X and is located on the short arm of chromosome 6.

Type IV (ecchymotic or arterial type) The skin is thin and not hyperextensible, with visible underlying veins prone to easy bruising. Joints are not hypermobile (except small joints of the hand). Bowel rupture, uterine rupture during pregnancy, arterial rupture (including aneurysms) which may lead to death also occur. Significant complications are rare before the 20s, but the mean of age death is in the early 30s. An autosomal dominant disorder, mutations in the COL3A1 gene result in abnormal type III collagen. New mutations are common: One-half of affected individuals have no family history.

Type V (X-linked) Similar to type II but transmitted as an X-linked recessive trait.

Type VI (ocular) Ocular fragility along with skin and joint features similar to type II, e.g., scoliosis (spinal curvature), poor muscle tone and motor developmental delay. An autosomal recessive disorder, it is caused by a defect in the enzyme lysl oxidase. This form is very rare with fewer than 60 cases having been reported.

Type VII Soft hyperextensible, easily bruisable skin that is not fragile and with nearly normal scarring. Marked joint hypermobility and congenital hip dislocation. It has been subclassified into three types: Types A and B are autosomal dominant and have mutations in the *COL1A1* and *COL1A2* genes respectively, while type C is autosomal recessive and due to a deficiency of the enzyme procollagen N-proteinase.

Type VIII (periodontal) Severe generalized periodontal (gum) disease with loss of most teeth by the early 20s accompany the characteristic thin, fragile, hypersensitive skin exhibiting abnormal scarring and easy bruising, and the mild to moderate joint laxity. It is an autosomal dominant disorder.

Type IX (occipital horns) Same as X-linked cutis laxa: lax, soft skin, bony growths (exostoses) at the back of the skull (occipital horns) and other skeletal abnormalities. Bladder diverticulae during childhood and mild chronic diarrhea are common. The X-linked recessive condition results from abnormal copper metabolism. Different mutations in the same gene cause MENKES SYNDROME. Thus, it is allelic (see allele) to that disorder.

Type X Features similar to type II with a disorder of platelet aggregation. Transmitted through autosomal recessive inheritance. A single affected family has been described.

Types I and II together are estimated to affect one in 20,000 to 40,000 people, and type III as many as one in 10,000 to 15,000 people. Type IV occurs in about one in 250,000 people. The other types are all very rare. Many cases may remain undiagnosed. Physicians may regard the continual bone breakage some affected individuals exhibit as attributable to clumsiness.

Contortionists (such as sideshow "Indian rubber man") generally have a form of this disorder. Niccolò Paganini, whose remarkable dexterity and virtuosity on the violin has been attributed by some to an unnatural (dis)ability wrought by MARFAN SYNDROME, has been suggested by others to have instead had EDS.

There is no accepted method of PRENATAL DIAGNOSIS for all forms of EDS, though theoretically AMNIOCENTESIS and CHORIONIC VILLUS SAMPLING can successfully detect those forms associated with identified genetic or biochemical defects.

Elephant Man See NEUROFIBROMATOSIS; PROTEUS SYNDROME.

elfin faceies with hypercalcemia See WILLIAMS SYNDROME.

elliptocytosis See HEREDITARY ELLIPTOCYTOSIS.

Ellis–van Creveld syndrome (chondroectodermal dysplasia) A rare form of short-limbed DWARFISM. First reported in 1940, it is named for Richard Ellis (1902–66), professor of pediatrics at the University of Edinburgh, and Simon van Creveld (1894–1971), a pediatrician in Amsterdam and authority on HEMOPHILIA. According to medical folklore, they met on a train while traveling to a medical congress and wrote a description en route of the syndrome that now bears their names.

While approximately 100 cases have been reported, half of them have been in an inbred religious group, the Old Order Amish, living in the vicinity of Lancaster, Pennsylvania.

In addition to short stature, the disorder is characterized by the presence of extra fingers (POLYDACTYLY) and congenital HEART DEFECTS, most typically atrial septal defect.

At birth, the head and face are normal, but there are frequent dental and oral abnormalities, such as NATAL TEETH, and a pseudocleft of the upper lip referred to as "partial hare lip" or "lip-tie." Dental abnormalities become more prominent with age. Fingernails and toenails are poorly formed. The upper and lower limbs are short, particularly in their middle (mesomelic) sections. The trunk and head size are relatively normal.

The disorder is inherited as an AUTOSOMAL RECESSIVE trait. Approximately half of patients die in early infancy due to cardiorespiratory difficulties. The majority of the survivors have normal intelligence. PRENATAL DIAGNOSIS has been accomplished by ULTRASOUND. Mutations in either of two genes, *EVC* and *EVC2,* have been identified as causing the disorder in some patients. The genes are located very close to each other on the short arm of chromosome 4. In families in which the gene defect has been identified, DNA analysis can allow carrier detection and prenatal diagnosis.

encephalocele   The protrusion of brain tissue through a congenital skull defect. Like SPINA BIFIDA and ANENCEPHALY, this is a NEURAL TUBE DEFECT (NTD), in this case a defect in the closure of the embryologic structure that leads to the brain, the membranes that surround it, and the bone that covers it, the skull. As the spinal cord protrudes through the bony defect in spina bifida, in encephalocele a portion of the brain is extruded through the skull defect. The brain pushes out with a bulging sac covered by skin and brain membranes (meninges) and containing cerebrospinal fluid that normally cushions the brain.

An encephalocele may form at the lower back of the head (occipital encephalocele), at the rear of the side of the skull (posterior parietal encephalocele) or in the front (anterior encephalocele) on the face. The most common type is the occipital, which may be associated with an abnormally small head (MICROCEPHALY), with the head flexed backward against the spine. An enlarged head caused by fluid accumulations (HYDROCEPHALUS) is also possible in some cases, especially with the posterior parietal type. An anterior encephalocele appears as a swelling at the base of the nose, which may progress and become associated with hydrocephaly, wide-set eyes (HYPERTELORISM), pulsating bulging eyes (exophthalmos) and difficulties with breathing, vision and feeding.

Mortality can range from 60% when hydrocephaly is present to 100% when there is a combination of massive occipital encephalocele and microcephaly. Treatment can involve surgery to close the skull opening and drain the cerebrospinal fluid from the sac. Among those who survive, about half will have various physical disabilities, including paralysis, BLINDNESS, seizures, retarded growth and defective muscular coordination (ataxia). MENTAL RETARDATION of varying degree can be as high as 40%.

Encephaloceles have a higher rate of associated anomalies than other forms of NTD. Frequency ranges from one in 2,000 to one in 5,000 live births. ULTRASOUND examination and detection of an elevated level of ALPHA-FETOPROTEIN produced by the FETUS is employed in PRENATAL DIAGNOSIS.

Encephaloceles may also be components of other syndromes, such as MECKEL SYNDROME and AMNIOTIC BAND SYNDROME. They have been reported in association with teratogenic insults, including maternal rubella (see TORCH SYNDROME), DIABETES MELLITUS and Warfarin embryopathy.

It is important to recognize those situations where the encephalocele is part of a larger syndrome when considering recurrence risks. When isolated, the risks of recurrence are likely to be the same as for the other NTDs.

enchondromatosis (Oilier disease)   Benign, slow-growing tumors of bone cartilage, resulting in a wide variety of skeletal deformities affecting primarily the long bones of the arms and legs. It includes bowing of bones, enlargement of the finger and toe bones, shortening of the limbs and deviation of the larger forearm bone (ulna) in its connection to the wrist. Bones may fracture easily, and the tumors may become cancerous (chondosarcoma) later in life. Enchondromes may also occur in other disorders.

The disorder is detectable after birth through clinical findings and X-ray examination. The growths appear near the ends of the long bones. Single or multiple bones may be involved. Typically the growths stop at the end of adolescence. Cancerous degeneration is rare. The exact cause of this disorder is not known, and most cases occur sporadically. Orthopedic procedures may alleviate some of the associated physical problems. Well over 100 cases have been reported.

endocrine neoplasias, multiple (MEN)   See MULTIPLE ENDOCRINE NEOPLASIAS.

enlarged vestibular aqueduct syndrome (EVA; dilated vestibular aqueduct [DVA]; vestibular aqueduct syndrome)   The most common anomaly of the inner ear, capable of causing progressive or fluctuating deafness.

The vestibular aqueduct is the bony conduit that connects the inner ear to the brain's cerebrospinal fluid. During normal gestation it develops from a short, wide shape into a narrow elongated form. But in some pregnancies the vestibular aqueduct never grows and remains in its short, enlarged or dilated form. The condition predisposes affected individuals to progressive deafness or episodes of impaired hearing. At birth, hearing is normal. It is thought that head trauma or changes in pressure on the inner ear, such as a rapid descent in an aircraft, can trigger the onset of deafness, which occurs suddenly. Both ears are typically involved and hearing is most affected in the higher frequencies. Loss of a sense of balance, or disequilibrium, is also common.

The condition is inherited as an autosomal recessive trait, and the gene thought to be responsible has been mapped to 7q31. This chromosomal region is also the locus of the genes responsible for Pendred syndrome, a hereditary form of deafness. Mutations in the *SLC26A4* gene, which is responsible for Pendred syndrome, a hereditary form of deafness, have been found in families exhibiting sensorineural hearing loss with EVA.

EVA is thought to account for at least 1–1.5% of cases of sensorineural hearing loss or balance problems. Studies have also concluded EVA is responsible for 5–7% of cases of sensorineural hearing loss of unknown origin The condition is usually diagnosed by radiological examination such as magnetic resonance imaging (MRI) or computerized tomography (CT) scan. However, not all individuals who have enlarged vestibular aqueducts exhibit hearing loss.

enuresis   More commonly known as bed-wetting and historically regarded as solely a psychological problem, a GENE linked to this condition was identified in 1995.

An estimated 5 to 7 million youngsters, mostly boys, are thought to be affected by persistent bed-wetting, or primary enuresis, defined as three or more bed-wetting incidents per week by a child seven years or older. This accounts for 75% of bed wetters.

The gene has been mapped to the long arm of chromosome 13, and appears to follow AUTOSOMAL DOMINANT inheritance patterns. The reason primary enuresis affects mostly boys is unknown. However, the gene may only be part of a larger behavioral SYNDROME.

enzyme   An organic catalyst required for a biochemical reaction; though enzymes do not enter into these reactions, they must be present for the reactions to occur. There are hundreds of enzymes in the human body. Composed of complex proteins, they are produced by RIBONUCLEIC ACID (RNA), which is a copy of a segment of DEOXYRIBONUCLEIC ACID (DNA); the DNA holds the master blueprint for the assembly of these enzymes. GENES are themselves segments of DNA. Thus, if there is a change or MUTATION in a gene, it is a change in the DNA, and this change in the blueprint may result in faulty enzyme assembly. This is the basis of hundreds of hereditary enzyme deficiency diseases. (See also BIOCHEMICAL ASSAYS.)

enzyme replacement therapy   The use of enzymes to treat diseases resulting from enzyme deficiencies.

Enzymes are required for catabolism, or metabolism of complex fat and protein molecules. Deficiencies may result from mutations of a gene or genes that render an individual unable to produce a necessary enzyme (as in Gaucher disease) or to provide enzymes the body can produce but which it cannot make use of (as in cystic fibrosis, where pancreatic enzymes are blocked by mucus buildup).

The therapy has been used since the 1960s when it was used to treat patients with Fabry disease by the intravenous (IV) infusion of normal plasma, which contains galactosidase, and the treatment of type 11 glycogen storage disease by infusion of glucosidase. Enzymes can also be taken orally for some disorders (e.g., cystic fibrosis). The therapy is also currently used to treat Gaucher disease and MPS 1 and 2.

epicanthal fold   See EPICANTHUS.

epicanthus (epicanthal fold)   Taken from the Greek *epi,* "upon or over," and *kanthos,* corner of the eye, this is a fold of skin that covers the inner corner of the eye; commonly seen in Asians, to a lesser degree among blacks and in a significant percentage of prepubertal whites. The small skin fold, joined to both the upper and lower eyelids, obscures the juncture of the lids. While primarily a benign condition of only cosmetic interest, it is also a frequent feature of many GENETIC DISORDERS, for example, DOWN SYNDROME.

There are three major theories about how this condition arises: That it is caused by excessive skin at the base of the nose, poor development of the bridge of the nose or retention of the fetal epicanthal fold, which is normally present in the fetus from the third to sixth month of prenatal life.

Epicanthus is variable in its expression. When present as an isolated characteristic rather than part of a larger SYNDROME, epicanthus is inherited as an AUTOSOMAL DOMINANT trait. It occurs in males and females with equal frequency. Approximately 70% of Asians and perhaps 50% of blacks exhibit epicanthus. It occurs in about 20% of white infants at age one, a figure that drops to an estimated 3% by age 12 as the fold of skin gradually disappears. In rare cases where the epicanthus is pronounced it may create vision problems by interfering with the field of view. Cosmetic surgery can remove the obstructing skin. Epicanthus may also make the bridge of the nose appear flat and give the usually mistaken impression that the eyes are misaligned. However, essentially this is a benign condition unless part of a larger syndrome.

epidermal nevus syndrome   The distinctive nevi (see NEVUS) that characterize this rare disorder may be present from birth, often forming in a line and most frequently appearing on the face. Seizures, mental and visual deficiencies, skeletal abnormalities and atrophy of the brain are common accompanying features.

The nevi exhibit excessive pigmentation and are usually found mid-face, from the nose to the forehead and scalp. At puberty the lesions develop wartlike elevations, sometimes accompanied by the growth of tumors caused by increased cell growth of the sebaceous glands. Reported skeletal deformities include backward or lateral curvature of the spine and foot and ankle malformations.

Approximately 450 cases have been reported, affecting males and females in an equal ratio. The cause is unknown. Two-thirds of the cases appear to be inherited as an AUTOSOMAL DOMINANT trait. Impact on lifespan is unclear.

epidermolysis bulossa (EB)   A group of 20 rare GENETIC DISORDERS characterized by blistering of the skin and mucosal membranes, ranging in expression from mild to lethal, depending on the specific type of the disorder. (Bullae are large blisters filled with fluids.) Copious blistering may occur after mild irritation or, in severe forms, without any skin friction, and may also form in the mouth, the gastrointestinal, genitourinary and respiratory tracts. In severe forms, blistering causes the loss of body fluids, blood and proteins, and may result in dehydration, anemia and growth retardation. Treatment is aimed at preventing the mechanical traumas that lead to blistering.

The basic defect that causes the disorders involves MUTATIONS in the GENES for various structural proteins found in the skin and connective tissues. The different forms involve different genes, including those for keratins, type VII collagen, laminins and integrins, among others. The overall incidence of EB is estimated at one in 20,000 live births, though it has also been estimated that between 25,000 and 50,000 Americans have some form of the disorder.

Relatively important forms of the disorder (which are classified on the basis of whether or not they lead to scarring, on their mode of inheritance and on their microscopic appearance) include the following:

Dominant simplex This autosomal dominant form usually appears soon after birth, or when the infant begins to crawl, and blistering most commonly affects the hands and feet. The severity of the lesions often lessen by puberty. There is no scarring. It is caused by point mutations in one of several keratin genes.

Dominant dystrophic A childhood form of EB, with onset before the age of one year in 20% of cases. Blistering appears on the ankles, knees, elbows, hands and feet. Oral blistering occurs in about one-fifth of the cases. It is inherited as an autosomal dominant trait, linked to the collagen VII, alpha 1 chain gene (*COL7A1*). Some improvement is common with age. This form has been diagnosed prenatally by a finding of elevated ALPHA-FETOPROTEIN levels in the AMNIOTIC FLUID.

Recessive dystrophic In this AUTOSOMAL RECESSIVE form, blistering begins soon after birth and can occur spontaneously. The eyes, teeth, mouth and esophagus are also commonly involved, in addition to blistering of the skin. Severe scarring occurs as the blisters heal, leading to hand deformities and obstruction of the esophagus. Death often occurs in childhood. It is caused by different mutations to the same gene (*COL7A1*) that causes the dominant diastrophic form of EB. (Thus, it is an allelic form of that type; see ALLELE.)

Recessive lethal (Herlitz type) Appears at birth, and complications (including excessive bleeding due to rupturing of blisters) cause death by the age of three months. Both of these latter forms have been detected prenatally by obtaining samples of fetal skin via FETOSCOPY for biopsy. A heterogeneous group of mutations in the genes encoding for alpha 6 or beta 4 integrin, collagen XVII or one of the three chains of laminin 5 all may cause this type of EB. All these genes are involved in the formation of hemidesmosomes or anchoring filaments, and defects in these cause junctional type epidermolysis bullosa. Junctional EB includes both Herlitz type and non-Herlitz type. (See HETEROGENEITY).

DNA-based PRENATAL DIAGNOSIS for EB has been accomplished and can be done in those families where the molecular basis of the disorder has been investigated and elucidated.

epidermolytic hyperkeratosis A hereditary, CONGENITAL skin disorder of variable severity characterized by thick, warty, blistering skin with large red patches (erythroderma) covering much of the body. Hyperkeratosis is an overgrowth of the horny layer of the epidermis. The skin at joint creases is particularly affected. Though scales may improve to localized disease after puberty, they are lifelong.

Transmitted as an AUTOSOMAL DOMINANT trait, the responsible GENE, keratin K1, is located on chromosome 12q and K10 (17q). About 3000 people in the United States are affected. Prenatal detection is possible via fetal skin biopsy or by DNA analysis when the MUTATION is known via AMNIOCENTESIS.

Application of keratolytics, agents that loosen the horny layer of skin, such as lactate lotion, can alleviate symptoms, as can emollients such as petroleum jelly. Long-term treatment with antibiotics is sometimes used to prevent secondary bacterial infection of the skin from forming pustules. Topical and systemic retinoids, vitamin A derivatives, are helpful for some patients, but care must be exercised in their use due to adverse side effects, particularly the risk to fetal development for pregnant women.

epigenetic modification The process by which a function of a gene is modified without an alteration of its DNA sequence. Epigenetic modification plays a key role in regulating gene expression, genomic imprinting and X chromosome inactivation. It also appears to play a role in aging and in the onset and progression of disorders including cancer, autoimmune diseases and psychiatric disorders.

epilepsy Any of numerous brain function disorders characterized by recurrent seizure attacks with sudden onset. (It is also the most common neurological condition complicating pregnancy.) Seizures occur when normal electrical signals between brain cells temporarily increase or otherwise act abnormally. One percent to 2% of the general population is estimated to have some form of epilepsy, and more males than females are affected. About 5% of the population will have a single seizure at some time in their lives.

There are over 20 different types of seizures that affect consciousness, movement and sensation. Seizures are also known as fits or convulsions, though the latter term is not always accurate because it implies movement. About 30–50% of epilepsy begins in childhood, most commonly in early childhood.

Seventy percent of epilepsy cases are idiopathic; no cause can be determined. With the other 30%, the epilepsy is secondary to an identifiable cause, often an underlying hereditary defect. A genetic cause may be involved in as much as 20% of cases. Epilepsy or seizures are associated with over 200 genetic conditions. However, these are individually rare and likely account for less than 1% of epilepsy patients. Two relatively common single-gene disorders that often cause seizures are TUBEROUS SCLEROSIS and NEUROFIBROMATOSIS. Other important conditions associated with seizures include ANGELMAN SYNDROME, Batten Disease (see NEURONAL CEROID LIPOFUSCINOSIS), and various metabolic disorder such as TAY-SACHS DISEASE and PHENYLKETONURIA.

Even when the cause of an individual's epilepsy is not identifiable, genetic factors undoubtedly influence predisposition to develop seizures. Trauma, infection and tumor are examples of environmental causes of seizures, which may still involve genetic predispositions. Indications that an individual's epilepsy is genetically influenced include a family history of seizures or the presence of additional abnormalities, such as MENTAL RETARDATION, metabolic disturbance, skin lesions, neurologic problems (including certain specific electroencephalographic abnormalities) and peculiar physical characteristics or anomalies.

In the ancient world, epilepsy was considered a divine affliction, and those affected were thought to be touched by the gods. However, Hippocrates (ca. 460–377 B.C.), the father of medicine, speculated that this, and other diseases, were actually hereditary: "But this disease seems to me to be no more divine than others . . . Its origin is hereditary like that of other disease . . . What is to hinder it from happening that where the father and mother were subject to this disease, certain of their offspring should be affected also?"

Considering all causes of epilepsy, a child with one epileptic parent is four to five times more likely than a child with non-epileptic parents to develop the condition. The risk is generally highest if the affected parent is the mother. Sons are slightly more likely than daughters to develop epilepsy, no matter which parent is affected. If one twin develops epilepsy, the risk of a fraternal twin developing it is 5% to 20%, and 40% to 90% for an identical twin.

Various anticonvulsant drugs or tranquilizers may prevent or reduce the severity of seizures in many forms of epilepsy. However, most ANTICONVULSANTS may potentially cause BIRTH DEFECTS if taken during pregnancy. In GENETIC COUNSELING of those with epilepsy, the possible teratogenic effects of anticonvulsant drugs are usually more important than the possibility of transmitting the tendency to have seizures to offspring. Most women with epilepsy will have an uncomplicated pregnancy and deliver a healthy newborn, but this requires specialized care and planning even before conception.

The more common forms of epilepsy include

Generalized tonic clonic seizures (convulsive seizures; grand mal epileptic seizures). The most common form of epilepsy, a generalized tonic clonic seizure often begins with a hoarse cry, leading to unconsciousness, body stiffening and jerking movements. If seizures begin before four years of age, there is a 7.5% chance that SIBLINGS or offspring will develop epilepsy before they are 20. If the age of onset is between four and 15 years, the risk drops to 4.3%.

Absence seizure (petit mal). An absence seizure lasts only a few seconds, occurs mostly in children and usually looks like daydreaming or blank staring, though it may be accompanied by blinking or chewing movements, turning of the head or waving of the arms.

Offspring and siblings of an absence epileptic have, in general, a 2% to 5% chance of developing the condition, though the risk may be as high as 10% for the daughter of an epileptic mother. Absence epilepsy is most likely polygenically inherited, with greater heritability in females.

Infantile spasms (hypsarrhythmic EEG pattern). These occur in infancy and childhood; in general, 5% of affected children have a family history of the condition. Some 15% of cases are idiopathic, and POLYGENIC factors are the likely culprit; in these, the general recurrence rate for siblings is 5% to 10%. Some studies suggest recurrence risks as low as 1.5% for siblings. Other studies suggest the general recurrence rate is in the 5–10% range. Infantile spasm seizures are also associated with genetic SYNDROMES, such as PHENYLKE-TONURIA and tuberous sclerosis, and there is an X-LINKED form as well. It has been reported that 25% of infants with infantile spasms develop tuberous sclerosis.

Myoclonic photosensitive epilepsy. Here, a neurologic hypersensitivity to flashes of light is dominantly inherited. In a small proportion of people with this abnormal EEG pattern, exposure to such light induces seizures. When seizures are present, they appear to be highly inheritable.

Nocturnal frontal lobe epilepsy. An AUTOSOMAL DOMI-NANT disorder, one of several in which specific single genes have been implicated. Age of onset is an average of 10 years, with clusters of seizures occurring during sleep. The seizure is preceded by an aura described as a shiver or a sensation of fear. The seizure begins with a moan or calling out and then this is often followed by a motor seizure with, for example, extension of the arms or unusual posturing of a hand. Rocking, thrashing and grabbing at bedclothes may follow. The seizure lasts about 15 to 45 seconds, and throughout it the individual is aware and staring, and following it, remains confused. It is often misdiagnosed as a nightmare or a psychiatric disturbance.

An EEG done during an episode is abnormal, revealing a focus of seizure activity in the frontal lobe of the brain. It is genetically HETERO-GENEOUS but in some cases MUTATIONS in a specific neurotransmitter receptor gene, CHRNA4,

found on the long arm of chromosome 20 have been observed. This gene codes for the alpha-4 subunit of the neuronal nicotinic acetylcholine receptor. Mutations in the *CHRNB2* gene, which encodes the beta-two subunit of this receptor, may also cause this syndrome. Other genes, not yet found, are also involved.

Benign familial neonatal convulsions. These typically start in an otherwise healthy baby on the second or third day of life but cease in the first weeks of life. There is an increased risk (10%) of the later development in epilepsy. The autosomal dominant disorder has been linked to the long arm of chromosome 20 in 80% of families, though in some it has been linked to the long arm of chromosome 8. In cases linked to chromosome 8, the gene involved is *KCNQ3*. In cases linked to chromosome 20, mutations have been found in a novel potassium channel gene found on 20q, named KCNQ2. A different potassium channel gene is involved in causing JERVELL AND LANGE-NIELSEN SYNDROME and in one form of long QT syndrome (see ROMANO-WARD SYNDROME).

Progressive myoclonic epilepsy of the Unverricht-Lund-borg type. This AUTOSOMAL RECESSIVE disorder is of particular prevalence in Finnish and Swedish populations. Onset is between six and 13 with myoclonus. It has been found to be caused by mutations in the cystatin B gene on chromosome 21.

These are the first specific genetic defects known to result in epilepsy. GENETIC LINKAGE has also been found in benign familial infantile convulsions, partial epilepsy with auditory features, and juvenile myoclonic epilepsy.

epiphyseal dysplasia, multiple See MULTIPLE EPIPH-YSEAL DYSPLASIA.

epispadias A malpositioned opening of the urethra, the duct that carries urine from the bladder. Similar to but rarer than HYPOSPADIAS, in this CON-GENITAL condition, the urethral opening is located above the normal position on the penis or vagina (rather than below it, as in hypospadias). Incidence is one in 100,000 live births. In severe forms it can interfere with urinary continence, sexual function and fertility.

EPP   See PORPHYRIA.

erythropoietic protoporphyria, EPP   See PORPHYRIA.

essential hypertension   Chronic elevated blood pressure in the arteries. Found in 20% or more of any large population group in the United States, if not brought under control, hypertension can lead to stroke, heart disease, kidney disease, vision disturbances and death. It is twice as common in blacks as in whites.

Between 90% and 95% of hypertension is classified as "essential" or "primary," and has no discernible cause. However, it is believed that many of these cases are due to MULTIFACTORIAL inheritance, that is, the result of the action of several GENES in concert with environmental agents such as diet, lack of exercise, smoking and stress. Genes in the renin-angiotensin system, which regulates blood pressure, in particular, the angiotensinogen gene, are suspected to be among the factors involved in essential hypertension.

Currently, there are no accurate figures that allow GENETIC COUNSELING or estimation of recurrence risks for relatives of affected individuals. Estimates of hypertension in children and adolescents range from 1% to 11%. Maternal hypertension during pregnancy is associated with increased health risks for both the mother and the FETUS.

Two rare forms of severe early onset hypertension are inherited in an AUTOSOMAL DOMINANT manner. These are referred to as glucocorticoid suppressible hypertension and Liddle syndrome. The single genes involved in both of these have been identified.

A MUTATION common among people with salt-sensitive hypertension has also been identified. This mutated form of the gene, angiotensinogen, is unusual in that it results in an overproduction, rather than an underproduction of a protein. The protein in this case controls constriction of the blood vessels.

ethics   Advances in human GENETICS have raised a host of ethical and legal issues. Efforts to address them lag far behind science's ability to move the questions from the realm of speculation to reality.

ABORTION issues have received the most attention, and extend beyond the question of a woman's right to abortion or society's right to limit access to this procedure. For example, if abortion is acceptable in cases when prenatal diagnosis discloses the presence of a disorder, what constitutes a disorder severe enough to warrant an abortion? To what extent should genetic analysis and abortion be used to "engineer" a family's offspring, or the population as a whole? While the practice of terminating a pregnancy due solely to the gender of the FETUS is abhorrent to virtually all, how will society handle desires by prospective parents to select gender prior to conception or embryo implantation, in the case of in vitro fertilization?

Non-abortion issues now receiving the attention of geneticists, lawmakers, philosophers, private citizens, employers and other interested parties include the following: May companies bar fertile women from jobs where they might be exposed to teratogenic chemicals that can harm unborn children? (See TERATOGEN; PROTECTIVE EXCLUSION.) Or, can a fertile woman demand to be transferred from a job, such as working at a video or computer monitor or with other electronic equipment, because she fears the reproductive effects of exposure? Additionally, with increased knowledge of the impact of maternal health on pregnancy, what level of lifestyle or behavior may be required by society in order to protect the unborn child from maternal neglect?

As genetic analysis becomes more sophisticated, it may be possible to screen individuals not only for potential defects in offspring, but also for their own predisposition to develop genetically influenced disorders, such as ALCOHOLISM and CORONARY ARTERY DISEASE. Thus, concerns have been expressed that genetic testing may become an instrument for discrimination in employment and insurance. Will predispositions to disorders or behaviors result in laws or practices that countenance genetic discrimination?

Diagnosis of some disorders may require tissue samples from several family members. Should family members be required to donate this material against their wishes? Should minors be tested for adult-onset disease such as HUNTINGTON CHOREA or ALZHEIMER'S DISEASE, which currently we can do nothing to prevent or treat? Should GENETIC COUNSELING be non-directive, that is, impart only facts without assisting with decision making? (For example, whether to try conceiving despite high risks of a resultant disorder or defect, or whether to terminate a pregnancy in uncertain situations?) Should genetic counseling be different from other medical counseling, where a doctor can be directive in pronouncing an appendix needs removal or a prescription for penicillin is needed?

It has been suggested that a woman who knows she is at reproductive risk for some genetic conditions may be liable if she fails to tell, for example, her sister about the risk, and the sister subsequently gives birth to an affected infant.

Also to be dealt with is the maintenance of severely deformed infants for the harvesting of organs and tissues (see ANENCEPHALY). If it is

TABLE X
ETHNICITY OF GENETIC DISEASE

Ethnic Group	Genetic Disorders
Acadian (Nova Scotia)	Niemann-Pick disease, Type D
American Indian	Congenital dislocation of hip, gallbladder disease
Amish (Pennsylvania)	Cartilage-hair hypoplasia, Ellis-von Creveld syndrome
Armenian	Familial Mediterranean fever
Blacks	Sickle-cell disease, alpha and beta-thalassemia, G6PD deficiency, polydactyly, hypertension
Chinese	Alpha-thalassemia, G6PD deficiency
Eskimo	Congenital adrenal hyperplasia, methemoglobinemia, pseudocholinesterase deficiency
French Canadian (Quebec)	Tyrosinemia, Morquio syndrome, Tay-Sachs disease
Finns	Aspartylglucosaminuria, congenital nephrotic syndrome, lysinuri protein intolerance
Hutterite	Meckel syndrome, Bowen-Conradi syndrome
Irish	Phenylketonuria, neural tube defects
Japanese	Acatalasia
Jews	
Ashkenazi	Abetalipoproteinemia, Bloom syndrome, Factor XI deficiency, familial dysautonomia, Gaucher disease (Type I), mucolipidosis IV, Niemann-Pick disease (Type A), pentosuria, spongy degeneration of the brain (Canavan disease), Tay-Sachs disease, torsion dystonia
Sephardic	Ataxia-telangiectasia (Morocco), congenital deafness (Morocco), cystinosis, cystinuria (Libya), familial Mediterranean fever
Oriental	Alpha-thalassemia (Yemen), beta-thalassemia (Kurdistan), G6PD deficiency (Kurdistan, Iran, Iraq), Dubin-Johnson syndrome (Iran), phenylketonuria (Yemen), thrombasthenia of Glanzmann (Iraq)
Lebanese	Dyggve-Melchior-Clausen syndrome, juvenile Tay-Sachs disease
Mediterranean (Italian, Greek)	Beta-thalassemia, G6PD deficiency, familial Mediterranean fever
Mennonites (Old Colony, Canada)	Congenital adrenal hyperplasia, hypophosphatasia, Leigh's disease, Tourette syndrome, diabetes mellitus
South African Afrikaaner	Porphyria variegata, Huntington disease
SE Asian (Laotian, Thai, Vietnamese)	Alpha and beta-thalassemia
Scottish	Cystic fibrosis, phenylketonuria

Source: Adapted from V. A. McKusick, *Mendelian Inheritance in Man*, 5th ed. (Baltimore: Johns Hopkins, 1978), pp. lix–lxi.

acceptable for fetal tissue to be used, is it acceptable for a woman to conceive precisely for this purpose? If this is acceptable for humanitarian purposes, such as supplying tissue to a family member who can only be helped this way, is it acceptable strictly for financial compensation?

The 1997 announcement by a British geneticist of the successful cloning of a sheep, Dolly, brought to the fore the possibility of human CLONING, or creating a human with the exact genetic makeup of an individual already alive. This has prompted questions over whether and how to control research and application of human cloning techniques.

Other reproductive technologies and techniques (e.g., surrogacy) and gene therapy raise additional issues. The issue of gender and trait selection will doubtless need to be addressed at some future point, as well.

Following the Supreme Court's lifting of most restrictions on abortion in 1973, the federal government in 1974 created an ethics advisory board for research involving human embryos and fetuses. The board was suspended in 1980. A number of medical schools and other organizations have committees and boards to deal with these issues. However, it seems certain that advances in science will continue to far outpace society's ability to answer the questions they raise.

ethnic groups   All ethnic groups, that is, populations sharing a common genetic and geographic heritage, demonstrate greater incidence of one or more inherited conditions than the incidence displayed by the general population. This increased incidence may be due to the isolated, inbred population, in which a mutant GENE is more common, or may simply be due to improved medical record keeping or research in a given area. Scandinavian populations, for example, are noted for increased incidence of several rare HEREDITARY DISEASES and this increase may be due to both of the factors cited above. (See Table X.)

The first to suggest inbreeding as a factor in higher rates of familial disorders found in population isolates was Joseph Adams in "A Treatise on the Supposed Hereditary Property of Disease," published in 1814.

Among the many disorders historically linked with particular ethnic groups are SICKLE-CELL ANEMIA in blacks, CYSTIC FIBROSIS in whites, THALASSEMIA in populations of Mediterranean ancestry, TAY-SACHS disease in Ashkenazi Jews and ACATALASIA in Japanese. (See also FOUNDER AFFECT; AMISH; JEWISH GENETIC DISEASES; MORMONS.)

ethnocephaly   See HOLOPROSENCEPHALY.

eugenics   The science or study of the genetic and prenatal influences that affect expression of certain characteristics in offspring. The term was coined by English scientist Francis Galton (1822–1911); he defined it as the improvement of a population by selective breeding of its best specimens. While this had long been practiced by farmers in plants and animals, Galton's concept of applying it to the human population was enthusiastically championed by many, initiating a eugenics movement that would hold sway for the next half century, until its ethical implications and practical problems, as well as Nazi policies and atrocities committed in its name, discredited it.

In the United States and Canada the movement was responsible for the passage of laws forbidding mentally deficient individuals from having children. These statutes were enforced through compulsory sterilization, and the laws remained on the books in some states and provinces until after World War II. The Cold Spring Harbor Laboratory on Long Island, New York, one of the most respected GENETICS research centers in the world, was founded as the Eugenics Records Office, and became a center for the promulgation of these policies. Tens of thousands of mentally deficient individuals were sterilized in the United States, mostly between the 1930s and the 1950s. In Virginia, approximately 8,300 were sterilized between 1924 and 1972, under a state law that was upheld in a landmark Supreme Court decision of 1927. In that ruling, Justice Oliver Wendell Holmes made a now notorious comment: "Three generations of imbeciles are enough."

In Nazi Germany, a system of eugenic health courts was established, and ordered the sterilization of more than half a million people between

1933 and 1940. These individuals were judged to be mentally retarded, psychologically disturbed, physically deformed or suffering from some other illness. Nazi physician Josef Mengele also conducted eugenic breeding experiments using 1,500 pairs of TWINS, both monozygotic and dizygotic (identical and fraternal).

China in 1988 began a program requiring individuals with an IQ of 49 or below to be sterilized if they were married or intended to marry.

euthanasia, passive   See PASSIVE EUTHANASIA.

eventration of the diaphragm   Difficulty in breathing is a hallmark of this disorder, an abnormality of the diaphragm, the muscular membrane separating the abdomen from the thoracic (chest) cavity. The lungs are in the thoracic cavity, and the motion of the diaphragm controls breathing.

An elevated diaphragm (eventration) creates problems because the lung may have only minimal room to expand on the affected side. This abnormality may cause the space between the lungs (mediastinum) to shift to the opposite side, which may further impair lung function by compressing the otherwise unaffected lung. This disorder is thought to be due to the failure of a FETUS to develop adequate muscle in the diaphragm. Complete CONGENITAL absence of muscle in the diaphragm is the rarest form of this disorder, and is incompatible with life.

The condition can also be acquired during delivery (see BIRTH INJURY) due to damage to the nerve controlling the diaphragm muscle and may be either temporary or permanent depending on whether the nerve is merely stretched or irreversibly damaged. Prognosis is excellent if surgery is performed before the infant has deteriorated from chronic oxygen insufficiency, prolonged failure of the lungs to expand (atelectasis) and associated pneumonia. (See also DIAPHRAGMATIC HERNIA.)

exercise   There is no evidence that physical exercise affects fetal health either positively or negatively in women with normal pregnancies.

A Brown University study of fetal cardiac response found no impact from exercise, except for a brief period of reduced fetal heartbeat rate following extremely strenuous workouts. In 1994, the American College of Obstetrics and Gynecologists recommended that women set their own exercise limits, rescinding more conservative exercise guidelines the group had adopted in 1985. The benefits of exercise for women during pregnancy appear to be primarily psychological.

Babies born to women who exercise tend to weigh about one-half pound less than babies born to sedentary women, but are within the normal range. No increased risk of miscarriage (see ABORTION), premature delivery (see PREMATURITY) or BIRTH DEFECTS is associated with exercise in a normal pregnancy. However, it is not advised for women with certain conditions, including pregnancy-induced hypertension, persistent bleeding, incompetent cervix, and cardiovascular and pulmonary disease.

expression profiling   Any of several methods used to analyze gene expression, or the degree to which a mutant gene will affect the individual who possesses it. Developed in the late 1990s, the technique is accomplished with microarray technology that allows comparison of gene expression between normal and cancerous or other diseased cells. It is used to analyze genetic material from tumors to identify individuals at increased risk of having a recurrence of tumors.

expressivity   The degree to which an individual who has inherited the GENES for a specific trait exhibits the characteristics of that trait. The term was coined by German neuropathologist Otto Vogt in 1926 (at the same time, he introduced a related term, PENETRANCE). (Vogt was an esteemed clinician of his time; he was summoned to Moscow from Berlin to attend Lenin after his first and second, and ultimately fatal, stroke. Critical of the Nazis as they came to power, Vogt was relegated to working as a stretcher-bearer in World War II.) Many inherited conditions have a variable degree of expressivity, that is, the characteristics of the condition vary from mild to severe. In others, expressivity has little variation, with all cases exhibiting uniform characteristics and prognoses.

Generally, expressivity in AUTOSOMAL DOMINANT disorders is variable, while the expressivity in AUTOSOMAL RECESSIVE disorders tends to be more uniformly severe.

exstrophy of bladder   The protrusion of the bladder through the abdominal wall, caused by the failure of the abdomen to close properly during fetal development. It was described in the cuneiform tablets of Chaldea dating from 2000 B.C. This surgically correctable condition occurs in about one in 30,000–50,000 births, affecting males three times as frequently as females. Recurrence in SIBLINGS is rare, empiric recurrence risk is about 1%. PRENATAL DIAGNOSIS can be accomplished with ULTRASOUND and maternal serum ALPHA-FETOPROTEIN (AFP) screening.

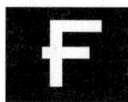

Fabry disease A hereditary ENZYME deficiency caused by the deficiency of alphagalactosidase A. Seen mostly in males, this SYNDROME is characterized by the accumulation of a glycosphingolipid (a derivative of a fat) trihexosyl ceramide, or GL-3, within the cardiovascular-renal system, the skin, eyes and mucous membranes in the mouth. Clusters of dark-red, raised, dot-like lesions of the skin (called angiokeratomas) usually appear during childhood and increase in size and number with age. They often appear in a "bathing suit" distribution, that is, on the buttocks, back, penis, scrotum, inner thighs and around the navel. The accumulation of GL-3 in the walls of small blood vessels leads to kidney disease, heart disease and stroke.

Named for J. Fabry (1860–1930), the German dermatologist who first described it in 1898. An English surgeon and dermatologist, W. Anderson (1842–1900), independently described it that same year.

In childhood affected males experience burning pain in the hands and feet (acroparesthesia). The pain may be triggered by exercise, fatigue, fever, emotional stress or change in temperature or humidity. They often have diminished ability to sweat. Nausea, vomiting, diarrhea and abdominal or side pain is common. There may also be swelling of the legs due to subcutaneous accumulation of lymph (lymphedema).

Retarded growth and delayed puberty are common. Ocular abnormalities include swelling and distortion of the blood vessels in the conjunctive and retina. A characteristic "whorl"-like deposit in the cornea is seen. These abnormalities do not interfere with vision. Cardiovascular and renal involvements increase with age.

The disorder exhibits X-LINKED recessive inheritance. Thus it is males who are primarily affected with the disorder. Female CARRIERS, however, often develop angiokeratomas and may have problems with burning pains. Some have kidney or heart problems. However, the characteristic eye changes are commonly noted. A rough estimate for the frequency of the disorder is one in 40,000 individuals.

In the past those affected by the disorder usually died by the fourth decade, either from kidney failure or cerebrovascular complications. Recent advances in kidney dialysis and transplantation have improved the outlook for affected individuals.

PRENATAL DIAGNOSIS is possible via AMNIOCENTESIS or CHORIONIC VILLUS SAMPLING. Previously, therapy was limited to symptomatic treatments, but enzyme replacement therapy (intravenous infusions of the deficient enzyme) is now available for this disease.

facio-scapulo-humeral dystrophy See MUSCULAR DYSTROPHY.

Factor V Leiden A form of THROMBOPHILIA that predisposes the blood to form clots, Factor V Leiden is the most common hereditary blood coagulation disorder in the United States, and perhaps the world. Like all hereditary thrombophilias, it is caused by variations in one or more of several genes that predispose an individual to develop the disorder, in concert with environmental factors.

An autosomal dominant trait with incomplete penetrance, the first mutation was identified in 1994. A protein, Factor V, made by the *Factor V* gene on 1q, plays a role in activating the blood clotting sequence. An allele of the gene results in the production of factor V Leiden, a defective form of the clotting factor. In some, but not all, affected individuals, the mutation results in thrombophilia, an increased risk of developing blood clots in the veins (venous thrombosis). Such clots can clog blood vessels and prevent blood from reaching an organ or body part and cause heart attack or stroke. Among Caucasians, 3–7% have a single mutant *Factor V Leiden* gene (heterozygotes), and about 0.1% have two (homozygotes). Factor V Leiden increases the risk of developing venous thrombosis three- to eightfold for heterozygotes, and 30–140-fold for homozygous individuals. The disorder is present in 20–50% of all patients under medical care for venous thrombosis and estimated to be 10 times more common than any other hereditary form of predisposition to thrombosis. Prevalence of the disorder in Western countries is estimated at one–three per 1,000 people. In the United States, about 1.2% of African Americans have a mutated *Factor V* gene.

Due to its incomplete penetrance, many individuals who have Factor V Leiden remain unaffected. Numerous environmental factors contribute to its onset, including smoking, obesity, pregnancy, oral contraceptives and hormone replacement therapy. Onset is usually in adulthood. Therapy typically involves minimizing exposure to environmental factors as well as use of anticoagulant drugs such as coumadin.

Testing for Factor V Leiden is possible by APC (activated Protein C) resistance assay or DNA analysis of the *Factor V* gene. However, as there is a high prevalence of this allele in the general population, interpretation of positive results requires careful evaluation. Prenatal testing for Factor V Leiden is typically not recommended.

failure to thrive   A general term for the inability of an infant to gain weight and grow appropriately. It is often seen in infants affected by a variety of CONGENITAL ANOMALIES and congenital or early-onset GENETIC DISORDERS. There are also a myriad of other non-genetic or non-congenital causes.

Fallot, tetralogy of   See TETRALOGY OF FALLOT.

familial adenomatous polyposis, FAP   See CANCER.

familial cirrhosis   Cirrhosis, a degeneration of the liver due to scarring and replacement with connective tissue, has been observed in multiple SIBLINGS in several families with non-affected parents. Familial cirrhosis most likely represents a heterogeneous (that is, of varying causes; see HETEROGENEITY) group of disorders, and in some instances non-genetic factors may be responsible for the familial aggregation. (These cases do not include, for example, WILSON'S DISEASE, type IV GLYCOGEN STORAGE DISEASE and GALACTOSEMIA), which are well-known causes of familial cirrhosis.)

In India, Indian childhood cirrhosis also affects multiple siblings. Onset usually occurs between six and 18 months of age. Progressive lethargy, jaundice, abdominal swelling and fever develop four to seven months before death.

familial disease   A disease that occurs in several individuals of the same family with greater frequency than would be dictated by chance. This would obviously include GENETIC DISORDERS (both single-GENE and MULTIFACTORIAL), but can also include environmentally caused diseases, as a family shares a common environment.

The fact that some disorders now known to be genetically influenced often appeared to run in families has been noted since antiquity. For example, Jews recognized that HEMOPHILIA affected only male members of a family. Among the familial conditions recognized by Hippocrates (ca. 460–377 B.C.), the father of medicine, were EPILEPSY, blue eyes and baldness, all of which are now known to be genetically influenced. (See also the Introduction.)

familial dysautonomia (Riley-Day syndrome)   A rare disorder of the autonomic nervous system and sensory system confined almost exclusively to Ashkenazi Jews (of Eastern European ancestry). As a result of defective development of the sensory system, individuals generally cannot feel pain or distinguish between hot and cold, and therefore are prone to injure themselves without realizing it. For example, they are unaware if a bone breaks or if they are being burned. Because of deficits in the autonomic nervous system, they have unstable blood pressure, body temperature (often with unexplained fever) and heartbeat. Ingested food or liquid may go into the lungs rather than the gastrointestinal tract, often leading to repeated attacks of pneumonia.

This disorder was first identified in 1949 by U.S. pediatricians C. M. Riley and R. L. Day, and for some time was identified as "Riley-Day syndrome," but familial dysautonomia is the current preferred designation. (Dysautonomia refers to the disturbed function of the autonomic nervous system.)

During fetal life, the autonomic and sensory nervous systems fail to develop properly. Babies born with familial dysautonomia are FLOPPY INFANTS with poor muscle tone (hypotonia) and have difficulty feeding because they do not have a normal suck reflex. Perhaps the most distinctive sign is the inability to produce tears when crying or when foreign objects get in their eyes. The resulting irritation can create ocular problems and is a serious consequence of the disorder.

Ninety-five percent develop lateral spinal curvature (SCOLIOSIS), often beginning early in life. Other associated features are stunted growth, clumsiness, speech difficulties, drooling and uncontrollable vomiting attacks. There is generally no mental impairment. The tongue of affected individuals lacks taste buds (fungiform papillae), and the resulting flat, smooth appearance of the tongue is useful in establishing the diagnosis. With age kidney function deteriorates. A frequently used diagnostic test involves the injection of histamine into the skin. Affected individuals will not get the characteristic redness (flare) around the injection.

The disorder is inherited as an AUTOSOMAL RECESSIVE trait, resulting from a mutation in the *2KBKAP* gene on the long arm of chromosome 9. About one in 30 Ashkenazi Jews is thought to be a CARRIER of the defective GENE. The incidence among the at-risk population is thought to be one in 3,600 live births, though a recent study in Israel found a higher incidence (one in 3,703). Virtually all individuals with this disease have two copies of the same mutation. Carrier detection and prenatal diagnosis are available using DNA analysis. Because of the increased frequency of this disorder in Ashkenazi Jews and the reliable detection of over 99% of the causative mutations, population screening using mutation

analysis of the *IKBKAP* gene is often offered to Ashkenazi Jewish individuals interested in preconception or prenatal genetic counseling.

In the past, approximately half of all cases succumbed to respiratory infections or other problems by the age of five, but now 80% are surviving beyond childhood, and about 1/2 of patients now reach adulthood. (See also INDIFFERENCE TO PAIN.)

familial Hibernian fever (FHF; Tumor Necrosis Factor Receptor-Associated Periodic Syndrome; TRAPS) A rare hereditary inflammatory disorder characterized by episodes of high fever, severe abdominal or chest pain, inflammation of the eyes and skin rash, features that closely mimic familial Mediterranean fever (FMF). First described in a family of Irish-Scottish descent by L. M. Williamson in 1982, FHF was identified in the course of studying FMF, after it was noted some affected subjects were not of Mediterranean stock. "Hibernian" differentiates it from the more common FMF.

The first mention in the literature of periodic inflammation disease, which was later identified as FMF, was likely in 1806, when British physician W. Heberden described a syndrome of periodic pain involving the abdomen, chest and extremities.

An autosomal dominant disorder, FHF is caused by mutations in a gene encoding a cell surface receptor for TNF (tumor necrosis factor), an inflammatory protein that plays a role in the body's defenses against infectious or other threatening agents. The gene's map locus is 12p13.2. This is the first disorder in which the TNF receptor was tied to a heritable trait. The mutation renders affected individuals predisposed to bouts of inflammatory reactions brought on by emotional stress, minor trauma or unknown causes. Subsequent studies found the mutation in genes for other TNF receptor groups, leading to its secondary designation, TNF Receptor-Associated Period Syndrome (TRAPS). It has been suggested the disorder could result from overproduction of TNF, which ultimately leads to over-signaling for an immune response.

There are no life-threatening complications associated with FHF, but its periodic episodes can have a major impact on affected individuals and their families, particularly if it remains undiagnosed, requiring repeated invasive attempts to determine the cause of the recurring symptoms. The identification of the mechanism behind the immune response may lead to the development of targeted cellular-level treatments. Steroids have been used to treat immune reactions in affected individuals, though they are associated with deleterious side effects. Etanercept, a fusion protein, has reportedly been used successfully to treat an affected infant who failed to respond to steroid therapy.

familial juvenile polyposis   This rare hereditary disorder predisposes affected individuals to develop polyps, or tumors, in the colon and gastrointestinal (GI) tract. "Juvenile" refers to microscopic characteristics of the polyps, rather than age of onset of the disorder, which can vary from infancy to adulthood. The tumors are primarily benign, but may bleed and cause anemia or eventually turn cancerous. The risk of individuals with FJP developing colon or GI cancers is unknown, but in a study of one large kindred, 55% of affected individuals had developed GI cancer, 38% had colon cancer and 21% had upper GI cancers.

Though not all juvenile polyposis can be traced to genetic causes, at least half of reported FJP cases result from this hereditary form. FJP is transmitted as an autosomal dominant trait. Mutations in at least three genes have been linked to FJP: *SMAD4* on chromosome 18 and *PTEN* on chromosome 10, and *BMPR1A*. *SMAD4* accounts for about 25% of affected families. The disorder exhibits anticipation; severity increases and age of onset decreases in successive generations. FJP also occurs as a result of de novo, or new, mutations. Testing for the presence of the *SMAD4* mutation and other mutations is possible. Clinical testing for some of the mutations is available. Initially, these tests were available only on a research basis, which took months or even years to yield results.

Unaffected family members of those with MJP have exhibited an increased risk for developing GI cancers, estimated at 9–50% greater than the general population's.

familial Mediterranean fever   This disorder is characterized by short, recurrent bouts of fever accom-

panied by pain in the abdomen, chest and/or joints, and a red rash. The attacks have their onset between the ages of five and 15 years, and frequency and duration of the episodes are unpredictable. They generally last up to 24 hours, but may go on for four days, and continue intermittently throughout life.

The disorder primarily affects North African Sephardic and Iraqi Jews (those who lived in Spain and left during the era of the Inquisition, settling in various countries bordering the Mediterranean), Armenians, Turkish and Levantine Arab populations. There have also been reports of clusters of the disorder in individuals of Irish and Italian descent.

While there is no specific treatment, the disorder is not life-threatening, though AMYLOIDOSIS, an accumulation of amyloid, a starch-like material, may accompany the disorder and damage internal organs. Amyloidosis particularly leads to kidney failure, and has occurred in almost 50% of Sephardic Jewish patients, but is rarer in other groups. The abdominal symptoms have caused many undiagnosed patients to undergo needless exploratory abdominal surgery.

The disorder is inherited as an AUTOSOMAL RECESSIVE trait. Frequency in some at-risk populations has been estimated as high as one in 2,700, with CARRIER frequency estimated at between approximately one in 25 and one in 50. The carrier ratio among North African Jews is 1:6, among Armenians 1:7. Males are affected more often than females. The GENE responsible is located on the short arm of chromosome 16 and appears to encode a protein, believed to control the activity of white blood cells, which combat infection. The gene, discovered independently in the United States and France, was named pyrin by its American finders, for the Greek word for fire, in deference to its role in fever. The French named it marenostrin, derived from the Latin name of the Mediterranean Sea and chosen because the ethnic groups affected with the disorder live around the Sea.

Identification of the molecular basis of the disease allows for better diagnostic tests for this disorder. Colchicine, a medicine prescribed for gout, has been used in treatment. It not only mitigates attacks but prevents both the attacks and development of amyloidosis.

familial nephritis (Alport syndrome) This is a group of hereditary renal diseases that present primarily with blood in the urine (hematuria) and progressive deterioration in kidney function leading to renal failure. In many cases it is associated with deafness and often visual problems as well. Hereditary nephritis is also known as Alport syndrome. In 1927, South African physician A. C. Alport (1880–1959) identified the combination of hematuria and sensorineural DEAFNESS (deafness caused by anomalies in the auditory nerves, rather than conductive deafness which is caused by anomalies in physical structures of the hearing organs) as a specific SYNDROME. The family he described had been the subject of reports dating to 1902.

Most cases of familial nephritis represent Alport syndrome, though forms of the disease without deafness have been described. The genetic basis of familial nephritis is quite HETEROGENEOUS, with different forms and different families demonstrating either X-LINKED dominant, AUTOSOMAL RECESSIVE, or perhaps AUTOSOMAL DOMINANT inheritance. The X-linked form is clearly the most common. It has been estimated that about one in 50,000 Americans carries the GENE for Alport syndrome, although not all will develop symptoms.

The hematuria is rarely severe, and the blood in the urine may require microscopic examination for detection. The kidney disease is generally more severe in males, leading to eventual kidney failure and death between the third and fourth decade of life if untreated. Females tend to have a relatively benign course, with no decrease in life expectancy.

In classic Alport disease, in addition to the progressive high frequency sensorineural deafness, there are generally also eye lesions, which may lead to visual deterioration. The kidney has specific changes evident on electron microscopy, and the defect appears to be related to an abnormality of type IV collagen, a component of connective tissue. This disorder is inherited in an X-linked manner, with males exhibiting more severe manifestations than females. The gene responsible appears to be on the middle of the long arm of the X CHROMOSOME. MUTATIONS causing this form are in the gene for the alpha-5 chain of type IV collagen (COL4A5). The alpha-3 (COL4A3) and alpha-4 chain (COL4A4) genes are found together on the long arm of chro-

mosome 2 and appear to be involved in at least some of the autosomal recessive forms of hereditary nephritis. Whether or not mutations in these genes can cause an autosomal dominant form has not been conclusively answered, and it is not clear whether an autosomal dominant form of classic Alport syndrome truly exists. Other mutations in the COL4A4 gene have been found to result in BENIGN FAMILIAL HEMATURIA.

familial panhypopituitary dwarfism See PITUITARY DWARFISM SYNDROMES.

familial polyposis of the colon, FPC See under COLORECTAL CANCER.

Fanconi anemia (Fanconi pancytopenia) SYNDROME characterized by multiple CONGENITAL abnormalities, bone marrow failure and CHROMOSOME ABNORMALITIES, and named for Swiss pediatrician Guido Fanconi (1882–1979), who described it in 1927. (It should not be confused with Fanconi syndrome of renal tubular dysfunction.) While the disorder is extremely variable in expression, the manifestations are potentially severe and life threatening. It is also a cancer predisposition syndrome.

Infants tend to have LOW BIRTH WEIGHT. The skin often exhibits abnormal pigmentation, consisting of generalized small patches of darkened skin and cafe au lait spots. The face is asymmetrical, with a small head (MICROCEPHALY), small eyes (microphthalmia), drooping eyelids (PTOSIS) and malformed ears. They may have various abnormalities of the thumb, congenital hip dislocation and deformities of the ribs and vertebrae. There are frequently abnormalities of the genitourinary tract and congenital HEART DEFECTS. Muscles on the upper trunk and shoulders may be underdeveloped. Some individuals (20%) have MENTAL RETARDATION, and DEAFNESS has been reported. Short stature is common. Another frequent set of malformations, in addition to heart and genitourinary, are those of the gastrointestinal system. Fifty percent of affected individuals have abnormalities of the thumb and/or radius (the bone on the "thumb side" of the forearm) ranging from a short thumb on one hand to absence of both the thumbs and radii.

Bone marrow failure develops at approximately seven or eight years of age, and involves the decreased production of the entire range of blood cells—red cells (resulting in anemia), white cells and platelets—due to abnormalities of the bone marrow, where the blood cells are produced. The decrease in number of blood cells is progressive and often lethal. There is also an increased tendency to develop leukemia and other CANCERS, and the CHROMOSOMES, upon examination, display a propensity for breakage.

Fanconi's anemia is generally inherited as an AUTOSOMAL RECESSIVE trait and occurs in approximately one in 100,000 live births. At least 13 subtypes of FA are known to exist, clinically indistinguishable and differentiated using laboratory testing. They each represent different genes that can cause this disorder. Type A is the most common subtype, found in about 2/3 of patients with FA. The gene for type A is located on the long arm of chromosome 16. Type B is X-linked. Type C is found in about 10% of patients, and the gene is mapped to the long arm of chromosome 9. Type C appears to account for the majority of patients in the Netherlands, and one specific MUTATION in the responsible gene accounts for most cases of FA in individuals of Ashkenazi Jewish descent. In fact this particular mutation has been found to be carried by about 1% of all Ashkenazi Jews, another example of FOUNDER EFFECT. The gene for type D1 is the *BRCA2* gene. The proteins produced by the various FA genes interact in a common cellular pathway involved in repair of breaks in DNA and control of the cell cycle, which governs how DNA makes copies of itself.

CARRIER screening is only available when the specific mutation is known, and only for populations in which the common subtype mutation has been identified. PRENATAL DIAGNOSIS has been accomplished in at-risk pregnancies by findings of increased chromosome breakage in fetal cells collected via AMNIOCENTESIS. In several instances, preimplantation genetic diagnosis has been used to test an embryo obtained by in vitro fertilization from a family with a previous child with FA. The embryo was found to be not only unaffected with FA, but

also HLA-identical to the affected sib, and was subsequently implanted and a pregnancy established. A normal child was born and, at birth, umbilical cord blood stem cells were collected. These stem cells were then successfully transplanted to treat the older sibling with FA.

Fanconi pancytopenia   See FANCONI ANEMIA.

Farber lipogranulomatosis   See LIPOGRANULOMATOSIS.

favism   Common in Sicily and Sardinia and recognized since antiquity, this is a hereditary deficiency of an ENZYME (glucose-6-phosphate dehydrogenase) in red blood cells, resulting in a sensitivity to fava beans (*Vicia fava*), which are staples of the diet in the population at risk. (Fava beans are also the main commercial source of L-dopa, a drug used in the treatment of PARKINSON DISEASE.)

It appears that the bean produces a substance that induces the breakdown (hemolysis) of enzyme-deficient red blood cells. Ingestion of as little as one seed of a fava bean, or inhalation of pollen, is enough to precipitate an attack. These episodes are characterized by malaise, headache, dizziness, fever, acute hemolytic ANEMIA, vomiting and diarrhea. Within approximately 24 hours, the skin takes on a yellowish tone (jaundice) and hemoglobin from the destroyed red cells is found in the urine (hemoglobinuria). It may lead to prostration and coma.

The sensitivity apparently diminishes over time, for children are more commonly affected than adults. The condition has been observed even in nursing infants whose mothers ingested the bean. (See GLUCOSE-6-PHOSPHATE DEHROGENASE DEFICIENCY)

febrile seizures   Infant and juvenile convulsive episodes associated with fever and often causing loss of consciousness and tremors. First described by the ancient Greeks, it was only late in the 20th century that febrile seizures were recognized as a syndrome distinct from epilepsy. Most of the seizures occur between six months and five years of age. Though no clear genetic basis has been found, a familial link exists; infants with first degree relatives who had febrile seizures have an above average chance of having febrile seizures.

The seizures usually last one to two minutes, though they can range in duration from a few seconds to 15 minutes. In the United States, between 2–4% of children have such a seizure by their fifth birthday. About 30% of those who have a febrile seizure will experience a recurrence. In addition to family history, risk factors associated with an elevated chance of recurrence are a young age at the time of first seizure a relatively low fever at the time of the seizure and a brief time lapse between the onset of fever and the initial seizure. Affected individuals with all four risk factors have a greater than 70% chance of having a recurrence. Those with none of these risk factors have a 20% chance of recurrence.

The great majority of episodes are harmless, with the greatest risk coming from secondary dangers such as choking on food or falling down and striking one's head. The episodes do not affect intelligence, and affected children develop normally.

A smaller percentage of affected youngsters (2–5%) develop epilepsy. Risk factors include seizures of a long length that only affect one part of the body or that recur within 24 hours. Children with development disabilities who have febrile seizures are also more likely to develop epilepsy. Infants and juveniles who have febrile seizures without any of the epilepsy risk factors have a 1% chance of developing epilepsy.

fetal alcohol syndrome (FAS) Though a link between excessive alcohol consumption during pregnancy and BIRTH DEFECTS has been noted since the time of the ancient Greeks, a specific SYNDROME of defects associated with fetal exposure to alcohol was identified only in 1973. Designated fetal alcohol syndrome (FAS), it is characterized by INTRAUTERINE GROWTH RETARDATION, typical facial features, MENTAL RETARDATION, and defects of the central nervous and cardiac systems. It is thought to be one of the most common causes of mental retardation, behind DOWN SYNDROME, FRAGILE X SYNDROME and SPINA BIFIDA. (Some health experts believe it is the number one cause.) The degree of mental retardation varies, with average IQ put at 63. Affected individuals exhibit poor hand-eye coordination, hyperactivity, trembling and poor attention span. Behavior problems such as poor judgment, distractibility and difficulties in recognizing social cues are common in adolescents and adults with FAS.

Characteristic facial features include a small head (MICROCEPHALY) and eyes, folds of the skin that obscure the inner juncture of the eyelids (EPICANTHUS), short, upturned nose (anteverted nares), thin upper lip and underdeveloped philtrum, the groove extending from the middle of the upper lip to the nose. Those affected may also exhibit dental abnormalities in childhood, including upper and lower teeth that fail to meet properly when biting (malocclusion).

Alcohol, a small molecule, easily passes through the placenta and enters the fetal bloodstream. It remains in the FETUS longer than in the adult. Drinking binges further exacerbate risks to fetal development. In addition to direct consequences of alcohol abuse, drinking may cause vitamin and mineral deficiencies in the mother, which may also contribute to fetal malformations.

Most infants with FAS are born to chronic alcoholics. Infants exposed to only two drinks a day showed primarily LOW BIRTH WEIGHT. At increasing levels of intake, additional clinical effects are seen and at intakes of at least eight to 10 drinks per day is where most children with full blown FAS are seen. Risk of FAS in the offspring of these chronically alcoholic women is estimated now to be 30–50%. The greatest risk is for some degree of mental HANDICAP. Some organizations, such as the National Institute on Alcohol Abuse and Alcoholism, recommend total abstinence during pregnancy.

FAS infants are of below average birth weight and at one year of age are typically only 65% of normal length. Those who don't have the full-blown syndrome, but exhibit some symptoms, are said to have fetal alcohol effects (FAE). FAE is often subdivided into and referred to as one of three entities: partial FAS, alcohol-related birth defects and alcohol-related neurodevelopmental disorder. Fetal alcohol syndrome is estimated to occur in approximately one in 700 to one in 2,000 live births. In various studies, FAE has been estimated to occur in from 1.7 per 1,000 live births to 90.1 per 1,000 live births. (See also ALCOHOLISM.)

fetal aminopterin syndrome   Aminopterin is a drug prescribed for treatment of CANCER. Taken during the first trimester of pregnancy, it can cause severe abnormalities and fetal death. Fetal exposure after the first trimester may induce a variety of bone deformities and MENTAL RETARDATION. (See also TERATOGEN.)

fetal face syndrome   See ROBINOW SYNDROME.

fetal imaging   Obtaining an image of the FETUS in the uterus. This can be of great help to the physician in determining the gestational age of the fetus and its general condition, as well as aiding in PRENATAL DIAGNOSIS of various disorders. The main techniques for fetal imaging are ULTRASOUND and FETOSCOPY. Fetoscopy carries certain risks and is not frequently employed.

Another method of fetal imaging is by X-ray. This is usually done to visualize the fetal skeleton at 17 to 19 weeks. The injection of a special water-soluble contrast dye provides information about the position of the fetus. Since some of the dye is swallowed by the fetus, this procedure also indicates its swallowing ability and the condition of its gastrointestinal tract. Risks are uncertain; some have speculated infants exposed to X-rays IN UTERO have higher incidence of childhood CANCER.

fetal surgery   Surgery performed on an infant prior to birth. Though most BIRTH DEFECTS are best treated after birth, a small and growing number are amenable to treatment prior to delivery. In most instances where surgery is performed, the infant would not survive without surgical intervention. Risk to the health of the mother, and her ability to have future pregnancies, are also considerations in fetal surgery decisions.

Among the conditions that may in some cases be suggested for surgery are HYDROCEPHALUS, herniated diaphragm (see DIAPHRAGMATIC HERNIA and

EVENTRATION OF THE DIAPHRAGM), hydronephrosis, an obstruction of the urinary tract, and multiple pregnancies, in which selected embryos are aborted to improve chances of survival of the remaining ones (see MULTIPLE BIRTHS; ABORTION).

The surgery may be performed through the amniotic sac while the infant is in the womb, or an incision may be made in the abdomen and the FETUS partially removed. In the latter operation, the fetus is usually out of the womb from three to 30 minutes.

It has been discovered that operations on infants before birth leave no scars. Some cosmetic surgeons suggest that facial deformities such as CLEFT LIP, or more serious conditions such as FAMILIAL NEPHRITIS could be successfully treated before birth and heal with no trace.

The first *human* fetal surgery in the United States was performed in 1981, by Dr. Michael R. Harrison of the University of California at San Francisco, on an infant with hydronephrosis. Currently, animals are being used to test experimental surgery and to practice surgical techniques for fetal repair of hernias of the diaphragm and SPINA BIFIDA, as well as for transplant techniques for fetal organs and fetal cells.

Non-surgical fetal treatments have been performed, including transfusions, and administration of drugs such as digitalis for heart failure or vitamin B_{12} for prenatally diagnosed methylmalonic acidemia.

fetal tissue sampling   Collection of a small amount of tissue from a developing embryo. Fetal tissue samples can currently be obtained by one of several methods: AMNIOCENTESIS, CHORIONIC VILLUS SAMPLING, FETOSCOPY or directly under ULTRASOUND guidance. Amniocentesis will provide tissue samples (essentially fetal skin and bladder cells) suspended in the amniotic fluid; chorionic villus sampling involves suction of tissue from tiny fronds at the edge of the placenta; and fetoscopy allows cutting out of a tiny tissue sample from the fetus itself. Newer techniques allow for direct sampling without the fetoscope under ultrasound guidance. The most common of these is CORDOCENTESIS and involves direct sampling of fetal blood from the umbilical vein. In this technique, also called percutaneous umbilical blood sampling or PUBS, a needle is placed in the vein under ultrasound guidance. Similarly, fetal skin or tissue biopsies can be done by use of a tiny biopsy forceps or needle directed by ultrasound. Risks are involved in all of these procedures, with amniocentesis being the safest and most commonly used technique.

fetoscopy Direct visualization of the FETUS, placenta and umbilical cord by the use of a fetoscope, a thin, flexible, fiberoptic tube that can be inserted into the uterus. This procedure has been largely replaced by ULTRASOUND and ultrasound-guided sampling techniques such as CORDOCENTESIS. Fetal skin, liver and muscle biopsies have all been performed using ultrasound guidance as well, making fetoscopy unnecessary. While direct visualization of the fetus is possible with fetoscopy, it offers only a limited field of view (about 2–4 cm^3). Given these limitations and the higher fetal mortality rates associated with fetoscopy—even in skilled hands, fetoscopy carries a 3% to 6% risk of fetal death and miscarriage and a 10% risk of premature birth—it is now rarely used.

fetus The developing offspring within the uterus. In humans, the developing infant is regarded as a fetus from the third month of pregnancy to birth; prior to the third month it is referred to as an embryo.

FG syndrome An uncommon, X-LINKED recessive hereditary disorder whose most common features include a large head, MENTAL RETARDATION, IMPERFORATE ANUS, CONGENITAL hypotonia and absence of the corpus callosum, the commissure of the brain between the cerebral hemispheres. Severity is variable, but affected individuals exhibit similar personality characteristics, typically friendly, outgoing and hyperactive. Their attention span is short, and they may be easily frustrated and prone to temper tantrums.

First described by John M. Opitz and E. G. Kaveggia in 1974, its name is derived from a classification system that employs the initials of the patients' surnames. Over 50 cases have been documented. Only males are affected. Female CARRIERS

may exhibit physical characteristics related to the SYNDROME, including a broad forehead, epicanthal folds (EPICATHUS), HYPERTELORISM (wide-set eyes) or abnormal placement of the anus.

One-third of affected infants succumb to cardiac defects or imperforate anus before two years of age.

fibrodysplasia ossificans progressiva, FOP (myositis ossificans) The formation of misplaced bony lesions (ossification) in soft tissues, such as connective tissue, skeletal muscle, tendons and ligaments. There are also typical foot and hand malformations associated with FOP: misaligned and shortened big toes, abnormally small thumbs and incurved fifth fingers. About 30% experience hearing loss, another 30% easy bruisabillity. Onset usually occurs before age four but may occur as late as puberty. Ossification typically begins in the head, neck, spine or shoulders, and goes on to involve many sites, including the chest, hips, ankles, wrists and, least commonly, hands. Each new lesion is painfully tender and swollen for several weeks until it becomes bony. As ossification continues, the individual finds it increasingly difficult to accomplish tasks unassisted, such as getting out of bed, dressing and bathing. Currently, no surgery or drug therapy affects the course of the disease. In fact any kind of trauma, including surgery, biopsy or intramuscular injection can be a site for abnormal ossification. In rare cases, ossification may begin during fetal life.

FOP is an AUTOSOMAL DOMINANT trait, though most cases have been SPORADIC. It is caused by a mutation in the *Activin A Receptor Type 1 (ACVR1)* gene, mapped to 2q23–q24. The causative gene, identified in 2006, makes a protein of the same name, ACVR1, which is involved in the creation of bone. It is believed that among those with the disorder, the protein is activated when it should not be, causing adult stem cells to become bone cells. About 600 cases have been reported. Approximately 90% appear to be new mutations. There is an increased incidence associated with advanced paternal age.

fifth disease Viral disease, caused by parvovirus 19, that takes its name from being the fifth of six pediatric disorders identified by scientists. The first four were rubella, MEASLES, scarlet fever and Dukes disease, which is a mild form of scarlet fever. The sixth disorder is exanthema subitum, also called roseola infantum.

Maternal infection with fifth disease during pregnancy can cause STILLBIRTH or miscarriage (see ABORTION), though the risk is thought to be small. The virus suppresses the fetal bone marrow, causing severe ANEMIA, congestive heart failure and fluid retention. Unlike rubella, there has been little evidence that fifth disease can cause BIRTH DEFECTS; however, this is not clear.

First reported in Europe in 1889, it usually occurs in the spring and winter among children from two to 12 years of age, and its most striking feature is a characteristic rash resembling a slap mark, usually found on the face and occasionally spreading to other parts of the body. Symptoms of fever and rash typically persist for about a week. Infection can be diagnosed via a sophisticated blood test. Some FETUSES that have been severely anemic due to maternal infection have been treated with blood transfusions IN UTERO.

Finnish diseases The Finnish population exhibits more than 30 disorders, some with a relatively high frequency of CARRIERS, which are either nonexistent or rare in other populations. Many of these disorders are seen only in highly localized areas. Several result from single MUTATIONS clearly occurring in a single founder individual. The rare cases of these disorders found outside Finland—Finnish type CONGENITAL nephrosis, for example—result from a variety of mutations. Conversely, AUTOSOMAL RECESSIVE disorders commonly seen in other European populations, such as CYSTIC FIBROSIS, PHENYLKETONURIA or GALACTOSEMIA are either rare or nonexistent in Finland.

Analysis of Y-chromosomal and mitochondrial genetic material (see MITOCHONDRIAL DISEASE) reveals that relatively few men and women contributed to the genetic lineage of today's Finnish population. This is thought to account for the so-called Finnish disease heritage. Analysis of mitochondrial mutations indicates the constriction in the population occurred about 4,000 years ago. This is thought to be when an agrarian culture moved into the area. Estonians and Basques are thought to exhibit similar FOUNDER EFFECTS.

Finnish-type sialuria See SALLA DISEASE.

fish odor syndrome (trimethylaminuria) A rare metabolic disorder imparting an odor of rotting fish upon affected individuals.

Onset occurs shortly after birth, and the odor may become more pronounced after puberty. Affected individuals often suffer from isolation and ridicule due to their odor. Incidence of the SYNDROME is unclear. A British study estimated it occurs in one in 25,000 births in that country, while rates in Ecuador and Papua New Guinea are said to be especially high. It appears the disorder is mentioned in ancient literature, and Shakespeare described a character with "a very ancient and fish-like smell" in *The Tempest*.

An AUTOSOMAL RECESSIVE trait, the responsible GENE was identified in 1991 by researchers at McGill University in Toronto and the University of London in England. The defect compromises the body's ability to produce the liver enzyme FMO3, which processes a smelly protein called TMA, or trimethylamine, produced by bacteria in the digestive system. The raw materials for TMA are found in food rich in choline, such as fish, eggs and liver. The unprocessed TMA seeps out of the body in perspiration and breath, creating the offensive odor.

Detection of CARRIERS may be possible by urinalysis after oral administration of trimethylamine. Avoidance of choline rich foods can reduce the odor, as can antibiotics that kill the intestinal bacteria that produce TMA.

FLK syndrome FLK stands for "Funny-Looking Kid," and was a general term for infants affected with various malformation SYNDROMES, particularly those involving multiple facial abnormalities. Considered demeaning and insensitive, it is no longer in use.

floppy infant An infant with poor muscle tone (hypotonia), exhibiting an inability to move limbs or other parts and presenting a limp, floppy appearance. It is common among newborns with many GENETIC DISORDERS and other CONGENITAL ANOMALIES.

fluorescence in situ hybridization (FISH)   A technique of CYTOGENETICS that uses fluorescently labeled DNA probes for specific CHROMOSOME regions. It is useful for revealing missing, duplicated or malpositioned (e.g., as in a translocation) chromosomal material that might not be obvious by routine cytogenetic investigation.

focal dermal hypoplasia   See GOLTZ SYNDROME.

focal dystonia   See DYSTONIA.

Forbes disease   See GLYCOGEN STORAGE DISEASE.

founder effect   The expression of a GENETIC DISORDER in a relatively large percentage of a distinct population resulting from a MUTATION transmitted from a single individual when the population group was small and isolated. For example, genetic disorders seen in much higher than average rates in populations such as Finns and Ashkenazi Jews result from the founder effect.

The term also refers to the difference in the genetic diversity of distinct, isolated samples of a given population group, and how these differences are manifest in subsequent generations. The concept of the founder effect was elucidated by A. R. Templeton in 1980.

fragile site   Specific points of the CHROMOSOMES that are prone to break, or at least to appear broken. When the chromosomes are "damaged" in this manner, the chromosomal aberrations that ensue may result in GENETIC DISORDERS. Translocations may occur at these sites, and they may have importance in the genetic changes underlying CANCER. Special techniques employed in laboratory testing are often needed to demonstrate the existence of these non-staining gaps, e.g., the use of a folate-deficient cell culture medium. (See also FRAGILE X SYNDROME; CHROMOSOME ABNORMALITIES.)

fragile X associated tremor ataxia syndrome (FXTAS)   A late-onset progressive neurological disorder characterized by severe tremor and impairment of walking and balance. Other symptoms can include short-term memory loss, cognitive decline, Parkinsonism, weakening of the lower limbs and dysfunction of the autonomic system.

FXTAS affects individuals who have a permutation of the same gene responsible for fragile X syndrome, *FMR1*. The normal allele of the *FMR1* gene has less than 40 CGG repeats. Individuals who develop FXTAS, or carriers of the premutation expansion, have from 55–200 CGG repeats. Those with fragile X syndrome have more than 200 CGG repeats. However, FXTAS and fragile X syndrome are completely different. FXTAS affects males. Individuals with the full-blown fragile X mutation are apparently not prone to the same molecular dysfunction that ultimately results in FXTAS. The fact that the same gene is involved in the two disorders opens new paths for research in the function of the fragile X gene.

A hallmark of the disorder is the presence of intranuclear inclusions in the neurons and astrocytes (star-shaped neurons that control branching) throughout the central nervous system. Individuals diagnosed with FXTAS are primarily grandfathers of children with fragile X syndrome. Symptoms typically appear in the 50s or 60s. Carriers of the permutation exhibit an increased level of *FMR1* messenger RNA. But studies have found that only 20–30% of individuals who have the premutation develop FXTAS. The disorder has often been misdiagnosed, as many neurologists are unaware of its existence. Due to suspected under- and misdiagnosis, prevalence is unknown.

fragile X syndrome   X-LINKED trait and the second most common identifiable cause of genetic MENTAL RETARDATION after DOWN SYNDROME. It was first identified by geneticist Herbert Lubs, who observed the chromosomal defect responsible for the SYNDROME in 1969.

Some people have CHROMOSOMES that when studied in the laboratory, have a tendency to "break" or "tear." The damage to these aberrant chromosomes typically occurs in particular regions, called FRAGILE SITES. Most of the time these fragile sites are not associated with medical problems, but a pronounced non-staining gap in one such region, at the end of the long arm of the X CHROMOSOME (referred to by cytogeneticists as Xq27–Xq28; see CHROMOSOME ABNORMALITIES), is associated with fragile X syndrome.

In addition to moderate to severe mental retardation, other characteristics in individuals with fragile X syndrome may include large ears, large testes (macroorchidism), large jaw (prognathism), speech delays, prominent forehead, double-jointedness, autistic symptoms and occasional self-mutilation such as hand biting. The features are subtle and the disorder is difficult to diagnose clinically; laboratory testing is required. Life span is normal.

Fragile X syndrome does not behave in the typical manner of an X-linked trait. Nearly 20% of fragile X males are silent CARRIERS, who are unaffected by the syndrome but can pass the fragile X chromosome to their female offspring. About one-third of female fragile X carriers, who would be expected to be asymptomatic, exhibit some symptoms of the disorder. The explanation for these unusual characteristics of inheritance can be found in the underlying nature of the disorder. The disorder results from a MUTATION in a GENE that has been named the FMR-1 gene. Within this gene is a TRINUCLEOTIDE REPEAT, a region of the gene containing a stretch of DNA with a variable number of repeated copies of the trinucleotide (three bases of genetic code), CCG. Normal individuals have from six to 54 copies of the repeat. Individuals with a slightly larger number of copies (54–200) are said to carry a premutation. Premutation carriers generally have no manifestations but are at risk for transmitting the mutation and of having affected offspring. Premutation carriers include normal transmitting males and unaffected carrier females. During the production of eggs during meiosis in females, expansion of a premutation to a full mutation can occur. Males with a full mutation with more than 230 copies (up to 1,000 copies) have the typical manifestations of the fragile X syndrome. Only about 1/2 of females with this "full" mutation have mental retardation (pre-

sumably because they also have another X chromosome with a "normal" copy of the gene). When the gene has the large number of repeats it undergoes a process known as hypermethylation, which causes it to be inactivated, rendering its normal function deficient and causing the disorder's manifestations.

In the expansion of a premutation, women with fewer repeats usually show smaller increases in the length of the repeat chain. Thus, women with small (60–79) premutations are more likely to have offspring who still have premutations rather than full mutations, but the premutations are likely to be larger than their mothers'. Women with a larger number of trinucleotide repeats (100–230) generally will have offspring with full mutations. It is extremely unusual for a normal copy number to expand to become a premutation (i.e., a new mutation).

Since the late 19th century it has been noted that males institutionalized for mental retardation outnumber females by five to four. The fragile X syndrome and other forms of X-linked mental retardation account for part of the difference.

Fragile X syndrome is estimated to affect one in 2,000 males and to be responsible for 4–8% of mentally retarded males. It has been described in blacks, Indians, Filipinos, Japanese, whites, Zulus, indeed, virtually all ethnic groups.

Molecular DNA based testing to determine the number of CCG repeats in the FMR-1 gene allows both identification of full mutations and of premutation carriers. It can be used for carrier detection and for PRENATAL DIAGNOSIS on fetal tissue samples obtained by CVS or AMNIOCENTESIS.

Folic acid is a form of vitamin B, and there have been attempts to treat fragile X individuals with vitamin B therapy, but the results thus far are generally considered inconclusive. Though numerous anecdotal reports suggest some behavioral improvement, many well conducted scientific trials have been unable to demonstrate any consistent benefit of folic acid therapy.

Fraser syndrome   See CRYPTOPHTHALMOS.

Freeman-Sheldon syndrome   See WHISTLING FACE SYNDROME.

Friedreich's ataxia   Ataxias are disorders characterized by neuromuscular disturbances resulting in the loss of coordination and balance, and Friedreich's ataxia (FA) is the most common inherited form. It is named for Nikolaus Friedreich, a German neurologist who, in the 1860s, published the first description of a mysterious inherited disease marked by progressive loss of coordination and nerve degeneration.

FA typically begins in the first or second decade of life. Clumsiness is exhibited in the upper or lower extremities, along with a peculiar swaying and irregular movements. As the disease progresses, there is further impairment of limb coordination, gradual loss of sensation in affected limbs, and muscle weakness. Eventually, speech can become affected, making communication difficult. Lateral curvature of the spine (SCOLIOSIS) usually develops, often with disabling results. Foot deformities and heart disease are also frequent features. As many as 40% of affected individuals have DIABETES MELLITUS. Within five years of onset, use of a wheelchair may be required. Complications are often fatal. The mean age of death is 37, though some that have come to medical attention appear to have a normal life expectancy.

The incidence is difficult to judge, as many affected individuals may be misdiagnosed. Estimates of the total number of affected individuals in the United States range from 2,000 to 3,000 to as many as 20,000 cases. It is inherited in an AUTOSOMAL RECESSIVE manner.

The location of the GENE responsible for FA is mapped to chromosome 9 and encodes a protein that has been named frataxin. It appears to be a protein involved in the function of mitochondria, the cellular organelle involved in energy metabolism. This gene carries a TRINUCLEOTIDE REPEAT (sometimes known as a triple repeat), a region of the gene containing a stretch of DNA with a variable number of repeated copies of the trinucleotide (three bases of genetic code), GAA. Normally there are only a small number of copies of this GAA repeat (5–33). Affected individuals have extended repeats (66–1,700) in both copies of their FA gene. (CARRIERS have one normal and one extended copy.) Most expanded alleles contain between 600 and 1,200 repeats. Premutation alleles are mutable but normal alleles and contain 34 to 65 repeats. These premutations do not cause Friedreich ataxia, but they may expand during transmission from either parent and result in disease-causing alleles and thus the disease. Rare patients have had point mutations in one copy of the gene and the expansion of the other.

This was the first AUTOSOMAL RECESSIVE disease found to be caused by a trinucleotide repeat mutation. Carrier detection, presymptomatic and PRENATAL DIAGNOSIS are all possible using direct mutation detection by DNA analysis. (There appear to be other very rare forms of the disease which involve a different gene.)

A number of drugs in development may help alleviate some symptoms of this disorder, but currently there is no cure.

frontometaphyseal dysplasia   Rare hereditary disorder marked by a peculiar facial appearance, dental abnormalities, multiple joint contractures (see ARTHROGRYPOSIS) and skeletal deformities.

The face is coarse, with wide nasal bridge, wideset eyes (HYPERTELORISM) and incomplete development of the sinuses. The ridges above the eyes (supraorbital ridges) tend to be prominent and the chin pointed and small. Onset of skeletal deformities begins in early childhood. Life span and intelligence are normal in most of those affected. It is inherited as an X-LINKED trait with severe manifestations in males and variable but generally more mild manifestations in females. Over 20 cases have been described.

Frontometaphyseal dysplasia is one of a heterogeneous group of disorders often referred to as the otopalatodigital spectrum disorders. The disorders include otopalatodigital syndrome types I (OPD1) and II (OPD2) (see entry) and Melnick-Needles syndrome (MNS) (see entry). Particularly in affected males, the severity of the disorders ranges from the mild manifestations seen in OPD1 to the more severe effects in FMD and OPD2. MNS is most commonly lethal before birth in affected males. All of these disorders are caused by mutations in the X-linked *FLNA* gene. Other mutations in this gene cause X-linked periventricular nodular heterotopia, a neuronal migration disorder that presents with seizures and nodules of neurons situated in the wrong place along the surface of the brain's lateral ventricles.

fructose intolerance (fructose-1-phosphate aldolase deficiency)   Fructose is a sugar present in foods such as fruits, sugar cane, corn syrup, honey and fruit juices. Table sugar or sucrose contains fructose and glucose. Fructose intolerance occurs when the body is unable to metabolize fructose because of the hereditary absence or deficiency of the ENZYME fructose-1-phosphate aldolase. Ingestion of fructose under these conditions results in the blocking of the formation of glucose, a sugar essential as a major source of energy for the body.

In infants born with fructose intolerance, the continued feeding of foods containing fructose will have serious complications, leading to nausea, vomiting, FAILURE TO THRIVE, seizures caused by an abnormally low level of blood sugar (hypoglycemia), enlarged liver (hepatomegaly), jaundice, excessive fluid in the tissues (edema), abnormal pooling of fluid in the abdominal cavity, malnutrition and wasting, eventual liver failure, dehydration and death. When the disorder is not discovered, infants who continue to be fed foods containing fructose often die between two and six months of age.

The disorder can be detected after birth by a fructose tolerance test or a liver biopsy that will disclose the enzyme deficiency. Once the determination is made, all fructose-containing foods must be completely avoided. Full recovery will follow with a normal life span.

This rare disorder is inherited as an AUTOSOMAL RECESSIVE trait. As the GENE for the deficient enzyme has been cloned, and several MUTATIONS causing the disease identified, DNA-based diagnosis is now possible. This can potentially be used as an alternative to loading tests (administering a substance to measure the ability to metabolize or excrete it), or liver biopsy for diagnosis, or for CARRIER detection and PRENATAL DIAGNOSIS in certain families.

fructose-1-phosphate aldolase deficiency   See FRUCTOSE INTOLERANCE.

fucosidosis   Very rare SYNDROME, identified in well under 100 children, caused by a deficiency of the ENZYME alpha-L-fucosidase, which results in abnormal intracelluar accumulation of fucose, a sugar containing compounds such as glypolipids, lipoproteins, oliogosaccharides and polysaccharides. There is variability in its presentation. Children with more severe forms of the disorder do not generally survive beyond six years of age.

In some patients, mental and motor development stop at age 10 months, followed by progressive deterioration of the nervous system and muscle weakness, followed in turn by the onset of spasticity and tremor and a loss of awareness of environmental contact, eventually resulting in a state of total unresponsiveness.

Frequently, physical characteristics include thick skin, short head with a prominent forehead, heavy eyebrows, wide-set eyes (HYPERTELORISM), flat nose and thick lips. The chest is broad, and lateral curvature of the spine (SCOLIOSIS) may be evident. The heart is often enlarged. Enlargement of the liver and spleen are evident (hepatosplenomegaly), giving affected infants an appearance resembling children with Hurler syndrome and other MUCOPOLYSACCHARIDOSES.

In some affected children, onset occurs later, between 18 months and three years. Spasticity and seizures can also be features. Deterioration of mental and motor skills and nervous system is less rapid. Skin lesions may develop, primarily in the pubic area. These lesions are termed angiokeratomas, dilated blood vessels whose walls are filled with accumulated substances and resemble those seen in FABRY DISEASE. Many affected individuals with only slow or minimal progression of their neorologic disease survive beyond adolescence and into young adulthood, and can live into their third or fourth decade.

A specific diagnosis may be made by low white blood cell or skin fibroblast activity of alpha-L-fucosidase. PRENATAL DIAGNOSIS may be made by examining fetal cells obtained via AMNIOCENTESIS or CHORIONIC VILLUS SAMPLING.

This disorder displays an AUTOSOMAL RECESSIVE inheritance pattern. There may be a higher frequency in children of Italian descent. The GENE is on the short arm of chromosome 1.

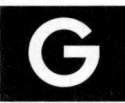

galactokinase deficiency Symptoms of this ENZYME deficiency are CATARACTS in early infancy, associated with an excess of the sugar galactose in the blood (GALACTOSEMIA). Affected individuals lack the Enzyme galactokinase, which helps metabolize galactose. A variant of galactosemia, the sole clinical significance of this deficiency is that the accumulation of unmetabolized galactose eventually leads to cataracts.

This disorder can be detected at any age by blood and urine tests. Newborns are routinely screened for galactosemia in many states, and depending on the test used, galactokinase deficiency may be found. A diet that excludes milk, milk products and other sources of galactose prevents cataract formation and can reverse cataracts that have just begun to form. Cataracts can also be removed surgically.

Life span is normal, although cataracts may recur, requiring further surgery.

Galactokinase deficiency is inherited as an AUTO-SOMAL RECESSIVE TRAIT. The GENE responsible is on the long arm of chromosome 17. First observed in three Gypsy families, well under 100 individuals with the disorder are known. Its frequency is estimated at one in 250,000. prenatal diagnosis can be accomplished by enzyme assay on AMNIOTIC FLUID cells. Pregnant mothers at risk should restrict their galactose intake to protect an affected FETUS.

galactosemia A rare hereditary metabolic disease observed in the newborn that can lead to MENTAL RETARDATION, BLINDNESS and ultimately death. It is caused by the inability to convert galactose (a milk sugar) into glucose (blood sugar), the body's fuel. This inability results from the absence of galactose-1-phosphate uridyl-transferase, the ENZYME responsible for this conversion. The condition was first described in 1908, and the enzyme defect demonstrated in 1956. (The GENE responsible has been mapped to chromosome 9.)

The disease usually appears within the first few days of life, following ingestion of breast milk or formula. Early symptoms include lethargy, feeding difficulties, vomiting, jaundice and an enlarged liver (hepatomegaly). Affected individuals may also exhibit irritability, FAILURE TO THRIVE, diarrhea and severe bacterial infections. Untreated, it may lead to death. Those who survive, even with prompt treatment, often fail to grow, may be mentally retarded, develop CATARACTS, and may suffer liver and kidney damage. Late manifestations include speech defects, learning difficulties, neurologic problems and ovarian dysfunction. Rare cases may have only mild or no symptoms and escape detection.

Galactosemia is the most common cause of cataracts in infancy. The elevated level of galactose and other sugars in the blood allows them to be absorbed into the cells of the lens of the eye. There, the sugars absorb water, swelling the eye to the extent that it loses transparency. Many states have mandatory neonatal screening programs for galactosemia.

Diagnosis is made on the basis of blood tests that measure the level of conversion enzyme activity in the infant's blood cells. Affected newborns exhibit no enzyme activity, while CARRIERS have about half the normal activity level. Galactose will also be present in the urine of those affected. PRENATAL DIAGNOSIS is possible via AMNIOCENTESIS. Though it has been recommended that pregnant women who are known carriers, or whose infants have been diagnosed in utero, should exclude galactose from their diets, it is not established that this is effective. Affected individuals may have to eliminate galactose from their diets for their entire lives.

Inherited as an AUTOSOMAL RECESSIVE trait, galactosemia is estimated to occur in approximately one in 20,000 to one in 60,000 live births.

gallbladder anomalies This group of ANOMALIES takes many forms. In its most extreme variation, the gallbladder is completely absent (gallbladder agenesis), usually in association with incomplete development of the bile ducts. In another, the gallbladder is duplicated. Other, very rare variations include: bilobed gallbladder, in which the gallbladder is partially divided (but not separated into two duplicate organs); diverticulum of gallbladder, in which a portion of the gallbladder herniates through a weak spot to form an extra pouch on the outside of an organ; floating gallbladder, in which the membrane (mesentery) that attaches the gallbladder to the body is greatly elongated; and anomalous location or ectopic gallbladder, in which the gallbladder is displaced to the left or the rear or is inside the liver. Other defects include abnormalities of the ducts of the gallbladder. Hypoplasia of the gall bladder is often seen in association with CYSTIC FIBROSIS.

Gallbladder duplication is common in animals (for example 1:8 cats) but rare in humans (1:3,000–1:4,000). These variations are also important during surgery when, for example, the anomalously positioned ducts can be accidentally severed or tied up.

The basic defect and genetic basis for the disorders are unknown. Normal life span is not affected, and the condition is usually asymptomatic except in circumstances where a floating gallbladder turns, twisting the mesentery, cutting off the organ's blood supply and causing pain, nausea and vomiting.

CONGENITAL absence of gallbladder occurs in approximately one in 3,300 live births, and duplications of gallbladder in one in 4,000 live births. Currently, there is no PRENATAL DIAGNOSTIC method available, though the gallbladder may be visualized by prenatal ULTRASOUND (fetal gallstones have been diagnosed in this way).

gampsodactyly See CLAWFOOT.

Gardner syndrome See COLORECTAL CANCER.

gastroschisis Comes from the Greek: *gastro*, "belly," and *schisis*, "separation." The failure of the abdominal wall to close completely before birth. As a result, the viscera are exposed at birth and usually protrude through the opening. Typically the opening is small (3–5 cm; 1.2–2 in) and to the right of the umbilicus, the point at which the umbilical cord joins the abdomen. The umbilicus is not affected, as contrasted with OMPHALOCELES. The intestines may be abnormally short. In some cases, the protrusion causes blockage of the intestines or abnormal attachment to other structures.

In contrast with omphalocele, in which 75% of individuals have associated ANOMALIES, in gastroschisis only about 20% do. The incidence is about 1:10,000 (estimates range from 1:6,000–1:15,000). Highest incidence occurs among young mothers (under the age of 20), where incidence is 7:10,000 births. Ten families with familial recurrence have now been documented. Ninety percent of infants with gastroschisis are liveborn. PRENATAL DIAGNOSIS is possible (and common) by ULTRASOUND or abnormal maternal ALPHA-FETOPROTEIN screening.

Gaucher disease (GD) Named for Dr. Philippe C. E. Gaucher, a French physician who first described the disease in 1882, Gaucher disease is an inherited metabolic disorder that leads to the accumulation of a particular lipid, a fatty substance, in internal organs.

GD, like other similar metabolic disorders, is referred to as a STORAGE DISEASE, due to the accumulation, or storage, of material in the body. The accumulation is the result of a deficiency of the ENZYME acid B-glucosidase, which is necessary to break down a particular lipid, glucosyl ceramide. As it accumulates, the glucosyl cerarnide is stored in the scavenger cells of the body, which, taking on a characteristic appearance unique to those affected with this disorder, are called "Gaucher cells." This lipid, which is normally present in only small amounts, accumulates in the spleen, liver and bone marrow and, in some cases, in the lungs. (It accumulates in the central nervous system only in types 2 and 3.)

Gaucher cells in the bone marrow can cause bone and joint pain, fractures and other orthopedic problems. Accumulation in the spleen and liver causes enlargement of these organs and can lead to blood abnormalities such as ANEMIA, easy bruising and impaired blood clotting.

Affected individuals experience pain, frequent nosebleeds, anemia, lack of energy, infections and extremely distended abdomens. At present, therapy for the disease is symptomatic. As the bones weaken, surgery may be required for hip or knee joint replacement. Surgical removal of the enlarged spleen may be necessary to correct the problems related to low blood counts.

There are three types of GD, differing in their severity, course and incidence. The three forms are differentiated by the absence or presence and severity of primary neurologic manifestations. All are inherited in an AUTOSOMAL RECESSIVE manner.

Type 1—Chronic (non-neuronopathic) form This is by far the most common form, with wide variability in the symptoms and severity. Features may include enlarged spleen and liver (hepatosplenomegaly), low blood count, bleeding episodes, bone deterioration, fractures and, rarely, acute liver complications. There is no mental or neurological involvement.

Symptoms of Type 1 GD usually appear in childhood or early adulthood, but diagnosis may be made as early as the first weeks of life, though some patients are not detected until mid- or late-adulthood. Some who come to medical attention have severe disease in childhood, while others may be completely asymptomatic when diagnosed at 60 or more years of age. The signs may be an enlarged abdomen, blood abnormalities or orthopedic problems. Due to the variability of this disorder, it is difficult to predict its severity in any given individual. There is no classic, predictable disease course.

Type 2—Infantile form This type is extremely rare, and shows no predilection for any particular racial or ETHNIC GROUP. Onset is in infancy, with diagnosis generally made by six months of age. The hallmark of this form is rapid nervous system deterioration, with death by the age of two years.

Type 3—Juvenile form This form is very rare, except in a particular region of Sweden, where most cases have been identified. It begins in childhood, with all the manifestations of Type 1 disease but has a neurologic component similar to Type 2,

except with a slower progression. Involvement of the brain creates the neurological problems, including retardation, seizures and abnormal body and eye movements, leading to death, often by 20 to 30 years of age.

Although GD affects all racial and ethnic groups, it is particularly prevalent in Ashkenazi Jews (of Central and Eastern European ancestry) and is the most common GENETIC DISORDER among this population: As many as one in 25 had been estimated to be CARRIERS of the GENE for this disease. Its incidence has been estimated to be approximately one in 2,500 live births among Ashkenazi Jews based on those individuals who were identified as being clinically affected. Less than one in 40,000 live births in the general population are identified. It has been estimated that there are approximately 20,000 affected individuals in the United States.

Carrier testing for GD is possible with a blood test to determine the level of the enzyme acid B-glucosidase. PRENATAL DIAGNOSIS for all forms of GD is possible with CHORIONIC VILLUS SAMPLING or AMNIOCENTESIS.

Significant research is currently under way on this disorder, as it is considered a model that may help unravel the mysteries of other storage and enzyme deficiency diseases, including specific therapy for these diseases by enzyme or gene replacement strategies.

The gene for this disorder is on the long arm of chromosome 1, and many MUTATIONS have been discovered. Five different mutations account for 96–98% of Gaucher disease in Ashkenazi Jews. DNA-based screening of this population has revealed that about one in every 10 to 15 such individuals is a carrier of a Gaucher disease mutation and about one in 400 to 600 is affected. Prior to the availability of this testing, it was thought that about one in 2,500 was affected, thus about 2/3 of those who have the disease have not been diagnosed. This is because their symptoms are vary mild, if they have any at all. Many patients who carry particular mutations may have only very late onset disease, very mild disease or no symptoms at all; but other individuals with this same mutation can have a quite serious, early onset disease.

Treatment involves enzyme replacement therapy, that is, infusions of the enzyme deficient in individuals affected with the disease. The enzyme is either purified from placental tissue or produced using RECOMBINANT DNA technology. The infusion must be given intravenously and is very expensive, costing in the hundreds of thousands of dollars a year per patient. Hundreds of patients are now receiving this therapy. Bone marrow transplantation is also an effective treatment but has many complications. Trials of gene therapy are under way. Carrier testing is available using both biochemical and DNA based methods. Screening for carriers (particularly in at-risk populations) is controversial though the disorder is frequent; though the test is reliable, and treatment available, individuals with identical mutations may have very different manifestations and prognosis. Many will be asymptomatic even without therapy. Prenatal diagnosis is available, but the same concerns have been raised regarding its use.

Other storage diseases include TAY-SACHS DISEASE, FABRY DISEASE, MUCOPOLYSACCHARIDOSIS and GLYCOGEN STORAGE DISEASE.

gene   The basic unit of hereditary traits. Chemically they are composed of DEOXYRIBONUCLEIC ACID (DNA), strings of complex, nucleic acid-based "super" molecules. Genetically, they are the determinants of the characteristics that identify living things as individuals and as members of a species. They are passed from generation to generation bundled within CHROMOSOMES, ever replicating and dividing in new combinations. Alterations in the genes result in genetic variations, which results in all our individual differences as well as in GENETIC DISORDERS.

The term *gene* was introduced in 1909 by Wilhelm Ludwig Johannsen (1857–1927), a pharmacist's apprentice from Copenhagen who went on to become a respected figure in genetics and botany. (He also introduced the term GENOTYPE). He defined a gene as an accounting, or calculating, unit of heredity. However, the concept of genes had already been accepted, called by names such as "physiological units," "gemmule," "idioplasm," "micellae" and "pangene."

Genes exist in pairs, strung together to form the 23 chromosome pairs found in the nucleus of every somatic, or non-sex, cell. It is estimated that if all this genetic material packed into each cell were unraveled, it would stretch 6 feet. If one were to have a written printout of all the individual's genes, including all the genetic material from both parents, using just one letter for each nucleotide (the individual molecules making up the DNA), the printout would fill the pages found in over 25 sets of *The Encyclopaedia Britannica.*

Each gene occupies a specific point (locus) on a chromosome, and each gene in a pair is called an ALLELE. Alleles are often dominant or recessive. Dominant genes are so named because their action will dominate, or override, the influence of a dissimilar allele in the pair. Recessive genes are so named because their action will be recessed, or overriden, by a dissimilar allele. Individuals who have identical alleles for a given trait, either both dominant or both recessive genes, are said to be HOMOZYGOTES, or homozygous for a given trait. Those who have dissimilar alleles, or genes, one dominant and one recessive, are said to be HETEROZYGOTES, or heterozygous for the trait. (The alleles for blood type are neither dominant nor recessive, but A, B and O, representing the three major blood types.)

Genes display great variety. Some control several functions. Others modify the workings of yet another. Some appear to be master genes regulating the action of several. And some turn on and off at different ages. Approximately half of the estimated 60,000 to 80,000 gene pairs found in each human cell have, as yet, no discernible function at all. Indeed, the concept of what constitutes a gene (as opposed to merely a small segment of genetic material) is not entirely clear.

Many HEREDITARY DISEASES are caused by genes that have been damaged or changed. (Damage or aberration in the chromosomes themselves, rather than in single genes, is also responsible for hereditary conditions. See CHROMOSOME ABNORMALITIES.) These changes are called MUTATIONS. Most mutations are harmless, but some have the ability to seriously affect the individual who possesses the mutation, whether acquired from inheritance or, in rare situations, from spontaneous mutation. Gene mutations may be either dominant or recessive. For a recessive condition to appear in an individual, he or she must be homozygous, that is, have two recessive mutant genes. For an individual to have a dominant condition, he or she needs only one gene for the disorder, that is, needs to be a heterozygote for the disorder to manifest. Homozygotes for dominant conditions, that is, those with two identical dominant mutant genes, often exhibit extremely severe symptoms of the condition, or die IN UTERO.

(See also AUTOSOMAL DOMINANT; AUTOSOMAL RECESSIVE; GENOME and the Introduction.)

gene mapping   The assignment of a GENE to a specific point on a CHROMOSOME. Knowing the location of genes that cause HEREDITARY DISEASES is an important tool in the diagnosis, and perhaps the eventual treatment, of these conditions. Mapping is also a critical tool in identifying the causes of GENETIC DISORDERS and screening individuals who may be at risk for developing them. By identifying the location of aberrant genes, researchers and clinicians can then look for the gene in that location in other individuals to confirm a diagnosis, or identify a CARRIER or those at risk for developing the disorder.

The first example of gene mapping was accomplished in 1911, when the gene for COLOR BLINDNESS was assigned to the X CHROMOSOME. It was another 50 years before genes could be mapped to autosomes, or non-sex chromosomes, but by the end of the 1990s, over 7,600 genes had been mapped, and tens of thousands of human gene fragments identified.

At the dawn of the 21st century, efforts were well underway to create maps of the human GENOME and identify all 60,000 to 80,000 genes that comprise it. The Human Genome Project (HGP), an international project largely funded by and conducted in the United States, projected a completion date of 2003. The Celera Corporation, a private venture between Perkin-Elmer, a manufacturer of gene-sequencing machinery, and Dr. J. Craig Venter of the Institute for Genomic Research of Rockville, Maryland, engaged in a parallel commercial effort. Major pharmaceutical companies operating as the SNP Consortium mounted a third mapping project in association with the HGP. (See RESTRICTION ENZYME for explanation of SNP acronym.)

gene splicing   See RECOMBINANT DNA.

gene therapy   The process of inserting a normal gene, or a portion of it, into cells and tissue to replace a missing or defective gene in an individual. Efforts to use gene therapy in the treatment of genetic disorders have focused on single-gene defects, such as cystic fibrosis, hemophilia, muscular dystrophy and sickle cell anemia. However, finding a method of inserting large sections of DNA to the right site on the genome has proved challenging. It is currently used to treat SCID, an immunodeficiency disease.

In the 1990s, scores of biotech companies were founded to create gene therapy products. However, in 1999, an 18-year-old died during gene therapy clinical trials at the University of Pennsylvania. The teenager, Jesse Gelsinger, had partial ornithine transcarbamylase deficiency, a rare liver disorder successfully controlled by medication. The death brought increased scrutiny to clinical research and the adequacy of patient safeguards and underscored society's difficulty in balancing regulation and research. Shortly thereafter, the National Institutes of Health disclosed it had received some 600 reports of adverse reactions in gene therapy trials going back to 1993, and the Food and Drug Administration suspended authorizations for several clinical gene therapy trials. In the half decade after, clinical gene therapy research remained largely dormant.

genetic code   The code whereby RNA (ribonucleic acid) creates AMINO ACIDS (from which proteins and polypepides are synthesized) or provides instructions for a step in creating a protein. The sequence of RNA used as the template for creating amino acids is determined by the DNA sequence upon which the RNA is made. The RNA is composed of nucleotide bases, linked together in groups of three called CODONS. Each individual codon of RNA specifies one of the 20 amino acids. For example, the three-base codon, CAG, in RNA codes for the amino acid glutamine. At any one of the three positions in the codon there are four possible bases and thus there are 64 possible triplet combinations ($4 \times 4 \times 4$). These different combinations code for the different amino acids (more than one combination specifies one amino acid as there are only 20 possible amino acids and 64 codons), and three of them code for a "stop" command signaling the end

TABLE XI
INDICATIONS FOR GENETIC COUNSELING

- Family history of a known genetic disorder or recurrent pathologic condition
- Birth defects—single anomalies, multiple defect patterns, metabolic disorders
- Mental retardation or developmental delay
- Chronic neurologic or neuromuscular childhood disorders
- Short stature and other growth disorders
- Dysmorphic features
- Ambiguous genitalia or abnormal sexual development
- Carrier status for a genetic disease with increased incidence in specific population groups—sickle-cell, Tay-Sachs, thalassemia
- Infertility, sterility, or fetal wastage
- Exposure to potentially mutagenic or teratogenic agents
- Pregnancy at age 35 or older
- Genetic risks in consanguinity
- Adult-onset disability of genetic origin
- Behavioral disorders of genetic origin
- Cancer, heart disease and other common conditions with a genetic component

Reproduced, with the permission of the National Genetics Foundation, Inc., from R. B. Berini and E. Kahn (eds.), *Clinical Genetics Handbook* (Oradell, N.J.: Medical Economics Co., Inc., 1987). All rights reserved.

of a protein sequence. Because there is virtually an infinite number of possible sequences of codons, all the different protein sequences can be encoded.

genetic counseling   The process of helping parents, prospective parents or others understand genetic information and issues that may have an impact on them and their families.

This counseling may be offered to prospective parents in helping them evaluate risks for hereditary or genetic conditions to their offspring based on familial history, age, lifestyle or other factors that may influence the health of their offspring. Counseling may be offered to parents following the birth of an affected individual. The goal of the counseling is to allow the parents or prospective parents to make informed decisions on their own, not to make decisions for them, as there is no option that is either right or wrong; the individuals being counseled must decide what is best for them. The information to be explained includes the diagnosis when a particular condition has been identified in an offspring, the prognosis, or outlook, for the future impact of the condition, and available treatment. When the condition is diagnosed prenatally, counseling includes information on options, such as termination of the pregnancy (see ABORTION) or, in rare cases, FETAL SURGERY. Assessing recurrence risks for future pregnancies is also a key component

TABLE XII
INCIDENCE OF GENETIC OR PARTIALLY GENETIC DISEASES PER 1,000 LIVE BIRTHS

Disease Category	British Columbia 1967–69 Study			UNSCEAR Reports			
	Minimal	Adjusted	Highest Rates	1966	1977[a]	1982	1986
Dominant[b]	0.6	0.8	1.4	10.0	10.0	10.0	10.0
X-linked	0.3	0.4	0.5	. . .	. . .	. . .	. . .
Recessive	0.9	1.1	1.7	2.0	1.1[c]	2.5	2.5
Chromosomal							
Numerical	1.6	2.0	1.9	4.0	4.0	4.0	3.4
Structural	. . .	. . .	. . .	. . .	. . .	. . .	0.4
Multifactorial							
Congenital	36.0	43.0	23.1	25.0	90.0	90.0	90.0[d]
Other	16.0	47.0	23.9	15.0	. . .	. . .	. . .
Genetic unknown	. . .	. . .	1.2	. . .	. . .	. . .	. . .
Total[e]	55.0	94.0	53.2	56.0	105.0	107.0	106.0

[a]The values used in the report of the BEIR committee in 1980 (8) were essentially identical to those in the 1977 UNSCEAR report.
[b]The figures from the UNSCEAR reports include autosomal and X-linked dominants.
[c]The change from 1.1 to 2.5 was made by UNSCEAR to include those disorders whose mutant genes are maintained by heterozygous advantage.
[d]Includes congenital anomalies and other multifactorial disorders.
[e]The sums are not exact owing to rounding.
Source: Patricia A. Baird, "A Population Study of Genetic Disorders in Children and Young Adults," *American Journal of Human Genetics* 42 (1988): 677–693.

of counseling, and may involve extensive diagnostic procedures, in an effort to determine the exact cause or nature of a BIRTH DEFECT or other anomalous condition. Counseling can also involve screening individuals from populations known to have an increased risk for some HEREDITARY DISEASES to determine if they are CARRIERS for the trait, when carrier detection is possible.

Genetic counseling began during the 1950s and 1960s, as advances in genetic research revealed the hereditary basis of a growing number of genetic conditions, and advances in diagnostic techniques, such as AMNIOCENTESIS (which was perfected by the end of the 1960s) allowed the identification of some of these disorders.

Genetic counseling may be offered by family physicians or by specialists trained in genetics. It is recommended for families in which an offspring exhibits birth defects, MENTAL RETARDATION, developmental delay, short stature or growth disorders, AMBIGUOUS GENITALIA or chronic neurologic or neuromuscular disorders.

It is also recommended in families with a known history of a GENETIC DISORDER, when parents are consanguineous (see CONSANGUINITY), and when maternal age is 35 years or older. (See Tables XI and XII.)

genetic disorder Any disorder with its origin in a variation of DNA (see DEOXYRIBONUCLEIC ACID), the genetic material in the cell nucleus that controls HEREDITY as well as the production of ENZYMES and other proteins. GENES, and the CHROMOSOMES on which they are found, are constructed from DNA.

Not all genetic disorders are hereditary, that is, passed from parent to offspring through the action of genes, though the majority are. For example, sporadically occurring chromosomal aberrations passed from parent to offspring, or variations that occur in the chromosomes soon after conception (see CHROMOSOME ABNORMALITIES), can cause disorders that are not hereditary, though they are genetic. Also, genetic disorders are not necessarily CONGENITAL, or apparent at birth (see BIRTH DEFECTS). They may have ages of onset ranging from early infancy to late adulthood.

Genetic disorders fall in three categories: MENDELIAN, or single-gene disorders; chromosomal disorders; and MULTIFACTORIAL disorders. Mendelian disorders result from the action of a single gene or gene pair. They are inherited in dominant and recessive fashion, following laws of inheritance first articulated by Gregor Mendel. More than 4,200 known or suspected single gene disorders have been reported to exist, and are estimated to occur in about 1% of the human population.

Chromosome disorders result from the addition or deletion of genetic material in the cell, or from an abnormal arrangement of the chromosomes. DOWN SYNDROME, for example, is a chromosomal disorder caused by the presence of an extra, third copy of chromosome 21. KLINEFELTER SYNDROME, a relatively common chromosomal disorder that occurs only in males, is caused by the presence of an extra X CHROMOSOME.

Multifactorial disorders are those caused by the action of several genes in concert with environmental influences. These make up the greatest number of genetic disorders by far, and include CLEFT LIP or CLEFT PALATE, CONGENITAL HEART DEFECTS, NEURAL TUBE DEFECTS (SPINA BIFIDA and ANENCEPHALY), SCHIZOPHRENIA and ESSENTIAL HYPERTENSION.

Genetic disorders are estimated to account for approximately 30% to 50% of all infant hospitalizations. More than 5% of all individuals under the age of 25 are believed to have a genetic disorder, and when late onset multifactorial disorders are included, about 60% of all individuals are thought to have genetically influenced conditions. Genetic influence also appears to play a strong role in premature adult death (below age 50) from all natural causes, including infections and cardiovascular disease. (See also the Introduction.)

genetic linkage The association of GENES located near each other on the same CHROMOSOME. As a result of this linkage, these genes are usually inherited together. (Linkage of traits was first seen in studies of coat color in house mice published by A. B. Darbishire in 1904.)

PRENATAL DIAGNOSIS of single gene disorders can be difficult or impossible if the underlying gene involved or the specific genetic defect or MUTATION is unknown. However, the diagnostic information desired may sometimes be obtained through

TABLE XIII
SAMPLE PRENATAL GENETIC SCREEN*

Name _____ Patient#_____ Date #_____

1. Will you be 35 years or older when the baby is due? Yes____ No____		

2. Have you, the baby's father, or anyone in either of your families ever had
   any of the following disorders?   Yes____   No____

   • Down syndrome (mongolism)   Yes____   No____
   • Other chromosomal abnormality   Yes____   No____
   • Neural tube defect, ie, spina bifida (meningomyelocele or open spine), anencephaly   Yes____   No____
   • Hemophilia   Yes____   No____
   • Muscular dystrophy   Yes____   No____
   • Cystic fibrosis   Yes____   No____

   If yes, indicate the relationship of the affected person to you or to the baby's father:_____
3. Do you or the baby's father have a birth defect?   Yes____   No____
   If yes, who has the defect and what is it? _____
4. In any previous marriages, have you or the baby's father had a child, born dead or alive, with a
   birth defect not listed in question 2 above?   Yes____   No____
   If yes, what was the defect and who had it?   Yes____   No____
5. Do you or the baby's father have any close relatives with mental retardation?   Yes____   No____
   If yes, indicate the relationship of the affected person to you or the baby's father: _____
   Indicate the cause, if known:_____
6. Do you, the baby's father, or a close relative in either of your families have a birth defect, any
   familial disorder, or a chromosomal abnormality not listed above?   Yes____   No____
   If yes, Indicate the condition and the relationship of the affected person to you or to the baby's father:_____
7. In any previous marriages, have you or the baby's father had a stillborn child or three or
   more first-trimester spontaneous pregnancy losses?   Yes____   No____
   Have either of you had a chromosomal study?   Yes____   No____
   If yes, indicate who and the results: _____
8. If you or the baby's father are of Jewish ancestry, have either of you been screened for   Yes____   No____
   Tay-Sachs disease?
   If yes, indicate who and the results: _____
9. If you or the baby's father are black, have either of you been screened for sickle cell trait?   Yes____   No____
   If yes, indicate who and the results: _____
10. If you or the baby's father are of Italian, Greek, or Mediterranean background, have either of
    you been tested for ß-thalassemia?   Yes____   No____
    If yes, indicate who and the results: _____
11. If you or the baby's father are of Philippine or Southeast Asian ancestry, have either of you been   Yes____   No____
    tested for a-thalassemia?
    If yes, indicate who and the results: _____
12. Excluding iron and vitamins, have you taken any medications or recreational drugs since being
    pregnant or since your last menstrual period? (include nonprescription drugs)   Yes____   No____
    If yes, give name of medication and time taken during pregnancy:

*Any patient replying "YES" to questions should be offered appropriate counseling. If the patient declines further counseling or testing this should
  be noted in the chart. Given that genetics is a field in a state of flux alterations or updates to this form will be required periodically.
Source: American College of Obstetricians and Gynecologists, *ACOG Technical Bulletin* 108 (1987), p. 3.

observation of gene linkage; the presence of the second marker gene, which may be perfectly normal, will disclose the presence of the linked defective gene. In order to use genetic linkage this way, the disease gene of interest must have been previously mapped and there must be GENETIC MARKERS linked to that gene available for use.

An advantage of this technique is that no special knowledge is required as to which specific gene, or what specific defect in a known gene, has caused the problem. If the linkage can be shown, then the diagnosis can be made with some degree of certainty. The major disadvantage of this technique is that linkage may be different for different families. Thus, many members of the family involved will have to be tested in order to known which genetic marker will work effectively to disclose the linkage. The family study must be undertaken prior to pregnancy or early in pregnancy, when linkage is to be used for PRENATAL DIAGNOSIS. In many cases, it is not possible to perform such an in-depth family study, and linkage analysis, therefore, will not be completely reliable.

Another potential problem is the possibility that the linkage relationship between the marker gene and the disease gene is altered due to recombination or crossing over. This occurs when the two chromosomes of a chromosome pair join together. When the chromosomes exchange material, if that exchange occurs between the marker and the gene of interest, they will not be inherited together. The frequency of this occurring is related to the distance between the two genes. The closer the two are, the less likely their linkage will be lost.

Knowledge that a gene is linked to another known gene also allows for mapping of the new gene (localization to a particular site or region on a specific chromosome) if the location of the first gene is known. This is an important step in identifying or cloning the new gene. With regard to cloning there must be a distinction made between cloning an organism (as in Dolly, the sheep cloned in England in 1998) and cloning a gene. Cloning an organism means making a complete copy while cloning a gene implies gene identification. (See also GENETIC MARKERS.)

genetic markers Indicators used to identify the presence of specific GENES or genetic defects. Often,

the genetic marker, or marker gene, will identify a DNA segment that indicates the presence of a particular GENETIC DISORDER without identifying the actual genetic defect, which may remain unknown. These markers are signposts linked to the disease gene. The marker gene and the disease gene, located close to each other on the same CHROMOSOME, are inherited together.

Some genetic markers involve specific biochemical variations, while other genetic markers depend on the variation among individual chromosomes that occurs when DNA is cut by RESTRICTION ENZYMES.

Restriction enzymes and DNA PROBES are often used in establishing genetic markers. DNA fragments produced by restriction enzymes, when mixed in solution with a DNA probe, will result in marking, or identifying, a particular segment of DNA that contains, or is close to, a specific gene.

Identifiable markers for genetic defects have aided in the PRENATAL DIAGNOSIS of disorders that previously could not be detected before birth. For example, FAMILIAL DYSAUTONOMIA could not be diagnosed prenatally until the discovery of a genetic marker closely linked to the gene for this disease. The gene that causes the disease isn't itself identified, but it is closely linked to the marker. If the marker is present, so too is the defective gene. Now, not only can it be diagnosed before birth, but also CARRIERS of this defect can be identified in families with familial dysautonomia, which enables parents who might conceive a child with familial dysautonomia to be made aware of this risk. (See also GENETIC LINKAGE.)

genetics The scientific study of heredity, the transmission of inherited characteristics from parent to offspring. The term was coined by English zoologist William Bateson, who formally suggested its adoption by the scientific community in 1906. (See also the Introduction.)

genetic screening Testing groups of individuals to identify defective GENES capable of causing HEREDITARY DISEASES. Screening is especially useful in populations known to be at increased risk for possessing mutant genes, such as blacks for SICKLE-CELL ANEMIA and Jews for TAY-SACHS DISEASE. In addition, newborn genetic screening programs exist for identifying infants with CONGENITAL disorders whose potentially devastating consequences, if diagnosed early, may be treatable. Examples are PHENYLKETONURIA (PKU) and CONGENITAL HYPOTHYROIDISM. (See Table XIII.)

genodermatosis   Any genetically influenced disease of the skin. These include EHLERS-DANLOS SYNDROME, PORPHYRIA, ICHTHYOSIS, EPIDERMOLYSIS BULLOSA, NEUROFIBROMATOSIS, TUBEROUS SCLEROSIS, ECTODERMAL DYSPLASIA, STURGE-WEBER SYNDROME and many others.

genome   The entire complement of genetic material found in the CHROMOSOMES. There are an estimated 20,000 to 25,000 GENES in the human genome. The human haploid genome (that is, the genetic material on one of each pair of chromosomes) contains 3 billion bases of DNA (see DEOXYRIBONUCLEIC ACID). Each gene is composed of a number of these bases. Just printing out this sequence, using one letter for each base of DNA, would occupy the equivalent of 13 sets of the Encyclopedia Britannica. The majority of the material is DNA that appears to have no role in the creation of proteins, the primary function of genes, and what role this material plays remains largely unanswered.

A preliminary map of the human genome was completed in 2003, created by the Human Genome Project (HGP). (Just a few years before completion of the map, it was thought the human genome contained as many as 100,000 genes, and previous estimates ran as high as 2,000,000.) The HGP began in 1986 and was formally launched in 1990, headed by the National Institutes of Health and the Department of Energy, with assistance from researchers in China, France, Germany, Japan and the United Kingdom. The $3 billion project was initially directed by Nobel laureate James Watson. In 1998, a privately funded effort to map the human genome was launched by Craig Venter and his company, Celera Genomics. The two groups collaborated on some aspects of the mapping and jointly announced completion of the preliminary map. In 2006, the project finished sequencing chromosome 1, the last and largest chromosome to be completely sequenced. The map of the genome will help researchers develop new approaches to the identification and potential treatment of genetic disorders.

genotype   The genetic makeup of an individual. This is contrasted to the PHENOTYPE, which refers to the physical appearance or characteristics of an individual. An individual will not always have characteristics that reflect his or her genotype. For example, some AUTOSOMAL DOMINANT disorders are not exhibited in all the individuals who possess the GENES for them. The degree to which the characteristics of a specific given gene (also referred to in a more limited sense as a genotype) are exhibited in an individual is referred to as EXPRESSIVITY, and the degree to which a genotype is manifest in a population is referred to as PENETRANCE. The term *genotype* was introduced in the 1900s by Wilhelm Ludwig Johannsen (1857–1927), a pharmacist's apprentice from Copenhagen who went on to achieve considerable renown in the fields of genetics and botany. He also introduced the terms *gene* and *phenotype*.

genu varum   See BOWLEG.

German measles   See TORCH SYNDROME.

geroderma osteodysplastica   See WALT DISNEY DWARFISM.

giant   See GIGANTISM.

gigantism   Excessive growth or development of any part of the body. Pituitary gigantism results from excessive growth hormone. Cerebral gigantism or SOTOS SYNDROME is a generally SPORADIC disorder of unknown cause resulting in large size, MENTAL RETARDATION and other problems.

Throughout history, there have been well-documented cases of "giants," individuals whose height and size was far above normal. Typically, these conditions are the result of hyperactivity of glands that regulate growth, are not visible at birth, and occur sporadically, the cause remaining unknown.

Gilbert disease Hereditary liver disorder, named for French physician and liver specialist Nicolas A. Gilbert (1858–1927) who first described it in 1901. A benign, congenital condition, it is characterized by a fluctuating elevation in serum bilirubin, a yellow pigment excreted by the liver. Bilirubin is produced by the breakdown of hemoglobin from red blood cells and is transported to the liver where it is chemically modified and excreted in the bile. In this disorder there is a defect in the liver's clearance of bilirubin.

Onset usually occurs during the teens or early adulthood. While symptoms are rarely significant, occasionally mild jaundice may appear, and the white of the eye may become yellow. Other than excess serum bilirubin, upon examination, all liver functions are normal. It requires no treatment and will not interfere with a normal life span. The importance of this condition lies in the fact that the mild jaundice may be mistaken for a more serious liver disease.

The estimated prevalence of Gilbert syndrome is reportedly as high as 3% to 7% of the adult population. Inherited in an AUTOSOMAL DOMINANT fashion, it results from deficient activity of the ENZYME glucuronyl-transferase in the liver.

Gilles de la Tourette syndrome See TOURETTE SYNDROME.

Glanzmann thrombasthenia See THROMBASTHENIA OF GLANZMANN AND NAEGELI.

glaucoma, congenital See CONGENITAL GLAUCOMA.

globoid cell leukodystrophy, GLD See KRABBE DISEASE.

glucose-6-phosphate dehydrogenase deficiency (G6PD) The most common inherited ENZYME deficiency, it results from a variety of MUTATIONS at a single GENE LOCUS. Over 300 such variations have been described. Transmitted as an X-LINKED recessive trait (the enzyme involved, G6PD, is produced by a single GENE on the X CHROMOSOME), it affects males primarily.

G6PD is involved in the repair of oxidation damage, which is critical in maintaining the membrane of red blood cells. The disorder is generally asymptomatic, though when triggered it results in episodes of hemolytic ANEMIA, a blood disorder caused by the premature destruction of red blood cells. The episodes may be triggered by exposure to certain drugs (e.g., quinine and derivatives), chemicals, infections, or ingestion of fava beans (see FAVISM). The chemicals present in fava beans that are believed to be responsible for triggering the episodes are divicine and isouramil.

There is a wide variability of severity among the forms of G6PD, depending on the severity of the inherited deficiency. Like SICKLE-CELL ANEMIA and THALASSEMIA, the disorder is common in populations originating in malaria-prone areas of the world, as the deficiency appears to bestow resistance to malaria.

Many newborns of Mediterranean or Asian ancestry with jaundice (neonatal hyperbilirubinemia) of unknown origin are found to be G6PD-deficient. Overall, G6PD deficiency is estimated to affect 400 million people worldwide. There are several common G6PD variants:

Type B. This is the usual form of the enzyme found in whites and in most black individuals. G6PD enzyme activity is normal.

Type A+. This variant, occurring in about 20% of black males in the United States, reduces normal G6PD activity only by about 10% and hemolysis does not occur.

Type A-. Found in about 12% of black males in the United States, it results in a reduction of G6PD activity by 10% to 20%. Enzyme activity declines as cells age. In type A-, the hemolysis is mild to moderate. If hemolysis occurs, it will affect older cells, leaving young red blood cells with normal enzyme levels, making diagnosis difficult. Hemolysis may occur after drug exposure.

G6PD Mediterranean. This is the most common abnormal variant found in white populations, particularly those of Mediterranean origin. Hemolysis is provoked by drugs or favism and can be severe. Activity is only 0–5% of normal.

Type B-. Two percent to 5% of U.S. males of Mediterranean ancestry have this variant. Enzyme activity is decreased a maximum of 5%, though it may not be decreased at all. Both young and old red blood cells may have reduced G6PD activity.

G6PD Chinese; G6PD Canton. These variants are common in Chinese populations and cause a reduction in enzyme activity of 4% to 25% of normal.

glutaric aciduria Affected individuals exhibit chronic problems with involuntary body movements. There is a wide variety of ceaseless, involuntary, rapid, highly complex, jerky motions or slow, writhing movements that are especially severe in the hands (choreoathetosis). Many of those affected contort themselves, holding one arm and shoulder back with the head drawn back to one side (dystonic posturing). They are usually mentally retarded. Some children have developed bleeding into the brain or in the eyes that could be mistaken for the effects of child abuse. Death is sometimes caused by an acute movement disorder episode.

At birth, infants appear normal, but within the first year they exhibit vomiting, diminished muscle tone (hypotonia) and abnormally high acid levels in the blood (acidemia).

Laboratory tests reveal elevated concentrations of glutaric and 3-hydroxy-glutaric acids in urine. Glutaric acid concentrations are also elevated in serum, cerebrospinal fluid and tissues. Glutaconic acids may occasionally be found in urine. The underlying abnormality is a deficiency of the ENZYME glutaryl-CoAdehydrogenase.

PRENATAL DIAGNOSIS is possible by enzyme assay testing of cultured amniotic cells obtained via AMNIOCENTESIS. At birth, the disorder can be detected by performing enzyme assay tests on white blood cells. Prenatal detection is possible by enzyme assay testing of cultured amniotic cells obtained via AMNIOCENTESIS. At birth, the disorder can be detected by performing enzyme assay tests on white blood cells. Infants affected with either type I or II (see below) may be identified in expanded newborn screening programs.

A rare disorder inherited as an AUTOSOMAL RECESSIVE trait, glutaric aciduria occurs in approximately one of every 30,000–40,000 births. It is much more common in the Amish community and in the Ojibway (First Nations) population in Canada. It is treatable with a special diet and with riboflavin (a B-complex vitamin). Carnitine replacement may also be used if levels are low. Most patients do not survive to childbearing age. The GENE is on the short arm of chromosome 19. Fewer than 100 cases have been reported in the United States.

Glutaric aciduria type II is a separate disorder in which not only glutaryl-CoAdehydrogenase is deficient, but also other enzymes involved in fatty acid metabolism—hence its more appropriate name, multiple acyl-CoAdehydrogenase deficiency. It varies in severity from overwhelming metabolic illness with death in the newborn period to milder cases with later onset in childhood with neurologic abnormalities, low blood sugar, hypotonia and heart abnormalities. GA type II is also autosomal recessive.

gluten-induced enteropathy (celiac disease; celiac sprue) Condition caused by an inability of the small intestine to digest and absorb nutrients, resulting from a hereditary sensitivity to gluten, a protein compound found in wheat and rye.

Onset is usually in late infancy or early childhood, but may begin in adult life. Symptoms include FAILURE TO THRIVE, passage of loose, pale, bulky, greasy and foul-smelling stools, and irritability. Affected individuals exhibit small stature, deficiencies of vitamin D, folic acid and iron, and increased risk of lymphatic system and gastrointestinal malignancies. There may also be an increased risk for DIABETES MELLITUS, autoimmune thyroiditis and lung diseases.

Both genetic and environmental factors have been implicated in the inheritance of celiac disease; the exact mechanism has not been clearly defined. The condition occurs in 1/1,000–1/2,000 live births. However, a wide variability of incidence is seen among various population groups, reflecting both genetic differences among these groups and differences in consumption of wheat. It occurs in 1/300 individuals in western Ireland. A MULTIFACTORIAL disorder, the genetic component includes at least some association with certain HLA genes. Gluten-free diets lead to improvement in symptoms within weeks in 75% of those treated.

glycogen storage disease (GSD) A group of inherited metabolic disorders of the liver and muscle, rendering the body unable to break glycogen down to glucose, the form of sugar needed to produce energy. As a result, there is an abnormal storage and accumulation of glycogen in tissues, especially the liver or muscle. One of the most common signs is a greatly enlarged liver (hepatomegaly). The other common symptom of some forms is muscle weakness.

Normally, the body stores excess sugar in the liver and muscles in the form of glycogen, a compound containing multiple branching chains of glucose molecules; these are molecules that are "branched" like a tree, rather than organized into a single long chain. Liver ENZYMES convert it back to glucose when the body needs energy. (Enzymes that control this activity are "debranching" enzymes.) The body can survive for days or weeks without eating, due to this conversion process. However, individuals with GSD cannot convert glycogen to glucose, and must be fed every few hours around the clock, to assure a constant supply of glucose from ingestion. Even with intensive dietary management, some individuals may suffer growth retardation, convulsions caused by low blood sugar, excessive bleeding, enlarged liver and abdomen, gout and increased susceptibility to infections. In severe cases, brain damage or early death may occur. The manifestations an individual exhibits depend on the specific type of the disease (see below). For example, in the forms affecting muscle, the muscle's ability to break down its stores of glycogen to get "fuel" for muscle contraction is impaired, resulting in fatigue and weakness.

The GSDs are inherited as AUTOSOMAL RECESSIVE traits (except for type IX, which may be either autosomal or X-LINKED recessive). There is a wide variability in the severity of the various types. However, even in mild forms, individuals may not achieve normal height, and may not be able to compete physically with other children their age.

Treatment generally consists of dietary management. In some forms (e.g., type I) nighttime infusion of glucose directly into the stomach is required, either through a drip tube inserted through the nose, or through creation of a surgical opening into the stomach from the abdomen. Liver transplants have been successful but are generally reserved for the most severe cases.

As a group, the GSDs affect about one in 40,000 individuals in the United States. Perhaps as many as 20 types of GSD have been identified, based on the specific enzyme deficiencies that cause each. Some of the most noted are the following:

Type I (von Gierke disease). Named for German pathologist Edgar O.K. von Gierke (1877–1945), who described it in 1929, this is the most common and severe form of GSD. Much of the above description relates to this disorder. It is caused by a deficiency of the enzyme glucose-6-phosphatase. The GENE for glucose-6-phosphatase is on chromosome 17. A number of MUTATIONS have been found, and CARRIER testing and PRENATAL DIAGNOSIS should be possible using DNA studies.

The liver and kidneys are most affected. There may be gross enlargement of the abdomen and kidneys, growth retardation, chronic hunger, fatigue and irritability. Low blood sugar (hypoglycemia) is a major associated problem. Gout and bleeding problems are less common features. In the past, individuals rarely survived into adulthood, but improved treatment makes survival beyond childhood the rule. However, liver tumors (both benign and malignant) may develop. In type I, a treatment that has been used as an alternative to constant nasogastric feeding is the use of uncooked cornstarch. Incidence is about 1:200,000.

Type Ib GSD refers to those children whose disease is indistinguishable from those with type I GSD but who have normal levels of glucose-6-phospatase. (If these enzyme levels are measured in fresh, not frozen, tissue it can be shown to be deficient.) These children suffer a severe form of the disease and also exhibit abnormalities of their white blood cells, causing recurrent infections. Treatment with granulocyte colony-stimulating factor (G-CSF) results in a reduction in the frequency of infections.

Type II (Pompe disease). This is generally a severe infantile form, first described by Dutch pathologist J. C. Pompe (1901–45) in 1932. Caused by a defect in alpha-1,4 glucosidase (sometimes called acid maltase), this autosomal recessive disorder is one of the forms affecting muscle and not the liver. Carrier testing and prenatal diagnosis are possible. The gene is located on the long arm of chromosome 17. Incidence is one in 40,000.

Type II GSD is actually a lysosomal STORAGE DISEASE and was the first disease to be recognized as such. In the other GSDs the glycogen that accumulates is not stored in the lysosomes, the digestive compartments of the cell, as in this form.

Involvement of organs is generalized, with the heart becoming greatly enlarged. Individuals present a FLOPPY INFANT appearance, with little muscle tone (hypotonia) and severe weakness. The tongue may also be enlarged (MACROGLOSSIA). The average age of death is five months, with survival beyond the first year highly unlikely, due to cardiorespiratory failure. Enzyme replacement therapy (intravenous infusions of the deficient enzyme) as a form of treatment is now available.

There is also an early childhood form of the disease characterized by slowly progressive muscle wasting with no heart abnormalities. It resembles a MUSCULAR DYSTROPHY and causes death before adulthood. An adult form with onset of muscle weakness after the age of 30 also exists. These forms exhibit some enzyme activity where the infantile form has none.

Type III (Forbes disease; Cori disease). This form is similar to type I, though with milder symptoms. Described by U.S. pediatrician G.B. Forbes in 1953, it is caused by a deficiency of the debranching enzyme in the liver and muscle tissue. The liver and heart and skeletal muscles are primarily affected. Diagnosis is usually based on liver and muscle biopsies. This condition is compatible with normal life expectancy, though individuals may develop muscle disorders as

they grow older. Treatment is dietary, with only rarely a need for continuous night feeds. Transmitted as an autosomal recessive condition, the gene is located on the short arm of chromosome 1. Incidence is approximately one in 200,000, but is much more common in Israel. There it accounts for 73% of all cases of glycogen storage disease and occurs almost exclusively among non-Ashkenazim, primarily those of North African extraction, with a frequency of at least one in 5,420. Prenatal diagnosis is possible.

Type IV (Andersen disease). In this very rare and severe form, described by U.S. pediatrician and pathologist Dorothy H. Anderson (1901–63) in 1952, cirrhosis of the liver occurs along with scarring of the affected muscles and heart. It is the result of a defect in the branching enzyme. Death usually occurs before the age of two years. Type IV is also autosomal recessive. The gene is located on the short arm of chromosome 3 and prenatal diagnosis has been accomplished.

Type V (McArdle disease). Named for British pediatrician B. McArdle, who described it in 1951, this is a mild form of GSD, involving only skeletal muscles. Individuals are essentially normal, though severe muscle cramping occurs during heavy exercise. Muscle fatigue is seen in the teenage years, and progressive weakness in adulthood. Muscle phosphorylase is the enzyme deficient in this form. An autosomal recessive disorder, the gene is located on the long arm of chromosome 11.

Type VI (Hers disease). Though extreme enlargement of the liver may accompany this form, it is considered mild. It results from a deficiency of liver phosphorylase. Individuals may exhibit short stature, but can lead normal lives without requiring any treatment. There are at least two forms of what has been called type VI. One is an X-linked form and another is autosomal recessive. These involve deficiencies in the enzyme phosphorylase in the liver or in one of the enzymes that leads to the activation of the liver's phosphorylase. The incidence of this subgroup of diseases, which includes types IX and X as well, is about one in 200,000.

Type VII. This mild form results from a deficiency of phosphofructokinase. It resembles type V.

GM1 gangliosidosis A rare GENETIC DISORDER characterized by the accumulation of a ganglioside, a carbohydrate-containing fatty substance, in nerves, spleen, liver, kidneys and other organs, with skeletal deformities. Generally evident at birth, the high level of ganglioside leads to cerebral degeneration, and affected infants rarely survive beyond two years of age. They often resemble infants with MUCOPOLY-SACCHARIDOSIS. Milder juvenile-onset and adult forms with primarily neurologic symptoms, without other organ involvement, are also known. A CHERRY-RED SPOT of the retina may be seen in about half of the affected infants. (TAY-SACHS DISEASE, a disorder with increased incidence in Ashkenazi Jews, is a different gangliosidosis, with storage of a related substance.)

First described in 1964, it is inherited as an AUTOSOMAL RECESSIVE disorder. The responsible GENE is located on chromosome 3. CARRIER detection and PRENATAL DIAGNOSIS are available by measurement of the ENZYME deficient in this STORAGE DISEASE, betagalactosidase.

Goldenhar syndrome (oculo-auricular-vertebral dysplasia; hemifacial microsomia) Syndrome characterized by varying degrees of facial abnormalities, DEAFNESS and, often, poor development (DYSPLASIA) of the spinal column. Named for physician M. Goldenhar, who published the first description in 1952, it is highly variable in its expression.

The facial abnormalities are often confined to one side of the face (hemifacial), though in severe cases there may be a major distortion of features involving the entire face. When the features are one-sided, it tends to be right-sided. A frequent abnormality is a lateral cleft on one side of the mouth, which may extend across the cheek. The facial bones and muscles are underdeveloped asymmetrically. The eye on the more affected side of the face may be lower than the other. Cysts (epibulbar dermoids) may be found on the eyeball.

Abnormalities of the ear are also commonly visible, though they usually are present only in one ear. The ears may be malformed, or there may be a missing outer ear or external canal. However, the most characteristic ear abnormality—small appendages or tags of skin adjacent to the ear (preauricular tags)—usually appear on both ears. The hearing problems resulting from this SYNDROME tend to be conductive, that is, due to ANOMALIES of the structure of the ear canal or bones involved with hearing, rather than due to sensorineural hearing loss, which results from abnormalities in the nerves that transmit impulses from the ear to the brain. The hearing loss, like the observable abnormalities, tends to be unilateral (affect only one side).

High arched palate, crowded teeth and, in some cases, CLEFT PALATE may also be present. The jawbone may be underdeveloped, as well. Spinal abnormalities may include SCOLIOSIS, extra vertebrae or poorly developed vertebrae, most often in the neck region. Congenital HEART DEFECTS may also accompany the syndrome. Mild MENTAL RETARDATION has been observed in some cases, but most patients are of normal intelligence. Oral surgery may correct some of the associated dental problems, and cosmetic surgery may lessen the degree of facial asymmetry or correct the ear malformations.

Goldenhar syndrome is estimated to occur in between one in 3,000 and one in 5,000 live births. It affects males more frequently than it affects females by a ratio of 3:2. Most cases are observed sporadically within families, although it has been suggested that in a few families there has been either AUTOSOMAL DOMINANT or AUTOSOMAL RECESSIVE inheritance in addition to MULTIFACTORIAL inheritance. Estimated risks of recurrence among SIBLINGS or offspring is about 2%. PRENATAL DIAGNOSIS is possible via ULTRASOUND.

Though various combinations of features have been given particular designations in the past (e.g., Goldenhar syndrome vs. hemifacial microsomia), these all seem to be variable gradations in the spectrum of severity of a similar malformation syndrome.

Goltz syndrome (focal dermal hypoplasia) Incomplete development (hypoplasia) and other abnormalities of the skin, bones, fingers and eyes. In its most severe form, the SYNDROME is lethal to males IN UTERO and greatly reduces fertility in females. It was first described in 1962 by Robert W. Goltz, head of dermatology at the University of Minnesota.

At birth, visible skin lesions include scarlike abnormalities, streaks of excess pigmentation, atrophy and prominent blood vessel markings (telangiectasia). In some cases, there are isolated areas with no skin at all. Often, there are soft yellow patches of subcutaneous fat along the line of the pelvic bones (iliac crest), groin and backs of the thighs. Benign skin tumors (papillomas) are common on and around the mouth, genitals, rectum, armpits and umbilicus. Hair, if it is present, is sparse and brittle.

Abnormalities of the bone include bone thickening (osteopathia striata), rib ANOMALIES and lateral curvature of the spine (SCOLIOSIS). Fingers are frequently webbed (SYNDACTYLY) and may show other abnormalities as well, including absent or anomalous fingernails.

Eyes are affected most commonly by fissures (COLOBOMA) in the iris and retina, although there may also be "crossed eyes" (STRABISMUS), jerky movements of the eye (nystagmus), obstructed tear ducts, failure of the eyes to develop to normal size (microphthalmia) and absence of one eye.

Other complications of Goltz syndrome include incomplete development of the ears, teeth, genitals, lips, palate and head, growth and MENTAL RETARDATION and DEAFNESS. In rare cases, there may be cardiac and kidney abnormalities.

The basic defect that causes this rare disorder is in the *PORCN* gene, encoding the human homologue of the fruit fly porcupine gene. It is transmitted as an X-LINKED dominant trait, due to the fact that it affects females much more commonly than males. (Under this hypothesis, a large proportion of affected male FETUSES are spontaneously aborted.) Most cases are new MUTATIONS. There is no known method of PRENATAL DIAGNOSIS.

Ratio of affected females to males is 150:11. More than 175 cases have been identified. The gene is on the short arm of the X CHROMOSOME. Males with the disorder are more severely affected than females.

goniodysgenesis   A CONGENITAL ocular defect with wide variability in expression arising from abnormal development of the anterior (front) parts of the eye. The defect may be an isolated ANOMALY or be part of a multiple anomaly SYNDROME, and

as an isolated defect may be an AUTOSOMAL DOMINANT trait. The vision of some members of a family may be severely affected while others are affected only slightly. Lifespan and intelligence generally are normal.

Posterior embryotoxon   The mildest form, in which a structure known as the Schwalbe line is displaced forward to resemble a prominent white ring on the border of the cornea. About 15% of the population has this defect in varying degrees. Posterior embryotoxon is also a feature of velocardiofacial syndrome and ALAGILLE SYNDROME.

Rieger anomaly/syndrome   The Rieger anomaly is a more serious defect in which the connective tissue supporting the iris is poorly developed or adheres to the displaced Schwalbe line. When this ANOMALY accompanies defects such as missing or cone-shaped teeth, the condition is known as RIEGER SYNDROME. This condition appears to have several genetic forms. One results from mutations in the *PITX2* gene, which codes for a homebox transcription factor and is located on the long arm of chromosome 4. A second locus is on the long arm of chromosome 13. Mutations in other genes, such as the *FOXC1* gene on chromosome 6, may also cause the Rieger anomaly or other forms of goniodysgenesis. GLAUCOMA and CATARACTS are common.

Peters anomaly   Faulty cleavage of embryonic structures results in clouding of the center of the cornea and adhesions of the iris (lens and cornea). Vision can be significantly impaired. It has been seen with a mutation in the PAX6 gene; other PAX6 anomalies cause ANIRIDIA. Familial forms are most often inherited in an AUTOSOMAL RECESSIVE manner. In a family with an individual with Peters anomaly and a PAX6 mutation, other family members had Rieger anomaly, suggesting that these are varying expressions of the same genetic defect. Peters anomaly may be seen with other anomalies such as short-limbed dwarfism. PRENATAL DIAGNOSIS should be possible in families with a known mutation. Peters anomaly may also result from mutations in one of several other genes, including *PITX2*, *FOXC1*, and *CYP1B1*.

Congenital anterior staphyloma   Characterized by gross disorganization of the structure between the pupil and the lens (anterior chamber). Severe GLAUCOMA is common.

Goniodysgenesis can be detected at birth. In all forms the defect may be isolated or may be associated with other anomalies or systemic abnormalities.

Gougerot-Carteaud syndrome   See ACANTHOSIS NIGRICANS.

gout   Gout has historically been identified as a condition afflicting the upper classes, particularly its obese (see OBESITY) and gluttonous members. It has been called "the disease of kings and king of diseases." Recognized since ancient times, those said to have been afflicted include Alexander the Great, Charlemagne, Isaac Newton, John Milton and Charles Darwin. The clinical features of gouty arthritis were first described by Hippocrates in the fourth century B.C.

Characterized by episodes of extreme pain in the foot (especially the big toe, though the instep, ankle, heel or wrist may also be affected), it is a disorder of purine metabolism causing a buildup of uric acid in the blood, resulting in the accumulation of crystals in joints. While most cases are idiopathic (of unknown origin), some (less than 1%) are known to have a genetic component. These cases are heterogeneous, that is, various GENE MUTATIONS all result in the same condition. X-LINKED forms have been identified, and AUTOSOMAL DOMINANT transmission has been suggested for some cases, as has MULTIFACTORIAL inheritance. Evidence has been found that both increased rates of uric acid production and impaired elimination of uric acid by the kidney may be involved. In some families studied in which both parents were affected, age of onset and symptoms in their children were unusually early and severe.

The origins of the cases of the early 18th to mid-19th centuries, which helped establish this disorder's reputation as an affliction of the upper classes, have been the subject of interesting speculation. Some suggest these cases were "saturnine gout," caused by the high levels of lead in the port wine favored by the upper classes of the time. Others suggest that dietary excess in general with increased purine intake was at the root of the disorder. Conversely, a hypothesis has been advanced that the power and influence enjoyed by these upper-class gout sufferers points to the influence of GENETICS, with genes transmitting the metabolic deficiency linked with genes associated with increased intelligence.

granulomatous disease, chronic   See IMMUNE DEFICIENCY DISEASES.

Grebe chondrodysplasia   A rare form of short-limbed DWARFISM (see CHONDRODYSPLASIA). The arms and legs appear progressively shortened along their length, so that the ends of the arms and legs exhibit greater dwarfing than the sections nearer the trunk. The legs are often more severely affected than the arms. Fingers may be very short, resembling toes, and the toes may be almost nonexistent. X-ray examination reveals severe developmental defects of the bones of the arms and legs (long bones). Extra digits may also be seen.

Inherited as an AUTOSOMAL RECESSIVE trait, this condition is observable at birth. STILLBIRTH and neonatal mortality rates (within the first four weeks of birth) are high, but long-term outlook is favorable for those who survive infancy. Intelligence is normal. Adult height is usually between 39 inches and 41 inches (99.1–104.1 cm). The disorder is named for H. Grebe, the physician who first described affected sisters in 1952.

CARRIERS of the trait, that is, those who possess a single GENE for the disorder, may exhibit mild shortness of the hands and feet.

Over 50 cases have been reported. It is caused by MUTATIONS in the CDMP1 (cartilage derived morphogenetic protein 1) gene, which is located on the long arm of chromosome 20. Other mutations in this same gene have been found to underlie other skeletal DYSPLASIAS (e.g., Hunter-Thompson type acromesomelic DYSPLASIA and type C brachydactyly).

Greig cephalopolysyndactyly syndrome (GCPS)   Large head, unusual facial features and multiple deformities of the hands and feet are the hallmarks of this rare hereditary disorder. Affected individuals have a high, prominent forehead, broad nose and wide-set eyes (HYPERTELORISM). Fingers and toes may be webbed (SYNDACTYLY) and thumbs and great toes are often abnormally large. An extra digit (POLYDACTYLY) may be on the little finger side of the hand and/or the big toe side of the foot. Mild MENTAL RETARDATION and HYDROCEPHALUS are occasionally associated. Males and females are affected equally.

Thought to be inherited as an AUTOSOMAL DOMINANT trait, the defective GENE (GL13) has been mapped to the short arm of chromosome 7 (7p13). Different MUTATIONS in this same gene cause the PALLISTER-HALL syndrome, which manifests with hypothalmic hamartoblastoma, hypopituitarism, IMPERFORATE ANUS and postaxial polydactyly. Other mutations have been linked to cases of isolated polydactyly.

grief   Emotions of grief, sadness and anger are common and healthy responses following the death of an infant affected by a GENETIC DISORDER or BIRTH DEFECT. Grief may be felt as intensely when a baby is lost before birth as when a death occurs in infancy, and a grieving process, and opportunities to express feelings, are important parts of coming to terms with the loss of an infant.

These same emotions often occur when an infant is born with a severe genetic condition or birth defect. Experiencing grief in these situations may be equally important.

Griffe des orteils   See CLAWFOOT.

GSD   See GLYCOGEN STORAGE DISEASE.

G6PD   See GLUCOSE-6-PHOSPHATE DEHYDROGENASE DEFICIENCY.

G syndrome   See OPITZ G/BBB SYNDROME.

Gunther's disease   See PORPHYRIA.

gynecomastia   The enlargement of the breasts in males. As a genetic condition gynecomastia with onset at puberty is associated with AMBIGUOUS GENITALIA, PSEUDOHERMAPHRODITISM, ADRENOGENITAL SYNDROMES, KLINEFELTER SYNDROME and other abnormalities of sexual differentiation. Familial cases have been reported in which gynecomastia is the only abnormality exhibited, and AUTOSOMAL DOMINANT, AUTOSOMAL RECESSIVE and X-LINKED transmission have all been proposed as the method of inheritance. As an isolated occurrence it is common among male adolescents. Reportedly as many as 60–70% exhibit mild, benign, transitory gynecomastia during puberty; it is self-limiting and self-resolving.

The lineage of the Egyptian pharoah Amenophis III, including Tutankhamun, may have been affected with isolated autosomal dominant gynecomastia. Others have suggested the pharoah may have had Klinefelter syndrome.

gyrate atrophy   Hereditary vision disorder with onset during the first decade of life. The retina (the inner surface of the back of the eye) and the choroid (the layer of tissue beneath the retina) degenerate. (Gyrate, meaning ring-shaped, refers to the circular pattern of atrophy or degeneration exhibited by the retina and choroid.) NIGHT BLINDNESS is progressive. All those affected are nearsighted (myopia). The visual field becomes increasingly constricted, leaving only a central tunnel of vision. Remaining vision deteriorates after the age of 30.

Inherited as an AUTOSOMAL RECESSIVE trait, over 70 different MUTATIONS have been identified in the GENE, located on the long arm of chromosome 10. This very rare condition is due to the deficiency of the ENZYME ornithine aminotransferase. A large proportion of the patients have been Finnish.

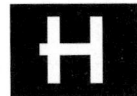

hairy ear Excessive growth of coarse hairs on the outer ear. This is the only trait (other than maleness) known to be Y-linked; that is, the gene for it is located on the Y CHROMOSOME. (See X-LINKED.) This trait has been observed in India, Israel and Malta.

Hallermann-Streiff syndrome A small face, mouth and jaw, large forehead and small, pinched, beaked nose give rise to the characteristic birdlike features that identify this disorder. In addition, there is always proporionate dwarfing, with adult height rarely exceeding 5 feet (see DWARFISM). It was described in 1948 by Wilhelm Hallermann, a professor of ophthalmology at Gottingen in West Germany, and in 1950 by Bernardo Streiff, professor of ophthalmology at the University of Lausanne, Switzerland. About 150 cases have been reported, virtually all SPORADIC.

Additional facial abnormalities include prominent scalp and nose veins, small mouth and double chin. Eyebrows, lashes and hair are frequently sparse (hypotrichosis), and the eyes are invariably smaller than normal (microphthalmia), with CATARACTS. Although the cataracts may disappear, there is a high incidence of eventual BLINDNESS. Whites of the eyes (sclerae) may be blue; other abnormalities of the eye include absence of the lens (aphakia), "crossed" eyes (STRABISMUS), jerky eye movement (nystagmus), presence of a membrane over the pupil and secondary glaucoma.

Head and facial bones may be somewhat smaller than usual or incompletely developed, and the palate is high and narrow. Teeth may be absent, incomplete or malformed. Overbite (malocclusion) is common, as are early severe cavities (caries). MENTAL RETARDATION has been reported in about 15% of cases. The genitals may be small or fail to develop completely.

The basic defect that causes Hallermann-Streiff syndrome is not known, nor has its genetic basis been identified. The condition is rare, and both sexes are affected equally. The greatest threat to life is in early infancy, when feeding difficulties and respiratory problems must be overcome. Surgery may be successful in correcting eye and mouth defects. In adults, the ability to reproduce is severely limited. There is currently no method of PRENATAL DIAGNOSIS available for this disorder.

hamartoma A CONGENITAL mass of slowly growing, abnormal tissue. They may appear in organs, blood vessels or other tissue. Hamartomatous tissues are similar to the organ they appear in, but the growth is abnormally organized. Hamartomas can cause complications due to the space they occupy, though they are not malignant.

handicap Many individuals who are affected by GENETIC DISORDERS and BIRTH DEFECTS are handicapped as a result of these conditions. Section 504 of the Rehabilitation Act of 1973 (Public Law 93-112) defines a handicapped individual as anyone with a physical or mental impairment that substantially impairs or restricts one or more major life activities. "Physical" or "mental impairment" includes, but is not limited to, speech, hearing, visual and orthopedic impairments, CEREBRAL PALSY, EPILEPSY, MUSCULAR DYSTROPHY, MULTIPLE SCLEROSIS, CANCER, DIABETES MELLITUS, HEART DEFECTS, MENTAL RETARDATION, emotional illness and specific learning disabilities such as perceptual handicaps, brain injury, dyslexia, minimal brain dysfunction and developmental aphasia.

The goal of the Rehabilitation Act of 1973 was to end discrimination against handicapped individuals in employment, housing and education, and assure their access to programs and facilities receiving government funds. The "American National Standard Specifications for Making Buildings and Facilities Accessible to, and Usable by, the Physically Handicapped" is the code that sets the requirements for accessibility.

Amendments to the Fair Housing Act require that any new multifamily rental or condominium building with four or more units be accessible to the handicapped.

The 1990 Americans With Disabilities Act extended the protection of the 1973 law, prohibiting discrimination in employment against disabled individuals, even in businesses and institutions that don't receive government funds. The law requires businesses to provide "reasonable accommodations" in their facilities for disabled customers and employees.

As government and society have sought to remove barriers that have prevented many disabled individuals from taking advantage of opportunities for recreation and employment they could otherwise enjoy, Americans have also been struggling with the language of disability. Concern about the effect of the terms and labels applied in the past to many disabling conditions has led to the use of less stigmatizing terminology, for example, *visually handicapped* instead of *blind*, or *physically challenged* rather than *paralyzed*.

happy puppet syndrome   See ANGELMAN SYNDROME.

harelip   A colloquial term for CLEFT LIP. (See also CLEFT LIP, CLEFT PALATE AND ASSOCIATED CLEFTING CONDITIONS.)

harlequin fetus (ichthyosis congenita gravis)   A rare and lethal disorder characterized at birth by thick, hardened plates of skin covering the entire body, cracked along lateral fissures where folds of skin would normally appear.

The first description, recorded in 1750 in the diary of Rev. Oliver Hart, a minister in South Carolina, stands as the definitive one:

On Thursday, April ye 5, 1750, I went to see a most deplorable object of a child, born the night before of one Mary Evans in "Chas" town. It was surprising to all who beheld it, and I scarcely know how to describe it. The skin was dry and hard and seemed to be cracked in many places, somewhat resembling the scales of a fish, The mouth was large and round and open. It had no external nose, but two holes where the nose should have been. The eyes appeared to be lumps of coagulated blood, turned out, about the bigness of a plum, ghastly to behold. It had no external ears, but holes where the ears should be. The hands and feet appeared to be swollen, were cramped up and felt quite hard. The back part of the head was much open. It made a strange kind of noise, very low, which I cannot describe. It lived about forty-eight hours and was alive when I saw it.

The most severe form of congenital ICTHYOSIS, the disorder takes its name from the diamond-shaped sections of cracked skin, which create the appearance of a harlequin's suit.

The basic cause of the condition is unknown. Inherited as an AUTOSOMAL RECESSIVE trait, it results from mutations in the *ABCA12* gene located on the long arm of chromosome 2. This gene is also responsible for lamellar ichthyosis type 2. Frequency is one in 500,000. It is very rare, with approximately 30 cases reported. Most infants die in the first week of life, though the longest surviving infant lived to nine months of age. PRENATAL DIAGNOSIS by fetal skin biopsy has been accomplished. Identification of the gene responsible should allow for early prenatal diagnosis in affected families where the gene mutation has been identified.

Hartnup disease   Symptoms of this condition, usually detected in newborns, are intermittent and variable, and include rashes on parts of the body exposed to sunlight (ultraviolet light), psychotic disturbances and impaired kidney and intestinal absorption of certain AMINO ACIDS, in particular tryptophan, an amino acid essential for metabolism. The defective absorption results from an inborn error involving the transport of these amino acids. Mutations in the *SLC6A19* gene on the short arm of chromosome 5, which encodes the transporter protein for these amino acids, can cause the disorder. As the rashes result from exposure to sunlight, they are more common from February to October.

Sudden attacks of ataxia, double vision and fainting may be seen. Untreated, it can lead to MENTAL RETARDATION, dementia and short stature. Many affected individuals are asymptomatic.

Although an exact cause for Hartnup disease is unknown, poor nutrition is thought to precipitate onset of symptoms, which resemble those of niacin, or B-complex, vitamin deficiency (pellagra). Good nutrition and niacin (nicotinic acid) supplements help to alleviate symptoms for most of those affected. Though affected individuals have a normal life expectancy and may remain asymptomatic, without treatment mental deterioration may occur in rare instances.

Hartnup disease is inherited as an AUTOSOMAL RECESSIVE trait. It is named for the first family identified as having the disorder, and was first described at London's Middlesex Hospital in 1956. It occurs worldwide in approximately one in 14,500 live births. Frequency in North American newborns is about 1:24,000. It is rare in areas where high nutritional standards prevent onset of symptoms.

heart defects (congenital heart defects, CHD) A variety of structural malformations of the heart and its major blood vessels resulting from abnormal embryonic development. Congenital heart defects (CHD) are the most common form of BIRTH DEFECTS (followed by renal, or kidney defects), and may appear as individual ANOMALIES or as part of a large number of specific SYNDROMES. These include HOLT-ORAM SYNDROME, NOONAN SYNDROME, ELLIS-VAN CREVALD SYNDROME, ASPLENIA SYNDROME, POLYSPLENIA SYNDROME, VATER ASSOCIATION and SMITH-LEMLI-OPITZ SYNDROME.

Although they exist as isolated malformations in most of those who come to medical attention, affected individuals are 10 times more likely than the general public to have a non-CHD major birth defect as well. The estimated frequency of the presence of non-heart (or cardiac) associated disorders ranges from less than 10% to more than 40%, with the presence of major non-cardiac malformations

put at about 25%. Early diagnosis is important in planning medical management. Some cardiac anomalies are incompatible with extended postnatal survival, and accurate diagnosis must be made in a timely fashion to allow appropriate medical decision making.

CHDs may result from hereditary, environmental and/or unknown factors. Approximately 3% are thought to be caused by single GENE disorders and 5% by CHROMOSOME ABNORMALITIES (primarily DOWN SYNDROME). The remainder are thought to be caused by the action of several genes in concert with environmental factors (MULTIFACTORIAL inheritance) (see HETEROGENEITY). Environmental factors include chemicals (drugs and toxic substances such as alcohol or some ANTICONVULSANT medications), biological agents (viruses such as rubella) and maternal conditions (2%), such as PHENYLKETONURIA and DIABETES (see TERATOGEN). The del 22q11 PHENOTYPE, the most common CHROMOSOME deletion syndrome (see CATCH 22), has been discovered to be an important cause of various heart defects.

In families in which an individual has been diagnosed as having CHD, GENETIC COUNSELING and diagnostic procedures can help establish the origin of the disorder, evaluate asymptomatic family members and determine the risk of recurrence in future pregnancies. In defined syndromes, the recurrence risk may be as high as 50%, while if the defect occurred as the result of an environmental insult the recurrence risk can be minimal. After the birth of an affected child with an isolated CHD of a presumably multifactorial basis, the risk of recurrence in a subsequent child is estimated to be about 2% to 5%.

Pregnant women with CHDs face potential health complications and increased risks for their infants: Not only may it put an additional strain on the heart, but in some studies, affected females were found to have a higher probability of transmitting CHDs to their offspring than affected males have. In addition, drugs taken for management of their CHDs may pose teratogenic risks.

A number of PRENATAL DIAGNOSIS procedures are available, depending on the particular form of CHD. Fetal cardiac ultrasonography (echocardiography) may detect certain abnormalities IN UTERO, and is becoming more widely available. Analysis of fetal chromosomes obtained via AMNIOCENTESIS may be useful in establishing diagnosis of CHDs associated with chromosomal abnormalities. ULTRASOUND may be used to look for associated malformations in syndromic cases.

CHDs occur in about eight per 1,000 births and account for approximately half of all deaths caused by CONGENITAL malformations and 15% of all infants deaths, affecting all ethnic groups about equally. Each year in the United States approximately 30,000 infants are born with a CHD. Many forms of CHDs have been reported, though approximately 10 to 15 varieties account for the majority of cases. These individual malformations may occur alone or in complex combinations.

Symptoms of CHD in the infant include cyanosis (the bluish color of the skin resulting from poor oxygenation), shortness of breath, feeding difficulties, excessive sweating, failure to grow appropriately or recurrent infections. A heart murmur may be heard on examination. Other laboratory investigations often help delienate the exact nature of the defect: chest X-rays, electrocardiography, echocardiography, cardiac catheterization and new imaging techniques including CT, MRI and nuclear screening.

Ventricular septal defect (VSD)   The most common form of isolated CHDs, these account for about 20% to 25% of all cases, occurring in about 22 to 25 per 10,000 live births. An abnormal opening in the wall (septum) between the bottom two chambers (ventricles) of the heart allows blood to flow directly from the left to right ventricle, and recirculate through the pulmonary artery and lungs. Recirculation of this already oxygenated blood puts a strain on the heart. Females are more often affected than males.

Severity is variable. There may be single or multiple openings, ranging in size from 1 mm to several centimeters across. Individuals with mild defects may be asymptomatic, and the septal defect may spontaneously heal. In more severe cases, symptoms include congestive heart failure, pneumonia, rapid breathing, FAILURE TO THRIVE, and restlessness and irritability. Surgery is required in about 20% of cases, and mortality rate in these situations is estimated at between 1% and 2%.

VSDs may be associated with chromosome abnormalities, particularly trisomy 18 (EDWARD SYNDROME).

Atrial septal defects (ASD)   These consist of an abnormal opening in the wall (septum) separating the two upper chambers (atria) of the heart. This causes an increased flow of oxygenated blood into the right side of the heart, and thus to the lungs. This may lead to heart failure. The severity of the condition is variable, and may be corrected surgically in most cases. ASDs account for 10% to 15% of all cases of CHD, occurring in approximately six to seven per 10,000 live births. In about 85% of all cases, it is an isolated malformation. It is the third most common defect after VSD and PATENT DUCTUS ARTERIOSUS. ASD affects females more commonly than males by a ratio of 2–3:1.

AUTOSOMAL DOMINANT and AUTOSOMAL RECESSIVE forms of the disorder have been documented. Individuals may remain asymptomatic, only developing symptoms well into adulthood. ASD is also a feature of the Holt-Oram and Ellis–van Creveld syndromes and thrombocytopenia-absent radius syndrome (see TAR SYNDROME).

Aortic stenosis (AS)   A narrowing of the aorta, the major artery leading from the heart, resulting in a reduced ability of the aorta to circulate blood from the left ventricle. The condition is classified by the site of the narrowing, which also determines the severity of the condition. Congestive heart failure, chest pain and fainting spells may result. AS occurs more often in males than females by a ratio of 4:1.

Valvular AS involves the point at which the aortic valve admits blood from the heart. It is often asymptomatic, but may lead to sudden death, due to abnormalities in the electrical impulses that control the valve's operation (conduction abnormalities). It accounts for about 5% of CHD.

The single most frequent isolated CHD is bicuspid aortic valve, in which the valve has only two leaflets rather than the normal three. This can lead to aortic stenosis or it may remain asymptomatic. It occurs in one in 100 births.

Supravalvular AS involves the section of the aorta that rises (ascending aorta) from the heart. There is an increased pressure due to the narrowing, increasing the risk for arteriosclerosis. It is also associated with WILLIAMS SYNDROME, a disorder characterized by coarse facial features, MENTAL RETARDATION and dental abnormalities. High calcium levels in the blood may be found. Males and females are equally affected. Mutations in the elastin gene have been found in cases of supravalvular AS, especially familial autosomal dominant cases and those that are part of Williams syndrome, where a deletion of chromosome 7 is observed in the region of this gene.

Subvalvular AS is an often asymptomatic disorder caused by a fibrous ring that encircles the left ventricular outflow tract at the point immediately before blood enters the aorta. Occurring twice as often in males as in females, it is suspected of being a rather common anomaly, possibly inherited as an autosomal dominant characteristic.

Pulmonic stenosis Like aortic stenosis, this condition may be subvalvular, valvular or supravalvular. It involves narrowing of the pulmonary artery, leading from the right ventricle to the lungs. The severity depends on the degree of narrowing, and whether or not there are accompanying septal defects. It may be asymptomatic, or the obstructions may result in heart failure and cyanosis by two to three years of age. In these cases, surgical intervention is usually required.

Pulmonic stenosis may be associated with fetal rubella syndrome (see TORCH SYNDROME) or other syndromes including NOONAN SYNDROME and LEOPARD SYNDROME.

Endocardial cushion defects (ECDS; atrioventricular canal) A variety of abnormalities resulting from defective development of the atrioventricular cushions, embryonic structures from which the walls (sepia) and valves of the upper heart chambers (atria) develop. Severity is variable. About one-third of cases are associated with trisomy 21 (DOWN SYNDROME), with the majority of the remainder due to multifactorial inheritance. They may also be associated with rare syndromes in which asplenia or polysplenia are features.

Mitral valve prolapse (MVP) A common but often undiagnosed condition in which the mitral valves fail to close properly, collapsing back into the upper left chamber (left atrium) of the heart when the lower chamber (ventricle) contracts during the cardiac cycle, allowing blood to flow back into the atrium. The condition is usually asymptomatic, though it may cause chest pains or an irregular heartbeat. The condition is not always present at birth. Incidence is estimated at 5% to 10% in the general population and a prevalence of 1% to 2% in children. The valve is also susceptible to infection and affected individuals need to take prophylactic antibiotics at the time of dental manipulations, for example, to prevent the development of infections.

As an isolated defect, MVP appears to follow an autosomal dominant hereditary pattern. It is also associated with MARFAN SYNDROME, OSTEOGENESIS IMPERFECTA, EHLERS-DANLOS SYNDROME, MUSCULAR DYSTROPHY and FRAGILE X SYNDROME.

Hypoplastic left heart syndrome Perhaps the most common cause of heart failure in the first week of life, this condition is characterized by the failure of development (hypoplasia) of the left ventricle. It may occur in conjunction with abnormalities of the aorta and mitral valves. Symptoms of the cardiac abnormalities, difficulty in breathing and failure to thrive, usually become apparent within 48 to 72 hours of birth. Prognosis is poor, though surgical repair is now attempted in some cases. Less than 10% of cases appear to be familial. Prenatal diagnosis has been accomplished frequently. Cardiac transplantation is a surgical option. (See TRUNCUS ARTERIOSIS.)

Coarctation of the aorta This is thought to be the most common cause of congestive heart failure from the second through fourth weeks of life, though most affected infants are asymptomatic. It consists of a constriction of the aorta, causing higher blood pressure on one side of the defect, and lower blood pressure on the other. This may result in an infant having high blood pressure in the arms and head, and low blood pressure in the legs. It is often associated with other CHDs, including patent ductus arteriosus and ventricular septal defects. It is three to four times more common in males and accounts for about 5% of CHDs, with a frequency of about five in 10,000 births.

Those who become symptomatic in childhood or later in life may exhibit dizziness, headaches, muscle cramps following exercise, nosebleeds and fainting. Surgery is usually recommended during childhood, due to life-threatening complications that may arise if left untreated, which include brain hemorrhage, heart failure, ruptured aorta and infections of lining of the heart (endocarditis). It is the most common heart defect in TURNER SYNDROME.

Congenital heart block Heart block results from abnormalities in the nerves responsible for conducting the electrical impulses that govern the heartbeat. This results in altered rhythm of the heart (arrhythmia). The condition may be present at birth as a result of defective fetal development, though it may also be caused by degenerative changes in the tissue wrought by toxins or infections. It is frequently seen in offspring of mothers with systemic LUPUS erythematosis. Conduction defects can also be caused by single-gene disorders such as the ROMANO-WARD SYNDROME and the JERVELL AND LANGE-NIELSON SYNDROME.

Other important CHDs include transposition of the great vessels (in which the aorta originates from the right ventricle instead of the left, and the pulmonary artery from the left instead of the right), truncus arteriosus (in which a single great vessel originates from the heart and gives rise to both the aorta and pulmonary artery), anomalous pulmonary venous return (where the blood from the lungs returns to the right side of the heart rather than the left) and tricuspid atresia (where the valve separating the right-sided chambers fails to perform properly). See also EBSTEIN ANOMALY; TETRALOGY OF FALLOT.

heart-hand syndrome   See HOLT-ORAM SYNDROME.

hemangioma   A benign, generally CONGENITAL malformation consisting of an abnormal growth or mass of blood vessels, which may be unusually large either in number or in degree of dilation. The growth may be flat or raised.

Hemangiomas of the skin are among the most common of ANOMALIES: They may be found in 40–45% of all infants. These include so-called strawberry marks, salmon patches and stork bites. These arteriovenous malformations occur in many SYNDROMES, and may occur as isolated MENDELIAN traits. When located near the skin rather than more internally, they impart a sharply delineated, reddish tone to the skin above. There have been some stud-

ies which have suggested an increase in frequency of hemangiomas in infants exposed to CHORIONIC VILLUS SAMPLING (CVS). (See also PORT WINE STAIN.)

hemangioma and thrombocytopenia syndrome (Kasabach-Merritt syndrome)   An association of a benign growth (tumor) that results from the proliferation of blood vessels (HEMANGIOMA) with a low number of platelets in the blood (thrombocytopenia). Hemangiomas may occur anywhere in the body but are most frequently noticed in the skin and tissue immediately below the skin, where they appear as reddish patches. The low number of platelets occurs partly as a result of their becoming trapped in the tumor. ANEMIA (low blood count) can also occur. There may also be a depletion of fibrinogen, a substance in the blood that aids coagulation. The type of hemangioma involved is not the type seen in about 40% of newborns—the so-called salmon patch or stork bite type—but rather capillary or cavernous hemangiomas that are present in about 1–3% of newborns and up to 10% of one year olds.

In this SYNDROME, a normal hemangioma may suddenly double in size, and purplish spots and patches caused by hemorrhaging appear on the skin. The original size of the hemangioma gives no clue as to possible development of the syndrome. It has been detected in persons ranging in age from newborn to 73 years, affects males and females equally and occurs in one in 500 persons with hemangiomas. (Hemangiomas appear in isolation in approximately one in 12 infants below one year of age.) The mortality rate is approximately 20%, usually due to internal hemorrhaging. The primary means of detection is by platelet count in the laboratory. The cause of the syndrome is unknown.

hematuria, benign familiar   See BENIGN FAMILIAL HEMATURIA.

hemifacial microsomia   See GOLDENHAR SYNDROME.

hemihypertrophy   Excessive growth or enlargement occurring on one side, or half (hemi), of the body. There is considerable individual variation both in severity and extent of the disorder. Unilateral, or one-sided enlargement can vary from a single digit or limb, or the face, to involvement of half of the entire body. Usually detected at birth, hemihypertrophy may increase with age, particularly with onset of puberty.

Total hemihypertrophy most often involves the right side of the body. Affected areas exhibit thickening of the skin, excessive glandular secretion, excessive hair growth (hypertrichosis) and extra nipples (polythelia). Additional characteristics may include enlarged bones in the involved area and various skeletal manifestations, including fused fingers (SYNDACTYLY), enlarged fingers (macrodactyly) or extra fingers (POLYDACTYLY). Between 20% and 30% of affected individuals have benign tumor-like nodules (HAMARTOMA) and various CONGENITAL defects and genitourinary ANOMALIES. MENTAL RETARDATION occurs in about 15%.

Where hemihypertrophy is restricted to the head, there may be enlargement of the tongue (MACROGLOSSIA), lips and palate. There is also usually premature loss of baby teeth and concomitant growth of permanent teeth on the affected side.

Hemihypertrophy may affect portions of both sides of the body. It may be limited to a single system (skeletal, nervous, vascular, muscular) or more frequency, affect multiple systems. It is also associated with development of cancerous growths (neoplasms), such as WILMS TUMOR or renal anomalies in young children, which can reduce life expectancy.

Treatment for hemihypertrophy consists of surgery to equalize leg lengths and plastic surgery to correct facial enlargement and deformities. Periodic examinations are recommended to detect development of neoplasms.

Hundreds of cases of hemihypertrophy have been reported. It appears to occur sporadically in the population, and may also be associated with a variety of GENETIC DISORDERS (Wilms tumor develops in about 4%). (See BECKWITH-WIEDMANN SYNDROME.) A few undocumented cases of familial occurrence have been reported. Occurring in approximately one in 15,000 live births, affected females have been reported more frequently than males. However, more males than females appear to be affected with total hemihypertrophy. PRENA-TAL DIAGNOSIS by ULTRASOUND, while theoretically possible, is generally difficult at best, as the disparity in limb sizes is generally subtle during the second trimester of pregnancy.

hemochromatosis (hereditary hemochromatosis)

Disorder characterized by the body's accumulation of iron. First described by Dr. A. Trousseau in 1865, it appears to be rather common and greatly under-reported, due to the asymptomatic nature of many cases. Variable symptoms make diagnosis difficult. Onset is usually between the ages of 40 and 60. Women tend to develop the disease later than men, as they normally lose significant amounts of iron during menstruation, pregnancy and lactation (which reduces iron levels). In severe cases the accumulation of iron leads to liver damage, which may eventually result in cirrhosis (see FAMILIAL CIRRHOSIS). Pancreatic damage may lead to severe diabetes (see DIABETES MELLITUS). Additionally, there may be endocrine and heart problems, ANEMIA, chronic fatigue and impotence. Abdominal pain is common.

One of the first signs of the disorder is a bronzish tint to the skin. If treated promptly, the condition can be controlled. Treatment usually consists of removing blood, as much as two pints a week, until iron levels reach a normal range. Early treatment can also prevent organ damage. Patients diagnosed after cirrhosis has occurred face an increased risk of liver cancer, even if iron stores are depleted with therapy. (The availability of early treatment makes this a preventable form of cancer.)

Inherited as an AUTOSOMAL RECESSIVE trait, studies in Europe, the United States and Australia indicate the frequency may be as high as one in 300 to one in 400 people. One in 10 to one in 20 individuals may carry the GENE for the disorder. It is said to affect an estimated 600,000 to 1.6 million Americans, with from 24–32 million CARRIERS. However, it is only rarely diagnosed: Fewer than 250,000 cases have been identified in the United States. Once thought to be a rare condition, it in now known as the most common genetic ANOMALY, more prevalent than CYSTIC FIBROSIS, PKU or hereditary MUSCULAR DYSTROPHY. A blood test can be helpful in diagnosing the disorder by measuring serum iron, total iron binding capacity (TIBC) and ferritin in the blood.

The defective gene is on the short arm of chromosome 6 near the HLA region. The protein it produces resembles the HLA proteins but appears to be involved in iron absorption in the intestine. Two MUTATIONS in this HLA-H gene account for about 90% of hemochromatosis. The basis for the remaining 10% is elusive.

Neonatal hemochromatosis appears to be a distinct disorder with a different genetic basis. There is also a juvenile form, beginning with abdominal pain in childhood and lack of adolescent sexual development in males (hypogonadatropic hypogonadism), and leading to heart failure between the ages of 20 and 30. A study in Finland identified a high iron level as second only to smoking as a cause for heart attack.

hemoglobin   The major component of the red blood cells, which carry oxygen from the lungs to the tissues. There are several normal types of hemoglobin, which is composed of heme, the iron-containing respiratory pigment that gives blood its red color, and globin chains. (Heme is also found in plants, where it gives chlorophyll its green color.) There are six known kinds of globin chains in man, designated alpha, beta, gamma, delta, epsilon and zeta. The specific combination of globin chains determines the type of hemoglobin. The latter two are found only in embryonic red cells.

Hemoglobin A is the major adult hemoglobin (approximately 92% of adult total hemoglobin). It is composed of two alpha chains and two beta chains. Hemoglobin A2 normally constitutes about 2.5% of the blood and is composed of two alpha and two delta chains. It may be increased in beta-THALASSEMIA and be decreased in iron deficiency. Hemoglobin F comprises the bulk of hemoglobin in the newborn, and is composed of two alpha and two gamma chains.

Hemoglobins are large molecules; due to their size, they have a propensity to exhibit a large number of MUTATIONS. More than 675 different types of abnormal hemoglobin have been identified. Many of the hemoglobin abnormalities cause no clinical abnormalities. Others may cause ANEMIA or decreased oxygen transport. Below are some of the more common abnormal hemoglobin conditions (hemoglobinopathies):

Hemoglobin alpha chain abnormalities. Abnormalities of the alpha chain of globins result in four forms of alpha-thalassemia, hemoglobinopathies with an increased incidence in Asian populations.

Hemoglobin C. This in an AUTOSOMAL RECESSIVE trait that results in a chronic hemolytic anemia, with symptoms including abdominal pain and an enlarged spleen (splenomegaly). It has an increased incidence in blacks in the United States, with an estimate of 3% carrying a single Hgb C gene at birth. Hgb C disease (2 copies) occurs in about one in 1,250 blacks. The disorder is sometimes associated with SICKLE-CELL ANEMIA. (See also hemoglobin S-C disease below.) This is a single base substitution in the GENE for betaglobin resulting in the substitution of lysine for glutamic acid in the sixth AMINO ACID position in the beta chain. This is the same position of substitution as in sickle-cell anemia, but a different amino acid is substituted.

Hemoglobin F, hereditary persistence of. This is not an abnormal hemoglobin. The F stands for "fetal" and is the primary type produced by the FETUS, due to its superiority in absorbing oxygen from maternal blood. During infancy, the body gradually replaces fetal hemoglobin with adult hemoglobin. However, the tendency for the body to continue producing fetal hemoglobin can be inherited as an AUTOSOMAL DOMINANT trait. It was first observed in blacks and has subsequently been seen in Greeks, Thais and other ethnic groups.

Hemoglobin H. This is a form of hemoglobin with only beta chains and no alpha chains. It is a form of alpha-thalassemia.

Hemoglobin M. This type of hemoglobin is called me/hemoglobin; it is associated with congenital cyanosis (BLUE BABY), a bluish or grayish tint of the skin caused by oxygen deficiency. In hemoglobin M disease, the iron in the methemoglobin is unable to combine with oxygen. While there is no effective therapy, it is not life threatening due to the compensating presence of normal hemoglobin.

Hemoglobin S. This abnormality causes sickle-cell anemia, which was the first disease discovered to be due to a molecular abnormality of hemoglobin. The hemoglobin S causes red blood cells to collapse and assume a sickle shape. The complications that result from this abnormal shape cause anemia. This is an autosomal recessive trait. Unless genes for hemoglobin S are inherited from both parents, the individual will rarely exhibit clinical manifestations from the characteristic sickling of red blood cells.

Hemoglobin S-C disease. If a gene for hemoglobin S (sickle cell) is inherited from one parent, and a gene for hemoglobin C from another, the individual will have hemoglobin S-C disease (sickle-cell-hemoglobin C disease), a mild form of sickle-cell anemia. Symptoms include blood in the urine (BENIGN FAMILIAL HEMATURIA) and pain in bones, joints, abdomen and chest. About one in 833 American blacks have S-C disease at birth. Onset is usually in the fourth decade, and the course of the disorder can be quite variable.

hemolytic disease of the newborn   A condition of the newborn characterized by ANEMIA, jaundice, enlargement of the liver and spleen (hepatosplenomegaly) and generalized swelling caused by excessive fluid in the tissues (edema; in newborns, this is called "hydrops fetalis"). It is caused by transplacental transmission of maternal antibody, usually provoked by incompatibility between maternal and fetal blood types. The first recorded case was described in 1609 by Louyse Bourgeois, a French midwife.

Incompatibilities of the ABO (blood) system are common but are not severe. Much more grave is Rh incompatibility, which may result in profound anemia in the FETUS, sometimes severe enough to cause death IN UTERO. The Rh factor was first discovered on the surface of mature blood cells (erythrocytes) of the rhesus monkey and subsequently found to be present to a variable degree in humans as well. Individuals who have this factor are said to be Rh positive (Rh+), and those without it are said to be Rh negative (Rh-). An Rh- mother who is carrying an Rh positive fetus may develop antibodies against the Rh factor (sensitization) for example,

as a result of fetal red cells entering the maternal circulation at the time of delivery. Rh sensitization is prevented by the administration of anti-Rh antibodies to Rh- mothers at the time of delivery to "block" the sensitization process if any fetal Rh+ cells enter the mother's circulation. Unless sensitization is blocked, these antibodies can cross the placenta in a future pregnancy and enter fetal circulation, where they may destroy the red blood cells of an Rh+ fetus.

The introduction of immunization with anti-Rh antibodies (immunoglobin) has been a major public health advance that has led to a dramatic decrease in the number of fetal and neonatal deaths from this disease. It is given not only after delivery of an Rh+ fetus to an Rh- mother, but also after a miscarriage, abortion, invasive procedures such as CHORIONIC VILLUS SAMPLING or AMNIOCENTESIS, or whenever there may be bleeding or leakage of blood from the fetal circulation into the maternal circulation.

Close monitoring of the pregnancy can minimize the consequences of this incompatibility. This involves prenatal testing, fetal transfusions and expert obstetrical care.

hemophilia   Any of several disorders of the blood clotting process that greatly prolong coagulation time. Coagulation, or clotting, is the body's mechanism to halt bleeding; it involves at least 14 sequential steps, each requiring a specific plasma protein or "factor," normally found in the blood. In hemophilia, one of the factors required for the clotting sequence is deficient or absent.

The condition known as hemophilia has been recognized for thousands of years. In ancient Egypt, women whose eldest child bled to death from a minor wound were forbidden to have more children. By A.D. 400, the Jews knew hemophilia to be an inherited disease, and male babies were permitted to go uncircumcised if they had two brothers who bled to death at circumcision. The pattern of inheritance characteristic of X-LINKED traits was even recognized by Jewish scholars, who also exempted a male infant from circumcision if his mother's sisters had had sons who died of bleeding following their circumcisions.

In the 19th and 20th centuries hemophilia was common in European royal families. Queen Victoria was a CARRIER, possibly the result of a new MUTATION inherited from her father or mother; she married her cousin, Prince Albert of Saxe-Coburg, and passed the GENE to several of her descendants, including Czarevich Alexis, son of Czar Nicholas II and the Czarina Alexandra. Alexandra turned to Rasputin to help cope with her son's disorder, ultimately ceding power to him, which may have helped precipitate the Russian Revolution.

In the United States, the first report of familial incidence was a 1792 newspaper account, and the transmission from unaffected mothers to sons was described in 1803.

The two most common forms of hemophilia are hemophilia A and hemophilia B. Hemophilia A and B have similar symptoms and were not recognized as separate disorders until 1952. Both are X-linked recessive disorders. While females carry the trait, they very rarely exhibit any symptoms.

Hemophilia A (classic hemophilia), is caused by the deficiency of antihemophilic factor, or AHF, which is most commonly called factor VIII. Hemophilia B (also called CHRISTMAS DISEASE, for the name of the family the disorder was first observed in) is caused by the deficiency of PTC (plasma thromboplastin component), or factor IX. Hemophilia A is four times as common, with an estimated incidence of one in 5,000 to one in 10,000 males. The Centers for Disease Control (CDC) reported there were 13,321 individuals with hemophilia A in the United States in 1997. About one-third result from new mutations. Hemophilia B is estimated to occur in one in 40,000 males. There were 3,638 individuals with hemophilia B in the United States in 1997, according to the CDC. Approximately one woman in 5,000 is a carrier for hemophilia A, and one in 20,000 is a carrier of hemophilia B. Only about one in 25,000,000 females has two copies of the hemophilia gene and is affected. Hemophilia B is one-fifth to one-tenth as common as A, with a prevalence of about one in 50,000 males.

Hemophilia C is the least common and least severe form of hemophilia. It is caused by the deficiency of factor XI (PTA, plasma thromboplastin antecedent) and is seen with greatest frequency in individuals of Ashkenazi Jewish descent. In contrast to hemophilia A and B it is inherited as an AUTOSOMAL RECESSIVE disorder. It often manifests as bleeding after a dental extraction or with heavy menstrual bleeding. Hemophilia C occurs in about one in 190 Ashkenazi Jews and about 5–13% of Ashkenazi Jews are carriers.

Hemophilia is typically divided into three classes: severe, moderate and mild, based on the level of clotting factor in the blood. In severe hemophilia, there is less than 1% of normal clotting factor. The degree of severity tends to be consistent from generation to generation.

Contrary to popular understanding, minor cuts and wounds do not present a threat to hemophiliacs. Rather, the gravest danger comes from spontaneous bleeding that may occur in joints and muscles. Episodes are most likely to occur during years of rapid growth, typically between the ages of five and 15 years. Repeated spontaneous bleeding in joints may cause arthritis, and adjacent muscles often become weakened. Pressure on nerves caused by the accumulation of blood may result in pain, numbness and temporary inability to move the affected area. In the past, this often led to permanent crippling disability by adulthood. The development of purified clotting factors in the 1970s, isolated from donated blood, significantly improved the long-term outlook for hemophiliacs. Severe hemophiliacs required transfusions of clotting factors as frequently as once a week.

However, transfusions of clotting factor, which may contain blood products from as many as 1,000 blood donors, created another major health problem for hemophiliacs. Prior to 1984, the clotting factor was not screened for the AIDS virus and most hemophiliacs who received blood products prior to 1984 were exposed to HIV. As many as 90% of heavily treated patients became HIV positive. Many of these have developed overt AIDS and about two-thirds died. This resulted in the mean life expectancy of hemophiliacs dropping from the age of 60–70 in 1980 to 49 by 1990. (In contrast it was about 11 in the early 1900s.) In 1997, the CDC reported just over 2,500 hemophiliacs taking part in federal health care programs were HIV positive. Many HIV-positive hemophiliacs have not yet developed AIDS. Gene therapy may offer a better treatment for hemophilia in the future.

Female carriers generally have lower clotting factor levels than non-carriers, facilitating carrier detection. Tests for factor VIII clotting activity can identify carriers of hemophilia A with 90% accuracy. DNA (see DEOXYRYBONUCLEIC ACID) analysis using gene probes can also be used to identify carriers of hemophilia A and B, but it may require that several family members be studied. In some families, not enough information is available to be useful. DNA-based diagnosis, either using direct analysis of the underlying mutation or using testing based on linked GENETIC MARKERS (see GENETIC LINKAGE), is available for carrier testing and PRENATAL DIAGNOSIS. A single common hemophilia A mutation (a large gene inversion) accounts for about 45% of severe cases.

Prenatal diagnosis of hemophilia is possible. The first step is to determine the gender of the FETUS via AMNIOCENTESIS or CHORIONIC VILLUS SAMPLING. Hemophilia can usually be detected in a male fetus through DNA analysis of fetal tissue or fetal blood sampling. (See also VON WILLEBRAND DISEASE.)

hemorrhagic disease of the newborn   Condition characterized by bleeding (hemorrhaging) in the newborn. Bleeding may be localized (frequently intestinal) or diffuse. It is caused by an inadequate supply of vitamin K–dependent coagulation factors: II, VII, IX and X (components of the blood involved in coagulation). This is usually due to depletion of coagulation factors derived from the mother during pregnancy and the delay in establishment of bacterial flora of the intestine that produce vitamin K. Maternal ingestion of drugs (e.g., dilatin or coumadin) may also cause it. The condition can be treated with vitamin K. Routine administration of vitamin K to infants at birth is now a standard part of neonatal care to prevent this disorder.

hepatitis   A viral disease that may result in inflammation of the liver and destruction of the liver cells, potentially leading to fatal scarring (cirrhosis) of the liver. It occurs in three recognized forms: hepatitis A, hepatitis B (HBV) and a more recently identified hepatitis C, which appears to be the most common. Of most concern during pregnancy is HBV.

Hepatitis B, often transmitted by contaminated needles, sexual contact or contact with contaminated blood, can be transmitted to a developing fetus by an infected mother. However, only an estimated 5% of affected infants are infected in the womb; the majority are infected during birth. Without treatment, an estimated 90% of infected infants will be chronic CARRIERS of the virus, perhaps showing no signs of the disease but capable of transmitting it to others. They also have a greatly increased risk of developing cirrhosis (see FAMILIAL CIRRHOSIS) and liver CANCER. An estimated 20,000 infants are born annually to infected women, and 3,500 become chronic carriers. Approximately 15–25% will ultimately die of liver cancer or cirrhosis. Maternal infection has also been associated with increased rates of miscarriage (see ABORTION), LOW BIRTH WEIGHT and premature delivery (see PREMATURITY). Over 100,000 Canadians are estimated to have chronic hepatitis B infection.

Estimates of chronic carriers range as high as 0.5–1% of the population and the U.S. Centers for Disease Control has recommended that all pregnant women be tested for hepatitis B. Vaccination with hepatitis B immune globulin soon after birth can prevent 85% to 90% of infected infants from becoming chronic carriers.

Hepatitis A is usually transmitted by contact with fecal material from an infected individual. Maternal infection during pregnancy is not associated with BIRTH DEFECTS, though if contracted during the last two weeks of pregnancy, the infant may be born with the infection.

Hepatitis C is believed to affect about 2% of the U.S. population. Incidence has fallen sharply from 180,000 new cases a year a decade ago, to about 35,000 cases a year now in the United States. It accounts for only a minority of acute hepatitis cases but is the most important cause of chronic hepatitis and liver disease. It is transmitted most commonly through IV drug, as well as through sexual contact and by transfusions of contaminated blood. Perinatal transmission is rare and estimated to occur in only about 5–6% of infected mothers. The safety of breast feeding is unresolved.

The virus that causes hepatitis C was not identified until the late 1980s; prior to that time there was no way to test for it, and cases were described simply as non A and non B hepatitis. Liver disease due to hepatitis C is the leading reason for liver transplantation in Canada. Diagnosis is possible by blood test. Research has also indicated that a drug, alpha interferon, can control the infection and prevent liver destruction in this form of hepatitis.

Other hepatitis viruses (D, E, F and G) have been found and account for a small percentage of hepatitis cases. The hepatitis E virus, like hepatitis A, is generally transmitted through fecal oral contamination, and the clinical course is also much the same, with fatigue, poor appetite, abdominal pain, joint pain and fever. It is often transmitted by contaminated water and is endemic in the developing world. Seen very infrequently in the United States or Canada (where cases have involved those who have traveled to developing countries), outbreaks have been seen in Asia and North and East Africa. Pregnant women seem to be exceptionally susceptible to severe disease and as many as 20% of pregnant women who develop hepatitis E may die from it.

hepatolenticular degeneration See WILSON DISEASE.

hereditary angiodema See HEREDITARY ANGIONEUROTIC EDEMA (HANE).

hereditary angioneurotic edema, HANE (hereditary angiodema) Affected individuals exhibit episodes of localized edema (an abnormal accumulation of fluid in body tissues), which can occur under the skin on the face, neck, lips, eyes, genitalia, hands and feet. The swelling is usually not painful, inflammatory or itchy.

Edema of a more serious nature can occur in the mucous membranes of the throat, stomach and intestines, accompanied by abdominal pain and vomiting. Unnecessary abdominal surgery has been performed in situations where the attending physician was not aware of the presence of this disorder, resulting in improper diagnosis of abdominal symptoms.

The greatest danger in this disorder is the occurrence of edema in the throat (larynx). Swelling of the laryngeal mucosa can obstruct the airway to the lungs, and has caused death in 10% to 30% of such cases. A tracheotomy, an incision in the throat to allow insertion of a tube that will permit breathing, is sometimes required.

The disorder can be detected in infancy. While present throughout life, symptoms are generally more severe in adolescence and tend to subside after 50 years of age.

Although first described and named medically in 1882, this disorder and its hereditary nature may have been noted earlier. It has been suggested that American author Nathaniel Hawthorne refers to this disorder in *The House of the Seven Gables,* published in 1851. The book describes members of a family who gurgled when excited and who sometimes died because of this, after a curse to choke on their own blood was placed on an ancestor. Hawthorne recognized that this was a HEREDITARY DISEASE and not a prophetic curse by noting that "this mode of death has been an idiosyncrasy with this family, for generations past . . . Old Maule's prophecy was probably founded on a knowledge of this physical predisposition."

Episodes of this disorder are recurrent and last from six hours to three days. There appears to be no precipitating event, although they are sometimes associated with menstruation, temperature extremes, physical trauma or emotional distress. The frequency of attacks and degree of disruption of daily living activities vary considerably. Some individuals may have only one episode in a lifetime, while others experience frequent episodes with abdominal pain or need repeated tracheotomies.

The basic cause of the disorder is the deficiency of an inhibitor to the activity of the ENZYME C1 esterase, which is believed to increase the permeability of blood vessels, bringing on the edema. In rare cases the underlying defect involves the production of an abnormal form of this enzyme. The GENE for the enzyme is found on the long arm of chromosome 11.

Inherited as an AUTOSOMAL DOMINANT trait, the disorder has been observed in a large number of ETHNIC GROUPS, including those originating in northern Europe, the Mediterranean area and Africa.

Periods of remission can be prolonged by therapy with the androgen danazol. It is an anabolic steroid with little masculinizing activity, which increases levels of C1 esterase inhibitor. Because this drug is teratogenic, it is not generally used in pregnancy. The use of other drugs to treat and prevent attacks of this disorder is also being investigated.

hereditary anonychia (absent [finger/toe] nails) The primary characteristic of this CONGENITAL disorder is a partial or complete absence of nails on fingers or toes and various abnormalities of the nails and finger or toe bones. Abnormalities may include underdeveloped nail beds (the portion of the fingers or toes normally covered by nails), or furrowing, thickening or thinning of the outermost layer or horny skin (nail plate) at the nail site. Flattening and spreading out (spatulation) of the bones at the ends of the fingers or toes, or shortening of the finger, toe or hand bones may be seen.

Both AUTOSOMAL DOMINANT and AUTOSOMAL RECESSIVE inheritance of this rare ANOMALY have been described. It is detectable at birth or may develop at a later age. Life span and intelligence are normal. Abnormalities of the nails may also be seen as part of malformation SYNDROMES, such as the ECTODERMAL DYSPLASIAS.

hereditary ataxias A group of hereditary disorders characterized by uncoordinated muscle movements (ataxia). Ataxias typically result from degenerative changes in the brain, and many of them are heritable disorders. Hereditary ataxias are classified by the mode of inheritance, either autosomal dominant or autosomal recessive, and the chromosomal location of the causative gene. Among the most common are Friedreich's ataxia and Machado-Joseph disease. Other forms of hereditary ataxias are associated with metabolic disorders, such as the Maple Syrup Urine disease, adrenoleukodystrophy and Refsum disease.

hereditary benign chorea An early onset, non-progressive form of chorea (involuntary movements), marked by involuntary twitching of the muscles of the limbs and face. In most cases onset is before the age of five. Mental function remains normal. It appears to be inherited as an AUTOSOMAL DOMINANT trait. Some patients with benign hereditary chorea have been found to have mutations in the gene encoding thyroid transcription factor-1 (*TITF1*). Other individuals with mutations in this gene have been found to present with CONGENITAL HYPOTHYROIDISM, along with more severe chorea-like movements, low muscle tone and respiratory difficulties in the newborn period.

Corticosteroids given to an affected individual to control non-associated asthma attacks have been found, coincidentally, to reduce the frequency and amplitude of the chorea.

It is important to distinguish this benign disorder from the more debilitating Huntington disease (HD), or HUNTINGTON CHOREA. The HD GENE is not involved in this much rarer condition.

hereditary coproporphyria See PORPHYRIA.

hereditary diffuse gastric cancer A hereditary predisposition to develop diffuse gastric, or stomach, cancer. "Diffuse" refers to the distribution of the cancerous material, spread within the stomach wall without forming a distinct tumor. Stomach cancer is the second most prevalent form of cancer after lung cancer. In Western Europe and the United States, incidence is 10–40 per 100,000. In Japan, incidence is 80 cases per 100,000 people. Rates are also high in Eastern Europe and parts of Latin America. Hereditary stomach cancers are estimated to represent 1% of all gastric malignancies.

Age of onset is from early teens to the late 60s, with an average of 38 years. Symptoms are variable in the early stages of the disease, and by the time of diagnosis the cancer is typically in its advanced stage. In this stage symptoms may include abdominal pain, loss of appetite, weight loss and nausea. For nonhereditary gastric cancer, the five-year survival rate is greater than 90% when diagnosed in the early stages, but in the advanced stage the five-year survival rate drops to less than 20%. Survival rates for hereditary gastric cancer may have a different stage-to-stage prognosis.

An autosomal dominant trait, the hereditary form of diffuse gastric cancer is caused by a mutation in the *CDH1* gene, mapped to 16q22.1, which encodes for the protein E-cadherin. A reduced level of E-cadherin has been shown to be involved in the development of a variety of cancers. Among those with the mutation, the chance of developing the cancer by age 80 is estimated at 67% for men and 83% for women.

Studies have found that 7% of individuals with gastric cancer have a *BRCA2* mutation. The link between this mutation and gastric cancer has not been established. Individuals who have hereditary nonpolyposis colorectal cancer (HNPCC) have an 11–15% risk of developing gastric cancer.

HDGC can be suspected if two or more first- or second-degree relatives have had diffuse gastric cancer, with at least one of them diagnosed before age 50. However, these criteria may be too broad to apply to Asian populations, such as Koreans and Japanese, where the incidence of gastric cancer is high.

Presence of the mutation can be tested via sequence analysis. Testing of an asymptomatic adult is possible if the mutation has been identified in a family member. Prenatal testing may also be available at some facilities. Typically, such tests are not administered for conditions that do not affect the intellect and for which treatments are available.

hereditary disease   A disease or abnormal condition that results from the influence of aberrant GENES inherited from the mother or father. Hereditary diseases may be transmitted as AUTOSOMAL DOMINANT, AUTOSOMAL RECESSIVE, X-LINKED, or POLYGENIC or MULTIFACTORIAL traits. This represents a vast number of disorders. More than 4,300 conditions have been linked to single-gene (autosomal dominant, autosomal recessive, X-linked) defects alone. The number of multifactorial disorders is thought to be much greater.

The fact that some disorders now identified as hereditary tend to run in families has been noted since antiquity. (See also GENETIC DISORDERS; FAMILIAL DISEASE; MENDELIAN and the Introduction.)

hereditary elliptocytosis   A benign hereditary condition in which the red blood cells are oval or elliptical, instead of exhibiting their normal round shape. In the general population, it is estimated to occur in one in 2,000 live births. However, it is extraordinarily frequent in Dyacks (aborigines of Sarawak) and other aboriginal groups in Malaysia and Melanesia, where the incidence is reported to approach 40% of the population. There are typically no clinical problems associated with this condition, but 10–15% of affected individuals may exhibit hemolytic ANEMIA.

It has been suggested that, like the other red cell disorders, such as hemoglobinopathies (e.g., SICKLE-CELL ANEMIA and THALASSEMIA), elliptocytosis may bestow an increased resistance to malarial parasites. It is inherited as an AUTOSOMAL DOMINANT TRAIT. (See ANEMIA.)

hereditary epilepsy   See EPILEPSY.

hereditary essential tremor   Familial disease, characterized by late-onset tremors, common in certain parts of Sweden and Finland. Onset is usually between the ages of 40 and 50, though it may appear in adolescence, early adulthood or, in exceptional cases, at birth. The tremors begin symmetrically in the hands and arms, and may progress to the facial muscles and tongue, and may cause speech difficulties (dysarthria). The trunk and legs are sometimes involved, and the gait may become rigid and stiff.

Tremors occur at the frequency of three to 12 per second, and are usually exacerbated by fatigue and emotion and relieved by consumption of alcohol. The tremor is unchanging for long periods following initial appearance of the disorder, but typically there is further progression late in life. Though progression of the disorder may cease, remission is rare.

Inherited as an autosomal dominant trait, one of the earliest documented cases of essential tremor was exhibited by Samuel Adams (1722–1803), the American revolutionist and brewer. The tremor, though mild, affected his hands, head and voice and was already evident when Adams was in his early 40s. A prolific writer, Adams experienced progressive difficulty with writing in his 50s and early 60s. By age 71, he had to dictate all his correspondence. His tremor was familial, affecting his daughter Hannah and her children.

It is estimated that in Sweden one in 10,000 individuals carry the gene for the disorder. However, in one parish, the gene frequency is estimated to be as high as one in 22. A study of 210 affected individuals found that all but two could trace their ancestry back to four couples. In parts of Finland, the disorder has been estimated to affect the remarkably high percentage of more than 55% of all persons over 40. Life expectancy for affected individuals appears to be greater than for their unaffected family members. Causative genes have been mapped to chromosomes 2 and 3, and there are likely others as well.

hereditary hemorrhagic telangiectasia   See OSLER-WEBER-RENDU SYNDROME.

hereditary motor and sensory neuropathy   See CHARCOT-MARIE-TOOTH DISEASE.

hereditary progressive arthroophthalmopathy   See STICKLER SYNDROME.

hereditary spastic paraplegia (HSP) (familial spastic paraparesis; Strumpell-Lorrain syndrome) A group of hereditary paraplegias characterized by progressive and severe spasticity of the lower extremities, either in isolation or in association with other neurological abnormalities. HSP is classified by its mode of transmission (autosomal dominant, autosomal recessive or X-linked recessive) and whether the spasticity occurs in isolation (uncomplicated HSP) or with other neurological effects (complicated HSP). These other effects can include ataxia, dementia, optic neuropathy, retinopathy, extrapyramidal disturbance, mental retardation, deafness and epilepsy.

Age of onset is variable, even within kindreds that have the same hereditary form. Most affected individuals exhibit their first symptoms in the second to fourth decade of life. However, it may have onset before the age of six years. The disorder often manifests with stiffness in the legs, stumbling and tripping, as motor control over the legs degenerates. Numbness below the knees often occurs, and

in some cases urinary incontinence may be a later manifestation. Muscle tone and strength of the upper body are unaffected. The severity is highly variable, with some affected individuals retaining ambulatory functions, while others are wheelchair bound and severely disabled. Lifespan is typically unaffected.

Mutations in any one of several genes can result in HSP. Three forms of an autosomal dominant form have been identified and the causative genes have been mapped to chromosome 2p, 14q and 15q. However, about 45% of the cases of dominant HSP appear to be caused by mutations in other genes. An uncomplicated autosomal recessive form has been mapped to chromosome 8q12-13. X-linked uncomplicated HSP, which is rare, is genetically heterogeneous; it can result from various mutations. Occasionally, affected kindreds have exhibited genetic anticipation, in that the age of onset is younger and symptoms more severe in succeeding generations.

Diagnosis is typically made based on neurological examination, but genetic testing and diagnosis are available at some medical facilities. No treatment is currently available, though physical therapy can help maintain muscle strength and range of motion.

heredity   The genetic transmission of characteristics from parent to offspring. That characteristics appear to pass from parent to offspring has been noted since antiquity. For example, Hippocrates (ca. 460–377 B.C.), the father of medicine, identified EPILEPSY, baldness and blue eyes as among hereditary conditions.

These characteristics may be inherited as single GENE traits (that is, AUTOSOMAL DOMINANT, AUTOSOMAL RECESSIVE or X-LINKED dominant or recessive), POLYGENIC (caused by the action of several genes) or MULTIFACTORIAL traits (caused by several genes in concert with environmental influences). Thousands of disorders in humans are hereditary; more than 2,200 different single-gene disorders alone have been confirmed, and more than 2,100 other suspected single-gene disorders have been reported. The number of multifactorial disorders is thought to be much greater. (See also FAMILIAL

DISEASE; HEREDITARY DISEASE; MENDELIAN and the Introduction.)

Hermansky-Pudlak albinism   See ALBINISM.

hermaphrodite (hermaphroditism)   An individual with the reproductive organs of both male and female. The concept of dual sexuality in one individual is common to many primal myths. Use of the term *hermaphrodite* dates to at least 300 B.C.; it is most likely taken from the son of Hermes and Aphrodite, Hermaphrodite. According to the Roman poet Ovid, he was a normal youth whose being was united with that of a water nymph, thus becoming both male and female. However, it has also been suggested that the term may refer to hermes, road markers and stone boundary columns that were dedicated to Hermes, god of the road, which were originally topped with the head of Hermes but were occasionally crowned with the head of Aphrodite.

Throughout the Hellenistic-Roman period, hermaphrodites were depicted on gems, vases and mural paintings, and references to hermaphrodites can be found in the works of the Greek and Roman historians Herodotus and Pliny. The first medical writings attempting to detail actual case histories appeared in the 16th century. However, until late in the Middle Ages, human hermaphrodites were considered monsters.

In affected individuals ovaries and testicles are both present, and the external genitalia and internal reproductive structures are highly variable in form. There may be both ovarian and testicular tissue on one side and either an ovary or a testis on the other; or ovaries and testes may be on both sides (bilateral).

Affected individuals have often been diagnosed in early infancy as the result of efforts to determine their sex in cases of AMBIGUOUS GENITALIA. Diagnosis is made by a variety of methods, including physical examination, endocrine studies, karyotyping and a variety of imaging techniques involving the genitals and reproductive system. GYNECOMASTIA develops in about 80% of affected individuals.

More than half have a 46XX KARYOTYPE, that of a normal female, and most of the remainder 46XY, that of a normal male. Thus, chromosomally the hermaphrodite's gender is definitive. However, a very small percentage have both 46XX and 46XY cells lines, and thus are both male and female chromosomally (see CHROMOSOMES; CHROMOSOME ABNORMALITY).

The cause of hermaphroditism is unknown. It has its genesis after the fourth week of pregnancy, when gonadal sex is established. (Prior to that time, though chromosomal sex of an embryo is determined, tissues that form the genitals and reproductive system remain sexually undifferentiated.) AUTOSOMAL DOMINANT and AUTOSOMAL RECESSIVE GENES have been proposed to be involved, as well as the Y chromosomal male-determining genetic material. Incidence is probably less than 1:50,000. An estimated 80% of hermaphrodites are capable, with surgical and hormonal therapy, of becoming fertile females, and giving birth. However, there are no reports of hermaphrodites raised as males ever siring children.

In the past, most hermaphrodites were raised as males. It has been suggested that it may be preferable to raise them as females, both due to the increased chance of reproductive viability, and because malignancies may develop in abnormal testicular tissue. These abnormal testes are often removed. Determining gender in such a situation is ultimately up to the parents in consultation with appropriate medical and personal guidance.

True hermaphroditism is rare in humans; little more than 525 cases have been documented. Much more common are conditions of ambiguous genitalia in which individuals appear to be of indeterminate gender, due to lack of development of external genitalia, such as PSEUDOHERMAPHRODITISM, a form of ambiguous genitalia with the presence of only a single type of gonadal tissue.

The term *hermaphrodite* is falling into disfavor, as it is felt to be stigmatizing and clinically problematic; the term *intersex* is preferred.

herpes simplex   See TORCH SYNDROME.

Hers disease   See GLYCOGEN STORAGE DISEASE.

heterochromia irides   Asymmetry of pigmentation of the irides (eyes of separate colors). Seen most frequently in WAARDENBURG SYNDROME and in PIEBALD SKIN TRAIT, it may also result from damage to autonomic nerves (cervical branches of the sympathetic nerves) as a result of birth injury. Cervical sympathetics are automatic nerves that govern pupil size, sweating and other functions. When these nerves are damaged, the iris may lose color.

Whether this condition ever occurs as an inherited condition independent of any other syndrome is not clear, though it has been suggested that it occurs in isolated cases as an AUTOSOMAL DOMINANT trait.

heterogeneity (heterogeneous) The ability of a single (or very similar) condition(s) to be caused by a variety of genetic or non-genetic causes. Many HEREDITARY DISEASES, Mendelian as well as MULTIFACTORIAL and POLYGENIC, are heterogeneous. The heterogeneity may involve different MUTATIONS in the same GENE (allelic heterogeneity) or may imply that different gene loci, or locations, are involved (locus heterogeneity). Even different patterns of inheritance may be found to underlie different cases of the same disorder.

heterozygote; heterozygous An individual with different ALLELES or unlike genes in a gene pair that controls a given characteristic. In the past, this generally indicated that an individual possessed one normal and one mutant, or one dominant and one recessive gene for a given characteristic. But the concept of heterozygosity has become more complex as geneticists have learned that there may be numerous forms (or alleles) of a recessive gene. Individuals who are heterozygotes for AUTOSOMAL RECESSIVE traits, and women who are heterozygotes for X-LINKED recessive traits, are often termed CARRIERS.

high scapula See SPRENGEL DEFORMITY.

hip, congenital dislocation of See CONGENITAL DISLOCATION OF THE HIP.

Hirschsprung disease (colon aganglionosis) A CONGENITAL dilation of the colon, which prevents feces from passing into the rectum and being excreted, causing constipation, vomiting, dehydration and FAILURE TO THRIVE. It results from the absence of the nerve cells (myenteric ganglia) in the colon that normally propel the movement of feces in the intestine. Surgical removal of the affected portion of the colon results in immediate recovery in 50% of those treated. Without treatment, those severely affected may die. (An estimated 20% die in infancy.)

Incidence is estimated at one in 5,000 live births, and males are more commonly affected than females by a ratio of approximately 4:1. It is named for Danish pediatrician Harald Hirschsprung (1830–1916), who published a description in 1888. This disorder is genetically heterogeneous (see HETEROGENEITY) and may be caused by dominant MUTATIONS in the RET oncogene on 10q (this mutation represents about 50% of cases; other mutations in this GENE cause MEN2) or by recessive mutations in the endothelin receptor type B gene on 13q (about 5%), both with reduced PENETRANCE. The genes for endothelin-3, on chromosome 20q; glial cell line-derived neurotrophic factor, found on 5p; the *Neurturin* gene on the short arm of chromosome 19; and endothelin-converting enzyme-1, which maps to 1p, have also been implicated in Hirschsprung disease. Other genes on chromosome 21 and the long arm of the X CHROMOSOME also appear to be involved in the development of the disorder. Mutations in these genes give dominant, recessive or polygenic patterns of inheritance.

Hirschsprung is also found as a feature of DOWN SYNDROME (accounting for about 10% of cases; Hirschsprung affects about 6% of Down individuals), WAARDENBERG SYNDROME, cartilage-hair hypoplasia, MEN2, SMITH-LEMLI-OPITZ SYNDROME and primary central hypoventilation syndrome (Ondine-Hirschsprung disease). Occurrence is most often SPORADIC.

hirsutism Excessive hair growth, typically at puberty and especially in females. The hair may appear on the face, chest, abdomen or extremities. Other secondary sex characteristics remain nominal.

histidinemia Histidine is a basic AMINO ACID found in many proteins and metabolized by the body. It is essential for optimal growth in infants. A deficiency of the ENZYME histidase, normally found in the liver and the thick outer layer of the skin (stratum corneum), results in a failure to metabolize histidine and produces an excess of histidine in the blood and urine of those affected, a condition known as histidinemia. For some years it was believed this resulted in emotional and behavioral problems, speech impairment, scholastic failure and mild to moderate MENTAL RETARDATION. However, it has become apparent that in the vast majority of cases histidinemia is a harmless biochemical abnormality. In only a small proportion of those with the enzyme deficiency (some believe less than 1%) does it cause significant neurologic dysfunction.

Inherited as an AUTOSOMAL RECESSIVE enzyme defect, histidinemia can be detected in the first week of life by a blood test for histidine or by a test for histidase activity in the stratum corneum. It occurs in approximately one in every 12,000 live births, a frequency approximating that of PHENYLKETONURIA.

In some states, the law has required testing of all newborns for histidinemia. Because of the question of whether histidinemia is really a "disease," the benefit of this screening is controversial.

HLA   See HUMAN LEUKOCYTE ANTIGEN.

holoprosencephaly   A group of facial malformations caused by defective development of the embryonic forebrain. Essentially, the forebrain fails to divide, or divide properly, into cerebral hemispheres. The type of holoprosencephaly exhibited is determined by the severity of this defective development.

In the most severe form, CYCLOPIA, there is a single eye-globe in the middle of the face and often CONGENITAL absence of the nose (arhinia), though there is usually a malformed nose-like structure with no connection to the postnatal space.

In ethmocephaly, another form of holoprosencephaly, there are two closely set eyes (HYPO-TELORISM) associated with absence of the nose, though, again, proboscis formation occurs.

Cebocephaly, a third form, is characterized by hypotelorism and a single nostril nose with a blind ending.

Other less severe forms have varying degrees of hypotelorism and abnormalities of the nose (e.g., a flat, boneless nose) and midline of the upper lip (e.g., clefts). The mild end of the spectrum of features includes a single central incisor (tooth).

Holoprosencephalic infants often have small heads (MICROCEPHALY) and their gestations are frequently abnormal, often with excess AMNIOTIC FLUID (polyhydramnios). About 25% require CESAREAN DELIVERY.

Holoprosencephaly is estimated to occur in one in 15,000 births. Among spontaneous ABORTIONS, the rate may be as high as one in 200.

This condition is often seen in CHROMOSOMAL ABNORMALITIES, particularly trisomy 13, 18p-, 13q and triploidy. Approximately 25–50% of individuals with holoprosencephaly have a numerical or structural chromosomal abnormality. Infants of diabetic mothers have a 1% risk (a 200-fold increase over the general population) for holoprosencephaly. It may also be seen in syndromes such as the MECKEL SYNDROME and in infants of mothers with fetal CMV infection. Overall, it has been estimated that about 18–25% of individuals with holoprosencephaly have a mutation in a single gene causing syndromic holoprosencephaly, and at least 25 different conditions have been described in which it can be a feature.

It is believed to be inherited as an AUTOSOMAL RECESSIVE characteristic in some cases, since there have been many instances of affected SIBLINGS, and an AUTOSOMAL DOMINANT form as well. Mutations in a specific gene on the long arm of chromosome 7 have been shown to result in autosomal dominant cases of holoprosencephaly. This gene encodes a protein known as the human sonic hedgehog homolog. This protein was so named because it is the human equivalent of a protein first identified in fruit flies and was given the fanciful name of a character in a children's video game. It is a signaling protein involved in embryonic development. Other genes involved include the zinc finger protein gene ZIC2 on chromosome 13q, the SIX3 gene on chromosome 2p, the TGIF gene on chromosome 18p and the PTCH gene (mutations in which can also cause NEVOID BASAL CELL CARCINOMA SYNDROME) on 9q. Most often, however, the defect is an isolated occurrence. If the case is sporadic, with normal chromosomal analysis and no identifiable syndrome, overall recurrence risk is about 6%.

Those with the most severe forms of holoprosencephaly do not survive infancy. Infants with milder forms often survive into childhood, though they exhibit moderate to severe MENTAL RETARDATION. PRENATAL DIAGNOSIS, especially in severe cases, may be accomplished with ULTRASOUND.

Holt-Oram syndrome (heart-hand syndrome)

Disorder characterized by defects in the thumbs, hands, arms and heart; first described in 1960 by Mary Holt and Samuel Oram, both cardiologists at Kings College Hospital in London.

The thumb may be absent or partially developed; It may also be finger-like, with three phalanx bones (triphalangeal) rather than the normal two, rendering it nonopposable. In the most severe cases, abnormal bones in the wrist (carpal bones) may further reduce rotation of the thumb as well as the wrist. The arms may be shortened, with the hand attached directly to the shoulder (PHOCOMELIA). The lower limbs are normal.

Atrial septal defect is the most common congenital HEART DEFECT seen among individuals with Holt-Oram syndrome. In addition, a duct that normally occurs only in the FETUS may decrease the amount of blood circulating in the lungs (PATENT DUCTUS ARTERIOSUS). Ventricular septal defect, transposition of the great vessels, and mitral valve prolapse may also occur.

In most cases both heart defects and upper limb abnormalities occur, although occasionally one may be seen without the other. The degree of the malformations varies among individuals with the SYNDROME, even within families with multiple affected individuals.

It is inherited as an AUTOSOMAL DOMINANT trait. MUTATIONS in a GENE found on the long arm of chromosome 12 cause most cases of this syndrome. Some, however are not linked to this LOCUS and the disorder must have HETEROGENEITY, that is, mutations in one of several genes can cause this syndrome, with other loci yet to be identified. The locus on 12q is the T-box 5 (TBX5) gene, a developmental gene that acts as a transcription factor. Mutations in the closely linked and structurally related T-box 3 (TBX3) gene result in the ulnar-mammary syndrome, in which defects of the ulna and little finger side of the hand are seen along with poor development of the breast and other malformations. Thus, the TBX5 gene is involved with the development of one side of the limb (thumb side), and TBX3 the other (little finger side).

Over 200 cases have been reported. The syndrome occurs in about one in 100,000 live births. It is detectable in infancy, with upper extremity abnormalities usually visible at birth. Life span depends on the severity of defects. Surgery can correct some of the heart and skeletal defects. Intelligence is normal. Prenatal ULTRASOUND may detect the syndrome if the abnormalities are severe.

homocystinuria Disorder that manifests in skeletal abnormalities, such as knock-knees (genu valgum), high foot arch (pes cavus), either a ridged or a funnel-shaped chest (pectus carinatum or excavatum) and SCOLIOSIS. The abnormalities may be detected visually or by X-rays. Restricted mobility of joints and osteoporosis, which leads to fracture, are common. The individuals have a tall, thin appearance, with long, thin extremities and digits resembling those of MARFAN SYNDROME.

Clotting (thrombosis) in blood vessels leading to the heart, lungs, brain and kidneys is also common and may cause death at any time from infancy. Some individuals may have flushed cheeks (malar flush). One-half to two-thirds are mentally retarded.

Most affected individuals who live past age 10 develop a displacement of the lens of the eye (ectopia lentis). This can lead to complications such as progressive nearsightedness, detached retina and GLAUCOMA.

Affected individuals lack the ENZYME cystathionine beta-synthase. This results in a buildup of toxic compounds that is assumed to cause the physical symptoms. The GENE for cystathionine beta-synthase is on chromosome 21 and many MUTATIONS have been found in affected patients including a common Celtic mutation.

Homocystinuria can be detected within two to four days of birth by urine or blood tests. In about half of cases, treatment with vitamin B$_6$ (pyridoxine) started in infancy prevents all signs of the disorder.

Another drug used in treatment is betaine. In other cases a low-methionine diet can minimize skeletal malformations and ocular changes and prevent MENTAL RETARDATION and thrombosis.

Incidence is below one per 100,000 in the general population, but slightly more prevalent in Ireland and among persons of Irish descent. In the United States it is about one in 58,000. Inherited as an AUTOSOMAL RECESSIVE trait, individuals may live past age 50, but the potential for thrombosis greatly reduces life expectancy.

Other rare, variant forms of the disease result from defects in vitamin B_{12} and folic acid metabolism. There appears to be a link between homocysteine metabolism and NEURAL TUBE DEFECTS, which is likely related to the protective effect of folic acid. The observation that thromboses are common in individuals with homocystinuria led to the observation that even mildly elevated levels of homocysteine increase the risk of thrombosis and vascular disease. These mildly elevated levels can result from the interplay of the genes involved in homocysteine metabolism and vitamin levels.

homozygote;   homozygous   Having   identical ALLELES or identical corresponding GENES for a given trait.

horseshoe kidney   A CONGENITAL abnormality in which both kidneys are united at their lower ends, creating a horseshoe-shaped mass rather than two individual kidneys. It occurs in an estimated one in 200–400 live births. Recurrence in families is rare. Usually SPORADIC, it can be associated with other ANOMALIES and seen as part of a number of SYNDROMES and CHROMOSOME ABNORMALITIES; e.g., 20% of infants with trisomy 18 (EDWARD SYNDROME) have horseshoe kidney. The condition is often entirely asymptomatic, but may lead to obstruction of urinary flow, and therefore to stones, infection or pain. Horseshoe kidney is generally detected by X-ray or ULTRASOUND.

human   leukocyte   antingen,   HLA (major histocompatibility complex)   The GENES of the major histocompatibility complex play a role in immunological response. In humans, the location (loci) of these genes is on the short arm of chromosome 6. The designation for this area on the CHROMOSOME is HLA (human leukocyte antigen).

HLA is used as a GENETIC MARKER in determining the compatibility of tissue for organ transplants. Proteins which are an integral part of the membranes of the body's cells, HLA is involved not only in transplant rejection, but also crucial to the maintenance of the immune system competence and integrity of the individual, and the body's recognition of self versus others.

If an individual is to receive an organ transplant, it is possible to test the compatibility of their HLA type with that of the potential donor. Complications associated with organ rejection will be minimized if the donor's HLA is compatible with the recipient's.

Certain HLA types are also associated with a susceptibility to develop a number of diseases. Thus HLA GENES appear to be one of the inherited "susceptibility factors" underlying the MULTIFACTORIAL inheritance of a number of common disorders, and may be responsible for the familial incidence of these diseases. The best known example of an association of HLA type with disease susceptibility is the association of ANKYLOSING SPONDYLITIS with HLA B27. Other disorders that are associated with specific HLA types include PSORIASIS, juvenile onset DIABETES MELLITUS, Graves disease, MYASTHENIA GRAVIS, celiac disease (GLUTEN-INDUCED ENTEROPATHY) and RHEUMATOID ARTHRITIS. Most of these associated disorders are autoimmune ones in which an immune reaction is directed against one's own tissues. Other diseases are closely linked to the HLA gene, and thus HLA types can be used as a marker for the presence of the disease gene. Such is the case for HEMOCHROMATOSIS and CONGENITAL adrenal hyperplasia (21-hydroxylase deficiency). (See also ADRENOGENITAL SYNDROMES.) HLA types are also used as markers for paternity testing.

humeroradial synostosis   The fusion of two bones of the arm (the humerus of the upper arm and the radius of the forearm) rendering the arm unable to bend at the elbow, or severely limiting its motion at the joint. The basic cause is unknown.

Other abnormalities have been associated with this condition in a few cases, and humeroradial synostosis may also be associated with a number of distinct SYNDROMES. THALIDOMIDE can also cause this malformation. In isolation, this rare condition may be inherited as either an AUTOSOMAL DOMINANT or AUTOSOMAL RECESSIVE trait.

humpback, hunchback An abnormal curvature of the spine that gives the back the appearance of having a lump or protuberance. Medically, this condition is referred to as kyphosis. A deformity associated with many CONGENITAL and HEREDITARY DISEASES affecting the skeletal system, it is perhaps best known as the affliction of Quasimodo, the fictional character in Victor Hugo's novel *Notre Dame de Paris* (1831) and in the Disney animated film of 1996 based on the book. It can be isolated or found as a feature of a number of SYNDROMES. The condition often occurs in combination with SCOLIOSIS, an abnormal lateral (sideways) curvature of the spine. When the two are seen together, it is referred to as kyphoscoliosis. Treatment when severe is surgical.

hunchback See HUMPBACK.

Hunter syndrome See MUCOPOLYSACCHARIDOSIS.

Huntington chorea (Huntington disease, HD) A progressive disorder of the central nervous system characterized by the development of bizarre, uncontrollable movements (chorea) of the arms, legs, torso and facial muscles, intellectual impairment and severe mental disturbances. Its arrival in the New World can be traced to the 17th century, and manifestations of the disorder may have been responsible for charges made against some men and women of consorting with the devil and of being witches.

In 1630, three men whose families had been persecuted for witchcraft immigrated to America. These men and their descendants had repeated problems with legal authorities, and several were executed for witchcraft. One of the three men sub-sequently settled in East Hampton, Long Island, in New York, and his progeny were notorious locally for a strange and frightening disease.

While growing up, George Huntington (1850–1916) visited patients from this family, accompanied by his father and grandfather, who were general practitioners. In 1872, after graduating from medical school, he published his first and only paper, "On Chorea," in which he described the disorder that now bears his name.

Approximately 25,000 individuals have been confirmed as having HD, and 150,000 are thought to be at risk for developing the disorder. Most cases in the United States can be traced to these three original settlers, though it is seen in other ETHNIC GROUPS as well. Cases in South Africa have been traced to Dutch immigrants who settled there in 1658, and in Venezuela to a German sailor who arrived about 1860. An extensive kindred near Venezuela's Lake Maracaibo has been well documented. It is one-third as prevalent among blacks, and rare in Japanese, Chinese and Finnish people.

The precise disease process in HD is unclear though identification of the HD GENE and development of animal models are beginning to shed some light on the mechanisms. The brains of affected individuals exhibit characteristic deterioration. An area that is important in motor control, the caudate nucleus, is severely shrunken, and spiny neurons, cells that carry impulses within the brain, are destroyed.

Onset is usually between the ages of 35 and 45, though it has appeared in children as young as two years of age and in adults as old as 80. In these unusual cases, differentiation from other neurologic diseases is imperative. Initial symptoms include irritability, clumsiness, depression and forgetfulness. Mood, personality change and uncontrollable movements may precede correct diagnosis by a decade. (Folk singer Woody Guthrie, who was affected, was first thought to be an alcoholic, and later a schizophrenic, before he was properly diagnosed.)

Progressive deterioration of the central nervous system leads to slurred speech, grimacing, compulsive clenching and unclenching of fists and flailing of arms and legs. Ultimately, those affected succumb to pneumonia, heart failure or other complications 15 to 20 years after onset.

HD is inherited as an AUTOSOMAL DOMINANT disorder with an incidence estimated at between from three and seven per 100,000 births. Age of onset and the rate of progression may be influenced by the gender of the parent from whom the disorder was inherited. When paternally inherited, the most common form of HD begins an average of three years earlier than when maternally inherited. For example, juvenile and adolescent forms are almost always paternally inherited. Late onset cases (age 50 or later) are twice as likely to be maternally inherited. New MUTATIONS are uncommon.

There is no cure, though drugs may alleviate some of the associated movement disorders. Antidepressants and counseling may be required due to the severe mental depression that often accompanies the disorder; by some estimates, as many as 25% of those affected are thought to attempt suicide.

Generally, those at risk or those affected have children before they learn whether they have inherited the condition and are thus capable of transmitting it to their offspring. A GENETIC MARKER, or a chromosomal signpost that indicates the presence of the HD gene, was discovered on chromosome 4 in 1983 as a result of studies of the large Venezuelan pedigree and other large families. The availability of the linked genetic marker made presymptomatic diagnosis possible using GENETIC LINKAGE testing techniques. In 1993 the HD gene itself was identified and the nature of the specific mutation causing HD clarified. The HD gene encodes a protein that has been named huntingtin. This protein is expressed in the neurons of the brain where it seems to play an important role in the functioning of the basal ganglia. It appears to have a role in the cell death of the neurons there, and malfunction of the gene caused by the HD mutation seems to impair that process. The HD gene contains a triplet or TRINUCLEOTIDE REPEAT, a region of the gene containing a stretch of DNA with a variable number of repeated copies of the trinucleotide (three bases of genetic code), CAG. Normal individuals have from eight to 35 copies of the repeat, while individuals affected with HD have expanded repeats with larger numbers of copies of the CAG sequence. Several interesting observations have been made: the longer the repeat length, in general, the earlier the age of onset. Expanded repeats are unstable and may enlarge, especially during the production of sperm. This explains why offspring of affected fathers may have earlier onset of HD. Definitive predictive testing became available with the identification of the specific genetic defect. Direct measurement of repeat length allows for the prediction of who will become affected with the disease either presymptomatically or even prenatally. The decision at-risk individuals must make of whether to undergo testing is a difficult and complex one. They must weigh the advantages of finding out they are at low risk against the possible negative effects of learning they will develop a disease for which there is no prevention or treatment. Extensive genetic and psychological counseling is an intrinsic part of the predictive testing protocol. While studies have shown that over the long term, predictive testing has had beneficial psychological results for at-risk individuals (whether they were found to have an increased or decreased risk), most people at risk have chosen not to be tested. Tests require blood or tissue samples from several relatives. Considered 99% accurate, testing is being done on a limited basis.

Huntington disease   See HUNTINGTON CHOREA.

Hurler syndrome   See MUCOPOLYSACCHARIDOSIS (type I).

Hutchison-Gilford progeria syndrome   See PROGERIA.

hydrocephalus   An abnormal increase of cerebrospinal fluid (CSF) within the cranial cavity accompanied by expansion of the ventricles of the brain, enlargement of the skull and atrophy of the brain. It may result in physical incapacity, MENTAL RETARDATION, BLINDNESS and death. The term is taken from the Greek words *hydros* (fluid) and *cephalus* (head).

Within the brain are four fluid-filled cavities called ventricles: two lateral ventricles (one in the center of each cerebral hemisphere) and smaller third and fourth ventricles (one atop the other in the middle of the brain, between the lateral ventricles). The ventricles are connected, or "communicate" through passageways that lead from the lateral ventricles into the third and fourth ventricles, and finally into the spinal column. Small, flower-like tufts within the ventricles, called the choroid plexus, produce CSF at a rate of approximately 350 to 500 cc. every day. (Most is produced in the larger lateral ventricles.) After circulating around the brain and spinal cord, the CSF is reabsorbed into the blood. In almost all cases, hydrocephalus is caused by a blockage somewhere in this CSF circulatory system. The body does not reduce CSF production, and the increase in cranial pressure caused by the buildup creates serious medical problems.

If upon examination there is no apparent blockage, and it appears that fluid is free to circulate throughout the ventricles, the hydrocephalus is referred to as "communicating." (That is, the ventricles remain in communication.) However, if blockage is observed within the CFS circulatory system, the hydrocephalus is said to be "non-communicating."

The signs of the condition are an enlarged head (macrocephaly), usually appearing first as a bulge of the anterior fontanelle, the soft spot on the forward top portion of the infant's head. Cranial sutures (the gaps or seams between the skull bones) may be widely separated, the scalp may appear to be stretched and glistening and scalp veins distended. In severe cases, the eyes may appear to deviate downward ("sunsetting") due to pressure on the optic nerve. Vomiting, irritability, lethargy and seizures are other symptoms.

In those born with the condition, the head may appear large from birth. When the condition develops before the bones of the skull have fused, the head will grow larger as the pressure builds. There will be less enlargement, but more intracranial pressure, when the skull bones have fused in approximately six to 12 months.

The condition is estimated to occur in one in 500 births. Seventy-five percent to 95% of cases have their origin in fetal development, the remainder develop hydrocephalus as a result of complications arising from other conditions. Males are somewhat more commonly affected than females. About 10% of cases have additional congenital anomalies.

Hydrocephalus can occur as an isolated condition, as part of a SYNDROME, or in association with other defects. An X-LINKED recessive form accounts for a significant proportion of male cases. It accounts for perhaps one-quarter of all hydrocephalus in males resulting from a narrowing of the communication between the third and fourth ventricles. Hydrocephalus may also result from intraventricular hemorrhages in premature babies. The blood clot that forms after the bleeding may block CSF circulation or reabsorption. X-linked hydrocephalus and the related MASA syndrome have been found to result from mutations in a particular GENE on the X CHROMOSOME which encodes a protein known as the L1 cell adhesion molecule. MASA (mental retardation, aphasia, shuffling gait and adducted thumbs) syndrome overlaps with isolated X-linked hydrocephalus and also includes flexed, clasped thumbs, mental HANDICAP, absent speech and a shuffling, spastic gait, as well as other cerebral malformations. Hydrocephalus can also result from certain infections such as TORCH SYNDROME infections or meningitis.

Children with hydrocephalus may have developmental delays, disorders of muscle tone and movement, feeding and speech difficulties, perceptual motor disturbances or sensory disorders, and occasionally ocular problems.

In about 30% of cases, an enlarged head is evident at birth. The majority of the remaining cases are diagnosed within the first few months of life, when a disproportionate increase in the size of the head becomes observable. Fifty percent of the cases are identified within the first four months of life and 80% within the first year.

The condition can be confirmed through CT scans of the brain and by measuring CSF pressure within the brain. PRENATAL DIAGNOSIS of the condition is sometimes possible using ULTRASOUND to detect an enlarged head. A positive finding may require delivery via CESAREAN DELIVERY due to the increased size of the cranium. Prenatal diagnosis can be difficult, however. Some enlargement of the ventricles evident on ultrasound in pregnancy may be a self-limited and nonprogressive abnormality compatible with normal functioning after birth. On the other hand, true severe hydrocephalus may only become evident after 16 to 18 weeks of gestation when ultrasound is generally performed.

The primary method of treatment is surgical implantation of a shunt, a tube that drains excess CSF from the ventricle of the brain. It typically runs under the skin along the scalp and neck and empties into the abdominal or peritoneal cavity, where it is absorbed into the body. Due to this procedure, affected individuals with proper diagnosis and treatment can live normal life spans relatively uncomplicated by the condition. Successful shunting operations have even been performed on hydrocephalic fetuses IN UTERO, but such operations remain experimental and the role of this procedure in future treatment is unclear.

As an isolated condition, the prognosis is least favorable when hydrocephalus is present at birth. Almost half of the cases of true CONGENITAL hydrocephaly are stillborn. One quarter die soon after birth, only 5% survive. Among the survivors, less than half have normal IQs, with the rest exhibiting mild to severe mental retardation.

Some infants with congenital hydrocephalus will also have additional abnormalities within the brain and other malformations that affect the brain or other organs of the body. These may be relatively harmless, such as CLEFT LIP and CLEFT PALATE, or may have serious consequences, such as heart disease and obstruction of the bowel. In addition, 80% of infants with SPINA BIFIDA may have hydrocephalus as a further complication.

hymen, imperforate   See IMPERFORATE HYMEN.

hyperammonemia, congenital   See UREA CYCLE DEFECTS.

hypercholesterolemia   See CORONARY ARTERY DISEASE.

hyperglyciremia, nonketotic   See NONKETOTIC HYPERGLYCINEMIA.

hyperimmunoglobulin E   See JOB SYNDROME.

hyperinsulinism   A condition of excessive levels of insulin in the blood in combination with low levels of glucose. Insulin regulates the blood glucose level and helps assure the body has energy available for metabolism at all times. The high levels of insulin that characterize this disorder interfere with this regulatory function.

Hereditary hyperinsulinism, though rare, is the most common cause of neonatal hypoglycemia (low blood sugar) in the first few hours of life. It is also an important cause of hypoglycemia in infants and children. Transient hyperinsulinism can also occur in babies born prematurely, those whose mothers have poorly controlled diabetes mellitus, or who suffered fetal distress due to lack of oxygen.

Infants exhibit cyanosis, respiratory distress, apnea, lethargy, hypothermia, sweating, seizures or irritability. Without proper treatment, the low blood sugar hyperinsulinism can cause brain damage and neurological problems. Brain damage occurs in about 50% of infants treated for hyperinsulinism.

Several hereditary forms of hyperinsulinism have been identified. Two autosomal recessive forms are caused by mutations in two adjacent genes on chromosome 11, *SUR* and *Kir6.2*. These genes control the potassium channel (KAPT channel) in the insulin-secreting beta cells in the pancreas, one stage in the control of the flow of insulin. Mutations in either of these genes render the potassium channel nonfunctional, allowing insulin to be released into the bloodstream unregulated. Mutations in the *SUR* gene are the most common. Mutations in the *Kir6* gene result in the classic, more severe recessive form of the two, KATP. These forms that affect the KAPT channel are called diffuse KATP.

Heterozygotes (carriers) who inherit only one mutation of the recessive form may also exhibit hyperinsulinism if the normal gene of the gene pair is missing in some pancreatic cells. This form is called focal KATP. Autosomal recessive forms are more common among Ashkenazi Jews and populations in Saudi Arabia.

A milder form of hyperinsulinism, transmitted in autosomal dominant fashion, is caused by mutations of either the *glucokinase* gene or the *glutamate dehydrogenase* gene (*GDH*). It can also occur sporadically, as a result of a new mutation. The mutation of the *glucokinase* gene increases the affinity of glucokinase for glucose, which leads to accelerated rates of glycolysis, which leads to increased ATP/ADP ratio and insulin secretion. Excessive glutamate dehydrogenase activity increases insulin release, and mutations of the *GDH* gene result in low blood glucose levels and persistent mild elevations of serum ammonia. Infants affected with this form typically exhibit symptoms later than onset of KATP, typically at three to four months of age. Other forms of hyperinsulinism also appear to follow autosomal dominant inheritance, but their molecular basis is unclear. An autosomal dominant form of diffuse KATP has also been identified.

Infants affected with either form of KATP require large infusions of glucose to normalize their blood glucose levels. Diagnosis is made on the basis of blood analysis of the levels of glucose, insulin, growth hormone, cortisol and other substances when the infant is hypoglycemic.

Incidence in the United States is estimated at one out of 50,000 live births. Worldwide, it is estimated to occur in 1:25,000 to 1:50,000 live births.

hypermobility   The ability to move joints beyond their normal range of extension; in colloquial language "double-jointedness." It is noted in disorders of the skeletal and connective tissues such as MARFAN SYNDROME and EHLERS-DANLOS SYNDROME. Benign hypermobility syndrome is an AUTOSOMAL DOMINANT disorder with hypermobility of the joints, which may dislocate, but with no skin involvement, as is seen in the Ehlers-Danlos syndrome.

hyperphosphatasia (hyperostosis corticalis deformans juvenilis)   Also known as juvenile Paget disease, this HEREDITARY DISEASE is characterized by numerous skeletal malformations, including easily fractured bones, bowed legs, short neck, an unusually prominent sternum or chest (pectus carinatum), abnormal curvature of the spine (kyphoscoliosis), an enlarged head and enlarged and pronounced brow (frontal bossing).

During the first year of life, infants exhibit fever and painful and swollen extremities, and between the ages of two and three years develop an enlarged head, often experiencing headaches and vision

and hearing loss. Affected individuals frequently have numerous bone fractures, though they heal normally. Growth is affected, but not seriously diminished. Activities such as running, walking or jumping are impaired due to muscle weakness; a movement such as extending the arm from the elbow is often impossible.

Laboratory tests reveal elevated serum acid and serum alkaline phosphatase levels with normal calcium and phosphorus levels. Elevated levels of the AMINO ACID hydroxyproline are found in connective tissue.

Hyperphosphatasia is inherited in an AUTOSOMAL RECESSIVE manner. It can result from osteoprotegerin deficiency caused by mutations in the *TNFRSF11B* gene, found on the long arm of chromosome 8. Bones remain weak since fibrous bone never strengthens or becomes compact as it should. Recombinant osteoprotegerin has been used in treatment of the disorder.

hypertelorism   An abnormally wide distance between the eyes. CONGENITAL ocular hypertelorism is very common in many GENETIC DISORDERS. As an isolated condition, familial cases have been noted, though the mode of inheritance is unclear.

hypertelorism-hypospadias syndrome   See G SYNDROME.

hypertension, essential   See ESSENTIAL HYPERTENSION.

hyperthermia of anesthesia   See MALIGNANT HYPERTHERMIA.

hypertriglyceridemia   See CORONARY ARTERY DISEASE.

hypochondroplasia   A form of DWARFISM caused by defective skeletal development (chondrodystrophy). A distinct disorder, for many years after it was first described in 1913 it was considered a form of ACHONDROPLASIA. Though it resembles achondroplasia, its features are milder, especially in the hands and spine as well as in the lack of craniofacial involvement. The degree of height reduction and disproportion of the physique is variable.

Birth weight may be low (see LOW BIRTH WEIGHT). The head appears normal, though the forehead may be prominent. Short stature may not be recognized for two to six years. Mildly affected individuals may remain undiagnosed. The body is thick and stocky with a relatively long trunk and short limbs. The elbows may not fully extend. The hands and feet are short and broad. Bowleggedness (genu varum, see BOWLEG) is sometimes present but often disappears with age. The abdomen may protrude slightly, and individuals may exhibit a swayback appearance (lumbar lordosis). As adults, individuals may experience pain in joints and lower back. Approximately 10% exhibit mild MENTAL RETARDATION. Life span is normal. Average height ranges from 51 inches to 57 inches (130 cm to 145 cm).

An AUTOSOMAL DOMINANT trait, familial incidence is well documented. Most cases appear to be SPORADIC, resulting from new MUTATIONS, in some cases related to advanced paternal age. It is estimated to occur approximately one-twelfth as frequently as achondroplasia. Diagnosis of this condition is often uncertain. Some cases are caused by mutations in the same GENE as achondroplasia, the FGFR3 (fibroblast growth factor receptor 3) gene. The mutations are, however, different ones. Thus achondroplasia and hypochondroplasia are allelic conditions (see ALLELE). Other mutations in the FGFR3 gene cause thanatophoric dysplasia. Some cases of hypochondroplasia involve genes other than the FGFR3 gene, but what this gene or genes are has yet to be discovered.

PRENATAL DIAGNOSIS may be possible in at-risk pregnancies based on ULTRASOUND findings of characteristic fetal skeletal deficiencies, and has been accomplished. However, because of the great variability of this condition it may not always be possible.

hypogammaglobulenemia See IMMUNE DEFICIENCY DISEASE.

hypophosphatasia A HEREDITARY DISEASE resulting in an abnormal balance of bone calcium and phosphate, causing the bone tissue to inadequately calcify or not calcify at all. It is caused by different MUTATIONS in the alkaline phosphatase GENE located on the short arm of chromosome 1, and occurs in infantile-, childhood- and adult-onset forms. Depending on the severity of the disorder, effects range from intrauterine death to modest HANDICAPS in childhood and adulthood.

The infantile form is the most severe, characterized by short, bowed limbs, soft and beaded ribs, deformed and enlarged joints, and poor skull formation. Seizures, vomiting and a high-pitched cry are common. Affected infants are often stillborn or die early due to respiratory problems. Some, however, spontaneously improve.

The childhood form is generally milder. Symptoms may appear after six months of age and include premature skull bone closure (craniosynostosis), growth retardation, narrow chest, enlarged wrists, knees and ankles and bowed legs caused by RICKETS. Additional features are premature loss of baby teeth and a weakened immune system. Calcification of the kidney and an excess of calcium in the blood (hypercalcemia) may accompany these symptoms.

The adult form is the mildest and appears as a reduction or thinning of bone mass (osteoporosis) and occasional bone fractures. Baby teeth are lost early and permanent teeth also loosen prematurely and often fall out.

Infantile and childhood forms of hypophosphatasia are AUTOSOMAL RECESSIVE traits. For the adult form, both AUTOSOMAL DOMINANT and autosomal recessive inheritance have been suggested. (It is possible that it only appears to be autosomal dominant in some families when affected individuals have actually inherited two different mild mutations, and it is really autosomal recessive, a circumstance described as pseudodominance.) One in 25 Manitoba Mennonites is a CARRIER of the adult onset form.

Occurrence is rare: Approximately 200 cases have been identified. The frequency of the lethal form is estimated to be about one per 100,000 live births. (Some classify the prenatal lethal form as a separate entity.)

PRENATAL DIAGNOSIS may be achieved by finding extremely reduced alkaline phosphatase activity (similar to that seen in the blood of affected individuals) in fetal cells obtained via AMNIOCENTESIS or CHORIONIC VILLUS SAMPLING. Prenatal diagnosis has also been accomplished by molecular testing. Prenatal ULTRASOUND has also been used to diagnose severe infantile cases before birth.

hypophosphatemia (X-linked hypophosphatemia; X-linked vitamin D–resistant rickets) Condition characterized by an abnormally low concentration of phosphate in the blood, detectable by laboratory testing at birth; it results from defective reabsorption of phosphate by the kidneys. In addition to the loss of phosphate through the kidneys, the body does not respond to dietary levels of vitamin D. Lacking these substances, bones become soft and easily deformed (RICKETS) as an affected child grows. Other symptoms, which may progress with age, include slow growth, short stature, dental abnormalities, spinal and skull deformities and joint limitations.

Exhibiting genetic HETEROGENEITY, the disorder can result from MUTATIONS in multiple GENES and several patterns of inheritance, including several X-LINKED as well as both AUTOSOMAL DOMINANT and AUTOSOMAL RECESSIVE forms have been described. The most common form is X-linked dominant, with the gene involved located on the short arm of the X CHROMOSOME. A number of different mutations have been identified.

Hypophosphatemia is estimated to occur in approximately one in 200,000 live births. It is partially responsive to early, continual treatment with oral phosphate and vitamin D supplementation.

hypoplastic congenital anemia See ANEMIA.

hypospadias Developmental defect of the urinary tract readily recognizable in the male at birth. The urethral opening, which is normally at the tip of the penis, is instead located on the underside of the penis. Also, there is a thin, deficient amount of foreskin on the upper surface of the penis. In approximately half of those affected, the penis also curves downward due to a fibrous band (chordee) that, combined with the urethral opening on the underside, forces the child to urinate in the direction of his feet rather than in the forward direction. If not corrected, chordee can cause painful erection later in life, and an inability to perform sexual intercourse and normal impregnation. Hypospadias can occur as an isolated ANOMALY or part of chromosomal or other SYNDROMES. Renal malformations are more common with more severe forms of hypospadias.

The location of the misplaced opening may be at the juncture of the head and shaft of the penis (60%); along the shaft (15%); at the point where the shaft joins the scrotum (20%); or in the perineum, the area between the scrotum and the anus (5%).

Complications of hypospadias can involve a narrowing (stenosis) of the urethral opening, disease resulting from this obstruction of the urinary tract (obstructive uropathy) and, ultimately, potential kidney failure.

Hypospadias is estimated to occur once in every 186 live births. The exact cause is unknown. It is primarily a male disorder, although a rare misplacement of the urethral opening inside the female vagina occurs about once for every 10,000 cases of male hypospadias.

Corrective surgery is almost always successful, and there is no shortening of the normal life span. Elective circumcision should not be done since the foreskin is used in the corrective surgery, which for psychological reasons is generally done prior to the age of 15 months.

It is the result of MULTIFACTORIAL inheritance in most cases. The risk of a second male being born with hypospadias has been estimated to be about 12%. This increases to 26% in those cases where the father also was born with hypospadias.

hypothyroidism, congenital See CONGENITAL HYPOTHYROIDISM.

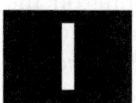

Iceland Individual members of ethnic groups and isolated populations share a genotype and exhibit common traits. These traits may include hereditary disorders that occur at incidence rates much, much higher than those seen in the general public. Iceland has long been recognized by geneticists as having a population that exemplifies these characteristics, which are invaluable in tracking the genetic roots of hereditary disorders. A nationwide commercial effort has been mounted to identify the genes for a variety of common genetically linked disorders including heart disease, diabetes, asthma and cancers. More than half of Iceland's adults donated DNA samples to the company conducting the research, DeCODE Genetics. The results will help in the development of diagnostic tests and treatments for these disorders. However, the efficacy of such treatments in the general population or whether these same genes are implicated in these disorders in populations outside of Iceland are unknown.

ichthyosis Any of several specific hereditary or CONGENITAL skin disorders. Taken from the Greek *ichthys,* for "fish," and o*sis,* for "condition," the skin of affected individuals is sometimes described as resembling that of a fish, due to its dry, scaly appearance. Ichthyosis occurs in AUTOSOMAL DOMINANT, AUTOSOMAL RECESSIVE and X-LINKED forms. Severity ranges from mild, easily treated cosmetic problems to severe, lethal conditions.

Ichthyosis vulgaris Inherited as an autosomal dominant disorder, onset occurs in infancy or later, with symptoms of mild scaling seen mainly on the extremities, particularly the palms and soles. This is the most common form of ichthyosis, accounting for 95% of all cases. Incidence is estimated at approximately 1% of the general population. A sig-

nificant proportion of those with dominant forms of ichthyosis who are under medical attention also have asthma, eczema or hayfever.

Lamellar ichthyosis Affected infants may be covered with a smooth layer of skin which is shed in two to three weeks after birth, often leaving the body covered with thick scales, which may persist or disappear spontaneously in early infancy. Inherited as an autosomal recessive trait and estimated to occur in one in 300,000 births, this form may result in death in the first months of life due to complications from severe skin lesions. However, individuals may heal completely or exhibit mild ichthyosis for the remainder of their lives. (See HARLEQUIN FETUS.) This form is most often caused by mutations in the GENE for keratinocyte transglutaminase, which has been mapped to the long arm of chromosome 14. Some other cases of the recessive form appear to result from a gene mapped to the long arm of chromosome 2. A rare dominant form has also been reported. PRENATAL DIAGNOSIS may be possible by fetal skin biopsy. HARLEQUIN FETUS, the most severe form of congenital ichthyosis, is caused by mutations in the *ABCA12* gene, which is the gene responsible for lamellar ichthyosis located on the long arm of chromosome 2.

X-linked ichthyosis As the name implies, this is an X-linked disorder seen only in males. It is similar to ichthyosis vulgaris, though it presents a more striking "fish-skin" appearance. It affects an estimated one in 6,000 males. The X-linked ichthyosis is linked to an inborn error of metabolism and is caused by deficiency of the enzyme steroid sulfatase. In about 85% of cases, this results from deletions involving a gene which is found on the short arm of the X CHROMOSOME. CARRIER females may have mild scaling but also may have low estrogen levels in pregnancy and can have a delay in the onset of labor due to failure of dilation of the cervix.

IDDM   See DIABETES MELLITUS.

imaging, fetal   See FETAL IMAGING.

immotile cilia syndrome   See KARTAGENER SYNDROME.

immune deficiency diseases   Those diseases that result in a breakdown of the immune system, the mechanism by which the body defends itself against viral and bacterial infection, parasitic disease, fungi and other microorganisms. The immune system is also responsible for allergic reactions, for rejecting transplanted organs and perhaps even for the prevention of the development of CANCER.

Immune disorders that result from defects within the immune system itself are called "primary" immunodeficiency diseases. ("Secondary" refers to disorders due to outside influences, such as AIDS.) Many primary immune deficiency diseases are genetically determined, and there is great variability in their severity and incidence. Over 70 of these disorders have been described, excluding a number of unusual variants in which only a few cases have been described.

The immune system operates by first recognizing foreign substances (antigens) and then reacting to them. A variety of different cell types and proteins are responsible for this activity. The major components of the system are B-lymphocytes, T-Lymphocytes, phagocytes, immunoglobulins and complement.

When stimulated by antigens, B-lymphocytes mature into plasma cells, which then produce antibodies, specialized serum protein molecules that attack specific antigens. The antibody proteins are called immunoglobulins or gammaglobulins. There are five major classes of these antibodies: immunoglobulins G (IgG), A (IgA), M (IgM), E (IgE) and D (IgD), each with its own special role in attacking antigens.

T-lymphocytes directly attack virus, fungi or transplanted tissue, and also act as regulators of the immune system. They develop in the bone marrow and migrate to the thymus gland, where they mature. (T stands for "Thymus.") Each T-lymphocyte reacts with a specific antigen, just as each antibody molecule does. Additionally, T-lymphocytes fall into three categories: "killer" T-lymphocytes actually destroy antigens; "helper" T-lymphocytes assist the killer T-lymphocytes and also help B-lymphocytes produce antibodies; and "suppressor" T-lymphocytes stop the activity of the helper T-lymphocytes. Without them, the immune system would continue reacting to antigens, even after an infection had been destroyed.

Phagocytes ingest and kill microorganism, and there are various types of these cells: All are either white blood cells or derived from them.

Complement is a group of serum proteins that assist in immune responses, from attracting phagocyte cells to the site of an infection, to coating microorganisms so they are more easily ingested by phagocytic cells.

A defect or deficiency in any one of these systems, or any part thereof, will result in an immune deficiency disease, making an individual more prone to infection.

Agammaglobulinemia (XLA; X-LINKED agammaglobulinemia; Bruton's agammaglobulinemia; congenital agammaglobulinemia)   This was the first identified immune deficiency disease, described by Dr. Ogden Bruton at Walter Reed Hospital in 1952.

Inherited as an X-linked recessive trait, it is caused by a deficiency or absence of immunoglobulins and results from the failure of B-lymphocytes to mature.

Affected individuals are prone to infections of the mucous membranes, such as the sinuses (sinusitis), respiratory tract (pneumonia in the lungs and bronchitis in the bronchial tubes), eyes (conjunctivitis), nose (rhinitis) and ears (otitis) and the gastrointestinal tract (gastroenteritis). Any of these infections may penetrate the mucous membrane and involve the blood stream or internal organs.

Individuals with this disorder are most prone to bacterial infection, from pneumococcus, streptococcus and staphylococcus, and to common viruses that cause diarrhea and respiratory infections such as colds and flu. In those affected, live vaccines can also cause the disease for which the vaccine is designed to protect against.

The presence of this disorder can be confirmed by testing of immunoglobulins in the blood. The levels will be abnormally low or absent in affected individuals. The test is difficult in infants under the age of six months, since they typically have low levels of these serum proteins. Other tests can establish the effectiveness of those immunoglobulins that are present.

The disease results from MUTATIONS in the Bruton tyrosine kinase (BTK) GENE, whose normal role is in the differentiation and activation of B-lymphocytes. Over 150 different mutations in the gene have been identified. Almost all are found in only a single family. Molecular techniques may be useful in individual families for CARRIER detection and PRENATAL DIAGNOSIS. A very rare form of agammaglobulinemia with AUTOSOMAL RECESSIVE inheritance also exists. This accounts for the cases of this disorder which occur in girls. Mutations in the mu heavy chain (immunoglobin) gene, found on chromosome 14, account for at least some of the cases of this autosomal recessive form.

At present, there is no cure. Treatment consists of transfusions of gammaglobulins culled from blood donations. Chronic or recurring infections may still occur, requiring laboratory identification of the specific microorganism causing the infection, in order to design a more specific antibiotic therapy.

Most affected individuals can lead relatively normal lives. Carrier females have normal levels of immunoglobulins, but there has been much recent research that may allow carrier detection in families with this disease.

Selective IgA Deficiency
This is the most common of the immunodeficiency diseases, with an incidence estimated as high as one in every 400 people. It is also one of the milder forms; there is a wide variability in expression, and many affected individuals are asymptomatic, and thus, not aware of their condition.

The disorder appears to be MULTIFACTORIAL. Some cases are familial and reports of both dominant and recessive inheritance have been published. Other cases appear to be acquired.

The most common features of this condition are recurrent or chronic infections and ALLERGIES. Immunoglobulin A (IgA) may be deficient or absent. Food allergies and asthma can occur with selective IgA deficiency. An additional complication is the development of autoimmune diseases, in which the immune system manufactures antibodies that attack the body's own tissues. Examples of associated autoimmune diseases are RHEUMATOID ARTHRITIS and systemic LUPUS erythematosus.

It is not possible to replace IgA in affected individuals. Gammaglobulin (such as administered for agammaglobulinemia) contains no IgA. Furthermore, if IgA is totally absent, introduction into the body (for example, by receiving blood transfusions) could trigger a massive allergic reaction, characterized by low blood pressure, difficulty breathing and collapse, as the immune system reacts to what it considers a foreign substance.

Long-term antibiotic therapy may be required. The prognosis is dependent on the severity of the individual case and its attendant complications, but generally the outlook is excellent.

Common variable immunodeficiency (hypogammaglobulinemia)
This disorder is characterized by frequent and unusual infections. They may first occur any time between infancy and the third or fourth decade of life. It is relatively common, caused by a variable deficiency of immunoglobulins, hence the name. There may be a deficiency in IgG by itself, or IgG and IgA, or IgG, IgA and IgM. Some patients have few or non-functioning B-lymphocytes, others lack helper T-lymphocytes, and another group has an excess of suppressor T-lymphocytes. The severity of this condition is also highly variable.

The cause is unknown, and while genetic factors appear to be involved, its inheritance pattern does not fit well-defined MENDELIAN patterns in all cases. A heterogeneous group of disorders (see HETEROGENEITY) rather than a single entity, familial clustering is seen, but the precise role of genetics is unclear. Mutations in the *TNFRSF13B* gene that encodes the transmembrane activator and CAML interactor (TACI) have been found in individuals with common variable immunodeficiency and in those with IgA deficiency.

Infections typically affect the ears, sinuses, nose bronchi and lungs. Repeated, severe infections may cause permanent damage to the bronchial tubes (bronchiectasis) or chronic lung disease. Gastro-intestinal complaints are also frequent, and may be caused by giardia lamblia, an intestinal parasite.

Infections of the joints, as well as painful joint inflammations (polyarthritis), may develop. Other autoimmune responses may also occur. For example, the body may destroy its own blood cells.

Immunoglobulin replacement can improve the condition and help control infection, though in some cases long-term treatment with a broad array of antibiotics may be required.

Severe combined immunodeficiency (SCID) This is the most serious of the primary immunodeficiency diseases. Infections begin in the first few months of life, and are typically severe and complicated. (The so-called BUBBLE BOY had this disorder.) If untreated, this disease is fatal by two years of age. Immunization with live viruses (for example, polio) can lead to serious complications and should be avoided. It occurs in about 1:100,000–1:500,000 live births.

Most cases of SCID are inherited. Both autosomal recessive and X-linked forms have been described.

The most common form in males is X-linked. It involves mutations in the gene for the gamma chain of the interleukin-2 receptor and can result from one of a number of mutations in this gene. Identification of the mutation in an affected boy can allow for carrier detection and prenatal diagnosis in his family.

There is also an ENZYME deficiency form of SCID (ADA deficiency, adenosine deaminase deficiency) that allows metabolic poisons to build up in the lymphocytes, slowly poisoning the cells. ADA deficiency was the first discovered molecular defect underlying an immunodeficiency disorder. It accounts for approximately half the cases of autosomal recessive SCID. The gene for ADA is on the long arm of chromosome 20, and about 30 different mutations in it have been found. Prenatal diagnosis is possible via CHORIONIC VILLUS SAMPLING.

Investigational treatments of this disorder include the use of PEG-ADA, a preparation of the enzyme coupled to polyethylene glycol. Injections of this drug appear to result in normalization of the enzyme level, correction of the immune defect, and recovery from infections. Long-term use is being evaluated. Trials of gene therapy for ADA

deficiency–SCID are at present under way. The normal ADA gene is placed into a virus which is used to carry the gene into the patient's immune cells (either circulating T cells or their precursor stem cells in the bone marrow). It is hoped that the transplanted gene will correct the enzyme and immune defect in those cells.

Rarer forms of SCID include purine nucleoside phosphorylase deficiency, an autosomal recessive disorder. The gene has been mapped to the long arm of chromosome 14 and isolated, and a number of mutations identified. Prenatal diagnosis in this form has been accomplished by CVS (chorionic villus sampling.)

Among the most dangerous infectious agents for those with SCID are chicken pox virus (VARICELLA), cytomegalovirus (TORCH SYNDROME), herpes simplex virus and MEASLES virus. Fungal or yeast infections are also very difficult to treat. Oral thrush (candida), a white fungus, is a common feature, as is diarrhea. The skin may become infected with the same fungus that causes oral thrush.

Tests to establish the diagnosis include lymphocyte counts in a blood smear, and tests to examine the effectiveness of those lymphocytes present. Usually, there is a decreased level of all classes of immunoglobulins.

Children with SCID typically endure repeated hospitalization and must be isolated from children outside the family. Usually they cannot be taken to public places, and contact with relatives should be limited. SIBLINGS exposed to chicken pox or other infectious agents may also present a potential source of infection. In some cases, they cannot absorb food normally, possibly requiring continuous intravenous feeding.

Gammaglobulin replacement therapy can be of some benefit. The most successful therapy is bone marrow transplantation. Bone marrow cells from a normal matched donor, once transplanted, can manufacture the immune system products missing in the SCID individual. The first such transplant was performed in 1968. The success rate after the first 100 of these operations was judged to be approximately 65%.

Without successful bone marrow transplantation, individuals are at constant risk of severe and fatal infection.

In 2007, Wisconsin began an experimental screening program to test all newborns for the presence of SCID, the first such effort in the United States. Several other states were considering instituting similar neonatal screening programs.

Chronic granulomatous disease (CGD) This form of immune deficiency is characterized by the inability of phagocytes to destroy certain microorganisms. While the phagocytic cells ("scavenger cells") can ingest the microorganisms normally, abnormal metabolism within the cell prevents them from killing the bacteria and fungi once ingested. The rest of the individual's immune system functions normally.

The infections often result in the formation of granulomas, or localized, swollen collections of infected tissue. These may block the intestine or urinary tract and require surgical treatment. The skin, lungs, lymph nodes, liver or bones are most frequently involved. Pneumonia is a recurrent problem.

CGD can be inherited as either an autosomal recessive characteristic or more commonly through X-linked recessive transmission (about 2/3 of cases). Affected males outnumber affected females by a ratio of 4:1.

The disease is usually recognized during infancy. Approximately 80% of those affected have unusually frequent or severe infections during the first year of life. Diagnosis is made by analyzing the function of phagocytic cells.

After identifying the chromosomal location of the X-linked CGD gene, this gene has been cloned and characterized. This has allowed understanding of the underlying defect in the disorder and has permitted prenatal diagnosis of the condition.

Continuous treatment with oral antibiotics is often recommended. Early treatment of infections is important. Treatment with recombinant interferon gamma significantly reduces serious infectious complications. Bone marrow transplantation has also been successfully used. Affected individuals are also generally advised to swim only in well-chlorinated pools, since organisms found in other waters may cause infections. They are also advised to refrain from smoking MARIJUANA, since the bacteria aspergillus is found in most samples and can cause lung infections in CGD patients. Dusty conditions, especially caused by spoiled or moldy grass and hay, should also be avoided. CGD occurs in an estimated one in 1 million live births.

The overall incidence of immunodeficiency (excluding IgA deficiency) is estimated to be about one in 10,000 with approximately 400 new cases annually in the United States.

Other immune deficiency disorders include DI GEORGE SYNDROME and ATAXIA-TELANGIECTASIA.

imparidigitate   Having an uneven number of digits (fingers or toes).

imperforate anus   A large group of anorectal malformations caused by a defect in the development of the tail end (terminus) of the embryo's hindgut, which forms the intestines and other organs of the lower abdomen. Conditions in this category include an external bowel opening that is (1) in the normal position but too small to function properly (anal stenosis); (2) in an unusual position (ectopic), such as the perineum or scrotum in males, the vulva, vestibule or vagina in females; or (3) not visible at all on examination. Most newborns in the two latter groups will show signs of intestinal blockage within 24 hours because the contents of their bowels at birth cannot be evacuated. Infants with anal stenosis usually develop constipation within days or weeks of birth.

About half of all cases of imperforate anus are accompanied by other abnormalities as well. The majority of associated problems are in the lower spine (lumbosacral malformations) or genitourinary system; other ANOMALIES may occur in the trachea or esophagus or in the central nervous, cardiovascular or gastrointestinal systems (see VATER ASSOCIATION). These other anomalies account for over 90% of all deaths associated with imperforate anus, which has an overall mortality rate of 10% to 30% in reported cases. It may be seen as a feature of a number of specific SYNDROMES including CAT EYE SYNDROME, FG SYNDROME, OPITZ G/BBB SYNDROME, and the TOWNES-BROCK SYNDROME as well as in association with a number of CHROMOSOME ABNORMALITIES. Prenatal exposure to THALIDOMIDE and maternal DIABETES have also been reported to cause this malformation.

Imperforate anus is seen in approximately one of every 5,000 live births, and males are 50% more likely than females to be affected (three to two ratio). Diagnosis in both sexes is usually made within days of birth. The majority of all cases are SPORADIC, but both AUTOSOMAL RECESSIVE and X-LINKED recessive inheritance have been suggested in some families with more than one affected child. Overall recurrence risk appears to be about 1%.

Treatment is usually surgical, with the immediate aim of relieving colon pressure. Enlargement of the external opening is all that is needed for correcting anal stenosis. When the external opening is in the perineum, scrotum, vulva or vestibule, however, plastic surgery to reposition the opening is required. If the external opening is in the vulva or lacking altogether, the newborn usually receives a colostomy until after the first year, when plastic surgery is performed to create an external opening in the appropriate location (anorectal reconstruction).

imperforate hymen The central portion of the hymen (which covers the vaginal opening) in this structural flaw fails to develop its normal opening. The external genitalia, vagina, cervix, uterus, fallopian tubes and ovaries are not affected. While it may be detected at birth through investigation of possible causes of accumulation of fluid in the vagina, it usually goes unnoticed until puberty when menstrual flow is blocked and accumulates. The hymen may bulge.

The incidence is believed to be as high as 0.3% in female newborns. Although it was reported that three sisters in one family were affected, heritable tendencies have not been frequently observed. The condition is not necessarily CONGENITAL; some cases may develop as the result of inflammation. It has no effect on fertility. Surgical correction is easily accomplished with no persistent problems.

imprinting (genomic imprinting) The differential expression of genetic material based on the gender of the parent from whom it was inherited. Now recognized as a phenomenon that affects the development of several GENETIC DISORDERS, imprinting constitutes a significant refinement of Mendel's laws of inheritance. It explains transmission and statistical aspects of inherited disorders that previously appeared to mock rules of genetics.

According to MENDELIAN theory, GENES inherited from each parent are equal in their influence, and will be expressed or masked depending on whether each is dominant or recessive, and on the ALLELE (the form of the gene inherited from the other parent) each is paired with. However, in some disorders the gender of the parent from whom the gene is inherited may also determine whether or not a gene will be expressed. For example, an aberrant gene inherited from the father may usually result in a specific disorder, while the same gene, inherited from the mother, will lie dormant. Imprinting is mostly associated with SYNDROMES that involve developmental abnormalities, CANCER, growth and behavior.

Among those who develop WILMS TUMOR, a childhood cancer, some individuals exhibit a deletion of material on one of their two chromosome 11s (see CHROMOSOME ABNORMALITIES). This damaged chromosome is almost always maternally inherited, that is, passed down from the mother. This suggests the maternal genes play some role in suppressing tumor development, and that loss of this suppressor function results in the development of Wilms tumor. Absence of the suppressor function is apparently not compensated for by genes on the chromosome 11 inherited from the father.

As another example, both the PRADER-WILLI SYNDROME and ANGELMAN SYNDROME, two very different disorders, are associated with deletions of the same area of the long arm of chromosome 15, q11-13. About 60% of Prader-Willi patients exhibit this deletion, and in these cases the deletion is always inherited from the father. In Angelman (happy puppet) syndrome, about 60% also exhibit a deletion of 15q11-13, but here the damaged chromosome 15 is inherited from the mother. It thus appears essential for normal development to have both maternally and paternally derived copies of at least some portions of some chromosomes.

Regardless of whether the genetic material is paternally or maternally imprinted, if an affected individual then transmits this genetic abnormality to a child, both sets of grandparental genetic material bear the imprinting of the affected parent's sex.

incontinentia pigmenti   One of a group of genetically linked neurocutaneous disorders, so named because they involve the nerves and cutaneous, or skin, tissue. Affected individuals have characteristic discolored skin, due to excessive deposits of melanin, along with abnormalities of the brain, eyes, nails and hair.

The skin begins to exhibit its characteristic discoloration of the trunk and extremities within the first two weeks of life. The discoloration appears as irregular marbled or wavy lines of gray, blue or brown. About 20% of affected children have slow motor development, mental retardation, hypotonia (low muscle tone) and seizures. Visual problems, included strabismus (crossed eyes), cataracts and severe loss of vision, are also common, as are dental abnormalities. The neurological problems may cause seizures, muscle spasms and mild paralysis. Skin discoloration typically resolves itself by adolescence or adulthood without treatment.

Mutations in the *NEMO* gene (*NF-KappaB essential modulator*) are responsible for about 85% of cases. *NF-KapaB* regulates genes controling immune and stress response and inflammatory reaction. Hypomorphic mutations of the gene are associated with anhidrotic ectodermal dysplasia with immunodeficiency. A more severe form, which osteopetrosis and lymphedema are also associated with, stops codon mutations of the gene.

Males are more severely affected than females. However, there is also an X-linked dominant form that affects mostly females and is lethal to males in utero.

index case   See PROBAND.

indifference to pain (congenital analgesis)   The first case of this rare HEREDITARY DISEASE is believed to have been reported in 1932, seen in an individual who made a living performing a human pincushion act. Though affected individuals can distinguish between feelings of sharpness and dullness, heat and cold, they do not experience feelings of pain. Otherwise, they are neurologically normal. Repeated fractures are common, with deformities often resulting. Some exhibit self-destructive behavior, such as biting the tip of the tongue. Indifference to pain is also a feature of FAMILIAL DYSAUTONOMIA. As an isolated anomaly, it is transmitted as an AUTOSOMAL RECESSIVE trait. Mutations in the *NTRK1* and *NGFB* genes account for the disorder in some families.

infantile autism   A potentially severely incapacitating and pervasive developmental disorder, characterized by unresponsive behavior and bizarre movements and speech, typically appearing during the first 30 months of life. The classic form was described by U.S. child psychiatrist Dr. Leo Kanner in 1943; he noted that in most cases behavior was abnormal from early infancy.

The effects of autism range from mild to severe. The developmental anomalies can be identified by three years of age and sometimes as young as 18 months. Clinical diagnostic criteria include quantitative impairment in social interaction, in communication, language and symbolic (imaginative) development, and a markedly restricted repertoire of activities or interests. There is slow development or lack of physical, social and learning skills, abnormal interpersonal communication and relations, immature rhythms of speech, poor comprehension of ideas and inappropriate use of words. Senses of sight, hearing, touch, pain, balance, smell and taste may also be abnormal. Individuals may exhibit inappropriate laughing or giggling, repeat phrases said by others (echolalia), have crying tantrums for no observable reason, act as though deaf, resist change in routine, engage in sustained odd play, develop inappropriate attachment to objects, indicate needs by gesture and fail to establish eye contact with others.

It is thought that in the past some affected infants, unwanted by parents, were abandoned in the wilds and later found and called "wild children" or "wolf children." One of the best documented cases was the "Wild Boy of Aveyron," a 12-year-old found wandering in the woods near Aveyron, France, in 1795. He did not speak and related poorly to humans. Modern examination of medical records of the case has led to the conclusion that he was most likely an autistic child. The case was dramatized in the film *L'Enfant Sauvage* by French director François Truffaut. A fictional portrait of an autistic adult, portrayed by Dustin Hoffman, was presented in the 1988 Academy Award–winning film *Rain Man.*

While many autistic children demonstrate skills in music, mathematics or use of spatial concepts (such as assembling jigsaw puzzles), they usually exhibit MENTAL RETARDATION. Sixty percent have IQ scores below 50; 20% score between 50 and 70; 20% score greater than 70. However, they may display a wide variability in performance on tests at different times.

Autism is believed to result from several causes, including fetal rubella infection (see TORCH SYNDROME), TUBEROUS SCLEROSIS, metabolic disorders such as PHENYLKETONURIA (untreated), CHROMOSOME ABNORMALITIES including FRAGILE X, and syndromes such as LESCH-NYHAN SYNDROME, CORNELIA DE LANGE SYNDROME, RETT SYNDROME or ANGELMAN SYNDROME. The hereditary disorders Asperger syndrome and Rett syndrome both include autism among their features. Chemical exposure in pregnancy and hereditary predisposition leading to disorders of brain development and central nervous system damage can also lead to autism. The cause of between 10% and 30% of cases may be identifiable. Contrary to earlier theories, it does not result from improper or cold, detached parenting.

Much research is being devoted to attempting to identify genes involved in autism, and genes on several chromosomes have been linked to the condition. These include genes on chromosome 2, the *GAT1* gene and *OXTR* gene on chromosome 3. The *GAT1* gene makes a protein that works with a neurotransmitter, GABA, which conveys messages between brain cells. The *OXTR* gene makes the oxytocin receptor protein that plays a role in brain development. On chromosome 7, the *FOXP2* gene is associated with speech and language development, *RELN* helps regulate how brain cells form and organize during fetal development and *WNT2* plays a role in the development of the nervous system. The *HOXA1* and *HOXB1* genes are involved in the development of the hindbrain, which exhibits abnormalities in some autistic individuals. Three GAGA receptor subunit genes, *GABRB3*, *GABRA5*, and *GABRG3*, make proteins that form the GABA receptors, and GABA (g-aminobutyric acid) is a chemical that carries messages between enver cells. Duplications of genetic material in a locus on 15q have also been suggested as playing a role in autism. As more males than females are affected, the X chromosome is also thought to have genes that could influence the development of autism.

One theory of the behavioral aspects of the disorder is that the autistic individual's brain is abnormally susceptible or vulnerable to overstimulation, and that withdrawal from the outer world is an attempt to limit stimulation. The repetitive actions they often engage in may have a calming effect on the cerebral cortex, and their abhorrence of change in routine can also be explained in this context. There is no cure, though symptoms may change or diminish over time. However, 75% function in the retarded range throughout life. Patients with autism may also have increased frequency of minor malformations.

Classic autism has been estimated to occur between two and six per 1,000 live births. However, some studies have found the prevalence of autism is increasing. In 2007, the Centers for Disease Control estimated autism affects almost one in 150 eight-year-old children in the United States. It is four times more common in males than in females, although females appear to be more severely affected and have a poorer prognosis. Recognizing the disorder as early as possible is important as intervention can have a dramatic impact on reducing symptoms and increase the affected child's ability to develop and learn new skills. (Autistic features are seen in about 20% of mentally retarded children.)

Most cases are SPORADIC. Recurrence risk is estimated overall as 3–8% in families with one affected child. In families with an autistic girl, researchers at the University of California found recurrence risk, or the possibility of a subsequent child being affected, of 14.5%; in families with an autistic boy, recurrence risk was 7%. In families with two affected infants, the figure rose to 35%. Speech delay is common in sibships (see SIBLING) containing autistic children.

There is no precise medical test for autism. Diagnosis is often made within the first two years of life, based on clinical observations and parental reports of the child's behavior. Computerized X-ray scans may reveal abnormalities in the ventricles of the brain in autistic children. The most favorable prognostic indicators are an IQ greater than 70 and speech present before the age of five years.

Treatment generally consists of special education programs, counseling and use of behavior modification and medication to control or decrease specific symptoms. In cases of autism identified as resulting from metabolic abnormalities, control of diet may be helpful in mitigating the symptoms. PRENATAL DIAGNOSIS of this disorder has not been achieved.

The prevalence of autism in adults is unknown. Autistic features continue into adulthood but outcomes vary from little speech and poor living skills to independent functioning and college graduation. Autistic adults may be labeled as being simply odd or reclusive, or may carry a psychiatric diagnosis such as obsessive compulsive, schizoid personality, SCHIZOPHRENIA or affective disorder or be labeled as mentally retarded or brain-damaged.

infantile lactic acidosis   See CONGENITAL INFANTILE LACTIC ACIDOSIS.

infantile osteopetrosis   Brittle, abnormally dense bones that fracture easily characterize this CONGENITAL condition. In fact, fractures may occur during delivery as well as throughout the child's life. Though the fractures tend to heal satisfactorily, deformities frequently develop in childhood. During the first year of life, the head becomes enlarged and square in shape with a prominent forehead. Hearing and vision grow progressively worse; ocular abnormalities may include drooping eyelids (PTOSIS), crossed eyes (strabismus) and CATARACTS. Progressive BLINDNESS and DEAFNESS result from pressure on the nerves from the encroachment of bone. Teeth may develop abnormally and are prone to decay. On X-rays, bones of the hand may have a "bone in bone" appearance, and ribs appear flared.

Other complications may include severe ANEMIA (resulting from bone encroaching on the blood-forming cells in the bone marrow) and enlargement of the spleen, liver and lymph nodes, and a predisposition to bone and marrow infection (osteomyelitis). While growth and developmental retardation are common in affected children, intelligence is usually normal.

A diagnosis of osteopetrosis can be made in the third trimester with X-rays. The basic defect of this relatively rare condition, which is inherited as an AUTOSOMAL RECESSIVE trait, appears to be heterogeneous. Some cases are caused by mutations in the *TCIRG1* subunit of the vacuolar proton pump gene. In other cases, the autosomal recessive infantile osteopetrosis can also result from a mutation in the *CLCN7* gene or from a mutation in the human equivalent of the mouse 'grey-lethal' gene (GL), also known as osteopetrosis-associated transmembrane protein-1 (OSTM1). CARRIERS cannot be detected. It occurs with unusual frequency in Costa Rica, and there and elsewhere it seems to strike offspring of blood relatives (see CONSANGUINITY). The condition occurs with equal frequency in males and females.

The prognosis for children with infantile osteopetrosis is poor. Anemia or a secondary infection often causes death in infancy or early childhood. Bone marrow transplants, however, have been successful in over 70 patients.

There is also an essentially benign AUTOSOMAL DOMINANT form of the condition. It has a later onset and has only the bony features without the other associated features. Height is normal but osteomyelitis is more common.

infantile subacute necrotizing encephalopathy of Leigh   Unusual eye movements beginning in infancy or early childhood, generally occurring in association with an infection, are usually the first signs of this rare inherited condition. Bearing the name of English neuropathologist D. Leigh, who published the first description in 1951, symptoms are variable from case to case but may include abnormal eye movements, sluggish pupils, degeneration of the optic nerve, tremors, weakness, numbness and unsteady gait. The irregular eye movements may stabilize or improve slightly when the infection clears but worsen with a second infection. In older children and adolescents the disease may be chronic and unremitting. Stress may also trigger episodes and cause periodic problems with walking. There may also be symptoms involving regulation of the heart, respiration, salivation and swallowing, and signs of cerebellar degeneration. Generally there is a progressive loss of neurologic functions, ultimately resulting in death.

Several different types of genetic metabolic defects can lead to Leigh disease. In most cases it appears to be inherited as an AUTOSOMAL RECESSIVE trait. Blood levels of lactate and pyruvate are generally elevated and in many cases biochemical defects in one of two ENZYMES, pyruvate dehydrogenase or pyruvate carboxylase, involved in the cell's energy metabolism, is found. Other deficiencies in enzymes involved in energy metabolism have also been seen. In some cases the underlying defect appears to be a MUTATION in the mitochrondrial DNA and may represent a mitochrondrial inheritance pattern. (see MITOCHONDRIAL DISEASES). The mechanism that produces the brain pathology remains unknown but may be related to the unusually high concentration of lactic acid in the body fluid and tissues (acidosis).

infertility The inability to conceive children. Worldwide, it's estimated between 2% and 7% of couples trying to conceive are unable. The National Center for Health Statistics estimated that in 1995 about 10% of the 60.2 million women of reproductive age in the United States were infertile. It may be caused by a variety of conditions in otherwise healthy men and women.

Examination of both chromosomal and DNA material indicates GENE defects and CHROMOSOME ABNORMALITIES can underlie infertility. These defects appear to have a more disruptive effect in the creation of viable germ cells in males than in females. A decade-long English study found 2.2% of men seeking services at an infertility clinic had a chromosome abnormality. A similar, though earlier study of women found 0.6% had a constitutional chromosome abnormality, while in the general population the rate was 0.4%.

A variety of treatments and assisted reproductive techniques are available though infertility clinics, including surgery to unblock reproductive organs, in vitro fertilization, egg donation and surrogacy. The use of fertility drugs, such as Clomid and Pergonal, can result in multiple embryos, which then face the potential complications associated with MULTIPLE BIRTHS.

Infertility is also a feature common to many genetic conditions that affect sexual development or differentiation. (See also KLINEFELTER SYNDROME; TURNER SYNDROME; ABORTION; ADRENOGENITAL SYNDROMES; CRYPTORCHISM; AMBIGUOUS GENITALIA.)

inguinal hernia A hernia is the protrusion of an organ through the wall of a cavity that usually contains it. In this common CONGENITAL developmental defect, a portion of the intestine protrudes through the inguinal canal, a passage in the abdominal wall (muscle, fascia and peritoneum) through which the testes descend to occupy the scrotum, causing problems in the development of reproductive organs and discomfort. Seen predominantly in males (approximately 90% of those brought to medical attention), it affects as many as one in 100 children. In males the intestine may push into the scrotal sac, blocking the testis from descending. Though it may be corrected surgically, in severe cases intestinal blockage may occur, resulting in intestinal perforation, shock and complications that may lead to death if not treated.

It is caused by the failure of an embryonic structure, the processus vaginalis, to close during fetal development. In 10% of cases the hernia is on both sides (bilateral). When on one side it is most commonly the right. Premature infants are more likely to develop an inguinal hernia than full-term babies. The condition may be diagnosed from early infancy to early childhood. Symptoms may include an accumulation of fluid (hydrocele) in the groin area, which can be felt during physical examination as a solid mass. Affected infants may exhibit signs of discomfort and distress.

Approximately half of those under medical attention for TESTICULAR FEMINIZATION SYNDROME have inguinal hernias. The cause of the developmental defect is unknown, and various modes of inheritance are suspected of being involved. Inheritance risks are complex. The observed recurrence risks in families is 30% in brothers of affected males and 27% in sisters of females. Inguinal hernias may also be seen as part of other SYNDROMES, particularly those involving connective tissue, such as MARFAN SYNDROME, EHLERS-DANLOS SYNDROME and CUTIS LAXA.

insulin-dependent diabetes mellitus, IDDM See DIABETES MELLITUS.

intestinal atresia or stenosis   Blockage (atresia) or narrowing (stenosis) of segments of the small intestine. Atresia is more common than stenosis. Characteristic sites of occurrence are the jejunum, the long segment of the small intestine leading from the stomach and duodenum, and the ileum, the long segment leading from the jejunum to the large intestine. In a small percentage of cases, atresia is found in both segments.

Symptoms of atresia—vomiting, constipation and swelling of the abdomen—are evident at birth or within the first week of life. Symptoms of stenosis—diarrhea or constipation—tend to occur later in infancy or may be delayed until childhood or even adulthood. X-ray studies can locate the specific sites.

Intestinal atresia and stenosis are always considered as secondary to other fetal disease processes. The immediate cause of both may be impairment of the blood supply to the membranous sac that contains the abdominal organs (mesentery). Associated ANOMALIES outside the gastrointestinal system are rare (<5%). Cardiovascular anomalies are the most common, occurring in 2% of cases. DOWN SYNDROME, an underlying condition in about 1/3 of infants with duodenal atresia, accompanies about 1% of nonduodenal intestinal atresias.

The incidence of the defect is between one in 330 and one in 1,500 live births. The risk of recurrence in other SIBLINGS or offspring can be high in cases in which atresia in a newborn is associated with meconium ileus, a defect characterized by thickening of the contents of the intestine (as is seen in CYSTIC FIBROSIS), which occurs in about 10% of all cases. The risk of recurrence in other forms of atresia is low. Except in cases associated with other disorders, (e.g., cystic fibrosis), affected persons have a normal life span. (See also DUODENAL ATRESIA.)

intracytoplasmic sperm injection (ICSI-assisted reproduction)   A method for fertilizing an egg as part of the in vitro fertilization (IVF) process, enabling a single sperm to be injected into the egg. It is typically used in situations where the prospective father's sperm count is low. First performed in 1992, ICSI involves micromanipulation using microscopy, extremely fine needles and pipettes. Oocytes, or eggs, retrieved by standard IVF stimulation and recovery techniques are held with a pipette, and the needles is used to inject a sperm into the egg. Fertilization occurs in 50–80% of injected eggs.

Genetic disorders are themselves a common cause of severe oligospermia (low sperm count) and azoospermia (no sperm). Where ICSI is used successfully in such cases, male offspring may have reproductive problems as adults.

intrauterine growth retardation (IUGR)   Growth retardation observable at birth. An estimated 3% to 7% of markedly small babies are classified under this broad category.

A baby born at term (the normal 40-week gestation period) and weighing under 5.5 pounds (2.5 kg) is said to be "small for gestational age," or SGA (as opposed to AGA-"appropriate for gestational age"). Among SGA infants are those with IUGR. Premature infants may or may not exhibit IUGR. Some infants, though born extremely prematurely, nonetheless have a normal weight for their gestational age (see LOW BIRTH WEIGHT; PREMATURITY).

Babies with IUGR have an increased risk during the newborn period of developing hypoglycemia (low blood sugar), hypocalcemia (low blood calcium) and polycythemia (thick blood due to a high number of red blood cells). They are also at increased risk for developing birth asphyxia due to lack of oxygen, infections and hypothermia (low body temperature). There is an increased frequency of CONGENITAL anomalies and a three- to 10-time increase in prenatal mortality. Long-term effects may include learning, behavior and neurologic problems.

Ninety percent of cases of IUGR are idiopathic, that is, the cause is unknown. However, several maternal, fetal and environmental factors are associated with the condition: Mothers who are themselves small tend to have smaller babies; first babies are generally smaller than subsequent babies; maternal nutrition can affect the infant's size at birth, as can maternal illnesses and infections. Also associated with an increased incidence of IUGR are multiple gestation, that is, carrying more than one FETUS; toxemia; abnormalities of the uterus or placenta; maternal use of drugs and especially tobacco; or living at high altitudes during pregnancy. CHROMOSOME ABNORMALITIES and various genetic SYNDROMES and DYSPLASIAS may also cause IUGR.

Some affected infants grow to normal size, while others remain below average throughout their lives. Generally, "catch up" growth, if it occurs, happens during the first year of life. In some infants, head size and, presumably, brain growth have been relatively spared.

in utero   Within the womb, or uterus.

isolated HGH deficiency   See PITUITARY DWARFISM.

isotretinoin   See ACCUTANE.

isovaleric acidemia   See SWEATY FEET SYNDROME.

Ivemark syndrome   See ASPLENIA SYNDROME.

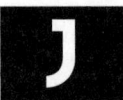

Jackson-Weiss syndrome CRANIOSYNOSTOSIS and foot abnormalities, varying from mild to severe, are the hallmarks of this HEREDITARY DISEASE. The craniosynostosis, or premature closure of the cranial sutures, results in characteristic craniofacial features: small jaw (micrognathia), flat nasal bridge and beaked nose (micrognathia); downslanting eyes, wide-set (HYPERTELORISM) with droopy lids (PTOSIS) and crossed eyes. High-arched or CLEFT PALATE is also common. A complicating factor is the often seen accumulation of excessive cerebrospinal fluid in the brain (HYDROCEPHALY). MENTAL RETARDATION and abnormalities of the digits have also been reported.

Surgery can correct craniofacial abnormalities as well as those of the hands and feet.

Jackson-Weiss syndrome is inherited as an AUTOSOMAL DOMINANT trait with incomplete PENETRANCE; that is, not all who inherit the gene for the disorder are affected by it. It is caused by a MUTATION in fibroblast growth factor receptor 2. This form of craniosynostosis is allelic (see ALLELLE) with CROUZON DISEASE, with mutations in the FGFR2 gene. More than 130 cases have been reported.

Jansen-type metaphyseal chondrodysplasia See NEURONAL CEROID LIPOFUSCINOSIS.

Jansky-Bielschowsky disease See BATTEN DISEASE.

Jarcho-Levin syndrome See SPONDYLOTHORACIC DYSPLASIA.

jaw winking syndrome (Marcus Gunn syndrome) Curious phenomenon consisting of a drooping (PTO-SIS) single eyelid which opens to a higher level than the non-drooping eyelid when the mouth opens. If the mouth is held open, the drooping recurs. If the jaw is moved to the side of the drooping lid, the ptosis increases. If the jaw is moved to the other side, the drooping decreases. Affected individuals also open their mouths whenever they look up. Its secondary designation bears the name of Scottish ophthalmologist R. Marcus Gunn (1850–1909), who described it in 1883. The drooping eyelid occurs more frequently on the left than the right, and though many variations have been observed, this phenomenon is rarely observed in both eyes (bilaterally).

This benign condition is detectable soon after birth because it is most noticeable during sucking. The basic cause is unknown. In some families it exhibits an irregular AUTOSOMAL DOMINANT inheritance pattern, but this leaves the origin of many cases unknown. The condition often grows less noticeable with age.

Jervell and Lange-Nielsen syndrome (cardioauditory syndrome; deafness and functional heart disease) Irregularities of heart rhythm, as a result of cardiac electrical conduction disturbances (which appear on electrocardiogram examinations as a prolonged QT interval), in association with profound CONGENITAL DEAFNESS, particularly at higher frequencies. It is named for Norwegian physicians A. J. Jervell and F. Lange-Nielsen, who described it in 1957.

The deafness is sensorineural, that is, involves the sensory nerves. The inner ear exhibits evidence of widespread degeneration of these nerves. While there may be some hearing of low tones, it is insufficient for normal learning of speech, and special education is necessary.

The conduction abnormalities cause heart arrhythmias that result in fainting spells. Fainting may begin in infancy or childhood and is often brought on by physical exertion or nervousness. The severity and frequency of attacks are highly variable. They range from mild spells to loss of consciousness for five to 10 minutes, with temporary disorientation following recovery. Intervals between episodes range from months or years between attacks to several a day. If this SYNDROME is not identified as the cause, the fainting may be mistaken for EPILEPSY or hysterical episodes. It has been suggested that CARRIERS of a single GENE may exhibit mild cardiac abnormalities upon electrocardiogram examination.

Transmitted as an AUTOSOMAL RECESSIVE trait, it has been estimated to have an incidence of 1.6–6 per million live births. Several genetic changes underlie this disorder. Most cases result from homozygosity (having two copies of mutant genes, one on each chromosome) for mutations in the *KVLQT1* gene found on the short arm of chromosome 11. The *KVLQT1* gene is also known as the *KCNQ1* gene and mutations in this gene account for more than 90% of individuals with Jervell and Lange-Nielsen syndrome. This gene encodes a potassium ion channel. Other mutations in this same gene, found only in a single copy in an individual (the heteroqygous state), lead to the Long QT syndrome (see entry), an autosomal dominant condition. Other cases of Jervell and Lange-Nielsen have been found to be caused by mutations in the *KCNE1* gene, found on 21q, which encodes other components of a potassium ion channel. Mutations in this gene, which is also called the *ISK* gene, account for less than 10% of individuals with Jervell and Lange-Nielsen syndrome.

Until recently, the cardiac complications caused death in half the affected individuals by the age of 15, and survival beyond the age of 21 was rare. The introduction of propranolol, a drug that controls characteristic cardiac rhythmic abnormalities, has reduced mortality from the disorder to less than 6%. In addition to use of antiarrythmic drugs, therapy in some cases has included use of an implantable automatic defibrillator.

Jeune syndrome (asphyxiating thoracic dysplasia) Rare CONGENITAL SYNDROME, named for French pediatrician M. Jeune, who described it in 1954, characterized by a narrow, immobile chest (thorax) and short arms and legs. In general, the long bones of the arms and legs are short and stubby and their ends irregular. The cartilage at the ends of hand and foot bones, the portion of the bone referred to as the epiphysis, is sometimes cone-shaped, and there may be extra fingers and toes (POLYDACTYLY). The ribs have an abnormally short and stubby appearance, and the lungs are often incompletely developed (hypoplastic).

Although this disorder is usually identified at birth by physical appearance and X-ray studies of the chest and pelvis, it may not be detected until weeks or months later when an upper respiratory infection causes acute respiratory distress. Narrowness and immobility of the thorax lead to rapid shallow breathing and cyanosis due to reduced oxygen in the blood. The condition is often rapidly fatal.

Transmitted as an AUTOSOMAL RECESSIVE trait, the basic defect that causes this disorder is unknown. It affects approximately one in 120,000 live births and occurs in two forms, one resulting in death within a few months of birth and a second, less fatal form characterized by later kidney disease. PRENATAL DIAGNOSIS may be possible via ULTRASOUND.

Jewish genetic disease Any one of several hereditary disorders that have a significantly increased prevalence among Ashkenazi Jews, those of Eastern European ancestry (as distinguished from Sephardic Jews, those from the Mediterranean area, and Oriental Jews, from Asia). More than 90% of Jews in the United States and Europe are Ashkenazim, as are 45% of Jews in Israel.

Jews have no higher rates of HEREDITARY DISEASE or aberrant genes than other ETHNIC GROUPS, but centuries of isolation within their own communities have produced distinct disorders whose GENETICS are easier to identify, thanks to the homogenous population.

For example, recent discoveries have shown that there are common MUTATIONS in the BRCA1 and BRCA2 genes that underlie familial breast and ovarian cancer among Askenazi Jews. As many as 1% of Ashkenazi Jews may have a particular BRCA1 mutation, 185de1AG, associated with BREAST CANCER, a high percentage for a GENETIC DISORDER. This mutation is thought to be present in about one in 800 non-Jews. A BRCA2 mutation, 6174delT (deletion of the letter "T" at position 6174) occurs in about 1% of Ashkenazi women. Thus, about one in 50 can have a gene predisposing them to breast or ovarian cancer. A specific mutation found in this population also predisposes it to colon cancer. The disorders include BLOOM SYNDROME; FAMILIAL DYSAUTONOMIA; GAUCHER DISEASE; MUCOLIPIDOSIS; NIEMANN-PICK DISEASE; TAY-SACHS DISEASE and TORSION DYSTONIA.

Some Ashkenazim have been reluctant to participate in or encourage study of these diseases, due to sensitivity regarding its suggestion of genetic inferiority, a charge that formed the basis for efforts to exterminate the Jews during the Holocaust.

Job syndrome (hyperimmunoglobulin E) According to the book of Job in the Bible (Job 2:7), "Satan . . . smote Job with sore boils from the sole of his foot unto his crown." Based on this description, in 1966 British Dr. S. D. Davis gave the name "Job syndrome" to a condition affecting two unrelated girls with lifelong histories of bacterial abscesses of skin (boils) and other organs, with little local inflammatory reaction. Since then, there have been several additional reports of this condition.

Other frequent sites of infection, in addition to the skin, are the middle and external ear, sinuses, gums and lungs. Most commonly, the bacterium involved in the recurrent infections is *Staphylococcus aureus.* There also may be decreased movement of white blood cells to sites of infection (defective chemotaxis). The most effective treatment is with antibiotics, though research into other therapies is under way.

Inherited as an AUTOSOMAL RECESSIVE trait, characteristics of this SYNDROME include coarse facial features, chronic eczema and elevated levels of immunoglobulin E.

Joseph disease See AZOREAN DISEASE.

Joubert syndrome A rare hereditary congenital brain malformation that causes mental retardation and lack of motor coordination. First identified by Marie Joubert in 1969, it results from the absence or underdevelopment of the cerebellar vermis, an area of the brain involved with coordination and balance. The brain stem is malformed, as well. Tremors and ataxia, irregular eye-rolling, crossing or other abnormal eye movements and periods of deep abnormal breathing during sleep may be observed. Other features can include Dandy Walker Malformation, renal cysts or retinal dystrophy.

Several variants of the disorder appear to exist. Expression is variable, ranging from mild to severe, depending on the degree of development of the cerebeller vermis. Affected individuals may also have extra fingers or toes (polydactyly), deformities of the tongue and cleft lip or palate.

Most cases of Joubert syndrome are sporadic, but autosomal recessive hereditary transmission has been seen in some families. It has been estimated that 10 affected infants are born in the United States annually. A gene involved, *AH11*, or Jouberin, was identified in 2004. Three other genes had also been identified by late 2007, but the genes involved in the majority of cases remain unknown. Prenatal diagnosis has been accomplished with ultrasound. Many affected individuals have a decreased lifespan.

Jumping Frenchmen of Maine Curious condition characterized by an exaggerated startle reflex. It was first studied by Dr. G. M. Beard in 1878, who noted a familial link (see FAMILIAL DISEASE) and reported his observations to the American Neurological Association. He found that some French-Canadian lumbermen from the Moosehead Lake region of Maine would respond abnormally to sudden sensory input. A sharp, unexpected sound or touch provoked a sometimes violent cry or movement in response (hence, the "jumping" appellation). Additionally, affected individuals would comply with quick, sudden commands, even if inappropriate. For example, if told to strike another person, they would do so without hesitation, even, according to Beard's 1880 account published in *Popular Science Monthly,* "if it was his mother and he had an axe in his hand." Often, they echoed the words of the command. If addressed quickly in a language foreign to them, some would repeat the phrase (echolalia). A tendency to blurt out whatever is being thought at the time of the stimulus has also been described.

This condition is now known to affect people of almost any nationality and geographic location. Transmitted as an AUTOSOMAL RECESSIVE characteristic, it manifests in childhood and lasts throughout life. The basic cause is unknown and there is no effective therapy.

A similar but unrelated disorder characterized by an exaggerated startle reaction has been termed *hyperexplexia* or *hyperekplexia,* and is also sometimes referred to as Kok disease after the author of a paper describing an affected family. Both AUTOSOMAL DOMINANT and autosomal recessive transmission of the characteristic have been observed. It manifests in childhood and lasts throughout life. Mutations in the gene (mapped to 5q) for the alpha-1 subunit

of the glycine receptor (a neurotransmitter receptor found in the central nervous system) appear to be responsible for both autosomal dominant and autosomal recessive forms of hyperexplexia. A mutation in the gene encoding the beta-subunit of the glycine receptor can also cause autosomal recessive hyperexplexia. Treatment with clonazepam has been effective in many patients.

Patients with hyperexplexia lack the echolalia, imitative actions and forced obedience response that are characteristic of the Jumping Frenchmen.

juvenile diabetes   See DIABETES MELLITUS.

juvenile Paget disease   See HYPERPHOSPHATASIA.

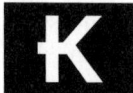

Kabuki syndrome (Kabuki makeup syndrome)
CONGENITAL MENTAL RETARDATION syndrome, first described in Japan in 1981 that takes its name from the peculiar facial appearance of affected individuals, particularly the elongated opening for the eyes between the eyelids (palpebral fissures), with the "aversion" (turning inside out) of the outer, or lateral third of the lower eyelids, which resembles the makeup of the actors of Kabuki, a traditional Japanese theatrical form.

Other facial features include a broad, depressed nasal tip, large, prominent earlobes and arched eyebrows. There is also recurrent inflammation of the middle ear in infancy. Skeletal features include dwarfing (see DWARFISM), SCOLIOSIS and a short fifth finger. Abnormalities of the vertebrae, hands and hip joints are observable in X-rays.

This rare disorder seems to be most prevalent in Japan, where it's estimated to occur in one in 32,000 newborns. Many non-Japanese patients have also been reported. The cause is unknown. Most patients identified to date have been SPORADIC with no other cases in the family, but some cases of parent-child transmission have been described. The findings to date are compatible with an AUTOSOMAL DOMINANT trait in which most affected individuals represent a new MUTATION.

Kallmann syndrome
Lack of genital development (hypogonadism) and absence of the sense of smell (anosmia) are the hallmarks of this hereditary disorder. It results from the abnormal development of the rhinencephalon, the area of the brain that controls the sense of smell. The maldevelopment interferes with communication between the hypothalamus and pituitary glands, reducing the secretion of lutenizing hormone and follicle-stimulating hormone.

Delayed puberty is the most characteristic manifestation, and anosmia is common. Males may have micropenis and CRYPTORCHISM (undescended testes). Females may have estrogen deficiency, dyspareunia (painful intercourse), osteoporosis and hot flashes. MENTAL RETARDATION and skeletal abnormalities may occur in more severe forms. Other abnormalities associated with the SYNDROME include COLOR BLINDNESS, hearing loss, CLEFT LIP or CLEFT PALATE, abnormal development of secondary sexual characteristics, and failure of the kidney(s) to develop (renal agenesis). Spastic paraplegia, a weakness and stiffness of the legs, is seen in a very rare form of the disorder.

Treatments with leutenizing hormone-releasing therapy can stimulate secondary sex characteristics, and fertility may be induced in both males and females with gonadotropin-releasing hormones. Production of sex cells can be obtained with injections of human chorionic gonadotropin in males and human menopausal gonadotropin in females.

The syndrome is inherited in AUTOSOMAL DOMINANT, AUTOSOMAL RECESSIVE and X-LINKED recessive forms. The X-linked form is believed to result from a deletion on the short arm of the X CHROMOSOME at the location of the *KALIG-1* GENE. It affects one in 10,000 males and one in 50,000 females.

Kartagener syndrome (immotile cilia syndrome)
The cilia—small hairline projections of some cells—do not move normally, or at all, in those affected by this syndrome, due to the cilia's defective structure. The consequences of the cilia's immotility on the respiratory system include thick mucoid nasal secretions, swelling of multiple nasal sinuses, recurrent respiratory infections, mouth breathing due to nasal polyps, and chronic bronchitis. These

occur during an affected child's first year in most cases. Chronic middle ear inflammation may result in some hearing loss, and coughing may become chronic.

Named for the Zurich internist who first described the SYNDROME in 1936, thick mucus blocks the sinuses, eustachian tubes and lobes of the lung, predisposing these areas to infection. Mucus collects because the cilia normally responsible for removing it from the tracheobronchial tract are impaired.

Other complications of Kartagener syndrome may include a partial or complete reversal of organ positions (situs inverses) (including a lower right, rather than left, testicle). The heart may be on the right side rather than the left (dextrocardia). Cardiac ANOMALIES may also be present, and their severity tends to be related to the degree of situs inverses. Adult males may be sterile due to immobile sperm. Semi-sterility in females has been observed.

Kartagener syndrome is inherited as an AUTOSOMAL RECESSIVE trait by about one in every 30,000 to 60,000 Americans, with incomplete PENETRANCE. Life expectancy is essentially normal, though respiratory problems, if severe, can limit rigorous physical activity. About 30% of patients undergo lung surgery. Antibiotic therapy is almost constantly required. Especially in infants, aerosols, postural drainage and decongestants are needed several times daily to assist breathing.

karyotype An individual's CHROMOSOMES, particularly when seen reproduced in a microphotograph and displayed in a standardized format, with the chromosome pairs arranged by size. The karyotype can reveal CHROMOSOME ABNORMALITIES responsible for several genetic ANOMALIES, such as DOWN SYNDROME and KLINEFELTER SYNDROME.

Kennedy disease A form of SPINAL MUSCULAR ATROPHY characterized by twitching of the muscles, progressing to muscle weakness and eventual atrophy. Onset occurs between the ages of 15 and 59 with involuntary muscular fasciculations, or twitching. Muscles of the face, trunk, arms and legs are typically affected, though they may be confined to one side of the body (unilateral). The lips, tongue, mouth, throat and vocal chords may also be affected. The muscles gradually begin to weaken and then waste. Difficulty in swallowing and speaking may ensue. The disorder may also result in impotence and INFERTILITY, as well as enlargement of the male breasts (GYNECOMASTIA).

A TRINUCLEOTIDE REPEAT DISORDER, it is inherited as an X-LINKED trait and affects only males. It is seen in about one in 50,000 births. The defective GENE has been mapped to Xq13-q22 (a region on the long arm of the X chromosome). The severity and age of onset is determined by the length of the trinucleotide repeat in the androgen receptor gene that is at the root of the disorder. The progression of the disease is generally very slow and may last many years with patients attaining old age. They may require a wheelchair, and speech may be impaired and difficult to understand.

King syndrome See MALIGNANT HYPERTHERMIA.

kinky hair disease See MENKES SYNDROME.

kleeblattschadel anomaly (cloverleaf skull) A severe form of CRANIOSYNOSTOSIS, a group of disorders characterized by premature closure of the gaps (sutures) between the skull bones, causing the skull to grow in aberrant directions. In this form, the skull bones fuse during fetal development, causing distorted growth that gives the head a cloverleaf appearance: a high, peaked forehead, with prominent bulges on both sides of the head. Those severely affected are typically stillborn or die in early infancy, while those who survive exhibit severe MENTAL RETARDATION due to central nervous system complications arising from intracranial pressure.

Generally arising sporadically, it may occur as an isolated malformation or as part of another condition (e.g., as a severe form of a craniosynostosis SYNDROME or other skeletal DYSPLASIA, such as THANATOPHORIC DWARFISM). When it is associated with thanatophoric dysplasia, it is caused by MUTATIONS in the FGFR3 (fibroblast growth factor receptor) gene, on chromosome 4p (*p* designates the short arm of the chromosome). When associated with craniosynostoses, other FGFR genes or other genes may be involved. (See also APERT SYNDROME; CARPENTER SYNDROME; CROUZON DISEASE; PFEIFFER SYNDROME).

Klinefelter syndrome   A genetic endocrine disorder that affects approximately one in 500 live-born males, characterized by the lack of normal sexual development, INFERTILITY and psychological adjustment problems. It bears the name of H. F. Klinefelter (b. 1912), a U.S. physician who observed several of the patients he first described (in 1942) while a Fellow at Harvard University under Dr. Fuller Albright, whose name is associated with several hereditary disorders.

The SYNDROME is caused by a CHROMOSOME ABNORMALITY, in which individuals have an extra X CHROMOSOME (XXY, instead of the normal XY male chromosomal complement, or KARYOTYPE). Approximately 10% of affected males have a mixture of cells with both normal and abnormal chromosome complements, a condition referred to as MOSAICISM. Klinefelter syndrome is probably the most common single cause of deficient sexual development and infertility found in humans. Affected individuals are reported to account for approximately one in 75 to one in 25 of all cases of male infertility.

The penis and scrotum are well differentiated, and the condition may remain unrecognized until puberty, at which time incomplete masculinization or development of some female characteristics, such as enlarged breasts (GYNECOMASTIA, seen in an estimated 50%) brings them to medical attention. At puberty there is decreased androgen (a male sex hormone) production. Infertility is complete. Body and pubic hair are sparse. The testes remain abnormally small. Legs are long in proportion to arms and trunk, and individuals tend to be about 2.5 inches (6.4 cm) above average height. Muscles fail to develop fully and the voice may remain high-pitched. Fat distribution about the body may give them a somewhat feminine physique. Individuals rarely develop acne.

As compared with normal males, individuals with this SYNDROME have a slightly greater incidence of physical disorders, including cardiac, hearing and dental ANOMALIES, as well as a variety of psychological problems including social maladjustment, emotional disturbances and alcoholism, and are reportedly at increased risk of incarceration. About 15% have below average intelligence. (One percent of all males with IQs of 90 or below are estimated to have Klinefelter syndrome.) Those of normal intelligence often have learning disabilities and may be passive and poorly motivated.

Life span appears normal, though breast tissue in affected men has a risk for developing CANCER 20 times greater than males in the general population.

Counseling and hormonal therapy can decrease the effects of the disorder. PRENATAL DIAGNOSIS is possible by chromosomal analysis of fetal cells gathered via AMNIOCENTESIS or CHORIONIC VILLUS SAMPLING.

Klippel-Feil sequence   Massive CONGENITAL fusion of neck vertebrae is the outstanding feature of this disorder, named for French neurologists Maurice Klippel (1858–1942), head of the department of medicine at the Hospital Tenon in Paris, and Andre Feil, his intern, who first described it in 1912. This developmental defect is associated with a variety of ANOMALIES, which can include a short neck with the child's head appearing to sit directly on the trunk, limited head movement, a very low hairline at the back of the head, low-set ears, crossed eyes, DEAFNESS, CLEFT PALATE, elevation of the shoulder blades (SPRENGEL DEFORMITY), flaring shoulder and back (trapezius) muscles, spinal deformation (SCOLIOSIS), congenital HEART DEFECTS and undeveloped kidneys.

Neurologic defects may also develop, and include involuntary muscle contractions (spasticity), brisker than normal reflex reactions (hyperreflexia) and paralysis of one side of the body (hemiplegia), of the lower portion of the body and both legs (paraplegia) or of all four extremities and the trunk (quadriplegic). Affected individuals may also exhibit an involuntary movement of one part of the body simultaneous with voluntary or reflexive movement of another part (synkinesis).

It has been estimated that this disorder occurs about once per every 35,000 individuals, with over 65% of severe cases occurring in females. The exact cause is unknown, though it has been suggested that faulty development of spinal segments along the neural tube in the embryo is a determining factor. Usually a SPORADIC occurrence, AUTOSOMAL DOMINANT inheritance with variable expression and reduced PENETRANCE has been described in some families, though this is thought to be rare. Research suggests a responsible GENE may be located on 8q (the long arm of chromosome 8). PRENATAL DIAGNOSIS may be possible in some cases by ULTRASOUND.

Klippel-Trenaunay-Weber syndrome Deformities of the limbs and digits, benign tumors composed of masses of blood vessels (HEMANGIOMAS) on and beneath the skin, swollen and twisted veins (varicosities), and enlargement (hypertrophy) of bones and tissue are the most notable characteristics of this SYNDROME.

Typically, one limb or one side of the body is predominantly affected. The deformities of the extremities, which can usually be seen at birth, include extra, missing, malformed or webbed digits, hemangiomas of the intestinal or urinary tracts, lymph tumors on the skin and general nonspecific enlargement of internal organs. Usually, but not always, the hypertrophied area has a hemangioma or other visible vascular (blood vessel) abnormality. Occasionally, abnormal communication between an artery and vein (arteriovenous fistula) is seen. In the unusual case, the vascular abnormality will most often affect another limb or, less frequently, the buttocks, lower back, flank or side of the chest.

Involvement of the head and face is rare; when it occurs, it is most frequently in the form of a PORT WINE STAIN. Facial involvement in this syndrome may be associated with MENTAL RETARDATION.

Most affected individuals have a reasonably favorable prognosis, though ulcers and chronic skin problems are not uncommon, and may impact on physical activities. Surgery may be necessary to remove a severely disproportionate digit, to amputate a limb if the vascular abnormality has been severe enough to cause clotting difficulties, or to correct an arterio-venous fistula.

The condition, first described in 1900, is named for Maurice Klippel (1858–1942), Paul Trenaunay (born 1875), who was Klippel's junior colleague in Paris when the first case was seen, and Frederick Parkes Weber (1863–1962), an eminent London physician who described numerous genetic SYNDROMES and further delineated this condition in 1907 and 1918.

In 1998, golfer Casey Martin, citing his affliction with this condition and the Americans with Disabilities Act, won a court battle over the Professional Golfers Association (PGA) for the right to ride a motorized golf cart rather than walk during tournament play, as stipulated by association rules.

The basic defect that causes Klippel-Trenaunay-Weber syndrome is unknown. It occasionally shows familial aggregation. Some cases are caused by mutations involving the *VG5Q* gene. Vascular nevi are found more frequently than expected in relatives of affected patients. PRENATAL DIAGNOSIS is possible with ULTRASOUND.

Kniest dysplasia A rare form of disproportionate DWARFISM. At birth the limbs appear disproportionately small, but the disproportion reverses as growth occurs, with the trunk appearing stunted as a result of spinal curvature (SCOLIOSIS). The long bones of the leg grow short and bowed. Characteristic facial appearance includes a flat "dish-face" countenance with a wide nasal bridge, large eyes and broad mouth. About half of the cases have CLEFT PALATE.

There may be developmental delays in walking and speech, but intelligence is usually normal. Recurrent respiratory distress in infancy is common. A swayback (lumbar lordosis) of the spine develops, as well as spinal curvature (kyphoscoliosis). The joints of the knees, elbows and hands are enlarged and prominent, and show a limited range of motion. Permanent bending of the joints (flexion contractures) occurs. Degenerative arthritis may leave affected individuals incapacitated by late childhood. Severe nearsightedness (myopia) may lead to retinal detachment. Frequent middle ear infections and loss of hearing are also common. Inherited as an AUTOSOMAL DOMINANT trait, life span is unaffected.

Most cases occur because of new MUTATIONS. This disorder in one of a spectrum of skeletal DYSPLASIAS that result from mutations in the GENE for type II collagen, COL2A1. Others include STICKLER SYNDROME, SPONDYLOEPIPYSEAL DYSPLASIA (CONGENITAL and late onset), and type II ACHONDROGENESIS.

koala bear syndrome See CHONDRODYSPLASIA PUNCTATA, rhizomelic type.

Krabbe disease (globoid cell leukodystrophy, GLD)
A rapidly progressive, fatal form of infantile LEUKODYSTROPHY. Onset is usually between the ages of three and six months, with irritability and hypersensitivity to external stimuli, feeding difficulties and sometimes stiffness of the limbs. Infants frequently cry without apparent cause. It quickly progresses to severe mental and motor deterioration, loss of muscle tone (hypotonia), seizures, BLINDNESS and DEAFNESS. There is no treatment. Death usually occurs before three years of age. (A late-onset form, which accounts for 10% of cases, develops between six and 18 months.)

The disorder was first described in 1916 by Danish neurologist K. H. Krabbe (1885–1961), who observed the condition in two SIBLINGS and noted the familial connection (see FAMILIAL DISEASE). Additionally, he described the globoid cells in the white matter of the brain that are considered the hallmark of the disorder. Globoid cells are large, irregular histiocytic (scavenger) cells that often contain multiple nuclei. The spinal fluid protein level is elevated and nerve conduction velocities reduced.

The underlying cause is a deficiency of galactocerebroside B-galactosidase, a lysosomal ENZYME that normally breaks down galactocerebroside, the main lipid component of myelin, into ceramide (a fat) and galactose (a sugar). (Myelin is the substance in the white matter that protects the axons, nerve fibers that transmit impulses in the nervous system.) As a result, galactocerebroside and its derivatives are thought to accumulate in cells of the brain, destroying the cells that produce myelin.

Inherited as an AUTOSOMAL RECESSIVE trait, overall incidence is about one in 40,000 newborns. There is a report of high frequency in Israel in an isolate of Druze, a religious group founded in Egypt in the 11th century.

Diagnosis is made either on the basis of abnormal enzyme activity consistent with the disorder, or on the finding of globoid cells in brain biopsies following death. A form of bone marrow transplantation has been shown to prevent or reverse manifestations of Krabbe disease. CARRIER detection is possible on the basis of deficient enzyme activity. PRENATAL DIAGNOSIS is possible by enzyme assay of cultured fetal cells obtained via AMNIOCENTESIS or CHORIONIC VILLUS SAMPLING.

This disorder has been reported in several mammalian species, and the "twitcher" mouse as well as a canine form are serving as models for studies of the condition.

Kuf's disease See NEURONAL CEROID LIPOFUSCINOSIS.

Kugelberg-Welander Disease See SPINAL MUSCULAR ATROPHY.

kyphosis See HUMPBACK.

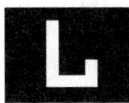

lactic acidosis (congenital infantile lactic acidosis) Lactic acid, a by-product of glucose metabolism, is an organic acid normally found in the tissues of the body. In this group of disorders, which occur in both hereditary and non-hereditary forms, lactic acid accumulates in the blood. Exact symptoms of the inherited form can vary from family to family, but may include convulsions, MENTAL RETARDATION and poor muscle tone (hypotonia), possibly leading to death. As a hereditary disorder, most forms are transmitted as an AUTOSOMAL RECESSIVE trait, but some may have other inheritance patterns, including X-LINKED and mitochondrial (see MITOCHONDRIAL DISEASES).

The accumulation of lactic acid that characterizes this rare disorder is believed to have numerous causes, including PYRUVATE CARBOXYLASE and DEHYDROGENASE DEFICIENCIES and other disorders of the mitochondria, the energy-generating organelle of the cells. Lactic acidosis can also result whenever there is poor blood supply and oxygen delivery to the tissues, as with low blood pressure or shock, and it may be seen with severe respiratory or cardiovascular disease. Lactic acidosis is also a feature of GLYCOGEN STORAGE DISEASE.

lactose intolerance The inability to digest lactose, a complex sugar found in milk, due to a deficiency of the ENZYME lactase, which triggers the breakdown of lactose into the more digestible simple sugars, glucose and galactose. Without such a breakdown, lactose is retained in the gut, resulting in bacterial fermentations and the influx of water into the intestine via osmosis.

After ingesting dairy products, individuals with this SYNDROME will experience symptoms ranging from bloating and abdominal cramps to severe diarrhea with frothy, sour-smelling stools. In milk-fed infants born with lactose intolerance, diarrhea can be followed by dehydration, malnutrition and even death if correct diagnosis is not made. Early detection by lactose loading test and, more important, by assay of intestinal enzyme through biopsy, followed by replacement of milk with a lactose-free preparation, can facilitate a normal life expectancy.

CONGENITAL lactose intolerance appears to be rare, but an adult-onset form can develop later in life, due perhaps to a gradual reduction in lactase production with aging. The late-onset form is common among most tropical and all subtropical and East Asian populations. So common is the intolerance in these groups that it is not considered a disorder so much as a variation, with both low and high intestinal lactase activities in healthy adults viewed as normal.

The exact risk of adult-onset lactose intolerance is unknown. However, more than 50% of American blacks are reported to suffer from this disorder. It is less life-threatening than the congenital form, possibly due to larger body size and less dependence on milk as a dietary element.

The GENE for intestinal lactase is on chromosome 2. However, the genetic basis and mode of inheritance of this disorder is not entirely clear. The lactase deficiencies should probably both be considered AUTOSOMAL RECESSIVE, though an AUTOSOMAL DOMINANT form of congenital lactose intolerance probably also exists.

Langer-Giedion syndrome Named for L. O. Langer and A. Giedion, who described it in 1974, this rare syndrome exhibits characteristic facial features recognizable at birth, including a bulbous nose, thin lips, sparse scalp hair, thick "tented" nostrils, large protruding ears with thickened edges, a small head (mild MICROCEPHALY) and a small lower jaw (micrognathia). During infancy, loose skin will produce excess skin folds about the neck, but this disappears as the child grows older. Other characteristics apparent as the child develops include abnormal curvature of the spine (SCOLIOSIS), thin ribs, uneven limb growth, excess joint looseness that permits an abnormal range of joint movement (HYPERMOBILITY), loss of muscle tone (hypotonia), wing-shaped shoulder blades, hearing difficulties, a fusion of two or more toes or fingers (SYNDACTYLY), abnormally short fingers with one or more permanently bent to the side (clinobrachydactyly), short stature, cone-shaped ends (epiphyses) of finger and toe bones rather than normally rounded ends, causing tapering of the digits, and many bony outgrowths on bone surfaces (multiple cartilaginous exostoses) that may require surgery. Also, many small areas of skin discoloration will be present on the upper trunk, legs, neck, scalp and face, some of which will be flat and smooth and others raised and solid (cutaneous maculopapular nevi).

Mild to moderate MENTAL RETARDATION is common to all affected individuals, with a marked delay in ability to speak. Upper respiratory tract infections are common in infancy but diminish as the child grows. The disorder shares many features with the TRICHORHINOPHALANGEAL SYNDROME.

Langer-Giedion is a CONTIGUOUS GENE SYNDROME involving deletions in the long arm of chromosome 8 (8q). The deletion involves at least two genes, EXT1 (a tumor suppressor gene) and TRPS1. Most cases are SPORADIC but AUTOSOMAL DOMINANT transmission can occur. The trichorhinophalangeal syndrome involves MUTATIONS in the TRPS1 gene alone and does not include the exostoses. Langer Giedion syndrome is often referred to as TRP syndrome, type II (see CHROMOSOME ABNORMALITIES).

Langer-Saldino type achondrogenesis See ACHONDROGENESIS.

Laron-type pituitary dwarfism See PITUITARY DWARFISM.

Larsen syndrome Named for Loren J. Larsen, chairman emeritus of the orthopedic surgery department at the Shriner's Hospital for Crippled Children in San Francisco, who first described it in 1950. This disorder is characterized by CONGENITAL joint dislocations involving the elbows, wrists, hips and knees, flat facial features with a depressed nasal bridge, wide-set eyes (HYPERTELORISM) and a prominent forehead. Abnormalities of the cervical spine, another hallmark, can have serious consequences as the vertebrae may impinge on the spinal cord. Other abnormalities include partial dislocation of the shoulders, spatulate thumbs, short hand bones, short nails, cylindrical nontapering fingers and clubfeet. Complications may involve respiratory difficulties in infancy, congenital HEART DEFECTS and CLEFT PALATE.

Both AUTOSOMAL DOMINANT and AUTOSOMAL RECESSIVE forms of this disorder have been identified. The GENE responsible for the dominant form, mapped to chromosome 3p, encodes for filamin B(FLNB). The SYNDROME may be diagnosed at birth by physical and X-ray examination. It is unusually frequent on the island of La Reunion in the Indian Ocean off the east coast of Africa. More than 40 affected children among the island's 600,000 inhabitants have been identified during the last 20 years, giving an approximate incidence of one per 1,500 births compared with a rate of one per 100,000 births in France.

Insufficient long-term data exists to provide a definitive prognosis. It appears, however, that the outlook can be relatively positive with aggressive orthopedic management.

laryngomalacia The most common CONGENITAL abnormality of the voice box (larynx), this condition makes breathing noisy and difficult for affected infants. The pyramid-shaped cartilage structures at the back of the larynx (arytenoids) and the cartilage flap that covers the entrance to the larynx (epiglottis) during swallowing are spongy and flutter excessively. An abnormal high-pitched breathing sound on inhaling (stridor) and a bluish tint of the skin due to lack of oxygen (cyanosis), especially during feeding, result. The stridor increases when the infant sleeps or cries vigorously.

The majority of affected infants worsen over the first two to three months of life and then improve near the end of the first year. Laryngomalacia can be detected one to six months after birth with direct examination of the larynx. In some patients it is caused by or accompanies a more general neurological dysfunction, and these infants may exhibit symptoms for a longer time.

To assist the infant's breathing, feeding must be frequently interrupted, and the position of least obstruction must be maintained. In severe cases, there may be a failure to gain weight, and a tracheotomy may be required.

Incidence is unknown and many milder cases do not come to medical attention or are not formally diagnosed. The cause of laryngomalacia is unknown, though it is more common in males. It is not generally considered to be genetic, though families have been reported in which AUTOSOMAL DOMINANT inheritance has been suggested. Life span and intelligence are not affected.

Laurence-Moon-Biedl syndrome   See BARDET-BEDL SYNDROME.

LCAT deficiency   See LECITHIN: CHOLESTEROL ACYL-TRANSFERASE (LCAT) DEFICIENCY.

lead   Fetal exposure to high levels of lead during pregnancy may result in stunted growth and MENTAL RETARDATION. However, the effects of exposure to low levels of lead during pregnancy are uncertain.

In the 1800s, women in the lead industry were frequently exposed to high levels of lead and frequently became sterile or had miscarriages. Currently, fetal lead poisoning is rare, though lead found in old house paint and in polluted soil or water may damage infants who ingest it. (See also TERATOGEN.)

learning disability   See MENTAL RETARDATION; DYSLEXIA; HANDICAP; EDUCATION.

Leber hereditary optic neuropathy (Leber optic atrophy)   First described by German ophthalmologist Theodore von Leber (1840–1917) in 1871, this rare hereditary disorder causes a sudden and rapidly progressive loss of central vision, the area of clearest acute vision in the eyes. The optic nerve atrophies (deteriorates), wasting away until central vision is destroyed.

It affects mostly males (85%) in their late teens to mid-20s, but has been reported in individuals from five to 65 years of age. Vision loss suddenly affects one eye and then the other. Headaches may accompany the onset of visual loss.

Leber hereditary optic neuropathy should be differentiated from LEBER'S CONGENITAL AMAUROSIS, an AUTOSOMAL RECESSIVE retinal dystrophy that presents with poor vision from birth.

This disorder is the first to be identified as resulting from a MUTATION in mitochondrial DNA, and it follows a mitochondrial inheritance pattern (see MITOCHONDRIAL DISEASES). All children of female CARRIERS are at risk, but none of the offspring of an affected is male. Prevalence is one in 50,000. PENETRANCE is estimated at 20–50% for men and 4–10% for women. Cardiac and neurologic manifestations (ataxia, peripheral neuropathy, hearing loss, a multiple sclerosis–like disorder) may occur. More than a dozen different mitochondrial MUTATIONS have been described in this disorder. Mitochondrial DNA analysis may help confirm the diagnosis in about 90% of cases. Further testing in the family is only of limited benefit, since all maternally related family members will share the mutation, but may not develop clinical features. Environmental factors (e.g., tobacco and alcohol use) may play a role in precipitating symptom onset. To date there is no treatment.

Leber's congenital amaurosis (LCA)   CONGENITAL retinal disease, named for German ophthalmologist Theodore von Leber (1840–1917), who first published a description in 1869. It causes moderate to severe BLINDNESS in infants due to a degeneration of the retina. (The term amaurosis means complete loss of vision, especially when it occurs for no apparent reason.) Signs of poor vision are usually evident in the first few months of life, although they can appear anytime during the first year and sometimes beyond that.

Infants may rub or poke at their eyes, sometimes vigorously enough to cause the eyeball to retract into the socket (enophthalmos).

Initial eye examination may disclose crossed eyes (STRABISMUS), constant and involuntary back-and-forth eye movements (pendular nystagmus), CATARACTS or an absent or minimal reaction of the pupils to stimulation by light (papillary reflex), in addition to retinal abnormalities.

Associated neurological disorders can include MENTAL RETARDATION, EPILEPSY, DEAFNESS, loss of muscle tone (muscular hypotonic) and an abnormal increase in cerebrospinal fluid (CSF), causing enlargement of the head (HYDROCEPHALY).

Two forms of the disease, which is a congenital form of RETINITIS PIGMENTOSA, are known: stationary and progressive. Those affected with the stationary form can retain fair vision. However, most common is the more severe, progressive form, which results in eventual blindness. A normal life span is possible, except in the cases where neurological disorders are severe enough to cause early death. The progressive form may often be associated with other problems such as skeletal or kidney abnormalities. For example, children with ZELLWEGER SYNDROME may exhibit this ophthalmologic abnormality. It may also occur with brain stem ANOMALIES in JOUBERT SYNDROME, with kidney anomalies in SENIOR-LOKEN SYNDROME, and with skeletal abnormalities in JEUNE SYNDROME.

The disorder is quite heterogeneous, with many different loci (probably 10 or more) involved. That is, mutations of a variety of genes all result in the same syndrome. Some patients with isolated LCA have defects in one of a number of retinal genes. These include *RETGC* (also called *GUC2D*), which maps to 17p; *RPE65,* located on 1p; and *CRX,* on 19q. These are genes that are active in photoreceptor cells. It affects both rod and cone photoreceptors. Other genes involved in different forms of this disorder include the *AIPL1* gene, which maps to 17p; the gene encoding the RPGR-interacting protein (RPGRIP1), on 14q; and the Crumbs homolog-1 (*CRB1*) gene on 1q. As an isolated defect, Leber's congenital amaurosis is inherited as an AUTOSOMAL RECESSIVE trait and occurs in approximately one in

33,000 live births. In cases where it occurs as part of a specific syndrome, it may have a different inheritance pattern.

lecithin: cholesterol acyltransferase (LCAT) deficiency (Norum disease) Deficiency believed to prevent the body from maintaining the normal balance between cholesterol and other cholesterol compounds called esters, resulting in an excess of fats in the blood (hyperlipidemia), a decrease in the red blood cell count (ANEMIA), some abnormal red blood cells (target cells) and excess protein in the urine (proteinuria). It results in progressive kidney failure. Opacity of the cornea is also seen with LCAT deficiency. All affected individuals have very low or absent levels of LCAT ENZYME in their blood plasma.

MUTATIONS in the gene for LCAT account for the symptoms of this disorder, sometimes referred to as Norum disease, after the first individual to report it in 1967. Another form of the disorder is called fish eye disease because the corneal opacities give the eyes of affected individuals the appearance of those of boiled fish. This disorder results from different mutations in the LCAT GENE (located on chromosome 16) and is inherited in an AD (AUTOSOMAL DOMINANT) manner.

The disease's progression may be prevented by frequent transfusions of plasma with normal levels of LCAT. Renal dialysis is available in the event of kidney failure.

Inherited as an AUTOSOMAL RECESSIVE trait, incidence is less than one in 100,000 people. It is probably detectable at birth by plasma enzyme determination. In a region in western Norway about one in 25 individuals may be carriers of this gene, but few cases have been seen elsewhere. In families where the mutation is known, molecular analysis should make CARRIER detection possible.

LEOPARD syndrome See MULTIPLE-LENTIGINES SYNDROME.

leprechaunism (Donahue syndrome) First described by W. L. Donahue in 1954, this rare disorder, evident at birth, is characterized by striking facial and physical features. Affected infants exhibit severe motor and MENTAL RETARDATION and progressive wasting. All have died between the ages of six months and one year.

The face has been described as "grotesque" and "elfin-like." The nasal bridge is flat, nostrils flared. The lips are thick and large, the eyes prominent and the ears low-set. Infants may have excessive facial hair (HIRSUTISM). The features are quite coarse, not cute as the leprechaun label might suggest. Excessive skin folds, lack of subcutaneous tissue and LOW BIRTH WEIGHT give infants an emaciated appearance. Breast enlargement is common in males and females, as are penile and clitoral enlargement. The hands and feet are also large. The striking physical appearance is usually sufficient for diagnosis.

Leprechaunism is inherited as an AUTOSOMAL RECESSIVE trait. The disorder is caused by a MUTATION in the insulin receptor GENE (found on 19p, the short arm of the chromosome), resulting in high insulin levels, insulin resistance and hyperglycemia. There is no effective treatment. To date, over 50 well-documented cases have been reported.

In affected families where the mutation has been found, CARRIER detection and PRENATAL DIAGNOSIS is possible and has been accomplished by molecular techniques.

Lesch-Nyhan disease SYNDROME, seen only in males, characterized by self-destructive behavior and severe motor and MENTAL RETARDATION. Unless affected individuals are physically restrained, they will engage in acts of self-mutilation, which may result in the tips of their fingers being chewed off and almost total detraction of the lips. (The lower lip is more frequently severely damaged.) However, the sensation of pain remains undiminished, and affected individuals are usually more comfortable when restrained.

At birth, infants appear normal and develop without incident for the first six to eight months of life. However, increased irritability may be noticed by three months of age. Gradually, motor control deteriorates. Infants become unable to sit or support their heads. Prominent spastic movements develop. Mental retardation is noted. Hand restraints become required to control self-destructive behavior, and sometimes selected baby (deciduous) teeth must be extracted to stop lip biting. (Lip biting decreases with age.)

The disorder was first described by M. Lesch (b. 1939) and W. L. Nyhan (b. 1926) of Johns Hopkins University in 1964. However, a pre-Incan ceramic figure excavated near Lima, Peru, is thought to display a representation of the characteristic self-mutilation of the lips and nose seen in this condition. Dr. Nyhan brought attention to this figure in a 1972 article in *Hospital Practice*.

Lesch-Nyhan syndrome is caused by the almost total absence of an ENZYME essential for the control of uric acid production, hypoxanthine guanine phosphoribosyltransferase (HGPRT). High uric acid levels can manifest as orange crystals in the diaper or as kidney stones. The HGPRT gene has been mapped to Xq26-27. Well over 50 MUTATIONS in the GENE have been described. Some cause only GOUT. This was the first condition identified in which a specific biochemical abnormality can be associated with a specific pattern of aberrant behavior.

While excessive uric acid production can be controlled with drugs, there is no decrease in self-mutilation or improvement in mental function. Death usually occurs during the teens or the 20s, primarily as a result of infection or kidney failure. Individuals with milder forms of deficiency of this enzyme exhibit elevated uric acid levels, gout, kidney stones and kidney failure.

Inherited as an X-LINKED trait, it is estimated to occur in one in 100,000 live births. CARRIER testing is available, and PRENATAL DIAGNOSIS is possible by the finding of reduced enzyme activity in fetal cells collected via AMNIOCENTESIS or CHORIONIC VILLUS SAMPLING. The possibility of gene therapy for the disorder is under investigation.

leukemia   See CANCER.

leukodystrophy Genetically determined, progressive disorders of the nervous system affecting the brain and spinal cord. The term is taken from the Greek *leuko,* for "white," referring to the white matter of the nervous system, and *dystrophy*, meaning "disordered growth."

The white matter of the nervous system contains a complex chemical substance called myelin. Composed of at least 10 lipids, complex fatty substances, the myelin forms a sheath that insulates the axon, a strand of nerve fiber that conducts nerve impulses. The nervous system contains billions of axons. The leukodystrophies destroy the myelin sheath, and sometimes the nerve cell (neuron) itself may be affected. This interferes with the conduction of electrical impulses, resulting in loss of function of the nervous system.

Each form of leukodystrophy affects one of the lipids that make up this myelin sheath, or destroys the axon itself. Most have their onset in infancy or childhood. First symptoms are often a loss of muscle tone (hypotonia), irritability, spasticity and weakness. There is a steady decline in mental function, motor activity and vision. The condition progressively worsens, impairing mental and physical abilities and resulting in death.

Bone marrow transplantation has been demonstrated to prevent or reverse the symptoms in some forms of leukodystrophy.

Most of the conditions, while affecting all populations, are quite rare. Inherited primarily as AUTOSOMAL RECESSIVE traits, some forms are X-LINKED.

For information on specific forms of leukodystrophies, see ADRENOLEUKODYSTROPHY, ALEXANDER DISEASE, CANAVAN DISEASE, KRABBE DISEASE, METACHROMATIC LEUKODYSTROPHY, PELIZAEUS-MERZBACHER SYNDROME and REFSUM DISEASE.

Li-Fraumeni syndrome   A rare autosomal dominant familial cancer syndrome that predisposes affected individuals to developing a wide variety of cancers. These cancers are noteworthy for their variety, early age of onset and potential for recurrences at multiple sites. This stands in contrast to the majority of familial cancer syndromes, which involve one or two types of tumors. Those affected are susceptible to malignancies in the breast, brain, bones, soft tissues, blood and glands. It is named for Frederick Li and Joseph Fraumeni, Jr., who identified five families with multiple tumors in 1969. Since then more than 100 families with the disorder have been identified.

The genetic basis for a significant percentage of the cases is a mutation in the tumor suppressor *TP53* gene on chromosome band 17p13, which was identified in 1990. The gene codes for a nuclear protein transcription factor are important in the DNA repair processes. Mutations of this gene in somatic cells (as opposed to germ cells or sperm and egg) are frequently seen in common cancers.

About 20–70% of families exhibiting classic LFS have detectable mutations in *TP53*, though current methods cannot identify potential anomalies in all areas of the gene. The type of mutation may affect the type of cancer that subsequently develops. Most mutations involve missense point mutations in the portion of the gene coding for the core DNA-binding domain of the protein.

An estimated two-thirds of the cases are inherited as an autosomal dominant disorder. LFS can also be caused by new (de novo) mutations in the developing embryo, or in one of the parents' germ cells.

Incidence is unknown. About five–10 cases of soft tissue sarcomas occur per 1 million children under the age of 15 years. An estimated 5–10% of these youngsters have family histories of cancers consistent with LFS or similar hereditary cancer syndromes. Estimates of gene carriers is about one in 50,000. Though individuals younger than 45 account for only 10% of cancers that occur in the general population, in families with LFS more than half the cancers affect family members below age 45. The risk of developing cancer in children who carry the gene has been estimated as 100 times that of the general population.

DNA analysis can identify mutations in the *TP53* gene. In families with members known to possess such a mutation, carrier testing is possible. Due to the inability to offer preventive treatment, some medical laboratories do not perform testing for *TP53* mutations nor report such mutations if found in minors who show no signs of tumors.

Therapy consists of standard treatment for cancers that occur. Due to improved treatment, long-term survival is high for most children diagnosed with LFS cancers, though they face the potential of developing future malignancies.

limb-girdle dystrophy   See MUSCULAR DYSTROPHY.

linkage, genetic   See GENETIC LINKAGE.

lipodystrophy, HIV   A syndrome that occurs in individuals with HIV treated with antiretroviral medications, most typically protease inhibitors. It is characterized by an accumulation of fat (lipohypertrophy) around the breasts, abdominal area and neck or the wasting of fat tissue (lipoatrophy) in the face, extremities and buttocks. Those with lipoherpertrophy may also develop a fat pad on the back of the neck referred to as a "buffalo hump." Changes in body shape may be accompanied by changes in laboratory measures of lipid levels and insulin resistance, both of which are associated with an elevated risk of heart disease and diabetes.

Various studies have reported the syndrome occurs in from 2–60% of patients who are HIV positive and in 13% of those taking protease inhibitors.

lipogranulomatosis (Farber lipogranulomatosis)   A very rare STORAGE DISEASE characterized by progressive and rapid physical and mental debilitation, resulting in death. Well under 100 cases have been diagnosed, with the majority succumbing by two years of age. (However, one patient survived to at least 17 years of age.) Its secondary eponymic designation is taken from U.S pediatrician S. Farber who first described the condition at the Mayo Clinic in 1952.

In infants, lumpy masses over the wrists and ankles (and other pressure-bearing areas) occur within the first few months of life. Signs of central nervous system disease are also evident. Other symptoms include hoarseness, noisy breathing, slowed development and chronic FAILURE TO THRIVE. Severe, painful joint swelling and restriction of movement is progressive, and there is gradual cerebral failure. Recurrent pulmonary infections are also common. In delayed-onset cases joint swelling is detected at age two or three years.

Inherited as an AUTOSOMAL RECESSIVE trait, the SYNDROME is the result of an inborn error of metabolism caused by a deficiency of the ENZYME acid ceramidase, resulting in the accumulation of the fat, ceramide. CARRIER detection is possible by enzyme assay, as is PRENATAL DIAGNOSIS using cells collected by CHORIONIC VILLUS SAMPLING or AMNIOCENTESIS.

lip pits or mounds   Small pits or openings on the exposed surface of the lips, appearing either in the angles at the juncture of the upper and lower lips (commissural lip pits) or adjacent to the midline of the lower lip (paramedian lip pits). Pits of the upper lip are very rare.

Commissural lip pits are reported to occur in approximately one in 80 to one in 500 whites, about one in 50 American blacks and approximately one in 110 Native Americans. Paramedian lip pits frequently are associated with CLEFT LIP or CLEFT PALATE, fusion of the eyelids or development of wing-like skin folds (pterygium) located behind the knees.

In 80% of affected individuals, lip pits occur as part of the VAN DER WOUDE SYNDROME, a hereditary disorder of lip pits in combination with cleft lip or palate. Van der Woude syndrome represents the most common single-gene cause of cleft lip and cleft palate. It is caused by mutations in the interferon regulatory factor-6 (*IRF6*) gene on the long arm of chromosome 1.

Lip pits are evident at birth. No treatment is prescribed for the commissural variety. Paramedian lip pits and pits of the upper lip may require surgery. Intelligence and life span are unimpaired.

Lip pits affect both sexes with equal frequency, and familial occurrences of commissural and paramedian lip pits suggest AUTOSOMAL DOMINANT transmission. Pits of the upper lip probably are of nongenetic origin.

lissencephaly   Lissencephaly means "smooth brain," and refers to the absence of gyri, or convolutions in the brain of affected individuals. It can be seen as an isolated abnormality or associated with other features in a number of SYNDROMES including Walker Warburg syndrome, MILLER-DIEKER SYNDROME being the most important. The specific GENE involved in isolated lissencephaly is the LIS-1 gene, which has undergone a point MUTATION. Diagnosis is made by CT, MRI or ULTRASOUND, demonstrating the smooth thin cerebral cortex.

Little's disease   See CEREBRAL PALSY.

live birth   A birth in which the infant exhibits signs of life, such as heartbeat, respiration or movement of voluntary muscle. In some countries, infants who die within 24 hours of delivery are not considered to be live births, a distinction that may have considerable impact on birth and neonatal mortality statistics.

localized absence of skin (aplasia cutis congenita)   Individuals with this rare disorder are born with skinless patches, usually limited to areas of the scalp. These patches have the appearance of ulcers, sometimes covered by a thin membrane. Usually, the affected area develops a scab that heals itself within a few weeks, leaving only a fine, depressed hairless scar. If the defective patch is large, skin grafts may be necessary. Such incomplete development of an organ, in this case the skin, is referred to as aplasia.

In more severe forms of this disorder (‹20%), the underlying skull, the covering of the brain (meninges) and brain may be included in the defect, and the trunk and limbs, particularly the lower legs, may be affected. In extremely rare cases, the SYNDROME is associated with CLEFT LIP or CLEFT PALATE, extra fingers or toes (POLYDACTYLY), eye abnormalities, tumors of the blood vessels (HEMANGIOMAS), SPINA BIFIDA, MENTAL RETARDATION, congenital HEART DEFECTS and CHROMOSOME ABNORMALITIES.

A very severe form of this disorder is associated with a form of lethal junctional epidermolysis bullosa and pyloric stenosis and can be caused by mutations in the integrin-beta-4 gene (*ITGB4*) or the integrin-alpha-6 gene (*ITGA6*).

A few hundred cases have been reported. Most occur sporadically. It can be seen in 50% of those affected with trisomy 13 (see PATAU SYNDROME) and 10% of those with 4p-.

Prognosis is favorable, except in those few cases with associated complications.

locus; loci (pl.)   In GENETICS, the location on a CHROMOSOME where a given GENE or other genetic material is found, or, as in the case of deletions, missing. The general locus of an abnormality is defined as being on either the long arm or the short arm of a chromosome, a position determined with reference to the centromere, the off-center point at which the two chromosomes of a pair join. The letter *q* designates a position on the long arm, the letter *p* (which stands for "petite") on the short arm. Thus, 13q designates a position on the long arm of chromosome 13. A number describing a band or region may be appended to the general location to define a specific point on the chromosome. For example, 13q14 describes the locus of the gene whose mutation results in retinoblastoma. However, one must be familiar with the banding and sequence of a particular chromosome to know where this places the locus on a given arm of a chromosome.

Lou Gehrig's disease   See AMYOTROPHIC LATERAL SCLEROSIS.

Louis-Bar syndrome   See ATAXIA-TELANGIECTASIA.

low birth weight   Weight of 2,500 grams, or 5.5 pounds or less, at birth. Approximately 5.7% of white and 13% of non-white liveborn infants in the United States are low birth weight, as are more than two-thirds of the 45,000 infants who die each year in the United States (see Table XIV). Low birth weight babies have at least five times the mortality rate of babies weighing 6.5 to 9.5 pounds, considered normal birth weight. Low birth weight infants are also more likely to suffer from long-term developmental disabilities than infants of normal weight.

Low birth weight is usually associated with PREMATURITY (birth before the 37th week of pregnancy; normal gestation is 40 weeks) but it can also be seen in full-term infants who exhibit fetal growth retardation. (All infants, whether born prematurely or at full term, can be classified as either "small for gestational age" [SGA] or "appropriate for gestational age," [AGA].) Lack of adequate development of their organ systems leaves low birth weight infants vulnerable to a host of health problems.

TABLE XIV

NUMBER AND PERCENTAGE OF LOW BIRTH WEIGHT BIRTHS BY STATE, U.S., 1994

State	Number	Rate %	Rank
Alabama	5,504	9.0	47
Alaska	588	5.5	6
Arizona	4,797	6.8	20
Arkansas	2,833	8.2	40
California	34,937	6.2	14
Colorado	4,617	8.5	42
Connecticut	3,146	6.9	22
Delaware	770	7.4	27
District of Columbia	1,403	14.2	51
Florida	14,753	7.7	36
Georgia	9,557	8.6	43
Hawaii	1,369	7.2	25
Idaho	958	5.5	5
Illinois	14,931	7.9	39
Indiana	5,638	6.8	21
Iowa	2,172	5.9	10
Kansas	2,417	6.5	19
Kentucky	4,056	7.7	36
Louisiana	6,521	9.6	49
Maine	822	5.7	8
Maryland	6,260	8.5	41
Massachusetts	5,332	6.4	17
Michigan	10,708	7.8	38
Minnesota	3,634	5.7	7
Mississippi	4,133	9.9	50
Missouri	5,569	7.6	33
Montana	691	6.2	15
Nebraska	1,416	6.1	13
Nevada	1,808	7.6	32
New Hampshire	772	5.1	1
New Jersey	8,900	7.6	34
New Mexico	2,018	7.3	26
New York	21,086	7.6	35
North Carolina	8,784	8.7	44
North Dakota	465	5.4	4
Ohio	11,622	7.5	29
Oklahoma	3,206	7.0	24
Oregon	2,214	5.3	3
Pennsylvania	11,630	7.4	28
Rhode Island	864	6.5	18
South Carolina	4,761	9.2	48
South Dakota	615	5.9	9
Tennessee	6,444	8.8	46
Texas	22,486	7.0	23
Utah	2,248	5.9	11
Vermont	439	6.0	12
Virginia	7,124	7.5	31
Washington	4,080	5.3	2
West Virginia	1,596	7.5	30
Wisconsin	4,349	6.4	16
Wyoming	564	8.8	45
United States	287,607	7.3	

Low birth weight is defined as less than 2500 grams (5 1/2 pounds)
Note: Rankings are based on more than one decimal place. A ranking of "1" represents the "best" rate.
Source: National Center for Health Statistics
Prepared by March of Dimes, 1996

There are different problems associated with premature infants when compared to SGA ones.

RESPIRATORY DISTRESS SYNDROME, an insufficiency of lung function, is one of the most common and acute problems associated with prematurity, accounting for 25,000 deaths a year in the United States.

Low body temperature causes additional problems. Instead of using energy from food for growth, low birth weight infants use it to maintain body warmth. Hypoglycemia, low levels of sugar in the blood, is frequently seen in these infants, and if untreated can lead to MENTAL RETARDATION and severe brain damage. Jaundice of the newborn is also common. RETINOPATHY OF PREMATURITY (ROP) may result in BLINDNESS.

Certain maternal factors are associated with increased incidence of low birth weight. Teenage mothers are more likely to have low birth weight infants. Twenty-five percent are born to teenagers, with the risk for a low birth weight infant greatest for those under 16. Women who have previously given birth to low birth weight infants are also at increased risk, as are those who will give birth to TWINS or any MULTIPLE BIRTH.

Maternal health can also have a profound impact on birth weight. Maternal GENETIC DISORDERS, DIABETES MELLITUS, high blood pressure, kidney and respiratory problems, have all been associated with low birth weight infants. Poor maternal nutrition also has been shown to have a potential negative impact on the infant's size at birth. Folic acid deficiency, which results from an insufficient amount of meats and leafy vegetables in the diet, can lead to megaloblastic ANEMIA of pregnancy, and may cause miscarriage.

Alcohol, CIGARETTES and drugs also appear to contribute to a birth weight that is considerably below that of infants in comparable groups who are not exposed to these substances (see TERATOGENS).

Since the mid-1980s, the proportion of low birth weight babies has been slowly but steadily increasing in the United States, from just under 7% in 1984 to 7.4% in 1996. Infants born at what is termed very low birth weight (VLBW), under 1,500 grams or 3 pounds, four ounces, accounted for 1.4% of births in 1996. Very low birth weight infants have at least 90 times the mortality rate of babies with normal birth weights.

Lowe syndrome / Named for U.S. pediatrician Charles U. Lowe, senior member of a group that in 1952 described three male children with the condition, a very rare disorder also called "oculo-cere-bro-renal syndrome," due to the three major organ systems involved: eye, brain and kidney.

Inherited as an X-LINKED trait, it appears almost exclusively in males, though a very small number of affected females have been reported. This may be due to a second mode of inheritance or a coincident CHROMOSOME ABNORMALITY, or may be like the situation for other X-linked disorders where females show a wide spectrum of variability of involvement. It occurs in all races, though most reported cases have been of white or Asian ancestry. The incidence is unknown, with estimates on the number of affected individuals worldwide ranging between a few hundred and a few thousand. By the mid-1980s, at least 150 cases had been reported in the medical literature.

At birth, affected individuals tend to have high, prominent foreheads, sparse hair and protruding ears. Undescended testicles are common. They often have a high palate and small mouth, which may result in extensive dental problems.

The ocular abnormalities include CATARACTS, glaucoma, corneal degeneration and crossed eyes (STRABISMUS). Any one of these may cause significant visual disability. Cataracts, a clouding of the lens, are present at birth or may appear in the neonatal period. Unless surgically treated soon after birth, the infant will not have the visual stimulation necessary to fully develop useful vision. Glau-

coma develops in about half of affected individuals, causing pressure within the eye to increase to the point that it damages the optic nerve, and may lead to total BLINDNESS. Scar tissue (keloid) may form on the cornea, the clear covering on the front of the eye, often causing progressive blindness.

Abnormalities in the central nervous system associated with this disorder include MENTAL RETARDATION, typically in the mild to moderate range, with some individuals exhibiting severe retardation. Some have seizures and serious behavioral problems, such as intense temper tantrums, hyperactivity and mild self-abuse. These abnormalities may be the result of abnormal brain development during fetal life.

Poor muscle tone (hypotonia) is another feature in most affected infants, resulting in a FLOPPY INFANT appearance. Poor head control and sucking reflex may cause feeding problems in infancy. Typically, motor development is significantly delayed.

Kidney abnormalities may not be present at birth, but are usually apparent by one year of age. The kidney is unable to reabsorb phosphate, potassium, AMINO ACIDS and other important substances from the blood, leading to a "wasting" of these substances. This can create serious metabolic problems.

Soft or broken bones and RICKETS are another common finding. Almost all affected individuals exhibit short stature and are prone to respiratory infections and constipation due to poor muscle tone. Joint swelling and arthritis may develop during teenage years.

The basic genetic defect involves MUTATIONS in the GENE which codes for production of inositol-polyphosphate-5-phosphatase. The symptoms arise out of the absence of this ENZYME. The gene has been localized to Xq25-26 (a region on the long arm of the X CHROMOSOME).

Diagnosis is made on the basis of the presence of the disorder's characteristic features. Female CARRIERS may have cataracts, which may aid in GENETIC COUNSELING. DNA probes are available for carrier detection and PRENATAL DIAGNOSIS. The main cause of death in infancy is chronic renal insufficiency. Deaths at all ages have been reported from kidney failure, dehydration and pneumonia. With no complications, affected individuals live into their 20s and 30s.

lung cancer   See CANCER.

lupus (lupus erythematosus, LE; discoid lupus erythematosus; systemic lupus erythematosus, SLE)   A widespread disorder that can affect either the skin (discoid lupus erythematosus) or multiple internal organ systems (systemic lupus erythematosus, SLE). Its prevalence (it is more common than MULTIPLE SCLEROSIS, MUSCULAR DYSTROPHY, leukemia and CYSTIC FIBROSIS) and the difficulty of diagnosing the more serious internal form due to the extreme variability of symptoms, make it a major health problem. While found in all races and ETHNIC GROUPS, it primarily affects women of childbearing years, though it can appear at any age.

Lupus is an autoimmune disease, that is, a disorder in which the immune system attacks the body's own tissue (see IMMUNE DEFICIENCY DISEASE). The exact cause is unknown, though it is thought to result from a combination of genetic, infectious (including viral), environmental, immunologic and hormonal factors. The pathogenesis of lupus is complex, resulting from both MULTIFACTORIAL and POLYGENIC influences. Genetic factors appear important as indicated by TWIN studies that show 60% CONCORDANCE in identical twins and the fact that familial aggregation of the disorder has been clearly demonstrated (see FAMILIAL DISEASE). Many relatives of affected individuals have abnormal proteins in their blood, though they may not have symptoms of the disorder.

Studies have found a 3%–12.8% incidence of SLE among first-degree relatives (parents, SIBLINGS, children) of patients with this disorder. In addition, there is accumulating evidence that specific HLA types (HLA-DR2 or -DR3; see HUMAN LEUKOCYTE ANTIGEN) are more common in patients with SLE than in the general population. The association with particular HLA types may be secondary, and the primary association may be with homozygosity for certain ALLELES (null alleles) of the complement GENES that lead to complement deficiency. The incidence is higher among American blacks than among American whites (three to four times higher), and certain North American Indian tribes (Sioux, Crow, Arapahoe) have an even greater predisposition. The female hormone estrogen may also play a role, as indicated by the preponderance of pre-menopausal female cases. (Ten percent of the cases are caused by adverse reactions to drugs.)

The first record of this disorder was probably made by Hippocrates in the fourth century B.C.; he described a disease characterized by the erosion and scarring of facial skin. Many centuries later the condition was given the name lupus, Latin for "wolf." There is disagreement over whether the name derives from the resemblance of the facial lesions to the bite of a wolf, or because the characteristic butterfly-patterned red rash across the bridge of the nose and cheeks resembles the markings on the face of a wolf. The word *erythematosus* (from the Greek word *erythema*, meaning "redness" or "flush") was added in the 1840s to distinguish this condition from other skin disorders. (At the time, physicians confused the condition with a form of tuberculosis, due to the rash's resemblance to tubercular lesions.) At the turn of the century, Canadian physician Sir William Osler added the word *systemic* to distinguish the form that involves internal organs from the form confined to the skin.

Ninety percent of patients are women, with half developing symptoms between the ages of 15 and 30. Lupus is estimated to occur in one in 400 to one in 500 women, affecting between 500,000 and 1 million Americans. Over 50,000 new cases are diagnosed, and 6,000 deaths are attributed to the disorder annually in the United States. Some suspect the disorder is even more prevalent, with many mild cases never coming to the attention of the medical community.

The symptoms can appear in any part of the body, though the most commonly involved areas are the skin, joints, blood, heart, lungs and kidneys.

Discoid LE   This mild form is generally confined to the skin and is characterized by a disc-shaped or butterfly-patterned rash that appears on the face. Raised, scaly red areas may also occur on the scalp, ears, chest and arms. Only about 2% to 5% of affected individuals exhibit internal symptoms of lupus, as well, though as many as 50% experience joint ache and fatigue. Seventy percent of patients with the disorder are women, with symptoms usually appearing between the ages of 20 and 40. Discoid lupus is diagnosed relatively easily by the characteristic skin rash.

Discoid lupus can be treated with corticosteroids, natural or synthetic hormones, that can suppress inflammation. Antimalarial drugs may be prescribed for cases that don't respond to corticosteroids.

Systemic lupus erythematosus (SLE) The baffling nature of this disorder has much to do with the extreme variability of expression. No two individuals display the same symptoms, and the symptoms often mimic other disorders, including RHEUMATOID ARTHRITIS, dementia, stroke, psychosis, EPILEPSY, kidney disease, ALLERGY and hypochondria. Its severity is also highly variable, ranging from mild to life-threatening. The writer Flannery O'Connor succumbed to complications of SLE, and four weeks before her death wrote: "The wolf, I'm afraid, is inside tearing up the place. I've been in the hospital 50 days already this year."

The facial lesion that characterizes the discoid form is observed in only 5% of newly diagnosed SLE patients. It may begin, like rheumatoid arthritis, with swelling of joints of the hands, feet, ankles or wrists. (Lupus is classified as a chronic inflammatory rheumatic disease of the connective tissue, in the same family as rheumatoid arthritis.) Additional symptoms may include fever, skin rashes, chest pain, extreme fatigue, loss of appetite, weight loss, sores in the mouth or vagina, increased susceptibility to infection and hair loss. Some affected individuals display RAYNAUD DISEASE, painfully cold fingers and toes caused by spasms of the small blood vessels resulting from cold or intense emotions. Sjorgren's syndrome, a dryness of the mucous membranes throughout the body, is exhibited in some cases.

The disease may begin in any of several organ systems and spread to others. The membranes surrounding the heart, lungs or abdominal organs may become inflamed. The gastrointestinal tract may be involved. In the cardiovascular system, SLE may mimic rheumatic heart disease or an arterial clot. Nerve damage may affect sensations and movement. Brain involvement may be misdiagnosed as a mental disturbance. In severe cases it may attack the kidneys, and cause kidney failure, a common cause of death among those who succumb to the disorder.

The diagnosis is based on medical history, physical examination and laboratory tests. The most reliable test involves screening for high levels of proteins called antinuclear antibodies (ANA) in the blood, which may indicate a problem in the immune system. However, due to the variability of symptoms, individuals suspected of having the disorder may be required to undergo a wide variety of diagnostic procedures.

While there is no cure, many symptoms can be treated and managed with corticosteroids and antimalarial drugs, in addition to aspirin, nonsteroidal anti-inflammatory and immunosuppresive drugs.

Though it is a lifelong condition, the symptoms appear and disappear unpredictably. Some individuals have no recurrence after the initial symptoms disappear. During periods of remission, flare-ups of symptoms can be triggered by insufficient rest, overwork, stress, irregular living habits and discontinuance of medication prescribed to control symptoms. About 40% of affected individuals are sensitive to ultraviolet radiation and must protect themselves from exposure to sunlight. Allergy-producing substances in hair colorings and cosmetics may also trigger reactions. In the mid-1970s, 80% of patients did not survive five years after diagnosis. Now, due to improved therapy, 80% to 95% of affected individuals live at least 10 years after diagnosis.

Currently there is no method of PRENATAL DIAGNOSIS. Many affected women who become pregnant will not experience any complications due to the disorder, though a slight worsening of their condition may occur. However, these women face an above-average risk of spontaneous ABORTIONS and STILLBIRTHS. This may be due to the presence of lupus anticoagulant, an acquired inhibitor of blood coagulation that circulates in the blood of patients with SLE. (See ANTIPHOSPHOLIPID SYNDROME.) This is not associated with bleeding but paradoxically with excessive clotting. The presence of the anticoagulant is associated with pregnancy loss.

In addition, the offspring of mothers with SLE are at risk for developing CONGENITAL heart block, a potentially life-threatening disturbance of cardiac rhythm. In this condition, the conduction of the electrical stimulus to cardiac contraction is delayed. So striking is the association between SLE and congenital heart block that it is recommended that all infants born to mothers with SLE be evaluated for heart block, and conversely that mothers of all infants with heart block, should be evaluated for evidence of lupus. Similarly, investigation for lupus anticoagulant has become a part of the evaluation of all couples with recurrent pregnancy loss.

lupus erythematosus, LE   See LUPUS.

Lyme disease   Though named for the town of Lyme, Connecticut, where it was first recognized by a team of Yale University medical researchers in 1975, this tick-borne bacterial infection occurs in many parts of the world. Symptoms include red, ring-like rashes, arthritis-like joint pain and swelling, and flu-like episodes. Untreated, it may damage the heart, brain, central nervous system and liver.

Individual case reports have been published suggesting that Lyme disease contracted during pregnancy can cause spontaneous ABORTION, congenital HEART DEFECTS, BLINDNESS and delayed develop-

ment. Additionally, at least two infants have been born with Lyme disease, apparently contracted from the mother IN UTERO. However, prospective controlled studies have failed to find evidence that intrauterine exposure to the Lyme disease bacterium causes CONGENITAL ANOMALIES or fetal death. Transmission from mother to FETUS does occur but is uncommon.

While a dearth of data prevents definitive conclusions about the potential teratogenic nature of the disease, pediatricians with experience with the infection recommend that pregnant women who develop any signs of Lyme disease seek immediate medical attention. It is possible for pregnant women to prevent tick bites in order to prevent infection (especially in areas where Lyme disease is common) by avoiding heavily wooded areas when possible or by wearing protective clothing. Lyme disease in the pregnant woman appears to pose "minimal risks" to the fetus if the mother is appropriately treated with antibiotics.

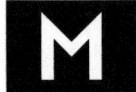

McArdle disease   See GLYCOGEN STORAGE DISEASE.

McCune-Albright syndrome   SYNDROME of skin and skeletal abnormalities first described in 1936 and 1937 by Donovan James McCune (1902–76), a pediatrician at Columbia University in New York, and Fuller Albright (1900–69), an endocrinologist at the Massachusetts General Hospital (Albright's name is attached to several skeletal disorders).

Irregularly shaped, coffee-colored splotches (café-au-lait spots) are observed on the forehead, neck, back and buttocks. Skeletal lesions are found throughout the long bones, especially the lower limbs, replacing bone tissue with sharp, gritty, glass-like splinters (fibrous DYSPLASIA). These result in pain, leg fractures, a limping, waddling gait, leg length discrepancies and a characteristic bowing or "hockey-stick" deformity. Bowing of the legs may appear as early as the first year of age, and nearly always prior to age 10. Multiple fractures may result in partial or complete disability. Rib fractures predispose some patients to pneumonia. Bony lesions of the skull and facial skeleton can cause bone overgrowth of facial passages, and may result in BLINDNESS or DEAFNESS. There may be protrusion of an eye associated with visual disturbances and enlarged distorted jaw and facial asymmetry in approximately 25% of the cases.

Accelerated skeletal growth in childhood produces adults of short stature. PRECOCIOUS PUBERTY is common in females, less frequent in males. Onset of menstruation (menarche) may occur as early as three months of age, but more often between one and five years. Development of breasts and secondary sexual characteristics follows, appearing between five and 10 years of age. Overactive thyroid glands are seen in 20% of these cases.

Reported cases have been SPORADIC and may be detected at birth by the characteristic pigmented skin blotches, or later by sexual prococity or bone deformities. Few convincing instances of familial occurrence have been reported.

The syndrome is caused by MOSAICISM for a MUTATION in the *GNAS1* GENE, which codes for the alpha sub unit of the stimulatory G-protein of adenyl cyclase. The new mutation arises not in the sperm, egg or fertilized egg, but in an embryonic cell that leads to a sub-population of cells in the body that has this mutation in it. The mutation leads to an overactive cyclic AMP pathway that stimulates the growth and function of certain tissues in the body, including bone forming cells (osteoblasts), the gonads, melanocytes (pigment cells of the skin), and certain pituitary gland cells.

The gene maps to 20q (the long arm of chromosome 20). Mutations in this gene have been found to lead to pituitary tumors, and other mutations in this gene cause ALBRIGHT HEREDITARY OSTEODYSTROPHY (pseudohypoparathyroidism), a distinct entity that should not be confused with McCune-Albright syndrome.

Hundreds of cases have been described. Life span may be normal except where there is extensive bone degradation. Bone deformities are treated by orthopedic surgery. The drug medroxyprogesterone is used to control sexual precocity.

Machado-Joseph disease   See AZOREAN DISEASE.

McKusick-type metaphyseal chondrodysplasia   See METAPHYSEAL CHONDRODYSPLASIA.

macroglossia An abnormally large tongue. It is associated with numerous CONGENITAL disorders and hereditary SYNDROMES, including DOWN SYNDROME, APERT SYNDROME, hypothyroidism, GREIG HYPERTELORISM, AMYLOIDOSIS, type 2 glycogen STORAGE DISEASE, STURGE-WEBER SYNDROME, HURLER SYNDROME and BECKWITH-WIEDEMANN SYNDROME. Macroglossia can interfere with feeding in infants and cause speech disorders as children mature, and may also result in improper dental development. Congenital cases may resolve as the infant grows, or the tongue may be reduced with surgery.

madarosis A very rare CONGENITAL condition characterized by underdeveloped eyelashes. Typically, those completely lacking eyelashes are also missing eyebrows and scalp hair. (Absence of eyelashes can also be seen in ECTODERMAL DYSPLASIAS.)

The cause of this disorder, which involves incomplete formation of hair follicles, observable with a microscope, has not yet been determined. The pattern of inheritance is uncertain, though in a few families it appears to be an AUTOSOMAL DOMINANT trait.

Madelung deformity A CONGENITAL deformity of the wrist resulting in pain and limited motion of the wrist and elbow. It is named for German physician Otto W. Madelung (1846–1926) who described it in 1878. Females are more frequently affected than males by a ratio of four to one. Inherited as an AUTOSOMAL DOMINANT trait, it is caused by the overgrowth of the ulna, one of the two bones of the forearm. Madelung deformity is also seen in individuals with the autosomal dominant disorder DYSCHONDROSTEOSIS. It can also occur due to trauma or infection, causing dislocation of the bones in the forearm.

Expression of dyschondrosteosis, or Leri-Weill syndrome, is not only more common but also appears to be more severe in females. The GENE for dyschondrosteosis, discovered in 1998, is called SHOX and is a so-called homeobox developmental gene. It is highly expressed in bone-forming cells. MUTATIONS in this gene have been known to be involved in growth retardation and short stature. The gene

is not located on an autosome, but on both the X CHROMOSOME and Y CHROMOSOME in what has been termed the pseudoautosomal region. It is called this because this portion of the X chromosome acts just like an autosome since the gene is located on both the X and Y (thus everyone has two copies, not just females) and this region on the X is not inactivated. (See MOSAICISM entry for a discussion of X inactivation.) Individuals possessing two copies of the gene, that is, HOMOZYGOTES for this gene, have a disorder named Mesomelic DWARFISM, Langer type.

major histocompatibility complex See HUMAN LEUKOCYTE ANTIGEN.

male pattern baldness Though not a disease or disorder, affected males have often sought a cure for this condition, characterized by the gradual loss of hair on the head. Severe early baldness is believed to be inherited as an AUTOSOMAL DOMINANT trait with expression only in males. However, women may also be affected if they inherit two copies of the GENE, that is, if they are HOMOZYGOTES for the baldness gene. However, the cause is likely more complex than a single autosomal dominant gene; genetic studies suggest it is likely caused by the action of multiple genes working together. A recent study demonstrated that genetic variation in the X-linked androgen receptor gene is a major component, but this does not explain the pattern resemblance of sons to their fathers as this gene is inherited from the mother.

Male pattern baldness is said to affect at least 50% of white men and 25% of white women. Blacks are less frequently affected, and baldness is relatively rare among Native Americans and Asians. In 15% of affected white men, the condition progresses until only a fringe of scalp hair remains. Women are rarely as severely affected, and the condition's appearance is usually different than that in men.

That baldness tends to run in families has been noted since the time of the Greeks, a link noted by Hippocrates (ca. 460–377 B.C.), the father of medicine. Specific patterns of balding can often be seen through successive generations, suggesting the operation of a single major GENE. The descendants of President John Adams are a well-known example among geneticists of an inherited pattern of baldness.

Treatment has traditionally consisted of the use of hairpieces and wigs to cover the bald areas. More recently, hair transplants and treatment with the drugs minoxidil and Propecia have helped alleviate the condition in some men. Minoxidil is a drug developed for the treatment of high blood pressure. Excessive hair growth (hypertrichosis) was noted as a side effect. This "side effect" has been capitalized upon and now the drug is more often prescribed for this than for its primary use. (See also ALOPECIA.)

malformation   See ANOMALY.

malignant hyperthermia, MH (hyperthermia of anesthesia; King syndrome)   Disorder that can cause death during or soon after surgery due to an at-risk individual's reaction to any of several commonly used general anesthetics. The administration of an anesthesia triggers a chain reaction in those affected beginning with increased metabolic rate and muscle rigidity. The body temperature may be elevated as high as, reportedly, 110 degrees Fahrenheit or more (hyperthermia). Death results from cardiac arrest, brain damage, renal shutdown or internal hemorrhaging. Those who survive an episode may exhibit impaired function of the brain, kidneys or other major organs.

The disorder was first described by Drs. Michael Denborough and Roger Lovell in 1960 in Australia. At the time, the mortality rate of those who had MH attacks in surgery was 80%. Since 1979, the drug dantrolene has been used as an antidote, reversing the course of these attacks, and mortality rate is now estimated at perhaps 10%.

MH occurs by itself, as an isolated entity, and has also been found in association with a number of other neuromuscular diseases, including MYOTONIC DYSTROPHY and myotonia congenita. The tendency to develop MH, as an isolated entity, is generally inherited as an AUTOSOMAL DOMINANT trait, though in some families (very rarely) it appears to be an AUTOSOMAL RECESSIVE or MULTIFACTORIAL trait. It is estimated that as many as one in 200 people may

carry the defective GENE that triggers these episodes. They may undergo surgery several times successfully without exhibiting any symptoms of the condition.

The disorder has been identified in almost all Western countries, as well as Japan, Australia and New Zealand. In the United States, it most commonly affects whites of Northern European ancestry. Attacks occur most frequently in older children and young adults. MH is seen in one in 50,000 anesthetized patients. Children appear to be at special risk with about one in 5,000–10,000 pediatric anesthetics having an MH complication. In about 50% of families with MH, a MUTATION in the gene for the ryanodine receptor, the skeletal muscle calcium release channel gene, found on 19q, accounts for the disease. (A mutation in this gene has also been found to underlie some cases of CENTRAL CORE DISEASE.) A mutation in a skeletal muscle calcium gene (CACNA1S), found on 1q, has also been identified in a family with MH.

Clearly MH is genetically heterogeneous with many loci, or gene locations, involved (see HETEROGENEITY; LOCUS, LOCI). For example, among others, MH loci have been mapped to 17q, 7q, 3q and 5p.

Some physical characteristics appear to be common in families susceptible to MH. They include a history of unexplained high fevers, unusual muscle weakness, spinal deformities, a history of muscle cramps and an inability to exercise in high heat.

Pigs have a similar disorder that is triggered by periods of stress, and there have been suggestions, though unproven, that in some individuals at risk for MH, episodes can also be triggered by intense stress or by exercise. It has also been suggested that there may be a link between MH and heat stroke.

Susceptibility for MH may be detected via a muscle biopsy with studies of muscle contraction after pharmacologic stimulation. However, these studies require removal of a significant amount of muscle tissue by an invasive procedure, are highly specialized, are available at only about 10 centers across the United States and do not reliably detect 100% of individuals at risk for developing MH. Thus, because of the potential catastrophic consequences, anyone with a first-degree relative (parents, offspring, SIBLINGS) who exhibited symptoms of MH during surgery must be considered at risk.

At-risk individuals undergoing surgery can be anesthetized with alternative agents, with special care taken to monitor them during and after the operation.

mandibulo-facial dyostosis See TREACHER COLLINS SYNDROME.

manic-depression (manic-depressive psychosis; affective disorders) An episodic psychological disturbance that manifests a tendency toward depression alternating with occasional periods of energized alertness, grandiosity and other signs of mania. It is called a bipolar disorder, indicating the presence of mania and depression or mania alone, as opposed to unipolar, which refers to depression alone. A familial aggregation and strong genetic predisposition to these disorders has long been recognized, both medically and popularly, as has been noted in the lyrics to a Memphis Slim song:

My mama had them
Her mama had them
Now I've got them, too
Folks, you've got to inherit the blues

It has been suggested that many famous artists, writers, and scientists may have had manic-depressive illness, including Vincent Van Gogh, William Blake, Walt Whitman and Edgar Allan Poe. If untreated, manic-depressive illness has been associated with a suicide rate of about 20%.

The mode of inheritance in most genetically determined cases is unknown. It is likely that a number of different GENE loci (see LOCUS, LOCI) are involved which may act on their own (genetic HETEROGENEITY) or together in a complex POLYGENIC manner. In some families it appears to be inherited in either an AUTOSOMAL DOMINANT manner or in an X-LINKED form. Other groups and affected individuals may have yet different forms. A major research effort is under way to map and isolate genes responsible. Some have been mapped to certain chromosomal regions but no individual genes have been isolated to date.

Two million in the United States are thought to be affected, and overall, the general population

risk for developing a unipolar or bipolar depressive disorder is about 1–2%. The risk to first degree relatives is put at 13–15%, or a 10-fold increase over incidence in the general population. Identical twins exhibit a nearly 40-fold increase of risk. Female first-degree relatives are 1.5 to two times as frequently affected as males. Risks approximately double if both a parent and SIBLING are affected. If the affected relative had the onset of disease at an early age (<40 years old), there is a higher risk to first-degree relatives than if the onset was at a later age. Adoption studies have shown that the risks for an adopted child correspond to that predicted based on their natural parents, not their adoptive ones.

The cause of bipolar disorders is unknown, but one theory holds that it may involve abnormalities in the transport of sodium and lithium in the brain. Thirty percent of affected individuals under medical supervision have such an abnormality in their blood cells; their affected relatives show similar signs, while unaffected relatives have no such defect. Antidepressant drugs alleviate some symptoms.

manic-depressive psychosis See MANIC-DEPRESSION.

mannosidosis A hereditary deficiency of the ENZYME alpha-mannosidase, this metabolic disorder results in accumulations of mannose-rich compounds.

The infantile onset form appears between three and 12 months of age. A progressive coarsening of facial features occurs, marked by a high forehead, prominent jaw bone, low flat nose, short neck, large tongue (MACROGLOSSIA), enlarged hands, feet and ears. DEAFNESS is common, as is delayed motor development. Growth is retarded and speech is delayed. MENTAL RETARDATION is characteristic, with IQs generally in the 50 to 70 range.

Other symptoms include spoke-shaped opacities in the lenses of the eyes, mild muscle weaknesses, spleen and liver enlargement (hepatosplenomegaly), HUMPBACK (kyphosis), demineralization of the long bones (osteoporosis) and umbilical or INGUINAL HERNIAS. Death usually occurs by age 10.

The SYNDROME is inherited as an AUTOSOMAL RECESSIVE trait, and there appears to be some concentration among Scandinavians. The GENE has been mapped to 19p (the short arm of chromosome 19). A less severe juvenile (with onset typically between one and four years of age) or adult-onset form of the disorder also exists. Diagnosis of mannosidosis is based on reduced levels of the enzyme alpha-mannosidase in blood constituents. A few hundred persons in the United States are affected.

CARRIER detection is not simple but PRENATAL DIAGNOSIS is possible through finding reduced enzyme levels in cultured AMNIOTIC FLUID (or chorionic villus; see CHORIONIC VILLUS SAMPLING) cells. Prognosis depends upon the form of the disease.

An animal model exists among cattle. A similar neurodegenerative disease due to a deficiency of beta-mannosidase has been described in goats and recently several cases have been found in humans.

maple syrup urine disease   An infant-onset metabolic disorder resulting in deterioration of the nervous system. First described in 1954, it is named for the urine's characteristic maple syrup odor. Untreated, death usually occurs before the age of one year.

Inherited as an AUTOSOMAL RECESSIVE trait, it is caused by defective metabolism of the AMINO ACIDS leucine, isoleucine and valine. These three amino acids are often referred to as the branched chain amino acids. Initial symptoms, evident soon after birth, include vomiting, lethargy, feeding problems and poor muscle tone (hypotonia). As the condition progresses, physical and MENTAL RETARDATION commonly result, as do coma and death if untreated. It can be managed by a controlled diet that excludes foods with the amino acids that cannot be metabolized. However, this dietary management is difficult and must be initiated within 10 days of birth.

Maple syrup urine disease is estimated to occur in one in 200,000 live births. However, among conservative Mennonites, a religious isolate in eastern Pennsylvania, frequency has been estimated as high as one in 176 live births. When the MUTATION is known in a family, CARRIER detection and PRENATAL DIAGNOSIS within the family can be accomplished by molecular techniques. Prenatal diagnosis

is accomplished by ENZYME assay of cultured fetal cells gathered via AMNIOCENTESIS or CHORIONIC VILLUS SAMPLING.

mapping   See GENE MAPPING.

Marcus Gunn syndrome   See JAW WINKING SYNDROME.

Marden-Walker syndrome   A hereditary disorder of the connective tissue that results in a variety of developmental abnormalities. Affected individuals have droopy eyelids (PTOSIS), a flat nasal bridge, low-set ears and a fixed facial expression. Other reported facial and cranial ANOMALIES include small head circumference, abnormally small eyes and mouth and a low hairline. Additional abnormalities include curvature of the spine, joint contractures, CLEFT PALATE or high-arched palate, growth retardation and slow muscle motion are other hallmarks. Heart abnormalities, anomalous sexual and urinary systems, a decrease in bone mass, and concave or protruding chest (pectus excavatum or pectus carinatum) may also be present.

About 20% of patients die at about three months of age from aspiration, infection or heart failure. Those who survive generally have been significantly mentally retarded. Transmitted as an AUTOSOMAL RECESSIVE trait, some 20 cases have been reported, with males affected more often than females.

Marfan syndrome   A GENETIC DISORDER of the connective tissue that primarily affects the skeletal, ocular and cardiovascular systems. It is named for Bernard-Jean Antonin Marfan (1858–1942), a founder of French pediatrics who in 1896 described a five-year-old girl with poor muscle development and abnormal spinal curvature, whose limbs, fingers and toes were long and thin.

In the skeletal system, the most distinguishing characteristic is excessive height with long extremities, including fingers and toes. Defects in the cardiovascular system, which become more threatening with age, are the major health consideration.

While the biochemical and molecular basis of the disease is known, the diagnosis of Marfan syndrome is still a clinical one. That is, identifying affected individuals is accomplished by testing suspected cases for signature indicators of the disorder, as well as ascertaining family history. Inherited as an AUTOSOMAL DOMINANT trait, it's believed to affect one in 10,000 individuals, making it more prevalent than CYSTIC FIBROSIS and HEMOPHILIA. An estimated 25,000–30,000 in the United States are affected. Twenty-five percent of the cases are the result of new MUTATION, and, as with many other dominant disorders, the rate of mutation appears to be linked to increased paternal age. Non-affected parents have an estimated one in 40,000 to one in 50,000 chance of giving birth to an infant with Marfan caused by a new mutation.

Expression is highly variable. Even within families with more than one affected member, the severity and specific features displayed can vary tremendously. Most of the characteristic features become more pronounced with age, making diagnosis generally easier at older ages.

Many Americans first became aware of the SYNDROME following the death of Olympic volleyball star Flo Hyman in 1986. At the age of 31, she collapsed and died of a ruptured aortic aneurysm during a tournament in Japan. She had never been diagnosed as having the disorder. Almost a decade earlier, collegiate basketball player Chris Patton died from the same manifestation of Marfan during a pickup basketball game.

Although the prognosis for this condition has improved dramatically in recent years due to new therapies, the difficulty in recognizing the disorder, and its often sudden, fatal consequences has led Dr. Reed Pyeritz, an expert on the disorder to say, "Often the first person to make the diagnosis of Marfan is the coroner."

Medical historians question whether the violinist Niccolò Paganini, noted as having exceptionally long fingers (a hallmark of the disorder), may have had Marfan syndrome. Additional attention has been focused on Abraham Lincoln, with some citing his excessive height and lean frame as evidence that he had the syndrome, and was likely to have died unnaturally early, even if spared an assassin's bullet. However, more recent historical examination notes that his hands were well proportioned, he had no spinal curvature or chest deformity, and he was exceptionally muscular, none of which is typical for affected individuals. Additionally, he was farsighted, which is extremely rare in the disorder.

Bones and ligaments are affected in many different ways. In addition to excessive height, arms and legs are often disproportionately long (dolichostenomelia), as are the fingers (ARACHNODACTYLY). The arms, when fully extended, may have a span considerably greater than body height. The joints may have the ability to bend beyond their usual limit (HYPERMOBILITY). This can cause clumsiness and precipitate repeated dislocations. Feet are usually flat. Spinal curvature (SCOLIOSIS) is common and may be severe. It can develop rapidly and may require surgical intervention. The breast bone may protrude (pigeon breast, pectus carinatum) or be indented (funnel chest, pectus excavatum).

The face, like the rest of the body, may be long and narrow, with a highly arched palate and crowding of teeth caused by a narrow jaw. There are a number of associated ocular abnormalities, as well. The most common is myopia, or nearsightedness. The lens may be dislocated (that is, off center). This is known as ectopia lentis and is seen in about 50% of patients with Marfan syndrome. Since this ANOMALY is observed in few other disorders, it is an important clue in diagnosing the syndrome. Retinal detachment may occur, requiring affected individuals to refrain from recreational activities that may subject them to blows to the head, which could precipitate detachment.

The cardiovascular characteristics, perhaps the most consistent features, are also the most serious. Most common is mitral valve prolapse. This occurs when the mitral valves, which separate the chambers of the heart, like the joints, are "floppy" and don't effectively cover the opening. The condition is found in 75% to 85% of cases. Complications of mitral valve prolapse can include abnormalities of heart rhythm (arrhythmia), infection of the valve (endocarditis) and, rarely, sudden death.

The aorta, the artery that carries all the oxygenated blood pumped from the heart, is the area most seriously affected. The wall of the aorta may become seriously weakened, even to the point where the vessel may suddenly rupture with fatal consequences.

(The bulging area caused by the weakened tissue is termed an aneurysm.) Furthermore, the dilation of the aorta that over time precedes this rupture may allow blood to flow back into the heart and can ultimately cause heart failure.

New surgical procedures for replacing this damaged section of the aorta are greatly increasing life expectancy among those who exhibit serious cardiac problems. Beta blockers, drugs that lower blood pressure, are also often prescribed to reduce the risk of ruptured aneurysms.

Cardiovascular abnormalities can be detected with an echocardiogram, a test that uses high frequency sound waves (ULTRASOUND) to create a sonar scan of the heart.

Marfan syndrome results from mutations in the fibrillin (FBN1) GENE, located on chromosome 15q. The mutation appears to be unique in each individual family, or at least there is no single common mutation known, making rapid genetic diagnosis or screening impossible. In families in which multiple members are affected, linkage analysis can be used for genetic testing and diagnosis.

Women with Marfan must be carefully monitored during pregnancy, due to the extra strain this places on their hearts. In addition, vigorous exercise and competitive sports should be avoided.

Some patients who have certain features of Marfan syndrome have a Marfanlike condition referred to as Marfan syndrome, type II, which is caused by mutations in the *TGFBR2* gene.

marijuana   Marijuana is a natural substance ingested for its psychoactive properties. Its main ingredient is delta-9-tetrahydrocannabinol, also available in an oral formation and used to treat nausea. Use during pregnancy is variously reported to be from 3% to 27%, but these figures are believed to be underestimates. Marijuana is most likely to be used in the first trimester, when pregnancy might not be expected, or for its anti-nausea properties.

Previously labeled as a suspected TERATOGEN, its effects on fetal development are unclear. Studies have been contradictory, and statistical data on incidence of BIRTH DEFECTS in marijuana users surveyed is hard to interpret due to the presence of other potential contributing factors, such as cigarette smoking, alcohol use and maternal health. Women who smoked marijuana have been reported to have had prolonged, difficult, or unexpectedly fast labor. In some studies, LOW BIRTH WEIGHT and PREMATURITY were associated with marijuana, while in others they were not. Infants born to marijuana users have been reported to have tremors and altered visual response in the first few days after birth, but these abnormalities have disappeared within a month.

No pattern of malformation has been observed that could be considered characteristic of fetal marijuana exposure (such as is seen in fetal alcohol syndrome). Growth retardation does seem to be associated with marijuana use during pregnancy. There is a possible association of IN UTERO marijuana exposure and acute nonlymphocytic leukemia in childhood. While sperm levels in male users have been reported to be reduced, it is not clear that this has any clinical significance as this reduction is not necessarily related to INFERTILITY.

markers, genetic   See GENETIC MARKERS.

Maroteaux-Lamy syndrome   See MUCOPOLYSAC-CHARIDOSIS.

MASS syndrome   A hereditary disorder of the connective tissue that takes its acronymic designation from the parts of the body affected: Mitral valve, Aorta, Skeleton and Skin. Transmitted as an autosomal dominant trait, it is caused by a mutation in the *FBN1*, or *fibrillin 1* gene, located at 15q21.1. This is the same gene involved in Marfan syndrome. More than 400 mutations of this gene have been described.

maturity-onset diabetes   See DIABETES MELLITUS.

MCAD deficiency (Medium-chain acyl-CoA dehydrogenase)   An autosomal recessive disorder characterized by an inability to properly metabolize fatty acids. This leaves those affected at risk for hypoglycemia, vomiting, lethargy, encephalopathy, respiratory arrest, seizures, apnea, cardiac arrest, coma and sudden death. Infants may exhibit developmental and behavioral disability, hypotonia, or chronic muscle weakness, failure to thrive and attention deficit disorder.

MCAD is an enzyme responsible for the metabolism of medium-chain fatty acids. Over a score of MCAD gene variants had been identified by 2005. The majority of affected individuals have the *K304E* MCAD mutation. The mutation has been found in 90% of all patients. The gene is responsible for producing a protein product that plays a role in the breakdown of fatty acids. The disorder renders the protein product abnormal, impairing oxidation of medium-chain fatty acids consumed in the diet or created within the cells.

Onset is typically between two months and two years of age, though patients as young as two days and as old as six years have been reported. The disorder is triggered by a precipitating event such as metabolic stress induced by infection, fasting or a seemingly innocuous illness that places high demands on fatty acid oxidation. Without prior recognition of metabolic irregularities, 20–25% of affected infants will succumb during the first episode of the disorder.

The gene responsible for MCAD deficiency has been mapped to 1p31. The disorder is most common among Caucasians of northern European descent. Carrier frequency in this population is estimated at 1:40–100, and the condition occurs in an estimated 1:6,500–20,000 live births. The penetrance of MCAD genotypes is unknown. Some fatal cases have been misdiagnosed as SIDs and account for an estimated 1% of reported cases in the United States, Europe and Australia.

Heterozygotes, or carriers, have below normal levels of dehydrogenase metabolic activity but are outwardly unaffected. Some individuals with both copies of the defective gene also remain asymptomatic.

Prenatal diagnosis is possible via amniocentesis, enzyme assayk, in vitro probe of fatty acid oxidation and DNA analysis for the *G985* mutation. The MCAD mutation can be identified through NDA-based PCR tests. Neonatal testing for MCAD deficiency is based on detecting abnormal metabolites. North Carolina and Massachusetts screen for MCAD deficinecy as part of their neonatal screening program. California, Pennsylvania and Wisconsin are among the other states instituting some form of newborn screening for MCAD deficiency.

measles (rubeola) A viral infection that, if contracted during pregnancy, can cause PREMATURITY, LOW BIRTH WEIGHT or miscarriage (see ABORTION). However, it has not been linked to BIRTH DEFECTS. If infection occurs near delivery date, the infant may be born with measles, with severity of symptoms ranging from mild to fatal.

Measles, also called rubeola, should be distinguished from rubella (German measles; see TORCH SYNDROME), a viral infection that can cause birth defects if contracted during pregnancy. (See also TERATOGEN.)

Meckel syndrome (Gruber syndrome) Invariably fatal SYNDROME characterized by multiple, severe physical abnormalities. The head is small (MICROCEPHALY) and the skull often has an opening at the back, or herniation, through which brain tissue protrudes (occipital ENCEPHALOCELE). The forehead is sloped, and the eyes may be small or completely absent (microphthalmia; anopthalmia). Other ANOMALIES include CLEFT PALATE, extra fingers or toes (POLYDACTYLY), polycystic kidneys and incomplete development of the genitalia. The abdomen and lower trunk may be swollen due to enlargement of the kidneys and liver, and may in some cases make delivery difficult. CLUBFOOT is common, as are other anomalies of the limbs. Infants are either stillborn or die soon after birth.

It is named for Johann Friedrich Meckel, who first described it in 1822. It is often referred to as Gruber or Meckel-Gruber syndrome for Dr. D. G. Gruber, who described it in 1934.

Inherited as an autosomal recessive trait, it is genetically heterogeneous: mutations in one of several genes may cause it. Two such genes have thus far been identified: the *MKS1* gene that lies on the long arm of chromosome 17 and the *meckelin (MKS3)* gene that is found on chromosome 8q. These genes are involved in the function of cilia. A third gene has been mapped to chromosome 11q. PRENATAL DIAGNOSIS is possible by ULTRASOUND with identification of either the encephalocele, enlarged cystic kidneys or polydactyly. An elevated alphafetoprotein level may also be seen in many cases with encephalocele. Incidence varies in different populations from 1:3,400 to 1:140,000 births and is said to be higher in India, Finland and among the Tartars in the former Soviet Union. The syndrome can vary among affected siblings.

median cleft face syndrome   A CONGENITAL developmental abnormality whose hallmark is a widened central portion of the face. The eyes are wide-spaced (HYPERTELORISM) and a CLEFT creates some degree of a vertical separation in the middle of the face. The skull itself may also be fissured. The severity of the median clefting ranges from broadening of the nasal tip to complete separation of the nose or nose and lip into two parts. Clefting of the palate also may be evident in severe cases. Other less common physical features include abnormally small eyeballs (microphthalmia), benign cysts located on the globe of the eye, fissures of the upper eyelid, CATARACTS, ear abnormalities, deformities of the fingers, and undescended testes. Also common is a "widow's peak" of the hair. Mild MENTAL RETARDATION is seen in approximately 12% of affected individuals, and severe mental retardation in 8%.

The basic cause of this rare SYNDROME is unknown, and most cases occur sporadically. Corrective and reconstructive surgery may repair some clefts. Life span is unaffected, and psychosocial therapy may help affected individuals adjust to their appearance.

Mediterranean anemia   See THALASSEMIA.

Mediterranean fever, familial   See FAMILIAL MEDITERRANEAN FEVER.

medium-chain acyl-CoA dehydrogenase deficiency (MCAD)   An infancy or early-childhood onset metabolic disorder caused by an inherited ENZYME deficiency, resulting in repeated episodes of metabolic acidosis (excessive acidity of bodily fluids), hypoglycemia (deficiency of blood sugar), lethargy and coma.

The enzyme medium-chain acyl-CoA dehydrogenase is necessary for the metabolism of fats, specifically for the oxidation of stored medium-chain fatty acids. Thus, the disorder renders affected individuals unable to metabolize stored fats. The liver may also be affected during periods of acidosis.

Symptoms can be avoided by assuring affected individuals do not go without food for a prolonged period, and in cases of affected children, may require waking them at night for feeding, or nocturnal intravenous or intestinal (enteral) feeding.

The disorder is diagnosed by detection of suberylglycine and phenylpropionylglycine in the urine. It is estimated to occur in about one in 15,000 live births, and is more common in individuals of northern European background. Males and females are equally affected. Inherited as an AUTOSOMAL RECESSIVE trait, the responsible GENE has been mapped to 1p, and a single common MUTATION accounts for about 85–90% of cases. Screening for the condition at birth has been advocated by many health care providers and has become part of the routine newborn screening in a number of states, provinces and countries.

melanoma   See CANCER.

Melnick-Needles syndrome   Abnormal bone development accompanied by characteristic facial features are the hallmarks of this congenital genetic disorder. Affected individuals have wide-set eyes (hypertelorism), small jaw (micrognathia), small facial bones and a slow-developing skull. Bones of the arms and legs may be bowed, and the humerus, phalanges, radius, fibula and tibia may be bowed, flared, or abnormally short.

The thoracic cage may be unusually small, the ribs irregular, shoulders narrow and the chest concave (pectus excavatum), which puts those affected at increased risk of respiratory infections. If the pelvis is involved, hip dislocation may occur.

Individuals typically achieve normal height, but may exhibit an unusual gait due to deformity of the hip joint (coxa valga).

This is one of a heterogeneous group of disorders often referred to as the otopalatodigital spectrum disorders, a group that includes otopalatodigital syndrome types I (OPD1) and II (OPD2) (see entry), and frontometaphyseal dysplasia (FMD). Particularly in males, the severity of these disorders range from the mild manifestations seen in OPD1 to the severe effects of MNS, which is most commonly lethal before birth in affected males. (As a result, more affected females than males have been reported.) All of these disorders are caused by mutations in the X-linked *FLNA* gene. Other mutations in this gene cause X-linked periventricular nodular heterotopia, a neuronal migration disorder that presents with seizures and nodules of neurons situated in the wrong place along the surface of the brain's lateral ventricles.

Mendel, Gregor   See MENDELIAN.

Mendelian   Genetic traits that follow patterns of inheritance described by Austrian monk Gregor Johann Mendel (1822–84). He was the first to

TABLE XV
MODES OF MENDELIAN INHERITANCE, RELATED SEX RATIOS AND RISKS OF RECURRENCE

Code	Mode of Transmission	Sex Ratio	Risk of Recurrence for	
AR	Autosomal recessive	M1:F1	Patient's sib:	1 in 4 (25%) for each offspring to be affected
			Patient's child:	Not increased unless mate is carrier or homozygote
AD	Autosomal dominant	M1:F1	Patient's sib:	If parent is affected 1 in 2 (50%) for each offspring to be affected; otherwise not increased
			Patient's child:	1 in 2
AD-85%± penetrance	Autosomal dominant with about 85% penetrance	M1:F1	Patient's sib:	If parent is affected 1 in 2 (<50%) for each offspring to be affected; otherwise not increased
			Patient's child:	1 in 2
AD-60%±	Autosomal dominant with about 60% penetrance	M1:F1	Patient's sib:	If parent is affected 1 in 3 (30%) or each offspring to be affected, 1 in 2 for inheriting mutant gene; otherwise not increased
			Patient's child:	1 in 3 (30%) for each offspring to be affected, 1 in 2 for inheriting mutant gene
X-linked R (rare)	X-linked recessive	M1:F0	Patient's sib:	If mother is a carrier 1 in 2 (50%) or each brother to be affected and 1 in 2 (50%) for each sister to be a carrier
			Patient's child:	1 in 1 (100%) for carrier daughters; not increased for sons unless wife is a carrier
X-linked D	X-linked dominant (rare)	M1:F2	Patient's sib:	If affected parent is female 1 in 2 (50%) for each sib to be affected. If affected parent is male 1 in 1 (100%) for each sister to be affected; not increased for brothers
			Patient's child:	If patient is female 1 in 2 (50%) for each offspring to be affected; if patient is male 1 in 1(100%) for daughters, not increased for sons

Source: Daniel Bergsma (ed.), *Birth Defects Compendium,* 2nd ed. (New York: A.R. Liss, 1979).

deduce correctly the basic principles of heredity. Mendelian traits are also called "single GENE" or "monogenic" traits, because they are controlled by the action of a single gene or gene pair. More than 4,300 human disorders are known or suspected to be inherited as Mendelian traits, encompassing AUTOSOMAL DOMINANT, AUTOSOMAL RECESSIVE and X-LINKED dominant and X-linked recessive conditions. Overall incidence of Mendelian disorders in the human population is about 1%. Many non-anomalous characteristics that make up human variation are also inherited in Mendelian fashion. (Non-Mendelian traits are inherited in POLYGENIC, caused by the action of several genes, or MULTI-FACTORIAL, caused by the action of several genes in concert with environmental influence, fashion.)

A monk in Brunn (now Brno), Moravia (now a part of the Czech Republic), Mendel, who had studied physics and mathematics, noticed that garden pea plants had varying traits. For example, some unripe pods were yellow, others green; some varieties were tall, others were dwarfed. The position of the flowers, whether clustered at the top, or distributed along the stem, also varied, as did the physical appearance of the peas themselves, being either smooth or wrinkled. In 1856 he began experiments in which he cross-bred pea plants, with the goal of studying the hereditary transmission of these and other characteristics, and the statistical relation of the subsequently appearing traits. Based on his observations, he hypothesized that each trait in the offspring is controlled by only two factors, one from the male and one from the female, and that these traits were either dominant or recessive: A dominant trait would override the influence of its complementary hereditary factor; the influence of a recessive trait would recede when paired with a dominant one. (See Table XV.) He presented his finding to the Natural History Society of Brunn, which published them in 1859, and was also in communication with Karl von Naegeli, one of the most respected botanists of the day. However, the importance of his work went unrecognized until 1900, when three researchers independently rediscovered his findings. (See also the Introduction.)

meningocele   A skin-covered, sac-like protrusion of the membranes (meninges) covering the brain or the spinal cord. It is one defect in the spectrum of NEURAL TUBE DEFECTS. Its origin in MULTIFACTORIAL (caused by several different GENES in concert with environmental factors), and it occurs in approximately one out of 20,000 live births, equally distributed between males and females.

In spinal meningocele, the neural material from the spinal cord does not extend into the sac, although there is usually an opening in the spine (SPINA BIFIDA), which requires surgical correction. In general, there is no paralysis or sensory loss with either cranial or spinal meningocele. It can occur in isolation or as part of another SYNDROME. With surgical repair during the first year of life, the prognosis is favorable.

Menkes syndrome (kinky hair disease)   A hereditary inability to absorb and use copper is the hallmark of this SYNDROME, first described by U.S. pediatrician/neurologist J.H. Menkes in 1962. Affected infants appear normal at birth, but near the end of the first year of life begin to show signs of drowsiness, increased difficulty with feeding, poor visual development and a tendency to have an abnormally low body temperature (hypothermia). By the age of three months, muscle spasms and seizures are evident.

As the disorder progresses, marked FAILURE TO THRIVE, severe MENTAL RETARDATION and a deficient physical growth are seen. The scalp hair is characteristically short, sparse, twisted and unruly; the hair abnormality gives the disorder its secondary name. Eyebrow hair is whitish and lacks color. Other symptoms include an abnormally small head (MICROCEPHALY) with a short, broad nose, full cheeks, small lower jaw (micrognathia) and a lack of facial expression. Loss of muscle tone (hypotonia) and a depressed sternum, or breast bone (pectus excavatum), are also characteristic. X-ray examination may disclose bone spurs on the long bones of the arms and legs and flaring of rib ends.

Degeneration of the central nervous system results in increased reflex reaction (hyperreflexia), muscle contractions and stiff, awkward movements (spasticity), and paralysis affecting all four limbs (quadriparesis).

Transmitted as an X-LINKED recessive trait, this rare disorder occurs only in males and has been estimated to occur once in every 35,000 to 298,000 live births. Death within the first or second year of life occurred in 90% of those initially identified. Some CARRIERS of the trait have been identified through examination of the scalp hair.

Many of the effects of the disorder result from lack of copper incorporation in a number of the bodys ENZYMES where it is important. The basic defect involves a GENE (at xq13) that encodes a copper transporter. (Different MUTATIONS in the same gene cause type IX EHLERS-DANLOS SYNDROME.) When a mutation is identified in a family, molecular techniques can be used for carrier detection and PRENATAL DIAGNOSIS. Research has also revealed elevated levels of copper in the AMNIOTIC FLUID of affected FETUSES. Carrier testing is difficult but prenatal diagnosis has been accomplished by studies of copper uptake in fetal cells obtained by AMNIOCENTESIS or CHORIONIC VILLUS SAMPLING.

mental retardation Impairments of learning, social adjustment and maturation, characterized by below-average intellectual function and behavioral development. A major health problem, it HANDICAPS more infants than any other childhood disorder; an estimated 150,000 infants a year are born with, or will later be diagnosed as having, mental retardation. It is thought to affect between 1% and 3% of the general population.

Mental retardation can result from genetic abnormalities, exposure to environmental agents, PREMATURITY, intrauterine or birth trauma, or a combination of these and other factors. However, in the majority of those affected (estimates of 40% to 80%), the cause cannot be determined.

As a genetic condition, mental retardation can be inherited as an AUTOSOMAL DOMINANT, AUTOSOMAL RECESSIVE, X-LINKED, POLYGENIC or MULTIFACTORIAL trait, or as a result of CHROMOSOME ABNORMALITIES. Approximately 5% to 15% of those affected are thought to have single-GENE (autosomal dominant, autosomal recessive or X-linked) forms. It is also a feature of hundreds of CONGENITAL conditions. Other GENETIC DISORDERS (for example, PHENYLKETONURIA, CONGENITAL HYPOTHYROIDISM, GALACTOSEMIA) can result in mental retardation if undetected and untreated following birth.

Studies in mental institutions indicate mental retardation of unknown origins occurs in multiple SIBLINGS in a considerable number of cases, and these may be due to rare recessive disorders. It has also been estimated that about a third of normal persons carry a recessive gene for a low-grade mental defect.

Though there are no precise means of measuring the extent of mental retardation, those with IQs below 70 are considered to be retarded, and their retardation is classified in one of four categories: mild, moderate, severe or profound. Ninety percent of affected children are in the mild range, with IQs in the range of 52 to 67. They are educable and may learn to function independently as adults, though they require special education. Mild retardation may be difficult to diagnose; since infants develop at different rates, diagnosis in these cases is often delayed until two to three years of age. Those in the moderate range (IQs of 36 to 51) may attain some degree of independence as adults and also require special education. In the severe range (IQs of 20 to 35) affected individuals can learn minimal conversation and self-care skills, though they require supervision throughout life; institutionalization may be necessary. Those with profound retardation (IQ below 20) may acquire only minimal self-care skills and toilet training. Language development is usually minimal, and total supervision is required. One percent of newborn infants are severely to profoundly retarded. However, many of them succumb to associated conditions, so that by seven years of age, only an estimated 0.3% to 0.4% of the population have IQs below 50.

Mild or moderate retardation is usually multifactorial in cause, that is, caused by the action of several genes in concert with environmental influences, while severe cases are more likely to be due to genetic defects alone; at least one-third of severely retarded individuals are believed to have genetic abnormalities. Perhaps half of the remainder are genetically influenced.

The risk of recurrence in family members and the possibility of PRENATAL DIAGNOSIS is dependent on the form of mental retardation. However, mild retardation is much more likely to be seen in multiple family members than severe retardation.

Among the more well-known conditions or SYNDROMES with which mental retardation is associated are CRANIOSYNOSTOSIS, DOWN SYNDROME, FRAGILE X SYNDROME, PHENYLKETONURIA, fetal exposure to rubella (see TORCH SYNDROME) and alcohol (see ALCOHOLISM; FETAL ALCOHOL SYNDROME), AMINO ACID disorder and STORAGE DISEASES. (See also EDUCATION; HANDICAP.)

mesomelic dwarfism   See MESOMELIC DYSPLASIA.

mesomelic dysplasia (mesomelic dwarfism)   A group of conditions of short-limbed DWARFISM characterized by shortening of the mesomelic or middle portion of the limbs. Several forms are recognized, differentiated by the clinical and, more important, radiographic (observable by X-ray) differences. Bones involved include the radius, ulna, tibia, and fibula.

Langer type   This form is named for radiologist L.O. Langer, who described it in 1967. It is characterized by severe shortening of the forearms and lower legs and malformations of the wrist (see MADELUNG DEFORMITY). The elbows may not extend fully. Intelligence and lifespan are normal. Adult height is about 51 inches (129.5 cm).

Inherited as an AUTOSOMAL RECESSIVE trait, individuals carrying a single copy of the GENE exhibit dyschondrosteosis—a short forearm with bowing at the radius, often with dislocation or limitation of movement at the elbow or wrist. Those with two copies of the gene (HOMOZYGOTES) have Langer type mesomelic dysplasia, with its significant dwarfism. The causative GENE, SHOX, was discovered in 1998. The so-called homeobox developmental gene, it is highly expressed in bone-forming cells. MUTATIONS in the gene are linked to growth retardation and short stature. The gene is not located on an autosome, but on both the X CHROMOSOME and Y CHROMOSOME in what has been termed the pseudoautosomal region. This portion of the X chromosome acts like an autosome, since the gene has a complement on the Y chromosome. Thus, males as well as females have two copies, and the region on the X is not inactivated. (See MOSAICISM for discussion of X inactivation). Patients with Langer type mesomelic dysplasia are homozygotes for mutations at this LOCUS.

Nievergelt type   Described by German physician K. Nievergelt in 1944, the forearms and lower legs are shortened and deformed from a mild to a severe degree. Dimpling of the skin on the forearms and lower legs may result from bony protuberances of the limbs. Motion of elbows and fingers may be limited. Intelligence and life span are normal. Adult height has been generally between 53 inches and 58 inches (134.6–147.3 cm) in the very few reported cases. It appears to be an AUTOSOMAL DOMINANT trait.

Reinhardt-Pfeiffer type   Described by German physicians K. Reinhardt and R.A. Pfeiffer in 1967, this is a moderate form of mesomelic short-stature, and has been described in only one family, with 14 affected individuals, demonstrating autosomal dominant inheritance. The lower legs are most affected, and the skeletal deformities may be progressive. Adult height was between 59 inches and 67 inches (149.9–170.2 cm), and intelligence and life span normal.

Werner type   Described in 1915 in Germany by gynecologist P. Werner, this form is characterized by extreme shortening of the lower leg, extra fingers or toes (POLYDACTYLY) and absence of thumbs. Bones of the ankles are also deformed. Forearms are normal, but the wrist bones may be deformed, and wrist movement may be limited.

Intelligence is normal, as is life span. Inherited as an autosomal dominant trait, the severity of the condition is highly variable.

metachromatic leukodystrophy (MLD)   Form of LEUKODYSTROPHY, a group of degenerative, progressive disorders of the nervous system. It takes its name "metachromatic" from the coloration of affected white matter cells after they are chemically stained during laboratory analysis; components of the same tissue take on various shades or colors, all differing from the color of the dye they are stained with.

The disorder is caused by the absence of the ENZYME arylsulfatase A (ASA), which normally breaks down sulfatides, a component of myelin, the protective sheath that covers the axons, nerve fibers that transmit electrical impulses. The sulfatides would normally be broken down into cerebrosides. The consequent accumulation of sulfatides in the brain, peripheral nerve, kidney, liver and gall-bladder causes the breakdown of myelin, though the reason for this destruction is unclear.

MLD occurs in three forms: late infantile, with symptoms appearing between about 14 months and two years of age; juvenile, with onset between the ages of four years and 16 years of age; adult, with onset after the age of 16.

In the late infantile form, first described in 1933, symptoms begin with poor muscle tone (hypotonia), unsteady gait, speech abnormalities and arresting of mental development. The disorder is progressive, with ultimate loss of voluntary muscle control (apraxia), inability to communicate (aphasia), dementia and BLINDNESS. Death usually occurs between the ages of three and six years. There is no generally recognized treatment, although successful treatment with bone marrow transplantation (BMT) has been reported. Those who are presymptomatic or are early in the course of their disease and with slow progression appear to be most likely to benefit from BMT.

The GENE has been identified on 22q (the long arm of chromosome 22) and several common MUTATIONS have been found. This can allow for CARRIER detection and PRENATAL DIAGNOSIS in families where the mutation is known, but general carrier screening by molecular techniques is not yet feasible. Some completely normal individuals have been found to have extremely low ASA levels, a situation termed pseudodeficiency. It results from a common variation (as much as 15–20% of the population may carry it) of the ASA gene that leads to production of an enzyme that functions normally in the body but appears to be deficient when studied by certain tests in the laboratory. This can cause difficulties in diagnosis.

The other two forms display wide variability of expression, though they are also progressive and lead to death. In the adult form, initial symptoms have usually, been psychiatric, leading to a diagnosis of SCHIZOPHRENIA, Disorders of movement and posture appear later. Until recently, most adult cases were diagnosed after death, though biochemical screening for indicative levels of enzyme activity now allows more timely detection. This method has found unsuspected cases among individuals institutionalized for mental disorders. Other diagnostic methods include computerized axial tomography (CAT) scanning, analysis of cerebrospinal fluid (CSF), and findings of low arylsulfatase A in tissue and white blood cells. (In another disorder, multiple sulfatase deficiency, the enzyme ASA is decreased as are many other sulfatases, resulting in a SYNDROME of MLD characterized by MUCOPOLYSACCHARIDOSIS, ICHTHYOSIS and DEAFNESS.)

MLD is inherited as an AUTOSOMAL RECESSIVE trait. Incidence has been estimated at between one in 40,000 and one in 50,000 live births in the general population. Successful treatment has been reported.

metaphyseal chondrodysplasia   Term describing several forms of short-limbed DWARFISM. "Metaphyseal" refers to the area of the bones involved, the metaphyses, the wide part at the end of the shaft of a long bone which contains the growth zone. "Dysplasia" refers to defective development, and "chondro" to cartilage. The defective development of the cartilage causes characteristic abnormal flaring of the metaphyses observable in X-rays. The bones of the arms and legs (long bones) show the most evidence of the abnormality. Several varieties have been identified. The Schmid type is relatively common, the McKusick type well known but uncommon and the remainder rare. Immunologic and endocrine abnormalities are important aspects of several forms.

McKusick type (cartilage-hair hypoplasia)   This disorder was first observed in the Old Order AMISH, a religious community in the area of Lancaster, Pennsylvania, where it is relatively common. It is also relatively common in Finland (one in 23,000 live births) and other groups. The McKusick referred to is Dr. Victor McKusick, a well-known geneticist at Johns Hopkins University in Baltimore, Maryland. Characterized by short-limbed short stature and abnormal development of long bone cartilage, adult height is usually between 41 inches and 57 inches (104.1–144.8 cm).

Body length is reduced but weight is normal at birth. The elbows have somewhat limited extension and ankles are deformed. As infants age, a single leg may bow inward or outward. Hands and feet are short and pudgy, and the fingers and toes show extreme flexibility of motion. By nine to 12 months of age, X-rays can detect the characteristic abnormalities.

The hair is light and sparse, and a distinctive feature is the small width of the hair shafts when examined microscopically. Immunity is deficient and individuals affected are prone to infections, particularly during infancy and early childhood. They have an increased susceptibility to chicken pox and other infections caused by the VARICELLA virus, due to a defect of the cellular immune system, and may be left with deep pocked scars. The infection may be severe and lethal.

Inherited as an AUTOSOMAL RECESSIVE trait, the condition is caused by mutations in the *RMRP* GENE, mapped to 9p.

Schmid type First described in 1949, this disorder is variable in its expression, with females being less severely affected than males. Increased paternal age has been associated with SPORADIC cases resulting from new MUTATIONS.

The dwarfing and short-limbed disproportion are usually seen by 18 months to 24 months of age. The first sign is a bowledgedness, and is usually noted when infants begin walking. As they age, the bowing increases, producing a waddling gait and contributing to degenerative arthritis in the hips. Shoulders, hips, wrists, knees and ankles are affected.

The abnormalities of the metaphyses of the bones revealed in X-rays are variable, from mild to gross. They appear to heal with bed rest, but reappear when weight is placed on them. Average adult height is 51 inches to 63 inches (129.5–160 cm). Caused by mutations in the type X collagen gene (COL10A1), located on 6q, it is an AUTOSOMAL DOMINANT trait.

Jansen type Named after the Dutch orthopedist and founder of that specialty in his country, this is a very rare form, inherited as an autosomal dominant trait. Permanent bending of joints (flexion contractures) is severe. Patients are severely dwarfed and disabled. Adult height averages about 47 inches (119 cm). High calcium levels (hypercalcemia) have been described. The disorder appears to be caused by mutations in the parathyroid hormone receptor gene, found on 3p. About 10 cases have been reported. Life span is normal.

metatropic dysplasia (metatropic dwarfism) Metatropic, from the Greek *metatropis,* meaning "changing pattern," refers to the reversal of the proportions of the dwarfing (see DWARFISM) observed in affected individuals. Cases of the disorder are believed to have been first described in 1892 in Germany.

At birth, infants appear to have relatively short limbs and relatively long, thin trunks. Craniofacial appearance is normal. Body length is usually normal during the neonatal period, but in late infancy, the spine begins to exhibit backward and lateral curvature (kyphoscoliosis), resulting in a short-trunk dwarfism. The kyphoscoliosis usually becomes severely incapacitating.

The limbs continue to exhibit dwarfing, and the bones of the arms and legs have a "barbell" shape upon X-ray examination. Additionally, the coccyx (the lower end of the spinal column) may be unusually long, resulting in what appears to be an almost tail-like appendage. Compression of the spinal cord can occur as a complication which can lead to paralysis or respiratory problems and death.

Generally inherited as an AUTOSOMAL RECESSIVE trait, metatropic dysplasia is relatively rare. While many affected individuals die in infancy, survival into the third decade of life is common, with height generally between 45 inches and 47 inches (114.3–119.4 cm). PRENATAL DIAGNOSIS is theoretically possible by findings of abnormal limb length via ULTRASOUND, but the dwarfism is usually diagnosed at birth. There is also a severe lethal autosomal recessive form of this disorder with extremely short bones and undermineralization of the spine with death before or shortly after birth. A less severe AUTOSOMAL DOMINANT form is also known.

methylation (DNA methylation) An enzyme-assisted biochemical process that adds methyl (CH_3) groups at selected sites on proteins, DNA and RNA. Methylation, or methyl "tagging," of these sites is a natural process, and methylation tags are believed to be involved in regulating gene expression and other chromosomal functions. In humans and most mammals, methylation is the only known natural alteration of DNA. In humans, methylation only occurs at some cytosine bases on the chromosomes, but 70 to 80% of all such sites are methylated.

Methylation patterns are established early in embryonic development and are an ongoing process as these sites add and lose methyl groups. Abnormalities in the methylation process have been linked to several genetic disorders.

Individuals with mutations that cause malfunctions in one of the methyltransferase enzymes involved in methylation exhibit ICF syndrome, characterized by immune system failures and other genetic anomalies. Abnormalities in one of the proteins involved in methylation is also responsible for Rett syndrome, a hereditary mental retardation syndrome affecting only females.

Methylation is also believed involved in imprinting, a genetic process that allows the expression of certain genes based on whether they were inherited maternally or paternally, in flagrant violation of Mendelian law. Anomalies in the methylation tags associated with imprinting are linked to Prader-Willi syndrome, Angelman's syndrome, and Beckwith-Wiedemann syndrome.

Abnormal increases and decreases in methylation tags are associated with most cancers. If some tags regulate genes that control cell proliferation, it is thought abnormalities in methylation could lead to the uncontrolled cell division that characterizes cancer.

methylmalonic acidemia A group of disorders characterized by the inability to metabolize methylmalonic acid or by a defect in the metabolism of vitamin B_{12}. The blood and urine exhibit an excessive level of the AMINO ACID glycine (hyperglycinemia), with an accompanying high level of ketones (ketoacidosis), which are substances normally processed by the liver from fats in food. Low blood sugar (hypoglycemia) is common. Methylmalonic acid, which is not normally found in the blood or urine, will also be detected. Also, an abnormally small number of circulating white cells in the blood (neutropenia) and a decrease in the number of blood platelets (thrombocytopenia) will be evident.

Repeated episodes of ketoacidosis may produce mental confusion, breathing difficulties, nausea, vomiting, dehydration and, if untreated, coma followed by death. MENTAL RETARDATION and marked growth retardation have been observed in those who survive the high rate of death in early infancy. Convulsions and fungal infections may also develop.

Inherited as AUTOSOMAL RECESSIVE traits, the incidence is about one in 50,000 live births. CARRIER testing and PRENATAL DIAGNOSIS using molecular genetic techniques is possible in families in which the mutations in the involved gene are known. Prenatal diagnosis is possible by testing for the presence of methylmalonic acid in the mother's urine or in the AMNIOTIC FLUID, as well as by detection of the ENZYME defects in fetal cells.

Treatment is complex, including dietary management with a low protein diet, often vitamin B_{12} supplements and possibly other agents such as carnitine.

Michelin tire baby syndrome First described and named in 1985, the SYNDROME was reported in two families. The first individual brought to medical attention was a three-year-old girl with deep skin folds on the back and on the arms and legs, reminiscent of the appearance of the Michelin Tire Man used in advertisements for the Michelin Tire Company. Some adult relatives had skin creases on wrists and forearms that apparently were remnants of similar skin folds in infancy. It is believed to be inherited as an AUTOSOMAL DOMINANT trait.

One researcher has suggested that this CONGENITAL ANOMALY has existed throughout human history; German pediatrician Hans-Rudolf Wiedemann, founder of the Society for Anthropology and Human Genetics, has called attention to a sculpture on a bronze door of the cathedral of Hildesheim in northwestern Germany, which depicts Eve nursing her infant son who appears to have features of this syndrome.

microarray (DNA microarray technology) A microarray is a small, solid support—a glass microscope slide, silicon chip or nylon membrane—onto which DNA sequences containing thousands of different genes can be attached at fixed locations so the DNA can be examined. Microarray also refers to the process such supports enable, a method of analyzing large numbers of genes at one time. The process identifies the expression level of individual genes, their purpose, interactions, gene health and other information of interest to researchers and clinicians.

Every cell in the human body with the exception of sperm and eggs has a complete set of chromosomes. Yet relatively few genes within the chromosome are active or expressed in any given cell. For example, some genes contain information on how to make growth hormone, but those genes are only expressed in the pituitary glands. Microarray allows thousands of genes from any cell to be analyzed simultaneously, enabling researchers to discover the roles of unknown cells and clinicians to identify genetic anomalies in their patients.

The process uses hybridization probing, in which fluorescently labeled nucleic acid molecules (messenger RNA, or mRNA) are used as mobile probes to identify complementary molecules. After incubating a DNA sequence with the nucleic acid the hybridization is complete. A laser scans the array, which stimulates the fluorescent tags, allowing a computerized microscope to measure the amount of mRNA bound to each site on the array. The degree of binding can be used to determine the expression of a given gene in that cell, help understand interactions among different genes, compare gene activity in two different samples or for a variety of other experimental and clinical purposes.

microcephaly   A small head, often with a receding forehead and large ears and nose. It is usually an associated feature of other disorders, rarely occurring in isolation, though infants with true hereditary microcephaly, an AUTOSOMAL RECESSIVE disorder, have only head and facial abnormalities as physical symptoms. It is not a primary malformation itself, but a sign of a small brain.

Microcephaly is sometimes visibly obvious in newborns by the characteristic forehead, flattened back of the head, and small or closed fontanels, the "soft spots" between the skull bones. It is often diagnosed by measuring the infant's head circumference.

Physical growth is generally retarded and children learn to walk more slowly than their normal counterparts. There is a delay in speech and mental development. Some patients experience seizures and spasticity and may exhibit cross eye (STRABISMUS). Personality and mood are variable and

may vacillate to extremes. Nearly 90% suffer from some form of prenatal brain damage. However, it is important to note that not all individuals with microcephaly will be retarded and have neurologic abnormalities; some are entirely normal.

This defect may be caused by a number of factors: GENETICS (20%), CHROMOSOME ABNORMALITIES, environment and factors of unknown origin. Environmental causes include prenatal radiation, infections (including rubella [TORCH SYNDROME] and toxoplasmosis) and drugs or agents (TERATOGENS), such as alcohol. Women with PHENYLKETONURIA (PKU) also give birth to microcephalic children. A number of multiple ANOMALY SYNDROMES have microcephaly as a feature.

Microcephaly may be inherited, but the GENE is considered extremely rare. In the general population, microcephaly due to genetic factors occurs in one in 30,000 to 50,000 live births, and in one per 10,000 births due to the other mentioned causes. In some population isolates, frequency may be as high as one in 2,000 births. In cases of isolated microcephaly with no other abnormalities and a negative family history, the recurrence risk is about 15–20%.

Attempts at PRENATAL DIAGNOSIS by ULTRASOUND should be undertaken with caution. Both false positive (diagnosing microcephaly when it isn't present) and false negative (failure to detect it) may occur. True hereditary microcephalics live an average-length life span, yet some die early due to other CONGENITAL defects or infectious diseases.

microdeletion 1p36 (monosomy 1p36)   One of the most common microdeletion syndromes, characterized by severe psychomotor retardation and developmental delays. Its name refers to the location on chromosome 1 of the chromosome band microdeletion. A microdeletion consists of a deletion of several contiguous genes too small to be seen in a microscope using conventional cytogenetic methods. Other anomalies associated with microdeletion 1p36 are microcephaly, seizures, hypotonia, feeding problems, behavior problems, self-injurious behavior and hearing and visual impairment. Patent ductus arteriosus (PDA) is also common. Characteristic facial features are a small, flat midface. The eyes are deep set and eyebrows straight. Preliminary diagnosis has been made on the basis of the distinctive facial features.

The condition is also called Monosomy 1p36. Monosomy typically refers to the absence of an entire chromosome from a chromosome pair, but in this instance it refers to the absence of a particular section of a chromosome. Prevalence is 1:5,000–10,000 live births. Prenatal detection is possible via amniocentesis, FISH and subtelomeric probe screening.

middle-ear infections (otitis media)   Among the most common illnesses in children, middle-ear infections occur when bacteria in the nose and throat migrate to the inner ear, causing irritation, inflammation and a buildup of fluid behind the eardrum. The condition, also termed otitis media, is painful and may be accompanied by temporary hearing loss.

A genetic contribution to susceptibility to otitis media is suggested by racial variations. The infections are more common among white or Native American than among black or Hispanic children. The frequency is not only unusually high in American Indians but also in Australian aborigines. About 10% of white children in one genetic study of the condition were affected. It appears to be a MULTIFACTORIAL trait.

(Children are also more prone to middle-ear infections than adults because their relatively short and horizontal eustachian tubes facilitate the migration of bacteria from the nose and throat to the ear.)

The infections can be easily treated with antibiotics. However, if left untreated, the buildup of fluid pressure can break the eardrum. Long-term problems with hearing and speech may result.

midget   Historically, this term has been used to describe short-statured individuals with normal body proportions, as opposed to "dwarfs," disproportionate short-statured individuals. (Actually, the body may not be proportionate, as upper/lower body segment ratios are not always in the truly normal range.)

The term *midget* is currently considered derogatory by short-statured individuals and its use is discouraged. The origin of the objection to this term is believed to be due to its circus-sideshow association and also to be a remnant of resentment from a time

when proportionate short-statured individuals were perceived by those of abnormal proportions as having fewer social disadvantages. Preferred terminology includes *dwarf,* and *small, little* or *short people.*

Proportionate short stature may be caused by CHROMOSOME ABNORMALITIES, hormone failure, primary growth disturbances, secondary growth failure, poor nutrition and inherited short stature.

For more information on proportionate short stature, see DWARFISM and PITUITARY DWARFISM.

Miescher's syndrome   See ACANTHOSIS NIGRICANS.

migraine headaches   Headaches accompanied by nausea and vomiting, often preceded by sensory disturbances, most commonly of a visual aura, such as a blind spot or twinkling lights. Migraines affect 5% to 10% of the population, and demonstrate an undoubted familial aggregation (see FAMILIAL DISEASES). In a study of 500 individuals who sought medical help for the condition, more than 98% had one parent who was similarly affected. Among offspring of one affected parent, more than 60% also had migraines, as opposed to less than 4% of the offspring of unaffected parents. Among offspring of two affected individuals, more than 80% were affected. While some specific forms of migraine appear to have an AUTOSOMAL DOMINANT (AD) inheritance, it appears most likely to be of MULTIFACTORIAL etiology.

Miller-Dieker syndrome (lissencephaly syndrome)   A brain malformation whose cardinal feature is the absence of gyri, or convolutions on the brain. (LISSENCEPHALY, its alternate designation, which means "smooth brain," may be seen in isolation or with other SYNDROMES.)

Infants affected with this rare developmental ANOMALY exhibit an abnormally small head (MICROCEPHALY), small mandible, unusual facial appearance, FAILURE TO THRIVE and retarded motor development. The most consistent facial features of MDLS are narrowing or hollowing at the temples, prominent forehead, often with vertical ridging and furrowing of the skin, especially when crying, short nose with upturned nostrils, prominent upper lip, thin border of the upper lip and small jaw. Newborns usually exhibit poor feeding, poor responsiveness, decreased muscle tone and early onset seizures. Lissencephaly is diagnosed by CT, MRI or ULTRASOUND demonstrating the smooth thin cerebral cortex. It is invariably fatal, either in infancy or early childhood.

Formerly considered an AUTOSOMAL RECESSIVE disorder, it is now known that the majority of familial cases result from chromosomal rearrangements. The causative GENE is located on 17p. Most cases arise from de novo (spontaneous) MUTATION. Most (90%) result from deletion in 17p, due to some CHROMOSOME ABNORMALITY. If the deletion is de novo, recurrence risk is negligible. Recurrence risk can be high where the rearrangement is familial rather than spontaneous. In this circumstance, PRENATAL DIAGNOSIS is possible. The deletion can be identified using FISH with genetic probes from the Miller-Dieker region of 17p.

The specific gene involved in isolated lissencephaly is the LIS-1 gene, which has undergone a point mutation. The facial dysmorphism and other features of Miller-Dieker syndrome result form the deletion of other contiguous genes. Thus Miller-Dieker lissencephaly syndrome (MDLS) is a CONTIGUOUS GENE SYNDROME.

Minimata disease   CONGENITAL mercury poisoning seen in the town of Minimata in southern Japan. Affected infants were among the offspring of pregnant women who ate fish from Minimata Bay, seafood that had high levels of mercury from industrial wastes discharged into the bay. Between 1953, when it was first observed, and 1971, 134 cases were reported. The mercury caused central nervous system disorders, resulting in death in an estimated 38% of affected infants and brain damage in more than 25% of the survivors. Affected infants had small heads (MICROCEPHALY) and severe brain damage manifest as CEREBRAL PALSY. A similar epidemic occurred in Niigata, Japan, in 1964.

miryachit   A "jumping disorder" reported in Siberia (in the present Russia) in the late 19th century, characterized by an exaggerated startle response, similar to JUMPING FRENCHMEN OF MAINE. Miryachit,

which means "to act foolishly," was characterized by extreme imitative behavior.

miscarriage   See ABORTION.

mitochondrial diseases (Kearns-Sayre syndrome; MELAS syndrome; MERRF syndrome)   A group of rare encephalomyopathies, disorders affecting the brain and muscle, characterized by defects in the mitochondria, the organelles inside cells that control metabolism. (See MITOCHONDRIAL INHERITANCE.) These disorders include Kearns-Sayre syndrome, MELAS syndrome and MERRF syndrome.

Kearns-Sayre syndrome is characterized by cardiomyopathy, neuropathy, ophthalmoplegia and retinal disease. The characteristic cardiac abnormalities may cause arrhythmias and heart block. Paralysis of the eye muscles (ophthalmoplegia) and droopy eyelids (PTOSIS) are characteristic ocular manifestations. Retinal degeneration may also occur resulting in impaired vision. Muscles in the arms and legs may also be abnormally weak. MENTAL RETARDATION, ataxia, DEAFNESS and short stature are also common.

Kearns-Sayre syndrome is caused by a mitochondrial deletion in most cases, but may also result from a point MUTATION in a nuclear GENE. Onset is before 20 years of age, and both sexes are affected equally.

MELAS syndrome takes its acronymic name from mitochondrial encephalopathy, lactic acidosis and stroke that characterize the disorder. The repeated stroke-like episodes have their onset between five and 15 years of age, and begin with sudden headaches followed by vomiting and seizures. Associated symptoms include hemiparesis, cortical blindness and hemianopsia (blindness in half the field of vision). LACTIC ACIDOSIS, progressive dementia and short stature are also common. The disorder results from a mutation in the mitochondrial DNA. Inheritance patterns are difficult to ascertain. Milder forms of the SYNDROME have been seen in relatives of affected individuals, and in some cases these individuals may be asymptomatic.

MERRF syndrome's acronymic designation is taken from the disorder's hallmarks: myoclonus epilepsy associated with ragged red fibers. The ragged, red fibers, seen in muscle tissue, are actually present in all three of these disorders. Myoclonic seizures are what sets this one apart. Affected individuals may also exhibit lactic acidosis, ataxia, muscle weakness, ocular deficiencies, short stature and hearing loss. Onset begins in childhood to early adulthood and symptoms become more pronounced over time. It is caused by a mutation in a mitochondrial gene.

Overlapping symptoms of the three disorders can complicate diagnosis and differentiation.

mitochondrial inheritance   The mitochondria are organelles inside the cell that perform a variety of metabolic functions, most important the synthesis of ATP by the process of oxidative phosphorylation, which provides the cell's energy. Mitochondria have their own DEOXYRIBONUCLEIC ACID, distinct from that of the cell's nucleus, all inherited maternally, from the mother. Prior to conception, the mitochondrial DNA is already in the egg; none is in the sperm. There are hundreds of mitochondria in each cell, and each mitochondrion has from two to 10 or more CHROMOSOMES. Mitochondrial DNA molecules encode for proteins that create ENZYME complexes required for oxidative phosphorylation.

MUTATIONS in mitochondrial genes are responsible for some GENETIC DISORDERS. Due to the maternal inheritance, any disorder caused by a mitochondrial genetic mutation is passed on only by females. Though males can be affected by these disorders, they cannot transmit them, nor are their children at risk of being CARRIERS (unless, of course, the mother also possesses a mitochondrial mutation). Females sometimes may be symptomless carriers, and all the offspring are at risk of developing the disorder, but only daughters of such carriers are at risk of transmitting it to their offspring.

The disorders suspected of being transmitted by this non-Mendelian inheritance pattern include MELAS, MERFF, Kearns-Sayre syndrome, rare forms of familial DEAFNESS and DIABETES MELLITUS, and various central nervous system degenerations. LEBER'S OPTIC ATROPHY has been clearly shown to be transmitted in this manner.

All relatives at genetic risk are likely to exhibit some degree of mitochondrial defect upon molecular analysis, but the correlation between the level of abnormal mitochondrial DNA found in the blood and the development of mitochondrial disorders is unclear. Each cell has many mitochondria, and some may exhibit mutations in their GENOME while others do not. Thus, PRENATAL DIAGNOSIS of these disorders is not possible.

mitral valve prolapse   See HEART DEFECTS.

Moebius sequence (congenital facial diplegia) Form of CONGENITAL facial paralysis first described by Dr. P. J. Moebius in 1888. It is caused by the abnormalities in the sixth and seventh cranial nerves or the portions of the brain from which they derive.

Patients often have a small jaw. The tongue may be small or immobile. About one-third may have CLUBFOOT (talipes equinovarus) and permanently bent fingers (flexion contractures; see CAMPTODACTYLY and ARTHROGRYPOSIS) have been associated with some cases. Feeding difficulties and problems with aspiration may lead to FAILURE TO THRIVE in infancy. Children have expressionless faces, which, along with speech impediments common in this condition, may lead to difficulties with social acceptance. In many cases the condition appears to result from insufficient blood supply to those structures that are supplied by the subclavian artery during intrauterine development. Tube feeding may be necessary. Facial surgery with muscle transfer may help correct abnormalities of the eyes and face. More external cranial nerve involvement or MENTAL RETARDATION is seen in about 15% of cases, and the SYNDROME may be associated with other non-neurologic defects as well.

Moebius sequence is very rare. Most commonly a SPORADIC occurrence, in some cases AUTOSOMAL DOMINANT inheritance is suspected.

Mohr syndrome   See ORAL-FACIAL-DIGITAL SYNDROME.

mongolian spots   Blue-gray areas of discolored skin seen on the lower back, thighs and sometimes shoulders of the newborn. These spots are benign and gradually fade. They are estimated to occur on 80% of non-white and 10% of white infants.

mongolism An archaic term previously used to describe individuals with DOWN SYNDROME, or trisomy 21, a CONGENITAL form of MENTAL RETARDATION. (See also CHROMOSOME ABNORMALITIES.) Its name was taken from the characteristic appearance of the eyes in this disorder: The eye slits (palpebral fissures) slant upward, away from the nose (mongoloid obliquity) and a small excess of skin adjacent to the nose obscures the juncture of the bottom and top eyelids. This is called an EPICANTHAL FOLD. Both mongoloid obliquity and epicanthal folds, while associated with numerous BIRTH DEFECTS and inherited congenital SYNDROMES in Western populations, are normal in Asians, hence the appellation.

monilethrix A defect of the hair shaft characterized by beaded and brittle hair. (The beaded appearance is observable under a microscope.) It usually appears by the second month of life and may result in ALOPECIA, the loss of scalp hair. The degree of hair loss among affected individuals is variable and may fluctuate over time. While there is no effective treatment, one affected individual reportedly responded to endocrine therapy.

Monilethrix is inherited as an AUTOSOMAL DOMINANT trait and has been studied extensively in several families. The disorder results from MUTATIONS in the type II hair cortex keratin GENE, mapped to chromosome 12q. These keratins are the major structural proteins of the hair shaft, and are also found in nails.

monosodium glutamate sensitivity See CHINESE RESTAURANT SYNDROME.

monosomy See CHROMOSOME ABNORMALITIES.

Mormon There are approximately 1 million Mormons in the religious community centered in the Salt Lake City, Utah, area. Most are descended from 20,000 pioneers who came to the area little more than a century ago. They tend to have large, extended families (some numbering in the thousands) and, due to church teachings, keep detailed records of their ancestors and ancestry. These provide perhaps the most extensive PEDIGREES available to genetic researchers. A computerized data base of these genealogical records has been created, as well. For these reasons, some Mormon families have been extensively studied by geneticists seeking data on the heritability of diseases, particularly CANCERS of the colon, breast and lung, and melanoma.

Morquio syndrome See MUCOPOLYSACCHARIDOSIS.

mosaicism The condition in which an individual has two different populations of cells, both derived from the same fertilized egg. (In contrast to a CHIMERA, where two populations of cells come from two fertilized eggs.) The cell populations may differ in KARYOTYPE—complement of CHROMOSOMES-or genotype—the GENES. Thus, an individual could have cells with a normal complement of chromosomes and cells with an abnormal complement, or cells with a gene MUTATION and other cells in which the gene mutation is absent.

The condition arises when an abnormality in chromosomal division or a gene mutation occurs soon after fertilization. Subsequently, this aberration is exhibited in those cells descended from this first chromosomally or genetically aberrant cell, while the remainder are normal. Among the conditions in which mosaicism is sometimes seen is DOWN SYNDROME.

Germline or gonadal mosaicism is said to exist when there are two or more genetically distinct or different populations of germline or gonadal (sex) cells, that is, sperm and eggs, resulting from a mutation during the production of these cells. The mosaicism in this case is limited to the sex cells and some of the cells will be "normal" and some will carry the mutation. This can lead to the situation where apparently unaffected parents have two children affected with an AUTOSOMAL DOMINANT disease. The birth of the first would have looked like a SPORADIC case due to a new mutation. However the birth of the second suggests that the new mutation occurred in a "precursor" cell in one of the parent's gonads (ovary or testes) within the cell line from which the gametes are produced. This has resulted in gametes being produced with the disease-causing mutation from an individual who does not have the mutation in the other cells of his or her body and is thus not affected with the disease him or herself.

In females, in any one cell, only one X CHROMOSOME (of the two) is active, and the other is inactivated. This process of X inactivation is random, and either X chromosome (paternal or maternal) may be "switched off" in each individual cell. This process occurs early in embryonic life and thus all females are in a sense mosaics since they have two populations of cells: one population with the maternal X active, one with the paternal X active. Therefore females are mosaic with respect to most X-LINKED genes.

Mowat-Wilson syndrome A rare hereditary developmental disorder characterized by mild to moderate mental retardation, delayed motor development, epilepsy, Hirschsprung disease and dysmorphic facial features. The association of these characteristics had been described for some 20 years before D. R. Mowat and M. J. Wilson provided the first detailed clinical description in 1998.

The facial features include small head (microcephaly), widely spaced eyes (hypertelorism) that are deeply set, turned-up ear lobes, small mouth and prominent chin. Other commonly observed congenital anomalies include congenital heart disease, hypospadias, genitourinary anomalies, agenesis of the corpus callosum and short stature.

An autosomal dominant trait, most, though not all, affected individuals have a deletion or truncating mutation of the *ZFHX1B* (or *SIP1*) gene mapped to 2q22. Prevalence is unknown. A total of 47 cases had been reported by 2004. Prenatal diagnosis may be possible, but would only be called for if a previous child had been affected.

mucolipidosis (ML) A group of rare hereditary ENZYME deficiency diseases. In each of these, the deficiency of a single enzyme causes various chemical substances to accumulate in cells throughout the body, resulting in progressive damage that ranges from problems in the joints leading to decreased mobility, to severe mental and physical retardation

with complications in all organ systems. Because the disorder involves the accumulation or "storage" of these compounds, it is one of a group of disorders called STORAGE DISEASES. However, what is stored is not actually a lipid in many cases, and therefore, some authorities have proposed changing the named mucolipidosis to oligosaccharidosis. (See MUCOPOLYSACCHARIDOSIS for a discussion of a group of storage diseases that share many of the features of ML; other disorders often grouped with the mucolipidoses are FUCOSIDOSIS, MANNOSIDOSIS and ASPARTYLGLUCOSAMINURIA.)

The combined incidence of the various forms of ML is estimated at one in 25,000 live births. There are four recognized types of this condition, all transmitted as AUTOSOMAL RECESSIVE traits. PRENATAL DIAGNOSIS is possible with AMNIOCENTESIS and CHORIONIC VILLUS SAMPLING.

Mucolipidosis I-sialidosis A disorder resulting from the deficiency of the enzyme neuraminidase, producing neurologic abnormalities (see NEURAMINIDASE DEFICIENCY).

Mucolipidosis II-I-cell disease Characterized by the early onset of severe psychomotor retardation and short stature, the face has a typical coarse appearance with thick hair, a high narrow forehead, heavy eyelashes, depressed nasal bridge, upturned nose (ante-verted nares) and low-set ears. The upper lip is thick, and the gums are very markedly enlarged. The teeth rarely erupt. The hands and feet are stubby, and the wrists widened.

Repeated respiratory infections are common during the first year of life, along with FAILURE TO THRIVE and lack of psychomotor development. Death usually occurs before the age of six years. The fundamental defect is in an enzyme that "targets" many other enzymes to the lysosomes (the "digestive" organelles of the cell). The affected enzyme is known as lysosomal phosphotransferase, and appears to map to 4q (the long arm of chromosome 4). These secondary enzymes' activities are deficient within the lysosome, allowing the molecules that these enzymes should have digested to accumulate. This accumulation has a characteristic appearance termed "I-cell," for inclusion cell.

HETEROZYGOTES cannot be detected, but prenatal diagnosis can be accomplished by AMNIOCENTESIS.

In the French-Canadian population of the Saguenay–Lac St. Jean region of the French province, it has been estimated that the prevalence at birth is 1/6,184, giving a CARRIER frequency of 1/39.

Mucolipidosis III (pseudo-Hurler polydystrophy) First described in 1966, and characterized by growth retardation and progressive stiffening of the joints, this is essentially a milder form of I-cell disease. Joint stiffness (unaccompanied by pain or swelling) begins by two to four years of age, primarily affecting the hands and shoulders. Clawhands, the extreme permanent bending of the joints at the ends of the fingers, become apparent by age six. Although less severe than MLII, most affected individuals do not survive beyond age 30.

The facial features are broad and coarse, the neck short. During formative years, the joints of the hips and elbows become affected. Carpal tunnel syndrome, a soreness and weakness of the thumb, may develop. The skin becomes tight and hardened. The corneas of the eyes show progressive clouding. As the mobility of the joints decreases, individuals may be unable to raise their arms above their heads. At eight to 10 years, they are usually below the third percentile in height for their age. Joint stiffness stabilizes around the time of puberty.

Additional common findings include mild MENTAL RETARDATION, congenital HEART DEFECTS and enlargement of the liver and spleen (hepatosplenomegaly).

By adulthood, joint stiffness results in a considerable HANDICAP. Surgery can often correct the carpal tunnel syndrome. The progressive destruction of the hip joints, which may be apparent by the late teens, is the most disabling aspect of the disorder.

As in ML II (I-cell disease), there is a deficiency or abnormality of glycoprotein nacetylglucosaminylphosphotransferase activity. In ML III the defect is partial, while in ML II it is complete.

Mucolipidosis IV First described in 1974, the features, which manifest during the first year of life are profound mental and motor retardation and visual impairment. Individuals' motor development never progresses beyond the age of 15 months. None can walk unsupported. Many cannot sit up without being supported. None can control utensils with their fingers. Language abilities also never progress beyond this developmental age. Some may verbalize five to 10 words, but most are completely uncommunicative. Corneal clouding is the usual first sign. Retinal degeneration and BLINDNESS are also features.

There are no abnormalities of the skeleton or internal organs, and there has been speculation that many cases may remain undiagnosed. The condition can be confirmed by electron microscopic examination of cells, which reveal the abnormal storage organelles (specialized areas within the cells) that typify the disorder. About 70% of individuals with mucolipidosis IV (MLIV) are of Ashkenazi Jewish background. The gene associated with MLIV is the *MCOLN1* gene. Two mutations account for 95% of mutations in individuals of Ashkenazi Jewish descent, permitting carrier detection in this population. The prognosis and life span of individuals are unknown, though patients have survived into their mid-20s.

mucopolysaccharidosis (MPS)   A group of hereditary STORAGE DISEASES; because of an ENZYME deficiency specific to each type, mucopolysaccharides are not properly metabolized, and therefore accumulate or are "stored" within the cells. This accumulation typically results in multiple problems, including severe skeletal deformities and MENTAL RETARDATION.

Mucopolysaccharides are components of various kinds of connective tissue, and include dermatan sulfate, an important constituent of skin and blood vessels, and heparan sulfate, typically found in the walls of blood vessels. Excess mucopolysaccharides leak from their storage sites into the urine and form the basis of several common screening tests for the disorder.

At least six basic types (most encompassing several sub-types) have been identified. All are inherited as AUTOSOMAL RECESSIVE (AR) traits, except for Hunter syndrome (MPS II), which is inherited as an X-LINKED recessive trait and is seen only in males. Overall incidence of MPS is estimated at one in 25,000 live births.

Enzyme replacement therapy, bone marrow transplantation (BMT) and GENE therapy are all being investigated as possible treatments for the MPS disorders. There appears to be some benefit in BMT but because of the high risk and uncertainties about the long-term neurologic outcome, the utility of this procedure is still not clear and is the subject of research.

Types of MPS include MPS I—Hurler syndrome, Scheie syndrome, Hurler/Scheie syndrome; MPS II—Hunter syndrome, mild and Hunter syndrome, severe; MPS III—Sanfilippo-A, Sanfilippo-B, Sanfilippo-C, Sanfilippo-D; MPS IV—Morquio-A, Morquio-B; MPS V—Vacant, formerly Scheie syndrome; MPS VI—Maroteaux-Lamy, classic severe; Maroteaux-Lamy, intermediate and Maroteaux-Lamy, mild; and MPS VII—Sly. Following are descriptions of the more prevalent forms of MPS.

Hurler syndrome (MPS IH)   The classic features of this disorder are growth failure after infancy, mental retardation, HUMPBACK and short, broad bones, especially in the hands, which lead to stiffness and limitation in movement of the joints. It is named for German pediatrician Gertrud Hurler (1889–1965), who described the condition in 1919.

Decelerated physical and mental growth becomes apparent during the latter part of the first year. Growth usually stops by two years of age. The face develops coarse features, including prominent forehead, thick earlobes, full lips and broad, low nasal bridge. Corneal clouding is present. The nostrils are upturned (anteverted nares), and a continual runny nose is common. The mouth is usually held open, especially after the age of three years. There is a protruding abdomen, deformity of the chest, shortness of the spine and enlargement of the liver and spleen (hepatosplenomegaly). Mental retardation becomes more severe with age. Death usually occurs by age 10 due to pneumonia or heart failure. It is caused by the deficiency of the enzyme alpha-L-iduronidase.

The gene has been mapped to 4p and identified, and though multiple MUTATIONS have been found, two account for 60–80% of cases. Molecular techniques can be used for CARRIER detection and PRENATAL DIAGNOSIS in families in which the mutation has been identified.

Prenatal diagnosis may be made based on studies of enzyme activity in cultured fetal cells obtained by AMNIOCENTESIS or CHORIONIC VILLUS SAMPLING.

Scheie syndrome (MPS I-S)   This form is characterized by moderately short stature, clouding of the corneas, and joint limitations leading to clawed hand. Intelligence is normal. No major abnormalities are seen in infancy until the appearance of progressive corneal clouding, which leads to decreased vision by the third or fourth decade. It is named

for Harold Scheie, professor of ophthalmology at the University of Pennsylvania, who described it in 1962. Patients tend to have moderately short, stocky and muscular physiques, with a short neck and broad, short hands. The same mucopolysaccharides accumulate as in Hurler syndrome and the same enzyme, alpha-L-iduronidase, is deficient.

MPS IH (Hurler) and MPS IS (Scheie) represent variable presentations at either end of a spectrum of severity of this enzyme deficiency. Affected individuals may also present with an intermediate form of the disorder and are said to have MPS IH/S. Individuals with this intermediate form have early-onset severe joint stiffness, difficulties with growth, chronic respiratory problems, progressive obstruction of the upper airway passages, clouding of the cornea, cardiac valvular disease, spinal cord compression and death in the third to fourth decades of life, usually from the cardiopulmonary complications of the disease. In the past, treatment of all forms of MPS I involved symptomatic, supportive treatment of the complications of the disease. Treatment with enzyme replacement therapy is now available. Patients with a very severe disease (MPS IH), who are diagnosed before the onset of severe mental retardation, are treated by bone marrow transplantation when a suitable donor is available. This has been shown to halt the primary neurologic deterioration seen in the disease.

Hunter syndrome (MPS II)   This syndrome, which has a mild and a severe form, has the symptoms of a less severe form of Hurler syndrome (MPS I), with onset typically between the ages of two and four years. It is named for Charles Hunter (1873–1955), a prominent physician in Winnipeg, Canada, who described it in 1917, calling it "gargoylism." During his military service in London in World War I, Hunter presented two brothers with the condition at the Royal Academy of Medicine. He intended the term gargoylism to describe the coarse facial features of affected individuals and to suggest the appearance of gargoyles decorating the architecture of churches such as Notre Dame cathedral. (It came to be used to describe other mucopolysaccharidoses as well.) However, similar features are common to many genetic conditions. Considered demeaning and insensitive, the term *gargoylism* is no longer used.

Characteristic facial appearance includes a flat nose with wide nostrils and depressed nasal bridge, thick lips, tongue and gums. Individuals often have excessive hair (hypertrichosis) and low hairlines. Breathing is noisy, accompanied by runny nose. The liver and spleen are enlarged. Mental deficiency often becomes apparent at approximately age five or six years. Deterioration is typically progressive after age five or six. In severe cases, physical activity decreases, speech is reduced, there is difficulty ingesting solid food and weight decreases. Respiratory infections may become more severe and frequent, and may cause death. Cardiac complications may also lead to death.

In the severe form, death usually occurs between the ages of five and 14 years, though survival to age 60 has been reported in the milder form.

Corneal clouding seen in MPS I is absent in this form. An X-LINKED recessive disorder, it results from iduronate sulfatase deficiency. The gene has been identified and a number of mutations found. The frequency of the disease appears to be about one in 100,000–130,000 live male births, although it appears to be more common among Israeli Jews (one in 34,000 live births). Female carriers can be detected by enzyme assay, and prenatal diagnosis is possible. Enzyme replacement therapy for the disorder is now available.

Sanfilippo syndrome (MPS III)   First recognized in 1963, this appears to be the most common form of MPS, manifest primarily as a neurologic disease. It bears the name of U.S. pediatrician Sylvester J. Sanfilippo, who described it in 1963. Growth is normal or accelerated for one to three years, followed by slow growth. Joint mobility is only mildly restricted in the elbows and knees. The face develops coarse features, including moderate enlargement of the head, sunken nasal bridge, heavy eyebrows and eyelashes, thick lips and abundant, coarse scalp hair. Behavioral problems include restlessness, aggressiveness, diminished attention span and sleep disturbances. These behavioral problems are often what bring individuals to the attention of physicians. Mental development slows and then deteriorates by 18 months to three years of age. Eventually individuals regress to a vegetative state.

Individuals may die during adolescence due to pneumonia, though one-third may survive into their thirties. Prenatal diagnosis is available through enzyme assay. There are, however, four types of this syndrome, each with different enzyme deficiencies. The exact form of the disease must be determined in each family for accurate diagnostic testing.

Morquio syndrome (MPS IV)   First described in 1929 by Luis Morquio (1867–1935), professor of pediatrics in Montevideo, Uruguay, this form of MPS is marked by growth failure and progressive spinal deformity. Essentially a skeletal dysplasia, there are two major types, each caused by a different enzyme deficiency.

The first symptoms, flaring of the rib cage, frequent upper respiratory tract infections, hernias and growth deficiency, become apparent by 19 months to two years of age. The facial features become coarse, with broad mouth, widely spaced teeth and upturned nose (anteverted nares). The neck is very short, and the head appears to rest directly on the shoulders. Abnormalities of the bones of the spine in the neck can lead to injury to the spinal cord. The extremities appear disproportionately long, as the trunk is shortened due to involvement of the bones of the spine. Individuals exhibit a semicrouching stance with "knock-knees." Corneal clouding occurs after age 10, and progressive DEAFNESS during adolescence. Adult height rarely exceeds 39 inches (about 1 meter). Intelligence is usually normal.

Prenatal diagnosis is available by studying cultured fetal tissue for enzyme activity. Though respiratory insufficiency or cardiac complications may result in death in adolescence, longer survival has been reported.

Maroteaux-Lamy syndrome (MPS VI)   This syndrome was originally described in 1963 by Pierre Maroteaux, the director of the National Center for Scientific Research at the Hospital des Enfants Malades in Paris, and Maurice Lamy (1905–75), the first professor of medical genetics at the University of Paris. Development is usually normal until approximately age six, when small stature and spinal deformities are noted. The chest is deformed with a prominent sternum, and the face exhibits coarse features common to MPS: large head, thick eyebrows and scalp hair, flat nasal bridge and upturned nose (anteverted nares), full cheeks and lips. In the more severe form, there is rapid progression to disability with short stature, marked facial and skeletal abnormalities, severely impaired vision and hearing, and prominent cardiac defects. While intelligence is normal, impaired vision and hearing, restricted mobility and psychological adjustment problems may impede the individual's abilities.

Individuals with the mild form have normal life spans. In the severe form, most succumb to cardiorespiratory problems by the end of the second decade. Enzyme replacement therapy for the disorder is under development.

The deficient enzyme is arylsulfatase B (ASB), the gene for which maps to 5q. Prenatal diagnosis is possible by assaying enzyme activity in fetal cells collected by amniocentesis or chorionic villus sampling.

Sly (MPS VII) Described in 1973 by U.S. pediatrician and genetics professor William S. Sly, symptoms of this more recently identified form are often visible at birth or appear within the first year of life and include growth retardation, joint contractures and spinal malformations. The characteristic coarse face, short stature and developmental retardation are also present, and there appears to be variability of severity of the symptoms among patients' as with the other forms of MPS. Because few cases have been described, long-term prognosis is unknown.

The causative gene has been mapped to 7q. Prenatal diagnosis is possible by analysis of fetal cells, as with other forms of MPS.

multifactorial A general term for disorders that have their origins in the effects of one or more

TABLE XVI
FREQUENCIES OF THE MOST COMMON MULTIFACTORIAL DISORDERS FOUND IN A SURVEY CONDUCTED IN BRITISH COLUMBIA, CANADA

Multifactorial Condition	1952–63		1964–73		1974–83		Total	
	N	Rate[a]	N	Rate[a]	N	Rate	N	Rate[a]
Diabetes mellitus	526	1,202.3	382	1,108.3	103	265.7	1,011	864.2
Schizophrenic psychoses	181	413.7	1	2.9	0	0.0	182	155.6
Affective psychoses	10	22.9	0	0.0	0	0.0	10	8.5
Borderline mental retardation	314	717.7	63	182.8	1	2.6	378	323
Mild mental retardation	181	413.7	37	107.4	5	12.9	223	190.6
Epilepsy	807	1,844.6	502	1,456.5	228	588.1	1,537	1,313.8
Strabismus	924	2,112.0	3,566	10,346.3	1,450	3,740.0	5,940	5.077.5
Asthma	124	283.4	53	153.8	71	183.1	248	212.0
Inguinal hernia	0	0.0	196	568.7	1,997	5,150.8	2,193	1,874.6
Eczema	37	84.6	4	11.6	3	7.7	44	37.6
Anencephaly	58	132.6	45	130.6	50	129.0	153	130.8
Spina bifida	214	489.1	117	339.5	67	172.8	398	3,40.2
Encephalocele	5	11.4	7	20.3	8	20.6	20	17.1
Congenital hydrocephalus	48	109.7	99	287.2	76	196.0	223	190.6
Congenital anomalies of heart and circulatory system	1,177	2,690.3	1,699	4,929.4	1,734	4,472.5	4,610	3,940.6
Cleft palate and cleft lip	468	1,069.7	445	1,291.1	431	1,111.7	1,344	1,148.8
Congenital hypertrophic pyloric stenosis	23	52.6	805	2,335.6	909	2,344.6	1,737	1,484.8
Hirschsprung disease, etc.	9	20.6	60	174.1	43	110.9	112	95.7
Hypospadias and epispadias	102	233.1	558	1,619.0	620	1,599.2	1,280	1,094.1
Clubfoot	679	1,552.0	1,433	4,157.7	1,967	5,073.4	4,079	3,486.7
Congenital dislocation of hip	197	450.3	878	2,547.4	1,322	3,409.8	2,397	2,048.9
Congenital dislocatable hip	0	0.0	12	34.8	622	1,604.3	634	541.9
Total	6,084	13,906.2	10,962	31,804.8	11,707	30,195.6	28,753	24,577.9

[a]Per 1 million live births.

Source: Patricia A. Baird, "A Population Study of Genetic Disorders in Children and Young Adults," *American Journal of Human Genetics* 42 (1988), pp. 677–693.

GENES, environmental influences and/or unknown factors acting in combination. (Though the term POLYGENIC is used interchangeably with multifactorial by some, polygenic properly refers to a disorder resulting from the action of two or more genes.) Multifactorial disorders often appear in familial clusters, though they do not conform to dominant or recessive patterns of heredity. They are the most common and least understood of genetic disorders; little is known regarding their exact cause. (See Table XVI.)

Multifactorial disorders include CLEFT LIP or CLEFT PALATE, congenital HEART DEFECTS, NEURAL TUBE DEFECTS (SPINA BIFIDA and ANENCEPHALY), SCHIZOPHRENIA and ESSENTIAL HYPERTENSION.

Risks of recurrence in a given family in which one member has a multifactorial disorder are low, generally estimated in the realm of 3%. Some multifactorial disorders are more common in one gender. In these gender-linked multifactorial disorders, risks for recurrence increase when the affected family member is of the sex in which the condition is typically less common. Recurrence risks also increase if multiple family members are affected or if the problem is more severe in the affected individual (e.g., bilateral cleft lip vs. unilateral). (See also AUTOSOMAL DOMINANT; AUTOSOMAL RECESSIVE; MENDELIAN.)

multiple acyl-CoA dehydrogenase   See GLUTARIC ACIDURIA.

multiple births   Giving birth to more than one child from a single pregnancy. Multiple births are associated with increased risks for miscarriage (see ABORTION), as well as greater risks for maternal and infant health and survival. BIRTH DEFECTS and LOW BIRTH WEIGHT are more common in multiple births, as well.

Multiple births have long been the object of interest and speculation. In his *History of Animals*, Aristotle wrote that five was the maximum of infants a woman was capable of producing in a single pregnancy (quintuplets). However, reports of women giving birth to six (sextuplets) and seven (septuplets) infants have been somewhat common

from Aristotle's time to the present. Yet no valid reports of such a birth were recorded until 1888, when the birth of septuplets was documented in Italy (and promptly criticized for contradicting Aristotle's teachings). In 1938 *Look* magazine reported finding a family of septuplets born in 1866, four of whom reached adulthood. In 1997, the world's first complete surviving set, the McCaughey septuplets, were born in Carlisle, Iowa. Due to the developmental problems associated with multiple births, at one year of age they exhibited the maturation of 10-month-old infants.

Multiple births, and their associated problems, have become more common as more women use fertility drugs in an effort to conceive. (Reliable statistics on women taking fertility drugs in the United States are difficult to acquire, but their numbers are believed to have grown substantially since 1990, when an estimated 20,000 women took such drugs; see CLOMIPHENE CITRATE.) These drugs may result in pregnancies in which as many as nine embryos begin to develop at one time. In these situations, intervention may attempt selectively to abort all but one or two of the developing embryos as none would otherwise survive to term. In 1997, the National Center for Health Statistics reported the number of U.S. women having triplets and multiple births more than quadrupled over the previous two decades. In 1994, 4,594 multiple births were recorded, compared to 1,034 registered in 1971. The rate was highest among married, college educated women aged 30 or older. (See also TWINS.)

multiple endocrine neoplasias (MEN)   Genetically influenced CANCERS of the endocrine glands. These rare conditions are classified into MEN I, II and III based on the site and characteristics of the tumors.

In MEN I, individuals may develop neoplasms or tumors that may appear in more than one gland, including the parathyroids (90%), pancreas (80%), pituitary (65%), adrenal cortex (35%) and thyroid glands (20%). By interfering with the hormonal secretion of these glands, the cancers may produce abnormalities in the bones, kidneys and mucous membranes, enlargement of extremities, headaches and visual disturbances. (The ZOLLINGER-ELLI-

SON SYNDROME of intractable peptic ulcer, caused by overproduction of the hormone gastrin from a tumor of the pancreatic islet cells is a common feature of MEN I.)

Predisposition to develop these cancers is inherited as an AUTOSOMAL DOMINANT trait. The tumors usually develop between the age of 10 and 60. The GENE for MEN I has been found on 11q and many different MUTATIONS identified. Once a specific mutation has been identified in a family, molecular testing can be used for presymptomatic (or prenatal) diagnosis. Even when the specific mutation is not known, if there is an extensive family history, linkage analysis can be used (see GENETIC LINKAGE).

Individuals with MEN IIA typically have specific cancers of the thyroid (medullary carcinoma) affecting the cells that produce calcitonin (a hormone important in calcium metabolism), as well as over-development of the parathyroid gland and tumors of the adrenal medulla or related nerve tissue (pheochromocytoma). Predisposition is inherited as an autosomal dominant trait. Onset may be anytime from early childhood to 60 years. MEN IIA results from a mutation in the RET proto-oncogene, which maps to chromosome 10.

MEN IIB also results from a mutation in the RET proto-oncogene, albeit a different one that is responsible for MEN IIA. Inherited as an autosomal dominant disorder, affected individuals often exhibit striking, small tumors (neuromas) of mucous tissues, appearing on the lips, tongue, gum, palate, nose and conjunctivae of the eyes. These tumors are usually evident by the age of eight years, and those affected typically have weak and thin physiques with severe muscular wasting and abnormal spinal curvature. They also often have medullary carcinoma of the thyroid or pheochromocytoma like those with MEN II. Onset is from early childhood to age 40.

Other cases of isolated familial medullary carcinoma of the thyroid (also autosomal dominant) are caused by different mutations in the RET gene, as are some cases of HIRSCHSPRUNG disease.

The tumors may become malignant in all forms of MEN, though early detection increases chances for survival. MEN is believed to result from errors in the development of the neural crest, the embryonic structure from which nerve tissue develops. PRENATAL DIAGNOSIS may be possible in families in which a mutation is known or when linkage analysis can be used. When molecular diagnosis is not possible, sensitive hormone assays can be used for early diagnosis.

It is recommended that first-degree relatives (parents, SIBLINGS, offspring) of affected individuals undergo annual examinations unless molecular testing has demonstrated that they have not inherited the MEN SYNDROME gene that is in the family.

multiple epiphyseal dysplasia A group of skeletal disorders affecting bone formation and resulting in DWARFISM. The epiphysis is a secondary bone-forming (ossification) center in the bones of infants, separated from the parent bone by cartilage. Normally, as skeletal growth proceeds, the epiphysis joins with the parent bone. In this group of disorders, the ossification of the epiphyses of the bones of the arms and legs is abnormal, resulting in mild shortening.

Generally, this form of dwarfism remains unrecognized until the ages of five to 10 years, when short stature begins to become apparent. The dwarfing is of the short-limbed variety, with trunk size remaining normal. The hands, and particularly the thumbs, may appear short and stubby. Affected individuals may exhibit a waddling gait, difficulty in running or climbing stairs, and experience pain and stiffness in the limbs and joints, particularly of the lower limbs. Degenerative arthritis of the hips is common in older individuals under medical care. Physical activities may be limited in those severely affected. Intelligence and life span are normal.

The various forms of multiple epiphyseal dysplasia may be inherited as AUTOSOMAL DOMINANT or AUTOSOMAL RECESSIVE traits, though most are dominant.

More severely affected individuals with autosomal dominant MED are referred to as having Fairbank disease. The milder form is often known as Ribbing type. Multiple epiphyseal dysplasia of the Fairbank type, as well as pseudoachondroplasia, is due to a MUTATION in the GENE for cartilage oligomeric matrix protein, found on 19p. Other families with autosomal dominant MED have been shown to have mutations in the gene for the alpha-2 chain of type IX collagen (COL9A2), found on

1p. Still other families with autosomal dominant MED have mutations in the *COL9A1, COL9A3* and *matrilin-3 (MATN3)* genes. Thus, mutations in five genes have been shown to cause dominant MED. However, in approximately 50% of all families with MED a mutation cannot be identified in any of these five genes; thus other genes must also be involved in causing dominant MED. Mutations in *SLC26A2 (DTDST)* gene cause autosomal recessive MED. Mutations in the DTDST gene in addition to recessive multiple epiphyseal dysplasia also cause diastrophic dysplasia, achondrogenesis type IB and atelosteogensis type 2. Thus this group of disorders exhibits much genetic HETEROGENEITY.

multiple exostoses   An exostosis is an extraneous, bony growth on a bone itself. In this disorder, exostoses appear at the end of the long bones, causing deformities of the forearms, knees, ankles, spine and pelvis. The shortened legs may cause short stature, and if the vertebrae are affected, the resulting compression of the spinal cord may cause numbness or paralysis.

Growth of the exostoses stops shortly after puberty. In a small number of cases (about 1–3%), the exostoses may turn malignant. Tumors that compress nerves, hinder movement or cause pain may be removed surgically.

Inherited as an autosomal dominant trait, two genes have been identified as being responsible for the vast majority of cases: the *EXT1* and *EXT2* genes on the long arm of chromosome 8 and short arm of chromosome 11, respectively. Another gene possibly involved may map to the short arm of chromosome 19. One hospital reported one in 90,000 patients have multiple exostoses. The Chamorros of Guam reportedly have a high incidence of this disorder.

multiple lentigines syndrome (LEOPARD syndrome)   The secondary name of this condition refers to the many freckles (lentigines) covering the face and body in 80% of cases, and is also an acronym for the features of this disorder. (Lentigines differ from freckles in that they are darker, present at birth and not related to exposure to the sun.) LEOPARD stands for lentigines, ECG abnormalities, ocular hypertelorism, pulmonic stenosis, abnormalities of genitalia, retardation of growth, and DEAFNESS. In addition, half of all affected infants display winged shoulder blades, and 35% show some degree of thick, webbed folds of skin from jawbone to mid-shoulder (pterigium coli).

About 95% of affected infants show electrocardiographic (ECG) changes indicating abnormalities in the transfer of heart impulses from one chamber to another (interventricular conduction). Equally common is abnormal narrowing of the heart valve leading to the blood vessel carrying blood to the lungs (pulmonary stenosis). Growth is retarded in 90% of cases, and 75% have very wide-set eyes (HYPERTELORISM).

About half of all affected males also have genital abnormalities such as failure of one or both testicles to descend (CRYPTORCHISM) or a urethral opening on the underside of the penis (HYPOSPADIAS). Deafness due to a lesion in the ear's cochlea occurs in about 35%.

Less common findings include triangular face with prominent forehead (bossing), drooping eyelids (PTOSIS) and other cardiac anomalies such as enlarged heart (hypertrophic cardiomyopathy), abnormal aortic valve (aortic valvular dysplasia) and a hole in the septum, which normally separates the heart's two atria (atrial septal defect).

LEOPARD syndrome is usually detected by age four or five, when lentigines become abundant, though some affected infants never develop lentigines. Detection is easy in cases with the characteristic lentigines, but even those without them can be screened with a detailed examination for accompanying symptoms. Life expectancy is usually not affected, nor is intelligence, unless hampered by deafness or severe pulmonary stenosis. Surgical correction of cryptorchism and cardiac lesions may be necessary in some cases.

Inherited as an AUTOSOMAL DOMINANT trait, LEOPARD syndrome can be caused by mutations in the *PTPN11* gene. (Other mutations in the same gene cause Noonan syndrome.) The prevalence of this variable disorder is uncertain.

multiple pterygium syndrome (Escobar syndrome)   Pterygia are fibrous malformations exhibiting a webbed appearance. In this disorder webbed folds of skin (pterygia) of the neck and armpit, inner part of the elbow, back of the knee and inner surface of the leg are evident at birth. Other associated defects include rocker bottom feet, deformed joints, webbed fingers (SYNDACTYLY), small penis and scrotum and undescended testicles in males (CRYPTORCHISM), and underdeveloped external genitalia in females. Affected individuals may also exhibit folds of skin at the inner corner of the eyes (EPICANTHUS), downward slanting at the outer corners of the eyelids and mouth, low hairline on the back of the neck, and crouched stance. Skeletal deformities include fusion of neck vertebrae and curvature of the spine. Adults are seldom taller than 4.5 feet.

A severe, lethal form of the disorder exists. A distinct genetic entity, this AUTOSOMAL RECESSIVE trait leads to STILLBIRTH or death in the immediate newborn period due to lack of development of the lungs. An X-LINKED form of the severe lethal type also exists, as do many other pterygium SYNDROMES.

multiple sclerosis (MS)
An autoimmune disorder that causes the immune system to attack myelin, the material that forms the protective sheaths surrounding nerve fibers. Mostly seen in females, onset is usually between the ages of 20 and 40 years. Variable symptoms and severity, and the episodic nature of attacks, make diagnosis difficult. Characteristic signs include blurring of vision, slurring of speech, muscle weakness, loss of balance, depression and frequently euphoria. Estimates of the number of those affected have been put as high as 250,000 in the United States (about one in 1,000 individuals).

Though first-degree relatives (parent, SIBLING, offspring) have been estimated to have a risk 15 times (1–2%) that of the general population's for developing MS, the genetic link is nonetheless weak, and the disorder follows no known pattern of inheritance. The recurrence of MS in sibs increases to 5% if two first-degree relatives are affected and higher still if more are affected. Even identical twins have only a 50% chance or less of both exhibiting the disorder if one of the pair has it. (However, there may be rare forms that are genetically caused.)

Genetic susceptibility to MS appears to be MULTIFACTORIAL. It is more common in whites than in African Americans and Asians, and is rare or absent among Inuits, Bantus and Native Americans. It appears to occur more often in temperate regions around the world.

While the disorder is not hereditary, susceptibility to develop MS appears to have a genetic component. Susceptibility has been linked to a number of different GENES or gene groups. Some of these genes or gene clusters are part of the HLA, complex (see HUMAN LEUKOCYTE ANTIGEN), which plays an important role in regulating the immune system, and others are also linked to immune system functioning. Virus infections and other environmental factors are also thought to contribute to the eventual onset of MS.

Renowned English cellist Jacqueline du Pre succumbed to the disorder at age 42 in 1987. Her story was recounted in a book, *A Genius in the Family*, and movie, *Hilary and Jackie*.

muscular dystrophy
A group of hereditary disorders characterized by progressive muscle weakness and wasting. The disease process causes healthy muscle cells to be replaced by fat and connective tissue. Muscular dystrophies may be transmitted as AUTOSOMAL DOMINANT, AUTOSOMAL RECESSIVE or X-LINKED traits, depending upon the particular form of the disease. New MUTATIONS can also be responsible for some cases.

Duchenne muscular dystrophy (DMD)
Named for Guillaume B. A. Duchenne (1806–75), a French neurologist who first described the disorder in 1861, this is the most common and severe form of muscular dystrophy. It is transmitted as an X-linked trait, though approximately one-third of new cases are thought to be the result of a new mutation. Incidence of DMD is estimated to be one in 3,000 to one in 4,000 male births, and there are about 15,000 DMD patients in the United States at any given time.

Symptoms of the disease become manifest between the ages of two and five years, and include waddling or walking on toes, stumbling, difficulty in running, climbing stairs or getting up from the floor. The wasting of muscles usually begins in the lower trunk and calves, and eventually affects all the major muscle groups. It is sometimes called pseudohypertrophic muscular dystrophy because the enlargement of the calf muscle that is characteristic of this disease is caused not by increased muscle tissue but by the accumulation of fat and connective tissue in the degenerating muscle fibers.

Progression of the disease is rapid. Walking becomes difficult, and skeletal contractures and muscle atrophy follow. Individuals generally require use of a wheelchair by adolescence. A number of children with this type of MD have MENTAL RETARDATION. Death due to respiratory failure usually occurs in adolescence.

Currently, the options for treatment are limited. Physical therapy can delay muscle atrophy and deformities. Orthopedic devices can help maintain mobility. Surgery to lengthen a contracted tendon is sometimes performed, and medication can help relieve muscle stiffness.

In 1986 scientists identified the defective GENE that causes DMD, located on the short arm of the X CHROMOSOME, and in 1987 isolated the protein the normal gene produces. The protein has been named "dystrophin," and is absent in the cells of those with DMD. In 1989 scientists successfully corrected a similar deficiency in mice unable to produce dystrophin by injecting immature muscle cells (myoblasts) into their tissue. Subsequently the mice were able to produce dystrophin. This research may ultimately provide avenues for treating DMD.

Prior to the identification of the defective gene, the primary screening test for DMD CARRIERS and individuals was the presence of highly elevated serum levels of creatine phosphokinase (CPK). This test can identify 60% to 70% of carrier females. About 5% of carriers have some muscle weakness.

Molecular DNA techniques or DNA analysis using the DMD gene have been used in PRENATAL DIAGNOSIS of DMD, as well as for carrier testing in families with individuals affected with DMD, but large scale population screening is not yet available. Antibodies to dystrophin are used in the diagnosis of this disorder by identifying the presence (normally) or absence (in DMD) of dystrophin in muscle tissue obtained by muscle biopsy.

Becker's muscular dystrophy   Similar in mode of transmission to DMD, it manifests itself later in life and progression is slower. Onset is usually in the second or third decade. The protein dystrophin is present in muscle cells of Becker's muscular dystrophy patients, but at levels far below those in unaffected individuals, or the dystrophin is abnormal. Abnormalities of the retinal blood vessels or hearing loss may also be seen. The responsible gene is on 4q, though other genes might also play a role in its onset. Becker and DMD result from different mutations in the same gene. Becker type is one-tenth as common as DMD.

Facio-scapulo-humeral dystrophy   This autosomal dominant form of muscular dystrophy, because of its mode of inheritance, can appear in nearly every generation among families with the disorder. It is the third most common form of dystrophy after DMD and myotonic dystrophy. Expression in families is highly variable; some individuals suffer no disability while others experience early incapacitation.

The dystrophy begins in muscles of the face (facio), shoulder (scapulo) and upper arms (humeral). Symptoms usually become evident in the teens, though they may appear at any time from infancy to middle age. There is facial weakness, such as difficulty in closing eyes, whistling and puckering lips. Abnormalities of the retinal blood vessels or hearing loss may also be seen. Progression is usually slow, though it may be rapid in some cases. Eventually trunk and leg muscles become involved, and individuals may be unable to walk.

As in Becker type and DMD, the causative gene has been mapped to 4q, though other genes may also be involved in this form. A high incidence has been found in Utah and Germany. Family studies are usually necessary to identify all affected individuals and establish the risks of recurrence.

Limb-girdle dystrophy   This dystrophy is generally inherited as an autosomal recessive trait. The symptoms, weakness in the shoulder or pelvis area, can begin to appear anytime from childhood through early adulthood.

The course of the disease is unpredictable. Progression tends to be slow, particularly if the disease begins in the shoulder, rather than pelvic area. Incapacitation occurs after 20 years or more. By middle age most individuals are unable to walk. Life expectancy is slightly diminished.

Genetically heterogeneous (see HETEROGENEITY), a number of different genes are involved, and several encode muscle proteins that are part of what is termed the sarcoglycan complex. Limb-girdle muscular dystrophy also includes rare dominantly inherited subtypes. Carrier testing and prenatal diagnosis may be available in those instances where the specific defect has been identified.

Emery-Dreifuss (rigid spine syndrome) This form, seen almost exclusively in males, affects the arms, legs, spine, face, neck and heart. Initially regarded as solely an X-linked disorder, more recent cases of affected females suggests another mode of inheritance may be involved as well.

Onset is typically four to five years of age. Progression is often slow. Toe walking is usually the first manifestation, followed by weakening of the leg muscles and pelvic girdle, causing a characteristic waddling. Wasting of the shoulder muscles occurs concurrently. Flexion contractures in the elbows and ankles are also seen. The effects on the heart muscle are a critical concern. Pacemakers are recommended for some with cardiac wasting. Heart transplants have been performed on some affected individuals.

Inherited as an X-linked disorder, the gene involved encodes a protein named "emerin."

Congenital (Fukuyama type) First described in 1960, it is seen mainly in Japan, where it is the second most prevalent form of muscular dystrophy. Infants are affected at birth. They are "floppy," with a lack of muscle tone. They often have difficulty sucking and swallowing, and their cries are weak. They may exhibit joint contractures in the elbows and knees, as well as mental retardation, seizures and developmental delays. Few learn to walk. The head is typically small and the brain is structurally abnormal. Death typically occurs by 10 years of age.

Inherited as an autosomal recessive trait, Fukuyama congenital muscular dystrophy is caused by a mutation in the gene encoding fukutin (*FCMD*), located on 9q. Slightly more males than females are affected.

mutagen Any substance capable of causing a genetic MUTATION. Many medicines, chemicals and physical agents such as ionizing radiation, cancer chemotherapeutic agents and ultraviolet light have this mutagenic ability. (See also TERATOGEN.)

mutation Any inheritable change or alteration in genetic material. GENETIC DISORDERS have their origin in mutations that have typically been passed down through generations. However, a proportion of affected individuals may be the result of a new mutation that occurred in the GENES of the sperm or egg of one parent or of the embryo. In some dominant genetic disorders that result in death in infancy, all affected individuals are the result of new mutations. (Mutations are distinct from CHROMOSOME ABNORMALITIES, which are also an important cause of BIRTH DEFECTS.) A point of mutation is a change in a single base pair of DNA. Mutations can also occur in the cells of the body after birth (somatic mutation) and may result in tumors.

The discovery that mutations could be artificially induced by exposure to heavy doses of X-rays, reported by Hermann J. Muller (1890–1967) in 1927, was a major advance in genetic research. Muller, then at the University of Texas, was awarded the Nobel prize in 1946 for his work. (See also RADIATION; TERATOGEN; and the Introduction.)

myasthenia gravis (MG) Translated from its Greek and Latin derivation, myasthenia gravis means "grave muscle weakness," and is characterized by weakness and loss of control over voluntary muscles, most often those responsible for eye movements and eyelids, chewing, swallowing, coughing and facial expression. Muscle control over breathing and the movement of arms and legs may also be affected.

Most cases of MG are not inherited but some show a familial aggregation (2% to 5% of cases) (see FAMILIAL DISEASES), and many of these are believed to be inherited as an AUTOSOMAL RECESSIVE trait, as they most often involve SIBLINGS, though they may not always conform to a simple MENDELIAN transmission pattern.

The familial form usually affects young children or adolescents and onset in adulthood is rare. The muscle weakness is static or only slowly progressive. Most frequently, onset of symptoms occurs in the first year of life, and it responds well to treatment with anti-cholinesterase drugs. The anti-cholinesterase drugs prolong the action of acetylcholine in impulse transmission at the motor end plate (where the nerve transmits the impulse to the muscle), by blocking the action of cholinesterase, which ordinarily stops it. Cases with onset between the age of two and 20 years resemble adult MG. (The adult form is the result of an autoimmune disorder that causes the body to destroy receptors between nerve endings and muscles that normally allow control over movement.)

There is also a familial infantile form of MG, "transient myasthenia gravis of the newborn." This form is caused by passive transfer of antibodies associated with the autoimmune disorder of adult MG to the fetus from a myasthenic mother. It occurs in 10% to 15% of babies born to MG mothers and is characterized by respiratory and feeding difficulties in the neonatal period. There is usually total remission after a few weeks, but it can be life-threatening if untreated during this time.

A GENE for familial infantile MG maps to 17p. A form of autosomal recessive CONGENITAL familial myasthenia gravis appears to be unusually frequent in Jews originating from Iran and Iraq. There is also an autosomal recessive form involving MUTATIONS in the acetylcholine receptor subunit-encoding genes.

myoclonus   A movement disorder characterized by sudden, uncontrollable spasmodic jerking of one or more skeletal muscles. It occurs independent of other symptoms and as part of a constellation of other ANOMALIES in several hereditary forms. In these types of myoclonus, the twitching is random and unpredictable (arrhythmic myoclonus).

Episodes can be triggered by sudden stimulus of sight, sound or touch, or by a voluntary movement. Anxiety, stress and fatigue can also precipitate a spasmodic episode. It is thought excessive neuronal discharge is at the root of most cases of myoclonus.

When appearing independently, hereditary essential myoclonus is an AUTOSOMAL DOMINANT trait. Progressive myoclonic EPILEPSY is distinguished by severe epilepsy combined with stimulus-sensitive myoclonus. Potentially disabling, dementia may be an associated feature. It is usually inherited as an

autosomal dominant trait, and may also be present in individuals with TAY-SACHS DISEASE, Kuf's disease (see NEURONAL CEROID LIPOFUSCINOSIS) and other GENETIC DISORDERS.

Ramsay-Hunt syndrome, in addition to epilepsy and myoclonus, includes neurologic abnormalities and cerebellar degeneration as its hallmarks. It is an autosomal dominant disorder.

Myoclonus can also be caused by a variety of non-genetic factors, including cerebral oxygen deprivation, brain infections or inflammation, metabolic disorders and exposure to toxins.

myopia   Commonly known as nearsightedness, this condition occurs when the eyeball is elongated so that the focal point of parallel light rays lies in front of, rather than on, the retina. It appears to have many possible genetic causes: Individual families have shown all the major types of MENDELIAN inheritance. There also appears to be an association between such factors as PREMATURITY, administration of oxygen after birth or maternal disease in pregnancy, and the incidence of myopia. A positive family history alerts parents to watch for mannerisms of nearsightedness, such as squinting. The actual diagnosis is usually made by age three.

On average, visual acuity among those affected ranges between 20/50 and 20/60. However, with corrective lenses, visual acuity may be correctable to 20/30 or better.

It is not unusual to also have a misalignment of the optic axis (STRABISMUS) associated with this condition. It has been suggested that children with myopia tend to have, on average, higher IQs than those without it, but this has not been convincingly demonstrated.

CONGENITAL myopia is a relatively rare disorder, affecting males and females equally. With corrective lenses prescribed as early as possible, the prognosis is favorable, since most cases of myopia do not deteriorate with age; it is rarely progressive.

There are some specific SYNDROMES with myopia (such as X-LINKED recessive syndrome of myopia and NIGHT BLINDNESS) and it may be a part of other disorders (e.g., MARFAN SYNDROME). For the child of an individual with an isolated case of severe myopia, a risk of 4% to 5% for similar severe eye problems has been suggested.

myositis ossificans   See FIBRODYSPLASIA OSSIFICANS PROGRESSIVA.

myotonic dystrophy (Steinert disease) First described by Steinert in 1909, this is the most common MUSCULAR DYSTROPHY of adult life. A combination of progressive weakening of the muscles (dystrophy) and muscle spasms or rigidity with difficulty relaxing a contracted muscle (myotonia) are hallmarks. It may also be associated with mild to severe MENTAL RETARDATION, CATARACTS, diminished endocrine function, including atrophy of the gonads, and decreased functioning of the pituitary, thyroid, adrenal cortex or pancreatic islets (the latter leading to a mild form of DIABETES MELLITUS). Affected males often exhibit frontal baldness.

Among the affected muscles is the heart, leading to cardiac irregularities and often death due to heart failure. The disease is highly variable in the expression of manifestations among different individuals. There is an enormous range of severity and age of onset, from prenatal to old age.

It appears to have three possible types, based on age of onset: during infancy; from early childhood to age 20 and after age 20. The average age of detection is in the second decade of life, but there are potentially recognizable symptoms early on-reduced fetal movements in pregnancy, poor sucking reflexes and muscle rigidity in infancy, drooping facial muscles and a characteristic sunkenness at the temples (temporal atrophy).

Symptomatic relief can be provided for the associated muscle weakness through physical therapy and orthopedic measures.

The GENE for myotonic dystrophy has been mapped to chromosome 19. Inherited as an AUTOSOMAL DOMINANT trait, in the infant-onset form, STILLBIRTH and infant mortality rates are high. Approximately one in 8,000 individuals are affected. A second rare form of the disease, myotonic dystrophy type 2, DM2, is caused by a CCTG repeat expansion in the gene *ZNF9* that encodes a protein termed zinc finger protein 9. Also transmitted in an autosomal dominant manner, its features include myotonia, cataracts, cardiac conduction defects, frontal baldness in males and diminished endocrine function.

An example of a TRINUCLEOTIDE REPEAT DISORDER, myotonic dystrophy results from an expansion in the trinucleotide repeats within the causative gene. The severity of the disorder increases and age of onset declines in subsequent generations as the trinucleotide repeat lengthens. This phenomenon is known as "anticipation" and is due to the expansion of the CTG repeat. This expansion is estimated to have a 93% chance of occurring whenever the abnormally long ALLELE is passed from parent to child. The size of the triplet expansion is thought to correlate with the severity of the disease and the age of onset. Thus infants with congenital myotonic dystrophy typically have the largest repeat sizes.

Confirmation of clinical diagnosis can be accomplished via DEOXYRIBONUCLEIC ACID (DNA) testing, which can also be used to evaluate at-risk, asymptomatic individuals with a family history of the disease, and for PRENATAL DIAGNOSIS.

myotubular myopathy This rare disorder, a congenital myopathy, occurs in three hereditary forms distinguished by severity and age of onset. Muscle samples in all three share a common appearance upon microscopic examination.

X-linked myotubular myopathy The most severe form, affecting only males, starts at birth or during early infancy. Affected infants exhibit poor muscle tone. Those of the jaw, lips, tongue, cheeks, mouth, throat and neck may be weak. Respiratory distress may be caused by deficiencies of respiratory muscles. Drooping upper eyelids (ptosis) and paralysis of the eye are also symptomatic. The poor muscle tone can also interfere with sucking and swallowing. The gene responsible, MTM1, has been mapped to Xq28. The protein product it encodes has been named myotubularin. Molecular genetic testing is available for confirmation of diagnosis, carrier detection and prenatal diagnosis.

Autosomal recessive myotubular myopathy This more moderate form has its onset in infancy or childhood, as muscles slowly being to weaken causing respiratory distress. As in the X-linked form, the jaw, tongue, lips, mouth, throat, neck and upper eyelid may be involved. By adolescence or young adulthood the muscle weakness is severe, often resulting in curvature of the spine. Described world-wide in all populations, a slight preponderance of females over males is affected. Blacks appear to exhibit a slightly higher incidence.

Autosomal dominant myotubular myopathy The least severe form, onset occurs between the first and third decade. A clumsy gait, one of the first symptoms, progresses to wasting of the leg muscles such that use of a wheelchair becomes necessary. Weaknesses of the shoulders and hips are also evident from onset. Though facial weakness may be present in some of those affected, the muscles of the throat and face are generally not involved. Males are affected twice as frequently as females.

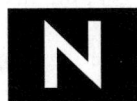

Naegeli syndrome   This rare hereditary SYNDROME, first described by Swiss hematologist O. Naegeli (1871–1938) in 1927, is a form of ECTODERMAL DYSPLASIA, a group of disorders characterized by abnormalities of the skin, teeth, hair and nails. (These form from embryonic ectodermal tissues during fetal development.) The soles of the feet and the palms of the hands appear thickened (plantar and palmar hypodrosis and hyperkeratosis). Affected individuals are unable to sweat normally and are especially sensitive to heat. Yellow spotting of the tooth enamel is another manifestation.

Inherited as an AUTOSOMAL DOMINANT trait, the disorder is caused by mutations in the *keratin-14* gene (*KRT14*). Life span and intelligence are normal.

Nager syndrome   Craniofacial abnormalities and radial limb and thumb anomalies are the hallmarks of this CONGENITAL SYNDROME. Affected individuals have a small jaw (micrognathia) and underdeveloped cheekbones, downward slanting eyes, absence of eyelashes, CLEFT PALATE and deformities of the internal and external ear structure.

The forearms are short and thumbs have little range of motion. Toes may be webbed (SYNDACTYLY), overlapping or absent, and CLUBFEET have been reported in some cases.

Affected infants may require the insertion of feeding and breathing tubes. Surgery can correct some craniofacial defects as well as deformities of the limbs.

The cause is unknown, though it is believed to be inherited in both AUTOSOMAL RECESSIVE and AUTOSOMAL DOMINANT forms.

nail-patella syndrome   As the name indicates, this disorder primarily affects the nails (fingernails more frequently than toenails) and the kneecaps (patellae). The deformities are apparent at birth. The nails are markedly reduced in size, often with the half toward the inner arm missing, and sometimes the white "moons" at the base of the nails are triangular. Thumbnails are most involved; changes progressively diminish from the index to the pinky finger. If the patellae are present at all, they are underdeveloped and likely to be dislocated. Hundreds of cases have been reported.

Other findings associated with nail-patella syndrome are fingers bent sideways (CLINODACTYLY), elbow joints that cannot be fully extended, SCOLIOSIS, underdeveloped shoulder blades, drooping eyelids (PTOSIS), CATARACTS and, in about 30% of affected individuals, kidney disorders. These renal complications (including kidney failure) are the only ones that may shorten life span. Affected individuals must be repeatedly tested to assure early diagnosis and treatment of any renal disease. (About 8% of affected individuals who come to medical attention succumb to renal disease.)

Nail-patella syndrome is an AUTOSOMAL DOMINANT trait with variable EXPRESSIVITY. The GENE that causes this disorder, identified in 1998, is the developmental gene *LMX1B*, which normally plays an essential role in the patterning and development of the skeleton and kidney. PRENATAL DIAGNOSIS may be possible using GENETIC LINKAGE studies or ULTRASOUND.

narcolepsy (narcoleptic syndrome)   A sleep disorder characterized by disabling daytime drowsiness, low alertness, loss of muscle tone (cataplexy), hallucinations, sleep paralysis and disrupted nighttime sleep. Daytime sleepiness occurs so suddenly and with such overwhelming power that some affected individuals refer to it as a sleep attack, with some experiencing several such episodes a day. Periods of sleep following these attacks generally last from a few seconds to 30 minutes, but may last several hours.

Familial narcolepsy was recognized as early as 1877, when an affected mother and son were described, but it was not until 1926 that the disorder was delineated as a specific entry (see FAMILIAL DISEASE).

The disorder seems to be caused by an imbalance in the brain's sleep/wake cycle. Rapid eye movement (REM) sleep and dreaming may occur when the individual is awake, often resulting in intense, vivid hallucinations, sometimes accompanied by frightening auditory, visual and tactile sensations. Occasionally they are difficult to distinguish from reality. Sleep paralysis, the momentary inability to move when waking up or falling asleep, may accompany these hallucinations.

Narcolepsy is a lifelong condition. There is no known cure and no confirmed reports of lasting remission. Symptoms usually become noticeable between the ages of 10 and 30. Subtle at first, they become increasingly severe over the years. The sleep attacks may become profoundly disabling, seriously disrupting social and professional lives. While narcolepsy by itself does not lower life expectancy, affected individuals must be careful to control symptoms while driving or engaging in other potentially dangerous activities.

Drug therapies can help control symptoms. Stimulants can stave off sleep attacks, and depressants are often prescribed to control cataplexy and hallucinations. Naps throughout the day may counter excessive sleepiness.

About half of all narcoleptics have cataplexy. Cataplectic attacks may be triggered by humor (hearing, or especially telling, a joke), competition (playing cards), excitement (viewing or participating in sports) and stress (asking for a pay raise). Individuals may abruptly lose muscle control and collapse into sleep. Attempts to control attacks by avoiding these feelings may restrict the individual's emotional development.

About 200,000 people in the United States are affected, according to the American Narcolepsy Association. The frequency of this disorder is about six in 10,000. About 4% are symptomatic by age 10, 25% after age 20 and 18% after age 30; onset after 40 is rare. Forty percent of patients in one study had at least one family member with an isolated daytime sleepiness complaint and 6% had a positive family history of narcolepsy. Inheritance may be MULTIFACTORIAL or AUTOSOMAL DOMINANT with incomplete PENETRANCE. A specific ALLELE of the GENE HLA-DQw6, namely DQB1-0602, or a gene located close to it, appears to be the susceptibility gene for narcolepsy. This specific HLA type has been found in nearly every narcolepsy patient. However, families with narcolepsy not linked to HLA have been reported.

natal teeth   About one in 3,000 liveborn infants have teeth at birth, a condition believed to be inherited as an AUTOSOMAL DOMINANT trait. They are most commonly lower central incisors. Historical figures who are reported to have been born with erupted teeth include Zoroaster, Hannibal, Richard III of England, and French cardinals and statesmen, Richelieu and Mazarin, revolutionary Mirabeau and 19th-century speech theorist Paul Broca. King Louis XIV of France was said to have been "a considerable vexation to his wet-nurses" as a result of this condition.

Natal teeth are also associated with genetic SYNDROMES, including ELLIS–VAN CREVELD SYNDROME and HALLERMANN-STREIFF SYNDROME.

nemaline myopathy   The word *nemaline* comes from the Greek for "thread." Fine thread-like structures, often referred to as nemaline rods, visible in the muscle fibers with a microscope, are the signature sign of this deficiency of the skeletal muscles. Floppiness may be evident at birth, though onset may not occur until middle age. In affected infants, trunk, thighs and upper arms may be very weak. Deep tendon reflexes may be absent, along with poor muscle tone and soft muscles. Deficiencies of the respiratory muscles, as well as those used in swallowing, can cause death before two years of age.

Affected individuals typically have a high-arched palate, thin face and prominent jaw. Though the disorder is progressive, youngsters may show general improvement through childhood due to the growth of muscle mass during this age. Adult onset cases may be marked by weakening of the shoulder, pelvic girdle, or facial muscles. The heart muscle may also be affected.

Inherited as an autosomal dominant trait, females are affected more frequently than males. An autosomal recessive form has also been reported. Mutations in five different genes have been identified as causing this disorder. All encode protein components of the muscle thin filament. The genes are: skeletal muscle alpha-1 actin *(ACTA1); nebulin (NEB); tropomyosin-3 (TPM3);* Troponin T1 (TNNT1); and tropomyosin-2 (TPM2). Other cases appear to involve as yet unidentified genes.

nephritis, familial See FAMILIAL NEPHRITIS.

nephrogenic diabetes insipidus (NDI) A rare hereditary kidney disorder that results in the passing of large quantities of water in the urine (polyuria). One of four types of diabetes insipidus, it renders the kidneys unable to respond to the antidiuretic effect of arginine vasopressin (AVP), a hormone that reduces urine output. AVP allows water passing through the kidneys to be reabsorbed in the collecting duct, concentrating the urine. In addition to the voiding of dilute urine, those affected exhibit chronic thirst (polydipsia) and are in constant danger of dehydration. Symptoms usually appear in the first few days to first weeks of life. The familial link was first noted in 1892 by G. H. McIlraith in the British medical journal *Lancet.*

There are three types of hereditary NDI: X-linked NDI is the most common type, representing 90% of the cases of hereditary NDI. It is caused by a mutation in the *Vasopressin-2 Receptor* gene *(V2R).* More than 70 mutations of the *V2R* gene have been identified. Males are more frequently affected than females. Females often remain asymptomatic. It occurs in about one in 250,000 live male births. A rare autosomal recessive form and a very rare autosomal dominant form also exist. Both are caused by a mutation of the *aquaporin-2* gene *(AQP2)* mapped to chromosome location 12q13. More than 13 mutations of the gene have been reported.

Diagnosis is made on the basis of tests for elevated plasma concentrations of AVP in the blood and low levels of osmotically active particles in the urine.

In addition to its hereditary forms, NDI may result from drugs or kidney disease. Non-hereditary forms of NDI are typically less severe in their manifestation.

nephrosis, congenital See CONGENITAL NEPHROSIS.

Neu-Laxova syndrome A very rare CONGENITAL disorder characterized by generalized edema, or swelling, a small head (MICROCEPHALY), unusual facial characteristics, joint contractures, scaly skin and abnormalities of the central nervous system. Growth retardation occurs IN UTERO.

The swelling usually occurs on the scalp, hands and feet. The unusual facial characteristics may include a short neck, small jaw (micrognathia) and eyes (microphthalmia), wide-set eyes (HYPERTELORISM), absent eyelids, a broad nasal bridge and sloping forehead.

Limbs may exhibit contractures and webbing of the toes and fingers (SYNDACTYLY). Additional associated features include malformed external genitalia, underdeveloped skeletal muscle and abnormal development of the brain.

Thought to be transmitted as an AUTOSOMAL RECESSIVE trait, about 20 cases have been reported. Most have been STILLBORN or died in the immediate newborn period.

neural tube defects (NTD) Term describing a variety of CONGENITAL defects of the spine or skull resulting from failure of the neural tube to close, or close completely, an ANOMALY that has its genesis in the fourth week of pregnancy. The neural tube is a region on the back portion of an embryo from which the brain and spinal cord develop. As the embryo grows, the top of the neural tube becomes the brain, and the bottom the spinal cord. When the neural tube fails to close properly, tissue associated with the brain or spinal cord remains exposed or incompletely protected, resulting in potentially severe developmental disabilities and infant death. Corrective surgery and physical therapy can help alleviate associated physical problems in some cases.

NTDs comprise the most frequent malformations of the central nervous system. The form and severity of an NTD depends on the location and the extent of the defect. They include SPINA BIFIDA (failure of the spinal cord to close), ANENCEPHALY (the failure of the cranium and brain to form or form completely) and ENCEPHALOCELE (protrusion of the brain through the skull, usually in the back of the head). Some NTDs are not open, and while the nerve tissue is incompletely shielded, the defect is covered by skin.

NTDs are caused by the action of several GENES either alone (POLYGENIC) or in concert with environmental factors (MULTIFACTORIAL). They may also be part of single gene disorders (e.g., encephalocele in MECKEL SYNDROME), or caused by CHROMOSOME ABNORMALITIES (e.g., trisomy 18; see EDWARD SYNDROME) or teratogenic exposure (e.g., spina bifida caused by valproic acid). There is also an increase in NTDs among offspring of diabetic women (DIABETES MELLITUS).

Dietary supplementation of folic acid (a B complex VITAMIN), before conception and during early pregnancy has been shown to reduce the risk of NTDs, though the mechanism of this preventive effect is not understood.

The link between vitamins, or nutrition, and NTDs had been noted for some decades; they are more common in the offspring of women in lower socioeconomic groups and women who have poor diets. Additionally, there was an "epidemic" of neural tube defects during the Depression, a time when many people, including women of child-bearing age, received substandard nutrition. However, the potential link between vitamin deficiencies and neural tube defects did not receive scientific attention until after World War II, when it was noted that women in England, Holland and Germany who had been malnourished gave birth to an unexpectedly large number of infants with these developmental defects. Yet it was only in the 1980s that the link was examined scientifically.

One early study found women who take multivitamins (including folic acid) at the time of conception had 60% less risk of giving birth to an infant with a neural tube defect than women who did not use vitamins. A later study by Boston University's Center for Human Genetics, published in 1989 and involving 23,000 pregnant women, found those who reported taking multivitamins in the first six weeks of pregnancy had rates of NTDs in their offspring only one-quarter the rates of women who did not use vitamins. (NTD incidence was 0.9 per 1,000 births among vitamin users vs. 3.5 per 1,000 births among non vitamin users.) A study by the National Institute of Child Health and Human Development published in 1997 found 100 micrograms of folic acid daily produced a blood folate level sufficient to reduce NTDs about 22%. A 200 microgram daily dose was associated with a 41% reduced risk of NTDs, and dosages of 400 micrograms with a reduction of 47%. Women who had one or more pregnancies affected by an NTD and who subsequently used supplemental folic acid significantly reduced their risk to have another child with an NTD to about 1%.

Folic acid is particularly important to fetal development in the first month, a time when many pregnancies are undetected. By the time the pregnancy is recognized, a shortage of folic acid could have led to a nascent NTD. The Institute of Medicine, a federal agency that sets nutritional guidelines, recommends pregnant women take 600 micrograms of folic acid daily. (Other adults are advised to take 400 micrograms.)

Neural tube defects occur in approximately one to two of every 1,000 live births in the United States,

TABLE XVII
NEURAL TUBE DEFECTS IN THE UNITED STATES (APPROX. 6,000/YEAR)

		Prognosis	
Type (Degree)	Incidence/ 1,000 Births	Neonatal Death (%)	Long-Term Disability (%)
Anencephaly	0.6–0.8	100	0
Spina bifida (open)	0.5–0.8	33	65*
Spina bifida (closed)	0.1–0.14	7	10*
Total	1.2–1.7	60	60*

*Disability has been reported to include lower limb paralysis, sensory loss, chronic bladder or bowel problems, clubfoot, scoliosis, meningitis, hydrocephalus and mental retardation.
Source: American College of Obstetricians and Gynecologists, *ACOG Technical Bulletin* 99 (1986), p. 1.

TABLE XVIII
RELATIVE RISKS OF OCCURRENCE OF NEURAL TUBE
DEFECTS IN THE UNITED STATES

Family History	Risk (Incidence/1,000 Births)
No family history of NTD	1
Positive family history	
Maternal	10
Paternal	5
One-parent with NTD	30
One prior infant with NTD	20
Two prior infants with NTD	60

Source: American College of Obstetricians and Gynecologists, *ACOG Technical Bulletin* 99 (1986), p. 1.

but the true rate of occurrence may be higher, as perhaps half of anencephalics are thought to be spontaneously aborted. Geography is also associated with variations in risk. In Wales and Ireland almost 1% of all newborns have NTDs. In the United States, incidence decreases from north to south and east to west. In New York the rate is approximately two per 1,000 live births, and in Los Angeles it is one per 1,000. NTDs are more common in whites than in other racial groups, and more common in first-born children. Affected females outnumber males by a ratio of between two to one and three to two. A woman who has had an infant with an NTD has a risk of recurrence estimated at between 1% and 5%, which rises to 4% to 9% after having two affected infants. (See Table XVIII.)

PRENATAL DIAGNOSIS of open NTDs is possible via findings of increased ALPHA-FETOPROTEIN levels found in AMNIOTIC FLUID collected with AMNIOCENTESIS. They may also be seen in utero with ULTRASOUND in some cases. Screening for NTDs is possible in low-risk pregnancies via measuring alpha-fetoprotein levels in maternal blood.

neuraminidase deficiency (sialidosis, mucolipidosis I) A group of rare hereditary deficiencies of an ENZYME responsible for the metabolism of some polysaccharides, sugar molecules found as components of larger complex molecules, leading to the accumulation of abnormal amounts of polysaccharides in the tissues. There are at least three forms.

In one form, onset is in childhood or early adulthood, characterized by seizure-like muscle spasms and progressive loss of vision. A CHERRY-RED SPOT is present on the retina of the eye. Intelligence remains normal. In another form, individuals may also have coarse facial features, bony abnormalities, enlarged livers and clouding of the cornea suggestive of MUCOPOLYSACCHARIDOSIS. In a third form, the kidney is also involved. The disorder is inherited as an AUTOSOMAL RECESSIVE trait. Definitive diagnosis is based on deficiency of the enzyme alpha-neuraminidase. CARRIER detection and PRENATAL DIAGNOSIS are possible by enzyme assay.

neurodermatosis See PHAKOMATOSIS.

neurofibromatosis (NF; von Recklinghausen disease) One of the most common inherited disorders, with an incidence from one in 2,500 to one in 3,300 births, this potentially disfiguring condition affects an estimated 100,000 Americans. It occurs in two forms, the more benign type 1 and the more severe type 2.

NF type 1 (NF1) exhibits great variability of expression, and 95% of cases are estimated to go unrecognized. In most cases, "café au lait" spots, irregularly shaped, coffee-colored splotches on the skin are the only symptom. Freckling about the armpits is another manifestation. Onset is usually in childhood, and progression may accelerate during puberty and pregnancy.

The disease derives its name from the thousands of neurofibromas, or tumorous growths, that disfigure severely affected individuals. Additionally, these tumors may be found in connective tissue, brain and spinal cord, eye, liver, stomach, bladder, kidney, larynx and intestine. Internal tumors can damage nerves and cause paralysis or BLINDNESS. In 3% to 15% of the cases, the tumors turn malignant. Learning disability is exhibited in 40% of the cases, and 2% to 5% are mentally retarded.

Type 1 is inherited as an AUTOSOMAL DOMINANT trait, with 50% of cases thought to be the result of new MUTATION. The defective GENE is on 17q and encodes a protein designated neurofibromin, which appears to function as a tumor suppressor.

The gene is extremely large, which accounts for the high frequency of new mutations. (The bigger the gene, the more places where something can go wrong.) Multiple individual mutations exist and there is no single common mutation. This form is also referred to as von Recklinghausen disease and von Recklinghausen neurofibromatosis for German pathologist F. D. von Recklinghausen (1833–1910), who published the first description in 1882. There is currently no method of PRENATAL DIAGNOSIS or identification of afflicted individuals who are asymptomatic.

NF type 2, or bilateral acoustic neurofibromatosis (also called central NF and NF2), the more severe form, occurs in one in 50,000 births. It develops at a later age, usually in the teens or 20s, and causes multiple tumors of the cranial and spinal nerves. This often results in ringing in the ears, DEAFNESS, balance disorders and paralysis, requiring multiple surgeries in adolescence or early adulthood. There are generally only a few café au lait spots and neurofibromas. Also an autosomal dominant disorder, the defective gene, which appears to be a tumor suppressor, has been mapped to 22q.

GENETIC LINKAGE techniques and family studies can be used for genetic testing in both types.

Neurofibromatosis came to greater public attention as a result of the popularity of the eponymous Broadway play and movie about Joseph Merrick, the grossly deformed 19th-century Englishman who was exhibited in a freak show as "The Elephant Man."

In an interesting twist, geneticists now postulate that the Elephant Man didn't suffer from neurofibromatosis at all, but rather from PROTEUS SYNDROME, a greatly disfiguring disease first described in 1976. They note that Merrick's skin and bone deformities (which included a head with a three-foot circumference) were too severe to be caused by neurofibromatosis. Additionally, Dr. Frederick Treves, Merricks's benefactor, never described neurofibromas in his case write-ups of the Elephant Man.

neuronal ceroid lipofuscinosis (NCL; Batten disease)   A group of invariably fatal childhood neurologic (nervous system) disorders. They comprise the most common childhood onset hereditary progressive neurodegenerative condition. The first symptoms are deteriorating vision or seizures, progressing to personality and behavior changes, loss of communication skills, increasing spasticity and loss of motor skills, facial grimacing, abnormal body movements and mental impairment. Affected children eventually become blind, bedridden and demented.

NCL is associated with a buildup of fatty pigment (ceroid lipofuscin) in cells of the brain, nervous system and other parts of the body. This pigment is thought to be the end product of a combination of metabolic derangements that mark the progressive deterioration of brain function. (This same pigment accumulates slowly during the normal aging process, but it is greatly accelerated in this disorder.) The accumulations are thought to be caused by the absence of ENZYMES necessary to break down fats and their associated sugars and proteins normally. The missing enzyme has been identified in at least one form and the causative GENES located in others.

Diagnosis requires numerous tests for confirmation, including blood tests, biopsies, electrophysiological examination of the brain (via electroencephalogram) and computer tomography of the head (CT scan). Characteristic cellular deposits ("curvilinear bodies") are seen when cells from biopsy are examined under the electron microscope.

Currently there is no treatment available. Research on animal models is being conducted. A similar disease has been found in English setters, dalmatians and New Zealand sheep, and several colonies have been bred for research purposes.

Inherited as an AUTOSOMAL RECESSIVE TRAIT, incidence has been estimated to be between one in 12,500 and one in 50,000 live births (about 3/100,000 of all types in the United States) PRENATAL DIAGNOSIS has been accomplished through electron microscope detection of curvilinear deposits in amniotic fluid cells.

While there are two very rare adult forms (Kuf's disease and Parry's disease), the great majority of cases appear in three childhood forms. Symptoms are similar, but age of onset and speed of progression vary.

Infantile NCL; Type 1 NCL (Santavuori disease)
Age of onset is about eight months and progresses

rapidly. Infants fail to thrive, head growth slows, resulting in an abnormally small head (microcephaly), and they exhibit shock-like muscle contractions (myoclonic jerks). Death usually occurs by age five, though some have survived a few years longer in a vegetative state. The underlying defect is in the enzyme palmitoyl-protein thioesterase (PPT1), which is involved in the breakdown of lipid modified proteins. Specific mutations have been identified in the gene responsible for manufacturing this protein, found on chromosome 1p. This makes prenatal diagnosis possible in affected families by biochemical and/or molecular techniques.

Late infantile (Jansky-Bielschowsky disease) Onset occurs at about three years of age, beginning with loss of muscle coordination and seizures. Symptoms progress rapidly, and death usually occurs between the ages of seven and 12. This form is common in Newfoundland, with a birth frequency of one in 5,000. The frequency in the general population is about one in 220,000. Mutations causing this form of the disorder have been found in five different genes: *PPT1;* the *TPP1* gene (which encodes the protein tripeptidyl-peptidase 1 and is also known as *CLN2*); and the *CLN 5, CLN6* and *CLN8* genes. In families in which the defect has been identified, prenatal diagnosis is possible.

Juvenile (Spielmeyer-Vogt-Sjogren disease; Batten disease) Age of onset is between five and 10 years. Progressive visual failure and seizures are the first signs. With a slower progression than the earlier-onset type, individuals survive into the late teens or early twenties. Some have lived longer. The responsible gene, *CLN3* has been found on chromosome 16, though the function of the protein it encodes is unknown. A number of mutations have been found, but one accounts for 73% of all mutations (90% of Finish patients): a 217-base pair deletion of the gene. Frequency of juvenile form is about one in 140,000. Prenatal diagnosis has been accomplished with molecular testing. Defects in the *PPT1* and *CLN2* genes have also been found in some cases of this form of the disorder.

The disorder was first described in Norway in 1826 by Dr. Christian Stengel, but its alternate appellation, Batten disease, honors English neurologist F. E. Batten (1865–1918), who first recognized the range of manifestations of the disease, publishing his findings in 1902. (Batten disease is synonymous with juvenile NCL.)

nevoid basal cell carcinoma syndrome (basal cell nevus syndrome; Gorlin syndrome) SYNDROME present in about one of every 200 patients with basal cell carcinoma (a skin tumor), characterized by eruptions of the skin and ANOMALIES of the ocular, skeletal, central nervous and endocrine systems. In addition, one in five among those in whom basal cell carcinoma develops before age 19 has the syndrome. Overall prevalence seems to be about one in 57,000.

At birth, ocular defects may include a deformity of the eyelid (dystopia, canthorium), abnormally wide spacing between the eyes (HYPERTELORISM) and congenital BLINDNESS. Numerous skeletal problems may also be present at birth, including anomalies of the ribs, spine, feet and digits.

In childhood, multiple jaw cysts begin to appear, followed by multiple basal cell carcinomas. The palms and soles may have small pits. The basal cell nevi first appear generally about the time of puberty. Early skin lesions start out as brownish, dome-shaped papules (raised skin areas) on the upper body. Later they may ulcerate. Adult patients develop a characteristic broad facial appearance due to a slightly protruding jaw, swelling around the forehead, sunken eyes and a broadening of the nose. By age 40, basal cell carcinomas and jaw cysts occur in more than 40%.

The prognosis for affected individuals is generally favorable, but is dependent on the location, number and severity of the tumors that characterize the syndrome. Radiation therapy should be avoided in patients with this syndrome as it tends to lead to the production of even more basal cell tumors.

The GENE involved, PTCH (located on 9q), is the human version of the patched gene, first identified in *Drosphila melanogaster* (the fly whose CHROMOSOMES have played a large role in genetic research), and acts as a tumor suppressor. The product of the patched gene acts as a receptor for a group of proteins called the hedgehog proteins, which are important in the normal regulation of development of various body structures.

Screening and PRENATAL DIAGNOSIS are possible via molecular techniques (direct detection of mutations or through GENETIC LINKAGE). About 40% of cases are new mutations.

The disorder's secondary appellation, Gorlin syndrome, takes its name from Robert J. Gorlin, a dentist, oral pathologist and eminent "syndromologist" who first reported the disorder in 1960. He was involved in the identification of many disorders and syndromes, some of which also bear his name.

nevus CONGENITAL discolorations or anomalous pigmentation of a well-defined area of the skin. Referred to as BIRTHMARKS and moles, they appear in various forms, some of which are hereditary.

Pigmented moles have long been observed to show a familial aggregation and are now known to be inherited as an AUTOSOMAL DOMINANT trait. Multiple pigmented moles are also a feature of one chromosomal aberration, TURNER SYNDROME. Multiple pigmented lesions may be seen in a variety of disorders such as NEUROFIBROMATOSIS (café au lait spots) or LEOPARD syndrome (see MULTIPLE-LENTIGINES SYNDROME). (See also PORT WINE STAIN.)

Niemann-Pick disease A group of disorders characterized by the accumulation of a phosphorus-containing lipid compound, sphingomyelin, in the lysosomes, the small digestive structures within cells. This accumulation in the cells of the central nervous system, liver and spleen leads to cell death, and in most cases has fatal consequences. The disorders are classified as STORAGE DISEASES, because they involve the abnormal storage of material in the cells.

Four major subtypes (A, B, C and D) have been identified. Type A occurs primarily in infants of Ashkenazi Jews (those of Eastern European ancestry), though it affects all ethnic groups. It was first described by Albert Niemann, a German pediatrician, in 1914. The features of the disorder were more fully detailed by the German physician Ludwig Pick in the 1920s, and the disorder now carries their names.

The primary metabolic defect in the first two forms (A and B) is the deficient function of the ENZYME sphingomyelinase, which normally helps metabolize the phospholipid, sphingomyelin. The

GENE for sphingomyelinase maps to 11p. The accumulation of lipids in the cells causes them to have a large, pale, "foamy" appearance. These "Niemann-Pick cells," which can be found in the bone marrow, liver, spleen, lymph nodes and lungs, are helpful in diagnosing the condition. The defect in types C and D appears to involve the processing of cholesterol and only secondarily results in any sphingomyelin accumulation. All forms are inherited as AUTOSOMAL RECESSIVE traits.

Type A This form is severe and rapidly progressive. The first signs, such as difficulty in feeding and failure to achieve normal developmental milestones, are usually noticed by four to six months of age. The spleen and liver become markedly enlarged (hepatosplenomegaly). About 50% of patients exhibit the retinal abnormality (cherry-red spot) characteristic of tay-sachs disease. As they age, infants lose control of motor function and mental capacity deteriorates. Infants take on an emaciated appearance with distended abdomens. The skin may have a brownish-yellow discoloration. Recurrent respiratory infections cause severe debilitation, and death usually occurs by three years of age. The disorder is estimated to occur in one in 25,000 to one in 30,000 infants of Ashkenazic Jewish ancestry. One in 85 to one in 100 Ashkenazi Jews is thought to be a carrier of the trait. Three specific mutations of the sphingomyelinase gene account for about 65% of the Ashkenazi Jewish type A patients.

Type B This rare form, which affects all ethnic groups, exhibits no mental or neurological involvement. Onset is in childhood, and other symptoms are consistent with type A, including presence of Niemann-Pick cells, severe enlargement of the liver and spleen and recurrent infections. There is also lung involvement in this form. Some patients have reached adulthood without significant disease-related complications. Life span may be normal. Enzyme replacement therapy for this form of the disease is under development.

Type C This rare form, which occurs in all ethnic groups, exhibits both neurological deterioration and organ involvement. The age of onset is highly variable and may be between one and two years of age or in adulthood, though it most commonly appears later in childhood. There is progressive loss of mental and motor skills. Liver and spleen are enlarged and Niemann-Pick cells are present. Gait abnormalities and ataxia, muscle weakness and seizures occur as the disease progresses. Death usually occurs between the ages of five and 15 years. The gene for type C has been mapped to 18q. Termed NPC1, it has some similarities in its genetic sequence to the patched gene that is mutant in nevoid basal cell carcinoma syndrome and others. There is a mouse model of this disease. Another gene, *NPC2,* located on the long arm of chromosome 14, accounts for about 5% of Type C cases.

Type D Resembles type C but is confined to individuals living in a coastal area of southwestern Nova Scotia with a common ancestor of French (Acadian) extraction. (An adult onset type E— including patients with disease resembling type C but with onset in adulthood—has also been suggested.) Type D is not a distinct type, but rather involves a particular mutation in the *NPC1* gene found frequently in this Acadian population, and thus the term type D is no longer used.

PRENATAL DIAGNOSIS of A and B subtypes is possible by observing deficient sphingomyelinase activity in cultured cells gathered through AMNIOCENTESIS or CHORIONIC VILLUS SAMPLING. Prenatal diagnosis, previously unreliable in type C, has been made more reliable by specifically measuring cholesterol esterification in fetal derived cells. As specific mutations become known, CARRIER testing and prenatal diagnosis by molecular techniques will also become more practical.

night blindness (nyctalopia)

night blindness (nyctalopia) The absence or deficiency of vision in darkness, caused by the absence or deficiency of visual purple, a pigment normally found in the retina of the eye and necessary for seeing in reduced lighting. Night blindness is usually inherited as an AUTOSOMAL DOMINANT trait, when occurring as an isolated non-progressive disorder.

A study of a French family, well known for the condition, was published in 1838. Their lineage was traced to Jean Nougaret, a butcher from Provence who settled in a small village near Montpellier in the south of France, and who was the common ancestor of everyone in the district with night blindness. A study of his genealogy found 629 persons, 86 of whom had night blindness.

There is also a variety commonly found in Japan, named Oguchi disease, for Japanese ophthalmologist Chuta Oguchi (1875–1945). Inherited as an AUTOSOMAL RECESSIVE trait, it is rare in the United States.

It is also a feature of other ophthalmalogic conditions, especially retinal degenerations, such as RETINITIS PIGMENTOSA.

nonketotic hyperglycinemia A hereditary CONGENITAL defect in the ability of the body to metabolize glycine, an AMINO ACID found in many animal and plant proteins. This results in nonketotic hyperglycinemia, a condition of excess glycine in the blood. This is to be distinguished from hyperglycinemia associated with increased ketone levels in the blood, a nonspecific feature of a number of organic acidurias such as PROPIONIC ACIDEMIA. In nonketotic hyperglycinemia, ketones are not elevated; it is a specific disorder of glycine breakdown. Incidence is one in 12,000 births in northern Finland.

This disorder is characterized by severe convulsions and MENTAL RETARDATION. Within the first few days of life, the affected infant will display lethargic behavior. Convulsions may appear from three days to six weeks after birth. Other complications may include irritability, marked muscular tension (hypertonia), increased reflex reactions (hyperreflexia), an abnormally small head (MICROCEPHALY) and abnormal cavity formation in the brain (PORENCEPHALY).

An AUTOSOMAL RECESSIVE trait, the disorder is caused by a defective glycine cleavage ENZYME, which has four different components (designated P, H, T and L proteins) coded for four different GENES. (Presumably defects in any of these can cause the disorder.) Genes that produce this enzyme are on the short arm of chromosomes 9 (P protein) and 3 (T protein), while the location of the others (H, L) are not known and defects in them have yet to be described. A blood test a few days after birth that shows an excess of glycine aids in the detection and diagnosis of this disorder. Glycine levels may be elevated in the urine and also in the cerebrospinal fluid. PRENATAL DIAGNOSIS has been accomplished by enzyme assay on fresh CHORIONIC VILLUS SAMPLING (CVS) samples.

Hyperglycinemia is very rare, and the prognosis for those affected is generally grave, with most dying in infancy. An atypical late onset form also exists. At present, there is no method for identifying CARRIERS of this disorder and no successful treatment that will allow normal development.

Noonan syndrome   Named for J. A. Noonan who described it in 1963, this SYNDROME is characterized by short stature, ovarian or testicular dysfunction, MENTAL RETARDATION and lesions of the heart or great vessels (blood vessels found primarily on the right side of the heart).

The first report in medical literature of an individual now thought to have Noonan syndrome was published in 1883 by O. Kobolinski. Facial features include wide-set eyes (HYPERTELORISM); downward slanting eyes; skin folds obscuring the inner juncture of the eyelids (EPICANTHUS); flat nasal bridge; upper and lower teeth that fail to meet properly (dental malocclusion); low-set ears with abnormal ear folds that may rotate backward; and short or webbed neck. In addition, the hair in white patients may be light in color and coarse in texture, and is often curly or kinky and extends low on the neck. Abnormalities of the shape of the chest, such as pigeon breast (PECTUS carinatum) or funnel chest (pectus excavatum), are common in addition to other skeletal abnormalities. In males, the testes may fail to descend (CRYPTORCHISM). The appearance of affected individuals is often similar to that of TURNER SYNDROME, though, unlike that syndrome (seen exclusively in females), either gender may be affected.

The severity of the Noonan syndrome is variable. Prognosis for life span, growth and reproductive ability depends on the severity of the specific abnormalities. Therapy may include surgery to correct cardiovascular defects or undescended testes. Hormonal substitution has been used in treating some individuals.

Noonan syndrome is inherited in an autosomal dominant pattern, though in most cases it occurs sporadically, that is, as a new mutation in the child of unaffected parents. A gene involved, *PTPN11*, has been mapped to 12q but there appears to be genetic heterogeneity (i.e., mutations in various genes can result in the same disorder). More than half of the individuals with Noonan syndrome have changes in the *PTPN11* gene. Mutations in the *RAF1* gene are found in 3–17% of affected individuals, in the *KRAS* gene in less than 5% of affected individuals and in the *SOS1* gene in about 10% of individuals with Noonan syndrome. Prevalence of the disorder may be as high as one in 1,000 and appears to occur with equal frequency in both genders. (See also HEART DEFECTS.)

Norrie disease   Characterized by total BLINDNESS in both eyes at birth, this rare X-LINKED hereditary condition occurs only in males. Eyeballs may be abnormally small (microphthalmia), and a gray or gray-yellow mass of tissue is visible behind the lens. This "tumor" must be differentiated from RETINOBLASTOMA. Often the pupil is dilated and does not react to light and the iris may be poorly developed. At first the lens may be clear, but CATARACTS may form. Eyeballs shrink by the age of 10. Most affected persons are also mentally retarded and frequently suffer severe DEAFNESS as they grow older.

There is close GENETIC LINKAGE of the disorder with certain marker GENES on the X CHROMOSOME, making CARRIER identification and PRENATAL DIAGNOSIS possible in some cases. Though the gene has been identified, there does not appear to be a single common MUTATION.

nuchal translucency screening (nuchal fold scan) A screening test that uses ultrasound to measure the clear (translucent) space in the tissue at the back of the neck of the developing fetus. It is used to assess the risk of Down syndrome and other chromosomal abnormalities. Developing babies with abnormalities tend to accumulate more fluid in the back of their necks during the first trimester of pregnancy, so the clear space is larger. Proper interpretation of the amount of clear space can identify these abnormalities in utero.

nucleoside phosphorylase deficiency An extremely rare AUTOSOMAL RECESSIVE immunodeficiency disease involving a deficiency of the ENZYME nucleoside phosphorylase. Patients show absent to severely depressed T-cell immunity, while maintaining normal B-cell immunity. However, B-cell immunity deteriorates with age, and patients increasingly suffer from infection, rarely surviving to the age of 10. The immune defect is often accompanied by a neurologic disorder with spasticity, weakness, paralysis, and movement (such as tremor) and behavior problems. Immunization with attenuated live viral vaccines, such as measles, can prove fatal. Very few patients have been identified and described. The GENE has been mapped to 14q, and several different MUTATIONS have been identified.

The enzyme abnormality is demonstrable at birth, though the immunologic function may at first seem normal. There is a possibility that diagnosis could be made IN UTERO by studying enzyme activity in fetal cells. At present, there is no known way to replace the missing enzyme and no effective treatment. (See also IMMUNE DEFICIENCY DISEASE.)

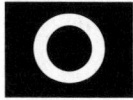

obesity The condition of being 20% or more above ideal body weight. Obesity results from an imbalance of energy (calorie) intake and energy expenditure. Research has found that some people inherit a strong tendency to become obese. TWIN studies, adoption studies and family studies all point to a role of GENETICS in obesity. Statistics in the Danish Adoption Register indicate a strong correlation between the weight class of adopted individuals and the body-mass index of their biologic parents, without any similar correlation between adoptees and their adoptive parents.

The prevalence of obesity is increasing, not from an increase in eating but from an increase in inactivity.

It appears to be a MULTIFACTORIAL trait. Over 16 different loci (see LOCUS, LOCI) that are apparently involved in obesity have been mapped. Obesity is also a component of many (›30) specific SYNDROMES, e.g. PRADER-WILLI SYNDROME, ALSTROM SYNDROME and COHEN SYNDROME. In the area of BIRTH DEFECTS, obesity is likewise important: Obese women are twice as likely as thinner ones to have babies with birth defects, and folic acid supplementation may not have the same protective effects. Mouse strains bred for obesity caused by genetic defects have been important in the study of obesity GENES and include the obesity, or ob mouse, and the tubby mouse. The ob mouse led to the discovery of leptin, a fat regulating hormone. It appears to regulate body weight and fat deposition primarily through effects on appetite and eating behavior. It also appears to play a role in determining intrauterine growth patterns and may be involved in the regulation of pubertal development. Defects in this gene, however, appear to be extremely rare as causes of human obesity, having been found only in one or two individual families.

obesity-hypoventilation syndrome See PICK-WICKIAN SYNDROME.

occipital horn syndrome See CUTIS LAXA.

ocular albinism See ALBINISM.

oculo-auricular-vertebral dysplasia See GOLDEN-HAR SYNDROME.

oculo-cerebro-renal syndrome See LOWE SYN-DROME.

oculocutaneous albinism See ALBINISM.

oculo-dento-digital dysplasia A CONGENITAL disorder characterized by defective development of the eyes, teeth, and fingers and toes. At birth, affected individuals exhibit microcornea, microphthalmia (small eyes), defective tooth enamel, and webbing (SYNDACTYLY) of the fourth and fifth fingers and third and fourth toes. The nose is slender with narrow nostrils, the hair is dry and slow growing. Other abnormalities include a prominent lower jaw, small head or teeth, crossed eyes (STRABISMUS), epicanthal folds (EPICANTHUS), and CLEFT LIP and/or CLEFT PALATE.

The disorder is inherited as an AUTOSOMAL DOMINANT trait. Among the 85 cases reported, many appear to be the result of a new SPORADIC MUTATION. The GENE responsible, the *connexia-43* (*GJA1*) gene, has been mapped to 6q. Additionally, an AUTO-

SOMAL RECESSIVE form exists which causes more severe ocular and skeletal abnormalities, including BLINDNESS, overgrowth of the lower jaw, excessive thickening of the cranial tissue, calcium deposits in the earlobes and an abnormally wide clavicle.

OFD syndrome   See ORAL-FACIAL-DIGITAL SYNDROME.

Oguchi disease   See NIGHT BLINDNESS.

olivopontocerebellar atrophy (OPCA)   See SPINO-CEREBELLAR ATAXIA.

omphalocele   In this CONGENITAL condition, defective embryonic development results in a hole in the abdominal wall, ranging in size from 1 cm (approximately 3/8 inch) to a massive area covering almost the entire abdomen. Portions of the intestinal tract, covered by a saclike membrane that is either skin or an extension of the inside of the abdominal wall (peritoneum), protrude through the hole at the base of the umbilical cord. Depending on the size of the defect, the contents of the sac range from a small loop of bowel to the entire intestinal tract, including stomach, liver and spleen. The sac may rupture during delivery.

Because elements of the intestinal tract are abnormally positioned, they may not function properly or the blood supply to them may be diminished. The intestine often is rotated and may require corrective surgery. The genitourinary system, cardiovascular system, and rarely the central nervous system may also be affected. The defect may be seen with CHROMOSOME ABNORMALITIES or as part of the BECK-WITH-WIEDEMANN SYNDROME. Associated ANOMALIES occur in 40–90% of cases: heart abnormalities in close to 50% and NEURAL TUBE DEFECTS (NTDs) in 40%. The recurrence risk for SIBLINGS after an isolated omphalocele is about 1%.

The greatest threats to life from omphalocele are infection of the peritoneum and starvation because the intestine is nonfunctional. However, most mortality in individuals with omphalocele is due to associated anomalies. Surgical correction is highly successful and is usually undertaken as soon after birth as possible. If the omphalocele is very large, the abdominal cavity may be too small to contain the viscera; in this case, the protrusion is covered by a pouch of synthetic material and returned to the abdominal cavity in stages as the cavity increases in size.

Although the basic defect that causes omphalocele has not been identified, it is known to occur in approximately one in 6,000 live births and to affect males more frequently than females by the ratio of three to two. ULTRASOUND may detect the presence of omphalocele. It may also be detected by elevated ALPHA-FETOPROTEIN (AFP) levels on maternal serum testing.

oncogene   GENES that appear to play a role in the development of CANCER, perhaps by orchestrating uncontrolled cell growth. First isolated in the 1980s, approximately 50 oncogenes had been identified by the end of the decade. A number of anti-oncogenes (tumor suppressor genes) have also been identified, which appear to inhibit the development of cancer. It is thought that several cumulative changes must occur before cancer develops. Among the changes, oncogenes must be activated and anti-oncogenes must be deactivated. Two or more oncogenes of different classes may also be required to cooperate before malignant cell growth is triggered.

It is likely that the action of oncogenes and anti-oncogenes underlies most if not all cancers, and it is only how these are triggered that differs from situation to situation. Viruses and other environmental agents are thought to play a part in activating oncogenes. Chromosomal rearrangements may also be involved: Oncogenes are located at the sites of CHROMOSOME rearrangements seen in various cancers, such as the Philadelphia chromosome observed in many leukemia patients. Many hereditary cancer SYNDROMES result from inherited MUTATIONS that inactivate tumor suppressor genes. Affected individuals inherit a single inactivated copy but still have one copy of the active gene. If a mutation occurs in a cell of that individual's body (e.g., the retina of the eye in a patient with familial RETINOBLASTOMA or breast cell in a woman with hereditary predisposition to BREAST CANCER) that inactivates the other copy, a cancer will result in that tissue of the body. Examples include breast cancer, retinoblastoma, NEVOID BASAL CELL CARCINOMA syndrome, familial polyposis, and NEUROFIBROMATOSIS. Examples of inherited oncogenes include abnormalities of the ret oncogene inherited in the MEN2 syndromes. Another type of cancer predisposing genetic change results from abnormalities in genes which normally function to repair damaged or mismatched DEOXYRIBONUCLEIC ACID (DNA). This has been found to be involved in colon cancers termed HNPCC, or hereditary nonpolyposis colon cancer. Mutations in DNA repair genes also underlie the cancer predisposition in disorders such as ATAXIA TELENGIECTASIA, BLOOM SYNDROME, FANCONI ANEMIA and XERODERMA PIGMENTOSUM.

Drs. J. Michael Bishop and Harold E. Varmus (later director of the National Institute of Health) shared a 1989 Nobel prize for their pioneering work in developing the oncogene hypothesis.

Ondine's curse (congenital central hypoventilation syndrome)   A dysfunction of respiratory regulation which may lead to brain damage and death in affected infants due to deficient breathing. When those affected with this disorder sleep, they do not automatically breathe. Affected infants may also exhibit restlessness, hypertension, poor muscle tone, apnea, stupor and coma. About 70% have epileptic seizures. Some also have HIRSCHSPRUNG DISEASE.

Most cases are thought to be inherited by AUTOSOMAL RECESSIVE transmission. Males and females are affected in equal numbers. The disorder can be associated with MUTATIONS in at least three GENES, *RET* (10q), *GDNF* (*glial cell line-derived neurotrophic factor*) on chromosome 5p, and *EDN3* (*endothelin-3*) on chromosome 20q. Acquired cases also exist.

The name "Ondine's curse" comes from the legend of an ondine, or water nymph, who married a mortal man with the understanding that he would never again marry a mortal woman. However, when the ondine later returned to the sea, he remarried. The punishment for forsaking his vow varies in different accounts of the legend, but always seems to include loss of breathing control. The play *Ondine*, by Jean Giraudoux, published in 1939, seems to be the basis for naming this condition. In Giraudoux's play, the husband, Hans,

explains: "a single moment of inattention, and I forget to breathe. 'He died,' they will say, 'because it was a nuisance to breathe . . .'"

Opitz G/BBB syndrome (Opitz-Frias syndrome; hypertelorism-hypospadias syndrome)   Originally reported as two separate entities, the G syndrome and the BBB syndrome, both in 1969, it has since been recognized that the two are one single entity, which has been referred to by various names. The name Opitz G/BBB syndrome seems to be favored.

The characteristic facial appearance of individuals with Opitz G/BBB syndrome includes asymmetric skull, wide-spaced eyes (HYPERTELORISM), flat bridge of the nose, prominent ridge on the side of the skull, slit-like eyelids that are often slanted either slightly upward or downward, a fold of skin that obscures the inner juncture of the eyelids (EPICANTHUS), upturned nose (anteverted nares) and abnormal development of the ear with some degree of backward rotation. Males may have IMPERFORATE ANUS. In terms of genital abnormalities, females may have splayed labia minora; typically, males have HYPOSPADIAS, the malposition of the urethral opening on the underside of the penis. Other features include CLEFTS of lip, palate and uvula as well as congenital HEART DEFECTS. The ANOMALIES in the SYNDROME are all midline defects.

Affected infants have a hoarse or harsh cry, and frequently the swallowing mechanism is faulty, both due to laryngotracheo-esophageal abnormalities. Swallowing difficulties may result in choking and coughing. If such a defect is present, alternative methods of feeding are essential to ensure survival. Swallowing capacity improves with time, usually a few months to one year, to the extent that individuals are able to eat a normal diet. Death, when it occurs, generally is due to aspiration or starvation. In mild cases, prognosis for life span and reproductive ability appears normal. About two-thirds of patients may have some mild to moderate MENTAL RETARDATION.

The "G" in G syndrome is taken from the first letter of the last name of the family in which this condition was initially observed. This is a method of naming disorders favored by geneticist Dr. John Opitz, who first identified the condition in 1969.

Both AUTOSOMAL DOMINANT and X-LINKED forms of the disorder exist, clinically indistinguishable. An autosomal dominant form is linked to chromosome 22q11 (see CATCH 22). The GENE for the X-linked form has been recently identified on the short arm of the X CHROMOSOME and seems to be involved in midline development. PRENATAL DIAGNOSIS has been accomplished with ULTRASOUND.

oral-facial-digital syndrome (OFD syndrome) A heterogeneous (of varying origins) group of disorders with nine recognized variants. All nine exhibit similar abnormalities, and sufficient overlap exists to make appropriate counseling and reliable prognosis difficult.

OFD I An x-linked dominant disorder, limited to females and lethal in males. It has distinct oral, facial and digital anomalies. Affected individuals have a small, short (partial) midline cleft in the lip with bands of fibrous tissue that connect the cheeks and lip to the gums and often cleft the tongue. In addition to cleft palate and a thin nose with a broad nasal root, the position where the upper and lower eyelid meet near the nose (canthi) may be displaced. The skin may be dry and there is thinning of the hair (alopecia) in over half the patients. White nodular cysts of the sebaceous glands and hair follicles (milia) are seen on the face. Central nervous system defects are common (approximately 20%) and mental retardation is seen in over half of those brought to medical attention. Asymmetric shortening of the digits with or without webbing of the digits (syndactyly), or extra digits (polydactyly), which may be unilateral or bilaterally asymmetric, may be seen. One-third of patients die in infancy. Survivors require surgery for the oral clefts and comprehensive dental care. The locus of the causative gene has been mapped to Xp22.3–p22.2.

OFD II (Mohr syndrome) This form is named for Otto Mohr (1886–1967), dean of the medical faculty at the University of Oslo and president of the Norwegian Academy of Science, who published a description in 1941. Recognizable at birth, distinctive facial features and the presence of extra fingers or toes (polydactyly) or webbing together of fingers or toes (syndactyly) characterize this rare disorder. Affected individuals commonly exhibit a cleft tongue with ankyloglossia (tongue-tie). In addition, the bridge of the nose is low, and the tip of the nose is broad, with an indentation. The point at which the upper and lower inner eyelids meet near the nose (canthi) may be displaced outward, and a cleft lip and underdeveloped cheek and jaw bones are common.

Often an additional finger after the fifth finger is present on both hands (bilateral manual ulnar hexadactyly) and the big toe is partially reduplicated; there are two great toes fused together. In some cases three or four fingers may be webbed together with extra bones in between.

Though nervous system defects may cause mental impairment, most patients are of normal intelligence. Hearing loss (conduction DEAFNESS) is frequent due to a defect in the incus, one of the small bones of the middle ear. Respiratory infections may cause death during infancy.

Oral-facial-digital syndrome II is believed to be inherited as an AUTOSOMAL RECESSIVE trait.

OFD III (Sugarman syndrome) Bulbous nose, extra and small teeth and polydactyly that is exclusively postaxial are among the distinguishing characteristics. Macular red spots associated with see-saw winking of the eyelids and/or myoclonic jerks are also symptomatic. It is transmitted via autosomal recessive inheritance.

OFD IV (Buru-Baraister syndrome) Cerebral atrophy, porencephaly and short stature are seen in this autosomal recessive form along with pre- and/or postaxial polydactyly of the hands and feet and short tibiae.

OFD V (Thurston syndrome) Postaxial polydactyly of the hands and feet, midline cleft lip and a duplication of the frenulum, a small fold of white matter on the upper surface of the covering of the medulla in the brain, are the hallmarks of this autosomal recessive form.

OFD VI (Varadi-Papp syndrome) Preaxial polysyndactyly of the toes and postaxial polydactyly of the fingers, a forked metacarpal (the bones in the palm of the hand) and cerebellar anomalies are characteristic of this autosomal recessive disorder. Growth hormone deficiency and anomalies of the sex organs and hypothalamus are sometimes associated.

OFD VII (Whelan syndrome) Reported in a mother-daughter pair, this form is characterized by congenital hydronephrosis, coarse hair, facial asymetry and weakness of the facial muscles. A mutation in the *OFD1* gene has been found in this family.

OFD VIII Absent or abnormal central incisors, a broad or sometimes split nasal tip, metacarpal forking and pre- and postaxial polydactyly of the hands, as well as short stature, abnormal tibiae and underdevelopment of the epiglottis are hallmarks of this X-linked disorder.

OFD IX Retinal abnormalities in conjunction with OFD abnormalities distinguish this form, reported in three males.

The basic cause of the OFD syndromes is unknown. PRENATAL DIAGNOSIS of either may be possible by finding hand and foot abnormalities (or perhaps clefts) with ULTRASOUND (or FETOSCOPY) in at-risk pregnancies.

organic acidemia, organic aciduria A group of congenital hereditary disorders characterized by the inability to properly metabolize amino acids. The severity of these disorders ranges from mild to lethal.

The amino acids that comprise protein we consume as food are broken down by numerous enzymes. The synthesis of each enzyme is controlled by a gene, and mutations in these genes can interfere with the production of a viable enzyme. Thus, there are numerous acidemias and acidurias. They are typically named for the enzyme that is missing or defective, and include: 2-Methyl-3-Hydroxybutyrl CoA Dehydrogenase deficiency (MHBD); 2-Methylbutyrl CoA Dehydrogenase deficiency (2-MBCD); 3-Hydroxy-3-Methylglutaryl CoA Lyase deficiency (HMG); 3-Methylcrotonyl CoA Carboxyl deficiency (3-MCC); 3-Methylglutaconyl CoA Hydratase deficiency (3-MGA); Glutaric aciduria Type I (GA-1); Isobutyryl CoA Dehydrogenase deficiency (ICBD); Isovaleric acidemia (IVA); Malonic aciduria (MA); Methylmalonic acidemia (MMA); Mitochondrial Acetoacetyl CoA Thiolase (3-Ketothiolase) (BKT); Multiple CoA Carboxylase (MCD) and Propionic acidemia (PA).

Affected individuals exhibit elevated levels of one or more acids in the blood and urine, and diagnosis is typically made by detecting an abnormal concentration of organic acids in the urine by tandem mass spectrometry. Newborns are routinely screened for organic acidemia. In some conditions, the urine is always abnormal, in others the characteristic substances are only present intermittently.

ornithine transcarbamylase deficiency See UREA CYCLE DEFECTS.

Osler-Weber-Rendu syndrome (hereditary hemorrhagic telangiectasia, HHT) A hereditary disorder of the capillaries, characterized by vascular lesions, or telangiectasias, occurring on the skin, mucous membranes and in many internal organs. Telangiectasias are clumps of dilated blood vessels caused by deficiencies in the capillary system; the vessel walls lack elastic tissue wherever the lesions occur. When occurring near the skin's surface, well-defined areas of red skin are visible above them. Complications are caused by bleeding from these lesions and by degenerative changes the lesions may undergo.

It is named for English physicians Sir William Osler (1849–1919), author of the landmark *The Principles and Practice of Medicine*, Frederick P. Weber (1863–1962) and French physician Henri J. L. Rendu (1814–1902). They independently published descriptions in 1901, 1936 and 1996, respectively.

The characteristic telangiectasias appear as red-to-violet lesions on the cheeks, ears, lips and tongue, as well as in the mucous membranes of the nose. Internally, they may appear in the gastrointestinal tract, bladder, the lungs, brain, spinal cord and liver.

Bleeding occurs spontaneously or as a result of trauma. Bleeding from the nose (epistaxis) and the gastrointestinal tract progresses with age, often leading to chronic ANEMIA. Internally, the lesions are believed to be capable of developing into arteriovenous fistulae (anomalous connections between arteries and veins) that may appear in the lungs, pulmonary arteries, brain and liver. These give rise to an increased frequency of hemorrhages. Brain hemorrhages may give rise to seizures, transient paralysis and vision or speech difficulties. Complications may lead to death in 10% of individuals.

Treatment is directed at preventing or stopping bleeding and removing large lesions. Blood transfusions may be used if symptoms of ANEMIA are exhibited. The disorder is generally worsened by pregnancy.

HHT, previously underestimated, is now thought to have an incidence of one in 16,000 live births. Inherited as an AUTOSOMAL DOMINANT trait, it is heterogeneous, i.e., MUTATIONS in several different GENES can all cause the same disease (see HETERO-GENEITY), and it exhibits variability in expression. The most frequent gene involved has been mapped to 9q and encodes a protein found in the cells that line blood vessels named endoglin. Mutations in this gene have been found in families with HHT, particularly those who have had pulmonary arteriovenous malformations. Other families have had mutations in the gene for the activin A receptor, type II-like kinase 1 (also called activin receptor-like kinase 1), a cell-surface receptor with a tissue distribution that parallels that of endoglin. This gene maps to 12q. A form of HHT that is combined with juvenile polyposis is caused by mutations in the gene *SMAD4*. Other families with HHT appear to have the disease caused by one or more other genes.

osteogenesis imperfecta (OI; brittle bone disease)

Translated from its Greek and Latin derivations as "imperfectly formed bones," in this HEREDITARY DISEASE of the connective tissue bones may be so fragile that, for example, a child can fracture a tibia (the large bone in the lower leg) merely by swinging his leg. Fractures may even occur during fetal development. In addition to fragile bones, the cardinal features are blue sclerae (that is, an abnormal blueness in the white fibrous tissue that covers the so-called white of the eye) and DEAFNESS. However, affected individuals do not always exhibit all the symptoms. There is marked variability of expression of features among patients with this disorder.

The face tends to be triangular-shaped, with yellowish-brown teeth. Stature is short and growth is stunted. Other associated features include abnormal lateral curvature of the spine (SCOLIOSIS), high-pitched voice, excessive sweating, loose joints, tendency to bruise easily, respiratory problems and constipation. Those affected are also reported to exhibit euphoria and a general sense of well-being. There is great variability in symptoms and their severity. It may be limited to a few fractures in childhood, cause 50 to 100 fractures by adulthood, or cause death in the fetus or newborn.

Most deaths caused by OI are the result of associated cardiopulmonary problems. Severely affected individuals who don't succumb to these complications usually require braces, crutches or a wheelchair for mobility.

Historically, this disorder has been described under numerous names. The first case suggestive of the disorder was the mythical Danish prince, Ivar Benlos (boneless; legless), who had to be carried into battle on a shield because he was unable to walk on his soft legs. Reports of a disorder with abnormal bone brittleness and multiple fractures date to the end of the 17th century. The first description of a family exhibiting the condition was reported by a Swedish military surgeon in 1788. At one time it was speculated that French painter Toulouse-Lautrec had this affliction, but that now appears to be incorrect; he most likely had PYCNODYSOSTOSIS.

OI is now recognized to represent at least four subtypes, with incidence estimated at one in 20,000 live births. There are approximately 30,000 affected individuals in the United States. Most cases are inherited as an AUTOSOMAL DOMINANT trait (90%), though a rare AUTOSOMAL RECESSIVE form exists. Some of these cases are the result of new MUTATIONS. The disorder results from the defective development of collagen, a major protein in skin and bone. Specific abnormalities of the collagen GENES have been demonstrated in some affected individuals. The different forms of OI all result from a decreased synthesis of type I collagen. Mutations in the COL1A1 gene on chromosome 17 or COL1A2 on chromosome 7 lead to reduced amounts of normal collagen I. In other families, OI demonstrates GENETIC LINKAGE to the genes for collagen.

Type I is characterized by fractures, but little or no deformity; 8% of patients have the first fracture noted at birth, 23% in first year of life, 45% in the preschool years and 17% at school age. After adolescence the frequency of fractures decreases, although it appears that inactivity, pregnancy and lactation are associated with an increased frequency of fractures. Patients have blue sclerae and 50% have hearing loss as adults.

Type II OI is lethal in infants, who are born with multiple fractures and marked deformities of the long bones. The patients are usually stillborn or die in early infancy because of respiratory failure. The vast majority of cases result from SPORADIC mutations. The recurrence risk in a family after the birth of a child with type II OI is about 6–7%. This is thought to be because of the possibility of germline MOSAICISM.

Patients with type III usually have multiple fractures present at birth. There is progressive bone deformity from birth through childhood and adolescence. Short stature is present from before birth. The sclera are typically somewhat blue in infancy but are usually normal when older. Hearing loss and tooth abnormalities are common. It is said to be about one-eighth as common as type I. It results from different autosomal dominant mutations in the same genes as types I and II in the vast majority of cases. Recurrences in families with unaffected parents appear also to result from germline mosaicism, but in some rare instances there may be an autosomal recessive form.

Type IV is similar to type I except that the sclerae are not blue. There may be more bone deformity and more pronounced short stature than in type I. Tooth abnormality is common but hearing loss is rare.

Several additional types of OI (types V, VI, VII and VIII) have been proposed based on their characteristic clinical features and underlying genetic causes.

PRENATAL DIAGNOSIS for some forms of the disorder is possible via ULTRASOUND, and in some families by measuring fetal collagen levels or examining the collagen genes in fetal tissue collected by CHORIONIC VILLUS SAMPLING (CVS).

osteopetrosis, infantile   See INFANTILE OSTEOPETROSIS.

otitis media   See MIDDLE-EAR INFECTIONS.

oto-palato-digital syndrome (Taybi syndrome; Andre syndrome)   This disorder, which affects only males, has as its hallmarks CLEFT PALATE and hearing loss combined with abnormalities of the thumbs and toes. It occurs in two forms: OPD-I (Taybi syndrome) and OPD-II (Andre syndrome), distinguished by their severity and mode of inheritance.

Males with OPD-I, generally the milder form, exhibit conductive hearing loss, mild MENTAL RETARDATION and short stature. Characteristic craniofacial features include prominent frontal bone, downward slanting palpebral fissures, broad nasal bridge and underdeveloped (hypoplastic) facial bones. The thumbs and great toes are short and broad. Fingernails are short, as well. Space between the toes is wide and sometimes webbed (SYNDACTYLY).

An X-LINKED recessive trait, expression of OPD-I is variable in females. Some females who carry a copy of the recessive gene for OPD-I have similar facial features, with wide-set eyes, prominent frontal bone, depressed nasal bridge and a flat midface.

Craniofacially, males with OPD-II, the more severe form, exhibit MICROCEPHALY (small head), HYPERTELORISM (wide-set eyes), small mouth and jaw, in addition to the features of type I. Mental retardation, however, may be less common than in type I. Significant development delays have been reported. Fingers are short, flexed and overlapping. The long bones of the forearms and legs are bowed. The majority of affected infants have been stillborn or died before five months of age due to respiratory problems.

OPD-II is an X-linked trait. Female CARRIERS may exhibit short stature, arched palate and a broad face with downward slanting palpebral fissures and low-set ears. Females with both copies of the gene may show mild expression of the disorder, but no cases of a female with full OPD (either type I or II) exist in the literature. (See also DEAFNESS.)

Both of these disorders are among a heterogeneous group of disorders often referred to as the otopalatodigital spectrum disorders. This group includes FRONTOMETAPHYSEAL DYSPLASIA (FMD) and MELNICK-NEEDLES SYNDROME (MNS). Particularly in affected males, the severity of the disorders ranges from the mild manifestations seen in OPD1 to the more severe effects in FMD, OPD II and MNS, which is most commonly lethal before birth in affected males. All of these disorders are caused by mutations in the X-linked *FLNA* gene. Other mutations in this gene cause X-linked periventricular nodular heterotopia, a neuronal migration disorder that presents with seizures and nodules of neurons situated in the wrong place along the surface of the brain's lateral ventricles.

otosclerosis   A slowly progressive hearing loss with its genesis in the middle and inner ear, unrelated to inflammation or disease of the middle ear. It is primarily a conductive form of DEAFNESS; that is, caused by abnormalities in the structure of the ear, rather than in the auditory nerves (sensorineural deafness). (However, abnormalities in the auditory nerves may occur and result in sensorineural deafness.) Hearing loss occurs as the ear bone composed of cartilage becomes progressively replaced by calcified abnormal bone. It occurs in young or middle-aged adults and due to slow onset is often not easily detected.

Nearly 75% of all cases affect both ears (bilateral). Those who come to medical attention may have a history of hearing best in noisy settings (paracusis Willisani) and may frequently complain about ringing in the ears (tinnitus), sometimes accompanied by an audible pulse. A small percentage experience dizziness.

The cause of this disorder is not clear, but is believed to be related to destruction of the thin membrane lining of inner surface of cochlea in the inner ear.

Inherited as an AUTOSOMAL DOMINANT trait, the disorder appears to be genetically heterogeneous, as studies suggest the presence of causative genes on a number of chromosomes, including at least: 15q, 7q, 6p and 3q. It affects about 25% to 50% of those who inherit the gene. Thus, PENETRANCE is 25% to 50%.

Estimates for disease prevalence differ according to racial groups. For whites, it is 0.2 to 1% among adults, making it the single most common cause of hearing impairment; for blacks, it is about one in 3,300, and for Asians, about one in 33,000.

Detectability is limited in younger individuals since symptoms manifest during young or middle adulthood. It may be exacerbated by pregnancy. Ten percent of cases are apparent at ages 11 to 15, and 50% become apparent by the ages 21 to 25. Mean age of onset is in the third decade and 90% of affected persons are under 50 years of age at the time of diagnosis. Approximately 10% of affected persons developed profound sensineural hearing loss across all frequencies. Although the sensorineural component of the hearing loss cannot be corrected, microsurgery in stages is highly successful in restoring the normal conduction mechanism and can improve hearing thresholds by as much as 50 dB. Life span and intelligence levels are unaffected.

overgrowth syndromes   A group of disorders characterized by advanced height and head circumference in association with a variety of medical and developmental problems. Affected individuals may be unusually large at birth and exhibit excessive postnatal growth. Increased risk of cancer is a feature of a number of these syndromes. They include Wiedemann-Beckwith syndrome, hemihyperplasia, Sotos syndrome, proteus syndrome, Klippel-Trenaunay syndrome, Sturge-Weber syndrome, Maffucci syndrome, neurofibromatosis and fragile X syndrome.

oxycephaly   See CRANIOSYNOSTOSIS.

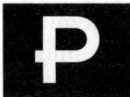

Pallister-Killian syndrome   A CHROMOSOME ABNOR-MALITY resulting in severe deveopmental retardation, seizures, lack of muscle tone (hypotonia) and distinctive facial features. The facial characteristics are visible at birth, and growth deficiency and lack of muscular deficiencies develop in infancy or early childhood. Severe developmental delays in psychomotor skills occur in later childhood, as do contractures and seizures.

All cases have appeared to be SPORADIC. Definitive diagnosis is made through genetic analysis. The KARYOTYPE of peripheral lymphocytes may be normal, but tetrasomy for 12p is seen in cultured fibroblasts and direct analysis of bone marrow. A number of other malformations may also be seen. A large number of those affected are stillborn or die in the newborn period. Incidence may be higher among the offspring of older mothers. PRENATAL DIAGNOSIS is possible by CHORIONIC VILLUS SAMPLING or AMNIOCENTESIS.

papyraceous fetus   A non-living FETUS that has been retained and not immediately and spontaneously aborted following death IN UTERO, and that exhibits a mummified appearance when ultimately delivered. This may occur, for example, when one of a pair of TWINS dies during fetal development, and is not delivered until the living twin is.

paramethadione   See ANTICONVULSANTS.

paramyotonia congenita (Eulenburg disease)   A very rare nonprogressive disorder characterized by intermittent weakness of the muscles, particularly those of the face, tongue and hands. Symptoms are usually first exhibited in infancy. The muscle weakness may be precipitated or exacerbated by exposure to cold. Low temperatures can also cause the muscles to stiffen or resist stretching.

Inherited as an AUTOSOMAL DOMINANT trait, this disorder is due to a MUTATION in the SCN4A GENE on 17q, the gene coding for the same sodium channel that is mutant in HYPERKALEMIC PERIODIC PARALY-SIS. Affected members of three large families have accounted for at least 60 cases.

paraplegia   Paralysis of both legs and the lower portion of the body, caused by damage or maldevelopment of the spinal cord. Infantile forms of paraplegia may be due to BIRTH INJURY.

Parenti-Fraccaro type achondrogenesis   See ACHONDROGENESIS.

Parkinson's disease (Parkinsonism)   Disorder characterized by tremors, mostly in the upper limbs, slow voluntary movements, stooped posture, shuffling gait and other physical symptoms that grow progressively more pronounced. A "masklike" facial expression is characteristic. It is named for London physician James Parkinson, who described it in "An Essay on the Shaking Palsy" in 1817, though this was not the first account of the disorder. The symptoms and suggested treatments are found in the *Ayurveda*, India's epic medical text, which dates to 5000 B.C., and in the *Nei Jing*, China's first medical text, which appeared in 500 B.C.

Parkinson's disease is the second most common neurogenic disorder after ALZHEIMER'S DISEASE, affecting approximately 1% of the population over age 50. Onset is typically between the ages of 50 and 65 years. Although occurring primarily in middle-aged and elderly populations, about 10%–20% of patients are under age 50. Some 500,000 Americans have Parkinson's disease and about 50,000 new cases are reported annually. Muhammad Ali and actor Michael J. Fox are among those affected, as was the late Pope John Paul.

While the origin of the disorder is unknown, some forms may be inherited, possibly as a MULTIFACTORIAL trait, and it has reportedly appeared in multiple generations in some families. Most cases are sporadic. There is a family history of Parkinson's disease in about 5–10% of affected individuals. In less than 1% of cases, it is clearly familial.

The disease can have more than one genetic and/or environmental cause. Lewy body Parkinson's disease appears to be a specific AUTOSOMAL DOMINANT disorder and juvenile Parkinsonism may be a specific autosomal dominant disorder, which has been described particularly in Japan. An X-LINKED recessive form of Parkinsonism occurs as part of at least two DYSTONIA syndromes, Segawa syndrome and the Filipino type of dystonia Parkinsonism. There is also evidence that mitochondrial MUTATIONS may cause or contribute to Parkinson disease (see MITOCHONDRIAL DISEASES).

In 1997, a GENE responsible for causing an autosomal dominant, early onset form of the disorder was mapped to the long arm of chromosome 4 (between genetic markers 4q21 and q23) by scientists at the National Human Genome Research Institute (see GENOME; GENE MAPPING). The gene, called PARK1, is a mutated form of the gene that codes for production of alpha synuclein, a protein involved in regulating the function of nerve cells. (A connection with Alzheimer's disease has been noted, as fragments of alpha synuclein have also been found in the amyloid plaques found in the brain of Alzheimer's patients upon autopsy.) Researchers believe this mutation accounts for a significant portion of this form of Parkinson's disease.

The gene was identified by studying a large Italian family, or kindred, in which some 50 members were affected. There is also a form of AUTOSOMAL RECESSIVE juvenile Parkinson's disease caused by mutation in a gene on 6q. This gene (*PARK2*) that encodes the protein parkin accounts

for about 50% of autosomal recessive Parkinson's disease.

Mutations in the *UCHL1 (PARK5)* gene, and *LRRK2* gene (which stands for *leucine-rich repeat kinase 2* and is also known as the *PARK8* gene) also cause autosomal dominant Parkinson disease. Mutations in the *DJ-1 (PARK7)* and *PINK1 (PARK6)* genes also result in autosomal recessive Parkinson's disease. In addition, there appear to be other susceptibility genes that can increase an individual's likelihood of being affected with Parkinson's disease that can be transmitted within a family. A specific mutation in the *LRRK2* gene is a major cause of Parkinson's disease among Ashkenazi (Eastern European) Jews. In addition, a group of North Africans of Arab descent have also been found to have a high frequency of this same gene mutation as a cause of Parkinson's disease. The *LRRK2* mutation may be found in both sporadic and in familial cases.

A study published by the American Medical Association in 1999 compared CONCORDANCE of Parkinson's diseases in monozygotic versus dizygotic TWINS, and concluded: "The similarity in concordance overall indicates that genetic factors do not play a major role in causing typical Parkinson's disease. No genetic component is evident when the disease begins after age 50 years. However, genetic factors appear to be important when the disease begins at or before age 50 years."

In families that do not have a Mendelian form of Parkinson's disease (that is, an autosomal dominant or recessive pattern), first-degree relatives of an affected individual have a lifetime risk of developing Parkinson's disease that is approximately 3–7%.

Treatment primarily consists of administration of levopoa (L-dopa) to patients, which makes up for the reduced levels of dopamine found in the brain of those with the disorder. Neural transplantation of dopamine-producing fetal cells directly into the brain has shown dramatic improvements in experimental treatment, but ethical issues regarding the use of fetal tissue make it unlikely this procedure will be widely used in the near future. A procedure used in advanced cases, pallidotomy, involves surgically cutting a lesion or scar in a portion of the brain.

Parkinsonism   See PARKINSON'S DISEASE.

Parry's disease See NEURONAL CEROID LIPOFUSCINOSIS.

passive euthanasia Allowing an individual to succumb to a fatal condition by withholding medical treatment. This sometimes occurs in the case of infants with severe CONGENITAL defects, generally at parental request. Opposition to passive euthanasia has, in some cases, led to legal efforts to compel medical treatment for affected infants. (See also BABY DOE.)

Patau syndrome (trisomy 13) A CHROMOSOME ABNORMALITY resulting from the presence of an extra chromosome 13. Named for U.S. geneticist K. Patau, who published the first description in 1960, it accounts for an estimated 1% of spontaneous ABORTIONS during the first trimester of pregnancy, and occurs in about one in 12,000 to one in 24,000 live births. It is slightly more common in females than in males.

The physical characteristics are so striking that diagnosis is often possible prior to the completion of CYTOGENETIC tests. These characteristics include a small head (MICROCEPHALY) exhibiting scalp lesions, sloping forehead, small eyes (microphthalmia) with sparse or absent eyebrows, CLEFT LIP or CLEFT PALATE, poorly formed ears and deformities of the hands and feet. The hand is often clenched and may have more than five fingers (POLYDACTYLY). The heel extends back abnormally.

Internally, there are frequently cardiac and renal (kidney) defects. Both males and females often display genital abnormalities, as well. The brain exhibits a malformation termed HOLOPROSENCEPHALY.

Only half of affected individuals survive the first month of life, only 25% survive beyond six months, 10% survive the first year, and 5% more than three years. However, survival to age 35 has been reported in a single case. PRENATAL DIAGNOSIS is possible by chromosome analysis of cells gathered via AMNIOCENTESIS or CHORIONIC VILLUS SAMPLING.

patent ductus arteriosus (PDA) Congenital HEART DEFECT resulting from the persistence after birth of a fetal duct that connects the pulmonary artery to the aorta. In the FETUS, the duct enables blood to bypass the lungs; no air enters them during fetal life. Soon after birth the duct ordinarily closes. PDA refers to the lack of this closure. This allows already oxygenated blood to flow back into the lungs, overloading the heart's ability to keep pumping blood, which may ultimately lead to congestive heart failure. The severity of the disorder is dependent on the size of the persisting fetal duct; the larger the opening, the more serious the consequences.

PDA is most common in premature infants, with females more often affected than males by a ratio of 2–3:1. It is also often associated with fetal rubella syndrome (see TORCH SYNDROME), TREACHER COLLINS SYNDROME and other single GENE disorders and CHROMOSOME ABNORMALITIES. It is usually not life-threatening and may spontaneously heal as the duct closes on its own. Infants are usually asymptomatic after one year of age. When the condition persists, affected infants are susceptible to bacterial infection of the heart (endocarditis) and may exhibit physical underdevelopment. In these cases the condition can be repaired surgically, generally resulting in complete recovery. If untreated, it may eventually cause cardiac failure and death.

PDA occurs in approximately one in 830 live births. Fifteen percent of those affected have additional cardiac abnormalities. The cause of the disorder is unknown, though MULTIFACTORIAL inheritance is suspected. Occasionally, patent ductus arteriosus occurs in so many members of multiple generations of a family that a simple AUTOSOMAL DOMINANT inheritance seems likely.

A SYNDROME first reported by Char in 1978, now referred to as Char syndrome, features patent arteriosus associated with unusual facial features: short philtrum (the midline groove between the nose and upper lip), duck-bill lips, PTOSIS (drooping eyes) and low-set ears. The inheritance pattern was consistent with autosomal dominant inheritance.

pectus From the Latin, pectus refers to the chest. Consistent deformities of the chest are seen in many GENETIC DISORDERS and CONGENITAL defects.

Pectus excavatum. Also called "funnel breast," this is an abnormally sunken chest. Some families have exhibited the condition in a pattern consistent with

AUTOSOMAL DOMINANT transmission. This deformity also occurs in hereditary disorders, including MARFAN SYNDROME.

Pectus carinatum. Popularly known as "pigeon breast" or "chicken breast," this is marked by an abnormal prominence of the sternum. It can also occur as part of malformation SYNDROMES such as Morquio disease (see MUCOPOLYSACCHARIDOSIS).

pedigree   A chart or schematic diagram detailing a family genealogy for the purpose of identifying and tracking the transmission of hereditary characteristics. The pedigree, or compendium of ancestors, is displayed through the use of symbols representing individual family members and lines representing their interrelationships.

The charts can be useful in determining if there is a genetic cause for an individual's anomalous condition, and if so, which form of MENDELIAN inheritance the trait follows: AUTOSOMAL DOMINANT, AUTOSOMAL RECESSIVE or X-LINKED. This information can then be explained to the affected individual and used as a means to assist in making family planning decisions.

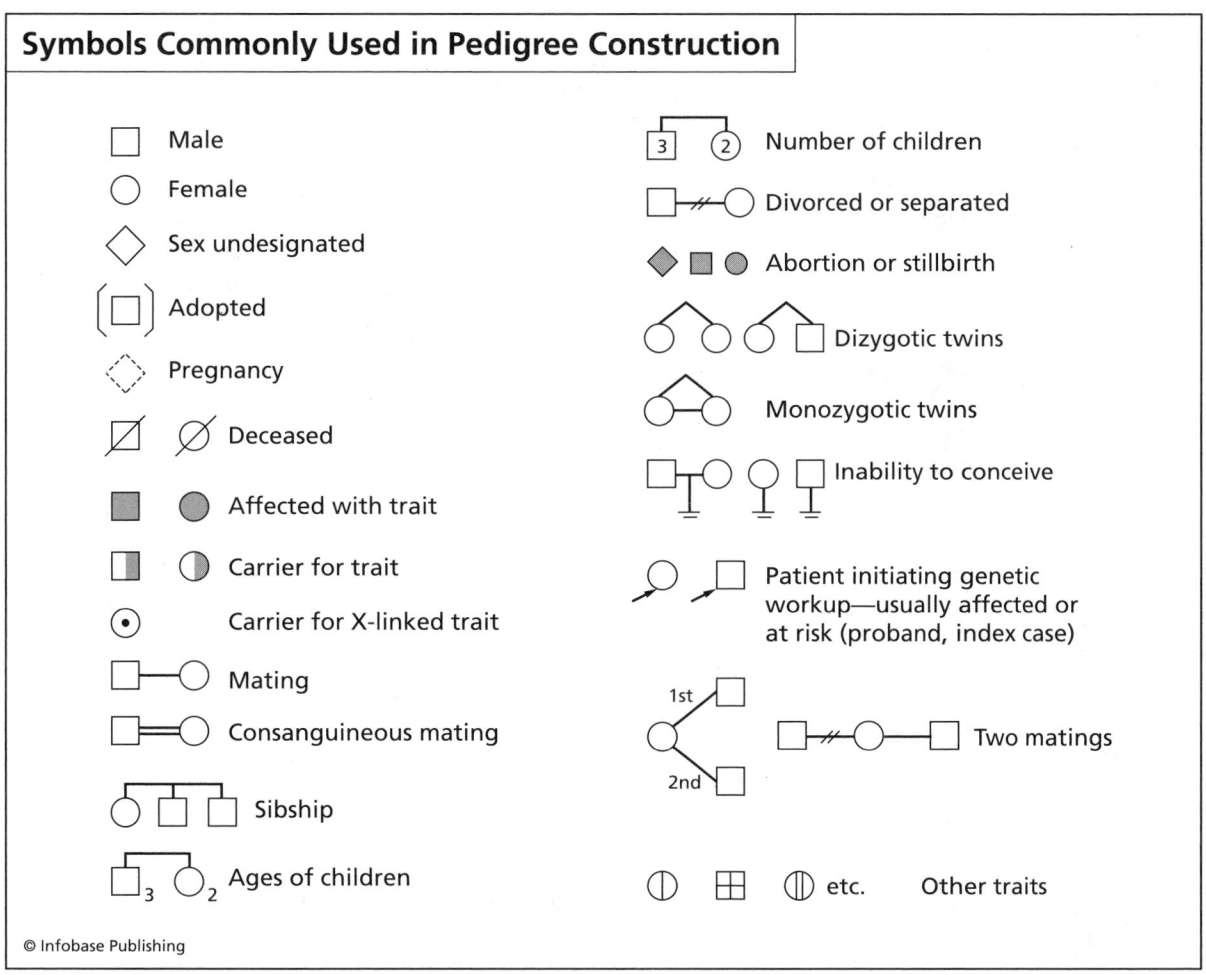

Symbols Commonly Used in Pedigree Construction

Male

Female

Sex undesignated

Adopted

Pregnancy

Deceased

Affected with trait

Carrier for trait

Carrier for X-linked trait

Mating

Consanguineous mating

Sibship

Ages of children

Number of children

Divorced or separated

Abortion or stillbirth

Dizygotic twins

Monozygotic twins

Inability to conceive

Patient initiating genetic workup—usually affected or at risk (proband, index case)

Two matings

etc.   Other traits

© Infobase Publishing

Adapted from the National Genetics Foundation, Inc., from R. B. Berini and E. Kahn (eds.), Clinical Genetics Handbook (Oradell, N.J.: Medical Economics Co., Inc., 1987). All rights reserved.

Sample Working Pedigree

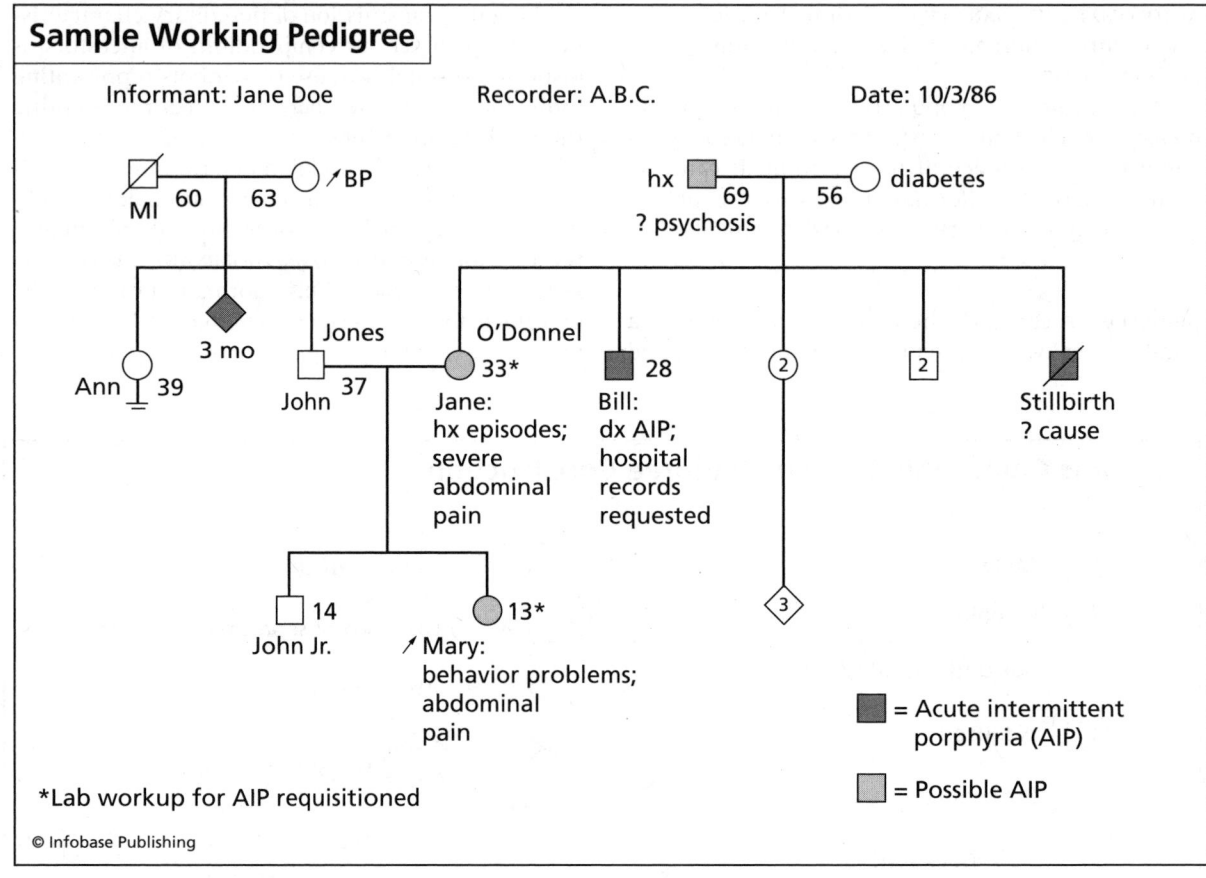

Informant: Jane Doe   Recorder: A.B.C.   Date: 10/3/86

*Lab workup for AIP requisitioned

■ = Acute intermittent porphyria (AIP)

▨ = Possible AIP

© Infobase Publishing

Information for preparing the chart is provided from interviews with the individual(s) undergoing counseling and from medical records, family photographs and examination of other family members.

Pelizaeus-Merzbacher disease   An infant-onset form of progressive spasticity named for German physicians F. Pelizaeus (1850–1917), who described the disorder in 1885, and L. Merzbacher (b. 1875), who described it in 1909.

Symptoms may appear from several days to six months after birth. It begins with a characteristic rolling motion of the head and eyes (nystagmus). This uncontrolled divergence and lack of coordination of the eyes is a common feature, and affected children are known in their families as "head nodders" and "eye waggers." (These symptoms may later, curiously, disappear.)

Developmental milestones of sitting and standing are delayed, and speech may be delayed as well. Mental abilities appear undiminished. The progression is gradual, with lower limbs and upper limbs showing increasing deterioration of muscular control. Movements of the arms become jerky and clumsy. Fine motor skills are especially affected. Dementia and Parkinsonian symptoms (see PARKINSON'S DISEASE) may develop over the first decade or two of life. Death often occurs between the ages of 16 and 25 years, often resulting from pneumonia brought on by respiratory complications resulting from the disorder. However, due to its slow progression, some individuals may survive much longer. Pelizaeus had one patient who lived to age 52.

The basic cause of the disorder is unknown, though it is associated with a loss of myelin, a fatlike sheath composed of lipids and proteins that surrounds some axons, the impulse-transmitting portions of nerve cells. The defect appears to be in the GENE for a component of myelin named proteolipid (PLP). A similar X-LINKED demyelination disorder occurs in the "jumpy" mouse.

This infant-onset disorder is inherited as an X-linked recessive trait and appears only in males. (Some heterozygous females, that is, CARRIERS of the recessive gene, may display symptoms of the disorder.) However, an adult-onset form has been identified as an AUTOSOMAL DOMINANT trait. In the autosomal dominant adult onset form, the signs and symptoms which begin in the third and fourth decade of life are often confused with those of MULTIPLE SCLEROSIS. There is also an AUTOSOMAL RECESSIVE acute infantile form that presents with muscle weakness and spasticity in the first weeks of life. CHORIONIC VILLUS SAMPLING (CVS) has been used for PRENATAL DIAGNOSIS of the classic X-linked form.

Pendred syndrome SYNDROME characterized by DEAFNESS in combination with an enlarged thyroid gland (goiter). While production of hormones in the thyroid is normal in most of those affected, those with deficiencies may experience a delay of skeletal maturation. A causal link between the thyroid disorder and the hearing deficit has not been established. (Hearing loss is associated with two other thyroid disorders: adult myxedema and endemic cretinism.)

The hearing impairment is sensorineural; it results from defects in the nerves involved in hearing, rather than blockage of hearing passageways or malformations of hearing organs (conductive deafness). The degree of impairment is variable, from mild to profound, though half exhibit severe to profound hearing loss. Usually both ears are affected identically (bilateral). It is present from early in life and may result in severe speech and language difficulties.

Pendred syndrome is inherited as an AUTOSOMAL RECESSIVE trait. Incidence has been estimated at between one in 12,500 and one in 100,000 live births, and it is believed to account for between 4% and 10% of all cases of sensorineural hearing impairment. The GENE has been identified and maps to 7q. The protein it produces, pendrin, appears to be a sulfate transporter. Its role in the development of the inner ear is unknown.

penetrance The proportion of individuals who exhibit an inherited trait for which they have inherited the necessary GENES. The term was coined by eminent German neuropathologist Otto Vogt in 1926 (who, at the same time, introduced a related term, EXPRESSIVITY). Implicit in this concept is the fact that not everyone who inherits the genes necessary to cause a hereditary disorder will exhibit the disorder. Penetrance is usually expressed as a percentage. If half of all those who possess the requisite gene(s) exhibit the disorder, penetrance is said to be 50%.

Taken as a whole, inherited conditions have a variable degree of penetrance. In disorders with a high degree of penetrance, virtually anyone who possesses the single dominant gene or the two recessive genes required for expression of the trait will exhibit it. In conditions with low penetrance, many who have the requisite genes may not exhibit any of the characteristic features of the trait. Interaction with other genes and with non-genetic factors may influence penetrance.

percutaneous umbilical blood sampling (PUBS) See CORDOCENTESIS.

periodic paralysis, familial A rare group of disorders, generally AUTOSOMAL DOMINANT in inheritance, characterized by attacks of weakness. The episodes may be accomplished by flaccid paralysis.

One form is associated with low potassium levels while others are associated with normal or high levels. The form with high potassium levels (hyperkalemic periodic paralysis) has been found to be due to MUTATIONS in a particular sodium ion channel GENE. This gene maps to 17q. Attacks in this condition often occur in the morning and last between 15 minutes and an hour and then improve spontaneously. Resting after strenuous exercise can provoke an attack of weakness. The frequency of attacks declines after the patient reaches mid-thirties to early forties.

Another LOCUS also may be involved in some cases. However, different mutations at this same locus cause other muscular disorders: PARAMYOTONIA CONGENITA and other myotonias. These disorders are characterized by muscle stiffness, which appears during exercise and worsens with continued exercise or exposure to cold. The muscles of the face, tongue, neck and head are most often involved. The symptoms are present from birth and persist through life.

The form of periodic paralysis with low levels of potassium (hypokalemic periodic paralysis) can be caused by mutations in a particular calcium ion channel gene mapped to 1q. It is genetically heterogeneous as at least one other gene must be involved; families with this disorder are known in which the gene is not involved. At least one family has demonstrated involvement of the sodium ion channel gene that usually causes hypokalemic paralysis.

The ion channel disorders include those such as spinocerebellar ataxia type 6 (SCA6) and rhythm disturbances of the heart such as prolonged QT syndrome (see ROMANO-WARD SYNDROME) and the JERVELL AND LANGE-NEILSON SYNDROME. Different ion channel diseases are involved in these disorders.

peroneal muscular atrophy   See CHARCOT-MARIE-TOOTH DISEASE.

pes cavus   See CLAWFOOT.

Peutz-Jeghers syndrome   See COLORECTAL CANCER.

Peyronie disease (bent stick syndrome)   A progressive deformity of the penis with onset in middle age; it results in an abnormal curvature (in any direction), especially during erection. François de la Peyronie (1648–1747), surgeon to King Louis XIV and a founder of the Royal Academy of Surgery in Paris, first published a description of the disorder in 1743. Inherited as an AUTOSOMAL DOMINANT trait, it is caused, as is DUPUYTREN CONTRACTURE, a condition with which it is associated, by the hardening of fibrous tissue. Although it is essentially benign and painless, it may interfere with intercourse. No effective treatment has been developed. Attempts to surgically remove fibrous masses typically result in generation of new hardened tissue.

Pfeiffer syndrome (acrocephalosyndactyly)   A form of CRANIOSYNOSTOSIS, skull malformations caused by premature closure of the gaps (sutures) between one or more skull bones. Growth is thus directed in aberrant directions. This form is named for R. A. Pfeiffer, who published a description in 1964.

The characteristic head shape, observable at birth is marked by a high forehead and squat skull (brachycephaly). Eyes are wide set (HYPERTELORISM) and the eye slits (palpebral fissures) are slanted down away from the nose (antimongoloid obliquity). The digits on hands and feet (particularly the second and third) exhibit webbing (SYNDACTYLY). The fingers are short, the thumbs and great toes are broad. However, facial features tend to attain a more normal appearance with age, and no treatment may be required. Intelligence is usually normal. This disorder is inherited as an AUTOSOMAL DOMINANT trait; many cases are new MUTATIONS.

Mutations in the GENE for *fibroblast growth factor receptor-1 (FGFR1)* cause one form of familial Pfeiffer syndrome. Other cases are caused by a mutation in the gene for *fibroblast growth factor receptor-2 (FGFR2)*: The original family reported by Pfeiffer (in 1964) was of this type. Yet other families cannot be related to either the *FGFR1* LOCUS on chromosome 8 or the *FGFR2* locus on chromosome 10 by GENETIC LINKAGE studies. Many different mutations (>50) in the *FGFR2* gene have been found, and specific ones result in one or more of the well-known craniosynostosis syndromes, such as APERT SYNDROME, CARPENTER SYNDROME and Pfeiffer. For example, one mutation has been found to underlie either Pfeiffer, CROUZON DISEASE or JACKSON-WEISS SYNDROME in different families. These disorders differ on the basis of the limb ANOMALY seen and in some cases may represent variable expressions of the same mutation. The Crouzon and Pfeiffer phenotypes usually "breed true" within families, and the finding of identical mutations in unrelated individuals giving different phenotypes was a highly unexpected discovery. (See also SAETHRE-CHOTZEN SYNDROME.)

phakomatosis (neurodermatosis)   Any one of a group of CONGENITAL and hereditary disorders characterized by skin (cutaneous) and nerve (neurological) abnormalities. They include NEUROFIBROMATOSIS, VON HIPPEL–LINDAU DISEASE, STURGE-WEBER SYNDROME and TUBEROUS SCLEROSIS.

phenobarbital   The barbiturate phenobarbital, prescribed to prevent epileptic seizures and as a sedative, has been named as a suspected TERATOGEN, a substance capable of causing BIRTH DEFECTS. However, it is often prescribed in combination with other drugs known to cause birth defects and there is disagreement on whether phenobarbital alone can induce fetal malformations. Some studies indicate that it magnifies the risks associated with some drugs it is frequently prescribed with.

Infants born to women taking barbiturates may exhibit drug withdrawal symptoms, and their blood may not clot normally. (See also ANTICONVULSANTS.)

phenotype   The observable or measurable characteristics associated with a GENE or genes. Most genetic conditions have characteristic physical or internal features, and the features exhibited by individuals with these conditions are said to be phenotypes. (This is in contrast to GENOTYPE, which refers only to having a particular gene or genes, not whether or how the associated traits are expressed in an individual; sometimes the gene does not manifest itself.)

The term *phenotype* was introduced in the early 1890s by Wilhelm Ludwig Johannsen (1857–1927), a pharmacist's apprentice from Copenhagen who went on to achieve considerable renown in the fields of GENETICS and botany. He also introduced the terms *gene* and *genotype*. (See also EXPRESSIVITY and PENETRANCE.)

phenylketonuria   An ENZYME deficiency disorder characterized by the inability to convert one AMINO ACID, phenylalanine, to another, tyrosine. (Amino acids are the building blocks of proteins.) Consequently, phenylalanine accumulates in the body, resulting in severe MENTAL RETARDATION. This disorder has been the prototype disease for newborn screening. If detected early enough through blood and urine tests, the disease can be halted. In most states it is routine to test for phenylketonuria in the first few days of life, after the infant has been exposed to a significant protein intake.

Symptoms may include severe vomiting and seizures during the first weeks of life, a "mousy" smell, dry skin or an eczema-like rash. Slightly smaller head (MICROCEPHALY), behavioral problems, abnormal hand movements and brisk reflexes may also be observed. Often, the brain-wave test (electroencephalogram or EEG) is abnormal.

Once diagnosed, the child can be treated with a diet that limits the intake of foods containing phenylalanine. With early treatment, the prognosis is excellent. Here again, this disease has been a prototype disorder for the treatment of inborn errors of metabolism through nutritional manipulation and dietary restriction. However, once mental retardation and seizures set in, the patient's life span may be shortened. It has been previously debated as to when and if the diet can be discontinued in an affected individual. Current recommendations are to continue the diet for life. Also, the metabolic dysfunction of women with PKU can have adverse effects upon the FETUS during gestation even if the fetus does not have the enzyme deficiency. Infants, with the maternal PKU syndrome exhibit microcephaly, mental retardation and congenital HEART DEFECTS.

Most children with the disorder have blond hair, blue eyes and fair skin. It is less likely to occur in blacks and Ashkenazi Jews (those of Eastern European ancestry). Inherited as an AUTOSOMAL RECESSIVE trait, it occurs in approximately one in 15,000 live births. The highest incidence occurs in Ireland and Scotland, lending support to the theory that the PKU gene is Celtic in origin. The PKU gene has been identified and mapped to chromosome 12.

Using molecular biologic techniques with the cloned PKU gene, PRENATAL DIAGNOSIS and CARRIER detection are possible in at-risk families.

The first case of PKU was identified by Asborn Folling in Norway in 1934. He detected and identified an abnormal substance in the urine of two mentally retarded SIBLINGS. (Coincidentally, it was later discovered that the children's mother was a distant relative of Folling's.) In a 1947 paper published in the *Journal of Biological Chemistry*, George A. Jervis identified the metabolic defect in the disease, and 20 years after Folling discovered the disease, German physician H. Bickel described the treatment of PKU. With the realization that PKU was a treatable form of mental retardation, if diagnosed early, Robert Guthrie, professor of pediatrics at the University of Buffalo, developed a simple screening test in 1963.

Today, millions of newborn children worldwide are screened for phenylketonuria, and thousands of children have been detected early, treated, and are leading normal, productive lives. PKU has served as an important example of the application of GENETICS in public health and in the prevention of mental retardation.

phenylthiocarbamide tasting   Common benign inherited trait that determines an individual's ability to taste phenylthiocarbamide (PTC). About 70% of the general population possess this trait and are said to be "tasters." A taste test using a strip of paper laced with PTC can determine the presence or absence of this trait in most individuals. PTC will taste bitter to those who possess the trait, and have no taste to those without it. Due to the ubiquity of this condition and the simplicity of the test, it is frequently used in high school science courses as a GENETICS demonstration.

Geneticists have attempted to link the GENE for this trait with genes for various inherited disorders in order to use it as a marker for simplified screening procedures, but thus far, these linkage efforts have been unsuccessful. Previously thought to be AUTOSOMAL DOMINANT, it may in fact be POLYGENIC. The incidence of inability to taste PTC is much lower in blacks than in whites in North America: 3% as compared with 30%.

phocomelia   A CONGENITAL malformation characterized by short, flipper-like appendages. The por-tions of the extremities nearest (proximal) to the body are poorly developed or absent, so hands and feet are attached almost directly to the trunk. An affected individual is said to be a "phocomelus."

This condition was associated with the use of THALIDOMIDE, a prescription sleeping pill marketed in Europe, Australia and Canada that was subsequently found to have teratogenic properties (see TERATOGENS). It can be seen in other conditions as well, including ROBERTS SYNDROME and HOLT-ORAM SYNDROME.

Pickwickian syndrome (obesity-hypoventilation syndrome)   A complication of extreme OBESITY that may result in death from interference with cardiac and respiratory functions (cardiorespiratory embarrassment). Its name is inspired by the obese character, Joe, in Charles Dickens's *The Pickwick Papers*. Individuals with PRADER-WILLI SYNDROME may develop and succumb to problems associated with this disorder.

The marked obesity causes obstruction to airflow and individuals may have restless and noisy sleep. Ultimately, as their obesity interferes with normal respiration to a severe degree, they may become so oxygen-deprived that they exhibit excessive sleepiness and may develop heart failure.

piebald skin trait   Piebald means spotted, or of different colors. Patches of skin of affected individuals are depigmented, thus giving them a spotted, piebald appearance. Depigmented areas are most common on the front of the body, such as the forehead, chest, abdomen and extremities. The borders of these patches may be hyperpigmented. There may be a white forelock of hair, and the eyebrows may be depigmented as well. Some individuals also have eyes of different color (HETEROCHROMIA IRIDES).

A piebald Mandan was painted by George Carlin (1796–1872), an artist known for his portraits of Native Americans, and the condition was said to have been common in the tribe. Though rare in other human populations, where it is inherited via AUTOSOMAL DOMINANT transmission, the piebald trait is common in the animal kingdom. A MUTATION in the KIT proto-oncogene causes the AUTO-

SOMAL DOMINANT form of piebaldism. It has been mapped to 4q11-q12.

Pierre Robin syndrome   See ROBIN ANOMALY.

pituitary dwarfism   The pituitary gland is a small organ, located in the brain, that controls the release of hormones (chemicals necessary for growth, reproduction, nutrition and metabolism) in the body. In pituitary DWARFISM, the pituitary gland fails to function properly, resulting in subnormal growth rate, and ultimately, stunted growth (proportional dwarfism).

Hereditary pituitary dwarfism is a genetically heterogeneous group of conditions including CONGENITAL defects of the pituitary, AUTOSOMAL RECESSIVE and X-LINKED panhypopituitary dwarfism, and peripheral unresponsiveness to growth hormone (see HETEROGENEITY).

These conditions cause slow growth rate after the first two years of life and may also result in low blood sugar (hypoglycemia), high-pitched voice and fat pads around the chest and abdomen (truncal obesity). Because the cheekbones and jaws are small, the face is distorted.

Additionally, if sex hormones are not produced by the pituitary, the child may not undergo puberty. Females will fail to menstruate or develop adult breasts or pubic hair. Males will have a small penis and testes and no facial hair.

Other organs affected are the thyroid gland, which plays a role in regulating growth and metabolism, and the adrenal gland, which, along with the pancreas, plays a role in the control of sugar levels in the body. As a result, the person may have low blood levels of sugar. (This condition improves as the child gets older.) Mild MENTAL RETARDATION can occur in some types of pituitary dwarfism.

There are four major types of pituitary dwarfism:

Familial panhypopituitary dwarfism. This is characterized by HGH (human growth hormone) deficiency and lack of one or more additional pituitary hormones, most typically gonadotropin (which regulates sexual development), ACTH (adrenocorticotropic hormone, which stimulates the adrenal gland) and TSH (thyroid-stimulating hormone). The features of this form depend on the specific hormones that are missing. Without gonadotropin, individuals will fail to mature sexually, and secondary sexual characteristics will not develop. Deficiency of ACTH may cause severe hypoglycemia. TSH deficiency may interfere with the functioning of the thyroid gland.

Most cases are not genetically influenced, though there are both autosomal recessive and X-linked recessive forms of the disorder.

This form of proportional dwarfing is believed to be the condition that affected TOM THUMB, the circus dwarf.

Congenital absence of the pituitary. Affected individuals are born without a pituitary gland, and there is a deficiency of HGH, ACTH and TSH. Individuals exhibit mental and physical retardation. The condition is inherited as an autosomal recessive trait.

Isolated HGH deficiency. Results from MUTATION in the GH gene on 17q. Inherited in both autosomal recessive and AUTOSOMAL DOMINANT fashion, different mutations account for either the dominant or recessive expression. Sexual development is generally normal as is the functioning of the adrenal and thyroid glands. Individuals with the recessive form have hypoglycemia attacks and insulin hypersensitivity. Growth hormone-releasing hormone (GHRH) acting through the GHRH receptor, plays a pivotal role in the regulation of GH synthesis and secretion in the pituitary. The molecular basis for the "little" (lit) mouse phenotype, characterized by a hypoplastic anterior pituitary gland, is a point mutation in the growth hormone releasing factor receptor, the GENE for which maps to 7p15-p14. In a consanguineous family (see CONSANGUINITY) with profound growth hormone deficiency, a nonsense mutation in the human GHRHR gene was demonstrated, and the phenotype in this family was comparable to that in the "little" mouse.

Laron-type pituitary dwarfism. Marked short stature and clinical GH deficiency are hallmarks of this autosomal recessive disorder. Caused by dysfunction of the growth hormone receptor (GHR), it could be termed GH insensitivity syndrome, or GH resistance. There are two types of GHR dysfunction. The first, type I, is associated with defects in GHR (the gene, mapped to 5p) while the second is apparently due to a defect in the process started once GH binds to the receptor.

Affected individuals are severely dwarfed, though normally proportioned. In females, there is normal female sexual maturation, while males exhibit delayed puberty. There may be mild MENTAL RETARDATION.

Combined pituitary hormone deficiency has been shown to be produced by MUTATIONS in the pituitary-specific TRANSCRIPTION FACTOR (PIT1;3p11). Furthermore, depending on the location of the mutation within the gene product, either autosomal dominant or recessive inheritance of the resulting PHENOTYPE can occur. Because these individuals typically have hypogonadism and are infertile, suspicion that it is an autosomal dominant trait is difficult to validate.

Administration of hormones can alleviate some of the features associated with hormone deficiencies.

Currently, there is no method of PRENATAL DIAGNOSIS for these conditions. The exception is those families with autosomal recessive isolated but complete HGH deficiency, where a gene deletion can be found. In these families molecular diagnostic techniques may be used for prenatal diagnosis. When a molecular defect is known in a family, for example in those families with autosomal recessive isolated complete GH deficiency where a gene deletion is found, molecular techniques may be used for prenatal diagnosis. The outlook for a normal life span is favorable.

plagiocephaly   See CRANIOSYNOSTOSIS.

pleiotropy   The ability of one GENE or gene pair to have numerous effects, or produce various characteristics. For example, the aberrant gene that causes MARFAN SYNDROME may manifest itself in abnormalities of the skeletal, cardiovascular, or other systems, and therefore exhibits pleiotropy.

poikiloderma atrophicans and cataracts   See ROTHMUND-THOMSON SYNDROME.

Poland sequence (Poland syndactyly)   Named for Alfred Poland (1822–72), this is a sporadically occurring developmental field defect involving muscles and tissue on one side of the chest and the hand on the same (ipsilateral) side. (A field defect is one with its origin in an isolated and localized area of the developing embryo.) Poland was a demonstrator of anatomy when he published the first account of this SYNDROME in 1841; he later became senior ophthalmologist at Guy's Hospital in London.

The syndrome is highly variable in expression. The constant features are abnormalities of the nipple, subcutaneous tissue and two of the major chest muscles, the pectoralis major and minor.

The breast and underlying tissue may be absent, or the nipple and breast may be displaced upward, located in the area of the armpit, for example. In both men and women, the affected breast will be smaller than the unaffected one. Portions of cartilage of the ribs may also be absent. There is usually no hair (hypotrichosis) on affected tissue. SPRENGEL DEFORMITY has been seen in some affected individuals.

The affected hand is usually smaller than the non-affected hand, and may exhibit several deformities. There may be absence of all or part of the hand. The middle bones of the fingers (phalanges) may be absent or fused with the first bone, and the skin between fingers may be webbed (SYNDACTYLY). The thumb is usually least affected.

Heredity generally does not appear to play a role in the condition, and most cases are SPORADIC. (However, cases have been attributed to AUTOSOMAL DOMINANT inheritance.) The syndrome has been estimated to occur in one in 20,000 live births. It has been estimated that about 10% of patients with syndactyly of the hand have the Poland sequence. It is three times as common in the male as the female, and 75% of the time involves the right hand. Since the vast majority of cases are sporadic, recurrence risk is negligible. The cause of the syndrome has been proposed to be the impairment of blood supply to the developing field structures.

Prenatally, if hand and chest deformities are severe, it may be possible to identify the condition via ULTRASOUND and FETOSCOPY.

polycystic kidney disease (PKD)   A group of disorders characterized by fluid-filled sacs (cysts) that slowly develop in both kidneys, eventually resulting in kidney malfunctioning. A high proportion of affected individuals develop kidney failure, requiring dialysis or kidney transplant. It is the third leading cause of kidney failure in the United States. It accounts for about 8–10% of cases of end-stage kidney disease.

One kidney can contain several hundred of these cysts, which form on the renal tubules, normal structures within the kidney. The cysts cause the kidneys to swell, often to several times their normal size, and can cause pain, blood in the urine, and kidney stones. They can also be associated with liver cysts and aneurysms in the brain or abdomen. Forty percent to 60% of PKD patients develop polycystic livers.

PKD is a GENETIC DISORDER and occurs in two forms: one inherited in AUTOSOMAL DOMINANT manner is slowly progressive, leading to chronic renal failure. It is a common disorder, estimated to affect as many as 300,000 to 500,000 Americans, and is found in all races and ETHNIC GROUPS. Some cases may be the result of new MUTATION. The less common AUTOSOMAL RECESSIVE form causes a severe kidney disease in infancy, with death in infancy or childhood. A study in Denmark showed that autosomal dominant PKD is one of the most common genetic diseases in humans (approximately one in 1,000 individuals affected), and is the most common genetic kidney disease.

In the dominant form, sometimes referred to as adult PKD, symptoms usually develop in the 30s, when abdominal pain or blood in the urine may appear. Calling it adult PKD is a misnomer, however, because the age of onset is variable and cysts have been found as early as on prenatal ULTRASOUND in some cases.

HYPERTENSION is found in about half of all PKD patients, apparently the result of increased production of the hormone angiotensin in the kidney, which elevates blood pressure, caused by the expanding kidney cysts. There is wide variability in expression of the disorder, with many affected individuals remaining unaware of the condition throughout their lives. However, there is generally consistency within families in the degree of severity and the age of onset. About half of all PKD patients ultimately develop kidney failure.

Diagnosis is made though a physical examination that may include CAT scan (computerized axial tomography) and sonogram to detect the development of cysts in the kidneys. Familial history can also play an important role in diagnosis.

The cause for the abnormal growth of kidney tubule cells that result in the disorder is unknown. However, it appears the cells that form the cysts operate in a way similar to simple benign tumors. But unlike tumors, these cells promote the accumulation of fluid as well as tissue mass.

More than one GENE LOCUS plays a role in the development of PKD. This is an example of genetic HETEROGENEITY, whereby a single disorder may result from any one of several defects. One gene that appears responsible for the most common form of PKD has been found on 16p. (A gene for tuberous sclerosis is located nearby.) The gene encodes a protein that has been termed polycystin-1. Detection of mutations in this gene is complicated and many mutations are known. A second gene on 4q has been identified and encodes polycystin-2. Some cases of autosomal dominant PKD do not appear to be caused by these two genes. In families where linkage to either gene can be demonstrated, GENETIC MARKERS can be used for presymptomatic or PRENATAL DIAGNOSIS.

The recessive form of PKD has been called infantile polycystic kidney disease. In addition to malfunctioning kidneys, infants may exhibit a characteristic "Potter's face" (squashed nose, small jaw and large, floppy, low-set ears), resembling a face pressed against a window pane, caused by the compression against the walls of the uterus due to lack of AMNIOTIC FLUID. (It is named for the physician who described the condition.) The amniotic fluid is mostly made up of fetal urine, which here is deficient because of the fetal kidney disease. Few affected newborns survive infancy. Affected infants with the recessive form of PKD also often have CONGENITAL fibrosis of the liver. Often the lungs have been underdeveloped. There have been reports of successful prenatal diagnosis in this form of PKD, using ultrasound. Incidence is approximately one in 40,000. It appears to be more common in Afrikaans-speaking families in South Africa. The gene, termed the *PKHD1* gene, has been mapped to 6p.

Polycystic kidneys are also associated with several genetic SYNDROMES, including EHLERS-DANLOS SYNDROME, TUBEROUS SCLEROSIS, MECKEL SYNDROME, ZELLWEGER SYNDROME and trisomy 13 (see PATAU SYNDROME).

polydactyly   Having more than the normal number of fingers or toes. This condition is seen in many GENETIC DISORDERS and also exists as an isolated malformation occurring in several forms, distinguished by the position and degree of definition of the extra digits. One inherited form, in which an extra digit after the fifth finger exists, is transmitted as an AUTOSOMAL DOMINANT trait. Ten times more frequent in blacks than in whites, a survey in Nigeria in 1976 found incidence of this form approximately 18 per 1,000 for females and 27 per 1,000 for males.

Polydactyly has an important place in the history of GENETICS. In the 1750s French naturalist Pierre Louis Moreau de Maupertuis (1698–1759) published the pedigree of Haboc Ruhe, a surgeon of Berlin, who had extra digits on all four limbs, a trait he inherited from his mother and grandmother, and which he transmitted to two sons out of six children. Maupertuis invoked "elementary particles" as the hereditary transmission agent, interpreting the PEDIGREE in terms that presaged Mendel's theories of inheritance, which came over a century later.

polygenic   An inherited trait caused by the action of two or more GENES. Though sometimes used interchangeably with MULTIFACTORIAL, multifactorial is more properly a term for disorders caused by the combined action of one or more genes, environmental influences and other unknown factors. In fact, most traits labeled polygenic are actually multifactorial; that is, environment plays a role in their expression.

polymastia   The growth of more than two breasts or nipples. Complete extra mammary glands are rare; more commonly extra nipples appear. It is usually detectable at birth, but in some cases development occurs only after puberty or pregnancy.

The majority of excess glands are located in the "milkline"—the area between the armpit and the groin, but, in rare instances, accessory breasts have appeared on the face, neck, arms, thighs, buttocks and back. They occur more frequently on the left side than on the right side of the body, and single additional breasts or nipples are more common than multiple ones.

Accessory breasts undergo the same cyclic changes as normal breasts and are prone to the same diseases, such as BREAST CANCER. It is not known, however, if tumors are more common in normal breasts or in accessory breasts. Extra breasts located above the normal breasts area typically are positioned toward the outside of the body; when located below the normal breast area, the extra breasts are positioned toward the midline of the body. The outer-positioned glands are usually well formed and can lactate, while the medial glands are imperfectly developed and cannot.

Occurrence is estimated at a remarkably high one in 100 in the general population, and reports of prevalence have ranged from one in 17 in New York females to one in 250 British children. In whites, nearly 90% of accessory breasts are located below the normal breasts and affect men more frequently than women. For the Japanese, however, about 90% of accessory breasts are located above normal breasts, and incidence for females is three times as great as males.

Polymastia is inherited as an AUTOSOMAL DOMINANT trait in some families, though the exact genetic basis in the majority of cases is unclear.

polymorphism   The multiple variations of a given GENE or genes; the ability of a GENETIC DISORDER to appear in more than one form.

A RESTRICTION FRAGMENT LENGTH POLYMORPHISM is a variation in DNA sequence (see DEOXYRIBONUCLEIC ACID). These polymorphisms are often useful as GENETIC MARKERS for linkage analysis. Individual fragments can be identified on the basis of the difference in length of DNA generated after the DNA is cleaved with a RESTRICTION ENZYME.

polyposis   See FAMILIAL POLYPOSIS SYNDROMES under CANCER.

polysplenia syndrome Malformation and duplication of internal organs characterize this rare CONGENITAL disorder. Affected individuals develop two spleens instead of the normal one, and may have one or more additional small spleens (splenules). This is a SYNDROME of bilateral "left-sidedness," i.e., right-sided organs or members of pairs of organs that are normally not symmetrical exhibit the structural characteristics of their left-sided counterparts, but in mirror images. For example, the right side of the lung normally has a distinctive branch of the bronchial tubes (the epiarterial bronchus), but in about 70% of individuals with this syndrome it matches the left lung. Likewise, the right and left lobes of the liver are of equal size, and the stomach may appear on either the left or right side (suits inversus). Intestinal defects are also common.

A range of heart malformations are usually present, such as abnormal return of venous blood to the right and left atria. Defects in the membranes of the heart that separate the chambers also occur (see HEART DEFECTS).

In asplenia, a condition of having no spleen, there is bilateral right-sidedness. Both bilateral left-sidedness (polysplenia) and bilateral right-sidedness (asplenia) have been seen in different members of the same family, suggesting two different presentations of an underlying primary genetic defect in body lateralization and symmetry. Asplenia/polysplenia are also known as isomerism sequence, or laterality sequence. Taken together, they have a frequency of about one in 22,000. Recurrence risks for SIBLINGS of about 5–10% have been suggested. Certain cases may be caused by mutations in the X-linked *ZIC3* gene, or the *CFC1* gene, encoding the CRYPTIC protein, on chromosome 2. Another locus for laterality abnormalities has been mapped to chromosome 6q.

Life span depends on the severity of heart defects. In extreme cases, insufficiency of oxygen (cyanosis), difficulty breathing and feeding, and congestive heart failure cause death within days or weeks of birth. When there are few or no cardiac abnormalities, individuals live to adulthood.

polysyndactyly The condition in which an individual has a greater than normal number of digits (fingers or toes) in association with fusion of the digits. The extra digits vary from well formed to mere skin tags, and the fusion varies from webbing of the skin between the digits to complete joining of bones of the digits. This condition is seen in a number of GENETIC DISORDERS. (POLYDACTYLY indicates having extra digits; SYNDACTYLY indicates the webbing of digits.)

Pompe's disease See GLYCOGEN STORAGE DISEASE, type II.

porencephaly Abnormal cavities within the brain. The condition may involve one side of the brain (unilateral) or both (bilateral).

The unilateral form usually results from birth trauma, infection or fetal vascular occlusions and lack of blood supply. As a result of these insults there is destruction and death of brain tissue. As these necrotic regions of brain dissolve, cavities remain and become cysts within the substance of the brain.

In the bilateral and symmetrical form, the abnormal cavities in the cerebral hemispheres mirror each other. This form represents a primary defect in the development of embryonic nerve tissue. A familial component of this form was first reported in 1983, with inheritance suggested as AUTOSOMAL DOMINANT. Increased access to computerized axial tomography (CAT) scans may enable the identification of more affected individuals. Individuals with porencephalic cysts may exhibit neurologic deficits (including seizures or CEREBRAL PALSY) or may be completely asymptomatic with relatively normal development. The cysts may be identified by prenatal ULTRASOUND.

porphyria Porphyrins are a group of nitrogen-containing organic compounds that form the basis of animal and plant respiratory pigments. In humans, they form heme, the iron-containing and oxygen-carrying portion of hemoglobin, and in plants, they form chlorophyll. "Porphyria" refers to a group of inborn errors of metabolism in which porphyrin is not converted to heme in a normal fashion, resulting in the accumulation of porphyrin or "porphyrin precursors" in the body. This causes disturbances in the nervous system or the skin. The symptoms may include acute episodes of abdominal pain, psychological disturbances and photosensitivity of the skin, causing burning, blistering and scarring of areas exposed to the sun. The dermatological eruptions are thought to result from the effect of long-wave ultraviolet light on porphyrins that have accumulated in the skin.

The name of the disorder is taken from the Greek *porphyrus*, meaning "purple," due to the tendency of some affected individuals to excrete purplish or reddish urine because of the presence of excess porphyrins. The urine may also darken after prolonged exposure to light.

The formation of heme is an eight-step process, each step requiring a specific ENZYME. Each form of porphyria (seven have been identified) results from a deficiency of the specific enzyme necessary for each step of this process.

Additionally, the porphyrins are subclassified in other ways. In hepatic porphyria, the excess porphyrins and porphyrin precursors originate mostly in the liver. In erythropoietic porphyria, they originate primarily in the bone marrow. Porphyrins that primarily affect the skin are referred to as cutaneous, while those involving the nervous system are referred to as acute.

There is great variability of severity among the forms of porphyria—and even of symptoms among individuals with a single form. It is believed that many who have enzyme deficiencies responsible for the disorder may never exhibit symptoms. These individuals are said to be latent, while those who exhibit symptoms are said to be active. The variability of symptoms often makes diagnosis difficult. While porphyrias are inherited, attacks are often triggered by non-genetic factors, an important example of genetic-environmental interaction. Environmental triggers can include drugs and other chemicals, foods, and exposure to the sun.

Diagnosis of the porphyrins generally involves measurement of urinary and fecal porphyrias and enzyme assay in red cells, liver or fibroblasts.

Acute intermittent porphyria (AIP) Active cases have their onset after puberty, and are more commonly seen in women than in men. Abdominal pain, which can be severe, is the most frequent symptom. There may also be nausea, vomiting, constipation, muscle weakness, urinary retention, pain in the back, arms and legs, heart palpitations, confusion, hallucinations and seizures. Symptoms usually resolve following attacks. The skin is not affected.

Inherited as an AUTOSOMAL DOMINANT trait, it is caused by the deficiency of the enzyme porphobilinogen deaminase (PBGD), also known as uroporphyrinogen I-synthase. The GENE is located at 11q. However, this deficiency alone will not cause the disorder, and must be accompanied by hormonal, drug or dietary changes in order to provoke symptoms. Most cases remain latent.

Incidence in all ETHNIC GROUPS is thought to be in the order of one in 10,000 to 20,000 live births. However, actual incidence may be much higher, due to the number of latent cases that remain undiagnosed. As many as 90% of individuals with AIP are thought never to be detected. It is most common in individuals of Scandinavian, Anglo-Saxon and German ancestry. This form of porphyria is known to also have a high incidence in northern Sweden, perhaps as high as one in 1,000 live births. The drug hematin has been effective in treating acute attacks.

It has been suggested that King George III of England suffered from AIP, traceable to Mary, Queen of Scots. However, many contemporary authorities doubt this contention. While he exhibited a disorder virtually indistinguishable from AIP, symptoms of skin involvement in other members of the royal family make it more plausible that "the royal malady" from which he suffered was variegate porphyria. It has also been suggested that Vincent van Gogh suffered from attacks of acute intermittent porphyria, exacerbated by malnutrition and absinthe abuse. This is said to explain the abruptness of the onset and the recovery from the attacks.

Management includes general supportive therapy, high carbohydrate intake, intravenous hematin and prevention through avoiding known precipitants.

Congenital erythropoietic porphyria (CEP) (Gunther's disease) Characterized by extreme photosensitivity, the disorder has its onset in infancy. Red urine may be present. Porphyrin accumulates throughout the body, and the teeth may also become red-stained. The skin may exhibit blistering, severe scarring and increased hair growth (hypertrichosis). Bacterial infection may occur at the site of skin lesions. The disease is mutilating; eventually facial features and fingers may be lost as a result of the disease process. Red blood cells have a shortened life span, and anemia may result. Prognosis is poor; few survive beyond 40 years.

The condition is considered extremely rare and fewer than 200 cases have been reported since it was first described in 1874. (H. Gunther published a more definitive description in 1911.) Inherited as an AUTOSOMAL RECESSIVE trait, the deficient enzyme is uroporphyrinogen III cosynthase. A similar disorder has been observed in several animal species, including cattle, swine and cats. It has been suggested that the "werewolves" of legend may have suffered from CEP or some severe cutaneous porphyria. It is felt that accounts of magical transformation into wolves were attempts to explain their subjects mutilated skin, hypertrichosis, red teeth and urine, and desire to avoid light exposure. (Others have suggested "werewolves" simply had hypertrichosis, an expression of an atavistic, long-dormant GENE that has survived in the genome from the time humans were covered with body hair.)

Porphyria cutanea tarda (PCT) A common form of porphyria, symptoms are confined to the skin. Onset is usually between the ages of 10 and 30. Blistering after minor trauma or exposure to sunlight may occur on the hands, face and other exposed areas, often developing into chronic ulcerating lesions. There may also be increased hair growth (hypertrichosis) and darkening (hyperpigmentation) and thickening of the skin.

PCT occurs in both hereditary (autosomal dominant) and acquired forms, and results from the deficiency of uroporphyrinogen decarboxylase (URO-D). It is a hepatic (involving the liver) form of porphyria, with huge amounts of porphyrins sometimes building up in the liver when the disease becomes active. However, in most individuals with the inherited enzyme deficiency, the disorder remains latent.

The acquired form may be triggered by alcohol or estrogens such as those found in oral contraceptives and drugs for treatment of prostate cancer.

While no reliable figures for incidence are available, it may be the most common form of porphyria, and is particularly common in the Bantu of South Africa.

Hereditary coproporphyria (HCP) This is a hepatic form, similar to acute intermittent porphyria, though generally less severe in its manifestation. Skin photosensitivity develops in some individuals (one-third). Inherited as an autosomal dominant trait, the deficient enzyme is coproporphyrinogen oxidase. Coproporphyria is the least common of the hepatic porphyrias.

Variegate porphyria Affected adults display variable photosensitive skin symptoms, including darkening of the skin (hyperpigmentation) and excessive hair growth (hypertrichosis). The skin symptoms resemble PCT, the acute attacks are similar to AIP, with severe abdominal pain, constipation, heart palpitations, hypertension, muscular paralysis, sensory disturbances, disorientation and psychosis. Attacks may be followed by prolonged disability.

This hepatic form is inherited as an autosomal dominant trait, and the deficient enzyme is believed to be protoporphyrinogen oxidase. While infrequent in the general population, it has a high incidence among the white population of South Africa. This disorder is a primary example of the FOUNDER EFFECT: It is believed that all those in South Africa suffering from the disorder inherited it either from Gerrit Jansz, a Dutch settler in the Cape, or his wife, Ariaantje Jacobs, who was one of a group of women sent from an orphanage in Rotterdam to provide wives for Dutch settlers. The prevalence among the white Afrikaans-speaking population of the Eastern Cape region may be as high as one in 250.

Erythropoietic protoporphyria (EPP) As the name implies, protoporphyrin accumulates primarily in the bone marrow and red blood cells (erythrocytes); poietic is a suffix that means "making or producing." In some cases it may accumulate in the liver as well. Onset is typically in childhood.

It is characterized by swelling, burning, itching and redness of the skin during or immediately after exposure to sunlight, even when the rays pass through a window. These symptoms typically disappear in 12 to 24 hours after exposure and leave no significant scarring or skin discoloration. However, the skin eruptions may progress to a chronic state, with lesions persisting for weeks and leaving slight scars upon healing. Attacks are usually more severe in summer and may last throughout life. Occasionally, affected individuals may have severe liver complications.

It is inherited as an autosomal dominant trait, and the deficient enzyme is ferrochelatase. The GENE for the enzyme maps to 18q.

porphyria cutanea tarda See PORPHYRIA.

port wine stain A BIRTHMARK of a well-defined patch of pink, red or purplish-colored skin, so named because the characteristic color resembles that of port wine. Most often seen on the face, it is caused by a collection of blood vessels beneath the skin that are abnormal either in their excessive number or in their degree of dilation. (Such an abnormal collection of vessels is called a HEMANGIOMA.) The increased blood flow this allows causes the discoloration in the skin over the affected area. The blood vessels are believed to be remnants of blood vessels present in the first month of embryonic life, though the cause of their retention is unknown.

Port wine stain may appear in isolation or as a feature of another condition or syndrome. It is commonly associated with STURGE-WEBER SYNDROME and KLIPPEL-TRENAUNAY-WEBER SYNDROME.

The size of the birthmark grows as the body does. After the age of 30, it may darken and become thicker than surrounding skin, and benign purplish skin growths may also appear.

Incidence of port wine stain is estimated at three per 1,000 live births. Mikhail Gorbachev, one-time president of the Soviet Union, has a port wine stain on his forehead. The majority of cases that are not associated with other conditions appear to be SPORADIC. Recently, laser surgery has been successful in treating affected areas of skin in some individuals.

posterior choanal atresia See CHOANAL ATRESIA.

post-term pregnancy A pregnancy that continues beyond the normal gestation period of approximately 40 weeks. Post-term pregnancies are associated with an increase in complications and fetal distress and death during delivery.

It is estimated that as many as 7% of pregnant women have not delivered two weeks after their due date. If the pregnancy lasts beyond 42 weeks, the placenta ages and becomes less efficient at supplying oxygen and nutrients to the fetus. As a result, postmature babies tend to be born long and thin.

Obstetricians generally begin testing a week after the anticipated delivery date to determine if it is safe to allow the pregnancy to continue. If labor does not occur spontaneously, it may be induced with drugs, or the baby may be delivered via CESAREAN DELIVERY.

Prader-Willi syndrome (PWS) A disorder characterized by OBESITY, MENTAL RETARDATION, poor development of the genitals and adult short stature. It is named for Swiss pediatricians Andrea Prader and H. Willi who described it in 1956, though it appears it was mentioned by Langdon Down (for whom DOWN SYNDROME is named) in 1887. In "Mental Afflictions of Childhood and Youth," describing a case of what he called "polysarcia" in a retarded 25-year-old, who, with a height of little more than 4 feet 4 inches (130.2 cm), weighed over 200 pounds, Langdon Down discussed the disparity between the small hands and feet and general obesity that is a hallmark of this condition. "Her feet and hands remained small and contrasted remarkably with the appendages they terminated . . . She had scarcely any (hair) on the pubis. She had never menstruated, nor did she exhibit the slightest sexual instinct."

At birth, individuals present a FLOPPY INFANT appearance (hypotonia), weigh a few hundred grams below average and exhibit feeding problems and poor swallowing and sucking reflexes. Their cry may be weak, and they may be unable to control their head and limbs. The face is also characteristic, with prominent forehead, poorly formed ears and a triangular-shaped upper lip. The eyes may be crossed, with uncoordinated focusing (STRABISMUS).

Small hands with delicate and tapering fingers and small feet are seen in most individuals with Prader-Willi syndrome. Individuals manifest severe skin-picking behavior and many children have scars from scratching due to itching. Less pigmentation relative to the familial background is a feature in about three-quarters of the patients. Another frequent and generally overlooked feature is the thick saliva at the edges of the mouth. Patients also tend to be relatively insensitive to pain (including that caused by taking blood samples).

The frequency of PWS is estimated at about one in 25,000 births; it may be the most common syndromal cause of human obesity. Seven clinicians experienced with PWS, in consultation with national and international experts, established consensus diagnostic criteria: one set for children aged 0–36 months and another for children aged three years to adult.

Developmental milestones (sitting, standing, walking, talking) are usually retarded. Physically, they lack large muscle strength and endurance and have poor balance and coordination. As infants grow, they become more lively and develop insatiable appetites. Compulsive overeating (hyperphagia) appears, on the average, at just under three years of age.

They may eat the food of house pets or food from the garbage. If eating is not controlled, obesity is usually prominent before five years of age, with a disproportionate amount of fat accumulating in the central body, lower trunk and buttocks.

The ravenous desire for food is due to a dysfunction of the central nervous system. Individuals will eat any time food is available and will not stop eating of their own accord. Additionally, they require fewer calories than average persons in order to gain weight. Exercise is difficult due to their poor muscle development.

Limiting access to food is of primary importance. In order to monitor consumption, parents are generally advised that refrigerators must be kept locked, and individuals must be monitored at all times. This becomes difficult as children age.

The degree of MENTAL RETARDATION is variable, with IQs typically in the 70s, though scores below 40 and above 100 have been found. Affected children are described as happy, friendly and cooperative, but capable of exhibiting extreme frustration, negativism and temper tantrums when denied unlimited food.

Genital abnormalities typically consist of a small penis and scrotum, often with undescended testes (CRYPTORCHISM) in males and poorly formed labia in females. Puberty is delayed and diminished. Males retain a high-pitched voice. Adult height is always below the 50th percentile.

DIABETES often appears during childhood or adolescence, and many individuals are said to exhibit excessive sleepiness (somnolence).

Independent living is rarely achieved. Life expectancy is diminished due to respiratory insufficiency. Death may also result from cardiorespiratory embarrassment (see PICKWICKIAN SYNDROME) or, more rarely, diabetic complications.

Chromosomal mechanisms are responsible for PWS; the SYNDROME is caused by lack of the paternal segment 15q11.2-q12. Considered to be an AUTOSOMAL DOMINANT disorder, the deletion can result from a defect in the paternal CHROMOSOME, or by maternal uniparental disomy, whereby both copies of the GENE, in this case 15, are inherited from the mother. The pattern of inheritance is complicated by the phenomenon of IMPRINTING, which refers to the suppression or expression of certain genes based whether they are transmitted by the mother or father. Thus, this represents a significant refinement of classic MENDELIAN theory, which holds that genes are simply either dominant or recessive.

It appears that certain genes at 15q-11q13 on the maternal chromosome are normally imprinted (suppressed) and expression of the paternally transmitted ALLELES is necessary for normal development. When these genes on the paternal chromosome 15 are absent or disrupted, the PWS phenotype results.

Absence of the analogous region in the maternally transmitted chromosome 15 leads to ANGELMAN SYNDROME; that is, the opposite maternal deletion (or paternal uniparental disomy) causes another characteristic PHENOTYPE, the Angelman syndrome.

The vast majority of PWS cases occur sporadically. The recurrence rate should be (and is) close to 0 when there is a 15q deletion not associated with a translocation (see CHROMOSOME ABNORMALITIES). There is no parental age effect in the deletion cases. Deletions of the paternal chromosome 15q11-q13 account for 70–80% of the cases. They are detectable either by high resolution chromosome analysis or by FISH. A minority consist of unbalanced translocations, mostly de novo, which are easily detected by routine chromosome examination. The remainder of cases are the result of maternal uniparental disomy. Results of cytogenetic examinations are typically normal in these latter cases, and molecular studies are needed to demonstrate disomy.

Prader-Willi syndrome is in effect a CONTIGUOUS GENE SYNDROME resulting from deletion of the paternal copies of the imprinted SNRPN gene, the necdin gene, and possibly other genes. Prenatal molecular investigation from chorionic villi should be recommended in every case despite very low recurrence risk (see CHORIONIC VILLUS SAMPLING). Prenatal ultrasonographic studies of fetal activity may be useful for a first screening since Prader-Willi fetuses will often show diminished fetal movement during the second trimester.

precocious puberty The appearance of sexual characteristics at a very early age, usually defined as before 10 years in males and 8.5 years in females. It has been reported as early as age three. Approximately one in every 10,000 children starts puberty prematurely. Boys grow facial, pubic and underarm hair, are prone to develop acne, and the penis and testicles enlarge. Viable sperm may be produced. Girls may develop breasts, grow pubic and underarm hair, menstruate and may ovulate. Children with precocious puberty are usually taller than their peers, but since maturation of the bones is typically accelerated and ends at an earlier age, both males and females may exhibit short stature in adulthood.

Various forms of precocious puberty exist. Isosexual precocious puberty results in feminization in girls and masculinization in boys. Heterosexual precocious puberty causes femininization in boys and masculinization in girls. Central precocious puberty involves the central nervous system. Gonadogtropin-dependent precocious puberty is marked by high gonadotropin levels in girls and may affect those with MCCUNE-ALBRIGHT SYNDROME. Gonadotropin-independent precocious puberty typically affects boys with low levels of gonadotropin as well as girls with McCune-Albright syndrome.

Though it is usually of unknown origin (idiopathic), familial cases of precocious puberty have been observed. The incidence in girls is about twice that of boys. Some 60% of cases in girls are idopathic, while disease underlies about 60% of the cases seen in boys. Sex hormone-secreting ovarian and adrenal tumors cause some of the cases seen in girls.

Male-limited precocious puberty (familial testotoxicosis), a sex-limited dominant trait, is caused by a MUTATION of the *LHRH* GENE, resulting in hypersensitivity to levels of leutinizing hormone (LH).

Precocious puberty may also be a feature of NEUROFIBROMATOSIS, RUSSELL-SILVER SYNDROME and disorders of the adrenal glands in addition to McCune-Albright syndrome.

Affected individuals may encounter psychological problems due to their accelerated growth and may feel alienated from their peers. They may exhibit increased aggressiveness and hyperactivity.

preimplantation diagnosis A method of PRENATAL DIAGNOSIS used in conjunction with in vitro fertilization. It involves the removal of one or two cells from the embryo when it is six to 10 cells in size, about three days after insemination. The genetic material is then analyzed by polymerase chain reaction (PCR) or FLUORESCENCE IN SITU HYBRIDIZATION (FISH) techniques. It is used to select healthy embryos for implantation. Initially used mainly to test for the presence of CYSTIC FIBROSIS, using PCR to look for known parental MUTATIONS, it has also been used to detect LESCH-NYHAN SYNDROME, TAY-SACHS DISEASE and DUCHENNE MUSCULAR DYSTROPHY. The identification of FRAGILE X SYNDROME and MYOTONIC DYSTROPHY, both of which are TRINUCLEOTIDE REPEAT DISORDERS, has also been reported. Chromosome abnormalities including both trisomies and unbalanced rearrangements, such as translocations, have also been diagnosed by this method. It has been used for HLA tissue typing as well, performed in an effort to bring to birth a child who could be a transplant donor to an affected sibling. It has also been used for sex selection, primarily to preclude X-linked disorders. Its use in sex selection for nonmedical purposes is controversial. Use for the diagnosis of adult onset diseases such as breast cancer or Alzheimer disease is also controversial. No negative effects of the procedure on subsequent implantation have been found in early studies.

premature birth See PREMATURITY; LOW BIRTH WEIGHT.

prematurity Birth before the completion of full gestational development or before the 37th week of pregnancy. (The normal human gestation period is 40 weeks.) Prematurity is associated with an increased incidence of infant health problems and death. Approximately 45,000 infant deaths are recorded annually in the United States, and two-thirds of these deaths are of infants who were born prematurely, though not all these deaths can be attributed to prematurity alone.

In 1981 the World Health Organization recommended replacing the designation "Prematurity" with LOW BIRTH WEIGHT. Low birth weight infants may be born early and thus be small, or may be born at term but be growth retarded.

prenatal diagnosis Any of a number of procedures for identifying the presence of a CONGENITAL or hereditary condition before birth.

A broad spectrum of prenatal diagnosis procedures is available, enabling physicians to confirm or rule out many fetal disorders. These diagnostic procedures can involve both invasive and noninvasive techniques. Invasive procedures include AMNIOCENTESIS and CHORIONIC VILLUS SAMPLING (CVS), which is followed by analysis using DNA PROBES, CHROMOSOME analyses and BIOCHEMICAL ASSAYS. In amniocentesis, a needle is inserted through the mother's abdominal wall and a sample of the AMNIOTIC FLUID is withdrawn for analysis. Chorionic villus sampling involves the use of either a catheter inserted into the uterus or a needle inserted through the abdomen to obtain tissue samples from projections on the membrane around the FETUS. (FETOSCOPY, now rarely used, involves inserting a thin tube through the abdomen into the uterus to visually inspect the fetus and collect fetal blood and tissue samples.) DNA probes, chromosome analyses and biochemical assays often depend on invasive procedures to obtain the fetal samples needed.

Non-invasive procedures primarily involve testing maternal blood for the serum levels of ALPHA-FETOPROTEIN (AFP), human chorionic gonadotropin (HCG) and unconjugated estriol (uE$_3$), and using ULTRASOUND to visualize an image of the FETUS in the uterus. X-rays may also be used for FETAL IMAGING. Maternal serum screening can indicate the possibility of DOWN SYNDROME, NEURAL TUBE DEFECTS (NTDs) or other CHROMOSOME ABNORMALITIES. More definitive diagnostic procedures, involving for example, testing of fetal tissue, could then be employed.

PREIMPLANTATION DIAGNOSIS, which is used in conjunction with in vitro fertilization, involves removing one or two cells from a six- to 10-cell embryo, and subsequently analyzing the genetic material with FISH or PCR prior to implanting the embryo in the uterus. Thus far it has been used to identify CYSTIC FIBROSIS, TAY-SACHS DISEASE, DUCHENNE MUSCULAR DYSTROPHY and LESCH-NYHAN DISEASE.

Which prenatal diagnostic procedure is used depends on the type of information being sought. The physician examines not only the patient herself but also carefully checks the previous medical history and available aspects of the family medical history of both parents for clues that may indicate the need for prenatal diagnosis. GENETIC COUNSELING is therefore a critical component of prenatal diagnosis.

Not all congenital and GENETIC DISORDERS can be diagnosed prenatally, and since prenatal diagnosis procedures involve some attendant risks to the fetus, it is usually indicated as a diagnostic tool only when certain conditions exist. (By the end of the 1990s, hundreds of congenital and genetic disorders could be diagnosed prenatally.) If the mother is 35 or older, prenatal diagnosis has often been offered because advanced maternal age increases the risk of conceiving a child with Down syndrome. In 2007, the American College of Obstetricians and Gynecologists recommended all pregnant women undergo prenatal screening for Down syndrome. Other conditions for which prenatal diagnosis is indicated include a previous birth of a child with a chromosomal ANOMALY or one parent known to have such an anomaly; a family history of children born with neural tube defects; a screening test that discloses elevated levels of alpha-fetoprotein or indicates a higher risk of Down syndrome or other chromosomal abnormalities; a previous birth of a SIBLING with a genetic or metabolic disorder; and parents who are confirmed or suspected CARRIERS of a genetic disorder. Prenatal diagnosis is considered as one of the reproductive options available for couples whose offspring are at risk for genetic or congenital diseases. (See also the Introduction.)

pretzel syndrome   The informal name given a specific genetic disorder characterized by skeletal deformity allowing hyperplasticity of the limbs, malformation of the brain, electrolyte imbalances, seizures and slowed mental development. Affected infants are born prematurely and their pregnancies are described as problematic, involving excess amniotic fluid. Malformed connective tissue and joints enable those affected to contort themselves into unusual positions, such as putting their feet behind their heads and giving the disorder its name. Affected individuals appear to have fewer nerve cells in their brains than normal and exhibit variable malformations of the heart and other organs. Renal problems result in persistent thirst and urination. There is no treatment. This disorder appears to be caused by a partial deletion of a gene located on chromosome 17. The syndrome has been observed among the Amish in Pennsylvania and Ohio.

primidone   See ANTICONVULSANTS.

prion disease   Proteinaceous infectious particles or prions (pronounced pree-ons), are proteins capable of acting as infectious agents and possibly underlying some hereditary disorders. The term prion was coined by Stanley Prusiner, who in 1984 proposed that a protein could act as an infectious agent at a time when it was thought genetic material was required for transmission of infections. Prions multiply by converting normal protein molecules into their shape. The known prion diseases are referred to as spongiform encephalopathies because they often cause the brain to become riddled with holes and "spongy," and all are fatal.

Widespread in animals, these disorders can take years to develop. The most common form is scrapie, found in sheep and goats. The animals develop an intense itch and scrape off their wool or hair, hence the name scrapie. In bovines, spongiform encepahlopathy is called mad cow disease. It can be spread by the use of food supplements that include the ground bonemeal from sheep infected with scrapie. There is concern that humans who consume the meat of cows infected with this disorder can develop a human form of the disorder.

Humans also exhibit prion disease. One is kuru, seen among Fore Highlanders in Papua New Guinea. First described in medical literature in 1957, it was called the "laughing death." Affected individuals exhibit ataxia (lack of coordination) and dementia. It is believed transmitted by ritual cannibalism, as the tribe reportedly consumed the brains of dead relatives. The practice has since stopped, and kuru has practically disappeared.

Creutzfeldt-Jakob disease, another prion disease, affects one per million, with age of onset about 60 years. It manifests as dementia. About 10 to 15 percent of cases are inherited, and some occur as a result of transmission during corneal transplantation, implantation of dura mater or electrodes in the brain, use of contaminated surgical instruments and injection of growth hormone derived from human pituitaries (before recombinant growth hormone became available). Gerstmann-Straussler-Scheinker disease and fatal familial insomnia, both hereditary disorders with midlife onset, are also prion diseases.

proband   The first person within a family who is identified as having a particular inherited disorder, or the individual who first presents a mental or physical disorder that prompts the study of the person's family in an effort to identify a potential genetic link to the abnormality. It is necessary to establish this link (if it exists) for proper diagnosis and treatment. (A synonym for the proband is the propositus, or index case.) (See also PEDIGREE.)

progeria (Hutchinson-Gilford progeria syndrome)   A rare genetic disorder resulting in premature aging. The name is derived from Greek, meaning "prematurely old." The classic type was first described independently by English surgeons Jonathan Hutchinson (1828–1913) and Hastings Gilford (1861–1941) in 1886. Gilford coined the term *progeria* in 1904.

The condition is characterized by DWARFISM, baldness, a pinched nose, small face and small jaw (micrognathia), delayed tooth formation and aged-looking skin. Intelligence is normal or above average. The voice is thin and high-pitched. Sexual maturation does not occur. Veins of the scalp are clearly visible. Joints are stiff. There is mild flexion of the knees, producing a "horse-riding" stance. As they age, there are frequent hip dislocations, generalized hardening of the arteries (atherosclerosis) and cardiac problems. Death from coronary artery disease is common and may occur before age 10. Over 80% of deaths are due to heart attacks or congestive heart failure. The average life expectancy is 12 to 14 years of age. One affected individual was still alive at age 29. At age 10, most affected children have the height of the average three-year-old. Lifetime height rarely exceeds that of a five-year-old.

The disorder first gained attention in the United States in 1981, when the news media reported on the meeting of two affected children, one from South Africa and one from Texas, at Disneyland.

Progeria is caused by mutations in the *lamin A (LMNA)* gene, which encodes the proteins lamin A and C, and is found on chromosome 1. A specific mutation in the *LMNA* gene has been found in most patients with progeria. The location of the mutation in the *LMNA* gene affects the production only of lamin A and not of lamin C. Different mutations in the *LMNA* gene have also been identified in a small number of other people with progeria. Progeria is inherited as an AUTOSOMAL DOMINANT trait, with virtually all cases being the result of new mutations occurring at the time of conception.

Some researchers believe an understanding of the disorder could provide clues to the aging process, since it mimics some aspects of natural aging. (However, unlike normal aging, affected individuals don't exhibit degenerative joint disease, CANCER, CATARACTS, DIABETES MELLITUS or senile dementia.)

The SYNDROME has an incidence estimated at between one in four million and one in eight million live births. More than 100 cases have been described around the world since it was first described.

Diagnosis is made on the basis of the physical appearance. It is usually diagnosed in the first or second year, when skin changes and failure to gain weight become apparent. (See also WERNER SYNDROME, an adult form of progeria.)

prolonged QT interval   See ROMANO-WARD SYNDROME.

propionic acidemia   A rare inherited deficiency of propionyl-CoA carboxylase, an ENZYME that breaks down ketoacids. As a result of the enzyme deficiency, ketoacids build up to toxic levels, as identified by an increased concentration of glycine in the blood, elevated concentrations of propionic acid and its precursors and metabolites in urine, and high concentrations of ketones in the urine. This is an organic aciduria (or acidemia).

Signs of the disorder early in infancy include recurring episodes of ketoacidosis, characterized by nausea and vomiting, "air hunger," or gasping for breath in an attempt to compensate for the acidosis, a fruity odor to the breath, abdominal tenderness and extreme thirst and dry mucous membranes. Ketoacidosis rapidly leads to coma and death, and few children with propionic acidosis survive infancy. Recently, a low-protein diet has shown some promise in treatment.

Those who do survive infancy exhibit MENTAL RETARDATION and a variety of neurological abnormalities. Neutropenia (a decrease in the number of blood granulocytes) leads to frequent infections, and thrombocytopenia (a decrease in the number of platelets) is associated with temporary episodes of purpura, a condition characterized by multiple hemorrhages just under the skin. There may also be thinning of the bones (osteoporosis) and subsequent fractures.

Incidence is estimated at one in 100,000 live births. Secondary carnitine depletion accounts for some of the adverse effects of the disorder. Inherited as an AUTOSOMAL RECESSIVE trait, two GENES are involved: One maps to 13q, the other to 3q. The definitive diagnosis is established by demonstrating the enzyme defects in cultured skin cells. Reduced activities have been observed in cell cultures from CARRIERS, and PRENATAL DIAGNOSIS has been carried out on cultured fetal cells collected by AMNIOCENTESIS and CHORIONIC VILLUS SAMPLING.

propositus   See PROBAND.

prostate cancer   A form of cancer affecting only males, characterized by the development of tumors, or neoplasms, in the prostate gland. It is the most common cancer in males, with rates comparable to that of breast cancer in women. Most cases develop after 50 years of age, and the average age of diagnosis is 70. Some 230,000 new cases of prostate cancer were diagnosed in 2005, and about 30,000 men died of the disease.

Part of the male reproductive system, the prostate gland makes and stores seminal fluid. The cancer, slow growing and initially asymptomatic, is often first detected due to high levels of prostate-specific antigen, or PSA, found during a routine physical examination blood workup. Elevated levels of PSA (above 4.0 ng/ml) are associated with an increased chance of the presence of prostate cancer. The PSA test, developed in the 1980s, has greatly improved detection of prostate cancer. Diagnosis is confirmed by examination of prostate tissue collected by biopsy.

The prostate gland is positioned in front of the rectum and surrounds part of the urethra, the tube which carries both urine and semen. Because the tumors can enlarge the gland, prostate cancer can interfere with urination, ejaculation and defecation. However, many men who develop prostate cancer remain asymptomatic. Autopsy studies conducted in populations around the world have found that approximately 30% of men in their 50s who succumbed to other causes of death and 80% of men in their 70s who died of unrelated causes had prostate cancer. Treatment options include surgery, radiation therapy, hormone therapy and chemotherapy. But the variable progression of the disease complicates selection of treatment. Should a tumor turn malignant, it can spread to the bones and lymph nodes, as well as other parts of the body.

The cause of prostate cancer is unknown. No single gene is responsible, but prostate cancer has a demonstrated genetic component, and numerous mutations have been linked to a predisposition to develop the disease. Studies of twins suggest that hereditary factors play a role in 40% of cases. Risk in families where a father or brother has had prostate cancer is doubled. Having an affected brother is associated with a higher relative risk than is having an affected father. With two first-degree relatives, a man's risk increases fivefold. With three or more close relatives, the risk for developing prostate cancer is very high—close to 100% in certain studies. African Americans are affected between 60% and 100% more frequently than Caucasians. Age, diet and lifestyle also influence the development of the cancer.

Genes associated with a predisposition to develop prostate cancer include the *HPC* gene (also called the *RNASEL* gene), the *MAX-interacting protein-1 (MXI1)* gene, the *PRCA1* gene on 1q and the KAI1 prostate cancer antimetastasis gene on 11p. PCAP on 1q is associated with early onset prostate cancer. *HPCX* on Xq and *CAPB* on 1p have also been implicated in early onset forms. Mutations in the gene encoding *macrophage scavenger receptor-1* (on 8p) and the *CHEK2 checkpoint homolog* (S. pombe) gene (on 22q) have been identified in both hereditary and nonhereditary (sporadically occurring) prostate cancer. A mutation that inactivates the *EphB2* gene on chromosome 1 has been found to increase the risk of prostate cancer in African Americans as much as three times. A promoter polymorphism in the *CDH1 gene* on 16q and mutations in the *HPC2/ELAC2* gene on 17p are linked to prostate cancer as well, as are mutations in the *PTEN* gene, located on 10q, the *MAD1L1* gene on 7p and the *ATBF1* gene on 16q. Point mutations in the *MXI1* gene on 10q have also been associated with prostate cancer. Mutations of the *BRCA1* gene on 17q and *BRCA2* gene on 13q, which are linked to increased risks of developing breast and ovarian cancer in women, also appear to be associated with an increased risk of developing prostate cancer in men.

In 2006, researchers identified a DNA-variant on chromosome 8 that increases the risk of developing prostate cancer among those who carry it by 60 percent. The variant is twice as common in black men as those of European extraction and was found in 16% of black men and 8% of men of European extraction who developed prostate cancer.

protanomaly   See COLOR BLINDNESS.

protanopia   See COLOR BLINDNESS.

protective exclusion   The workplace policy of excluding women who are pregnant, fertile or of child-bearing age from jobs that may endanger fetal health. The policy has been adopted by some manufacturing and chemical companies. Studies have found increased rates of miscarriage (see ABORTION) and BIRTH DEFECTS in certain workplace environments, such as in manufacturing processes involving toxic chemicals. Protective exclusion has also been practiced in hospitals and research labs, the semiconductor industry and among workers using VIDEO DISPLAY TERMINALS.

Reproductive disorders rank in the top 10 work-related illnesses and injuries, according to data from the National Institute of Occupational Safety and Health, and more than 14 million workers a year may be exposed to known or suspected reproductive hazards on the job. While the extent of the reproductive risks for males in these environments is unknown, few companies exclude them from jobs from which they bar women for reproductive reasons.

The Equal Employment Opportunity Commission estimates at least 100,000 jobs in the United States are closed to women due to the risk to fetal health. The legality of the policy is unclear. Title VII of the Civil Rights Act prohibits sex discrimination in employment, but court decisions on the permissibility of protective exclusion have varied. The issue first came to public attention in the latter 1970s, when several women sued the American Cyanamid Company for violating their civil rights, claiming they had to undergo sterilization to keep their high-paying jobs in the company's West Virginia lead pigment plant. They settled their claims for $200,000. Subsequently, federal courts have barred companies from excluding women from

workplace environments that present reproductive risks. More recently, however, in a case involving a Milwaukee manufacturer that prohibited all fertile women from working in its battery-making operations, appeals courts have reached contradictory verdicts.

Where companies have no policy of protective exclusion, workers have sometimes demanded the right to transfer out of jobs they perceive as presenting reproductive risks. For example, several unions, including the Communications Workers of America, have won the right for their pregnant members to temporarily transfer away from video display terminal work without a loss of pay or seniority.

proteomics   The study of the structure, function and interactions of proteins produced by genes. The field takes its name from *proteome,* the entirety of the proteins produced in the life cycle of a cell or an organism. The term was coined as a nod to *genomics,* its predecessor field of genetic inquiry. The proteins produced by genes are constantly changing. While about 22,000 human genes are involved in protein production, the genes produce about 200,000 different proteins. These proteins can express themselves in radically different ways depending on the part of the body, the part of the life cycle, and an organism's environment an international effort to catalog all human proteins and their functions is currently under way.

proteus syndrome   This disorder, possibly first described in 1976, was named in 1983 by German pediatrician Hans Rudolf Wiedemann, and is characterized by grossly enlarged hands and feet, multiple nevi (see NEVUS) on the skin, distorted abnormal growth of half of the body (hemihypertrophy) and gigantism of the head. Mental deficiency occurs in about 20% of cases. It is named for the Greek god Proteus, "the polymorphous," presumably because of the variable manifestations in the four unrelated boys first identified as having the SYNDROME. While it is apparently a GENETIC DISORDER, its mode of inheritance is unknown, though AUTOSOMAL DOMINANT transmission has been suggested. All cases to date have been SPORADIC. Some individuals with proteus syndrome have mutations in the *PTEN* gene. Cystic malformations of the lungs, while rare, can be life-threatening.

It is believed this is the condition that afflicted the Elephant Man, rather than NEUROFIBROMATOSIS, as had been generally accepted.

prune-belly syndrome   The most obvious manifestation of this CONGENITAL disorder in newborns is a large, thin-walled protuberant abdomen covered with many loose folds of skin (hence the name "prune belly"); caused by an abdominal muscle development deficiency (hypoplasia). The internal abdominal organs can be felt and examined with the fingers, and the wavelike and rhythmic movement (peristalsis) of the intestines can be seen through the thin abdominal walls. The two other associated major congenital defects are undescended testicles (CRYPTORCHISM) and urinary tract abnormalities, which include dilation of the bladder (megalocystis), gross distension of the ureter (hydroureter) caused by blockage of urine, swelling of the collecting systems of the kidney due to blocked urine (hydronephrosis), and abnormal development (DYSPLASIA) of the kidneys.

First described by F. Froelich in 1839 in Wuerzburg, Germany, it is a generally SPORADIC, etiologically heterogeneous (having several causes) disorder. (See HETEROGENEITY.) It can result from a urethral obstruction or from pooling of fluid in the fetal abdominal cavity (ascites). Familial cases have only rarely been reported, and AUTOSOMAL RECESSIVE and X-LINKED recessives have been suggested.

Hip dysplasia is common. Approximately 40% of affected infants have CLUBFEET (talipes equinovarus), 30% have congenital HEART DEFECTS and 30% show intestinal abnormalities such as failure of the bowel to develop normally during embryonic growth, and hardening (calcification) of tissue in the colon.

This disorder occurs about once in every 50,000 births and affects mostly males; only about 5% are females, who are mildly affected and have no severe urinary tract involvement. The exact genetic cause is not clear. It is suspected that it results from a localized defect in the mesoderm, a cell layer in the embryo that develops into connective tissue.

About 20% of those affected are stillborn or die within a month of birth. Fifty percent die within two years, mainly due to urinary tract infection or kidney failure. ULTRASOUND examination may detect an abnormally small amount of AMNIOTIC FLUID (oligohydramnios), an enlarged bladder, or ascites.

pseudohermaphroditism   A general term for several forms of AMBIGUOUS GENITALIA, ANOMALIES of the external sex organs. Unlike true HERMAPHRODITES, these individuals have the internal sexual organs of only one gender. Females exhibit various degrees of external sexual ambiguity, depending on the form, and may be raised as males. Males exhibit the same spectrum of variation and crossgender rearing. Individuals usually come to medical attention due to abnormalities of pubertal development. (See also ADRENOGENITAL SYNDROMES; TESTICULAR FEMINIZATION SYNDROME.)

pseudo-Hurler polydystrophy   See MUCOLIPIDOSIS.

pseudohypoparathyroidism   See ALBRIGHT HEREDITARY OSTEODYSTROPHY.

pseudo-thalidomide syndrome   See ROBERTS SYNDROME.

pseudoxanthoma elasticum   A chronic degenerative skin and arterial disease, signs of which can become apparent anytime from birth to the 30s or 40s. General characteristics of the disorder include skin alterations, failing vision brought on by retinal hemorrhages, weak pulses in the limbs, persistent high blood pressure (HYPERTENSION), severe chest pain from lack of blood flow to the heart due to CORONARY ARTERY DISEASE (angina pectoris) and dizzy spells. There are also visual and speech disturbances and other stroke symptoms (transient cerebral ischemic attacks) brought on by thickening of artery walls (arteriosclerosis). Abdominal pain is common due to constriction of the celiac artery, which supplies the abdominal region, as is severe pain in calf muscles while walking (intermittent claudication) and gastrointestinal bleeding caused by degeneration of the elastic fibers in the arteries of the walls of the gastrointestinal tract.

The skin alterations include a thickening and loss of elasticity, with raised, yellowish, pebble-like areas (nodules) appearing in mucous membranes of the mouth, cheek and inner lips, and also in the armpits, groin, around the navel and on the neck, where the skin will be loose and folded.

Pseudoxanthoma elasticum is an AUTOSOMAL RECESSIVE disorder. The prevalence is approximately one in every 70,000 to 100,000 live births. Females are diagnosed with the disorder twice as frequently as males. Intelligence is normal, though life span is significantly shortened by complications of internal bleeding and arterial blockages. The disorder involves abnormalities in connective tissue whereby the elastic fibers become fragmented and calcified, though the basic defect involved is unknown.

Mutations in the *ABCC6* gene (also known as the *MRP6* gene), which is located on the short arm of chromosome 16, are responsible for this disorder. This gene encodes the ATP-binding cassette protein multidrug resistance-associated protein 6. In some families affected with this disorder, an affected individual has one affected parent and one apparently unaffected. In these families the disorder appears to be inherited in an autosomal dominant manner, in which one copy of the altered gene is sufficient to cause the disorder. But the inheritance pattern is actually autosomal recessive in these families, because the normal-appearing parent can be shown to be a carrier of an *ABCC6* mutation. The affected offspring thus has inherited two mutations, one from each parent. This phenomenon is called pseudodominance.

psoriasis Inflammation of the skin (dermatitis) characterized by pink or dull red lesions covered by silvery scales. Demonstrated to occur in a hereditary form, it is the most common scaling skin disease, affecting 1% to 3% of the white population (and a smaller percentage of blacks) and may be severe and disabling. It is rare in Eskimos, American Indians and Japanese. Though all forms of inheritance have been reported, except for those families in which it is clearly inherited as an AUTOSOMAL DOMINANT trait, MULTIFACTORIAL inheritance seems to be the most likely cause. A survey in Denmark's Faeroe Islands found that more than 90% of those receiving medical care for the condition had affected relatives, and a large kindred exhibiting the disorder has been studied in North Carolina.

As with other "common" diseases, what is likely inherited are GENES conferring susceptibility to develop the disorder. Several have been mapped, including an association with certain HLA ALLELES. Between 5–8% of patients with psoriasis have psoriatic arthritis.

If one first-degree relative (parent, SIBLING, offspring) is affected, the recurrence risk appears to be approximately 7.5% to 17%. With both parents affected the risk may exceed 50%. The expression is variable and may be more or less severe than other affected relatives. The lesions may erupt periodically or they may be chronic. Onset is usually sometime in adulthood.

A form of arthritis may accompany familial psoriasis, resulting in painful crippling contractures of the hands or other joints, along with the eruptions of the skin. Called psoriatic arthropathy, the disorder was the model for the disease that afflicted the protagonist of a public television series of the 1980s produced in England, *The Singing Detective*. The creator of the series, Dennis Potter, a highly regarded writer, suffered from the disorder himself.

ptosis The dropping or drooping of an organ or part of the body. Most commonly it is seen in the upper eyelids, which demonstrate a tendency to droop in many GENETIC DISORDERS and other disease conditions. As an isolated phenomenon, CONGENITAL ptosis of the eyelids may have a genetic basis, often demonstrating AUTOSOMAL DOMINANT transmission.

pycnodysostosis A mild form of short-limb DWARFISM, first identified in 1962. Its name, taken from the Greek *pyinos,* meaning "thick," refers to the increased thickness and density of the bones. A characteristic appearance results from underdevelopment of the facial bones and abnormally large cranial sutures (the gaps between the bones of the skull). This creates a relatively large head with a prominent forehead and a small face with parrot-like hooked nose, receding chin, dental and oral anomalies and bulging eyes.

French doctors Pierre Maroteaux (b. 1926) and Maurice Lamy (1895–1975), who first described it, speculated that this may have been the affliction of French artist Henri de Toulouse-Lautrec (1864–1901). He had consanguineous parents (first cousins) (see CONSANGUINITY). His dwarfism was marked by multiple bone fractures, and the top hat he habitually wore may have been an attempt to hide the marked prominence of the forehead that is a hallmark of this disorder, as well as to cover a patent fontanelle (the "soft spot" atop an infant's head that has been retained into adulthood). Similarly, his beard may have been grown to cover a receding chin.

The increased density makes the bones, particularly long bones in the limbs, prone to fracture easily and fail to grow together properly, exacerbating the natural tendency of stunted development of the limbs that is characteristic of this condition. The jawbone is also prone to breakage; for example, it can be fractured by a tooth extraction.

Though the trunk is not shortened, abnormalities of the trunk are typically present. The shoulders are narrow. The chest may be sunken (PECTUS excavatum) and the breasts may be underdeveloped in females. The spine may be curved abnormally (SCOLIOSIS) or may be humped (kyphosis) or swaybacked (lumbar lordosis). The tips of the fingers and toes may appear bulbous, and the nails may be poorly formed.

Infants display a FAILURE TO THRIVE. The persistence of the milk teeth gives an appearance of a double row of teeth in childhood. The permanent teeth are poorly formed and prone to cavities. The eyes are prone to vision problems. Adult height is usually under five feet. Life span is normal. MENTAL RETARDATION has been reported in about one in six cases.

Pycnodysostosis is inherited as an AUTOSOMAL RECESSIVE trait. It is caused by MUTATIONS in the cathepsin K gene which maps to 1q. Osteoclasts are the cells that normally are involved in the resorption of bone, and in this disorder it appears that because of cathepsin K deficiency the osteoclasts don't adequately degrade the bone.

pygmy Studies conducted in the Central African Republic indicate the short stature observed in African pygmies may be the result of their failure to respond to somatomedin C or insulin-like growth factor I (IGF 1), a human hormone growth mediator. It has been suggested that a GENE for this unresponsiveness is on chromosome 12, and that the short stature of the pygmies is inherited as an AUTOSOMAL RECESSIVE trait (with almost all pygmies carrying only the recessive genes due to inbreeding). However, other research suggests that the inheritance of short stature in pygmies is MULTIFACTORIAL in nature. Whether the mouse MUTATION called pygmy (pg), a recessive mutation that maps to mouse chromosome 10, has anything more than similarity of name and reduced size to the human pygmy is uncertain. Levels of growth hormone are normal as in the human pygmy. (See also DWARFISM.)

pyloric stenosis CONGENITAL narrowing of the opening between the stomach and small intestine, the pylorus. Characteristically, an affected infant begins projectile vomiting (ejecting the stomach contents with great force) at three to four weeks of age, and as the obstruction becomes nearly complete, the infant suffers weight loss, constipation and imbalances in levels of sodium and potassium in the blood. Eagerness to nurse after vomiting is common. The enlarged and thickened pylorus can be felt through the abdominal wall as a movable mass about the size of an olive. These signs and symptoms can be confirmed by X-ray or ULTRASOUND studies.

The defect is a MULTIFACTORIAL trait involving several GENES and environmental influence. It occurs in approximately one in 300 live births and is most common in whites. Males are affected four times as frequently as females. Recurrence risks are higher for SIBLINGS of females. The prognosis after surgical repair is excellent. There is some evidence that survivors have a higher incidence of peptic ulcer later in life. Though prenatal ULTRASOUND has demonstrated distension of the stomach in congenital pyloric stenosis, the reliability of sonography for PRENATAL DIAGNOSIS of this condition has not been established.

pyruvate carboxylase deficiency

Rare progressive neurological disorder resulting from an absence of pyruvate carboxylase, an ENZYME that is important in the cycle by which the body derives energy from food. It is a cause of primary LACTIC ACIDOSIS.

Newborns and infants appear normal, but their development is slow, and abnormalities are evident by one year of age. They exhibit symptoms such as FAILURE TO THRIVE, vomiting, irritability, apathy, inactivity, poor muscle tone (hypotonia), absent reflexes (areflexia), spasticity, inability to coordinate muscular movements (ataxia), abnormal eye movements and seizures.

Although the signs and symptoms of the disorder are nonspecific and inconsistent, diagnosis has been made within several months of birth in some cases. It is detected by higher-than-normal lactate and pyruvate levels.

Neurological and intellectual deterioration is progressive, and death generally occurs within several years.

It is inherited as an AUTOSOMAL RECESSIVE trait and the causative GENE is located on 11q. PRENATAL DIAGNOSIS is possible by measuring the amount of the enzyme in fetal cells.

pyruvate dehydrogenase deficiency

Symptoms of this group of disorders vary from excessive production of lactic and pyruvic acid (acidosis) and rapidly progressive, fatal illness within the first few days of birth to uncoordinated muscle movements, growth and MENTAL RETARDATION, and muscle weakness in later infancy or childhood, often after a respiratory infection.

Both AUTOSOMAL RECESSIVE and X-LINKED forms exist. The disorder is caused by the absence of the ENZYME pyruvate dehydrogenase. This is actually an enzyme complex of multiple individual enzymes. Each is encoded by a different GENE, each of which maps to a different chromosome. Both autosomes and the X CHROMOSOME are involved, hence both AR and X-linked recessive inheritance is observed.

The degree of enzyme deficiency corresponds to the severity of manifestations. Meals high in carbohydrates may exacerbate acidosis, a decreased alkalinity of the blood and tissues marked by sickly sweet breath, headache, nausea and vomiting, and visual disturbances. Severity of acidosis varies; LACTIC ACIDOSIS may cause early death.

Pyruvate dehydrogenase deficiency can be diagnosed shortly after birth by analysis of skin fibroblast cells, but the age at which it is detected is likely to depend on its severity. PRENATAL DIAGNOSIS is theoretically possible. Irreversible neurologic damage and mental retardation usually occur by the time of diagnosis.

pyruvate kinase deficiency

Rare hereditary ENZYME deficiency, detectable at birth and manifested as ANEMIA caused by destruction of red blood cells (hemolytic anemia). The severity of the anemia is variable, even within the same family. In addition, blood bilirubin levels are often above normal (hyperbilirubinemia).

Gallstones from chronic hyperbilirubinemia are a common complication. Infections may exacerbate anemia by preventing red blood cells from developing (erythroid hypoplasia). In severely anemic cases surgical removal of the spleen reduces or eliminates the need for blood transfusions.

A study of the prevalence in the province of Quebec found it to be higher in eastern Quebec (1/81,838) than in western Quebec (1/139,086), and the estimate of the prevalence at birth of PK deficiency is 1/16,490 in the French-Canadian population of the Saguenay–Lac St. Jean region of the Quebec province.

The basic defect in this disorder is a low level of the enzyme pyruvate kinase in red blood cells, or production of the enzyme with an abnormal structure so that it has a low level of activity. Similar forms of this enzyme exist in different tissues of the body, an almost identical form being present in the liver. A DNA PROBE for the liver type of pyruvate kinase was used to clone and sequence the defective GENE, which was subsequently mapped to 1q.

Inherited as an AUTOSOMAL RECESSIVE trait, most individuals with the disorder survive to adulthood, and those with mild anemia may have near-normal life spans, depending on complications.

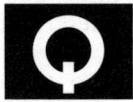

quinacrine Fluorescent dye used for banding (staining) CHROMOSOMES in CYTOGENETIC analysis. The Y CHROMOSOME, for example, is highly fluorescent when stained with this dye. Q banding, as this technique is called, was initially described by Torbjorn Caspersson and colleagues at the Karolinska Institute in Stockholm, Sweden, in 1970; it was the first banding technique and served as the first reference for identifying individual chromosomes. (See also the Introduction.)

quinine Substance used as a "folk remedy" for inducing ABORTION. It is not effective for this purpose. Large doses kill both mother and FETUS. Children exposed to smaller doses as an abortifacient (any substance used to induce abortion) have had damaged nervous systems, malformed arms and legs, BLINDNESS, DEAFNESS or other vision and hearing defects. Although quinine was once the only medication for malaria, BIRTH DEFECTS were not associated with its use for this purpose (most likely due to the lower dosage used). The overall risk for serious abnormalities of fetal development appears to be relatively low when standard doses of quinine or related agents are used in pregnancy; less toxic drugs are now prescribed for malaria. Individuals with G6PD DEFICIENCY are susceptible to hemolytic anemia when exposed to quinine.

RA See RHEUMATOID ARTHRITIS.

radial defects A range of defects involving arrested development and absence of bones of the thumb-side of the forearm, hand and wrist. In the mildest form, the thumb and bone in the hand leading to it (first metacarpal) are incomplete. In the next degree of severity, the first metacarpal is absent and the thumb is attached to the index finger only by soft tissue rather than by bone. In a more severe form, the radius, the bone on the outer or thumb side of the forearm is incomplete or absent with varying degrees of arrested development of the first metacarpal bone and thumb. In the most severe form, both bones of the forearm (radius and ulna) are missing, and the upper arm bone (humerus) is defective.

Though knowledge of limb defects such as absent fingers dates back to Aristotle, radial defects are rare. The frequency at birth of radial defects has been estimated as one in 30,000. About 20% of affected persons have no other defects, and among two-thirds of these persons only one arm is affected. Most cases in which the affected person has no other defect or ANOMALY originate sporadically, that is, there is no familial or genetic tendency. Intelligence and life span are not affected.

Radial defects also occur as part of many other SYNDROMES, including the VATER ASSOCIATION, FANCONI ANEMIA, TAR SYNDROME and HOLT-ORAM SYNDROME, as well as being associated with CRANIO-SYNOSTOSIS, congenital HEART DEFECTS or CHROMO-SOME ABNORMALITIES.

radiation Exposure to some forms of electromagnetic radiation has potentially serious consequences for fetal development. Of major concern is ionizing radiation, which includes gamma and X-rays. (Questions have also been raised regarding the consequences of long-term exposure to electromagnetic fields surrounding high-tension power lines and household appliances; these questions are the subject of current research. Suggestions that radiation emitted from VIDEO DISPLAY TERMINALS may have an adverse impact on fetal development have not been demonstrated or verified.)

The discovery that X-rays are capable of inducing MUTATIONS was a major advance in genetic research. It was reported by Hermann J. Muller in a 1927 paper, "Artificial Transmutation of the Gene." Prior to that time, researchers, whose primary research subject was the fly *Drosophila melanogaster,* had to wait for natural mutations to appear, a rare occurrence. Muller reported he could increase mutation rates 15,000 times by exposure to heavy doses of X-rays; he called these changes "mutations." (He was awarded the Nobel Prize in 1946 for his work.) The following year, Lewis Stadler reported similar findings using maize (a corn plant) and barley.

Knowledge of the impact of radiation on human development comes primarily from studies of the infants, exposed IN UTERO, and of survivors of the atomic bombings of Hiroshima. An unexpectedly large number of these individuals had abnormally small heads (MICROCEPHALY), ocular abnormalities and mental and physical growth retardation. Additionally, high levels of radiation formerly used in CANCER treatment of some pregnant women were also associated with an increase in CONGENITAL ANOMALIES.

Ionizing radiation appears to disrupt fetal development by interfering with the rapid cell division that characterizes early embryonic development. The extent of the damage is dependent on the size of the dose and the period of fetal development when exposure occurs. Dosage is commonly measured in rems or rads, a unit of ionizing ability. The average American is exposed to 200 millirems, or one-fifth of a rad, annually. Fetal exposure to more than 10 rads is considered to increase risks for developmental abnormalities, according to standards published by the American Academy of Radiologists in 1975. This is a level much higher than that received in diagnostic X-ray examinations. In the first two weeks of pregnancy, large doses (well above 50 rads) will either kill the fetus or have no impact at all. Exposure at two to four weeks is associated with multiple organ system malformations. Growth retardation is associated with later exposure, while the central nervous system is vulnerable throughout pregnancy.

In addition to interfering with cell division, radiation can damage GENES and CHROMOSOMES as well, creating a mutation or CHROMOSOME ABNORMALITY that may affect an individual in a later generation. However, little is known about the risks of transmitting these aberrations following adult exposure to radiation. It has been recommended that women who receive direct pelvic exposure to radiation (as in radiotherapy, a therapeutic cancer treatment) defer conception for a period of several months to a year, and men are advised to wait at least a year.

The low levels of radiation associated with diagnostic X-ray procedures used during pregnancy are also considered to pose no risk to fetal development. Exposure to a dose exceeding five rads would be unusual, and thus the risks of malformations or mutations due to radiation exposure are considered to be minimal. (See TERATOGEN.)

radioulnar synostosis   The term *synostosis* means the fusion of separate, adjacent bones. In this rare CONGENITAL deformity, inherited as an AUTOSOMAL DOMINANT trait, the bones of the forearm, the radius and the ulna are fused, restricting the twisting motion of the forearm to less than half of the normal range and resulting in limited function of the hand. The condition is exhibited in both forearms (bilateral) in more than 80% of those affected. It is also often seen in individuals with an XXXXXY chromosomal constitution, a rare CHROMOSOME ABNORMALITY.

Raynaud disease   Named for French physician Maurice Raynaud (1834–81), who published a description in 1862, this disorder is characterized by constriction of the blood vessels in the hands and feet upon exposure to cold or emotional stress. It is most frequently seen in females between the ages of 18 and 30. During episodes, the extremities, especially the fingers, may become white as the constricted blood vessels prevent blood from reaching the underlying tissue. The condition in itself is benign (except for the possibility of gangrene of the finger tips in extreme cases). However, it has been associated with the development of RHEUMATOID ARTHRITIS and SCLERODERMA.

A hereditary form was first identified in England in 1933 in an English working-class family, some of whose members had periodic attacks in which their fingers turned white and became numb. This form is transmitted as an AUTOSOMAL DOMINANT trait.

recombinant DNA (gene splicing)   The process and result of splicing a segment of DNA (see DEOXYRIBONUCLEIC ACID) from one source into the DNA of another. When the newly combined genetic material replicates itself, the transplanted genetic material will also be copied. This technique is useful in examining the properties and action of specific GENES. It is the basis for molecular diagnostic tests using DNA markers.

It is also anticipated that it may be possible to treat some GENETIC DISORDERS in the future by replacing defective segments of genetic material via this process. It is already being used for the manufacture of certain biochemical products such as insulin and growth hormone.

Refsum disease (phytanic acid storage disease)   A rare inherited disorder first described by Norwegian physician S. Refsum in 1946, characterized by three symptoms: deep pigmentation of the retina of the eye (RETINITIS PIGMENTOSA), weakening of the nerves of the limbs (peripheral neuropathy) and poor coordination resulting in a staggering gait (cerebellar ataxia). It is caused by the body's inability to break down (metabolize) phytanic acid, which is present in dairy products, beef, lamb, white bread, white rice, boiled potato, egg yolk and some seafoods. This results from deficiency of ENZYME phytanic acid alpha-oxidase, also known as phytanoyl-CoA hydrolase. The oxidation of phytanic acid is a function of a subcellular organelle called the peroxisome.

Inherited as an AUTOSOMAL RECESSIVE trait, the disorder is generally detected during the first 20 years of life. NIGHT BLINDNESS is usually the first symptom, due to the chemical's effect on the eye. Other symptoms include tunnel vision, muscle weakness, muscle shrinkage (atrophy) and decreased sensitivity to pain. Mapped to 10p, the GENE and its MUTATIONS have been identified.

Because the disease affects most of the specialized nerves of the brain (cranial nerves) and spinal cord, it also results in DEAFNESS, tingling sensation in the limbs, toes and fingers (paresthesias), difficulty perceiving smells, abnormal responses of the pupil to light, and slowed reflexes. Other parts of the body affected are the heart, which may be enlarged, and the kidney. The skin may have a scaly quality, especially on the palms and soles of the feet.

Onset is anywhere from childhood to age 50, but first features are generally seen by age 20. In rare cases, affected individuals will die in childhood, but a substantial number survive beyond 40 years of age. Death usually results from irregular heart rhythm (arrhythmia) or respiratory difficulties. Once diagnosed, it can be treated by limiting the intake of foods that contain phytanic acid and removing it by plasmapheresis, a technique of filtering the patient's blood plasma. Persons of Scandinavian descent seem to be most frequently affected.

The effects of phytanic acid can also be minimized by supportive therapy, such as physical therapy, orthopedic devices and CATARACT removal, if necessary.

Infantile Refsum disease is a more generalized disturbance of peroxisome function and resembles mild forms of ZELLWEGER SYNDROME or neonatal ADRENOLEUKODYSTROPHY.

regional ileitis　See CROHN DISEASE.

renal agenesis unilateral　See UNILATERAL RENAL AGENESIS.

respiratory distress syndrome (RDS)　Respiratory insufficiency, formerly called hyaline membrane disease, is one of the most common health problems among newborns, affecting approximately 40,000 annually in the United States. It is frequently associated with LOW BIRTH WEIGHT due to PREMATURITY. The lungs (as well as other organs) of these infants tend to be underdeveloped and often cannot provide a sufficient supply of the lecithin-rich "pulmonary surfactant," a lubricant that helps the air sacs in the lungs to inflate and prevents them from collapsing and sticking together after each breath. Without it, the alveoli collapse, leading to oxygen starvation (hypoxia) characterized by a blue or gray tint to the skin (cyanosis). Symptoms, which are usually exhibited at birth, include gulping for air (dyspnea), rapid breathing, expiratory grunt, limpness, cardiac failure and arrest. If death occurs, it is almost always within the first three days of life.

Progress has been made in diagnosis and treatment of RDS. The level of surfactant in fetal lungs can be measured by analysis of AMNIOTIC FLUID, and several hormones have been developed that may accelerate fetal lung development when taken by the mother shortly before birth. New respirator technology is helping prolong infant survival for the three to five days necessary for the lungs to produce enough surfactant for normal respiration. Surfactant replacement therapy is now used to prevent or treat RDS, which involves instilling a synthetic preparation of surfactant into the premature newborn's respiratory tract. It appears to improve survival rate and reduce the severity of RDS.

restless legs syndrome　A neurological disorder characterized by sensations of irritation and aching in the legs, particularly at night, causing affected individuals to continuously move their feet and legs to alleviate the discomfort. Approximately one-third of cases are hereditary, transmitted as an AUTOSOMAL DOMINANT trait. Research indicates it may be caused by a defect in the brain's ability to control sleep. It affects males and females with equal frequency and severity.

Onset of attacks typically begins in adolescence, and the episodes usually occur when the legs are at rest, such as when sitting or in bed. Sensations of intense itching and aching occur between the ankle and knee, and the discomfort and efforts to ameliorate it can interfere with sleep. Affected individuals reportedly exhibit myoclonic leg jerks just before falling asleep, and even when awake, with greater frequency than the general population. (See MYOCLONUS.) Restless legs syndrome can also be seen in pregnancy, as well as ALCOHOLISM, iron deficiency ANEMIA and DIABETES MELLITUS.

restriction enzyme (restriction fragment length polymorphism, RFLP) Proteins that chemically cut DNA strands into specific fragments for use in identifying genetic defects. The first, found in 1970, was produced by the bacteria *Hemophilus influenzae* and capable of slicing the DNA of some viruses and bacteria at specific points.

There are hundreds of restriction ENZYMES available for DNA analysis. Each of these enzymes will cut DNA at different locations, resulting in fragments of varying but reproducible lengths. These are termed restriction fragments. A genetic MUTATION may cause the restriction enzyme to cut an individual's DNA (or fail to cut it) at a location other than the "normal" site, producing a fragment length that differs from normal, thus indicating the presence of a genetic variation.

These variations in fragment length are called restriction fragment length polymorphisms (RFLP). (A mutation in a single nucleotide that gives rise to such a fragment is called a "single nucleotide polymorphism" [SNP, or snip].) By comparing the patterns of the fragments with reference patterns of genetic fragments of known length, scientists are often able to pinpoint which genetic abnormality is present. Even if the specific GENE involved is not known, or what the specific defect is, diagnosis may be possible using tests involving GENETIC LINKAGE. Use of restriction enzymes has enabled more accurate PRENATAL DIAGNOSIS of a variety of genetic defects, including those that cause CYSTIC FIBROSIS and SICKLE-CELL ANEMIA. (See also DNA PROBES and the Introduction.)

restriction fragment length polymorphism (RFLP) See RESTRICTION ENZYME.

retinitis pigmentosa (RP) A group of hereditary ocular disorders that comprise the most common forms of retinal degeneration. More than 200 inherited disorders lead to retinal degeneration, and at least 10% of inherited diseases involve the retina directly or indirectly. The retina, which forms the inner wall on the back of the eyeball, is the area where light coming into the eye registers on the photo receptor cells, called rods and cones, and is then transmitted to the brain. In RP, the retina undergoes progressive degeneration as the rods and cones stop functioning. On examination, the retina appears abnormally pigmented. The cause of this degeneration is unknown, but research has found some individuals with RP may have defective metabolism of docosahexaenoic acid, a lipid (or "fatty acid") found in high concentrations in the retinas of individuals with normal vision.

The earliest symptoms are decreased night vision (NIGHT BLINDNESS), followed by a gradual constriction of the peripheral visual field. Eventually, only a small, central portion of vision remains, as though the individual was looking through a tunnel. This progression usually occurs over many years or several decades. Onset usually occurs during childhood or young adulthood. This condition may create a sense of isolation as night driving becomes impossible, eliminating many opportunities for socializing.

Prevalence is estimated at between one in 2,000 and one in 7,000 individuals. It is estimated that RP affects 100,000 individuals in the United States. More than 20,000 persons in the United States with this disorder are classified as legally blind, though individuals generally retain some vision.

At one time it was thought that exposure to bright light speeded the progression of the disorder, but that now appears to be incorrect. Treatment consists of visual aids to maximize the use of remaining vision. There is no cure, and ongoing ophthalmological health care is important.

RP is inherited in AUTOSOMAL DOMINANT, AUTOSOMAL RECESSIVE and X-LINKED recessive forms. There is a great degree of variability in the expression of the disorder, though within families the rate and severity of vision loss is generally similar. Mutations in the *rhodopsin* gene on 3q are associated with about 20% of autosomal dominant cases of RP. Many other genes (over 39 have been mapped for isolate RP, and 30 identified as of 2006) have been found to be involved. Mutations in the *USH2A* gene may be the most common cause of nonsyndromic autosomal recessive retinitis pigmentosa. Other mutations in this gene, which is located on the long arm of chromosome 1, cause USHER SYNDROME, type 2. Usher syndrome is one of several hereditary disorders in which RP is a feature. These include BARDET-BIEDL SYNDROME, MUCOPOLYSACCHARIDOSIS, ALSTROM SYNDROME, and Refsum's disease (see PHYTANIC ACID STORAGE DISEASE). At least 50 other disorders show retinal involvement similar to RP, along with other features.

More than one-half of RP cases are isolated. When inherited without other features, all forms of inheritance have been seen. AUTOSOMAL RECESSIVE inheritance is found in about 20% of cases, AUTOSOMAL DOMINANT in 20% and X-linked in about 15%. In 50% of cases, there is no family history and the inheritance pattern is unknown. Female CARRIERS of the X-linked form can often be identified. When the mutation is known in a family, carrier testing, predictive and prenatal testing may be possible. (See also BLINDNESS.)

retinoblastoma A childhood malignant CANCER of the retina of the eye. Retinoblastoma was first described by a Dutch physician, Pawius, in 1597. It is estimated to develop in approximately one in 18,000 liveborn infants. Incidence is equal in blacks and whites, though other ETHNIC GROUPS may have rates four times as high. Between 10% and 45% of the cases are hereditary, transmitted as an AUTOSOMAL DOMINANT trait, with PENETRANCE of over 90% (more than 90% of those who inherit the gene for the condition will develop the associated retinal malignancy).

Hereditary cases tend to affect both eyes (bilateral). If not treated early, it may lead to death, though in some cases the cancer may go into spontaneous remission. It was not until treatment progressed to the point that affected individuals lived into adulthood and had children that the hereditary basis of many cases became clear. Treatment options include irradiation or removal of the affected eye(s), cryotherapy, photocoagulation (laser), and chemotherapy.

Some cases have been associated with cytogenetically detectable abnormalities or chromosome 13q. This led to the discovery of the GENE involved in the development of retinoblastoma. In inherited cases a MUTATION in this gene is transmitted from a parent, whereas in spontaneous cases the mutations occur anew in the retina cells of the individual. The gene on chromosome 13 that plays a role in retinoblastoma may also be involved in other cancers; mutations that inactivate a tumor suppressor gene can lead to the development of cancer. Affected individuals also have a risk for developing bone cancer, later in life, estimated to be 500 times that of the general population. (See also BLINDNESS; ONCOGENE.)

retinopathy of prematurity, ROP (retrolental fibroplasia, RLF) An excessive growth of blood vessels on the retina, the light-sensitive tissue on the back of the eyeball. The growth usually occurs between four weeks and 14 weeks of age, and can lead to retinal bleeding, scarring, retinal detachment and BLINDNESS. It is estimated that 8,000 infants born annually in the United States develop the disorder, causing vision loss in 2,600 and blindness in 650.

In the early 1950s, it was discovered that the condition may occur in premature infants receiving too much oxygen in incubators. As a result, incubator oxygen use was monitored more closely, and cases of blindness caused by ROP dropped. However, increased survival rates of extremely premature infants in recent years has led to an increase in this condition. It has also become clear that multiple factors related to PREMATURITY (and not just oxygen) are the cause of this disorder.

ROP may be treated with cryotherapy, a surgical procedure in which areas of the white (sclera) of the eye's outer surface are briefly frozen with a probe cooled to approximately minus 316 degrees Fahrenheit. The procedure stops or slows the growth of the excessive blood vessels on the retina. It has been estimated that this treatment can reduce by half the risk of severe vision loss from ROP.

retrolental fibroplasia See RETINOPATHY OF PREMATURITY.

Rett syndrome   A neurological disorder observed only in females; first described in 1966 by Dr. Andreas Rett of Vienna, Austria, it was not until 1983 that the disorder came to the attention of the medical community at large.

Affected females develop normally until six to 18 months of age, at which time developmental stagnation occurs. As the condition manifests, the growth of the head lags behind the rest of the body, and behavioral, social and psychomotor skills begin to deteriorate. Typically, within a year and a half of onset, the condition progresses to severe to profound MENTAL RETARDATION, INFANTILE AUTISM, loss of purposeful use of the hands, and shaking of the torso and possibly the limbs, especially when the individual is upset or agitated. They may grind their teeth (bruxism) and grimace. Crying and screaming spells are sometimes exhibited and may continue intermittently over a period of days. They do not develop meaningful language skills.

One of the most striking symptoms is repetitive hand movements, such as hand "washing," wringing and clapping and putting the hands in the mouth. These may become almost constant during waking hours.

About half can walk, exhibiting an unsteady, wide-based, stiff-legged gait, sometimes walking on their toes. Seizures develop after the age of five in about 80% of cases.

Other associated medical problems include lateral curvature of the spine (SCOLIOSIS) and respiratory problems such as lung congestion and repeated respiratory infections. Abnormal respiratory control, characterized by periods of disorganized breathing and ineffective respiratory effort often resulting in poor oxygenation, is characteristic during waking hours. Deterioration typically halts by the age of 10.

While approximately 1,500 cases have been identified worldwide, incidence is thought to be as high as one in 12,000 to one in 15,000 live female births. The condition may often be misdiagnosed as autism or CEREBRAL PALSY.

Rett syndrome is inherited in an X-linked dominant fashion. It is caused by mutations in the *MECP2* gene on the X-chromosome. The mutation is lethal in utero to affected males. Almost all cases result from new mutations in the *MECP2* gene and occur in people with no familial history of the disorder, though a small number of familial recurrences have been reported. Prenatal testing is available to families when the *MECP2* mutation has been identified in a family member.

RFLP   See RESTRICTION ENZYME.

Rh blood factor   See HEMOLYTIC DISEASE OF THE NEWBORN.

rheumatoid arthritis (RA)   Rheumatoid arthritis is a common autoimmune disease in which the body attacks its own tissue. First described by the father of medical GENETICS, Archibald Garrod (see the Introduction), it is characterized by inflammation, swelling and stiffness in the joints, causing pain and potential crippling. Occasional families show a considerable number of individuals affected with this disorder, and it has been suggested that it is transmitted as an AUTOSOMAL DOMINANT trait in these cases. However, simple MENDELIAN inheritance (dominant or recessive) has not been proven. It has a prevalence of about 1% in the general population. As many as 15% of first-degree relatives may be affected when the PROBAND is severely affected. Certain HLA-types (see HUMAN LEUKOCYTE ANTIGEN) are more frequently seen in affected individuals, and one particular type (HLA-DRW4) may be a major determinant of susceptibility to the disease in familial cases.

rhizomelic dwarfism   See DWARFISM.

ribonucleic acid (RNA)   Genetic material that controls the synthesis of protein. RNA forms on a template of DEOXYRIBONUCLEIC ACID (DNA) in the nucleus of cells. Genetic errors, or MUTATIONS, present in the DNA will be reflected in the RNA and possibly cause errors in protein synthesis, which may result in GENETIC DISORDERS.

rickets   A childhood condition primarily caused by vitamin D deficiency, which results in abnormal, stunted bone development. Other symptoms may include delayed eruption and poor development of teeth, large head and thin skull bones. It is an associated complication of many CONGENITAL and infant onset hereditary disorders, including disorders of vitamin D metabolism such as HYPOPHOSPHATEMIA.

Rieger syndrome A SYNDROME, first described by ophthalmologist Herwigh Rieger in 1935, consisting of an association of eye malformations and non-ocular abnormalities. The eye abnormality—known as the Rieger ANOMALY, the Rieger eye malformation sequence, goniodysgenesis or mesodermal dysgenesis of the iris—is a structural defect of the anterior (aqueous) chamber of the eye, the fluid-filled portion of the eye between the cornea and the iris and lens. There is defective development (hypoplasia) of the iris along with other abnormalities of the aqueous chamber, including a band that runs from the iris to the cornea. The defective development of the iris may be associated with CONGENITAL absence of all or part of the iris (aniridia) or a fissure, or cleft, of the iris (COLOBOMA). Other ocular defects include unusually large or small corneas, corneal clouding or GLAUCOMA. In most cases affected individuals have slit-like pupils.

The association of this eye anomaly with hypodontia, a reduced number of teeth, has been termed the Rieger syndrome. The Rieger anomaly may also be a feature of other syndromes (see GONIODYSGENESIS).

As affected individuals grow, they tend to show common facial features. The top of the nose (nasal root) is broad and flat. A prominent jaw that juts beyond the projection of the forehead (prognathism), protruding lower lip and short phittrum (the narrow groove between the top lip and the nose) are characteristic. Teeth may be peg or cone-shaped. There is also protrusion of the skin around the umbilicus.

More than one genetic form of Rieger syndrome exists. Rieger syndrome type 1 is caused by MUTATIONS in a homeobox TRANSCRIPTION FACTOR GENE, PITX2, which maps to 4q. Linkage studies (see GENETIC LINKAGE) indicate that a second type of Rieger syndrome maps to chromosome 13q14.

Though affected individuals may have poor vision (requiring ocular surgery in some cases), there is no impairment of intelligence, and life span is not affected.

Inherited as an AUTOSOMAL DOMINANT trait with an extreme variability of expression, Rieger syndrome is estimated to occur in approximately one in 200,000 live births. Currently, there is no method of PRENATAL DIAGNOSIS for this disorder.

In recent years Rieger has come under criticism due to his affiliation with the Nazi Party and his service in the Wehrmacht in World War II. He assumed a professorship in ophthalmology at the German University of Prague where he identified this syndrome after his predecessor had been fired for having a Jewish wife.

Riley-Day syndrome See FAMILIAL DYSAUTONOMIA.

RNA See RIBONUCLEIC ACID.

RNA interference (RNAi) The mechanism by which fragments of double-stranded RNA interfere with the expression of a particular gene that shares the same DNA sequence as the RNA. The process plays a role in regulating gene activity. It was previously referred to as post transcriptional gene silencing or transgene silencing.

The life cycle and replication of many viruses involves a double-stranded RNA stage, so it is thought this process evolved as a defense against viruses.

Roberts syndrome (pseudothalidomide syndrome; SC syndrome) Named for John B. Roberts (1854–1924), a distinguished plastic surgeon in Philadelphia who, in 1919, described the condition in three affected SIBLINGS of first-cousin Italian parents, this SYNDROME is characterized by severe malformations of the head and limbs.

The head is small (MICROCEPHALY), the ears are malformed and the eyes protrude abnormally (exophthalmos). Bilateral CLEFT LIP with or without CLEFT PALATE is almost always present. The skull may be shortened, and scalp hair is sparse.

The limb malformations are striking, and tend to be symmetrical. Bones of the arms and legs may be missing or severely deformed, resulting in shortening of the limbs. Hands and feet may be attached directly to the trunk (phocomelia), and digits on the hands and feet are often missing. In almost all cases, the number of digits missing is greater in the hands than in the feet. Undescended testes (CRYPTORCHISM) is seen in most males. There may be penile or clitoral enlargement. LOW BIRTH WEIGHT (less than five pounds) is common.

Other associated defects include HYDROCEPHALUS, SPINA BIFIDA, short neck, atrial septal defect, polycystic kidneys and horseshoe-shaped kidney.

Most affected infants are stillborn (see STILLBIRTH) or die in early infancy. Those who survive have marked growth deficiency, and many exhibit MENTAL RETARDATION.

Roberts syndrome is caused by mutation in the *ESCO2* gene, which maps to the short arm of chromosome 8. This gene encodes a protein that is involved in chromosome behavior during the cell cycle. While most cases have been sporadic, affected siblings and parental consanguinity have been observed, and the disorder is inherited in an autosomal recessive manner. Prenatal diagnosis has been accomplished using ultrasound. Prenatal testing and carrier detection is possible in families where the *ESCO2* mutation has been identified.

Robin anomaly (Pierre Robin syndrome)

A strikingly small jaw (micrognathia), protruding tongue (glossoptosis) and CLEFT PALATE are the three cardinal features of this SYNDROME, caused by an abnormality of embryonic development. Although described in medical literature as early as 1911, it bears the name of French dental surgeon Pierre Robin (1867–1950), who published a description in 1923.

The most dangerous result of this condition is interruption of breathing at birth, due to obstruction of the newborn's airway. If artificial means of breathing are not provided immediately, the lack of oxygen reaching the brain may cause severe MENTAL RETARDATION.

Associated features in some cases are congenital HEART DEFECTS, crossed-eyes (STRABISMUS), and GLAUCOMA. The cleft palate may be repaired surgically after the infant is 18 months old. By age six, the jaw reaches normal size, though it may continue to have an unusual shape.

Affecting males and females equally, it occurs in an estimated one in 2000 to 30,000 live births.

PRENATAL DIAGNOSIS is currently not routine, though it may be possible with ULTRASOUND. However, the anomaly may not be evident until late in gestation. The mode of inheritance is unknown, though it appears to be caused by the action of several GENES in concert with environmental influence (MULTIFACTORIAL). In addition, the Robin anomaly may be one feature of a number of associated syndromes, most importantly the STICKLER SYNDROME, which may account for as much as 30% of infants born with this anomaly. It may also be seen among the spectrum of anomalies seen with deletion of chromosome 22 (see CATCH 22 and VELOCARDIOFACIAL SYNDROME).

Robinow syndrome (fetal face syndrome)

A rare disorder, described by American physician M. Robinow in 1969, and also known as the fetal face syndrome because the face resembles that of a FETUS of about eight weeks gestation. These features include a disproportionately large skull, bulging forehead, curving, S-shaped lower eyelids, short, upturned nose (anteverted nares) and flat face. The mouth may turn down at the corners, and the teeth may be misaligned or crowded. Arms may be short and the fingers and toes short and stubby. As the affected person grows, fused vertebrae and sideways curvature of the spine (SCOLIOSIS) may become apparent. There is moderate dwarfing and the forearm bones are shortened. External genitalia may be underdeveloped, often to a severe degree. Early death secondary to cardiac or pulmonary complications occurs in about 10% of patients.

In some cases, the syndrome is transmitted as an AUTOSOMAL DOMINANT trait. The autosomal recessive form of Robinow syndrome has been shown to be caused by homozygous mutations in the *ROR2* gene. Heterozygous mutations in the same gene, which is found on the long arm of chromosome 9, cause autosomal dominant BRACHYDACTYLY type B.

Romano-Ward syndrome (prolonged QT interval)   Defect characterized by sudden losses of consciousness triggered by an insufficient supply of blood to the brain (syncope). These episodes may be brief and apparently harmless, or lengthy, severe and even fatal. It was first described in Italy in 1963 by C. Romano, and in the United States in 1964 by B. C. Ward. The QT interval refers to a portion of the electrical activity of the heartbeat as measured by the electrocardiogram.

Usually the syncope is brought on by violent emotion or strenuous exercise. The underlying cause is an irregular or inappropriate heartbeat. Electro-cardiography may show that the heart fails to increase its rate of contractions rapidly enough to meet the work demand placed on it. Frequency of these episodes ranges from several per month to only one or two in a lifetime.

Genetically heterogeneous, mutations in the *ANK2, KCNE1, KCNE2, KCNH2* (also known as *HERG*), *KCNQ1* (also known as *KVLQT1*) and *SCN5A* genes cause Romano-Ward syndrome. The gene known as *KCNQ1* is the chromosome 11p-linked LQT (long QT) gene. *KCNQ1* is strongly expressed in the heart and codes for a protein with structural features of a voltage-gated potassium channel. Homozygosity for different mutations in this same gene is responsible for Jervell and Lange-Nielsen syndrome. The gene on chromosome 7q has homology, or is analogous, to the Drosophilia "ether-a-go-go" gene, which encodes a calcium-modulated potassium channel. Its discoverers called the gene *HERG* (for human ether-a-go-go related gene).

Mutations in the *KCNQ1* gene appear to be the most frequent cause of this disorder, followed by mutations in *KCNH2* and then the cardiac sodium channel gene, *SCN5A*.

Ventricular fibrillation is estimated to cause over 300,000 sudden deaths annually in the United States. In approximately 5–12% of cases (15,000–36,000) no cardiac or noncardiac causes for the episodes are found, which is therefore classified as idiopathic ventricular fibrillation (IVF). Mutations in the SCN5A gene have been found in some cardiac patients who exhibit an electrocardiographic pattern characteristic of IVF. Individuals with this distinctive pattern may account for 40–60% of all cases of IVF. Mutations have also been found in the ISK gene on chromosome 21 among this population. (As for *KCNQ1*, other mutations in this gene have also been found in Jervell and Lange-Nielsen syndrome families.)

This rare defect is inherited as an AUTOSOMAL DOMINANT trait. Affected individuals can be identified by characteristic electrocardiographic findings. Historically, the prognosis has been poor, with about half of those affected dying before reaching adolescence. However, modern drug therapy has improved the long-term prognosis. (In 1990, all-American college basketball star Hank Gathers collapsed and died on the basketball court from long QT syndrome.)

The disorder is similar to Jervell and Lange-Nielsen syndrome but distinguished from the latter by the absence of DEAFNESS as a feature. New therapies include implantable defibrillators and QT sensitive pacemakers.

Rothmund-Thomson syndrome (RTS; poikiloderma atrophicans and cataract)   Disorder whose primary features are abnormalities of the skin and eyes. It was first described in 1868 by August von Rothmund (1830–1906), professor of ophthalmology and head of the state eye clinic in Munich, Germany. Matthew S. Thomson (1894–1969), senior dermatologist at Kings College Hospital in London, described what is believed to be the same condition in 1936, and it now bears both their names.

Abnormalities of the skin may be present at birth, but usually appear between three and six months of life. Large, reddened patches caused by the dilation of capillaries near the surface of the skin (erythema) appear on the face and later involve the ears, buttocks, extremities and ultimately the entire body, and lesions form on these areas. The progression stabilizes after the first few years of life. However, skin lesions may turn cancerous in adulthood. Other skin abnormalities include brown pigmentation, depigmentation and telangiectases (prominent, dilated blood vessels). There may be sensitivity to sunlight resulting in blistering, though this is more common early in life.

About half of affected individuals have sparse hair, eyebrows and eyelashes, and some have total loss of hair (ALOPECIA). Nails of the hands and feet may be malformed. Teeth may be small, malformed or fail to erupt.

CATARACTS are the most common ocular manifestation, and usually are found in both bilateral eyes. They develop rapidly over a period of a few weeks or months. They may appear as early as four months of age, and in most cases appear by the age of five years. However, in some cases they have appeared as late as age 40.

Other associated features include short stature, SCOLIOSIS and malformation of the hands and fingers. MENTAL RETARDATION has been reported in some affected individuals. While there are no consistent skeletal deformities, maldevelopment of the arms and pelvis have been reported. Although sterility is frequent, pregnancy has been reported on several occasions.

In both sexes, the development of secondary sex characteristics is poor. Inherited as an AUTOSOMAL RECESSIVE trait, most cases of Rothmund-Thomson syndrome are caused by mutations in the DNA helicase gene *RECQL4*, which is located on the long arm of chromosome 8 and encodes a protein that unwinds double-stranded DNA into single-stranded DNAs. Although there is evidence to suggest that mutations in another gene must cause this disorder, no other gene has yet been identified. It is a rare condition; only 80 cases have been reported. Seventy % of reported cases are female, but the reason for the seeming sex predilection is unknown. Currently, PRENATAL DIAGNOSIS of this condition is not possible.

rubella   See TORCH SYNDROME.

rubeola   See MEASLES.

Rubinstein-Taybi syndrome   A highly variable disorder first described in 1963 by U.S. physicians J. H. Rubinstein and H. Taybi, as a SYNDROME of broad thumbs and toes, and facial abnormalities.

The facial abnormalities consist of a small head (MICROCEPHALY), prominent forehead, eyes that slant downward away from the nose (antimongoloid obliquity), a broad nasal bridge and a beaked nose. Eyebrows may be heavy, eyelashes may be long, eyelids may droop (PTOSIS) and the eyes may be wide-set (HYPERTELORISM). The ears may be abnormally shaped, low-set or rotated. Grimacing and an unusual smile are frequently observed. A high-arched palate and dental malocclusion are also common.

In addition to the thumbs, the ends of the fingers tend to be broad, as well. An incurving (CLINODACTYLY) of the little finger and overlapping toes are other digital malformations seen in more than 50% of cases.

Skeletal abnormalities include short stature, concave chest (PECTUS excavatum) and curvature of the spine (kyphoscoliosis). Growth deficiency and mental retardation are common. Average IQ is about 50.

It is caused by MUTATION in the GENE encoding the transcriptional coactivator CREB binding protein, found on 16p. This is an example of a specific set of multiple congenital malformations with mental retardation being caused by a generalized dysregulation of gene expression. Affected patients are HETEROZYGOUS (involving only one gene of a pair) for point mutations and deletions involving this gene. About 25% of cases are due to microdeletions detectable by FISH. It can thus be considered an AUTOSOMAL DOMINANT disorder in which most cases result from new mutations. More than 550 cases have been reported. The recurrence risk in sibs (see SIBLINGS) is low, but would be 50% for offspring of an affected individual.

Russell-Silver syndrome   A rare form of DWARFISM identified in about 100 cases, named for Alexander Russell, professor of pediatrics at the Hebrew University in Jerusalem, and Henry Silver, professor of pediatrics at the University of Colorado, who published descriptions in 1954 and 1953, respectively. Its most distinctive feature is asymmetry of the body. In some individuals, this asymmetry is limited to the skull or a single limb. In others, one entire side of the body is significantly larger than the other. At birth, affected individuals are unusually small for full-term infants, though head size is normal, giving the appearance of a large head in comparison to the rest of the body. Throughout childhood they exhibit a pattern of growth at the lower end of the normal range. There may be CLIN-ODACTYLY of the fifth fingers, which are short and incurving.

The facial characteristics can be quite distinct: prominence of the forehead (pseudohydrocephaly, frontal bossing), prominent eyes with long eyelashes and blue tint to the white of the eye (bluish sclerae), marked underdevelopment of the jaw (micrognathia) and thin lips with the corners of the mouth turned down. Other findings include the presence of café au lait spots (coffee-colored flat birthmarks), bending or fusion of the fingers or toes, poor muscle development and retarded early motor performance. In about one- third of the cases, mild MENTAL RETARDATION is also seen. Some children have had low blood sugar after short periods of fasting or have had deficiency of growth hormone.

The cause of this disorder is unknown. It is believed that the basic genetic defect underlying this SYNDROME may be a new MUTATION in the affected individual. It appears to be genetically HET-EROGENEOUS. Maternal uniparental disomy for chromosome 7 has been found in a number of cases (see CHROMOSOME ABNORMALITIES). Most occur sporadically.

PRENATAL DIAGNOSIS by ULTRASOUND of the growth retardation has been reported. Evaluation for growth hormone deficiency should be considered and the use of growth hormone theraphy has been advocated by some. The prognosis for affected individuals depends on the degree of asymmetry. Most patients lead normal lives.

Ruvalcaba syndrome Signature facial abnormalities are the most unifying feature of this developmental disorder. It causes varying degrees of short stature and MENTAL RETARDATION in over half of affected individuals, and may also be associated with other musculoskeletal or other abnormalities, including hernia, CRYPTORCHISM, short hands and feet and broad hips.

The head is small (MICROCEPHALY), the face oval, with a hooked nose, downslanting eyes, and a turned down mouth. The sides of the nose may be underdeveloped. The jaw is pointed and the ears low set.

Common skeletal abnormalities include narrow chest (PECTUS carinatum), SCOLIOSIS and kyphosis in the trunk. Believed to be inherited as an AUTO-SOMAL DOMINANT trait, cases have been reported in North America, Japan and Europe.

S

sacrococcygeal teratoma Tumors in the area of the buttocks, usually appearing during the first two months of life. "Sacrococcygeal" refers to the portion of the end of the vertebral column where these cancerous masses, or teratomas, appear. The tumors begin to develop IN UTERO, and may displace or disrupt function of the bowel and bladder. Benign tumors consist of tissues similar to normal structures. The tumors may contain skin, hair, muscle, lung or pancreatic tissue and even bowel loops, and teeth or limb components, such as digits. Malignant tumors are generally of "yolk sac" origin, having their genesis in early embryonic development. While most of the tumors are benign (55% to 75%), virtually all of the infants with malignancies die in infancy.

The cause of these teratomas is unknown; they occur in an estimated one in 40,000 births. Females are affected four times as frequently as males. It is the most common tumor seen in newborns. Most occur sporadically. (See also CANCER.)

Saethre-Chotzen syndrome A form of CRANIOSYNOSTOSIS, a group of disorders caused by premature closure of the gaps (sutures) between the cranial bones, resulting in an abnormal shape of the skull. It bears the names of physicians Haakon Saethre and F. Chotzen, who published descriptions in 1931 and 1932, respectively. Saethre, a Norwegian psychiatrist, reported it in a patient after initially being sought for consultation regarding a suspected case of SCHIZOPHRENIA.

In this form of craniosynostosis, the shape of the skull deformity is variable. Most typically, the head is pointed (acrocephaly), though it may be elongated (dolichocephaly) in some cases or somewhat squat (brachycephaly). Although the skull abnormality may not be evident at birth, typical facial characteristics are often present: The face tends to be lopsided, the eyes wide-set (HYPERTELORISM), the nose beaked and the ears low-set and rotated somewhat backward. Head circumference is reduced, and the hairline may be low.

This condition is also associated with vision problems and mild hearing loss. The eyes may not be coordinated, resulting in difficulty focusing (STRABISMUS). Individuals may be nearsighted (MYOPIA) and the eyelids may droop (PTOSIS).

Digital abnormalities are also common, especially a partial joining of the skin between the second and third fingers, so that the two digits appear somewhat joined (SYNDACTYLY). Shortened fingers (BRACHYDACTYLY) have also been reported. Short stature, undescended testicles (CRYPTORCHISM) and renal (kidney) ANOMALIES have also been associated with this condition. Intelligence is usually normal, but mild to moderate MENTAL RETARDATION may occur.

Inherited as an AUTOSOMAL DOMINANT trait, it is caused by MUTATIONS in the twist transcription factor gene located on 7p that result in its diminished function. In cases attributed to new mutation, an increased paternal age may play a role.

Theoretically, in an at-risk pregnancy, ULTRASOUND may be able to detect cranial abnormalities exhibited in severe cases.

Salla disease (Finnish type sialuria) HEREDITARY DISEASE first reported in northeastern Finland in 1979 and named for the geographic area where the affected families lived. It is characterized by progressive deterioration of mental and physical abilities, with onset by 12 to 18 months of age. Children who have already learned to walk lose this skill. Growth is retarded in about half of those under medical care, and cardiac abnormalities have been noted. Spasticity and impaired speech are other features.

One of the hallmarks is the increased urinary excretion of free sialic acid. It is a STORAGE DISEASE and the free sialic acid (a complex sugar that is a component of mucopolysaccharides and glycoproteins) is stored in many cells of the body. It appears to result from a defect in transmembrane transport in the lysosome, leading to lysosomal storage of fatty acid.

Inherited as an AUTOSOMAL RECESSIVE trait, the responsible GENE maps to 6q. CARRIER detection has not been accomplished but PRENATAL DIAGNOSIS has been reported.

Sandhoff disease   First described by German biochemist Konrad Sandhoff in 1968, this condition is extremely similar to TAY-SACHS DISEASE and may be indistinguishable from it without laboratory testing. It is likely that some non-Jewish children diagnosed as having Tay-Sachs before the availability of definitive diagnostic procedures actually had Sandhoff disease. However, unlike Tay-Sachs, bones and abdominal organs (e.g., liver) may show signs of abnormalities.

Motor weakness begins in the first six months of life. There is an exaggerated startle response to sound, and early BLINDNESS, along with progressive motor and mental deterioration. The face is doll-like, the head is large and the CHERRY-RED SPOT in the eye, characteristic of Tay-Sachs, is also present. The loss of swallowing ability is progressive, causing difficulty in feeding (food may be inhaled) and an increased risk of lung and chest infections, which usually lead to death by three years of age.

This disorder is caused by an ENZYME deficiency of hexosaminidase A and B, which are essential for metabolizing GM2 ganglioside, a fatty material. It results from MUTATIONS in the GENE for the beta subunit of hexosaminidase, which lies on chromosome 5q. (In Tay-Sachs disease, only hexosaminidase A is absent.) Due to the enzyme deficiency, this fatty substance (GM2 ganglioside) accumulates in the child's brain cells. This is therefore a STORAGE DISEASE, caused by an abnormal accumulation or storage of material in the cells.

The disorder is inherited as an AUTOSOMAL RECESSIVE trait. Adult CARRIERS can be identified through careful screening procedures. PRENATAL DIAGNOSIS is possible through the finding of almost total absence of hexosaminidase activity in fetal tissues collected via AMNIOCENTESIS or CHORIONIC VILLUS SAMPLING (CVS).

Sanfilippo syndrome   See MUCOPOLYSACCHARDOSIS, type III.

scaphocephaly   See CRANIOSYNOSTOSIS.

Scheie syndrome   See MUCOPOLYSACCHARIDOSIS.

Schimke immuno-osseous dysplasia (SIOD; spondylo-epiphyseal dysplasia)   A hereditary disorder characterized by disproportionate dwarfing in association with kidney anomalies and immune system deficiencies. It was first described by R. N. Schimke in 1971. Severity is variable. Growth failure may begin in utero. Individuals with severe early-onset symptoms typically succumb early in life. Individuals who exhibit less severe symptoms with a later onset often survive into adulthood. Adult height for men is 53.5–62" and for women 39–56". Facial features are dysmorphic, and the neck and trunk are disproportionately short. Intelligence and neurological development are normal.

Progressive nephropathy (kidney failure) usually begins between one and 12 years of age and results in fatal renal disease. The kidney involvement is typically identified within five years of diagnosis of growth failure. T cell deficiency, another feature of the disorder, predisposes affected individuals to opportunistic infections, which are a common cause of death. Central nervous system (CNS) symptoms, including migraine headaches and strokes, have been reported in about half of those affected. Half of patients have hypothyroidism, and one-tenth exhibit bone marrow failure. However, these CNS and immune system symptoms are confined to early onset cases. Diagnosis is made on the basis of clinical observation of the characteristic constellation of anomalies.

SIOD is an autosomal recessive disorder caused by mutations in the *SMARCAL1 (SW1/SNF2-related, matrix-associated, actin-dependent regulator of chromatin, subfamily a-like 1)* gene, mapped to 2q34-q36. It is thought that the degree of mutation in this gene is linked to the severity of its expression in affected families and individuals. In families with the severe, early onset form, affected individuals have been found to have two alleles with nonsense, frameshift or splicing mutations. The milder form is associated with a missence mutation on each allele.

The prevalence of SIOD is unknown. Sequential analysis of the gene has been accomplished on a research basis. Prenatal testing may be available for at-risk families in which the mutation has been identified.

Schinzel-Gideon syndrome A collection of ANOMALIES involving the kidneys, heart, brain and skeleton accompanied by a characteristic flat mid-face (mid-face retraction). Ears are low set, nose is short and low and eyes are wide set. There is excessive space in the cranial sutures. Hair is excessive (hypertrichosis), and the neck is wide with excessive loose skin (CUTIS LAXA). The lower arms and legs are short. EPILEPSY, vision and hearing difficulties, and MENTAL RETARDATION are also frequent features.

Hydronephrosis, excessive fluid in the kidneys, results from an obstructed ureter, one of the signs of the disorder. The heart may exhibit atrial septal defects. Both may be treated surgically. Anticonvulsant drugs can help control epileptic seizures. Thought to be inherited as an AUTOSOMAL RECESSIVE trait, males and females are affected equally.

schizophrenia Term describing a variety of diseases characterized by hallucinations, delusions, disorders of thinking and irrational behavior. It is thought to affect almost 1% of the population at some time in their lives.

Schizophrenia appears to have a significant genetic component. The mode of inheritance is unclear but MULTIFACTORIAL inheritance seems most likely. A familial link has long been noted; studies of affected identical (monozygotic) TWINS reared apart further suggest that the disorder has a genetic basis, as do adoption studies: The incidence in adopted children is close to that predicted for their natural rather than their adoptive parents. It may not be a single entity. In some families a single major GENE may be involved and it may appear as an AUTOSOMAL DOMINANT trait. Chromosomal locations for possible genes involved have been suggested, but much of the initial research was inconclusive.

The risks for additional family members developing schizophrenia range from 2% to 3% if an aunt, uncle, nephew, niece or first cousin is affected, to 40% to 60% if an identical twin is affected. The risk if one parent is affected is 13% and 40% if both are.

Anticipation appears to be inherent in the transmission of familial schizophrenia. The findings support investigations of unstable MUTATIONS (i.e., trinucleotide repeat mutations; see TRINUCLEOTIDE REPEAT DISORDERS) and other mechanisms that might contribute to true anticipation in schizophrenia. There is a reported excess of sex-chromosome aneuploidies (e.g., XXY and XXX) among patients with schizophrenia, and it is also seen in certain disorders such as velocardiofacial syndrome (see CHROMOSOME ABNORMALITIES).

In addition to genetic factors, substantial evidence exists for environmental factors in the origin of schizophrenia. Numerous studies have found an excess of schizophrenia births in the winter months in the Northern hemisphere, particularly in the low genetic risk group. Variations in incidence related to birth dates may be due to certain infections and perinatal brain damage which may also vary seasonally, or nutritional deficiencies.

The diagnosis of schizophrenia can be difficult, complicating genetic studies. There is no universally accepted definition of the disorder for a variety of reasons including the lack of a central feature (such as the mood change seen in manic depression) and of characteristic pathology (such as neurofibrillary tangles seen in ALZHEIMER'S DISEASE).

Effective antipsychotic drugs used to treat schizophrenia have their primary site of action in competing for dopamine receptors in the brain, leading to suspicion that an abnormality in dopamine metabolism or dopamine receptor sensitivity may be involved in the disorder. Hereditary factors may play a role in this abnormality or sensitivity. There is, at present, no method of identifying those at risk for developing schizophrenia by presymptomatic or PRENATAL DIAGNOSIS.

Schmid-type metaphyseal chondrodysplasia   See METAPHYSEAL CHONDRODYSPLASIA.

Schwartz-Jampel syndrome   Symptoms of this rare SYNDROME, characterized by distortion of the facial features, short stature, muscle spasms and rigidity, and ocular problems, initially occur after the first year of life. It is thought to be caused by an interruption of the embryo's muscular and skeletal development. U.S. physicians O. Schwartz and Robert S. Jampel published the first description in 1962.

The most common skeletal effects of the disease are short neck, protruding chest (PECTUS carinatum), curvature of the spine, and small hips, which can make walking difficult. The eyes may be small in size, set far apart (HYPERTELORISM) and may have two or more rows of eyelashes. There may be drooping of the eyelids (PTOSIS), MYOPIA or CATARACTS. The chin and mouth may be small. Speech may be high-pitched or difficult to understand due to arching in the roof of the mouth. Muscles of the limbs may be thick and small, and some children may have bulges in the stomach or groin due to weak muscles (hernias). Because the muscles of the face are contracted, affected individuals appear to have no expression.

Intelligence and life span are normal. Surgery may help correct ocular or skeletal problems, and orthopedic devices may be useful as well. Some children exhibit spontaneous improvement of their muscle contractions. MALIGNANT HYPERTHERMIA is a potentially lethal complication during anesthesia.

The syndrome is inherited as an AUTOSOMAL RECESSIVE, caused by mutations in the gene encoding perlecan.

SCID   See IMMUNE DEFICIENCY DISEASES.

scleroderma   A chronic disease that causes hardening (sclerosis) of the skin (dermis) and internal organs, including the gastrointestinal tract, lungs, heart and kidneys. It occurs in women four times as often as in men. The skin feels taut and leathery and is firmly bound to subcutaneous tissue. It may itch and later become hyperpigmented. Involvement of internal organs may lead to fatal complications.

The cause is unknown. Familial occurrence has been reported and it has been suggested that a familial form may be inherited as an AUTOSOMAL DOMINANT trait. Many of the clinical features of this disorder resemble those of chronic graft versus host disease (CGVHD) (which results from donor cells "attacking" the recipient after transplants, such as bone marrow transplants). This led to the hypothesis that fetal immune cells, which are known to cross the placenta and enter the maternal circulation, persist as "micro-transplants" and lead to a form of CGVHD. Persistent male DNA has been demonstrated in many female patients years after the delivery of a male infant, but not in a matched group of unaffected women. Another theory suggests that infection with CMV (cytomegalovirus; see TORCH SYNDROME) may be involved in the cause of this disorder. An underlying genetic predisposition, as has been suggested in systemic lupus erythematosus (see LUPUS) and RHEUMATOID ARTHRITIS, may also be involved.

scoliosis   A lateral, or sideways, curvature of the spine. While it is often a secondary feature of many SYNDROMES (e.g., MARFAN SYNDROME, DYSAUTONOMIA NEUROFIBROMATOSIS, MUSCULAR DYSTROPHIES and FREDREICH'S ATAXIA), scoliosis occurs most frequently as an independent disorder of the musculoskeletal system.

It may be CONGENITAL, that is, present at birth, due to defective embryonic spinal development. However, much more common is idiopathic scoliosis, which represents 80% to 90% of cases. Idiopathic (of unknown cause or origin) scoliosis is believed to be inherited as a MULTIFACTORIAL, or POLYGENIC, trait, that is, several GENES may be responsible for its transmission, with expression and severity partly dependent on environmental factors. This form of scoliosis demonstrates a familial tendency, though the degree of the severity shows wide variability within affected family members. A child whose SIBLING has scoliosis has approximately double the general population's risk of developing the disorder.

Idiopathic scoliosis is classified by the age at which it appears: infantile (0–4 years), juvenile (4–9 years) and adolescent (10 years to skeletal maturity). Most cases fall into the adolescent category, perhaps owing to hormonal influence on development of the condition.

An estimated 4% to 10% of the adolescent population has some degree of scoliosis. Females develop the disorder more frequently than males, by a ratio of 8:1.

One of the most common signs of scoliosis is a prominent shoulder blade, most frequently the right one. One shoulder also tends to be higher, and affected children tend to list to one side. Hips may be uneven, with one higher than the other. Clothing may appear to fit improperly. This is most obvious in girls by observing an uneven hemline in skirts or dresses.

Mild cases may be unnoticeable or require no treatment. However, severe cases may result in significant skeletal deformity, and require the wearing of a brace to straighten the spine, or surgery to correct the spinal curvature.

Currently there is no method of detecting the disorder by PRENATAL DIAGNOSIS, or identifying families at high risk for having affected family members.

SC syndrome   See ROBERTS SYNDROME

Seckel syndrome (bird-headed dwarfism)   "Bird-headed dwarfism" was the name used for this inherited disorder by Helmut P. G. Seckel (1900–61), professor of pediatrics at the University of Chicago School of Medicine, who wrote the definitive description of it in 1960. Principal characteristics include LOW BIRTH WEIGHT, DWARFISM, abnormally small head (MICROCEPHALY), large eyes, a large, prominent nose with a beaklike protrusion, narrow face, receding lower jaw, small brain size, CLUBFOOT, lateral spinal deformation (SCOLIOSIS), underdeveloped thumbs, dislocation of the heads of the thigh bones out of the hip sockets, crossed eyes (STRABISMUS), malformations in the genitourinary system and MENTAL RETARDATION.

Although a normal life span is possible, mental retardation and associated body malformations make functioning difficult. Affected children tend to be friendly and pleasant but are easily distracted and hyperactive.

Inherited as an AUTOSOMAL RECESSIVE trait, this disorder appears to show genetic HETEROGENEITY, that is, a mutation in any one of several genes can cause it. A mutation in the *ATR* gene, which encodes a protein called the ataxia-telangiectasia and RAD3-related protein, is responsible for one form of Seckel syndrome. This gene maps to the long arm of chromosome 3. Other genes for Seckel syndrome have been mapped to chromosomes 18p and 14q. The incidence is estimated to be approximately one in 10,000 live births.

selective IgA deficiency   See IMMUNE DEFICIENCY DISEASES.

selective termination   See ABORTION.

Senior-Loken syndrome   An inherited disorder characterized by the wasting of the kidney (nephronophthisis), which may or may not be accompanied by medullary cystic disease and progressive ocular disorders.

The disorder usually becomes apparent during the first year of life. Onset of kidney problems is gradual, but tubular degeneration leads to progressive kidney failure. Nausea, weight loss, fatigue and ANEMIA precede kidney failure. Progressive atrophy of the retina occurs simultaneously.

Senior-Loken syndrome is inherited as an autosomal recessive trait. Homozygous mutations (i.e., identical mutations in both genes of a gene pair) in any of a number of genes may cause this disorder. Thus, it shows genetic HETEROGENEITY. Genes involved include the *NPHP1* gene, which is mapped to chromosome 2q and encodes the nephrocystin protein; the *NPHP4* gene, which maps to chromosome 1p and encodes the nephroretinin protein; and the *IQCB1* gene (also known as the *NPHP5* gene), which maps to chromosome 3q and encodes the nephrocystin 5 protein. More than 150 cases have been reported, affecting males and females equally.

severe combined immunodeficiency   See IMMUNE DEFICIENCY DISEASES.

sex chromosome   The X CHROMOSOME and Y CHROMOSOME. These CHROMOSOMES determine gender and carry GENES for sex-linked characteristics. In the 23 pairs of chromosomes found in the normal human KARYOTYPE, the sex chromosomes are the 23rd pair. All the non-sex chromosomes are called autosomes.

The sex chromosomes were observed as early as 1891, by German zoologist Herman Henking (1858–1942), who noted them while studying the chromosomes of the fire wasp (phyrrho coris). Their function remained unrecognized until after the rediscovery of Mendel's laws. (See also X-LINKED; AUTOSOMAL DOMINANT; AUTOSOMAL RECESSIVE.)

sex limited   Expression of a genetic characteristic or trait in one sex only, in which the primary MUTATION does not involve the SEX CHROMOSOMES. These characteristics often involve a structural defect for which there is no anatomical counterpart in the opposite sex. An example is HYPOSPADIAS in the male. (See X-LINKED.)

sex-linked   See X-LINKED.

sex reversal   See XX MALE SYNDROME.

short stature   See DWARFISM.

SHOX (short stature homeobox)   One of a family of genes that orchestrates production of a protein that regulates the activity of other genes. (Such a gene is termed a transcription factor.) Early in embryonic development, the *SHOX* gene helps control the formation of body structures and develop-

ment of the skeleton and plays a key role in the growth of the bones of the arms and legs.

The *SHOX* gene is located on the short arms of both the X and Y chromosomes, in an area called the pseudoautosomal region. Unlike other regions of the X and Y (or sex) chromosomes, where only one copy of a gene exists, in this region there are gene pairs as there are in the 22 autosomal chromosome pairs.

Mutations or other anomalies involving the *SHOX* gene typically result in skeletal abnormalities caused by the disruption of the production of the SHOX protein. Leri-Weill dyschondrosteosis and the more severe Langer mesomelic dysplasia are examples. A mutation in one *SHOX* gene results in the Leri-Weill dyschondrosteosis, while a mutation in both copies of the *SHOX* gene results in Langer mesomelic dysplasia. Both disorders are characterized by unusually short stature, with the bones of the forearm and lower legs particularly affected.

Turner syndrome, which affects only females, results from the absence of one sex chromosome. Thus, affected individuals have only one *SHOX* gene, which may play a role in the short stature and skeletal abnormalities observed in this disorder. Some individuals with unusually short stature have been found to have mutations within or the deletion of the *SHOX* gene.

Mutations of the *SHOX* gene have also been found in 2.4% of children with idiopathic (of unknown origin) short stature (ISS) without other skeletal anomalies. Conversely, overactivity of the *SHOX* gene has been suggested to result in long limbs and tall stature, as in Klinefelter syndrome.

A *SHOX* mutation is estimated to be present in at least one in 2,000 children. Growth hormone has been used to treat individuals with ISS and Turner syndrome successfully.

Shwachman syndrome (metaphyseal dysplasia with pancreatic insufficiency and neutropenia)   First described in five children by H. Shwachman in 1963, the SYNDROME consists of pancreatic insufficiency and abnormally low level of white blood corpuscles (leukopenia) in conjunction with metaphyseal chondrodysplasia, a form of DWARFISM.

During embryonic development the exocrine pancreatic cells are replaced by adipose, or fatty tissue. Due to this abnormal development, the ENZYMES amylase, lipase and trypsin normally created by these cells are absent. Intestinal lipase is thought to compensate for the lack of pancreatic lipase. Diarrhea and FAILURE TO THRIVE from malnutrition can result from the pancreatic problems.

Short-limb dwarfism is present at birth. Infants exhibit failure to thrive, most commonly between two and 10 months of age. The luekopenia may occur intermittently, often accompanied by bacterial infections. Mild MENTAL RETARDATION is seen in about one-third of those affected. IQ is significantly lower than that of SIBLINGS.

Pancreatic enzyme therapy has achieved dramatic results in some patients but has little effect in others.

Inherited as an AUTOSOMAL RECESSIVE trait, Shwachman syndrome is caused by mutations in the *SBDS* gene, located on the long arm of chromosome 7. Numerous cases have been reported. Scott Hamilton, 1984 Olympic Gold Medalist figure skater, was affected with Shwachman syndrome as a child.

sialidosis   See MUCOLIPIDOSIS; NEURAMINIDASE DEFICIENCY.

sialuria, Finnish type   See SALLA DISEASE.

Siamese twins   See CONJOINED TWINS.

sibling (sib)   A brother or sister; multiple children of identical parents. Sibling actually refers to a younger brother or sister, though in common usage the two are often used interchangeably. Siblings have half of their GENES in common, and siblings of those affected with hereditary or CONGENITAL disorders may have increased risks of developing or being born with the same disorder, depending on the condition and its cause, whether the result of genetic or environmental influences or a combination of the two. Unaffected siblings of those with hereditary or congenital disorders may experience feelings of neglect and guilt as a result of familial or personal response to the affected sibling, further complicating the interpersonal dynamics in these families.

sickle-cell anemia   This hereditary, chronic form of hemolytic ANEMIA (an anemia characterized by breakdown of the red blood cells) takes its name from the characteristic sickle, or crescent, shape of the red blood cells (erythrocytes) seen in those with the disorder.

Red blood cells get their color from hemoglobin, an iron-based molecule that carries oxygen in the blood, nourishing tissues throughout the body. The sickling of the red blood cells that characterizes this disorder is caused by the change in a single AMINO ACID within the hemoglobin molecule, changing it to hemoglobin-S, which makes the red blood cell collapse when deprived of oxygen. Blood cells are most likely to sickle in the capillaries, or small blood vessels, after the oxygen has been released to the body. The sickle shape causes the blood to clog these vessels, depriving organ tissue of oxygen, in turn causing more blood sickling, more oxygen deprivation, creating pain and leading to organ damage.

The identification of the basis of sickle-cell anemia, made by U.S. chemist Dr. Linus Pauling (1901–94) in 1949, was one of the seminal events in molecular genetics. Working at the California Institute of Technology, he found the flaw in the hemoglobin molecule responsible for the condition. This change in the molecule altered its electric charge. Thus, it behaved differently in an electrical field than normal hemoglobin, a fact Pauling used to detect the abnormal molecules. This was also the first condition linked (in 1978) to variations within a family of specific segments of DNA containing the aberrant GENE (SEE RESTRICTION ENZYME). Dr. Pauling was awarded the 1954 Nobel Prize in chemistry for his work. (An opponent of U.S. nuclear policy, he was also awarded the Nobel Peace Prize in 1963.)

The expression, or severity, of the disorder among individuals with sickle-cell anemia is highly variable, ranging from mild to severe. Symptoms may include growth retardation, delay in secondary sexual development, leg ulcers, fatigue, ocular abnormalities, gallstones and stroke. Affected individuals may experience recurrent attacks of pain.

These episodes may require several hospitalizations a year. Life span is somewhat shortened.

The spleen is among the first internal organs affected. Sudden blood pooling in the spleen may cause death. The spleen is also important in the body's immune response to bacteria. As a result of damage to it, affected infants are prone to bacteremia, a severe infection often caused by the bacteria pneumococcus, and may develop fevers and die within 12 hours. About a third of infants with bacteremia below the age of three years succumb to it. They may also develop pneumonia or meningitis, an infection of the membrane that covers the brain.

These infections have been a major cause of mortality among infants with sickle-cell anemia, but daily doses of penicillin in at-risk infants have been found to be helpful in preventing death.

Inherited as an AUTOSOMAL RECESSIVE trait, the disorder has a high frequency among blacks, with an incidence of approximately one in 500 to one in 625 live births. Overall, 2,000 infants a year are born with sickle-cell anemia. It is estimated that one in 1,875 African Americans has the disorder. One in 10 to one in 12 are thought to be CARRIERS of the gene. These carriers, who exhibit no symptoms, are said to have the sickle-cell trait. While carriers generally do not express any abnormalities of the blood, it is possible for their cells to exhibit "sickling" if subjected to prolonged oxygen deprivation, such as altitudes of 10,000 feet or more, or extreme physical exertion.

Frequency of sickle-cell anemia is also somewhat elevated in Mediterranean and other populations originating in malaria prone areas. It is believed that the gene for several red blood cell abnormalities (hemoglobinopathies; see HEMOGLOBIN) including sickle-cell trait, confers an increased resistance to malaria, and therefore may have been an advantage in a time and place when malaria was a greater threat than anemia.

Currently there is no cure for sickle-cell disease. Treatment includes transfusions of normal red blood cells and medications to control pain and infections. Bone marrow transplantation can be curative but carries the risks of death from the procedure and complications such as chronic graft versus host disease (CGVHD), sterility and other complications. The drug hydroxyurea has been found effective in reducing the number of crises. It appears to act by increasing the production of fetal hemoglobin which acts to prevent the red cells from becoming rigid.

Due to its prevalence and its potentially serious consequences, it is often recommended that all newborn infants be tested for both the sickle-cell trait and sickle-cell anemia. Carriers of the sickle-cell gene (sickle-cell trait) can be easily detected using a simple blood test. Because the specific MUTATION causing this abnormality is known (there is a single base change in the GENETIC CODE), new DEOXYRIBONUCLEIC ACID (DNA) diagnostic tests have made PRENATAL DIAGNOSIS relatively straightforward. These tests identify the change in the DNA of the M-globin gene by analysis of that gene in fetal cells obtained by CHORIONIC VILLUS SAMPLING or AMNIOCENTESIS. A new test, the polymerase chain reaction (PCR) allows this test to be performed rapidly.

For other forms of anemia, see also ANEMIA, THALASSEMIA, GLUCOSE-6-PHOSPHATE DEHYDROGENASE DEFICIENCY.

SIDS   See SUDDEN INFANT DEATH SYNDROME.

simian crease   A single crease on the palm of the hand, resembling the transverse flexion crease found in some monkeys. Normally, at birth the palm of the hand contains several flexion creases, areas where the skin folds when the palm is manipulated. Two of these creases are separate and run generally crosswise (transverse) over the palm. When these two appear to fuse and form a single transverse crease in the middle of the palm, it is termed a simian crease.

Simian crease is often present in a variety of developmental abnormalities, including DOWN SYNDROME, FETAL ALCOHOL SYNDROME, CORNELIA DE LANGE SYNDROME and many others. It is also found on one hand in about 4% of normal babies and in both hands in 1%. It is twice as common in males as in females.

sirenomelia   Taking its name from the mermaid-like lower extremities of the sirens in Homer's

Odyssey, this rare CONGENITAL deformity is characterized by the fusion of the legs. The cause of this developmental ANOMALY is unknown, though it may be due to an alteration in early blood vessel development whereby blood is diverted away from the developing lower portion of the embryo. In addition to the single lower extremity, affected infants also may have other defects of the gastrointestinal and genitourinary tracts. It occurs in one in 60,000 to 100,000 births.

situs inversus   A congenital reversal of the normal position of the organs of the abdominal cavity (the viscera). The heart, lungs, arteries and other visceral organs are positioned as mirror images of their proper location. The liver and gallbladder, for example, are transposed to the left side of the body, while the heart, spleen and stomach are on the right. The position of blood vessels, nerves and intestines are also reversed. (The correct positioning of the organs is termed *situs solitus.*) Scottish anatomist Matthew Baillie first published a description of situs inversus in 1793.

If the heart as well as other organs have been transposed, the condition is termed situs inversus with dextrocardia, or situs inversus totalis. In rare instances (one in 22,000 cases of situs reversus) the heart remains on the left side of the chest, though the other organs are transposed, a condition known as situs inversus with levocardia. Congenital heart defects (CHDs) are seen in 5–10% of individuals with situs inversus totalis.

Dextrocardia, that is, the heart transposed to the right side of the chest, can occur without situs inversus, and this condition, as well as situs inversus levocardia, exhibits much higher rates of congenital heart defects than situs inversus totalis. Congenital heart disease affects as many as 95% of individuals with situs inversus levocardia.

Situs inversus is a common feature of KARTAGENER SYNDROME, which is characterized by frequent respiratory infections due to immotility of the cilia, which clear mucous from the bronchial tract. About half of all those affected by Kartagener syndrome have situs inversus, while some 20–25% of patients with situs inversus have Kartagener syndrome.

Inherited as an autosomal recessive trait, situs inversus is present in about 0.01 percent of the U.S. population. Many affected individuals are diagnosed when they seek attention for an unrelated medical problem. The condition may also go unrecognized by physicians who assume the X-ray revealing the anatomical anomaly has been mislabeled. Most affected individuals have a normal lifespan and the organ reversal has no medical consequences. However, there are associated CHDs or respiratory complications among those with Kartagener syndrome.

skin cancer   See CANCER; NEVOID BASAL CELL CARCINOMA SYNDROME

skin tag   A small outgrowth of skin, which is usually joined on the neck, armpit, or groin. It is often present at birth.

Sly syndrome   See MUCOPOLYSACCHARIDOSIS.

Smith-Lemli-Opitz syndrome   First described in 1964 by U.S. pediatrician D. W. Smith and geneticists L. Lemli and J. M. Opitz, this SYNDROME is characterized by multiple CONGENITAL abnormalities, including a long narrow skull (scaphocephaly), an abnormally small head (MICROCEPHALY), drooping eyelids (PTOSIS), crossed eyes (STRABISMUS), skin folds over the inner corners of the eyes (EPICANTHUS), CATARACTS, wide-set eyes (HYPERTELORISM), a broad nasal bridge and tip, upturned nostrils (anteverted nares), increased distance between the nose and the lips, low-set ears, small jaw (micrognathia) and a short neck. Prevalence is estimated at one in 20,000 to one in 40,000 live births. In some regions, the disorder may occur as often as one in 10,000, while the incidence appears to be much lower in Asian and African populations.

Other characteristics include hand clenching, incurving fifth fingers (CLINODACTYLY), fusion of the second and third toes (SYNDACTLYL) and a distinct single crease across the width of the palm (SIMIAN CREASE).

Male infants may have a markedly small penis, undescended testicles (CRYPTORCHISM) and a urinary opening on the underside of the penis (HYPOSPADIAS). Moderate to severe MENTAL RETARDATION has been observed in all infants affected with this syndrome.

Affected infants are moderately small at birth and exhibit FAILURE TO THRIVE. During the first 28 days after birth, the affected infants exhibit vomiting, shrill screaming and susceptibility to infection. About half of those affected die within 18 months.

An AUTOSOMAL RECESSIVE disorder, the responsible GENE is located on 7q. The basic defect involves an ENZYME deficiency causing a block in the conversion of 7-dehydrocholesterol to cholesterol. This leads to a deficiency of cholesterol, an essential building block of all cell membranes and the white matter of the brain. Thus the disorder appears to be caused by abnormally low levels of the enzyme 7-dehydrocholesterol reductase, which converts 7-dehydrocholesterol into cholesterol. Affected children with the lowest cholesterol levels tend to have the most severe forms of the disorder and often die at birth or in the first few months. The discovery of this defect has led to attempts for treatment via dietary supplementation with large doses of cholesterol. The efficacy of this treatment appears to have some beneficial effects in patients.

Diagnosis of the syndrome can be made by specialized measurement of 7-dehydrocholsterol. CARRIER detection and PRENATAL DIAGNOSIS can now be accomplished through biochemical testing.

SNP (singular nucleotide polymorphism)   Pronounced "snip," a SNP is a natural DNA variation that occurs when a single nucleotide (A, T, C or G) in a genome sequence is altered. The variation must occur in at least one % of the population to be accepted as a SNP. SNPs comprise 90% of all human genetic variation. About 3 million SNPs are believed to exist in the human population. Many have no effect on cell function, but others may predispose individuals to disease or influence their reaction to drugs or environmental influences.

The onset of Alzheimer's disease, for example, appears to be influenced by SNPs in the *apolipoprotein E (ApoE)* gene. *ApoE* contains two SNPs, which can result in three different alleles, or alternative forms of the gene: *ApoE2, ApoE3* and *ApoE4*. The protein these alleles produce differs from each other by one amino acid. Individuals who inherit at least one *ApoE2* allele appear to have a reduced chance of developing Alzheimer's, while individuals who inherit at least one *ApoE4* allele have a greater chance of developing the disease.

SNPs may also be involved in polygenic disorders, such as cancer, diabetes, vascular disease and some forms of mental illness, in which multiple genes influence the onset or course of disease.

Efforts to develop an SNP map of the human genome are have been undertaken by the Human Genome Project and the SNP Consortium (TSC), which is comprised primarily of pharmaceutical companies.

solar sneeze reflex syndrome   See ACHOO SYNDROME.

sonography   See ULTRASOUND.

Sotos syndrome (cerebral gigantism)   The primary features of this disorder are advanced height, weight and bone age, characteristic facial appearance and mental deficiency. It is named for Juan F. Sotos, who published a description in the *New England Journal of Medicine* in 1964.

At birth, average weight is over nine pounds. Head, hands and feet are disproportionately large. Head circumference and height are typically above the 97th percentile for age, and bone age, two to three years beyond chronological age.

The characteristic face consists of a large skull, prominent forehead, receding hairline, wide-set eyes (HYPERTELORISM), large jaw (prognathism) pointed chin and upturned nose (anteverted nares). Teeth are present at birth in over half of the affected infants (see NATAL TEETH).

Walking is usually delayed until after 15 months of age, and speech until after 2.5 years. Neurological dysfunction, unusual clumsiness and episodes of aggressive behavior are common. The average IQ is

60. Growth is rapid in the first years of life, though final height is often in the normal range.

Sotos syndrome is caused by a mutation in the *NSD1* gene, which is located on chromosome 5q. Sotos syndrome is inherited in an autosomal dominant manner. More than 95% of individuals have a new mutation. Children with this disorder may be at an increased risk for developing tumors, though less than 5% have developed either benign or malignant tumors. Over 100 cases have been reported, with males outnumbering females by a ratio of 2:1.

Prenatal diagnosis is potentially available for those families in which a mutation has been identified. ULTRASOUND may indicate abnormal size for fetal age.

spherocytosis   See ANEMIA.

sphingolipidosis   Any one of a group of hereditary disorders characterized by defective metabolism and storage of sphingolipids. They may result in severe neurological deterioration beginning in the first few months of life, or in other significant medical problems. The disorders include SANDHOFF DISEASE, FABRY DISEASE, TAY-SACHS DISEASE, GAUCHER DISEASE, KRABBE DISEASE and NIEMANN-PICK DISEASE.

spider fingers   See ARACHNODACTYLY.

Spielmeyer-Vogt-Sjogren disease   See NEURONAL CEROID LIPOFUSCINOSIS.

spina bifida   Meaning "split spine," spina bifida is a CONGENITAL condition that results from abnormal fetal development of the spinal cord. It is the leading disabler of newborns in America.

The condition falls into the class of disorders known as NEURAL TUBE DEFECTS (NTDs). The neural tube is the embryonic structure that evolves into the brain and spinal cord. Spina bifida has its genesis in the first four weeks of pregnancy, when the neural plate, a precursor to the neural tube, is forming. Normally, the edges of the neural plate curl toward each other, joining together to form the neural tube. As the neural tube develops into the spinal cord, bone (the spine) and muscle form a protective barrier around it.

In spina bifida, part of the neural plate fails to join together, and bone and muscle are unable to grow over this open section of the developing spinal column. Nerves that relay sensation and control movement in the legs, bladder and bowel are damaged or incompletely developed. The severity of symptoms is determined by the particular nerves involved and their degree of damage or maldevelopment.

Until the 1960s, many affected infants died soon after birth due to HYDROCEPHALUS or infections of the nervous system. Today, an estimated 80% to 95% survive and grow to maturity.

The incidence of spina bifida is between one and two of every 1,000 live births in North America. In the United States, more infants with spina bifida are born in the eastern and southern states than in the West. In western Great Britain and Ireland the incidence is four in 1,000. (It was previously as high as eight in 1,000).

The cause is unknown. It is believed to be a MULTIFACTORIAL trait, that is, one in which both genetic and environmental factors play a role. Evidence supporting a genetic component is ample. Parents with one child with spina bifida have an increased risk of giving birth to another. More females than males are born with the condition. Variation is incidence is seen among ethnic and racial groups. Blacks, Asians and Ashkenazi Jews have lower rates than people of Northern European origin or Egyptians.

Dietary supplementation of folic acid (a B complex VITAMIN) before conception and during early pregnancy has been shown to reduce the risk of NTDs, though the mechanism of this preventive effect is not understood.

The link between vitamins, or nutrition, and NTDs had been noted for some decades; they are more common in the offspring of women in lower socioeconomic groups and women who have poor diets. Additionally, there was an "epidemic" of neural tube defects during the Depression, a time when many people, including women of child-bearing age, received substandard nutrition. However, the potential link between vitamin deficiencies and neural tube defects did not receive scientific attention until after World War II, when it was noted that women in England, Holland and Germany who had been malnourished gave birth to an unexpectedly large number of infants with these developmental defects. Yet it was only in the 1980s that the link was examined scientifically.

One early study found women who take multivitamins (including folic acid) at the time of conception had 60% less risk of giving birth to an infant with a neural tube defect than women who did not use vitamins. A later study by Boston University's Center for Human Genetics, published in 1989 and involving 23,000 pregnant women, found those who reported taking multivitamins in the first six weeks of pregnancy had rates of NTDs in their offspring only one-quarter the rates of women who did not use vitamins. (NTD incidence was 0.9 per 1,000 births among vitamin users vs. 3.5 per 1,000 births among non–vitamin users.) A study by the National Institute of Child Health and Human Development published in 1997 found 100 micrograms of folic acid daily produced a blood folate level sufficient to reduce NTDs about 22%. A 200 microgram daily dose was associated with a 41% reduced risk of NTDs, and dosages of 400 micrograms with a reduction of 47%. Women who had one or more pregnancies affected by an NTD and who subsequently used supplemental folic acid significantly reduced their risk to have another child with an NTD to about 1%.

Folic acid is particularly important to fetal development in the first month, a time when many pregnancies are undetected. By the time the pregnancy is recognized, a shortage of folic acid could have led to a nascent NTD. The Institute of Medicine, a federal agency that sets nutritional guidelines, recommends pregnant women take 600 micrograms of folic acid daily. (Other adults are advised to take 400 micrograms.)

There are two major forms of the disorder. Spina bifida occulta ("hidden") is the mildest form, with the opening of the spinal cord covered by skin. In some cases, it may manifest itself as no more than a small cavity (dermal sinus) between two adjacent vertebrae, indicating that they have not fused properly. A hairy patch or birthmark may be above the defect. In another form of spina bifida occulta, the spinal cord ends in fatty tissue, which extends through the spinal column and forms a bulge under the skin. If the abnormality is mild enough, there are usually no symptoms. But if several vertebrae are involved and a fatty area, hairy patch or dimple in the skin over the defect is noticeable, bowel, bladder or motor problems may eventually develop.

The other form is spina bifida manifesta (also called "aperta" or "cystica"), in which a sac is immediately noticeable ("manifest") on the infant's back. This form is itself divided into two categories. In the less severe, the spinal cord develops normally but bulges out through incompletely developed vertebrae, forming a sac (meningocele—meningo refers to membranes, cele means a swelling or cavity). There can be minor muscle paralysis or incontinence if nerves protrude into this sac.

The much more common and severe form of spina bifida manifesto occurs when a portion of the undeveloped spinal cord itself protrudes through the back and forms a sac (myelomeningocele—myelo refers to the spinal cord). This accounts for perhaps 90% of all cases and is what is generally referred to when spina bifida is discussed.

Generally, the higher up on the back this sac is located, the more severe the case, since all the nerves lower on the back are usually affected. If it occurs high on the spinal column, the lower limbs may be totally paralyzed. A sac on the bottom of the spine may result only in relatively mild paralysis and bladder and bowel problems.

The exposed sac is usually surgically closed between 24 and 48 hours after birth. Hydrocephalus is a common complication seen in between 70% and 90% of spina bifida infants, either at birth or within a few days of it. This may require additional surgery.

After the age of one, chronic bladder infections and kidney deterioration pose the greatest danger, due to the individuals' inability to control many aspects of their excretory functions. Between 8% and 15% are born with a forward bending of the lower spine (kyphosis), creating a hunchbacked appearance (see HUMPBACK). Some are born with CLUBFEET and dislocated hips. A lateral bend of the spine (SCOLIOSIS) may develop in childhood. Many are confined to wheelchairs or can walk only with the assistance of braces or crutches. Approximately 30% exhibit slight to severe MENTAL RETARDATION. Muscle imbalance caused by lack of muscular control may create deformities of the hip, knee and foot joints.

Though the need for medical care is most acute during the early years, the problems created by the condition require some level of lifelong professional attention. However, with proper assistance and access to opportunities, affected individuals can lead productive and fulfilling lives.

PRENATAL DIAGNOSIS is often possible. A series of tests including ALPHA-FETOPROTEIN screening, ULTRASOUND and AMNIOCENTESIS can identify approximately eight to nine out of 10 cases of neural tube defects. (See also ANENCEPHALY.)

spinal muscular atrophy (SMA) Any of a group of muscular atrophies (muscle wasting), almost always genetic in origin, characterized by degeneration of neurons (nerves) of the spinal cord. These neurons control voluntary movement and the disorder is characterized by progressive weakness, loss of tendon reflexes, involuntary twitching of muscle fibers (fasciculation), and contractures, or permanent flexion, of joints.

Intelligence and sensory organs are unaffected. Overall, spinal muscular atrophy is the second most common lethal, AUTOSOMAL RECESSIVE disease in Caucasians (after CYSTIC FIBROSIS), occurring in about one in 6,000–10,000 live births. It is estimated that one in 40 to one in 80 individuals is a CARRIER of a GENE for one of these conditions.

More than 80% of these disorders are classified as proximal spinal muscular atrophies, because they begin in muscles closest (proximal) to the affected nerves, later spreading to the muscles farther away (distal). While several varieties have been described, subclassification is considered somewhat arbitrary. Most are inherited as autosomal recessive traits.

Inherited by autosomal recessive transmission, SMA Types I–IV are caused in many cases by disruption of copies of a duplicated gene called SMN1 for "survival motor neuron," located on 5q. This gene is missing in a majority of SMA patients and small MUTATIONS in it have also been associated with spinal muscular atrophy.

Identification of these genes has permitted carrier detection and PRENATAL DIAGNOSIS through molecular analysis. However, the molecular genetic diagnosis of SMA is complicated.

Werdnig-Hoffman disease (SMA Type 1 This is an infantile form of spinal muscular atrophy, with general muscle weakness beginning either before birth or during the first week of life. It is named for Austrian neurologist G. Werdnig, who published a description in 1891, and German neurologist Johann Hoffman (1857–1919), who published in 1893.

Infants present a characteristic "frog" position with hips raised and the knees flexed. Other symptoms may include hypotonia (decreased muscle tone), weakness, swallowing and feeding difficulties, and respiratory problems. The disease's progression is rapid and inexorable, with death occurring usually by one year of age, typically due to pulmonary infection or respiratory insufficiency. However, some infants have survived as long as six years. It is estimated to occur in between one in 20,000 and one in 25,000 live births. There may be a lack of fetal movement during pregnancy.

SMA Type II (intermediate spinal muscular atrophy) Usually apparent within the first six months to two years or life. While not as severe as Type 1 SMA, its features may include inability to sit unsupported, stand, crawl or walk, hypotonia, decreased or absent deep tendon reflexes, and muscle fasciculations (involuntary contractions or twitching of groups of muscles). Frequent respiratory infections may occur and shorten life expectancy.

Kugelberg Welander disease (SMA Type III) A childhood or adolescent-onset form first described in 1956 by Swedish neurologists E. Kugelberg and M. Welander. Early symptoms include a waddling gait and difficulty in climbing stairs. Resembling Becker's or limb-girdle muscular dystrophy, the weakness spreads to the shoulders and the extremities. Some individuals may lose the ability to walk during their late teens, but others remain ambulatory for decades.

SMA Type IV This form occurs in adulthood, usually after age 30. Symptoms are generally mild to moderate and include muscle weakness and twitching, as well as tremor.

Other non-proximal spinal muscular atrophies include juvenile progressive bulbar palsy (childhood facial palsy), distal spinal muscular atrophy, characterized by infant weakness in the distal muscles of the legs, and facioscapulohumeral spinal muscular atrophy. These differ from the proximal forms in their highly localized muscle weakness.

There is also an adult-onset form (spinal and bulbar muscular atrophy) known as KENNEDY'S DISEASE, inherited as an X-LINKED trait. Affecting only men, onset may occur between 15 and 60 years of age. Features of this type may include weakness of the facial and tongue muscles, dysphagia (difficulty in swallowing), and dysarthria (impairment of speech), as well as the GYNECOMASTIA (excessive development of the male mammary glands). The course of the disorder varies but generally tends to be slowly progressive. It is not associated with increased mortality.

spinocerebellar ataxia (SCA; spinocerebellar atrophy; olivopontocerebellar atrophy, OPCA) A rare group of disorders characterized by a wasting of portions of the brain; the cerebellum, which lies below the larger cerebrum and behind the spinal column and controls muscular coordination and equilibrium; the pons cerebelli, a bridge-like structure of the brain stem connecting with the medulla oblongata (the enlarged portion of the spinal column at the base of the brain); and the olivary body, which lies on the medulla oblongata.

The nomenclature of this group has been changing and the once-preferred designation OPCA is no longer accepted. The disorders are among the inherited ataxias (disorders characterized by a loss of coordination). They have been termed spinocerebellar atrophies, or perhaps most preferably, spinocerebellar ataxias (SCA). This is because in these conditions in addition to the changes seen in the portions of the brain listed above, changes are also seen in basal ganglia, spinal cord, cerebral cortex, and peripheral nerves. The pathological changes may vary even among affected members of the same family. Most of these are AUTOSOMAL DOMINANT in inheritance (FRIEDREICH'S ATAXIA, another important inherited ataxia, is AUTOSOMAL RECESSIVE) and are clinically and genetically heterogeneous

(see HETEROGENEITY). Families show variability in expression and often decreased PENETRANCE.

Symptoms usually begin to appear when the affected person is about 30 years old, but may appear as early as childhood in some forms, or as late as the 50s or 60s in others. Beginning with a slowly developing unsteadiness of gait, the impairment eventually involves all the limbs. An affected person experiences a slowly progressive loss of muscular coordination (ataxia). Control is lost over muscles used in speaking (dysarthria). Tremors and involuntary movements follow. Muscles may be rigid. In some forms of the disease there may be sensory impairment, mental deterioration, paralysis of eye movement or retinal degeneration with loss of vision. Affected persons may die of pneumonia or other debilitating disease in their fourth to seventh decade of life. (See also AZOREAN DISEASE.)

The GENES for a number of these disorders have been discovered and typically involve TRINUCLEOTIDE (CAG) REPEAT expansion. As a result, with some exceptions, the autosomal dominant SCAs share a number of common characteristics. Primarily, the repeat is unstable and tends to enlarge with transmission from one generation to the next, which causes the phenomenon of genetic anticipation, whereby age of onset declines and severity increases as the CAG repeat becomes larger in succeeding generations. The repeat tends to enlarge particularly when transmitted from a male. Genes with CAG repeats have been found for SCA1, (gene involved is ataxin-1, mapped to 6p), SCA2 (ataxin-2, 12q), SCA3/Machado-Joseph disease (14q), SCA6 (caused by expansion of a CAG repeat in the coding region of one isoform of the alpha(1A) calcium channel subunit (CACNL1A4) on 19p whose repeat is stable), SCA7 (3p), and dentato-rubral-pallido-luysian atrophy (seen mostly in Japan, which maps to 12p). Loci (see LOCUS, LOCI) for SCA4 and SCA5 map to 16q and 11 respectively. For SCA5 there is a very large kindred in which 56 of 170 individuals distributed over 10 generations were affected by a dominant ataxia. The family had two major branches, both of which descended from the paternal grandparents of President Lincoln.

The gene involved in SCA5 is the *SPTBN2* gene that encodes the spectrin beta chain, brain 2 protein. The *SCA8* gene maps to chromosome 13q and involves a CTG expansion. The *SCA10* gene maps to chromosome 22q and involves a ATTCT pentanucleotide (five nucleotide) repeat expansion. The *SCA12* gene maps to chromosome 5q and involves a CAG triplet repeat expansion within the *PPP2R2B* gene. Overall, more than 30 different loci for AUTOSOMAL DOMINANT spinocerebellar ataxias have been suggested and several other genes are known, including those for *SCA14* and *SCA15,* as well as those for several forms of episodic ataxia. In addition to FRIEDRICH'S ATAXIA there are several other AUTOSOMAL RECESSIVE disorders, and individual families have been described with ataxia inherited in an X-linked pattern.

Predictive testing is now available via DEOXYRIBONUCLEIC ACID (DNA) analysis of repeat size, and many of the issues (psychosocial and ethical as well as genetic) seen in predictive testing for HUNTINGTON CHOREA come into play with these disorders as well.

spinopontine atrophy   See AZOREAN DISEASE.

spondylocostal dysostosis   See SPONDYLOTHORACIC DYSPLASIA.

spondyloepiphyseal dysplasia   The name of this form of short-trunk DWARFISM is taken from the Greek *spondylos* for "vertebra," and *epiphyseal,* referring to the bone-forming area separated from the parent bone by cartilage. As infants normally grow and mature, the cartilage is gradually replaced by bone. In this disorder, these secondary bone-forming areas of the vertebrae exhibit DYSPLASIA, or abnormal tissue development. The condition has both a CONGENITAL and late childhood of form.

Spondyloepiphyseal dysplasia congenita This condition is present at birth. The ossification (formation of bones from cartilage) of the spine is retarded, causing the vertebrae to appear flattened and abnormal. Ossification of other bones may be more grossly retarded or totally absent. The hands are of normal size and shape, though ossification of the bones is retarded.

Lack of muscle tone (hypotonia) presents a FLOPPY INFANT appearance. The face tends to be flat. CLEFT PALATE or CLUBFOOT may be present. There may be moderate hearing loss, and about half of affected infants have visual defects, including MYOPIA (nearsightedness) and retinal detachment, which may lead to BLINDNESS. The chest is barrel-shaped. The bones of the limbs may be severely bent. Legs may be knock-kneed (genu valgum) or BOWLEGGED (genu varum). Individuals walk with a waddling gait. Fully grown males are usually between 33.5 inches and 51 inches (85.1–129.5 cm) in height.

Inherited as an AUTOSOMAL DOMINANT trait, affected individuals exhibit a wide variability in the severity of the characteristic defects. Incidence is about one in 100,000.

This disorder is one of a spectrum of skeletal dysplasias that result from MUTATIONS in the GENE for type II collagen, *COL2A1,* found on 12q. (Collagen II is sometimes called "cartilage collagen.") Others include STICKLER SYNDROME, KNIEST DYSPLASIA and type II ACHONDROGENESIS.

Spondyloepiphyseal dysplasia tarda This is a delayed onset, usually x-linked form (the gene is on Xp), exhibited only in males. Rare autosomal dominant and autosomal recessive forms have also been reported, clinically indistinguishable from the X-linked variant. Prevalence of this type overall is one in 100,000.

Infants appear normal at birth. The failure of normal growth is noted between the ages of five and 10 years, when growth of the spine appears to stop. The shoulders take on a hunched-up appearance, the neck appears shortened, the chest enlarged. There is premature deterioration (osteoarthritis) of the bones of the spine and hips, which may limit movement. Adults are mildly dwarfed, with height usually between 4 feet 4 inches and 5 feet 2 inches (130.2–155.1 cm).

spondylometaphyseal chondrodysplasia   A group of at least seven forms of moderate, juvenile-onset DWARFISM, mostly affecting the trunk, differentiated on the basis of minor X-ray differences and inheritance patterns. The name is taken from the Greek *spondylos* for "vertebra," and *metaphyseal,* referring to primary growing area of a bone. Normally, as infants grow, cartilage (chondro) turns to bone. However, in these disorders, the bone-forming process of the cartilage of the vertebrae exhibits DYSPLASIA, or abnormal tissue development.

The most common and well-known form was first described by Dr. K. Kozlowski in 1967, and is sometimes referred to as spondylometaphyseal chondrodysplasia, Kozlowski type.

Dwarfing usually becomes apparent between ages one and four years and is progressive. There are deformities of the spine, including pronounced hump (kyphosis), lateral bend (SCOLIOSIS) or both (kyphoscoliosis). Joints may exhibit severe deterioration. Individuals have a waddling gait. Adult height is about 4 feet 7 inches (147.8 cm). Life expectancy and intelligence are normal.

Inherited as an AUTOSOMAL DOMINANT trait, more than 40 cases have been documented. Most are new MUTATIONS.

spondylothoracic dysplasia (Jarcho-Levin syndrome; spondylocostal dysostosis)   A rare and generally lethal form of CONGENITAL DWARFISM characterized by a markedly shortened trunk, protuberant abdomen and limbs that may appear relatively long, though they are of normal length. The face is round and appears puffy. The neck is short, and the chin appears to rest on the chest.

The name of the disorder is taken from *spondylo,* Greek for "vertebra," and *thoracic,* referring to the chest. Both the vertebral column (spine) and the rib cage exhibit DYSPLASIA, or abnormal development. First described by Jarcho and Levin in 1938, the typical appearance of the chest on X-ray is called "crab-like." Death is usually from respiratory insufficiency or pneumonia as a result of a small chest.

Most cases are believed to be inherited as an AUTOSOMAL RECESSIVE trait. Mutations causing autosomal recessive forms of spondylothoracic dysplasia have been identified in 3 genes in the Notch signaling pathway: *DLL3, MESP2* and *LFNG* (which stands for the Lunatic Fringe Gene). The majority of affected individuals have been Puerto Rican, with more female than male cases in the literature. There is probably also an AUTOSOMAL DOMINANT form with milder manifestations. PRENATAL DIAGNOSIS may be possible by ULTRASOUND, though the characteristic changes may not be obvious until late in gestation.

spongy degeneration of the brain   See CANAVAN DISEASE.

sporadic   The random appearance of a BIRTH DEFECT or CONGENITAL condition that results from an unknown cause or from a new MUTATION; an isolated case.

Sprengel deformity (high scapula)   The scapula is the large, flat, triangular bone that forms the back of the shoulder, the "shoulder blade." In this rare developmental abnormality, named for German surgeon Otto Sprengel (1852–1915), the scapula is poorly formed and displaced higher and more toward the midline of the back than when normally positioned. This, in turn, may restrict the ability to raise the arm. The condition may be in one (unilateral) or both (bilateral) of the scapulae. Surgery may help alleviate both restrictions of movement and cosmetic aspects of the disorder.

About two-thirds of the cases exhibit associated abnormalities, including lateral curvature of the spine (SCOLIOSIS), fused vertebrae, missing ribs and poor development of the shoulder muscles.

Most cases are SPORADIC, but some are believed to be transmitted as an AUTOSOMAL DOMINANT trait.

Stargardt disease   A hereditary, early onset form of macular degeneration, and one of the most frequent causes of macular degeneration in childhood. Affected children and young adults exhibit progressive deterioration of the macula, the portion of the retina that controls central vision. As a result, they lose central vision, rendering them legally blind. Though they retain peripheral vision, they are unable to read, drive or see straight ahead.

Inherited as an autosomal recessive trait, onset is between six and 15 years of age. It affects about one in 10,000 people in the United States. The causative gene, *ABCA4,* mapped to chromosome 1p, is one of a family known as ABC transporters. It codes for a protein used to pump material—typically a single type of molecule—out of a cell. The material it transports has not been identified. Abnormal transporters are involved in several diseases, including cystic fibrosis. This is a disease of the rods of the retina, and the particular mutant ABC transporter is expressed in rod photoreceptors. In addition to mutations in the *ABCA4* gene, the recessive form of this disorder has also resulted from mutations in the *CNGB3* gene, which is located on chromosome 8q. Other mutations in this gene lead to achromatopsia. An autosomal dominant macular dystrophy resembling Stargardt disease can be caused by mutations in the *ELOVL4* gene, which is located on chromosome 6q and appears to be involved in fatty acid metabolism in the retinal photoreceptor cells.

Thus far, a link to adult onset macular degeneration has not been established. It has been suggested that being a CARRIER for Stargardt disease may increase the risk of developing the disorder later in life.

Steinert disease   See MYOTONIC DYSTROPHY.

Stein-Leventhal syndrome   Named for U.S. gynecologists Irving F. Stein, Sr. (b. 1887) and Michael L. Leventhal (1901–71), who published a description in 1935, this disorder is characterized by the development of multiple cysts in the ovaries (polycystic ovaries). Affected females are usually infertile (see INFERTILITY), and some may have excessive body hair (hirsutism). Fathers of affected individuals also tend to have excessive body hair, and sisters and mothers may exhibit menstrual irregularities.

Believed to be inherited as an AUTOSOMAL DOMINANT trait, there is evidence that variation at the CYP11A LOCUS on 15q is involved in the cause of this SYNDROME, at least in some cases. This GENE encodes a portion of the ENZYME involved in the initial and rate-limiting step in the pathway leading from cholesterol to the production of steroid hormones which takes place in the adrenal cortex, testis, ovary, and placenta.

stem cell   An undifferentiated cell that has the ability to develop into other cell types. Theoretically, stem cells could be used to repair specific tissues or grow organs, if and when researchers learn how to trigger their transformation to a specific cell type. Cancers, spinal cord injuries, Parkinson's disease and muscle damage are among the conditions researchers speculate stem cells could one day be used to treat.

Several types of stem cells exist. Adult stem cells are found among differentiated cells and, contrary to their name, can be found in children or umbilical cords as well as adults. Adult stem cells are used in the treatment of more than 100 disorders. Cord blood stem cells come from the blood of the placenta and umbilical cord and are used to treat Gunther's disease, Hunter syndrome, Hurler syndrome, acute lymphocytic leukemia and other genetic disorders seen most in children. Embryonic stem cells are cultured cells obtained from the undifferentiated inner mass cells of a human embryo early in its development, when the embryo consists of 50 to 150 cells (blastocyst). Embryonic stem cells, first isolated from a human embryo in 1998, are believed to have greater potential to differentiate into other cells types than adult stem cells.

Stem cell research, particularly using human embryonic stem cells, has generated intense controversy, as harvesting these cells requires destruction of an embryo, though the potential benefits of the therapeutic use of stem cells appears great.

sterility   See INFERTILITY.

Stickler syndrome (hereditary progressive arthroophthalmopathy)   Rare hereditary SYNDROME of progressive near-sightedness (MYOPIA) and abnormalities of the joints. The myopia, beginning in the first decade of life, often eventually results in retinal detachment and BLINDNESS. First recognized in 1965 by Gunnar B. Stickler, chairman of pediatrics at the Mayo Medical School in Minnesota, it is estimated to affect one in 10,000 people. (Thirty percent to 40% of patients with Pierre Robin sequence have Stickler syndrome.)

Enlarged ankles, knees and wrists, as well as a developmental defect involving a small jaw, relatively large tongue and CLEFT PALATE (ROBIN ANOMALY), are among the first signs of this disorder in newborns. Typically, affected individuals have rounded, asymmetrical faces, depressed bridge of the nose, folds of skin at the inner corners of the eye (EPICANTHUS) and a marked undergrowth of one side of the jaw compared to the other. They may also have a flat midface and cleft palate. Other clinical feature include mitral valve prolapse and sensorineural hearing loss.

During childhood, stiffness and soreness in the joints may occur after overuse, accompanied by swelling and redness, leading to temporary locking of the joints. Crepitation, a soft, fine crackling sound, may be heard over the joints through a stethoscope.

If the thigh bone is involved, the individual may experience difficulty walking. Frequently there may also be problems of premature and progressive arthritis. About 25% of all patients experience problems with outward curvature of the spine (thoracic kyphosis) or sideward curvature (SCOLIOSIS) and 40% will have excessive joint mobility.

Prognosis for a normal life span in favorable, though affected individuals must be particularly careful of ocular problems such as GLAUCOMA, CATARACTS and retinal degeneration.

Genetically heterogeneous (see HETEROGENEITY), a variety of MUTATIONS in different GENES are responsible for this disorder. Many cases result from mutations in the gene for type II collagen, COL2A1, found on 12q, one of a spectrum of skeletal DYSPLASIAS that result from mutations in this gene. Others include SPONDYLOEPIPHYSEAL DYSPLASIA, KNIEST DYSPLASIA and type II ACHONDROGENESIS. The disorder in the kindred in which Stickler fist noted the syndrome had a mutation in this gene, for example. The family was a large Minnesota kindred which had been examined at the Mayo Clinic as early as 1897 by Dr. C. H. Mayo.

About half of the Stickler syndrome families do not demonstrate linkage with COL2A1 and, therefore, probably have mutations in some other gene. Some families have been found to have mutations in the gene for alpha-2 chain of type XI collagen (COL11A2), which maps to 6p. These families do not have the eye problems of Stickler syndrome, as this chain of this type of collagen is not used in the eye. Mutations in the COL11A1 gene (the gene for the alpha-1 chain of type 11 collagen), which maps to 1p, can also cause the full disorder. PRENATAL DIAGNOSIS by molecular analysis may be accomplished in families in which the mutation is known.

stiff man syndrome Extreme rigidity (hypertonia) of the voluntary muscles of the neck, trunk, shoulders and upper portions of the limbs give this very rare neurologic disorder its name. About 70% of affected individuals are male.

The first signs of the disorder are an aching and tightness in the muscles, progressing to rigidity. The condition can be painful and some affected individuals have difficulty making sudden movements. In severe cases, bones have been broken as a result of the muscle contractures. Eventually, the muscles of the back and abdomen are involved, and may bend the spine, causing HUMPBACK (kyphosis) or abnormal convexity (lordosis).

Muscle spasms can be provoked by sudden noise and emotional stimulation. Sleep can alleviate muscle contractions, and diazepam (Valium) has been found effective in treating the spasms.

The disorder appears to be familial, though the GENETICS involved has not been elucidated. It often occurs as an acquired disease and has been suggested to be an autoimmune disorder. It has also been suggested that hereditary stiff man syndrome, which results from a MUTATION in the GENE for the alpha-1 subunit of the glycine receptor, found on 5q, and startle disease (hyperplexia; see JUMPING FRENCHMEN OF MAINE) are identical.

stillbirth The birth of a dead infant. This may be caused by CHROMOSOME ABNORMALITIES, lethal GENETIC DISORDERS, physical conditions within the uterus or injuries associated with childbirth. In many cases the cause may be unclear.

Approximately 20% of stillbirths or neonatal deaths have CONGENITAL ANOMALIES, compared with incidence in the general newborn population of between 2% and 3%. An estimated 5% to 10% have chromosome abnormalities, while only 0.5% of all newborns do (trisomy 18—EDWARD SYNDROME—is the most common). However, these are not necessarily the cause of death. Postmortem examinations can sometimes reveal the cause and be of assistance in GENETIC COUNSELING and management of future pregnancies.

storage disease Genetic disorders caused by ENZYME deficiencies. Due to these deficiencies, the body is unable to metabolize, or break down, substances that then accumulate, or are stored, within cells. Examples include TAY-SACHS DISEASE, GAUCHER DISEASE, FABRY DISEASE, MUCOPOLYSACCHARIDOSIS and GLYCOGEN STORAGE DISEASE.

strabismus   The inability to direct the axis of the eyes in tandem; each appears to be looking in a different direction. In common terminology, it is referred to as being "cross-eyed."

Strabismus is seen in many GENETIC DISORDERS. As an isolated ANOMALY, a familial link has been recognized in medical literature since Hippocrates. No simple MENDELIAN inheritance pattern (dominant or recessive) is established, and it is thought to be a POLYGENIC (caused by the action of several GENES) trait. SIBLINGS of affected infants have a 15% chance of exhibiting the disorder. If a parent is affected as well, risk rises to 40%.

strawberry mark   See NEVUS.

Sturge-Weber syndrome   A non-familial CONGENITAL condition characterized by large areas of facial discoloration and neurological abnormalities. Abnormalities of the eye and internal organs may also be present.

The disorder bears the names of English physicians W. A. Sturge (1850–1919) and F. P. Weber (1863–1962). Sturge, who sometimes attended Queen Victoria, described the disorder in 1879, and Weber, the son of noted physician H. D. Weber, published a description in 1922.

The facial discoloration (PORT WINE STAIN; NEVUS) typically involves at least one upper eyelid and the forehead, though there is great variability among affected individuals. It is usually on one side (unilateral) of the face but may be on both (bilateral). The nevus can extend down the neck and onto the chest or back. The color, which rarely fades with age, ranges from light pink to deep purple and is caused by an overabundance of aberrant capillaries just beneath the surface of the skin. (Laser treatments have shown promise in reducing skin discoloration.)

Excessive blood vessels also develop on the surface of the brain (angiomas), usually on the back of the brain on the same side as the facial discoloration, and can cause abnormal brain activity. Seizures often begin by one year of age, with convulsions occurring on the side of the body opposite from the affected side of the face. MENTAL RETARDATION occurs in 30% of cases, most typically in individuals with frequent seizures.

Common visual problems include GLAUCOMA (in 30% of those under medical care), a buildup in pressure within the eyeball that damages the optic nerve. It is usually confined to the side of the face with the characteristic BIRTHMARK. The eye may also become enlarged (buphthalmos), and there may be opacity or clouding of the lens (CATARACT). The neurologic and ocular complications occur only in those patients where the lesion is on that part of the face that gets its stimulation from the first branch of the fifth cranial nerve (trigeminal nerve).

The condition has its origins in the sixth week of fetal development. A mass of blood vessel tissue forms in the area that develops into the head, beneath the layer of embryonic tissue that will become facial skin. Normally, this mass of blood vessels diminishes during the ninth week of gestation, but in this condition it remains.

All cases of this rare SYNDROME have been SPORADIC, with no gender or ethnic predilection, or clear evidence of hereditary factors. There is no method of PRENATAL DIAGNOSIS. Theoretically, an extensive nevus could be observed via FETOSCOPY. (See also KLIPPEL-TRENAUNAY-WEBER SYNDROME.)

stuttering (stammering)   A hesitant or faltering speech disorder, apparently genetically influenced. Mentioned in Mesopotamian clay tablets, Chinese poems and Egyptian hieroglyphics, it is said to be unusually frequent in Japanese, infrequent in Polynesians and virtually absent in American Indians. A family from India was described in 1979 in which there were 12 stutterers in five generations. In the United States, it is estimated that at least 4% of children and 1.1% of adults stutter. Among identical TWINS, CONCORDANCE for stuttering is between 76% and 90% (that is, in from 76% to 90% of identical twins, if one stutters, the other will also). Among fraternal twins, concordance is 20%. These figures suggest hereditary transmission. It has also been suggested that, in some cases, this is an AUTOSOMAL DOMINANT trait. Synonyms: anarthria literalis; spasmophemia.

subtelomeric probes The telomere is the end portion or tip of the arm of a chromosome. Rearrangement of chromosomal material that occurs at these locations (termed *telomeric translocations*) is associated with mental retardation, congenital abnormalities and other genetic disorders. These rearrangements are difficult to detect by conventional screening methods and hence are also called cryptic translocations.

Subtelomeric probes are advanced DNA probes used in FLUORESCENCE IN SITU HYBRIDIZATION (FISH), cytogenic tests used to locate and identify specific telomeric translocations. More than 40 specific probes for the 46 human subtelomeres (one telomere each end of the 23 chromosomes) have been created.

Comparative cytogenic studies of individuals with mental retardation of unknown origin and unaffected individuals suggest that cryptic translocations may be a major cause of idiopathic (of unknown origin) mental retardation. Telomeric translocations have also been linked to specific mental retardation syndromes including Wolf-Hirschhorn, cri-du-chat, and Miller-Dieker syndromes. Such translocations have also been implicated in autistic disorders and recurrent miscarriages.

sudden infant death syndrome (SIDS; crib death) The sudden and unexplained death of an infant with no apparent disease. This is the leading cause of death in infants between one month and 12 months of age in North America, claiming up to one out of every 1,000 live-born babies, or an estimated 7,000 to 8,000 lives annually in the United States. It affects blacks three times as frequently as whites. Ninety percent to 95% die before six months of age, with the peak incidence between two and four months. Most deaths occur during the winter months and between the hours of midnight and 8 A.M. (In most cases, the infants die during

normal sleep periods. This is the origin of its secondary name, "crib death.") Premature and LOW BIRTH WEIGHT infants, those born to teenagers, smokers and drug addicted mothers, and those with a SIBLING who succumbed to SIDS, are all at increased risk. SIDS is slightly more common in males.

The cause of SIDS is unknown. Recognized since biblical times, it was once thought to be caused by inadvertent suffocation of the infant by the mother while sleeping, a belief now known to be incorrect. (The Old Testament story of King Solomon ordering a baby cut in half to learn the identity of its true mother is thought to represent an account of both SIDS and this erroneous suffocation assumption. Each of the women had a baby, but one of the infants died during the night. As related in the Bible: "and this woman's died in the night because she overlaid it . . . And she arose at midnight and beheld it was dead" [I Kings 3:19].) Other suspected causes have also been ruled out, including choking, allergic reactions, infection, parental neglect and immunizations. Periodic cessation of breathing (apnea) during sleep has been suggested as a cause, though the true nature of SIDS appears to be more complex. Current hypotheses are focusing on defects in the interplay of several regulatory systems required to maintain life. Abnormalities in the brainstem tissue, which have been found in SIDS infants, may also play a role. Subtle defects in the medulla, the area of the brainstem that regulates breathing and heart rate, have been found posthumously in infants who have succumbed to SIDS. The cells in this region of SIDS babies' brains are less sensitive to serotonin, a brain chemical associated with mood and arousal, than in those of unaffected babies. The defects were most noticeable in male infants, which, if these anomalies indeed play a role in SIDS, may account for their higher risk of SIDS.

Studies in Europe and Australia have suggested that the risk of SIDS drops by more than 50% if children sleep on their backs. This has led to widely accepted recommendations on the positioning of babies. The American Academy of Pediatrics, for example, now recommends that healthy infants sleep on their backs to reduce the risk of SIDS. J. Bruce Beckwith has been quoted as calling this finding the most significant he has seen since he coined the term SIDS in 1969. This advice has not led to the elimination of SIDS, but does reduce the risk. Between 1992 and 1998, incidence of SIDS in the United States declined approximately 20% to 30%, a decline attributed in part to these recommendations. In countries where the prone sleeping rate has been reduced to no more than 5% to 10%, the reduction in the SIDS rate has approached 70% to 80%.

Since the institution of the American Academy of Pediatrics's "Back to Sleep" campaign, which encourages placing babies to sleep on their backs, there has been an increase in the incidence of positional plagiocephaly (see CRANIOSYNOSTOSIS). In positional plagiocephaly, infants develop a flattened spot on the back of their heads from spending too much time lying on their backs. This condition may be easily treated and prevented by changing the infant's position frequently. There is now the accompanying advice to allow for more "tummy time" when the child is awake.

Some infant deaths may be improperly attributed to SIDS. The most notable example involved a 1972 paper that described "the H. family," in which all five children died of apparent SIDS. The paper was widely interpreted as evidence of a familial link in SIDS, until the H. family in question came to the attention of the criminal justice system. After a lengthy investigation, Waneta E. Hoyt confessed to murdering her five babies between 1965 and 1971 and in 1995 was sentenced to 75 years in prison.

Exposure to tobacco smoke during and after pregnancy has also been shown to increase the risk for SIDS. Overheating, for example due to too much clothing, too heavy bedding and too warm a room, may also increase the risk for SIDS, particularly for an infant with a cold or infection. A 1998 study found an association between prolongation of the QT interval (see ROMANO-WARD SYNDROME) in the first week of life and SIDS.

A number of previously unrecognized defects in fatty acid and organic acid metabolism have been discovered to be the cause of some instances of SIDS. Inherited through AUTOSOMAL RECESSIVE transmission, the frequency of these disorders among SIDS cases, while still unknown, is probably not high. The disorders can lead to sudden death, but occur more often among children older than infants, and therefore are not regarded as true SIDS.

supernumerary teeth Having more than the normal number of teeth. Approximately 2% of the population have extra teeth, almost always upper incisors. This condition is also associated with dental developmental abnormalities, such as CLEFT PALATE.

sweaty feet syndrome (isovaleric acidemia) A characteristic odor resembling that of sweaty feet, apparent within the first few weeks of life, gives this rare SYNDROME its name. It is caused by the inability of the body to metabolize adequately the AMINO ACID leucine. As a result, infection or ingestion of protein produces abnormally high levels of isovaleric acid in the blood.

Signs of this disorder usually become apparent within the first few weeks of life. In addition to the characteristic odor, they include intermittent acute attacks of vomiting, loss of muscular coordination (ataxia), seizures, lethargy and coma. Half of affected infants die within a few weeks of birth. Infants who survive the newborn period will often have intermittent episodes or attacks of illness precipitated by an infection as trivial as a cold or by excessive intake of high protein foods. Many affected children with this disorder develop a natural aversion to foods containing protein from an early age. Treatment includes dietary restrictions of protein and supplementation with glycine and carnitine.

The defect, the inability to degrade leucine, is probably due to a flaw in the ENZYME isovaleryl-CoA dehydrogenase. Inherited as an AUTOSOMAL RECESSIVE trait, the GENE maps to 15q. Laboratory tests can reveal the defective ENZYME in a newborn, and PRENATAL DIAGNOSIS by enzyme assay of fetal cells is possible.

Interestingly, about 1.4% of Caucasians and 9.1% of blacks cannot smell the sweaty odor of isovaleric acid. Thus, the inability to smell isovaleric acid is also a genetic trait.

syndactyly Fusion of the digits of the fingers or toes. The extent of the fusion varies from webbing of skin tissue between the digits to complete joining of the bones of adjacent digits.

Syndactyly is a common feature of many CON-GENITAL conditions, and it is also believed to occur in five hereditary forms as an isolated or featured characteristic. Most are believed to be AUTOSOMAL DOMINANT traits, though recessive forms also exist.

A survey of approximately 600,000 consecutive births in Latin America conducted in 1980 found incidence of syndactyly at approximately three per 10,000 live births. (See also ZYGODACTYLY.)

syndrome A recognizable pattern or group of multiple signs, symptoms or malformations that characterize a particular disorder. The word is derived from the Greek *syn,* meaning "together with," and the Greek *drome,* meaning "to run." A syndrome is a collection of specific features, all of which "run together," resulting from a common cause. Syndromes are thought to arise from a common origin and result from more than one developmental error during fetal growth.

synophrys The joining together of the eyebrows over the bridge of the nose, giving the suggestion of one long, continuous eyebrow. This condition is seen in many GENETIC DISORDERS, including CORNELIA DE LANGE SYNDROME, Sanfilippo syndrome (see MUCO-POLYSACCHARIDOSIS) and WAARDENBURG SYNDROME.

syphilis A venereal disease caused by the spirochetal bacteria, treponema pallidum. Though usually transmitted sexually, syphilis can be passed from an infected mother to the FETUS through the placenta from the fourth month of pregnancy until birth.

Syphilis progresses in three stages: The first symptoms are painless skin sores, often on the genitals. Three months or longer after the sores heal, a rash appears, accompanied by swollen glands, headache and fever. The final stage begins three to 10 years after the first infection and damages most organs and tissues in the body.

Risk to the fetus depends on which stage of the disease the mother is in. Those in the first stage who are more than four months pregnant are assumed to have transmitted the infection to the fetus. Treatment with penicillin and erythromycin can cure the fetus before birth. As many as half of the infants born to syphilitic women in the second and third stages of the disease may be healthy, but the chances of STILLBIRTH or premature birth (see PREMATURITY) are high, and 10% to 40% are born with syphilis. Ninety-eight percent of those who receive treatment after birth survive.

Syphilitic infants may have skin sores, particularly around the mouth, genitals or anus, though physical signs of infection often are not manifest for months or years. Other early symptoms include mucus discharge from the nose and throat ("sniffles"), bone problems, skin rash, enlarged liver and spleen, and ANEMIA. Ocular problems, including GLAUCOMA, as well as DEAFNESS, abnormal teeth and bones, a deformed nose, MENTAL RETARDATION and central nervous system disorders, develop if the disease remains untreated.

Although largely brought under control after World War II with the ready availability of penicillin, rates of CONGENITAL syphilis began to rise in the late 1980s. This trend has been attributed to promiscuity and lack of prenatal health care among female abusers of crack and cocaine. In 1988, the U.S. Centers for Disease Control reported 691 cases of congenital syphilis, more than 50% above the previous year, and the highest since the advent of penicillin. New York City alone reported 1,000 cases of congenital syphilis in 1989, compared to 57 in 1986.

systemic lupus erythematosus See LUPUS.

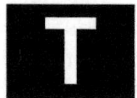

talipes   See CLUBFOOT.

talipes callus   See CLUBFOOT.

tandem mass spectrometry   An analytical instrument used in the screening process for hereditary disorders. First used as a neonatal screening tool in the early 1990s, the technology allows more than 20 disorders of body chemistry to be detected in a single analysis of a small blood sample collected in the first few days of life.

Tangier disease (analphalipoproteinemia)   Rare disorder named for Tangier Island in the Chesapeake Bay, whose inhabitants exhibit a higher than normal incidence of this hereditary condition. The primary defect is an abnormally low level of high-density lipoprotein (HDL) due to the complete absence of a protein component of HDL, termed apolipoprotein A-I. This protein, found in blood plasma, carries cholesterol and other fats from the blood to the tissues. The defect is presumably present at birth, though the disease may first be detected at any time during infancy to late adulthood. Affected individuals can absorb and store dietary fat in the form of triglycerides, a fatty substance, but there is a delay in clearing the triglycerides from the blood once they are made, and high triglyceride blood levels result. Though elevated triglyceride and diminished HDL blood levels suggest increased risk for premature heart disease, life span expectations for affected individuals are not reduced.

The hallmark of the disorder is enlarged orange tonsils. The rectum may also appear orange. Other symptoms include enlarged spleen (splenomegaly) and liver and lymph glands and, in many cases, neurologic symptoms such as muscle wasting and loss of sensation in the skin.

Inherited as an AUTOSOMAL RECESSIVE trait, CARRIERS have half the normal lipoprotein levels, allowing for carrier detection. Probably fewer than 50 people worldwide are affected. (See also CORONARY ARTERY DISEASE.)

TAR syndrome (thrombocytopenia-aplasia of radius syndrome)   First described in 1956, at birth this SYNDROME is easily recognizable due to deformities of the upper and lower limbs. They include absence or shortening of the outer forearm bone (radius), often accompanied by malformation or absence of the inner forearm bone (ulna) and upper arm bone (humerus), as well as deformity of the wrist, hands, legs or feet. The thumbs are always present. The defects are usually bilateral, that is, affect the limbs on both sides of the body.

Small, purplish spots (petechiae) appear on the body from bleeding due to the abnormal decrease in the number of platelets (thrombocytopenia). The platelets are the blood cells involved in initiation of blood clotting. Internal examination often discloses an enlarged liver and spleen (hepatosplenomegaly), and a host of other abnormalities may be found; about one-third of affected infants have a CONGENITAL HEART DEFECT. Testing of the blood and bone marrow reveals defects, including a deficiency in the large bone marrow cells that produce the platelets (megakaryocytes), a decrease in red blood cells (ANEMIA) and an abnormal increase in certain white blood cells (granulocytosis and eosinophilia).

Approximately 40% of those affected die in infancy because of hemorrhaging. Cow's milk allergy is said to be common and can be a significant problem, as ingestion of cow's milk can result in hematologic problems. The severity of the platelet problem lessens over time and adults with this syndrome usually have few if any problems related to the hematologic features. The basic defect causing the syndrome is unknown, although AUTOSOMAL RECESSIVE inheritance is suspected. Use of ULTRASOUND prenatally may disclose the upper limb defects.

Tay-Sachs disease (TSD) A fatal degenerative disease of the nervous system found primarily, but not exclusively, among Ashkenazi Jews, those of Eastern European ancestry. (There is a noticeable incidence of TSD among non-Jewish French Canadians living near the St. Lawrence River.) It is named for Warren Tay (1843–1927), a British ophthalmologist who in 1881 first described the CHERRY-RED SPOT on the retina of the eye that is one of the characteristic symptoms of the disorder, and Bernard Sachs (1858–1944), a New York neurologist who described the cellular changes of Tay-Sachs and noted its increased prevalence in the Eastern European Jewish population in 1887.

Inherited as an AUTOSOMAL RECESSIVE trait, TSD is one of a group of STORAGE DISEASES: Due to a deficiency of the ENZYME hexosaminidase A (Hex-A), there is an accumulation of GM2 ganglioside, a fatty substance, in the nerve cells of the brain. (The Hex-A GENE is located on chromosome 15q.) Storage of this substance causes nerve degeneration. Though the process begins during pregnancy, the child appears healthy at birth and develops normally until about six months of age.

Among the first symptoms are a slowing of development, loss of vision, abnormal startle response and convulsions. Examination of the retina reveals the characteristic cherry-red spot. As the disease progresses, there is a deterioration of all functions, leading to BLINDNESS, MENTAL RETARDATION, paralysis and death, usually by the age of three to four years.

Researchers have concluded that the proliferation of the TSD gene occurred after the second Diaspora (70 A.D.) and before the major migrations to regions of Poland and Russia (1100 A.D. and later).

Some researchers believe that CARRIERS of the TSD gene may be at some selective advantage for resistance to tuberculosis, though this is a controversial hypothesis. TSD affects about one in every 2,500 newborn Ashkenazi Jews, and it is estimated that approximately one in every 25 Jews in the United States is a carrier of the TSD gene. The carrier rate in the general population as well as in Jews of Sephardic origin is about one in 250. There is also an increased incidence of TSD in the Cajun community of Louisiana. At present, there is no cure or effective treatment for TSD. Bone marrow transplantation has been attempted but to date has not been successful in reversing or slowing damage to the central nervous system in babies with TSD.

TSD screening has been the prototype for carrier screening programs designed to permit the prevention of GENETIC DISORDERS. Carriers can be identified through GENETIC SCREENING. By 1992 almost 1 million persons had been screened (953,000) and over 36,000 carriers identified.

At-risk women should be tested before pregnancy. The standard biochemical test used to test males and non-pregnant women cannot be used in pregnant women because of changes in serum enzyme levels during pregnancy. Pregnant women must instead be tested using white blood cells. This test is as reliable as the serum test, but is considerably more complex and costly. DNA-based carrier testing is also available; it looks for specific MUTATIONS in the gene that codes for Hex-A.

Since 1985, when the Hex-A gene was isolated, over 50 different mutations in this gene have been identified. Some are more common than others, some occur more frequently in certain populations, and a few are associated with a later-onset variant form of the disease, rather than with the infantile form. The limitation of DNA-based carrier testing is that not all known mutations in the Hex-A gene are detected by the test, and others have yet to be identified. The tests currently available detect about 95% of carriers of Ashkenazi Jewish background and about 60% of non-Jewish individuals. Therefore, some people who are carriers will not be identified by DNA analysis alone.

PRENATAL DIAGNOSIS is possible by assay for Hex-A activity in cultured fetal cells obtained via AMNIOCENTESIS or CHORIONIC VILLUS SAMPLING. DNA-based testing is also used in prenatal diagnosis. Recently, new assisted reproductive technologies have become available to at-risk couples who wish to have children but for whom ABORTION is not an acceptable option. One option is artificial insemination using a sperm donor who has been demonstrated to be a non-carrier. Another option, which is available only for couples with identified DNA mutations in the Hex-A gene, is termed PREIMPLANTATION DIAGNOSIS. This involves in-vitro (test tube) fertilization using the couple's own eggs and sperm. Then, in-vitro fertilization is followed by an analysis of the DNA of the newly formed embryos to determine which carry two copies of the TSD gene and which do not. Only those embryos determined not to be affected with TSD are implanted in the woman. This technique is very complex, not widely available and quite expensive. The availability of GENETIC COUNSELING, screening and prenatal diagnosis have had a major impact on the incidence of this disease. Since 1970 there has been a dramatic decrease in the number of babies born with TSD, and more cases of TSD are now identified in non-Jewish than in Jewish babies.

teratogen   With its etymological origin in the Greek word *teras,* meaning "monster," a teratogen is any substance (drug, chemical, infectious or environmental agent) that can trigger malformation of the fetus. Maternal medical conditions associated with BIRTH DEFECTS, such as DIABETES MELLITUS or PHENYLKETONURIA, are also considered teratogens. (The term *teratology,* which refers to the study of human malformations, was coined by zoologist Isidore Geoffroy Saint-Hilaire (1805–61), who was among the first to scientifically investigate these conditions.)

A teratogen may damage the embryo directly or by disrupting normal functioning of the placenta by which the fetus receives nutrients, thereby creating an abnormal uterine environment.

The impact on fetal development is in general dependent on the amount of exposure to a given teratogen and the stage of fetal development at which the exposure occurs. The greater the exposure, the greater the risk to the FETUS. However, the susceptibility to the effect of a given teratogen varies greatly from individual to individual.

The first two weeks after conception is called the "all-or-none" period; exposure to a teratogen at this critical period will generally either result in the death of the embryo (and a miscarriage; see ABORTION) or have no impact at all. During the third through eighth weeks of pregnancy, the embryo's cells begin to develop characteristics of specific organ systems, and exposure to teratogens during this period can result in damage to specific organs. The central nervous system in susceptible to teratogens throughout pregnancy.

Most substances recognized as teratogens produce a particular pattern of defects. The drug THALIDOMIDE, for example, led to missing limb bones; in some cases the entire limb failed to develop so that the hand or foot was attached directly to the body. Epileptics who take ANTICONVULSANTS during pregnancy sometimes give birth to babies with distinctive facial features and heart defects caused by the drugs. Some infections during pregnancy can also lead to birth defects. Rubella (German measles; see TORCH SYNDROME) can cause CATARACTS, DEAFNESS, congenital HEART DEFECTS and MENTAL RETARDATION in the infant exposed IN UTERO.

Teratogens may also cause birth defects in concert with genetic influences in families predisposed toward certain malformations. CLEFT LIP, CLEFT PALATE, NEURAL TUBE DEFECTS, such as SPINA BIFIDA and ANENCEPHALY, PYLORIC STENOSIS (an abnormally small passage between the stomach and the intestine), CONGENITAL HIP DISLOCATION and some congenital heart defects are examples. About 20% of birth defects are estimated to be caused in this MULTIFACTORIAL (combination of genes and environmental agents) manner.

For information on specific agents, see ACCUTANE, AGENT ORANGE, CAFFEINE, CIGARETTES, COCAINE, FETAL ALCOHOL SYNDROME, LEAD, MARIJUANA, MEASLES, PHENOBARBITAL, QUININE, RADIATION, SYPHILIS, VARICELLA, VIDEO DISPLAY TERMINALS and WARFARIN EMBRYOPATHY.

teratoma of head and neck   See DERMOID CYST.

testes, absent   See ABSENT TESTES.

testicular feminization syndrome (androgen insensitivity syndrome, AIS; complete androgen insensitivity)   A form of PSEUDOHERMAPHRODITISM. This is an intersex condition, in which the reproductive organs differ from the genetic sex of the person. Affected individuals are born with female external genitalia and are thought to be females at birth. At puberty, their breasts develop, and though they usually have little body hair, they otherwise have normal female appearance. However, the CHROMOSOMES are those of a male: an XY chromosome pair, rather than the XX found in normal females.

Every FETUS, whether genetically male (XY) or female (XX), starts life with the capacity to develop either a male or female reproductive system. All fetuses have undifferentiated, non-specific genitals for the first few weeks after conception. After a few weeks, in an XY fetus (without AIS), these non-specific genitals develop into male genitals. In AIS, the child is conceived with male (XY) sex chromosomes. Embryonic testes develop inside the body and start to produce androgens. In AIS, these androgens cannot complete the male genital development due to a rare inability to use the androgens that are being produced by the testes. The problem lies in the androgen receptor GENE on the X CHROMOSOME received from the mother. This affects the responsiveness, or sensitivity, of the fetus's body tissues to androgens. The development of the external genitals continues along female lines, but another hormone produced by the fetal testes acts normally and suppresses the development of female internal organs. Thus a person with AIS has external genitals that are completely female. However, internally there are testes instead of a uterus and ovaries.

Affected individuals typically come to medical attention when they fail to begin menstruating at the time of puberty. Upon examination, the vagina is shallow, and there are no Fallopian tubes or uterus. The testicles may be in the abdominal area and are incapable of producing viable sperm.

The testes are generally removed, and plastic surgery can enlarge the size of the vagina, enabling continued female gender identification. (Some physicians suggest that affected males never be told their true genetic sex for psychological reasons. However, most professionals now view the withholding genetic and gonadal information as an old-fashioned and paternalistic attitude and recommend full disclosure with psychological support and counseling.)

Following treatment and continued estrogen therapy, affected individuals live as normal women, although they are sterile. Life span and intelligence are normal.

It has been proposed by one genetic researcher that Joan of Arc was actually a male with this SYNDROME. The suggestion is based on examination of ex tensive documentation of her physical characteristics presented at her trial for heresy in 1431 and at her posthumous Trial of Rehabilitation in 1456. This documentation includes accounts by those who lived in close quarters with her that while she had well-developed breasts, she had no pubic hair and did not menstruate. This hypothesis has led to speculation concerning elevated testosterone levels and her behavior. The same suggestion has been made with regard to Queen Elizabeth I, England's "Virgin Queen" (1533–1603).

A nationwide registry of Danish patients suggested an incidence of one in 20,400 male births. The androgen receptor gene is located on the X chromosome, and the disorder is therefore an X-LINKED trait. In about two-thirds of cases, AIS is inherited from the mother. The other third result from spontaneous MUTATION in the fetus. CARRIER females can be detected by biochemical means and PRENATAL DIAGNOSIS has been accomplished by CHORIONIC VILLUS SAMPLING.

tetrahydrobiopterin deficiencies   A rare CONGENITAL neurological disorder that can result in delayed motor development, seizures, lack of coordination, muscle tone and neurologic disturbances. It is caused by the deficiency of a tetrahydrobiopterin (a cofactor that is needed for certain ENZYMES to work properly) due to defects in an enzyme involved in its synthesis.

Tetrahydrobiopterin is used by the enzyme involved in converting the AMINO ACID phenylalanine to tyrosine, as well as in the reactions involved in the synthesis of neurotransmitters, important chemicals involved in brain function. The deficiency of tetrahydrobiopterin leads to defective activity of these enzymes which reduces the level of neurotransmitters. It also results in an abnormally high concentration of the amino acid phenylalanine in the blood. Thus, it causes a variant form of PHENYLKETONURIA.

Inherited as AUTOSOMAL RECESSIVE traits, the deficiencies are believed to affect 1–3% of all infants diagnosed with phenylketonuria (PKU) at birth. In the United States, PKU occurs in one in 11,600 live births.

The disorder can be treated somewhat with the administration of tetrahydrobiopterin to normalize phenylalanine levels along with various neurotransmitter-like drugs. Without diagnosis and treatment, neurologic damage is irreversible.

tetralogy of Fallot   A complex of four associated congenital HEART DEFECTS (CHD): ventricular septal defect; an enlarged (hypertrophied) right ventricle; a malpositioned aorta, the major artery leading from the heart; and a narrowing (stenosis) of the pulmonary artery.

Named for French physician Etienne L. A. Fallot (1850–1911), this is the most prevalent form of cyanotic heart disease. Males are more often affected than females by a ratio of 3:2.

About 1% of all newborns have CHDs, and of these about 10% have tetralogy of Fallot. About 25% of affected individuals also have another associated non-cardiac CONGENITAL abnormality. This defect has also been seen in patients with DI GEORGE SYNDROME or velocardiofacial syndromes, leading to the realization this is among the types of heart defect found in patients with deletion of 22q11.

Affected infants exhibit bluish skin (cyanosis), feeding difficulties and FAILURE TO THRIVE. Older children display a characteristic squatting position, although standing, and clubbed fingers and toes. Without surgery to correct the cardiac defects, prognosis is poor.

Besides occurring in isolation, this condition may be associated with GOLDENHAR SYNDROME and KLIPPEL-FEIL ANOMALY, as well as with exposure to some TERATOGENS, such as THALIDOMIDE, maternal PHENYLKETONURIA and TRIMETHADIONE.

thalassemia (Cooley's anemia; Mediterranean anemia)   The thalassemias are a group of inherited disorders involving defective production of HEMOGLOBIN, the oxygen-carrying component of red blood, resulting in ANEMIA, a generally debilitating condition marked by weakness and fatigue. Thalassemia is taken from the Greek *thalassa,* meaning "sea." The names "thalassemia" and "Mediterranean anemia" are indicative of its high incidence in populations bordering on the Mediterranean Sea, particularly in Italy and Greece. As in other red blood cell disorders with origins in populations from malaria-prone areas, it appears that asymptomatic CARRIERS of the trait have an increased resistance to malaria. The disorder is also prevalent in Southeast Asia, India, the Middle East and parts of Africa.

Hemoglobin occurs in several forms. It is composed of heme, the oxygen carrying respiratory pigment that gives blood its red color, and globin chains, designated alpha, beta, gamma and delta. Specific combinations of globin chains determine the form of hemoglobin.

The thalassemias have their origin in abnormal production of hemoglobin A, the main form of adult hemoglobin, which normally contains two alpha and two beta globin chains. Beta-thalassemias, the most common type, involve abnormalities in the beta chain synthesis. These were among the first human GENETIC DISORDERS to be examined by RECOMBINANT DNA analysis techniques.

The World Health Organization estimates that at least 6.5 percent of the population are carriers of GENES for one of the hemoglobinopathies (disorders affecting hemoglobin, including the thalassemias and sickle cell disease).

The thalassemias are inherited as AUTOSOMAL RECESSIVE traits. Thalassemia has been cured using bone marrow transplantation, but the treatment is possible only for a small minority of patients who have a suitable bone marrow donor, and the transplant procedure carries risks and can result in death.

Cooley's anemia (beta-thalassemia major)   This is the most severe form of beta-thalassemia, first described in 1925 by Dr. Thomas Benton Cooley (1871–1945), an American pediatrician. In this disorder, beta chains are absent from hemoglobin A, or their synthesis is greatly reduced.

Infants appear normal at birth. Onset is usually in the first few months of life. Early signs are paleness, fatigue, irritability and FAILURE TO THRIVE. There may also be fever, feeding problems, diarrhea and gastrointestinal complications. Symptoms become progressively more severe, leading to an enlarged spleen (splenomegaly), severe anemia, enlargement of the heart, slight jaundice and leg ulcers.

Under examination, the red blood cells appear pale, thin and misshapen, and most are unusually small. While normal red blood cells survive for four months, these break down within a few weeks. The need for more red blood cells causes the bone marrow, where they are produced, to expand dramatically, thinning the surrounding bone, especially the bones of the skull and face. This gives affected infants a characteristic facial appearance, with prominent cheek bones, eyes slanted toward the nose, overgrowth of the upper jaw and dental malformations of the upper teeth. Bones fracture easily.

Additionally, the iron and waste products from the breakdown of the red blood cells accumulate in organs, damaging the spleen, liver and heart. The iron overload that results causes many of the life-threatening problems of the disease. Without treatment, Cooley's anemia is invariably fatal. Current management consists of blood transfusion of packed red blood cells in concert with iron chelators, agents that bind with excess iron in the body so that it can be excreted. Removal of the spleen (splenectomy) may be necessary in some cases. The prognosis for life expectancy using these modern treatment methods is currently unknown, though some affected individuals are surviving into their 20s and 30s. Experimental research on the effectiveness of bone marrow transplantation as a means of stimulating healthy red blood cell production is in progress. In general, the younger the child is when the disease appears, the more unfavorable the prognosis.

In the United States, it is estimated that one in 800 to one in 2,500 individuals of Greek or Italian descent have this disorder. The GENE for the beta globin chain is on 11p. Carrier screening is available. PRENATAL DIAGNOSIS is now possible using recombinant DNA techniques through analysis of the globin chain genes in fetal cells obtained by CHORIONIC VILLUS SAMPLING or AMNIOCENTESIS. Since a variety of different MUTATIONS cause thalassemia, the specific mutation in a given family must be known before prenatal diagnosis is possible.

Beta-thalassemia minor (thalassemia trait) This is a mild, often completely asymptomatic trait that results from having only one recessive gene for the condition, rather than the two recessive genes necessary for full expression of the disorder. It is estimated that over 2 million Americans, and 4% of all individuals of Greek or Italian descent, are carriers of this trait. The incidence of the gene is also higher among blacks than in the general population, and may play a role in the expression of sickle-cell anemia. While blacks may have an increased incidence of beta-thalassemia minor (the beta-thalassemia trait), they rarely have thalassemia major.

Alpha-thalassemia This disorder is seen mainly in Asian populations and involves defective synthesis of alpha chains in hemoglobin. As with beta-thalassemias, it appears in major and minor forms. Alpha-thalassemia major frequently results in fetal death.

Alpha-thalassemia commonly results from the deletion of one or more of the four genes that code for alpha chains, located on 16p. If all four are deleted, it is lethal IN UTERO, or affected infants are stillborn (see STILLBIRTH) with hydrops fetalis. If there are three deletions, hemoglobin H disease results, with hemolytic anemia of variable severity. Only one or two deletions results in alpha-thalassemia minor, the carrier state, with no clinical abnormalities.

thalidomide A sedative widely prescribed in the late 1950s in Europe, Australia and Canada to prevent nausea in pregnant women and subsequently found to cause severe limb deformities. One dose is sufficient to induce deformities. Affected infants typically had incompletely developed arms or legs, with hands or feet attached almost directly to the trunk (PHOCOMELIA). Although 10,000–12,000 thalidomide babies were born, initial suggestions of a link between the drug and the defects were discounted; prior to that time, it was believed the placenta protected the FETUS from harmful influences, and therefore that drugs could not cause birth defects. Though animal studies had been conducted with thalidomide, the drug did not have the same effect on laboratory animals as on humans.

It was never approved for use in the United States by the Food and Drug Administration, due to concerns about its sole known side effect, numbness of the hands and feet (peripheral neuropathy). Only 17 affected infants were born in the United States. Thalidomide's use as a sedative was halted in 1961 in Europe and 1962 in Canada. Some 5,000 thalidomide babies survived into adulthood. They refer to themselves as "thalidomiders."

While banned as sedative, thalidomide remains in use as an immunosuppressive agent, treating autoimmune disorders (see IMMUNE DEFICIENCY DISEASES) by suppressing the immune system. In England it is used for treating some skin diseases, discoid lupus (see LUPUS) and RHEUMATOID ARTHRITIS. It has also been renamed in England due to the negative associations of the name thalidomide; it is now known as "sauramide." In Canada it is available as an "emergency status" agent, requiring special permission from the Health Protection Branch for use.

Thalidomide is also a major medication for a form of leprosy, erythema nodosum leprosum, a use for which it was prescribed for a limited number of leprosy patients in the United States under the "compassionate use" program. In 1997, the Food and Drug Administration approved thalidomide for use for treating this form of leprosy, making the drug available in the United States for off-label use, such as in treating cancers and some AIDS-related illnesses. It is used in the treatment of multiple myeloma as well.

In order to prevent the birth of affected infants, women of child-bearing age in the United States who are taking thalidomide must have proof they are using contraception and have a pregnancy test at least once a month. Some physicians have been reluctant to prescribe thalidomide for female patients who could benefit from it due to concerns about possible BIRTH DEFECTS and legal liability. (See also TERATOGEN.)

thanatophoric dwarfism　A severe form of short-limbed DWARFISM that results in death soon after birth. This is the most common neonatal lethal skeletal DYSPLASIA. Death is primarily due to respiratory insufficiency caused by the abnormally small rib cage. Named in 1967, and incorporating the Greek *thanatos*, "death," in its designation, the first report of a condition that fits this description was published in 1898.

Believed to be inherited as an AUTOSOMAL DOMINANT disorder, with all affected infants resulting from new MUTATIONS, it is divided into two types. Type I, the most common, is characterized by curved long bones (especially the femora, or thigh bones) and flat vertebrae. Type 2 is characterized by straight femora and tall vertebrae. Some cases of type 2 are associated with a severe cloverleaf skull malformation, KLEE-BATTSCHADEL ANOMALY. Affected infants have mutations in the fibroblast growth factor 3 receptor GENE, located on 4p. Different mutations in this *FGFR3* gene cause ACHONDROPLASIA.

Incidence has been estimated at between one in 6,400 and one in 8,900 births.

Thomsen disease (Thomsen-Becker myotonia; myotonia congenita)　A rare and nonprogressive neuromuscular disorder that causes stiffness in the muscles. This disorder was first described in 1876 by Danish physician Julius Thomsen in his own family. Onset is usually at birth or in infancy. Muscles become rigid when efforts are made to move, and once a movement has been made, the muscles exhibit an inability to relax. The muscle may remain in its contracted state for 30 seconds. Movements such as talking, walking, chewing and swallowing are typically slow.

Affected infants' muscles are often large and well-developed for their age. As they grow older, the condition may improve. Inherited as an AUTOSOMAL DOMINANT disorder, it is caused by a MUTATION in the GENE for a skeletal muscle chloride channel (*CLCN1*), located on chromosome 7. Males appear to be more frequently affected than females. Life span is unaffected.

thrombasthenia of Glanzmann and Naegeli (Glanzmann thrombasthenia, GTA)　Taken from the

Greek *thrombos,* for "clot," and *asthenia,* for "weakness," thrombasthenia is a hemorrhagic (bleeding) disorder characterized by prolonged bleeding and abnormal platelet function. When viewed microscopically, blood smears show little evidence of platelet aggregation. It was first described by Swiss pediatrician E. Glanzmann (1887–1959) in 1918. It also bears the name of Swiss hematologist Otto Naegeli (1871–1938).

Multiple blood factors (in the platelets, plasma and tissues) have been identified as being necessary for proper platelet function. In this disorder, the factor that makes platelets adhere to the walls of injured vessels is missing. This factor is a complex of platelet membrane proteins called GP IIb and GP IIIa. (VON WILLEBRAND DISEASE is caused by the absence of another plasma factor.) A variety of defects have been identified in the *GP IIb* and *GPIIIa* GENES, which are located adjacent to one another on chromosome 17q.

While almost all cases are considered the result of AUTOSOMAL RECESSIVE inheritance, there is likely more than one form of the disorder. It has been reported as being the second most common bleeding disorder in Jordan, and frequent among Iraqi Jews.

Affected individuals have a lifelong tendency of mild to severe bleeding from mucous membranes (e.g., nosebleeds, gums etc.) and prolonged bleeding after injury.

HETEROZYGOTES (CARRIERS), those who have only one of the two genes required for the expression of this disorder, may exhibit mild clotting abnormalities, though upon examination their blood appears normal.

thrombocytopenia-aplasia of radius syndrome   See TAR SYNDROME.

thumb sign   The protrusion of the thumb, when bent, across the palm and beyond the clenched fist. It is seen in children with MARFAN SYNDROME. It is sometimes called the Steinberg thumb sign for I. Steinberg, who described it in 1966 as a "simple screening test" for Marfan syndrome.

thymic alymphoplasia   See DI GEORGE SYNDROME.

tobacco   See CIGARETTES.

Tom Thumb   "General" Tom Thumb, born Charles Stratton, was the most famous dwarf of the 19th century, an era in which there were a great many "prodigies" whose physical abnormalities formed the basis of performing careers that often brought them considerable renown and fortune. The name "Tom Thumb," is taken from a legend, probably Scandinavian in origin but common to several European countries, of an extremely small person. This mythical person is limned in the 1630 poem "Tom Thumbe: His Life and Death."

> In Arthur's court Tom Thumbe did live
> A man of mickle might,
> The best of all the table round,
> And eke a doughty knight;
> His stature but an inch in height
> or quarter of a span;
> Then thinke you not this little knight
> Was prov'd a valiant man?

Born January 11, 1832, Stratton reached 25 inches in length at five months, and then stopped growing for several years. His condition is believed to have been panhypopituitary dwarfism (see PITUITARY DWARFISM). His parents were first cousins (see CONSANGUINITY) and thus he probably had an AUTOSOMAL RECESSIVE disorder interfering with the synthesis of growth hormone. He was first exhibited by P. T. Barnum at his American Museum in New York and created an immediate sensation, drawing 30,000 attendees. A crowd estimated at 10,000 saw him off when he set sail for his first European tour in January of 1844, and his reception in Europe was even more tumultuous than in New York. He was received by Queen Victoria and other European heads of state.

His act consisted of posing himself in the attitude of various famous Greek statues, or impersonations of Cupid with wings and bow, the gladiator Hercules and Napoleon Bonaparte. In this last role, he would appear in deep meditation or strut about the stage in a miniature uniform. He was presented to the Duke of Wellington, who asked what he was thinking about while seeming so lost in thought during the impersonation. "I was thinking of the loss of the battle of Waterloo," Tom replied.

After his last visit to Europe in 1878, Tom Thumb retired and lived on the large fortune earned from his European tours.

tongue folding or rolling   The ability to fold the tongue backward or roll it into a tubular shape, two independent traits, are inherited by AUTOSOMAL DOMINANT transmission. The conditions are benign. In samples of various population groups, the majority of those surveyed were able to roll their tongues. In males, an association with the ability to move, or "wiggle," one's ears has been noted.

The ability to move one's ears is inherited as a somewhat irregular dominant trait. One study found 19.9% of men and 9.57% of women could move their ears.

tongue-tie   See ANKYLOGLOSSIA.

tooth-and-nail syndrome (dysplasia of the nails with hypodontia)   As the name implies, this disorder involves underdevelopment of the teeth and nails. Though rare, it has been reported as being frequent among Dutch Mennonites in Canada. Some teeth are absent (most often the mandibular incisors, second molars and maxillary canines). Nails on fingers and especially toes form poorly. (Nails grow normally following childhood.) The condition has usually been detected when teeth failed to erupt. It is inherited as an AUTOSOMAL DOMINANT trait.

The group of disorders that are characterized by ANOMALIES of dental development and skin appendages (nails, hair, sweat glands) are termed ECTODERMAL DYSPLASIAS (ED). Tooth-and-nail syndrome is distinguished from other forms of ED by little involvement of sweat glands or hair: Eyebrows and eyelashes are normal but the scalp hair is fine.

TORCH syndrome   An acronym for four infectious diseases known to cause similar birth defects: toxoplasmosis, rubella and infections with cytomegalovirus (CMV) and herpes simplex virus. PRENATAL DIAGNOSIS of fetal infection with these organisms is now possible using new invasive diagnostic techniques of fetal blood sampling, such as CORDOCENTESIS.

Toxoplasmosis

A common infection caused by the parasitic microscopic organism *Toxoplasma gondii*. Humans contract the disease by eating or handling raw meat or coming in contact with cat feces containing the organism. Outdoor cats that hunt are more likely to be infected.

Women who have had the infection before pregnancy (about 35%) are immune to it, and they confer this immunity to their unborn child. However, if a woman becomes infected during pregnancy, particularly between the 10th and 24th weeks, the FETUS may be affected. Infection in early pregnancy carries a lower risk of the infection spreading to the fetus than infection later in pregnancy; however, early infection carries a higher risk of severe abnormalities. In the United States, the incidence of CONGENITAL toxoplasmosis is approximately two to six per 1,000 live births. Premature birth (see PREMATURITY) is common among such infants, although only 10% to 20% of infected infants show signs of illness.

Among those with severe infection, over 80% suffer MENTAL RETARDATION and have seizures. Other abnormalities include ocular defects, such as inflammation of the retina (see in about 25% of cases), accumulation of fluid in the brain (HYDROCEPHALUS), convulsions, calcium deposits in the brain, an abnormally small head (MICROCEPHALY) and yellowish skin color (jaundice). However, about 60% of infants born with toxoplasmosis exhibit no, or only minor, health problems.

The mainstay of diagnosis of infection is antibody testing. However, since most pregnant women with acute toxoplasmosis infections are asymptomatic, toxoplasmosis is not usually suspected until after the birth of an affected infant.

Prompt treatment of CONGENITAL toxoplasmosis is important. In cases where maternal infection early in pregnancy is documented, decisons about treatment must weigh the relative benefits, consequences and risks (e.g., the apparently small teratogenic potential of the drugs used to treat the infection). There is no vaccine against toxoplasmosis. The best preventive measure is avoidance of infection by avoiding raw meat (especially red meat) and exposure to cat feces.

Rubella

Maternal infection with rubella (German measles) during pregnancy may cause CATARACTS and GLAUCOMA, congenital HEART DEFECTS, DEAFNESS, delayed motor development or CEREBRAL PALSY, and mental retardation. It may also result in miscarriage (see ABORTION) or STILLBIRTH. Infants with rubella often develop other infections, such as pneumonia, meningitis and encephalitis. Endocrine abnormalities such as DIABETES MELLITUS may result. The abnormalities seen vary with the time in gestation during which infection occurred.

Between 15–25% of infants infected during first trimester can be recognized as having congenital rubella in early infancy. After the first trimester the incidence of severely affected children drops off substantially. However, some manifestations such as hearing loss and developmental delay are still seen in children exposed in the fourth and fifth months of gestation.

About 10% to 20% of infants with congenital rubella die within their first year. It is preventable by immunization against rubella prior to pregnancy.

Rubella epidemics used to occur approximately every six to nine years, with major epidemics occurring at intervals of up to 30 years. The most recent of these major outbreaks occurred between 1962 and 1965. Beginning in Europe, it reached the United States in 1964. This 1964–65 epidemic in the United States resulted in an estimated 12.5 million cases of rubella, and more than 11,000 cases of fetal death by miscarriage or therapeutic abortion. Approximately 20,000 infants were born with congenital rubella syndrome. Of these, an estimated 2,100 died in early infancy and almost 12,000 were deaf. The economic cost of this epidemic was placed at approximately $1.5 billion.

The development of a live attenuated rubella vaccine in 1969 greatly reduced the incidence of this viral infection. No large epidemics have subsequently occurred in areas where the vaccine is in wide use, though limited outbreaks continue to occur in settings such as schools, where large groups of susceptible individuals are in close contact with one another. The vaccines have not been associated with evidence of any increased risk to the fetus. All 50 states require rubella vaccinations prior to school entry.

Cytomegalovirus (CMV)

A very common and usually asymptomatic infection, this is a variety of herpes virus. Nearly everyone has been infected by the age of 40, but unlike rubella and measles, CMV can recur. Contracting CMV for the first time during pregnancy presents a greater risk to the fetus than a recurring infection. The mother can transmit the virus to her newborn before birth through the placenta as well as during the birth process or through breast milk.

With the exception of rubella epidemics, this is the most common congenital infectious cause of mental retardation and nervous system damage (including DEAFNESS). Approximately 1% of infants in the United States are born with CMV. About 90% are asymptomatic at birth. In those who show signs of infection, enlarged liver and spleen (HEPATOSPLENOMEGALY), a purplish rash from multiple areas of bleeding (purpura), a yellowish skin color (jaundice) and a form of ANEMIA are common. Mental retardation, seizures and hearing loss may also occur.

No treatment is available but most infants with mild cases recover completely. As with the previous two infections, the effects vary depending on the time of infection.

Herpes Simplex Virus (HSV)

There are two types of this common infection; one primarily causes sores around the mouth, the other, transmitted sexually, primarily causes genital sores. Herpes can be transmitted from mother to infant during birth. If a woman contracts herpes during pregnancy, the risk of miscarriage or stillbirth is greatly increased.

Symptoms of herpes at birth include blisters on the skin or eyes (cutaneous or conjunctival vesicles), fever, jaundice and seizures. About half of infants with herpes die within a week of birth. Of those who survive, 25% to 30% have eye defects, abnormal motor development or mental retardation.

Birth by CESAREAN DELIVERY can prevent infection of the newborn in women known to harbor the virus in their genital tracts.

torsion dystonia   See DYSTONIA.

Tourette syndrome (Gilles de la Tourette syndrome)   Named for Georges Gilles de la Tourette, who first described and noted the familial nature of the SYNDROME in 1885, Tourette syndrome (TS) is a neurological disorder characterized by rapidly repetitive multiple movements called tics and by involuntary vocalizations.

The tics may include eye blinking, shoulder shrugging, head jerking, facial twitches or repetitive movements of the torso or limbs. The vocalizations may include repeated sniffing, throat clearing, coughing, grunting, barking or shrieking. Some affected individuals repeat other people's words (echolalia), stutter, repeat their own words (palilalia) or utter inappropriate or obscene words (coprolalia). (Though coprolalia occurs in only 5% to 40% of patients, it is the most well-known symptom of the disorder.) These body movements and vocalizations are the result of a chemical imbalance in the brain.

The disorder usually appears between the ages of two and 16 years and lasts throughout life. It occurs relatively frequently in Ashkenazi Jews and rarely in blacks. About three-quarters of patients are male, and 10% of affected individuals have a family history of the disorder. Those most at risk are sons of mothers with TS, where the percentage who develop it may be as high as 30%. The specific mode of genetic transmission has not been established. Some hold susceptibility to TS is conveyed by a single major GENE in combination with a MULTIFACTORIAL background. Familial cases suggest that TS is an AUTOSOMAL DOMINANT trait with sex thresholds that affect the expression of the disorder. However, many SPORADIC cases have been reported. The incidence of full-blown cases of TS is estimated to be one in 2,000 live births. Mild cases may appear as frequently as one in 200 or one in 300 live births. It is said to be unusually frequent in a Mennonite religious isolate population in Canada.

Compulsive behaviors, seen in 40% of cases, include repeated touching, rubbing, incessant thoughts, imitating other people's movements, distractibility, ritualistic actions, and self-mutilation. Some compulsive behavior may be dangerous, such as the compulsion to run across the street before oncoming cars. Learning disabilities are present in 60% of cases.

Affected individuals rarely exhibit all the symptoms. There may be tremendous variability over time in the symptoms, their frequency and severity. In mild cases, a few tics or twitches may be confined to the face or eyes. In more severe cases, individuals may exhibit arm flapping, foot stamping or stomach jerks. It has been suggested the great scholar-lexicographer Samuel Johnson (1709–84), known for his tics, mannerisms, postures and verbal repetitions, may have had Tourette syndrome.

The symptoms wax and wane, usually over three- to four-month periods. New symptoms may join old symptoms or take their place. Stress usually aggravates the condition. Events like birthdays, holidays, the beginning of a new school year may exacerbate the disorder. Symptoms also tend to get worse during puberty and sometimes stabilize during adulthood. However, it's estimated that 5% to 16% of cases go into remission at puberty.

While the vocalizations or body movements are involuntary, some affected individuals can suppress them, or substitute less socially inappropriate tics for brief periods of time, such as in a classroom, at work or when being examined by a physician. However, their symptoms usually emerge more explosively when they return to less threatening surroundings. A variety of medications may be useful in suppressing the symptoms.

Currently, there is no method of PRENATAL DIAGNOSIS or CARRIER screening.

It should be noted that perhaps 15% of all children exhibit transient tic disorders during their early school years, such as eye blinking, nose puckering, grimacing or squinting, and it may be especially noticeable with excitement or fatigue. Therefore, tics by themselves should not be taken as an indication of the presence of TS.

Townes-Brocks syndrome Described in 1972 by U.S. physician Philip L. Townes (b. 1927) and his colleague, E. R. Brocks, this malformation SYNDROME was first observed in one family, affecting a father and five of his seven children. All six had IMPERFORATE ANUS (failure of development of the opening of the end of the intestinal tract to allow passage of the bowel contents), malformed ears and MENTAL RETARDATION. Most also had malformations of the thumb and other digits and mild to moderate DEAFNESS.

Inherited as an AUTOSOMAL DOMINANT trait, it is caused by a MUTATION in the SALL1 putative TRANSCRIPTION FACTOR GENE, a developmental regulator, on 16q. Over 50 cases have had been reported.

Marked variability in expression and severity is characteristic. Kidney and urinary tract ANOMALIES may also be seen. The syndrome's features overlap with those of the VATER ASSOCIATION.

The anomalies of the anus and rectum and malformed thumbs and ears can be surgically treated. The outlook for a normal life span appears to be favorable.

toxoplasmosis See TORCH SYNDROME.

tracheoesophageal fistula An abnormal opening, present at birth, between the branches of the esophagus leading to the lungs and the digestive system. As a result, ingested liquids and foods may enter the lungs, causing respiratory infections and feeding difficulties. Once diagnosis is made, it can be repaired surgically.

Tracheoesophageal fistula frequently accompanies esophageal stenosis, a CONGENITAL narrowing of the esophagus, or esophageal atresia, where the esophagus ends in a blind pouch and doesn't continue through to the stomach.

The maldevelopment has its genesis in the fourth week of embryonic development, though the cause is unknown. Over 50% of the fistulas are associated with other malformations, including those in infants with the VATER ASSOCIATION or in some CHROMOSOME ABNORMALITIES such as trisomy 18 (see EDWARD SYNDROME).

It is thought to occur in one in 3,000–3,500 births. Recurrence risks are generally likely to be low. PRENATAL DIAGNOSIS by ULTRASOUND is possible.

transcription factor Proteins that initiate the transcription, or copying, of a segment of DNA (DEOXYRIBONUCLEIC ACID) into a complementary segment of RNA (RIBONUCLEIC ACID), from which a protein or proteins are synthesized.

Treacher Collins syndrome (mandibulo-facial dysostosis) Inherited condition evident at birth due to its characteristic facial appearance. It is named for Edward Treacher Collins (1862–1932), an ophthalmologist at the Royal Eye Hospital in London, who described the condition in 1900, although a case may have been described in 1846. Its secondary name refers to malformations of the individual bones (DYSOSTOSIS) of the jaw and face (mandibulofacial).

The slits of the eyes (palpebral fissures) slant downward away from the nose (antimongoloid obliquity). The outer portion of the lower eyelid may be fissured (COLOBOMA), with a deficiency of eyelashes on the lower lid.

The cheek bones are underdeveloped, giving the nose a large appearance. The nasal bridge may be raised, the nostrils narrowed and the jaw very small (micrognathia). The ears may show several developmental abnormalities; the outer ear may appear grossly malformed or misplaced. The auditory canal may be missing, or the bones of the inner ear may be anomalous. CLEFT PALATE, dental malocclusion and high-arched palate are common.

Nonfacial features occasionally associated with this primarily craniofacial disorder include congenital HEART DEFECTS, deformities of the spinal cord, CONGENITAL ANOMALIES of the extremities, undescended testicles (CRYPTORCHISM) and renal (kidney) abnormalities.

Plastic surgery can correct some of the cosmetic manifestations of the SYNDROME.

The syndrome is inherited as an AUTOSOMAL DOMINANT trait and displays a high degree of variability in severity of expression. It is caused by MUTATIONS in the *TCOF1* GENE on 5q which encodes a protein that has been named "treacle." Over half of the cases are thought to arise from new mutation. Life span is normal, except in rare occasions where severe cardiac or renal abnormalities are present, leading to potentially fatal complications. Intelligence appears normal. (Reports of MENTAL RETARDATION in some cases may be due to the hearing disorder that usually accompanies this syndrome.)

Both ULTRASOUND and molecular analysis have been used for PRENATAL DIAGNOSIS.

tremor, hereditary essential See HEREDITARY ESSENTIAL TREMOR.

trichorhinophalangeal syndrome This SYNDROME involves abnormalities of the face, hair and joints of the fingers. At birth, affected infants have sparse scalp hair, eyelashes and eyebrows, a bulbous nose with tented (dilated) nostrils, large protruding ears and a thin upper lip. The infant may also have a high forehead, a long indentation between the nose and the mouth (philtrum) and a horizontal groove on the chin.

From mid-childhood until puberty the fingers and possibly the toes become progressively deformed due to abnormal growth of the bones. The fingers appear tapered. Flat feet are also common. Bone age is often several years behind chronological age and many adults with this disorder tend to be short, with approximately 40% below the third percentile in height.

Other features may include small teeth, problems with the bite (dental malocclusions), abnormal curvature of the spine (SCOLIOSIS), winging or prominence of the shoulder blades and congenital HEART DEFECTS.

The syndrome involves MUTATIONS in the TRPS1 GENE on the long arm of chromosome 8. Both AUTOSOMAL DOMINANT and RECESSIVE forms of the disorder exist, though most cases are dominantly inherited.

Life expectancy is normal. However, during infancy and early childhood affected individuals have an increased susceptibility to upper respiratory tract infections. A degenerative hip disease often develops in young adulthood.

LANGER-GIEDION SYNDROME is often referred to as TRP syndrome, type II. It is distinguished by the presence of multiple exostoses, or bony outgrowths. A CONTIGUOUS GENE SYNDROME, it involves deletions in the long arm of chromosome 8.

trigonocephaly See CRANIOSYNOSTOSIS.

trimethadione See ANTICONVULSANTS.

trinucleotide repeat disorders Any of a group of diseases whose molecular basis is a GENE's abnormal trinucleotide repeat sequence. In normal genes, these sequences repeat five to 50 times, but once they reach a critical length they become unstable and are prone to expansion during replication, ultimately interfering with the normal operation of the gene and resulting in GENETIC DISORDERS.

This mechanism of genetic MUTATION was first noted in 1991 in KENNEDY DISEASE and FRAGILE X SYNDROME, identified in MYOTONIC DYSTROPHY in 1992 and in HUNTINGTON disease in 1993. Among the other disorders, it is recognized as the basis for are FRIEDREICH ATAXIA, SPINOCEREBELLAR ATAXIA I and MACHADO-JOSEPH DISEASE.

In these disorders, the sequences may repeat hundreds of times, or in the case of CONGENITAL myotonic dystrophy, thousands. Huntington and Kennedy diseases and a number of hereditary ataxias belong to a group caused by the expanded trinucleotide sequence of CAG, which codes for glutamine. It is thought the abnormal properties of the expanded polyglutamine built by the gene as a result of the expanded template causes these disorders. The abnormal polyglutamines cause neurological degeneration.

The primary similarity among trinucleotide repeat disorders is the phenomenon of anticipation, whereby successive generations exhibit increasing severity and decreasing age of onset, as the repeat sequence becomes longer with successive generations.

Another common characteristic is that during sexual cell division, the degree of instability of a given repeat sequence differs between males and females, a characteristic called differential expansion. Recognition of anticipation and differential expansion has helped elucidate the genetic mechanisms at work in formerly puzzling phenomena, such as the appearance of new cases of HUNTINGTON CHOREA arising from paternal transmission, and of new cases of congenital myotonic dystrophy arising from maternal transmission.

triploidy The condition of having a complete extra set of CHROMOSOMES, that is, having three rather than the normal complement of two of each of the 23 chromosomes. Therefore, instead of having 46 chromosomes (2 × 23), individuals with triploidy have 69 (3 × 23) (see CHROMOSOME ABNORMALITIES). Pure triploidy can result from the fertilization of one egg by two sperm (dispermy) or a failure of disjunction during meiosis, the process whereby pairs of chromosomes split during the formation of sperm and egg. However, some individuals may exhibit triploidy in only some cells of the body (see MOSAICISM), resulting from an error in cell division shortly after conception.

Approximately two-thirds to three-quarters of triploidy cases result from dispermy. About one-quarter of cases arise from fertilization of a normal ovum by a diploid sperm, and about 10% are the result of a diploid ovum. Mosaic cases of triploidy are very rare. There is no evidence of an increase in risk of recurrence or that maternal or paternal age affects incidence.

Pure triploidy is generally lethal, resulting in spontaneous ABORTION, STILLBIRTH or death within days of birth. However, individuals who have mosaic triploidy may have prolonged survival, though they usually exhibit MENTAL RETARDATION.

Newborns with pure triploidy as well as mosaics are typically premature and exhibit LOW BIRTH WEIGHT. Abnormalities of skull development are common, as are wide-set eyes (HYPERTELORISM) that are unusually small (microphthalmia). The ears are often low-set and malformed. The tongue may be enlarged (MACROGLOSSIA) and protrude from the mouth, and the chin is small (MICROGNATHIA). Fine, downy hair (lanugo) may be visible on the cheeks and forehead.

Some of the fingers and toes may be webbed (SYNDACTYLY), the feet may be clubbed (talipes equinovarus) and in males the external genitalia may be small. Part of the intestine may protrude through a defective wall of the abdomen (OMPHALOCELE). A host of other internal malformations may be found of nervous system, heart, kidney, digestive tract or genitalia.

This condition may occur as frequently as one in 2,500 live births and in approximately 2% of conceptions. Most are lost as miscarriages and account for approximately 20% of all chromosomally abnormal spontaneous abortions.

While there is no specific prenatal diagnostic procedure for this condition, FETUSES with omphalocele or NEURAL TUBE DEFECTS will cause elevated maternal ALPHA-FETOPROTEIN levels. Triploidy can then be detected prenatally by chromosome analysis of fetal cells obtained via CHORIONIC VILLUS SAMPLING or AMNIOCENTESIS.

trisomy An individual or organism that has three rather than the normal complement of two CHROMOSOMES in a given pair. A number of genetic disorders in humans result from CHROMOSOME ABNORMALITIES characterized by the presence of trisomy. The most noted in DOWN SYNDROME, or trisomy 21, in which affected individuals have three copies of chromosome 21. Others include PATAU SYNDROME (trisomy 13), EDWARD SYNDROME (trisomy 18) and KLINEFELTER SYNDROME, in which males have three sex chromosomes present (XXY) rather than the normal two (XY).

trisomy 13 See PATAU SYNDROME.

trisomy 18 See EDWARD SYNDROME.

trisomy 21 See DOWN SYNDROME.

tritanopia See COLOR BLINDNESS.

tuberous sclerosis An AUTOSOMAL DOMINANT HEREDITARY DISEASE characterized by epileptic seizures, MENTAL RETARDATION, tumors that may appear on internal organs, and a variety of skin manifestations. Affected individuals may exhibit one or more of these symptoms.

Seizures occur in more than 85% of cases. Lesions and tumors are often found in the brain, kidneys and retina. They may also occur in the heart, bone, lungs and liver. A common skin manifestation in growing children consists of reddish, seed-like bumps that appear in a butterfly pattern across the cheeks and nose (angiofibroma). Depigmented areas on the skin (hypomelanotic macules), commonly called "White spots," or "ash leaf spots," are present at birth in 60–90% of affected infants.

Café au lait spots (coffee-colored patches of skin) may also be evident. Collagenous patches of slightly elevated, yellowish-brown skin with the texture of an orange peel (shagreen patches) may also be present. Nail beds of the fingers and toes may have wart-like growths.

Affected individuals may display unusual behavior or exhibit delayed speech, slow motor development and learning disabilities. Mental retardation of a moderate to severe degree is seen in about two out of three patients.

There is a great variability in expression of this disorder, even within a family with a history of the condition. While some affected individuals lead normal and productive lives and may remain undiagnosed, severe cases may result in premature death due to seizures, tumors or infections.

There seems to be a correlation between the age of onset and the severity of seizures and the degree of mental retardation. For that reason, early diagnosis and treatment with anticonvulsant drugs is important in reducing the potential severity of the condition.

The disorder is inherited as an autosomal dominant trait, with 50–80% being the result of a new MUTATION. Unlike what is seen in other dominant disorders such as ACHONDROPLASIA and APERT SYNDROME, no increase in parental age has been linked to these SPORADIC cases. When first identified in 1862 by F. D. von Recklinghausen, it was considered to be rare, but now incidence is estimated at approximately 1:5,000–6,000 newborns. An estimated 40,000–80,000 in the United States and over 1 million worldwide are thought to have tuberous sclerosis. The wide range reflects the possibility that many cases remain unrecognized.

Diagnosis is made on the basis of seizures, behavioral symptoms and computerized axial tomography (CAT) scanning, which can reveal hallmark internal manifestations of the disorder. TS demonstrates genetic HETEROGENEITY in that mutations in more than one GENE can cause the disorder. The *TSC1* gene is mapped to chromosome 9q. It encodes a protein that has been named hamartin. It appears to act as a tumor suppressor. There appears to be a reduced risk of mental retardation in *TSC1* as opposed to *TSC2* disease. The *TSC2* gene maps to chromosome 16p. It too seems to function as a tumor suppressor gene. It sits immediately adjacent to the *PKD1* polycystic kidney disease gene. In fact, it appears that renal cystic disease occurring in tuberous sclerosis probably reflects mutational involvement of the *PKD1* gene, with large deletions involving both *TSC2* and *PKD1*. The protein encoded by the *TSC2* gene has been named tuberin. *TSC2* mutations seem to account for a slightly larger number of cases than *TSC1* mutations. It was previously thought that there were also genes for *TS* on chromosomes 11 and 12, but this does not seem to be the case. PRENATAL DIAGNOSIS using molecular techniques may be possible in certain families but is not generally available.

Turcot syndrome   A rare hereditary disorder characterized by tumors in the lining of the lower gastrointestinal tract (colon) and brain tumors (astrocytoma, glioblastoma or spongioblastoma). It was first identified by J. Turcot, who in 1959 described the disorder in a brother and sister whose parents were third cousins. Onset usually occurs in the second decade of life. The gastrointestinal polyps may number from the hundreds to the thousands, and while usually confined to the colon, in some cases may be seen in the stomach and small intestine. The polyps may cause diarrhea, rectal bleeding, abdominal pain, fatigue and weight loss. They may also turn malignant and result in death from the second to the fifth decade. Brain tumors may result in neurological symptoms and may be malignant and lethal, their severity influenced by the tumor's type, size and location.

It has been suggested that Turcot syndrome is actually a variant of familial adenomatous polyposis (FAP). It is thought to result from a mutation in either the *adenomatous polyposis coli gene (APC)* or in the mismatch repair genes *MLH1* or *PMS2*. Autosomal recessive inheritance is suspected.

Turner syndrome   This condition, exclusively seen in females, is characterized by short stature, failure to develop secondary sex characteristics and INFERTILITY. It is caused by the total absence of one of the two X CHROMOSOMES normally found in all of a female's cells, or the structural alteration of one of the two X chromosomes in some or all of a female's cells.

It carries the name of U.S. physician Henry H. Turner (b. 1892), who first identified the characteristics of the disorder in 1928. The chromosomal aberration that causes it was discovered by Dr. C. E. Ford in 1959.

Turner syndrome is estimated to occur in one of every 2,500 live female births, though only about 2% of Turner's fetuses survive to full term. In addition to the features described above, there may be malformations and/or health problems in the eyes and ears. Cardiac defects (most often coarctation of the aorta) and urinary tract malformations (such as horseshoe kidney) may also be seen, along with an increased frequency of hypothyroidism, an underactive thyroid gland.

Typical physical characteristics include low-set ears, low hairline, webbed neck, broad chest with wide-spaced nipples, puffy hands and feet and pronounced bending out of the elbows. The average height at full growth is 4 feet 8 inches (150.3 cm).

Turner syndrome does not affect intelligence, but affected individuals tend to have poor spatial perceptual abilities and an increased incidence of specific learning disabilities. The need for psychological care and support for those affected can be as important as medical attention for the physical complications arising out of this disorder.

Most affected individuals do not have ovaries. Hormone therapy can replace the estrogen normally produced in these reproductive organs. However, while infertility is the rule, there have been exceptions, with isolated cases of women with Turner syndrome giving birth. Though the risk in such cases has been said to be high, with an increased risk of miscarriage (see ABORTION), STILLBIRTH, CHROMOSOME ABNORMALITY and malformations, some of this increased risk may be due to ascertainment bias. That is, the mother was found to have Turner syndrome only after investigation because of the adverse outcomes of childbirth.

New reproductive technologies have also been used to help women with Turner syndrome become pregnant should they so desire. A donor egg is used for in vitro fertilization to create an embryo that is carried by the Turner syndrome woman.

Approximately one-third of those identified are diagnosed in the neonatal period (the first six weeks of life), one-third during childhood and one-third during the late teens when they fail to sexually mature. Diagnosis is made by chromosomal analysis, which reveals the chromosomal aberration that causes the disorder. Growth hormone, which improves growth velocity and probably final adult height, is approved by the Food and Drug Administration for treatment of Turner syndrome.

PRENATAL DIAGNOSIS is accomplished by chromosome analysis, which may be prompted by an elevated maternal serum ALPHA-FETOPROTEIN or abnormal ULTRASOUND. Individuals with Turner syndrome have normal life expectancies and can lead full and productive lives.

turricephaly   See CRANIOSYNOSTOSIS.

twins   The result of the simultaneous gestation of two embryos in one mother. Twins occur in approximately one in 70 to one in 100 deliveries and may be either identical or fraternal. About 30% are identical and 70% fraternal. Twinning is also associated with increased risks for fetal development or structural defects due to uterine crowding.

Identical twins are monozygotic (MZ), the product of a single egg that divides into separate embryos soon after conception. Therefore, the twins share identical genetic endowments: All their GENES are the same. (Genetically, the children of identical co-twins are half-siblings, rather than cousins.) Identical twins occur in 3.5 to four of every 1,000 deliveries in all populations and ETHNIC GROUPS.

Fraternal twins are dizygotic (DZ). They originate from two separate eggs: Genetically, they are no more alike than SIBLINGS and may be either of the same or opposite sexes. The frequency of fraternal twins ranges from 16 per 1,000 in blacks to eight per 1,000 in white and four per 1,000 in Asians. There is also a familial tendency: Women who have had fraternal twins have a 3% chance of having fraternal twins again, about four times the rate found in the general population. The incidence of fraternal twins also increases with maternal age. Conceptions that occur soon after puberty have essentially a 0% chance of producing fraternal twins, rising to 15 per 1,000 births by the age of 37 and falling to 0% again shortly before menopause.

It has been suggested that the familial tendency toward dizygotic twinning is transmitted preferentially through the female line. Ethnic differences in the rate of dizygotic twinning is also evidence of genetic factors. In interracial marriages the rate follows that of the mother's ethnic group. An AUTOSOMAL DOMINANT gene has been found in sheep, that leads to higher concentrations of a hormone that stimulates ovulation and which leads to multiple ovulation.

Twins have commanded attention in cultures around the world throughout history. Mythical twins have often been depicted as healing gods or magicians, and in many fables they have the power to foretell the future, control fire and flood, promote fertility and cure disease. Mystical powers were imputed to the twins Castor and Polydeuces (Pollux among Romans) of Greek legend, who are represented in the constellation Gemini. The mythical founders of Rome, Romulus and Remus, were twins as well.

In some primitive societies, however, twins were considered dangerous aberrations, and mothers of twins, and in some cultures one or both twins as well, were immediately killed.

Genetically, twins are important in determining genetic components of traits, particularly those that do not demonstrate clear MENDELIAN inheritance patterns, such as CLEFT PALATE and blood pressure. (The degree to which twins both exhibit any given trait exhibited in one is called CONCORDANCE and is expressed as a percentage. If the trait is always present in both members of a twin pair when it is present in one, concordance is 100%.) Yet the potential importance of twin studies was not recognized until 1875, when Galton raised the question of the comparative influence of "nature and nurture" in twins' physical and mental character. Since that time, studies of twins have indicated that hereditary factors often exert more influence than environmental factors in shaping behavior.

In a twin pregnancy, any genetic risks faced will be considerably higher than if it were a singleton pregnancy. PRENATAL DIAGNOSIS in that setting is also more complicated. Techniques for selective ABORTION are possible when only one of a twin pair is found to be abnormal. Monozygotic twins (but not dizygotic ones) have an increased overall malformation rate of around 5%, double that for a singleton pregnancy. The increase is for a variety of structural abnormalities including NEURAL TUBE DEFECTS. MULTIPLE BIRTHS are seen with increased frequency following various reproductive techniques such as in vitro fertilization.

tyrosinemia   A group of disorders of the metabolism of tyrosine, an AMINO ACID.

Tyrosinemia type I, hepatorenal tyrosinemia, manifests in early infancy with FAILURE TO THRIVE, vomiting and diarrhea, and enlargement of the liver (hepatomegaly). Liver CANCERS are also characteristic. Death results from liver failure. Some patients have a more chronic form, with chronic liver disease (cirrhosis), kidney abnormalities and RICKETS. This form is thought to be due to the deficiency of the ENZYME fumaryl acetoacetase. Measurement of the enzyme allows PRENATAL DIAGNOSIS. The causative AUTOSOMAL RECESSIVE GENE is located on 15q.

Though it is rare in the general population, tyrosinemia I has been reported to have an incidence as high as one in 1,500 births in an isolated French Canadian population.

Drug therapy with the agent NTBC results in improvement of many of the metabolic abnormalities and improvement in liver function. It may also prevent the development of liver cirrhosis and abolish or diminish the risk of liver cancer. Liver transplantation offers definitive therapy.

Tyrosinemia type II is caused by a deficiency of the enzyme tyrosine aminotransferase. The gene is located at 16q. Termed oculocutaneous tyrosinemia, it is characterized by skin and ocular lesions and MENTAL RETARDATION in some individuals. In this form, skin lesions (patchy thickened areas of skin) primarily affect the palms and soles. The ocular findings include increased tearing, intolerance to bright light (photophobia) and inflammation and ulceration of the cornea. There is no liver or kidney disease. Many cases are of Mediterranean origin, particularly Italian. As in type I, inheritance is autosomal recessive.

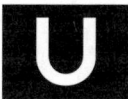

ultrasonography See ULTRASOUND.

ultrasound (ultrasonography) An imaging procedure for viewing a developing FETUS in the womb using high-frequency sound waves. It is one of the most common prenatal diagnostic procedures in use today. The sound waves, above the range of human hearing, are directed into the uterus. The echoes, reflected by the various densities of the fetal tissues encountered, are displayed on a TV-like monitor, forming an image. This image, interpreted by a skilled operator, can be useful for PRENATAL DIAGNOSIS, by itself or as a component of other prenatal diagnostic procedures.

Diagnoses using ultrasound are based on the images displayed and concern mostly structural details, although fine distinctions can be made in this respect. Ultrasound has proved useful, for example, in prenatal diagnosis of the enlarged skull caused by excessive fluid in the cranium (HYDROCEPHALY) and of an absence of brain tissue accompanied by a failure of the skull to close (ANENCEPHALY). Also, stunted limbs and some heart, kidney and intestinal defects can be disclosed by ultrasound. However, the inherent nature of ultrasound does not allow for genetic determinations through ultrasound itself.

Ultrasound is of vital importance in guiding the movement of the instruments employed in prenatal diagnostic procedures that are invasive in nature: AMNIOCENTESIS, CHORIONIC VILLUS SAMPLING, FETOSCOPY and fetal blood and tissue sampling.

Other uses of ultrasound fetal images include evaluating the age of the fetus, locating the placenta, determining fetal size, monitoring fetal growth, evaluating the amount of AMNIOTIC FLUID in the sac, determining if the pregnancy will produce twins or triplets and indicating the sex of the fetus.

The small exposure to ultrasound, as used, has not proved dangerous to either the mother or the fetus, and this procedure is considered relatively safe. However, physicians have cautioned that it should not be routinely performed unless suspected defects or other medical conditions warrant its use. Using ultrasound to determine the sex of the fetus or to show the mother an image or provide educational demonstrations is not generally recommended.

unilateral renal agenesis Affected individuals are born with only one kidney (usually on the right side). It may remain undiagnosed in the absence of other CONGENITAL ANOMALIES or future dysfunction of the remaining kidney. However, there is a reported 30–50% increased risk for problems in the remaining kidney. First-degree relatives (parents, children, SIBLINGS) of affected individuals should be examined for this condition as it demonstrates a familial aggregation, though the cause and mode of transmission are unknown. It should be distinguished from Potter syndrome, a fatal condition in which infants are born without either kidney (bilateral renal agenesis). First- degree relatives of a child with bilateral renal agenesis have a 13% chance of having silent unilateral renal agenesis. This increases to 30% in families in which two infants with Potter syndrome are born. In families in which unilateral renal agenesis has occurred, there is an increase in bilateral agenesis, as well. In other words, though the two defects are distinct, in families in which one of these anomalous conditions occurs, there is also an increased incidence of the other condition, in addition to other developmental abnormalities of the kidney. In females the fallopian tube may be missing on the same side, and there may be uterine and vaginal abnormalities.

Estimates of incidence range from one to two per 1,000 to one per 4,000. PRENATAL DIAGNOSIS can be accomplished by ULTRASOUND.

uniparental disomy Having both CHROMOSOMES in a pair inherited from one parent. The possibility that one parent could contribute both chromosomes was first suggested in 1980 by E. Engle and subsequently confirmed by molecular genetic analysis. Both copies of many different chromosomes have been found to be inherited this way, and specific abnormalities are associated with uniparental disomy at various regions of the chromosomes.

PRADER-WILLI SYNDROME and ANGELMAN SYNDROME, which are usually associated with chromosomal deletions (-15q) of paternal or maternal origin, respectively, can likewise result from uniparental disomy, so that genetic material from only one parent is expressed in those chromosomal regions.

Uniparental disomy also carries the risk of expressing a recessive disorder, if identical copies of a chromosome with a mutated recessive GENE make up the uniparental pair. CYSTIC FIBROSIS, BLOOM SYNDROME, OSTEOGENESIS IMPERFECTA, SPINAL MUSCULAR ATROPHY and congenital chloride diarrhea have all been inherited from a single carrier parent this way.

The condition has its genesis in TRISOMY, where both copies of one parent's chromosomes and a single copy of the other's are present at conception. Studies indicate 2–3% of all pregnancies may begin as a trisomy. Usually these result in non-viable pregnancies. However, through a process called "trisomy rescue," early in embryonic life, a cell line in which one of the extra chromosomes is eliminated, may develop, allowing survival of the embryo. One-third of such trisomy rescues result in uniparental disomy.

Uniparental maternal disomy for chromosome 7 is associated with severe pre- and postnatal growth retardation, accounting for about 10% of prenatal growth retardation. Uniparental paternal disomy for chromosome 11p is associated with BECKWITH-WEIDEMANN SYNDROME and various tumors (see CHROMOSOME ABNORMALITIES).

urea cycle defects A group of rare hereditary ENZYME disorders characterized by the accumulation of very high levels of ammonia in the blood and tissues (hyperammonemia). Symptoms include vomiting, lethargy, seizures, respiratory distress and coma, possibly leading to death in the first weeks of life, though some may be less severely affected. MENTAL RETARDATION and neurologic defects are common resultant disorders in the survivors.

Ammonia is a by-product of the metabolism of protein and its constituents, the AMINO ACIDS. The only way the body can eliminate ammonia is by converting it to urea (through the urea cycle) so that it can be excreted in urine. Most of this activity occurs in the liver. Several enzymes are necessary for this conversion, and an inherited deficiency of any one of the enzymes will result in a specific urea cycle disorder. These disorders, in total, have an estimated incidence of approximately one in 30,000 births.

Treatment for urea cycle disorders is individualized, based on the specific enzyme deficiency and the severity of the child's symptoms. In general, it involves the restriction of dietary protein and the use of medications which provide alternate pathways for ammonia removal from the blood. Frequently, the medications are accompanied by amino acid therapy and other special dietary supplements. In some cases, liver transplantation has been done successfully as a cure for the disorder.

Argininemia This deficiency of the enzyme arginase may result in mental retardation, seizures and progressive spastic diplegia. It is diagnosed by the finding of elevated levels of arginine in the urine and blood, which may be reduced by low protein diets. Inherited as an autosomal recessive trait, the gene maps to 6q. Parents of affected infants have been reported to have subnormal arginase activity in red blood cells, which may allow carrier detection and prenatal diagnosis in some cases.

Argininosuccinic aciduria Characterized by severe symptoms of hyperammonemia in the majority of affected infants, a significant proportion may be less severely affected and may come to medical attention due to mild mental retardation and a natural aversion to protein. Affected individuals often have hair and skin abnormalities as well.

Inherited as an autosomal recessive trait, it results from deficiency of the enzyme, argininosuccinic acid lyase, the gene for which maps to 7q.

Both prenatal diagnosis and carrier detection are possible.

Carbamyl phosphate synthetase deficiency (CPS-I) In general, one of the more severe forms of UCD. Diagnosis is made based on examination of enzyme activity of CPS-I in liver tissue. A low-protein diet and complex regimen of drug therapy may be beneficial for some affected. Inherited as an autosomal recessive trait, the gene maps to 2q. Prenatal diagnosis may be possible using genetic linkage studies.

Citrullinemia This may manifest with severe symptoms soon after birth, or may have onset in later childhood and exhibit a much more benign course. The variations are thought to be due to varying levels of reduced enzyme activity among affected individuals. Protein-restricted diets are recommended. Diagnosis is easily made from the massive amounts of citrulline excreted in the urine and its higher levels in the blood.

Inherited as an autosomal recessive disorder, it results from deficiency of the enzyme argininosuccinate synthetase. The gene maps to 9q. It may be diagnosed prenatally.

Ornithine transcarbamylase (OTC) deficiency This X-LINKED disorder is often lethal in males during early infancy. They may have a complete absence, or less than 1% of normal levels of the enzyme OTC. Surviving males are treated similarly to those with CPS deficiency. Females are much more mildly and variably affected. Enzyme activity is 10% to 40% of normal level. They may be entirely asymptomatic, have lethargy and nausea after eating a high protein meal, or be as symptomatic as affected males.

Affected females are typically placed on low-protein diets. Carrier identification for females is possible in some cases, and prenatal diagnosis is now available using molecular analysis with the cloned OTC gene.

Usher syndrome (retinitis pigmentosa and congenital deafness)

A group of inherited disorders characterized by hearing loss and deteriorating vision. The hearing loss is usually profound and present at birth, but may be milder and occur soon after birth. If the DEAFNESS is not profound, it usu-

ally does not deteriorate beyond the deficit first exhibited. The loss of vision is a result of RETINITIS PIGMENTOSA, a group of disorders resulting in retinal degeneration and possibly leading to BLINDNESS. The retinal problems begin with NIGHT BLINDNESS, followed by blind spots, then slowly progressive tunnel vision in daylight. Both rods and cones deteriorate. RP may result in what is classified as legally blind in cases of Usher, but most individuals retain some vision.

The relationship of hearing loss to RP is not well understood. The association was first reported in 1858 by A. von Graefe, but is named for the Scottish opthalmologist Charles H. Usher (1865–1942), who first emphasized the hereditary nature of the disorder in 1914. Approximately 30% of all RP patients report some degree of hearing impairment.

The major forms of Usher syndrome are classified as type 1, 2 or 3, based on severity and age of onset, with 1 being the most severe. It is characterized by complete (profound) hearing loss, poor balance and vision loss in early childhood. Infants respond only to very loud, low tones.

In type 2, infants are born with moderate to severe hearing deficits, from mild loss in low frequencies to severe-to-profound loss in the high frequencies. Balance is normal in some but reportedly affected in others. Vision problems develop in late childhood or adolescence, and individuals are legally blind by early adulthood.

Individuals with type 3 are believed to be born with minor to mild hearing loss which deteriorates over a decade or more, with auditory deficits similar to type 2. Some progressive balance disturbance has been suggested as occurring. Type 3 has been estimated to comprise only 2% of all Usher syndrome cases. However, over 40% of patients with Usher syndrome in Finland appear to have type 3, and they have been the subject of a study to learn more about this form.

There are an estimated 10,000 individuals with Usher syndrome in the United States. It is believed responsible for about 50% of deaf-blindness in adults. Occurring in the order of one in 15,000 and one in 30,000 live births, it accounts for 3–6% of all deaf children and perhaps an equal percentage of hard-of-hearing youngsters. A relatively higher frequency of type 1 has been found in

French Canadians, Louisiana Cajuns, Argentineans of Spanish descent, Ashkenazi Jews and Nigerians.

All forms of Usher syndrome are inherited by autosomal recessive transmission, but genes at several different loci have been found to be capable of causing the disorder, even among those with the same subtype. Mutations in at least 10 different genes, the *CDH23, MASS1, MYO7A, PCDH15, USH1A, USH1C, USH1E, USH1G, USH2A,* and *USH3A* genes, cause Usher syndrome. At least seven different genes appear to be involved in type 1. The most frequent, the gene for myosin *VIIA,* is on 11q. (Different mutations in this same gene cause nonsyndromic autosomal dominant and autosomal recessive sensorineural hearing loss.) The other genes that can cause Usher syndrome, type 1, include the *CDH23* gene on chromosome 10q, the *PCDH15* gene, also on 10q, and the *USH1C* gene on 11p. Other mutations in any of these genes can also lead to autosomal recessive nonsyndromic deafness. A particular mutation in the *PCDH15* gene is the most common cause of Usher syndrome, type 1, in Ashkenazi Jews. Mutations in the *USH1A* gene on 14q, the *USH1E* gene on 21q and the *USH1G* gene on 17q also can cause type 1, Usher syndrome.

Most people with type 2 appear to have a mutation in the *USH2A* gene, which encodes the usherin protein, on the long arm of chromosome 1. Usher syndrome, type 2, can be caused by mutations in at least four genes, which in addition to the *USH2A* gene include the *MASS1* (also called *VLGR1*) gene, which is located on the long arm of chromosome 5. Other mutations in the *USH2A* gene cause RETINITIS PIGMENTOSA. About 25% to 50% of patients with retinitis pigmentosa have an *USH2A* mutation. Mutations in the *USH3A* gene (located on the long arm of chromosome 3) cause Usher syndrome, type III. Mutations in another gene, as yet unidentified but believed to be located on 3q, also appear to cause type 3.

There is no cure for the loss of hearing, which results from an inner ear problem, or for the loss of vision. The hearing of some patients has reportedly benefited from cochlear implants.

The combination of deafness and blindness creates problems both in diagnosing the condition and coping with psychological implications. Deteriorating vision, which typically begins in the late teen years, may go unrecognized for a long period of time. Individuals have no way of knowing that what they see is different from what others see. Individuals may exhibit clumsiness and bump into people and objects. They may have many small auto accidents, be labeled as inattentive and stupid and be unable to follow group conversations in sign language because of the inability to see more than one person at a time. There is a strong tendency toward denial of visual problems among those first diagnosed with Usher, and care must be taken to help individuals cope with the eventual condition of deaf-blindness. Patients require extensive counseling and information about the condition.

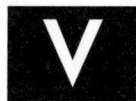

Van der Woude syndrome   A SYNDROME of LIP PITS in combination with CLEFT LIP or CLEFT PALATE; 80% of all cases of lip pits are seen with this disorder, and it is a significant source of facial clefts.

Great variability of expression is a hallmark of this SYNDROME. A mildly affected parent may have a severely affected child and vice versa. Overall risk to inherit a CLEFT from an affected parent is about 20%. Among those affected, 33–44% have pits without a cleft; 26–66% have pits with a cleft, depending on whether mild clefts of palate are included; 10% have a cleft without pits; and perhaps as many as 20%, though probably less, have neither. Less than 1% of patients with cleft lip and palate have lip pits.

Inherited as an autosomal dominant disorder, the gene for Van der Woude syndrome, *IRF6*, is located on 1q. *IRF6* encodes interferon regulatory factor-6. Incidence is estimated to be one in 35,000 to one in 100,000. Thirty % to 50% are new mutations. In all cases of clefts, the child and parents should be examined for lip pits.

Different mutations in the *IRF6* gene cause the more severe and much rarer popliteal pterygium syndrome, which presents with cleft lip and palate and webbing of the lower extremities, as well as external genital abnormalities, anomalies of the skin around the nails and adhesive folds of skin connecting the jaws or eyelids.

varicella (chicken pox; congenital varicella syndrome)   Fetal exposure during the first two trimesters of pregnancy to varicella, the virus that causes chicken pox, is associated with severe BIRTH DEFECTS.

One to seven women in 10,000 will develop chicken pox during pregnancy. (About 3.9 million cases of varicella are estimated to occur annually in the United States, most in otherwise healthy children under age 10.) CONGENITAL varicella syndrome occurs in about 2% of infants born to women who contract varicella in the first or second trimester of pregnancy. It is extremely rare if infection occurs after 20 weeks. Congenital varicella syndrome is associated with profound abnormalities of the skin, limbs, eyes and central nervous system and can include scars, defects of muscle and bone, malformed and paralyzed limbs, a smaller-than-normal head, BLINDNESS, seizures and MENTAL RETARDATION. Another risk is a severe chicken pox infection in the newborn which occurs when the mother develops the rash from five days before to two days after delivery. Without preventative treatment, about 25% of newborns become infected and develop a rash between five and 10 days after birth. Up to 30% of infected babies die if not treated. A susceptible pregnant woman should avoid anyone with this highly contagious disease, and any susceptible individual who has been in contact with an infected person.

A susceptible (that is, not immune) pregnant woman who has been in close contact with someone who has chicken pox, should receive varicella zoster immune globulin (VZIG), which is safe for mother and baby. When given within 96 hours after exposure, VZIG helps prevent chicken pox, or at least lessens its severity. This is important for the pregnant woman, as complications of chicken pox, such as pneumonia, are much more common in adults than in children. It is not yet known whether giving VZIG to a pregnant woman helps to protect the FETUS from infection. Shingles (herpes zoster) is caused by a limited reactivation of the chicken pox virus, usually years later. It causes painful, localized clusters of blisters. Doctors believe it is unlikely that shingles during pregnancy can cause birth defects.

In 1995, the Food and Drug Administration approved a chicken pox vaccine. The American Academy of Pediatrics recommends the chicken pox vaccine for all children between 12 and 18 months who do not have a history of chicken pox. Older children should be immunized at the earliest opportunity. If a woman has never had chicken pox and blood tests show that she is not immune to chicken pox—and she is not yet pregnant—she should ask about getting vaccinated. Pregnant women should not be vaccinated and women should postpone attempts to conceive for at least three months after vaccination. (See also TERATOGEN.)

variegate porphyria   See PORPHYRIA.

VATER association   The acronym VATER describes a group of abnormalities that are found together more frequently than would be expected at random: vertebral anomalies; anal malformations (IMPERFORATE ANUS); an abnormal passage from the trachea to the esophagus (tracheoesophageal fistula); and thumb and forearm (radial limb) abnormalities. At least three of these abnormalities must be present to be considered an example of the VATER association.

About 60% of affected individuals also have congenital HEART DEFECTS. Kidney abnormalities (most often absence of one kidney) are also common. In addition, half-formed vertebrae and spinal deformities near the pelvis frequently occur, as well as an absent or malformed radius bone in the forearm. Because of the kidney and cardiac involvement, the acronym VACTERL, with *c* for cardiac, *r* for renal and *l* for limb anomalies, is sometimes used. The features overlap with those of the TOWNES-BROCKS syndrome.

About 75% of affected individuals survive infancy. Heart failure is the most common cause of death. Although surviving infants tend to be small and usually require surgery, they grow to the normal range of height and weight by four or five years of age.

Almost all cases have been SPORADIC, and it is probably etiologically heterogeneous; that is, different defects result in the same disorder (see HETERO-GENEITY). The basic cause of the abnormalities is not known, although they are believed to result from an event during the second month of gestation, when differentiation of organ systems (morphogenesis) takes place in the fetus. No drug or virus has been implicated, and no CHROMOSOME ABNORMALITY has been found in the majority of cases, but the components of the association can be found in some infants with chromosome ANOMALIES. It is seen more frequently in offspring of diabetic mothers. PRENATAL DIAGNOSIS of this disorder is currently unavailable, but ULTRASOUND may detect skeletal, kidney or heart defects.

VDT   See VIDEO DISPLAY TERMINALS.

ventricular septal defects   See HEART DEFECTS.

video display terminals (VDTs)   By 1998 some 50 million American workers were using computers, many of them women of childbearing age. The potential link between maternal exposure to video display terminals during pregnancy and an increased risk of miscarriage (see ABORTION) has received a great deal of attention, though there is no clear consensus on the actual danger.

Suggestions that use of VDTs can have an adverse impact on pregnancy are based on their radiation emissions. Additionally, several small "clusters" of miscarriages and BIRTH DEFECTS have been reported among women who used VDTs during pregnancy. Subsequent animal studies with chicken eggs and pregnant mice exposed to similar electromagnetic radiation were inconclusive. Studies of reported clusters have found the variety of defects indicated no common source, nor were they of the type associated with high radiation levels. Reliable epidemiological studies have concluded that the incidence of adverse pregnancy among women who use VDTs in pregnancy and those who don't are not statistically different.

A 1988 study in California reported the risk of miscarriage was almost doubled for women in clerical positions who worked with VDTs 20 more hours per week, though none for women in management who worked with VDTs for the same amount of time. However, a 1991 study by the National Institute for Occupational Safety and Health, one of the largest and most comprehensive on the subject, found the risk of miscarriage among women who worked with VDTs all day and those who didn't was identical. The study also found the level of radiation users were exposed to was no higher than that found in most homes.

Both the American College of Obstetricians and Gynecologists and the American Medical Association have concluded that the levels of radiation emitted by VDTs are insufficient to cause birth defects or miscarriage.

However, animal studies have found that very low frequency, pulsed, non-ionizing electromagnetic radiation emitted by VDTs can interfere with embryonic cellular growth. Little is known about the effects of this type of radiation; furthermore, most of the radiation is emitted from the back and sides of the terminal, so that the individual sitting in front of the terminal may be less exposed than an individual in back of it.

Pregnant women who are concerned about VDT use can minimize their exposure by sitting an arm's length away from the front of the computer screen. The strength of VDT emissions drop off quickly after about 24 inches. Neither lead aprons nor any other type of radiation shield stops the emissions.

Many VDT workers complain about neck, back, wrist, hand and shoulder pain, termed repetitive strain injury, as well as eye strain. Psychological stress is also frequently reported, and some studies have suggested that high levels of stress may adversely affect pregnancy. Many of the other physical and psychological stresses of VDT work can be eliminated or reduced by appropriately timed work breaks and good workplace design. The VDT workstation may have to be modified during pregnancy because of changing body proportion.

Legislation has been introduced in a number of states in the United States to regulate exposure to VDTs for all workers, and include provisions for pregnant women. Additionally, some unions representing clerical workers have negotiated contracts allowing women to transfer to jobs that don't involve VDT exposure should they become pregnant.

vitamins Use of some vitamins in pregnancy has been shown to have an impact on fetal development. Most noteworthy is folic acid, a B vitamin, whose use has been shown to decrease NEURAL TUBE DEFECTS (NTDs), which include SPINA BIFIDA and ANENCEPHALY. The Institute of Medicine, a federal agency that sets nutritional guidelines, recommends pregnant women take 600 micrograms of folic acid daily. (Other adults are advised to take 400 micrograms.)

The link between vitamins, or nutrition, and NTDs has been noted for some decades. NTDs are more common in the offspring of women in lower socio-economic groups and women who have poor diets. Additionally, there was an "epidemic" of neural tube defects during the Depression, a time when many people, including women of childbearing age, received substandard nutrition. However, the potential link between vitamin deficiencies and neural tube defects did not receive scientific attention until after World War II, when it was noted that women in England, Holland and Germany who had been malnourished gave birth to an unexpectedly large number of infants with these developmental defects. Yet, it was only in the 1980s that researchers examined the link scientifically.

One early study found women who take multivitamins (including folic acid) at the time of conception had 60% less risk of giving birth to an infant with a neural tube defect than women who did not use vitamins. A later study by Boston University's Center for Human Genetics, published in 1989 and involving 23,000 pregnant women, found those who reported taking multivitamins in the first six weeks of pregnancy had rates of NTDs in their offspring only one-quarter the rates of women who did not use vitamins. (NTD incidence was 0.9 per 1,000 births among vitamin users vs. 3.5 per 1,000 births among non–vitamin users.) A study by the National Institute of Child Health and Human Development published in 1997 found 100 micrograms of folic acid daily produced a blood folate level sufficient to reduce NTDs about 22%. A 200 microgram daily dose was associated with a 41% reduced risk of NTDs, and dosages of 400 micrograms with a reduction of 47%.

In its natural state, folic acid is found in foods including citrus fruits, dark green leafy vegetables, dried beans and liver. Due to dietary deficiency, the Food and Drug Administration (FDA) recommends pregnant women take vitamin supplements to be assured of receiving the recommended daily requirement. However, folic acid is particularly important to fetal development in the first month, a time when many pregnancies are undetected. By the time the pregnancy is recognized, a shortage of folic acid could have led to a nascent NTD. For that reason, in 1998 the FDA mandated fortifying all enriched foods with folic acid, representing the first new fortification of foods since 1943, and the first addition aimed at reducing BIRTH DEFECTS. It is added to enriched breads and flour, cornmeal, rice and pasta products. Levels are set to keep daily intake below 1 milligram, as doses above that can mask the symptoms of pernicious ANEMIA (which primarily affects the elderly).

A study at the University of Aberdeen in Scotland found that children of mothers who had an insufficient intake of vitamin E during pregnancy were at a higher risk of developing asthma by age five and more prone to wheezing. The children of women in the lowest 20% of prenatal vitamin E intake in the study group were five times as likely to develop asthma by this age as the children of women in the top 20%.

Some vitamins can cause birth defects when taken in large quantities. Concern has been raised regarding vitamin A, particularly since a vitamin A derivative, ACCUTANE, is known to be teratogenic. A study published in *The New England Journal of Medicine* in 1995 found consumption of vitamin A at or above 10,000 IU (international units) was linked to birth defects. That is twice as high as the recommended daily value (a term that replaces U.S. RDAs) for vitamin A. The type of vitamin A linked to the defects is pre-formed vitamin A found in animal products (especially liver), fortified breakfast cereals and some vitamin supplements. Pre-formed vitamin A is immediately available to the body. Babies born to mothers who took more than 10,000 IU of pre-formed vitamin A per day showed an increased rate of a variety of birth defects including those of the heart, neural tube, brain, limbs, kidneys and genitals.

Many prenatal supplements now provide vitamin A as beta-carotene, because this form of the nutri-

ent is not linked with birth defects. Carotenoids, including beta-carotene, are plant-based vitamin A sources that are transformed into an active form of vitamin A once they have been digested. The American College of Obstetricians and Gynecologists recommends 5,000 IU of vitamin A as the maximum intake prior to and during pregnancy. Eating fruits and vegetables rich in beta-carotene is also recommended, some of the best sources being broccoli, carrots, sweet potatoes, cantaloupe and winter squash.

vitiligo   A benign condition characterized by well-defined patches of depigmented skin. Similar to PIEBALD SKIN TRAIT, its only impact is cosmetic. However, vitiligo is distinguished from the piebald trait by its onset after birth and tendency to progress or regress.

The etiology is unknown and the exact mode of inheritance is unclear, though familial aggregation has been seen. One study found 20% of PROBANDS reported one or more first-degree relatives also affected. Offspring of probands were found to have the highest relative risk for developing vitiligo, followed by SIBLINGS, parents and grandparents. It is 10 to 15 times more common in patients with immune disorders.

von Gierke disease   See GLYCOGEN STORAGE DISEASE.

von Hippel–Lindau syndrome (VHL)   The hallmark of this hereditary disorder is the abnormal growth and proliferation of blood vessels (HEMANGIOMA) on the retina of the eye and the cerebellum of the brain. Onset is in early adulthood, with initial symptoms of headaches, dizziness and visual disturbances, progressing to uncontrolled clumsy movements on one side of the body (unilateral ataxia), BLINDNESS and permanent brain damage. The disorder is frequently associated with cysts and CANCERS in the kidneys and pancreas. Hemangiomas of lung and liver and adrenal tumors (pheochromocytomas) may also be seen. Variability in expression is great; that is, the SYNDROME expresses itself differently in every patient. Even in the same family, affected members may show only one, or several features of VHL.

Cryotherapy (a surgical procedure involving ultra-cold temperatures) of the retina may alleviate some ocular symptoms. Cysts may be treated with conventional surgical techniques.

The estimated incidence is one in 36,000 live births. Inherited as an AUTOSOMAL DOMINANT trait, it is named for Eugen von Hippel (1867–1939), a German ophthalmologist, and Swedish pathologist Arvid Lindau (b. 1892), who published descriptions in 1895 and 1926, respectively. The VHL GENE, a tumor suppressor gene, is mapped to 3p. The types of MUTATIONS responsible for VHL without pheochromocytoma differ from those responsible for VHL with pheochromocytoma. More than 300 different mutations have been identified. Presymptomatic detection of affected individuals by DEOXYRIBONUCLEIC ACID (DNA) analysis is now possible for more than 80% of VHL families. Somatic mutation or inactivation of the VHL gene has been found also in 85% of the random kidney cancers in the general population. About 5% of VHL cases are the result of new SPORADIC mutations.

von Recklinghausen disease   See NEUROFIBROMA-TOSIS.

von Willebrand disease   The first hereditary bleeding disorder distinguished from HEMOPHILIA. Inherited (usually) as an AUTOSOMAL DOMINANT trait, this relatively common disorder is characterized by prolonged bleeding and easy bruising, which manifests at an early age, and as excessive bleeding after dental extractions or surgery, and excess blood loss during menstruation. The severity of symptoms decreases with age. It is named for Finnish physician Eric A. von Willebrand (1879–1949), who found the condition among the inhabitants of the Aland Islands in the Sea of Bothnia between Sweden and Finland. He published a description of the condition in 1926, calling it "pseudohemophilia."

It has been demonstrated that the platelets responsible for clotting are normal, but they have reduced adhesiveness due to a factor VIII deficiency. The GENE responsible for the von Willebrand factor is on 12p.

Mild von Willebrand disease may affect as much as 1% of the population. The frequency of new MUTATIONS in this gene is low. Most mutations in the gene act in an autosomal dominant manner, with reduced (an estimated 60%) PENETRANCE. In rare cases, different mutations in the same gene have AUTOSOMAL RECESSIVE inheritance. PRENATAL DIAGNOSIS has been accomplished in some families with a partic ularly severe form of the disease. A variety of blood factor replacement measures may treat bleeding episodes successfully.

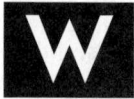

Waardenburg syndrome (WS) The most striking features of this inherited condition are the abnormal pigmentation seen in the hair, skin and eyes, though its most serious feature is CONGENITAL sensorineural DEAFNESS. Named for Dutch physician P. J. Waardenburg, who first described it in 1951, it is estimated to account for 2% of congenital deafness.

In its classic form there is a white forelock of depigmented hair, premature graying, milky white patches of skin (VITILIGO) and eyes of differing colors (HETERO-CHROMIA IRIDES). The white forelock may be present at birth and later disappear. The inner portion of the eye slits (palpebral fissures) may not extend toward the nose as far as would normally be expected (lateral displacement of inner canthi). The eyebrows may grow together (SYNOPHRYS) over a broad nasal bridge. CLEFT PALATE may also be present.

Two primary forms of this disorder, labeled as type I and type II, have been documented. In type I there is lateral displacement of the inner canthi; in type II, there is not. Mild to profound sensorineural hearing loss is reported in an estimated 25% of those affected with type I and 50% of those with type II. White forelock and skin patches are more frequent in type I. Heterochromia irides are more common in WS type II. Diagnosis may be made at birth, or soon after, based on pigmentary and facial manifestations. Hearing aids and educational assistance are usually recommended when hearing impairment is present. Life expectancy and intelligence are unaffected, though apparent MENTAL RETARDATION may be associated with significant hearing impairment.

Another form has been called WS type III and has also been referred to as the KLEIN-WAARDENBURG syndrome. A very severe disorder, it includes pronounced upper-limb defects. A disorder designated type IV, or Waardenburg-Shah syndrome, or Waardenburg-Hirschsprung disease, combines features of Waardenburg syndrome and HIRSCHSPRUNG DISEASE.

Inherited as an AUTOSOMAL DOMINANT trait, Type I is caused by MUTATIONS in the *PAX3* GENE located on chromosome 2q. It encodes a TRANSCRIPTION FACTOR. The *PAX3* protein directly regulates another transcription factor, called the microphthalmia associated transcription factor or *MITF*. Mutations in the *MITF* gene (located on 3p) are found in about 20% of Waardenburg syndrome type II. This transcription factor (*MITF*) has been shown to activate the gene for tyrosinase, a key ENZYME for the generation of the melanin pigment (see ALBINISM), and is involved in the differentiation of melanocytes, or pigment cells. Absence of melanocytes affects pigmentation in the skin, hair, and eyes and hearing function in the cochlea (inner ear.) Thus, the pigmentation abnormalities and hearing loss in many cases of type II are likely to be the results of an anomaly of melanocyte differentiation caused by *MITF* mutations, and failure of the regulation of *MITF* due to *PAX3* mutations causes the auditory and pigmentary symptoms in type I. Other cases of type II appear to be caused by another gene that maps to 1p. WS type III appears to be a homozygous (see HOMOZYGOTE) form of Waardenburg syndrome (with homozygous *PAX3* mutations), and in other cases, it appears to be a CONTIGUOUS GENE SYNDROME with deletion of *PAX3* and other adjacent genetic sequences. Type IV results from mutation in the endothelin-B receptor gene (13q), in the gene for endothelin-3 (20q), or in the *SOX10* gene (22q). Mutations in the *endothelin 3 gene (EDN3)* can also cause type IV. Other mutations in this gene can cause HIRSCHSPRUNG DISEASE without Waardenburg syndrome. In some cases of Waardenburg syndrome, type II, both copies of the *SNAI2* gene (located on the long arm of chromosome 8) are missing. One copy of the *SNAI2* gene is missing in some cases of PIEBALD SKIN TRAIT, another condition characterized by a white hair forelock and depigmented patches of skin.

Waardenburg syndrome is estimated to occur in about one in 40,000 live births, though there is a wide variability of severity and expression. Not all gene CARRIERS will have the distinctive pigmentary abnormalities, and not all will be deaf; affected, yet apparently asymptomatic individuals can transmit the disorder to offspring. (As for the signature white forelock and premature graying, these conditions are common in the population and are not in themselves an indication of WS.) Advanced paternal age has been associated with SPORADIC mutations.

WS has been reported in American blacks, Maoris (aboriginal New Zealanders) and whites. In South Australia, this is a leading cause of deafness and holds a position similar to that of PORPHYRIA in South Africa, having been introduced by early settlers (with many descendants).

Walt Disney dwarfism (geroderma osteodysplastica) First described in a Swiss family in 1950, in addition to short stature, characteristic features of this disorder include changes in the skin that suggest premature aging, and osseous (bone) changes, including osteoporosis, susceptibility to fractures and multiple lines on bones that appear like growth rings of trees.

A physical appearance similar to the characters in *Snow White and the Seven Dwarfs*, Walt Disney's animated film, was noted in affected family members, hence the name of the disorder. Inherited as an AUTOSOMAL RECESSIVE trait, it is very rare.

wandering spleen One or more of the ligaments that normally hold the spleen in place are absent or underdeveloped in this rare CONGENITAL BIRTH DEFECT. The untethered organ may shift position, or "wander" into the lower abdominal or pelvis area. The movement may interfere with the function of the spleen or other organs, and may also complicate diagnosis of the underlying cause. Twisting of the spleen and compression of its blood vessels may cause it to enlarge.

Some affected children may experience acute or chronic abdominal pain, accompanied by vomiting and fatigue, though others may remain asymptomatic. The episodes may be provoked by spontaneous movement of the spleen. The malposition of the spleen has led, in some cases, to its misidentification as an abdominal mass. In severe cases, blood flow to the spleen is reduced and excessive amounts of platelets and red blood cells collect in the greatly enlarged spleen.

In suspected cases, the spleen can be externally pushed into its normal position. Definitive diagnosis is made with ultrasonography and CT scans.

The cause of congenital wandering spleen is unknown, but may arise from defective development of the mesogastrium dorsum, the embryonic structure from which the ligaments that anchor the spleen originate. Males are more frequently affected than females during the first two years of life, though from age two to 21 they are affected equally. About half the cases have had onset below age 10.

The disorder also occurs in a non-hereditary, adult onset form, which affects females 20 times more frequently than males. Pregnancy is believed to exacerbate laxity of the ligaments.

warfarin embryopathy Warfarin is an anticoagulant that is prescribed to treat and prevent blood clots, certain cardiac conditions and strokes. Taken during the first trimester of pregnancy, warfarin increases the risk of miscarriage (see ABORTION and STILLBIRTH), and causes a SYNDROME of CONGENITAL defects in 5% to 25% of infants exposed IN UTERO. Infants with warfarin embryopathy have an abnormally small nose with deformed cartilage. Nasal passages are small and in some cases blocked, creating breathing difficulties. LOW BIRTH WEIGHT, slow development, BLINDNESS and other ocular problems, and bone deformities such as shortened fingers are also seen.

Features resemble the AUTOSOMAL DOMINANT or X-LINKED forms of CHONDRODYSPLASIA PUNCTATA. The only difference may be the absence of skin and hair changes. Warfarin inhibits the activity of an ENZYME named arylsulfatase E (ARSE), and this appears to cause the features of the syndrome. MUTATIONS in the ARSE GENE cause the X-linked form of chondrodysplasia punctata.

Though exposure during the sixth to ninth weeks after conception carries the greatest risk of ANOMALIES, when taken during the second and third trimester of pregnancy, warfarin still may cause MENTAL RETARDATION, an abnormally small head (MICROCEPHALY) and vision problems.

Watson-Alagille syndrome   See ALAGILLE SYNDROME.

Werdnig-Hoffmann disease   See SPINAL MUSCULAR ATROPHY.

Werner syndrome (WS)   Also called "PROGERIA of the adult," WS has several features resembling premature aging. Affected individuals appear normal during childhood but stop growing during their early teenage years. There is a premature graying or whitening of hair, early CATARACT formation, development of aged-looking skin with hard, scaly patches (SCLERODERMA), a high-pitched voice, weakening of muscles, poor wound healing, chronic leg and ankle ulcers, hardening and loss of elasticity of the walls of the arteries (atherosclerosis), loss of calcium from bones (osteoporosis) and DIABETES MELLITUS. Affected individuals have the appearance of old age by 30 to 40 years of age. About 10% develop CANCERS. Mean age of survival is 47, with a range of 31 to 63.

The SYNDROME is named for Otto Werner (1879–1936), a general practitioner in Eddelak, Germany, who first described it in 1904 when he made it the subject of his doctoral thesis.

While there is no specific diagnostic test, affected individuals exhibit elevated levels of hyaluronic acid in their urine, as do individuals with progeria. Currently, there is no method to identify CARRIERS or for PRENATAL DIAGNOSIS of this disorder.

Incidence estimates range from one in 1,000,000 to 20 per 1,000,000. More than 400 cases have been reported. Inherited as an AUTOSOMAL RECESSIVE trait, it results from a MUTATION in a DEOXYRIBONUCLEIC ACID (DNA) helicase GENE mapped to 8p. DNA helicases have been implicated in a number of molecular processes, including unwinding of DNA during replication, DNA repair, and accurate chromosomal segregation.

whistling face syndrome (Freeman Sheldon syndrome; craniocarpotarsal dysplasia)   Taking its name from its characteristic facial appearance, features consist of a mask-like, immobile expression, with a flat mid-face, deeply set, widely spaced eyes (HYPERTELORISM), a long philtrum (the groove extending from the upper lip to the nose), small nose, receding chin and small mouth (microstomia) fixed in a puckered position, as if whistling. Additional abnormalities are flexion contractures of the hands and CLUBFOOT deformities: The ankles are twisted inward, and the sole turned upward, so that the heel is the lowest part of the foot (talipes equinovarus).

The SYNDROME was first described in 1938 by Ernest A. Freeman (1900–75) and Joseph H. Sheldon (1893–1972), senior orthopedic surgeon and senior physician at the Royal Wolverhampton Hospital in England. They called the condition "craniocarpotarsal DYSPLASIA" in their original report of two unrelated children that they presented at the Royal Society of Medicine in London. It is sometimes referred to by that name, or as Freeman-Sheldon syndrome.

The basic defect that causes this disorder is unknown. Most cases have been SPORADIC, but there is evidence it can be inherited as an AUTOSOMAL DOMINANT trait with variable EXPRESSIVITY. An AUTOSOMAL RECESSIVE form has also been reported.

The diagnosis of the condition is made by the distinctive facial appearance combined with the characteristic musculoskeletal abnormalities, although some cases have been mistaken as ARTHROGRYPOSIS multiplex congenita.

Intelligence and life span are normal. However, vomiting and swallowing difficulties may lead to FAILURE TO THRIVE in infancy, and retarded growth and short stature are common features. Surgical treatment may improve facial appearance and functioning of the hands and feet.

There is no accepted method of PRENATAL DIAGNOSIS, though ULTRASOUND and FETOSCOPY have been used in some pregnancies to detect severe skeletal abnormalities.

Williams syndrome (elfin facies with hypercalcemia)

The two major features of this SYNDROME are a characteristic, elfin facial appearance and CONGENITAL HEART DEFECTS. Affected individuals often have LOW BIRTH WEIGHT and exhibit FAILURE TO THRIVE and developmental delays in sitting, walking, talking, as well as in development of motor skills. Adult height is generally slightly smaller than average.

The classic characteristics were first described in 1961 by Dr. J. C. P. Williams of New Zealand. The facial features include flat mid-face with full cheeks, thick, wide lips with open mouth, upturned nostrils (anteverted nares), broad forehead, widely spaced teeth, small chin, puffiness around the eyes and depressed nasal bridge. The head tends to be small. The ears may be prominent. These features become more striking with age.

Ocular findings may be present, including a star-like pattern in the iris (stellate iris pattern) of blue- and green-eyed children, and sometimes corneal opacities or crossed eyes (STRABISMUS).

Any of several cardiovascular abnormalities may be present, and include narrowing (stenosis) of the aorta just above the aortic valve, narrowing of the pulmonic valve or pulmonary arteries, and atrial or ventricular septal defects. Some infants with Williams syndrome have elevations in their blood calcium level. When hypercalcemia is present, it can cause irritability or "colic-like" symptoms. In most cases, the problem resolves on its own during childhood, but occasionally dietary or medical treatment is needed and a lifelong abnormality in calcium or vitamin D metabolism may persist.

Children with Williams syndrome may also be hypersensitive to sound and exhibit friendly, talkative, impulsive personalities. They are typically unafraid of strangers and show a greater interest in contact with adults than with their peers. They usually read and write poorly and struggle with simple arithmetic. Yet they display a facility for spoken language and for recognizing faces. As a group, they tend to be empathetic, loquacious and sociable. They often have remarkable musical abilities, though patients with Williams syndrome are often described as having a harsh, brassy or hoarse voice.

MENTAL RETARDATION and attention-deficit disorders are common features, and perceptual and motor functions may be impaired.

The basic cause of Williams syndrome is unknown, though the inability to handle calcium, demonstrated by some patients, may play a role. Williams syndrome appears to be a CONTIGUOUS GENE SYNDROME with affected patients exhibiting a submicroscopic deletion of the long arm of chromosome 7; that is, they are missing some genetic material from 7q. The deleted area includes the gene that makes the protein elastin (a protein which provides strength and elasticity to vessel walls.) It is likely that the elastin gene deletion accounts for many of the physical features of Williams syndrome, including the involvement of the heart and blood vessels.

Some of the other medical and developmental problems are probably caused by deletions of additional genetic material near the elastin gene on chromosome 7. Another gene involved in its pathogenesis is that for LIM-kinase-1 (LIMK1). The absence of a copy of the LIMK1 gene has been proposed as the basis for the impaired visuospatial cognitive abilities in this disorder.

The incidence is estimated to be approximately one in 20,000 live births. In most families, the child with Williams syndrome is the only one to have the condition, and it has been a SPORADIC occurrence. However, the individual with Williams syndrome has a 50% chance of passing the disorder on to each of his or her children as it follows an AD pattern of inheritance. PRENATAL DIAGNOSIS can be accomplished using FLUORESCENCE IN SITU HYBRIDIZATION (FISH) analysis on cells obtained by CHORIONIC VILLUS SAMPLING (CVS) or AMNIOCENTESIS.

The clinical diagnosis of Williams syndrome can be confirmed using the FISH technique. This test of the DEOXYRIBONUCLEIC ACID (DNA) detects the elastin deletion on chromosome 7 in 95% to 98% of individuals diagnosed as having the disorder. The presence of two copies of the elastin locus in a patient does not rule out the diagnosis.

Treatment for the various conditions that comprise the syndrome often require a team approach that includes physician, speech and language therapist, occupational and physical therapy, and vocational training. Surgery may be required for correction of cardiac abnormalities.

Wilms tumor Infant-onset CANCER of the kidney(s). One of the most common forms of childhood cancer, Wilms tumor accounts for 15% of all tumors diagnosed before the age of 15 years. Fifty percent of cases occur before age three and 90% are diagnosed before the age of 10. Approximately one-third of those affected have inherited the tendency to develop the tumor. Incidence is estimated at between one in 10,000 and one in 25,000 live births in the human population, with no ethnic or other predilection. Despite its ubiquity, it was only after effective therapy became available that affected families were noted with regularity. A little over 60% of those who inherit the tendency develop the disorder. (One inherits a predisposition to develop cancer rather than the cancer itself.) Its eponymic designation refers to German surgeon M. Wilms (1867–1918), who published the seminal description in 1899.

Wilms tumors are believed to result from malignant transformation of abnormally persistent renal stem cells which retain embryonic differentiation potential. Familial cases (see FAMILIAL DISEASE) have a greater likelihood than SPORADIC cases of affecting both kidneys (bilateral) and tend to have an earlier onset than sporadic cases. Initial symptoms include abdominal distension, an abdominal or flank mass, weight loss and hypertension.

It is associated with BECKWITH-WIEDEMANN SYNDROME, HEMIHYPERTROPHY, male PSEUDOHERMAPHRODITISM and other abnormalities. It is also seen in one-third of individuals affected with absence of the iris of the eye (ANIRIDIA) and is one of the cardinal disorders of WAGR syndrome, a SYNDROME involving two or more of the following: Wilms tumor, aniridia, genitourinary abnormalities and MENTAL RETARDATION. The genitourinary abnormalities include AMBIGUOUS GENITALIA, GONADOBLASTOMA, CRYPTORCHIDISM and HYPOSPADIAS. Wilms tumor (without aniridia) is also a feature of Denys-Drash syndrome, a rare condition in which severe urogenital aberrations result also in renal failure and PSEUDOHERMAPHRODITISM.

Some affected individuals exhibit a deletion of chromosomal material on the short arm on one of their two chromosome 11s. The deletion involves the tumor suppressor GENE *WT1* in which MUTATIONS can cause not only Wilms tumor, but others as well (e.g., mesothelioma) and are involved in some of the other syndromes with kidney and genitourinary abnormalities. There appears to be a second gene locus on 11p that also can cause Wilms tumors and other genes on 16q and 17q. The deletion may serve as a basis for chromosomal analysis for PRENATAL DIAGNOSIS.

It also appears that the gender of the parent the damaged chromosome 11 was inherited from may influence development of the disorder, through the process of IMPRINTING. When found in those affected, the chromosome 11 exhibiting the deletion (see CHROMOSOME ABNORMALITIES) is almost always inherited from the mother. This suggests that a maternally inherited copy of the *WT1* gene normally plays some role in suppressing tumor development, and that the loss of this suppressor function is apparently not compensated for by the gene(s) carried on the paternally derived chromosome 11.

The long-term outlook for affected individuals was previously uniformly poor. Currently, with early diagnosis and treatment, there is a high probability of cure.

Wilson disease (hepatolenticular degeneration) A genetic disorder characterized by the accumulation of copper in body tissues, particularly in the liver, kidneys, brain and cornea of the eyes. Essentially, it results in chronic copper poisoning.

The liver is the first organ to store copper. Rising levels in the liver can cause loss of appetite, nausea, fatigue, dark urine, clay-colored stools and jaundice, as in an atypical or prolonged case of hepatitis. It may lead to enlargement of the liver and can lead to cirrhosis and liver failure. Eventually, the buildup of copper causes degenerative changes in the liver, brain and nerves, resulting in incoordination, drooling, slurred speech, tremors, muscular rigidity, spastic movements, lack of balance, double vision, difficulty in swallowing (dysphagia) and mask-like facial appearance. The symptoms progress over months, and in the most advanced stages, weakness and emaciation leave affected individuals totally helpless, unable to walk or talk.

Psychiatric manifestation may be prominent and differ from case to case. They include depression, bizarre behavior, mania, psychosis, hysteria or even SCHIZOPHRENIA. Drugs typically prescribed to control these psychic disturbances may only exacerbate neurologic and psychiatric problems in individuals with Wilson disease.

Left untreated, or if diagnosed too late, the condition is ultimately fatal. However, with early diagnosis and therapy, affected individuals can recover fully. Therapy typically consists of drugs known as chelators, which have the ability to combine with metals. Copper binds with the drugs and is eliminated in the urine. Treatment must continue throughout the individual's life. Liver transplants have been successful in some patients with severe liver damage who haven't responded to drug therapy.

The first case was possibly described as early as 1861, with later reports calling the disorder "pseudosclerosis." It is named for British neurologist Samuel A. Kinnier Wilson, who made the first detailed study of the disease and provided the classic description of the condition in 1912.

The scientific name "hepatolenticular degeneration," refers to the degenerative effects on the liver (hepato), which mimic cirrhosis, and lenticular nuclei, a region of the brain.

Wilson disease has been observed in all races and ETHNIC GROUPS. Symptoms typically begin between the ages of six and 20, though they may appear as early as four or as late as 40. Unfortunately, it is difficult to diagnose, as the symptoms present themselves in many different ways and are similar to several different neurological and psychiatric disorders, liver diseases, and blood, kidney and bone disorders. The corneal accumulation of copper is one of the most indicative signs of the disorder, creating a rusty brown ring in each eye, known as a Kayser-Fleischer ring. However, this may not be present in early stages of the disease process, and it is difficult to observe in brown-eyed individuals.

Inherited as an AUTOSOMAL RECESSIVE trait, incidence is estimated at one in 100,000 live births. However, due to the difficulty of diagnosing the condition, some studies suggest that the incidence may be much higher, perhaps as much as one in 35,000 live births, with one in 100 people being CARRIERS of the disorder. Some 2,000 individuals have been diagnosed in the United States.

The GENE that causes Wilson disease is a copper transporting protein, on the long arm of chromosome 13. It is a relatively large gene and many MUTATIONS have been found, some more common in certain populations. Due to the number of mutations, genetic testing is difficult and costly. Carrier detection and presymptomatic and PRENATAL DIAGNOSIS can be accomplished using molecular techniques with either direct detection of mutations known to be in the family or using linked GENETIC MARKERS.

Wiskott-Aldrich syndrome A severe hereditary IMMUNE DEFICIENCY DISEASE with onset in infancy or childhood. It is named for German pediatrician A. Wiskott, who first reported the disorder in 1937, and U.S. pediatrician R. A. Aldrich, who published a second report in 1954.

Affected children also have platelet abnormalities and eczema. Death usually results from repeated infections or massive bleeding. Those who survive infancy often succumb to various CANCERS of the lymph system, though some have lived into their teens. An X-LINKED recessive disorder, it is exhibited only in males, and occurs in about four per million live male births in the United States. The GENE responsible has been named *WASP* for Wiskott-Aldrich syndrome protein.

Molecular techniques can be used for CARRIER detection and PRENATAL DIAGNOSIS and the condition can be corrected with bone marrow transplantation.

Wolf-Hirschhorn syndrome (4p-) A CHROMOSOME ABNORMALITY caused by the deletion of the most distal, or end, portion of the short arm of chromosome 4. It is characterized by severe motor, growth and MENTAL RETARDATION. Birth weight is low (see LOW BIRTH WEIGHT), generally well under five pounds. Infants have seizures and exhibit poor muscle tone (hypotonia) from birth.

The SYNDROME is named for German geneticist Dr. Ulrich Wolf and United States geneticist Dr. Kurt Hirschhorn (b. 1926) of Mt. Sinai Medical Center in New York City, who simultaneously published separate descriptions in *Humangenetik* (now *Human Genetics*) in 1965. (Dr. Hirschhorn also published an earlier description in 1961.)

The head is markedly small (MICROENCEPHALY), the trunk is long and the limbs thin. The face is often described as resembling a "Greek warrior helmet." Facially, the forehead is high, the eyes wide-set (HYPERTELORISM) and often down-slanting and the eyelids may droop (PTOSIS). The eyebrows are sparse, the nasal bridge wide, the corners of the mouth down turned. The groove extending from beneath the nose to the top lip (philtrum) is short and deep. The ears are lowset, and the ear lobes adhere to the side of the head. CLEFT LIP and CLEFT PALATE are noted in over half of the cases, as are CONGENITAL HEART DEFECTS.

Occurring in about one in 50,000 live births, it affects females twice as often as males. A very small region of the short arm of chromosome 4 appears to be the critical region, and even deletions too small to be detectable by standard chromosomal analysis can result in this SYNDROME. Those cases can be detected using fluorescence in situ hybridization (FISH) with probes that map to that critical region. In 80% of cases caused by a deletion, the deletion involves the paternally derived chromosome; this suggests that IMPRINTING plays a role in its inheritance. In approximately 10% to 15% of cases the deletion is due to a translocation. At least one-third of affected infants die within two years of birth, though some survive into adulthood.

Wolman disease   An inborn error of lipid metabolism (lysosomal acid lipase [LAL] deficiency) causing lipids (fatty substances) to accumulate in the spleen, liver and other organs, with fatal consequences. Inherited as an AUTOSOMAL RECESSIVE trait, it is caused by a MUTATION in the LAL GENE, resulting in an absence of LAL ENZYME activity. Onset occurs in the first few weeks of life, beginning with vomiting and diarrhea. The liver and spleen enlarge (hepatosplenomegaly) due to the accumulation of lipids. Death usually occurs by two to four months of age, due to nutritional failure.

Israeli pathologist M. Wolman (b. 1914) co-authored a report in 1956 describing the disorder, which now bears his name.

CHOLESTEROL ESTER STORAGE DISEASE, a more benign form of this STORAGE DISEASE, is caused by a different mutation of the LAL gene.

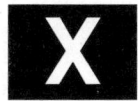

X chromosome The "female" SEX CHROMOSOME. Females have only X chromosomes and no Y chromosomes, and the presence of two X chromosomes is responsible for their gender. A pair of X chromosomes can be found in every somatic cell of the normal female, and characteristics transmitted on the X chromosome are said to be X-LINKED, or sex-linked. However, only one of the two X GENES is active; the other is inactive, and it can be identified by a small dark mass within the nucleus of the cell called a "Barr body" for its discoverer, Canadian anatomist Murray L. Barr.

X chromosomes were observed as early as 1891 by German zoologist Hermann Henking (1858–1942), who noted them while studying chromosomes of the fire wasp (*pyrrhocoris*). Henking was unable to identify the nature of these chromosomes, hence he labeled them "X" chromosomes. Their function remained unrecognized until after the rediscovery of MENDEL's laws. The X (and Y) chromosomes were first identified as sex chromosomes in 1910, from a study of sex-linked traits in the fly *Drosophila melanogaster* by Thomas Hunt Morgan at Columbia University.

X inactivation The process by which one of the two X chromosomes a female inherits is inactivated. Unlike the active X chromosome, the inactive X chromosome does not express the majority of its genes. The inactivation first occurs early in embryonic development, when the embryo has perhaps 32 cells. In each cell, one of the X chromosomes is inactivated. The inactivated X chromosome may be inherited maternally or paternally. Thereafter, all cells that arise from the division of these cells will have one X chromosome inactivated. Such a change, in which the function of a gene changes without an alteration of its DNA, is called an *epigen-etic* change. The process is also termed lyonization, in honor of English geneticist Mary Lyon who first suggested the concept in 1961. This process also occurs in males with Klinefelter syndrome, who, like females, have two X chromosomes, along with a single Y chromosome. If one of the X chromosomes wasn't inactivated, the cells would produce excess proteins from the extra copy of the gene. This would result in abnormalities, as is seen in Down syndrome, in which individuals have three copies of chromosome 21. The excess protein production is responsible for the characteristic anomalies seen in Down syndrome.

xeroderma pigmentosum A rare, progressive disorder characterized by sensitivity to sunlight, abnormal pigmentation and freckling of the skin, and the development of numerous growths, lesions and tumors on areas of the skin exposed to the sun. Degenerative changes also occur in the eyes.

The condition was first described in Vienna by Hungarian dermatologist Moriz Kaposi in 1863. He called it "xeroderma," or parchment skin, and added the term *pigmentosum* in 1882 to emphasize the striking pigmentary abnormalities.

Inherited as an AUTOSOMAL RECESSIVE trait, several different forms exist. It appears that eight different GENES may cause this disorder, all the MUTATIONS resulting in defects in the repair of DEOXYRIBONUCLEIC ACID (DNA) damaged by ultraviolet radiation from sunlight.

Overall incidence is about one in 60,000 to 100,000 live births. (One in 250,000 in Europe and the United States and one in 40,000 in Japan.) Malignant melanoma has been associated with affected individuals from Europe and the United States, but not from Japan.

Onset is typically in the first years of life. Acute sun sensitivity occurs in early infancy, with minimal exposure to sunlight causing severe blistering. Copious freckles begin to appear on the skin, especially on sun-exposed areas, prior to the age of two years. Hyperpigmented areas may also appear on the lips, tongue, palms and soles. The skin becomes dry, wrinkled, scaly and parchment-like. It may tighten, especially at the center of the face, making severely affected individuals unable to fully open their mouths. Benign growths, warts and lesions appear on exposed areas, especially the face. Lesions may become malignant over a period of years. Similar growths may occur on the surface of the eye.

In acute forms, the first exposure to sunlight triggers the development of malignant growths on the skin, which lead to death in childhood. The basic defect involves the inability of DNA to repair damage done by ultraviolet radiation from the sun or other sources.

Affected individuals must be constantly protected from exposure to sources of ultraviolet radiation, including sunlight, germicidal lamps, sunlamps and to a small extent from common, unfiltered, cool white fluorescent lamps. Light from incandescent lamps or sunlight passing through windows is not known to be harmful.

There is a delayed onset form of the disorder, with slow progression, in which individuals may live to an old age, as well as a severe form, which includes progressive neurological abnormalities and degeneration, MENTAL RETARDATION and dwarfing. This is also known as the De Sanctis–Cacchione syndrome, first reported in 1883 by Albert Neisser of Breslau, Germany (discoverer of the bacterial cause of gonorrhea, the agent Neisseria).

PRENATAL DIAGNOSIS is possible by cultivating fetal skin fibroblasts obtained at AMNIOCENTESIS to test their reaction to exposure to ultraviolet radiation. CARRIER detection by similar assays is not always reliable.

X-linked (sex-linked) A mode of genetic transmission of hereditary traits. It is the confirmed or suspected form of hereditary transmission of approximately 350 genetic disorders. Like non-X-

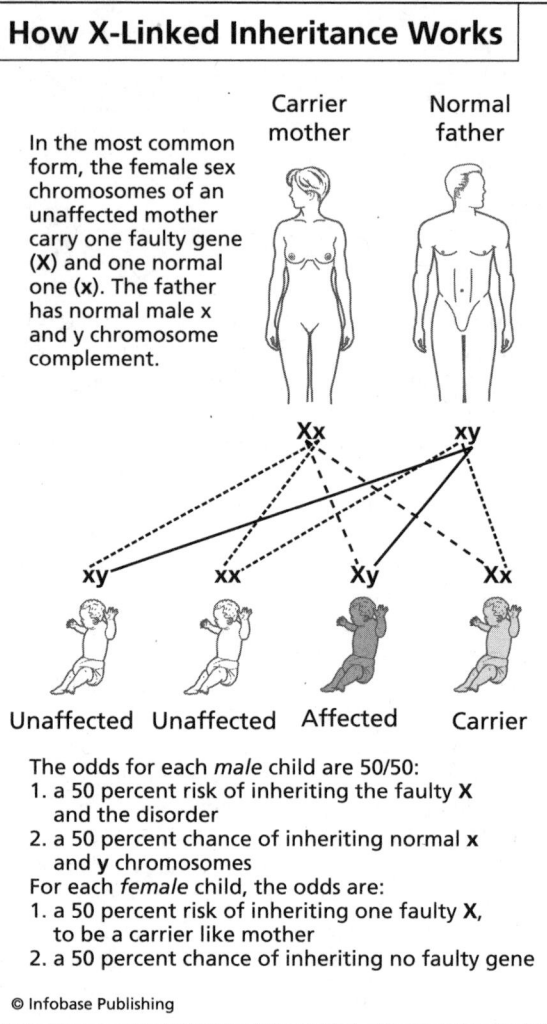

How X-Linked Inheritance Works

In the most common form, the female sex chromosomes of an unaffected mother carry one faulty gene (**X**) and one normal one (**x**). The father has normal male x and y chromosome complement.

Carrier mother — Xx

Normal father — xy

xy — Unaffected
xx — Unaffected
Xy — Affected
Xx — Carrier

The odds for each *male* child are 50/50:
1. a 50 percent risk of inheriting the faulty **X** and the disorder
2. a 50 percent chance of inheriting normal **x** and **y** chromosomes

For each *female* child, the odds are:
1. a 50 percent risk of inheriting one faulty **X**, to be a carrier like mother
2. a 50 percent chance of inheriting no faulty gene

© Infobase Publishing

Adapted from March of Dimes Birth Defects Foundation, Genetics Counseling (January 1987).

linked traits (that is, autosomal traits), X-linked disorders may be either dominant or recessive, though the majority are recessive. (Some X-linked disorders have not yet been clearly fit into either dominant or recessive categories.)

These disorders are called X-linked because they have their origins in MUTATIONS, or defects in individual GENES, found on the X CHROMOSOME, which is found in the 23rd chromosome pair in humans. Due to the nature of this chromosome pair, many X-linked disorders are exhibited only in males, while only females are silent CARRIERS. Classic X-linked disorders include COLOR BLINDNESS and HEMOPHILIA.

Though inheritance of X-linked traits such as color blindness and hemophilia had been recognized for some time, the link between sex chromosomes and X-linked traits was established in 1910 by Thomas Hunt Morgan in experiments with the fly *Drosophilia melanogaster* (see the Introduction).

Females have two X chromosomes while males have one X and one Y CHROMOSOME. The Y chromo-

some has fewer genes than the X chromosome, and in X-linked disorders, a recessive, aberrant gene on the X chromosome has no normal counterpart on the Y chromosome to override its influence. Any male that inherits an X chromosome with such a mutation will therefore exhibit the trait. (Individuals who possess only one gene of a given gene pair are termed "hemizygous" for that trait or gene.) A female, with two X chromosomes, will almost always have a normal gene to mask the influence of the aberrant recessive one. These women are

TABLE XIX
FREQUENCIES OF THE MOST COMMON X-LINKED DISORDERS FOUND IN A SURVEY CONDUCTED IN BRITISH COLUMBIA*, CANADA

X-Linked Condition	1952–63		1964–73		1974–83		TOTAL	
	N	Rate[a]	N	Rate[a]	N	Rate[a]	N	Rate[a]
Other testicular dysfunction	8	18.3	0	0.0 7	18.1	15	12.8	
Disorders of urea-cycle metabolism	1	2.3	0	0.0	3	7.7	4	3.4
Disorders of calcium metabolism	0	0.0	2	5.8	0	0.0	2	1.7
Mucopolysaccharidosis	3	6.9	3	8.7	0.	0.0	6	5.1
Deficiency of humoral immunity	6	13.7	2	5.8	0	0.0	8	6.8
Anemia due to disorder of glutathione metabolism	3	6.9	2	5.8	14	36.1	19	16.2
Congenital factor VIII disorder	28	64.0	24	69.6	14	36.1	66	56.4
Congenital factor IX disorder	7	16.0	10	29.0	1	2.6	18	15.4
Functional disorder of neutrophil polymorphs	0	0.0	0	0.0	3	7.7	3	2.6
Mental retardation	13	29.7	5	14.5	5	12.9	23	19.7
Hereditary progressive muscular dystrophy	43	98.3	34	98.6	13	33.5	90	76.9
Color-vision deficiencies	29	66.3	32	92.8	14	36.1	75	64.1
Nephrogenic diabetes insipidus	3	6.9	2	5.8	4	10.3	9	7.7
Congenital anomalies of posterior segment	2	4.6	2	5.8	3	7.7	7	6.0
Anomalies of skull and face bones	2	4.6	1	2.9	3	7.7	6	5.1
Other specified congenital anomalies of skin	3	6.9	3	8.7	7	18.1	13	11.1
Other specified congenital anomalies	1	2.3	0	0.0	3	7.7	4	3.4
All other X-linked conditions[b]	5	11.4	10	29.0	11	28.4	26	22.2
Total	157	358.9	13.2	383.0	105	270.8	394	336.8
Sum of highest individual rates								532.4

*Statistics reflect local population bias.
N = Number of patients.
[a]Per 1 million live births.
[b]Each individual rate was used to get the sum of highest individual rates for these conditions.
Source: Patricia A. Baird, "A Population Study of Genetic Disorders in Children and Young Adults," *American Journal of Human Genetics* 42 (1988), pp. 677–693.

said to be carriers. (Inheritance of two recessive genes or two dominant genes for an X-linked disorder may be lethal IN UTERO for females.)

Classic X-linked disorders can never be passed from father to son, since the aberrant gene is on the X chromosome, and the affected father must pass on the Y chromosome to have male offspring. However, all daughters will be carriers. Screening can identify carriers in some of these disorders. (See Figure V.)

X-linked dominant disorders are very rare. In some, they follow inheritance patterns of AUTOSOMAL DOMINANT transmission, with no transmission from father to son. Some may be seen only in females, as inheritance of the single dominant mutant gene is lethal IN UTERO for males. HYPOPHOSPHATEMIA, ORAL-FACIAL-DIGITAL SYNDROME, type I and incontinentia pigmenti are among them.

Female carriers may exhibit mild symptoms in some X-linked disorders. In females, in any individual cell, only one X chromosome is active (see MOSAICISM).

X-linked agammaglobulinemia   See IMMUNE DEFICIENCY DISEASES.

XX male syndrome (sex reversal)   Individuals exhibiting the PHENOTYPE, or typical appearance, of a normal male, though chromosomally (GENOTYPE) they are females, having two X CHROMOSOMES instead of one X and one Y CHROMOSOME found in males. The penis, scrotum and testes are usually small but well differentiated, but the individuals fail to exhibit normal pubertal development. Breasts develop (GYNECOMASTIA) in about one-third of those affected. Pubic hair may grow in a characteristic female pattern, and body and facial hair is decreased. Affected individuals are infertile, as well.

A translocation (see CHROMOSOME ABNORMALITY) of a particular region of the Y chromosome, which contains the TDF, or testis determining factor, GENE, is involved in causing this disorder. TDF had been theorized as the "master switch" for determining male characteristics. The TDF gene is synonymous with the SRY (sex-determining region on the Y)

gene, and its discovery made it possible to demonstrate the presence of Y chromosome material on one X chromosome in most XX males.

Some familial cases of this SYNDROME have been reported. In some cases there is evidence of a translocation of chromosomal material from the Y chromosome onto a chromosome other than the X chromosome.

XXXXX   A rare CHROMOSOME ABNORMALITY exhibited only in females in which individuals have 49 CHROMOSOMES, with five X CHROMOSOMES. It results from failure of chromosomal separation, generally in the formation of egg cells. MENTAL RETARDATION (of varying severity), failure to mature sexually at puberty, and sterility are the hallmarks. (For the male equivalent of this disorder, see XXXXY.)

At birth, the external genitalia appear normal. Non-genital physical characteristics are similar to those exhibited by males with XXXXY. Infants display poor muscle tone (hypotonia) and are short, with height often below the third percentile. The head tends to be mildly undersized. The face is usually rounded. They may resemble babies with trisomy 21 (DOWN SYNDROME). The eyes are often wide-set (HYPERTELORISM) and frequently exhibit ocular abnormalities, including inability to focus the eyes in concert (STRABISMUS, or crossed eyes), nearsightedness (MYOPIA) and mild upward slant (obliquity) of the eye slits (palpebral fissures).

As infants age, the roundness of the face disappears, but mid-face growth is retarded, creating a rather pronounced, jutting jaw (mandibular prognathism), particularly after puberty.

The breasts and uterus remain infantile, and there is scant pubic hair growth at the time of puberty. In some individuals, microscopic examination of the ovaries reveals no abnormalities. Life span is normal.

XXXXY   A rare CHROMOSOME ABNORMALITY, exhibited only in males, in which individuals have 49 CHROMOSOMES, with four X CHROMOSOMES and one Y. It results from failure of chromosomal separation, generally in the formation of egg cells. MENTAL RETARDATION (of varying severity), poor development of external genitalia and STERILITY are the hall-marks. It is believed to occur at the least 10 times more frequently than XXXXX. (For the female equivalent of this disorder, see XXXXX.)

At birth, infants exhibit poor muscle tone (hypotonia) and are short, with height often below the third percentile. The head tends to be mildly undersized. The penis, scrotum and testes are very small, and the testes are undescended (CRYPTORCHISM). The face is usually oval. Most infants exhibit wide-set eyes (HYPERTELORISM), frequently accompanied by ocular abnormalities, including inability to focus the eyes in concert (STRABISMUS, or crossed eyes) and mild upward slant (antimongoloid obliquity) of the eye slits (palpebral fissures). The neck is short and webbed.

As infants age, mid-face growth is retarded, creating a rather pronounced, jutting jaw (mandibular prognathism), particularly after puberty. Abnormalities of the upper limbs are characteristic, especially inability to bend the elbow. Life span is normal.

XY syndrome   The normal male GENOTYPE. It has semi-facetiously been suggested by one genetic researcher that this is a SYNDROME in which affected individuals have an increased susceptibility to stroke, hypertension and cardiovascular disease, as well as a tendency to exhibit aggressive behaviors associated with increased mortality rates.

XYY syndrome   CHROMOSOME ABNORMALITY characterized by the presence of an additional Y CHROMOSOME, the SEX CHROMOSOME that determines male gender. Affected individuals are sometimes referred to as "hypermasculine" or "supermales."

It occurs as frequently as one in 840 live male births but may remain undiagnosed throughout life, as the features are subtle. They include accelerated growth in mid-childhood, potentially explosive, antisocial behavior, relative weakness, poor coordination of fine motor skills and low intelligence; IQ is usually 10 to 15 points below unaffected SIBLINGS. Physically, affected individuals tend to be tall and thin, with mildly sunken chests (PECTUS excavatum). Severe acne may develop in adolescence.

It has been suggested that individuals with this KARYOTYPE are more prone to criminal behavior, but studies have not corroborated this speculation, though among institutionalized male juvenile delinquents, incidence has been reported as much as 24 times above that in the general population.

Affected individuals have passed the condition on to their sons only in very rare instances, though the majority of XYY individuals are fertile.

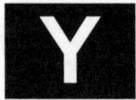

Y chromosome The "male" SEX CHROMOSOME. Males have one X CHROMOSOME and one Y sex chromosome, and the presence of the Y chromosome is responsible for their gender. (Females have two X chromosomes.) While only an X chromosome can be inherited from the mother, the father may pass on either an X or Y chromosome. If he passes on a Y chromosome, the offspring will be a male. The XY chromosome pair can be found in every somatic cell of the normal male.

In addition to the male determining factor (termed TDF, or testis determining factor), a number of GENES have been mapped to the Y chromosome involved not only with male sex determination, but also with spermatogenesis. Several other Y-linked genes are homologues of genes that map to the pseudoautosomal region of the X chromosome. The existence of a Y-linked gene for hairy ears has also been suggested. A gene associated with stature appears to be on the Y, as well; this growth-related gene also has dental growth factor properties and determines tooth size.

The Y and X chromosomes were first identified as sex chromosomes in 1910, arising from a study of sex-linked traits in the fly *Drosophila melanogaster* by Thomas Hunt Morgan at Columbia University.

Zellweger syndrome (cerebro-hepatorenal syndrome, CHRS)   First described in 1964 by Hans V. Zellweger (b. 1908) and colleagues at Johns Hopkins University, this disorder is marked at birth by LOW BIRTH WEIGHT, a FLOPPY INFANT appearance due to lack of muscle tone (hypotonia), and characteristic facial features. Most infants are relatively motionless. The forehead is high and bulging, the face is round, the eyes are wide-set (HYPERTELORISM) and slanted toward the nose (mongoloid obliquity) with epicanthal folds (see EPICANTHUS). The eyelids are puffy, and other ocular abnormalities may include GLAUCOMA, corneal clouding and CATARACTS. The nose is upturned (anteverted nares) and ears are poorly formed, low-set and rotated slightly backward. The jaw is small (micrognathia).

The liver is almost always enlarged (hepatomegaly). Microscopic cysts develop in the kidney and can only be confirmed by biopsy. There are also stippled calcifications, dot-like flecks of calcium deposits, seen on X-rays of the knees. Fingers and knees may exhibit permanent bending (flexion contractures). Mental and physical development is extremely limited, and seizures are common. Death, most often from pneumonia, usually occurs before the age of six months. There is no effective therapy.

The features of CHRS overlap with those of neonatal ALD (see ADRENOLEUKODYSTROPHY) as well as with infantile REFSUM DISEASE. The basic defects in the three disorders overlap as well. All are caused by MUTATIONS in any of several GENES involved in the synthesis, or biogenesis, of peroxisomes. Peroxisomes are organelles in the cells that serve as storehouses for ENZYMES used in metabolism. The responsible genes encode proteins called peroxins, with *PEX* being the gene acronyms. Genes involved in CHRS include *PEX1* (chromosome 7q), *PEX2* (8q), *PEX5* (12p) and *PEX6* (6p).

CHRS is inherited as an AUTOSOMAL RECESSIVE trait. Initially estimated to occur in one in 100,000 live births, discoveries of new cases indicate the incidence may be as high as one in 25,000 to one in 50,000 newborns. Twice as many affected females as males have been identified. PRENATAL DIAGNOSIS can be accomplished using biochemical and in some cases molecular techniques.

Zollinger-Ellison syndrome   Gastric distress is the hallmark of this GENETIC DISORDER. Peptic ulcers, gastric hyperacidity, and small tumors that secrete gastrin, a digestive acid, are common symptoms. MULTIPLE ENDOCRINE NEOPLASIA, Type 1 (MEN1) is a feature of the SYNDROME. Benign or malignant tumors may develop in the pancreas or the stomach, duodenum, spleen or abdominal lymph nodes. About 40% of patients develop such tumors, of which about 50% are malignant. The cause of these tumors is unknown. Life-threatening internal obstructions, perforations and bleeding may also occur.

Onset may occur during childhood but diagnosis is usually between the ages of 20 and 70. Two forms are currently recognized: SPORADIC and AUTOSOMAL DOMINANT. Males and female are affected in equal numbers. Sporadic cases usually have a later onset.

Control of gastric acid secretion with antacids and drugs is the primary treatment. Surgical removal of tumors or portions of the stomach has been helpful in some cases.

zygodactyly   The fusion of the second and third toes or the third and fourth fingers by a web of skin. It is the mildest form of SYNDACTYLY (the fusion of the digits). It may be SPORADIC or inherited in an AUTOSOMAL DOMINANT manner and may be seen in normal children as well as those with associated problems.

Studies on the prevalence of the malformation has yielded rates of 17 per 100,000 to as high as one per 200 to 1000 (0.5–0.1%). It is twice as common in males as females.

APPENDIXES

APPENDIX I
CONGENITAL DEFECTS SURVEILLANCE DATA

The data in Appendix I is from the Metropolitan Atlanta Congenital Defects Program (MACDP), administered by the Centers for Disease Control and Prevention. Established in 1967, MACDP is a source of case data for numerous studies of birth defects and birth defects prevention and serves as the model for many state-based birth defects surveillance programs as well as those in many other countries.

TABLE 2

NUMBER OF LIVE BIRTHS STRATIFIED BY DESCRIPTIVE CHARACTERISTICS, FIVE CENTRAL COUNTIES OF METROPOLITAN ATLANTA, 1968–2003

	Total		1968–1972		1973–1978		1979–1983		1984–1989		1990–1993		1994–1998		1999–2003	
Characteristic	Count	Percent	Count	Percent	Count	Percent	Count	Percent	Count	Percent	Count	Percent	Count	Percent	Count	Percent
Total	1,232,191	100.0	137,202	100.0	143,532	100.0	135,541	100.0	202,760	100.0	154,325	100.0	208,832	100.0	249,999	100.0
Maternal age (years)																
<25	491,355	39.9	78,224	57.0	73,143	51.0	60,535	44.7	78,616	38.8	54,662	35.4	67,334	32.2	78,841	31.5
25–29	352,867	28.6	37,218	27.1	44,345	30.9	42,068	31.0	63,417	31.3	44,992	29.2	55,300	26.5	65,527	26.2
≥30	386,404	31.4	21,742	15.8	25,383	17.7	32,871	24.3	60,599	29.9	54,616	35.4	86,117	41.2	105,576	42.2
Unknown	1,065	0.1	18	0.0	661	0.5	67	0.0	128	0.1	55	0.0	81	0.0	55	0.0
Maternal race/ethnicity*																
White	670,150	54.4	98,496	71.8	92,965	64.8	83,024	61.3	122,593	60.5	79,415	51.5	98,060	47.0	95,597	38.2
Black or African American	420,173	–	–	–	49,088	34.2	50,566	37.3	75,764	37.4	64,215	41.6	84,293	40.4	96,247	38.5
Hispanic or Latino	64,985	–	–	–	–	–	–	–	–	–	5,906	3.8	16,587	7.9	42,492	17.0
All Other Races	76,058	–	38,706	28.2	1,479	1.0	1,918	1.4	4,355	2.1	4,728	3.1	9,596	4.6	15,276	6.1
Unknown	81	0.0	–	–	–	–	33	0.0	48	0.0	–	–	–	–	–	–
Birth weight (grams)																
<2500	105,498	8.6	12,059	8.8	12,341	8.6	11,721	8.6	16,264	8.0	13,379	8.7	17,882	8.6	21,852	8.7
≥2500	1,123,927	91.2	124,448	90.7	129,495	90.2	123,709	91.3	186,361	91.9	140,878	91.3	190,922	91.4	228,114	91.2
Unknown	2,766	0.2	695	0.5	1,696	1.2	111	0.1	135	0.1	68	0.0	29	0.0	33	0.0
Gestational age (weeks)																
20–36	114,390	9.3	10,577	7.7	12,083	8.4	12,331	9.1	19,747	9.7	15,900	10.3	19,465	9.3	24,287	9.7
≥37	1,054,396	85.6	116,000	84.5	120,469	83.9	113,064	83.4	167,372	82.5	130,112	84.3	185,220	88.7	222,159	88.9
Unknown	63,295	5.1	10,625	7.7	10,980	7.6	10,146	7.5	15,641	7.7	8,313	5.4	4,125	2.0	3,465	1.4
Sex																
Male	629,847	51.1	70,191	51.2	73,831	51.4	69,444	51.2	103,904	51.2	78,794	51.1	106,516	51.0	127,167	50.9
Female	602,311	48.9	67,011	48.8	69,682	48.5	66,096	48.8	98,852	48.8	75,528	48.9	102,312	49.0	122,830	49.1
Ambiguous/Unknown	33	0.0	–	–	19	0.0	<5	0.0	<5	0.0	<5	0.0	<5	0.0	<5	0.0
Parity																
1 Live birth	541,589	44.0	52,146	38.0	72,254	50.3	63,477	46.8	89,574	44.2	66,837	43.3	91,842	44.0	105,459	42.2
2 or more live births	671,253	54.5	71,973	52.5	71,278	49.7	72,064	53.2	109,484	54.0	87,050	56.4	116,183	55.6	143,221	57.3
Unknown	19,349	1.6	13,083	9.5	–	–	–	–	3,702	1.8	438	0.3	807	0.4	1,319	0.5
Gravidity																
1 Pregnancy	463,728	37.6	48,628	35.4	67,027	46.7	65,487	48.3	70,570	34.8	52,058	33.7	72,931	34.9	87,027	34.8
2 or more pregnancies	746,818	60.6	75,491	55.0	76,505	53.3	70,054	51.7	128,333	63.3	101,699	65.9	134,683	64.5	160,053	64.0
Unknown	21,645	1.8	13,083	9.5	–	–	–	–	3,857	1.9	568	0.4	1,218	0.6	2,919	1.2
Plurality																
Singleton	1,200,719	97.5	134,708	98.2	140,601	98.0	132,829	98.0	198,132	97.7	150,240	97.4	202,615	97.0	241,594	96.6
Multiple	31,232	2.5	2,494	1.8	2,702	1.9	2,712	2.0	4,625	2.3	4,082	2.6	6,214	3.0	8,403	3.4
Unknown	240	0.0	–	–	229	0.2	–	–	<5	0.0	<5	0.0	<5	0.0	<5	0.0

* Black or African American race is included in the All Other Races category for 1968–1972. Data on Hispanic or Latino ethnicity were available beginning in 1990. Therefore, percentages of the total are not calculated for these subgroups. Race/ethnicity data for 1990–2003 were obtained from a vital records file with slightly fewer live births than that used for the other strata. Therefore, the sums of the race/ethnicity strata do not equal the total number of live births in the corresponding column.

TABLE 3

ANNUAL PREVALENCE (PER 10,000 LIVE BIRTHS) OF SELECTED BIRTH DEFECTS, MACDP, 1968–2003

Birth defect	Total		1968		1969		1970		1971		1972		1973		1974	
	Cases	Prev*	Cases	Prev	Cases	Prev	Cases	Prev	Cases	Prev	Cases	Prev	Cases	Prev	Cases	Prev
All defects	32,938	267.31	543	205.18	566	206.22	642	216.26	600	214.01	521	203.78	624	248.10	625	252.27
Spina bifida	706	5.73	38	14.36	34	12.39	41	13.81	35	12.48	33	12.91	23	9.14	23	9.28
Conotrucal heart defects‡	849	9.74														
Dextrotransposition of the great arteries‡	211	2.42														
Tetralogy of Fallot‡	399	4.58														
Atrioventricular septal defect‡	326	3.74														
Coarctation of the aorta‡	338	3.88														
Atrial septal defect‡	730	8.37														
Ventricular septal defect‡	2,490	28.56														
Perimembranous ventricular septal defect‡	707	8.11														
Cleft lip with or without cleft palate	1,177	9.55	28	10.58	24	8.74	36	12.13	26	9.27	37	14.47	25	9.94	33	13.32
Cleft palate alone	672	5.45	8	3.02	10	3.64	15	5.05	24	8.56	15	5.87	14	5.57	18	7.27
Pyloric stenosis	1,656	13.44	20	7.56	34	12.39	36	12.13	29	10.34	36	14.08	40	15.90	47	18.97
Anal or rectal atresia or stenosis	457	3.71	9	3.40	12	4.37	18	6.06	12	4.28	7	2.74	8	3.18	13	5.25
Hypospadias	3,730	30.27	44	16.63	50	18.22	63	21.22	62	22.11	52	20.34	70	27.83	65	26.24
Congenital dislocation or dysplasia of the hip	959	7.78	19	7.18	20	7.29	24	8.08	20	7.13	14	5.48	30	11.93	26	10.49
Clubfoot without a neural tube defect	2,099	17.03	70	26.45	65	23.68	92	30.99	64	22.83	53	20.73	70	27.83	69	27.85
Polydactyly	1,913	15.53	28	10.58	38	13.84	22	7.41	34	12.13	33	12.91	28	11.13	24	9.69
Transverse limb deficiency	377	3.06	12	4.53	12	4.37	13	4.38	11	3.92	6	2.35	9	3.58	10	4.04

* Prev = Prevalence.
‡ Numbers of cases and prevalence estimates are not provided for congenital heart defects prior to 1982 because not all of these cases have been reviewed by pediatric cardiologists.

TABLE 3

ANNUAL PREVALENCE (PER 10,000 LIVE BIRTHS) OF SELECTED BIRTH DEFECTS, MACDP, 1968–2003

Birth defect	1975 Cases	1975 Prev*	1976 Cases	1976 Prev	1977 Cases	1977 Prev	1978 Cases	1978 Prev	1979 Cases	1979 Prev	1980 Cases	1980 Prev	1981 Cases	1981 Prev	1982 Cases	1982 Prev
All defects	710	308.35	661	291.46	638	271.43	676	277.09	716	280.33	755	275.93	806	300.35	785	281.71
Spina bifida	18	7.82	15	6.61	21	8.93	16	6.56	18	7.05	22	8.04	17	6.34	14	5.02
Conotrucal heart defects‡															32	11.48
Dextrotransposition of the great arteries‡															11	3.95
Tetralogy of Fallot‡															12	4.31
Atrioventricular septal defect‡															13	4.67
Coarctation of the aorta‡															7	2.51
Atrial septal defect‡															6	2.15
Ventricular septal defect‡															32	11.48
Perimembranous ventricular defect‡															9	3.23
Cleft lip with or without cleft palate	27	11.73	28	12.35	17	7.23	28	11.48	32	12.53	32	11.70	27	10.06	28	10.05
Cleft palate alone	21	9.12	14	6.17	15	6.38	17	6.97	22	8.61	10	3.65	7	2.61	11	3.95
Pyloric stenosis	51	22.15	36	15.87	18	7.66	29	11.89	38	14.88	31	11.33	32	11.92	29	10.41
Anal or rectal atresia or stenosis	12	5.21	8	3.53	9	3.83	11	4.51	10	3.92	11	4.02	10	3.73	8	2.87
Hypospadias	80	34.74	68	29.98	70	29.78	76	31.15	87	34.06	60	21.93	75	27.95	67	24.04
Congenital dislocation or dysplasia of the hip	26	11.29	25	11.02	16	6.81	31	12.71	29	11.35	25	9.14	17	6.34	13	4.67
Clubfoot without a neural tube defect	80	34.74	65	28.66	64	27.23	53	21.72	62	24.27	63	23.02	55	20.50	43	15.43
Polydactyly	28	12.16	43	18.96	30	12.76	37	15.17	39	15.27	48	17.54	151	56.27	142	50.96
Transverse limb deficiency	10	4.34	10	4.41	8	3.40	8	3.28	5	1.96	10	3.65	6	2.24	11	3.95

* Prev = Prevalence.
‡ Numbers of cases and prevalence estimates are not provided for congenital heart defects prior to 1982 because not all of these cases have been reviewed by pediatric cardiologists.

TABLE 3

ANNUAL PREVALENCE (PER 10,000 LIVE BIRTHS) OF SELECTED BIRTH DEFECTS, MACDP, 1968–2003

Birth defect	1983 Cases	Prev*	1984 Cases	Prev	1985 Cases	Prev	1986 Cases	Prev	1987 Cases	Prev	1988 Cases	Prev	1989 Cases	Prev	1990 Cases	Prev
All defects	738	264.17	744	254.45	989	319.08	1,024	312.29	904	258.26	939	256.22	1,011	265.47	981	252.97
Spina bifida	21	7.52	21	7.18	20	6.45	23	7.01	17	4.86	21	5.73	18	4.73	19	4.90
Conotrucal heart defects‡	24	8.59	29	9.92	25	8.07	23	7.01	26	7.43	40	10.91	32	8.40	36	9.28
Dextrotransposition of the great arteries‡	8	2.86	9	3.08	6	1.94	7	2.13	7	2.00	11	3.00	7	1.84	7	1.81
Tetralogy of Fallot‡	11	3.94	15	5.13	17	5.48	12	3.66	12	3.43	18	4.91	20	5.25	19	4.90
Atrioventricular septal defect‡	11	3.94	10	3.42	11	3.55	13	3.96	12	3.43	14	3.82	11	2.89	8	2.06
Coarctation of the aorta‡	14	5.01	11	3.76	12	3.87	10	3.05	13	3.71	15	4.09	20	5.25	12	3.09
Atrial septal defect‡	14	5.01	16	5.47	10	3.23	19	5.79	17	4.86	25	6.82	34	8.93	32	8.25
Ventricular septal defect‡	42	15.03	56	19.15	59	19.04	83	25.31	80	22.85	79	21.56	102	26.78	85	21.92
Perimembranous ventricular septal defect‡	14	5.01	18	6.16	8	2.58	18	5.49	11	3.14	20	5.46	21	5.51	23	5.93
Cleft lip with or without cleft palate	37	13.24	27	9.23	34	10.97	26	7.93	30	8.57	34	9.28	29	7.61	46	11.86
Cleft palate alone	12	4.30	16	5.47	11	3.55	22	6.71	20	5.71	18	4.91	19	4.99	18	4.64
Pyloric stenosis	30	10.74	43	14.71	53	17.10	50	15.25	63	18.00	58	15.83	54	14.18	58	14.96
Anal or rectal atresia or stenosis	10	3.58	10	3.42	16	5.16	13	3.96	18	5.14	8	2.18	17	4.46	15	3.87
Hypospadias	78	27.92	79	27.02	102	32.91	114	34.77	110	31.42	128	34.93	149	39.13	134	34.55
Congenital dislocation or dysplasia of the hip	14	5.01	18	6.16	19	6.13	25	7.62	33	9.43	28	7.64	40	10.50	41	10.57
Clubfoot without a neural tube defect	42	15.03	42	14.36	54	17.42	56	17.08	51	14.57	48	13.10	53	13.92	45	11.60
Polydactyly	94	33.65	39	13.34	52	16.78	45	13.72	53	15.14	46	12.55	50	13.13	48	12.38
Transverse limb deficiency	6	2.15	10	3.42	8	2.58	10	3.05	5	1.43	8	2.18	11	2.89	10	2.58

* Prev = Prevalence.
‡ Numbers of cases and prevalence estimates are not provided for congenital heart defects prior to 1982 because not all of these cases have been reviewed by pediatric cardiologists.

TABLE 3
ANNUAL PREVALENCE (PER 10,000 LIVE BIRTHS) OF SELECTED BIRTH DEFECTS, MACDP, 1968–2003

	Year															
	1991		1992		1993		1994		1995		1996		1997		1998	
Birth defect	Cases	Prev*	Cases	Prev	Cases	Prev	Cases	Prev	Cases	Prev	Cases	Prev	Cases	Prev	Cases	Prev
All defects	995	260.18	953	249.38	965	246.88	1,070	268.59	1,165	289.38	1,188	290.46	1,144	266.65	1,315	292.66
Spina bifida	12	3.14	14	3.66	12	3.07	19	4.77	7	1.74	12	2.93	17	3.96	21	4.67
Conotrucal heart defects‡	29	7.58	37	9.68	41	10.49	39	9.79	44	10.93	47	11.49	31	7.23	42	9.35
Dextrotransposition of the great arteries‡	9	2.35	10	2.62	8	2.05	12	3.01	15	3.73	9	2.20	6	1.40	7	1.56
Tetralogy of Fallot‡	17	4.45	16	4.19	19	4.86	14	3.51	18	4.47	23	5.62	17	3.96	21	4.67
Atrioventricular septal defect‡	18	4.71	12	3.14	10	2.56	15	3.77	19	4.72	24	5.87	12	2.80	17	3.78
Coarctation of the aorta‡	14	3.66	9	2.36	8	2.05	19	4.77	24	5.96	16	3.91	14	3.26	19	4.23
Atrial septal defect‡	33	8.63	23	6.02	36	9.21	28	7.03	43	10.68	28	6.85	38	8.86	34	7.57
Ventricular septal defect‡	99	25.89	90	23.55	85	21.75	120	30.12	120	29.81	119	29.10	129	30.07	139	30.93
Perimembranous ventricular septal defect‡	22	5.75	29	7.59	28	7.16	51	12.80	43	10.68	36	8.80	42	9.79	36	8.01
Cleft lip with or without cleft palate	30	7.84	35	9.16	31	7.93	37	9.29	43	10.68	37	9.05	29	6.76	46	10.24
Cleft palate alone	18	4.71	24	6.28	15	3.84	16	4.02	24	5.96	27	6.60	14	3.26	25	5.56
Pyloric stenosis	62	16.21	55	14.39	49	12.54	38	9.54	62	15.40	60	14.67	63	14.68	58	12.91
Anal or rectal atresia or stenosis	13	3.40	7	1.83	19	4.86	16	4.02	12	2.98	9	2.20	19	4.43	20	4.45
Hypospadias	120	31.38	108	28.26	121	30.96	135	33.89	153	38.00	142	34.72	140	32.63	135	30.04
Congenital dislocation or dysplasia of the hip	57	14.90	37	9.68	26	6.65	29	7.28	33	8.20	20	4.89	28	6.53	30	6.68
Clubfoot without a neural tube defect	53	13.86	52	13.61	52	13.30	68	17.07	57	14.16	57	13.94	54	12.59	69	15.36
Polydactyly	50	13.07	31	8.11	38	9.72	62	15.56	60	14.90	55	13.45	53	12.35	64	14.24
Transverse limb deficiency	10	2.61	17	4.45	11	2.81	11	2.76	18	4.47	16	3.91	11	2.56	11	2.45

* Prev = Prevalence.
‡ Numbers of cases and prevalence estimates are not provided for congenital heart defects prior to 1982 because not all of these cases have been reviewed by pediatric cardiologists.

TABLE 3

ANNUAL PREVALENCE (PER 10,000 LIVE BIRTHS) OF SELECTED BIRTH DEFECTS, MACDP, 1968–2003

Birth defect	1999 Cases	1999 Prev*	2000 Cases	2000 Prev	2001 Cases	2001 Prev	2002 Cases	2002 Prev	2003 Cases	2003 Prev
All defects	**1,362**	**289.69**	**1,385**	**276.89**	**1,418**	**279.43**	**1,473**	**291.44**	**1,307**	**252.92**
Spina bifida	5	1.06	10	2.00	14	2.76	19	3.76	16	3.10
Conotrucal heart defects[‡]	45	9.57	55	11.00	62	12.22	63	12.46	47	9.10
Dextrotransposition of the great arteries[‡]	9	1.91	15	3.00	14	2.76	13	2.57	11	2.13
Tetralogy of Fallot[‡]	19	4.04	24	4.80	20	3.94	35	6.92	20	3.87
Atrioventricular septal defect[‡]	20	4.25	19	3.80	18	3.55	18	3.56	21	4.06
Coarctation of the aorta[‡]	21	4.47	17	3.40	20	3.94	23	4.55	20	3.87
Atrial septal defect[‡]	53	11.27	51	10.20	59	11.63	61	12.07	70	13.55
Ventricular septal defect[‡]	171	36.37	173	34.59	194	38.23	199	39.37	234	45.28
Perimembranous ventricular septal defect[‡]	54	11.49	48	9.60	68	13.40	52	10.29	56	10.84
Cleft lip with or without cleft palate	39	8.30	42	8.40	36	7.09	45	8.90	36	6.97
Cleft palate alone	33	7.02	41	8.20	32	6.31	25	4.95	21	4.06
Pyloric stenosis	57	12.12	61	12.20	76	14.98	57	11.28	43	8.32
Anal or rectal atresia or stenosis	13	2.77	19	3.80	18	3.55	16	3.17	11	2.13
Hypospadias	174	37.01	159	31.79	143	28.18	180	35.61	137	26.51
Congenital dislocation or dysplasia of the hip	19	4.04	30	6.00	33	6.50	31	6.13	33	6.39
Clubfoot without a neural tube defect	68	14.46	46	9.20	55	10.84	58	11.48	51	9.87
Polydactyly	68	14.46	63	12.60	80	15.76	78	15.43	59	11.42
Transverse limb deficiency	6	1.28	18	3.60	18	3.55	11	2.18	10	1.94

* Prev = Prevalence.

‡ Numbers of cases and prevalence estimates are not provided for congenital heart defects prior to 1982 because not all of these cases have been reviewed by pediatric cardiologists.

TABLE 4

THREE-YEAR PREVALENCE (PER 10,000 LIVE BIRTHS) OF SELECTED BIRTH DEFECTS, MACDP, 1968–2003

Birth defect	Total		1968–1970		1971–1973		1974–1976		1977–1979		1980–1982		1983–1985	
	Cases	Prev*	Cases	Prev	Cases	Prev	Cases	Prev	Cases	Prev	Cases	Prev	Cases	Prev
Anencephalus	446	3.62	81	9.69	64	8.13	35	4.97	42	5.72	33	4.02	31	3.52
Encephalocele	190	1.54	14	1.67	12	1.52	11	1.56	17	2.31	24	2.92	18	2.04
Hydrocephalus†	256	4.77												
Congenital cataract	265	2.15	6	0.72	8	1.02	16	2.27	37	5.04	21	2.56	17	1.93
Complete atrioventricular septal defect‡	196	2.32											22	2.5
Valvar pulmonary stenosis‡	353	4.18											26	2.95
Hypoplastic left heart syndrome‡	212	2.51											22	2.5
Aortic stenosis‡	93	1.10											9	1.02
Secundum atrial septal defect‡	499	5.91											21	2.38
Muscular ventricular septal defect‡	1,167	13.83											6	0.68
Single ventricle	79	0.94											6	0.68
Partial and total anomalous pulmonary venous return‡	72	0.85											7	0.79
Esophageal atresia or stenosis‡	266	2.16	17	2.03	15	1.9	18	2.55	14	1.91	25	3.05	23	2.61
Duodenal atresia or stenosis	199	1.62	11	1.32	8	1.02	12	1.7	7	0.95	15	1.83	14	1.59
Jejunal and/or ileal atresia or stenosis	201	1.63	12	1.44	13	1.65	12	1.7	8	1.09	14	1.71	14	1.59
Hirschsprung disease	227	1.84	7	0.84	5	0.63	13	1.84	11	1.5	16	1.95	14	1.59
Bilateral renal agenesis or dysgenesis	169	1.37	8	0.96	10	1.27	11	1.56	16	2.18	13	1.58	19	2.15
Any cystic kidney disease	507	4.11	19	2.27	19	2.41	18	2.55	15	2.04	19	2.32	39	4.42
Craniosynostosis	481	3.9	18	2.15	18	2.29	31	4.4	31	4.22	26	3.17	24	2.72
Skeletal dysplasia	226	1.83	15	1.79	6	0.76	9	1.28	9	1.23	19	2.32	14	1.59
Diaphragmatic hernia	280	2.27	18	2.15	15	1.9	19	2.7	12	1.63	17	2.07	11	1.25
Omphalocele	337	2.73	25	2.99	32	4.06	30	4.26	26	3.54	31	3.78	25	2.84
Gastroschisis	244	1.98	6	0.72	8	1.02	6	0.85	17	2.31	13	1.58	15	1.7
Down syndrome, maternal age 35 years or older	419	3.4	19	2.27	19	2.41	11	1.56	10	1.36	14	1.71	12	1.36
Down syndrome, maternal age younger than 35 years	874	7.09	44	5.26	65	8.25	48	6.81	43	5.85	68	8.29	70	7.94
Any autosomal trisomy, maternal age 35 years or older	528	4.29	20	2.39	23	2.92	13	1.84	13	1.77	15	1.83	19	2.15
Any autosomal trisomy, maternal age younger than 35 years	1,156	9.38	58	6.94	71	9.02	59	8.37	51	6.94	83	10.11	96	10.89

* Prev = Prevalence.
† Numbers of cases and prevalence estimates are not provided for hydrocephalus prior to 1992 because a specific definition for this defect was not applied to all cases prior to that time.
‡ Numbers of cases and prevalence estimates are not provided for congenital heart defects prior to 1983 because not all of these cases have been reviewed by pediatric cardiologists.

TABLE 4

THREE-YEAR PREVALENCE (PER 10,000 LIVE BIRTHS) OF SELECTED BIRTH DEFECTS, MACDP, 1968–2003

	Three-year period											
	1986–1988		1989–1991		1992–1994		1995–1997		1998–2000		2001–2003	
Birth defect	Cases	Prev*	Cases	Prev	Cases	Prev	Cases	Prev	Cases	Prev	Cases	Prev
Anencephalus	32	3.06	27	2.35	21	1.79	30	2.42	35	2.47	15	0.98
Encephalocele	20	1.91	14	1.22	12	1.02	18	1.45	14	0.99	16	1.05
Hydrocephalus†					43	3.67	59	4.76	83	5.85	71	4.64
Congenital cataract	20	1.91	21	1.82	22	1.88	29	2.34	33	2.32	35	2.29
Complete atrioventricular septal defect‡	34	3.26	25	2.17	22	1.88	33	2.66	32	2.25	28	1.83
Valvar pulmonary stenosis‡	28	2.68	31	2.69	42	3.59	66	5.32	91	6.41	69	4.51
Hypoplastic left heart syndrome‡	23	2.2	39	3.39	22	1.88	34	2.74	35	2.47	37	2.42
Aortic stenosis‡	18	1.72	9	0.78	11	0.94	10	0.81	19	1.34	17	1.11
Secundum atrial septal defect‡	25	2.39	40	3.48	63	5.38	85	6.85	109	7.68	156	10.2
Muscular ventricular septal defect‡	22	2.11	75	6.52	132	11.27	203	16.36	300	21.13	429	28.05
Single ventricle‡	11	1.05	7	0.61	11	0.94	16	1.29	18	1.27	10	0.65
Partial and total anomalous pulmonary venous return‡	7	0.67	22	1.91	6	0.51	10	0.81	10	0.7	10	0.65
Esophageal atresia or stenosis	19	1.82	23	2	28	2.39	32	2.58	23	1.62	29	1.9
Duodenal atresia or stenosis	13	1.24	19	1.65	19	1.62	26	2.1	25	1.76	30	1.96
Jejunal and/or ileal atresia or stenosis	18	1.72	19	1.65	18	1.54	22	1.77	25	1.76	26	1.7
Hirschsprung disease	17	1.63	28	2.43	24	2.05	26	2.1	31	2.18	35	2.29
Bilateral renal agenesis or dysgenesis	10	0.96	15	1.3	15	1.28	21	1.69	14	0.99	17	1.11
Any cystic kidney disease	41	3.93	46	4	65	5.55	68	5.48	75	5.28	83	5.43
Craniosynostosis	29	2.78	66	5.73	69	5.89	60	4.84	53	3.73	56	3.66
Skeletal dysplasia	24	2.3	18	1.56	31	2.65	30	2.42	25	1.76	26	1.7
Diaphragmatic hernia	30	2.87	30	2.61	25	2.13	25	2.02	30	2.11	48	3.14
Omphalocele	24	2.3	31	2.69	29	2.48	27	2.18	34	2.39	23	1.5
Gastroschisis	26	2.49	33	2.87	27	2.3	19	1.53	36	2.54	38	2.48
Down syndrome, maternal age 35 years or older	23	2.2	28	2.43	49	4.18	43	3.47	80	5.64	111	7.26
Down syndrome, maternal age younger than 35 years	71	6.8	96	8.34	73	6.23	92	7.42	101	7.11	103	6.73
Any autosomal trisomy, maternal age 35 years or older	28	2.68	37	3.21	60	5.12	62	5	105	7.4	133	8.69
Any autosomal trisomy, maternal age younger than 35 years	97	9.29	120	10.43	106	9.05	133	10.72	139	9.79	143	9.35

* Prev = Prevalence.
† Numbers of cases and prevalence estimates are not provided for hydrocephalus prior to 1992 because a specific definition for this defect was not applied to all cases prior to that time.
‡ Numbers of cases and prevalence estimates are not provided for congenital heart defects prior to 1983 because not all of these cases have been reviewed by pediatric cardiologists.

TABLE 5

TOTAL PREVALENCE (PER 10,000 LIVE BIRTHS) OF SELECTED BIRTH DEFECTS, MACDP, 1968–2003

Birth defect	Total	
	Cases	Prevalence
Anophthalmia	62	0.50
Truncus arteriosus[‡]	48	0.55
Pulmonary atresia[‡]	41	0.47
Levotransposition of the great arteries[‡]	29	0.33
Vascular ring[‡]	89	1.02
Ebstein anomaly[‡]	45	0.52
Choanal atresia or stenosis	152	1.23
Large intestinal atresia or stenosis	25	0.20
Biliary atresia	98	0.80
Exstrophy of the bladder	19	0.15
Posterior urethral valves	137	1.11
Intercalary limb deficiency	40	0.32
Longitudinal limb deficiency	176	1.43
Split-hand and/or split-foot malformation	49	0.40
Other and unspecified limb deficiency	26	0.21
Urethral obstruction sequence	50	0.41
Trisomy 13, maternal age 35 years or older	27	0.22
Trisomy 13, maternal age younger than 35 years	104	0.84
Trisomy 18, maternal age 35 years or older	71	0.58
Trisomy 18, maternal age younger than 35 years	150	1.22
Turner syndrome	110	0.89
Conjoined twins	15	0.12

‡ Numbers of cases and prevalence estimates are not provided for congenital heart defects prior to 1982 because not all of these cases have been reviewed by pediatric cardiologists.

TABLE 6A

ALL DEFECTS: PREVALENCE (PER 10,000 LIVE BIRTHS) STRATIFIED BY DESCRIPTIVE CHARACTERISTICS, MACDP, 1968–2003*

Characteristic	Total		1968–1972		1973–1978		1979–1983		1984–1989		1990–1993		1994–1998		1999–2003	
	Cases	Prev**	Cases	Prev	Cases	Prev	Cases	Prev	Cases	Prev	Cases	Prev	Cases	Prev	Cases	Prev
Total	32,938	267.31	2,872	209.33	3,934	274.09	3,800	280.36	5,611	276.73	3,894	252.32	5,882	281.66	6,945	277.80
Maternal age (years)																
<25	12,632	257.08	1,521	194.44	2,020	276.17	1,853	306.10	2,231	283.78	1,278	233.80	1,729	256.78	2,000	253.68
25–29	9,052	256.53	806	216.56	1,192	268.80	1,064	252.92	1,684	265.54	1,118	248.49	1,494	270.16	1,694	258.52
≥30	11,140	287.93	485	223.07	709	279.32	881	268.02	1,686	278.22	1,496	273.91	2,647	307.37	3,236	306.51
Unknown	114	–	60	–	13	–	<5	–	10	–	<5	–	12	–	15	–
Maternal race/ethnicity†																
White	18,972	283.10	2,244	227.83	2,821	303.45	2,225	267.99	3,397	277.10	2,210	278.28	3,060	312.05	3,015	315.39
Black or African American	10,838	257.94			1,085	221.03	1,542	304.95	2,098	276.91	1,428	222.38	2,196	260.52	2,489	258.61
Hispanic or Latino	1,628	250.52									142	240.43	383	230.90	1,103	259.58
All Other Races	1,391	182.89	628‡	162.25	26	175.79	26	135.56	111	254.88	109	230.54	222	231.35	269	176.09
Unknown	109	–			<5	–	7	–	5	–	5	–	21	–	69	–
Birth weight (grams)																
<2500	7,858	744.85	686	568.87	872	706.59	905	772.12	1,277	785.17	947	707.83	1,493	834.92	1,678	767.89
≥2500	24,851	221.11	2,107	169.31	3,028	233.83	2,878	232.64	4,312	231.38	2,933	208.19	4,360	228.37	5,233	229.40
Unknown	229	–	79	–	34	–	17	–	22	–	14	–	29	–	34	–
Gestational age (weeks)																
20–36	7,379	645.07	498	470.83	730	604.15	803	651.20	1,156	585.41	932	586.16	1,489	764.96	1,771	729.20
≥37	25,227	239.26	2,360	203.45	3,189	264.72	2,984	263.92	4,340	259.30	2,934	225.50	4,335	234.05	5,085	228.89
Unknown	332	–	14	–	15	–	13	–	115	–	28	–	58	–	89	–
Sex																
Male	19,574	310.77	1,677	238.92	2,382	322.63	2,219	319.54	3,250	312.79	2,334	296.22	3,564	334.6	4,148	326.19
Female	13,292	220.68	1,193	178.03	1,539	220.86	1,573	237.99	2,349	237.63	1,543	204.3	2,307	225.49	2,788	226.98
Ambiguous/Unknown	72	–	<5	–	13	–	8	–	12	–	17	–	13	–	8	–
Parity																
1 Live birth	14,794	273.16	1,212	232.42	1,820	251.89	1,780	280.42	2,357	263.13	1,825	273.05	2,705	294.53	3,095	293.48
2 or more live births	17,259	257.12	1,210	168.12	2,084	292.38	1,984	275.31	2,954	269.81	2,060	236.65	3,136	269.92	3,831	267.49
Unknown	885	–	450	–	30	–	36	–	300	–	9	–	41	–	19	–
Gravidity																
1 Pregnancy	10,789	232.66	1,109	228.06	1,490	222.30	1,342	204.93	1,753	248.41	1,169	224.56	1,778	243.79	2,148	246.82
2 or more pregnancies	21,978	294.29	1,732	229.43	2,412	315.27	2,441	348.45	3,832	298.60	2,717	267.16	4,065	301.82	4,779	298.59
Unknown	171	–	31	–	32	–	17	–	26	–	8	–	39	–	18	–
Plurality																
Singleton	31,580	263.01	2,793	207.34	3,793	269.77	3,675	276.67	5,389	271.99	3,719	247.54	5,603	276.53	6,608	273.52
Multiple	1,336	427.77	79	316.76	141	521.84	123	453.54	203	438.92	175	428.71	279	448.99	336	399.86
Unknown	22	–					<5	–	19	–					<5	–

TABLE 6B

ALL DEFECTS: PERCENTAGE OF CASES BY DESCRIPTIVE CHARACTERISTICS, MACDP, 1968–2003*

	Total		1968–1972		1973–1978		1979–1983		1984–1989		1990–1993		1994–1998		1999–2003	
Characteristic	Cases	Percent	Cases	Percent	Cases	Percent	Cases	Percent	Cases	Percent	Cases	Percent	Cases	Percent	Cases	Percent
Birth outcome																
Live birth	31,616	96.0	2,676	93.2	3,768	95.8	3,683	96.9	5,442	97.0	3,732	95.8	5,610	95.4	6,705	96.5
Stillbirth	978	3.0	195	6.8	163	4.1	113	3.0	159	2.8	100	2.6	131	2.2	117	1.7
Elective termination	341	1.0	–	–	<5	–	<5	–	10	0.2	62	1.6	141	2.4	123	1.8
Unknown	<5	–	<5	–	–	–	<5	–	–	–	–	–	–	–	–	–
Age at diagnosis																
Prenatally or <7 days	25,702	78.0	2,419	84.2	3,165	80.5	3,157	83.1	4,490	80.0	3,079	79.1	4,396	74.7	4,996	71.9
8 days–6 months	4,891	14.8	394	13.7	652	16.6	508	13.4	909	16.2	627	16.1	920	15.6	881	12.7
6 months–1 year	982	3.0	55	1.9	108	2.7	117	3.1	174	3.1	127	3.3	214	3.6	187	2.7
1–5 years	502	1.5	<5	–	<5	–	8	0.2	11	0.2	32	0.8	157	2.7	289	4.2
>5 years	38	0.1	–	–	–	–	–	–	<5	–	7	0.2	17	0.3	13	0.2
Unknown	823	2.5	<5	–	7	0.2	10	0.3	26	0.5	22	0.6	178	3.0	579	8.3
Socioeconomic status§																
Upper	7,615	23.1	–	–	–	–	1,069	28.1	1,882	33.5	1,528	39.2	1,957	33.3	1,179	17.0
Middle	7,371	22.4	–	–	–	–	1,145	30.1	1,665	29.7	1,246	32.0	1,993	33.9	1,322	19.0
Lower	7,172	21.8	–	–	–	–	1,491	39.2	1,989	35.4	1,059	27.2	1,638	27.8	995	14.3
Unknown	10,780	32.7	2,872	100.0	95	2.5	75	1.3	61	1.6	294	5.0	3,449	49.7		

* Cells containing fewer than 5 cases are indicated as "<5". Prevalence estimates based on these cells are indicated as less than the prevalence based on 5 cases in Table A. Percentages based on these cells are not provided in Table B. Cells containing zero cases are indicated as "–". Counts are provided, but prevalences are not estimated, for strata with unknown values in Table A. Counts and percentages are provided for strata with unknown values in Table B.
** Prev = Prevalence.
† Data on Hispanic or Latino ethnicity were available beginning in 1990.
‡ The category of All Other Races includes 619 cases of Black or African American race.
§ Information about socioeconomic status was available only for 1979–2001.

TABLE 7A

ANENCEPHALUS: PREVALENCE (PER 10,000 LIVE BIRTHS) STRATIFIED BY DESCRIPTIVE CHARACTERISTICS, MACDP, 1968–2003*

Characteristic	Total		1968–1972		1973–1978		1979–1983		1984–1989		1990–1993		1994–1998		1999–2003	
	Cases	Prev**	Cases	Prev	Cases	Prev	Cases	Prev	Cases	Prev	Cases	Prev	Cases	Prev	Cases	Prev
Total	**446**	**3.62**	**123**	**8.96**	**81**	**5.64**	**61**	**4.50**	**60**	**2.96**	**37**	**2.40**	**45**	**2.15**	**39**	**1.56**
Maternal age (years)																
<25	215	4.38	71	9.08	44	6.02	32	5.29	25	3.18	15	2.74	19	2.82	9	1.14
25–29	136	3.85	34	9.14	18	4.06	21	4.99	22	3.47	10	2.22	13	2.35	18	2.75
≥30	93	2.40	17	7.82	19	7.49	8	2.43	13	2.15	12	2.20	12	1.39	12	1.14
Unknown	<5	–	<5	–	–	–	–	–	–	–	–	–	<5	–	–	–
Maternal race/ethnicity†																
White	317	4.73	111	11.27	61	6.56	51	6.14	39	3.18	17	2.14	23	2.35	15	1.57
Black or African American	91	2.17	–	–	19	3.87	9	1.78	19	2.51	17	2.65	15	1.78	12	1.25
Hispanic or Latino	16	2.46	–	–	–	–	–	–	–	–	<5	<8.47	<5	<3.01	10	2.35
All Other Races	20	2.63	12‡	3.10	<5	<33.81	<5	<26.07	<5	<11.48	<5	<10.58	<5	<5.21	<5	<3.27
Unknown	<5	–	<5	–	–	–	–	–	<5	–	–	–	<5	–	–	–
Birth weight (grams)																
<2500	341	32.32	91	75.46	60	48.62	47	40.10	49	30.13	27	20.18	37	20.69	30	13.73
≥2500	71	0.63	20	1.61	18	1.39	9	0.73	6	0.32	6	0.43	5	0.26	7	0.31
Unknown	34	–	12	–	<5	–	5	–	5	–	<5	–	<5	–	<5	–
Gestational age (weeks)																
20–36	277	24.22	69	65.24	42	34.76	32	25.95	46	23.29	25	15.72	36	18.49	27	11.12
≥37	164	1.56	53	4.57	39	3.24	28	2.48	11	0.66	12	0.92	9	0.49	12	0.54
Unknown	5	–	<5	–	–	–	<5	–	<5	–	–	–	–	–	–	–
Sex																
Male	154	2.45	39	5.56	26	3.52	18	2.59	19	1.83	15	1.90	20	1.88	17	1.34
Female	286	4.75	84	12.54	53	7.61	42	6.35	40	4.05	21	2.78	24	2.35	22	179
Ambiguous/Unknown	6	–	–	–	<5	–	<5	–	<5	–	<5	–	<5	–	–	–
Parity																
1 Live birth	186	3.43	54	10.36	42	5.81	28	4.41	23	2.57	12	1.80	13	1.42	14	1.33
2 or more live births	235	3.50	48	6.67	38	5.33	33	4.58	34	3.11	25	2.87	32	2.75	25	1.75
Unknown	25	–	21	–	<5	–	–	–	<5	–	–	–	–	–	–	–
Gravidity																
1 Pregnancy	150	3.23	48	9.87	37	5.52	20	3.05	17	2.41	9	1.73	9	1.23	10	1.15
2 or more pregnancies	294	3.94	75	9.93	43	5.62	40	5.71	43	3.35	28	2.75	36	2.67	29	1.81
Unknown	<5	–	–	–	<5	–	<5	–	–	–	–	–	–	–	–	–
Plurality																
Singleton	417	3.47	119	8.83	76	5.41	56	4.22	56	2.83	32	2.13	42	2.07	36	1.49
Multiple	29	9.29	<5	<20.05	5	18.50	5	18.44	<5	<10.81	5	12.25	<5	<8.05	<5	<5.95
Unknown	–	–	–	–	–	–	–	–	–	–	–	–	–	–	–	–

TABLE 7B

ANENCEPHALUS: PERCENTAGE OF CASES BY DESCRIPTIVE CHARACTERISTICS, MACDP, 1968–2003*

	Total		1968–1972		1973–1978		1979–1983		1984–1989		1990–1993		1994–1998		1999–2003	
Characteristic	Cases	Percent	Cases	Percent	Cases	Percent	Cases	Percent	Cases	Percent	Cases	Percent	Cases	Percent	Cases	Percent
Birth outcome																
Live birth	166	37.2	34	27.6	30	37.0	33	54.1	29	48.3	13	35.1	14	31.1	13	33.3
Stillbirth	230	51.6	88	71.5	50	61.7	27	44.3	28	46.7	13	35.1	11	24.4	13	33.3
Elective termination	49	11.0	–	–	<5	–	<5	–	<5	–	11	29.7	20	44.4	13	33.3
Unknown	<5	–	<5	–	–	–	–	–	–	–	–	–	–	–	–	–
Age at diagnosis																
Prenatally or <7 days	432	96.9	123	100	81	100	60	98.4	58	96.7	35	94.6	43	95.6	32	82.1
8 days–6 months	<5	–	–	–	–	–	<5	–	–	–	<5	–	–	–	–	–
6 months–1 year	<5	–	–	–	–	–	–	–	–	–	<5	–	–	–	–	–
1–5 years	–	–	–	–	–	–	–	–	–	–	–	–	–	–	–	–
>5 years	–	–	–	–	–	–	–	–	–	–	–	–	–	–	–	–
Unknown	11	2.5	–	–	–	–	–	–	<5	–	–	–	<5	–	7	17.9
Socioeconomic status§																
Upper	73	16.4	–	–	–	–	25	41.0	22	36.7	10	27.0	10	22.2	6	15.4
Middle	75	16.8	–	–	–	–	19	31.1	16	26.7	14	37.8	14	31.1	12	30.8
Lower	79	17.7	–	–	–	–	17	27.9	22	36.7	13	35.1	18	40.0	9	23.1
Unknown	219	49.1	123	100.0	81	100.0	–	–	–	–	–	–	<5	–	12	30.8

* Cells containing fewer than 5 cases are indicated as "<5". Prevalence estimates based on these cells are indicated as less than the prevalence based on 5 cases in Table A. Percentages based on these cells are not provided in Table B. Cells containing zero cases are indicated as "–". Counts are provided, but prevalences are not estimated, for strata with unknown values in Table A. Counts and percentages are provided for strata with unknown values in Table B.
** Prev = Prevalence.
† Data on Hispanic or Latino ethnicity were available beginning in 1990.
‡ The category of All Other Races includes 12 cases of Black or African American race.
§ Information about socioeconomic status was available only for 1979–2001.

TABLE 8A

SPINA BIFIDA: PREVALENCE (PER 10,000 LIVE BIRTHS) STRATIFIED BY DESCRIPTIVE CHARACTERISTICS, MACDP, 1968-2003*

Characteristic	Total		1968–1972		1973–1978		1979–1983		1984–1989		1990–1993		1994–1998		1999–2003	
	Cases	Prev**	Cases	Prev	Cases	Prev	Cases	Prev	Cases	Prev	Cases	Prev	Cases	Prev	Cases	Prev
Total	706	5.73	181	13.19	116	8.08	92	6.79	120	5.92	57	3.69	76	3.64	64	2.56
Maternal age (years)																
<25	301	6.13	97	12.40	58	7.93	35	5.78	53	6.74	21	3.84	20	2.97	17	2.16
25–29	217	6.15	49	13.17	30	6.77	31	7.37	39	6.15	16	3.56	28	5.06	24	3.66
≥30	183	4.73	30	13.80	28	11.03	26	7.91	28	4.62	20	3.66	28	3.25	23	2.18
Unknown	5	–	5–	–	–		–		–		–		–		–	
Maternal race/ethnicity																
White	514	7.67	161	16.35	95	10.22	65	7.83	84	6.85	38	4.78	52	5.30	19	1.99
Black or African American	138	3.28	–	–	20	4.07	25	4.94	33	4.36	18	2.80	20	2.37	22	2.29
Hispanic or Latino	27	4.15	–	–	<5	–	<5	–	–		<5	<8.47	<5	<3.01	22	5.18
All Other Races	26	3.42	20‡	5.17	<5	<26.07	<5	<11.48	–		–		–		<5	–
Unknown	<5	–	–		–		–		–		–		–		–	
Birth weight (grams)																
<2500	205	19.43	49	40.63	29	23.50	19	16.21	36	22.13	20	14.95	34	19.01	18	8.24
≥2500	484	4.31	122	9.80	84	6.49	72	5.82	82	4.40	36	2.56	42	2.20	46	2.02
Unknown	17	–	10	–	<5	–	<5	–	<5	–	<5	–	–		–	
Gestational age (weeks)																
20–36	192	16.78	31	29.31	28	23.17	19	15.41	33	16.71	23	14.47	37	19.01	21	8.65
≥37	506	4.80	149	12.84	86	7.14	73	6.46	83	4.96	33	2.54	39	2.11	43	1.94
Unknown	8	–	<5	–	<5	–	–		<5	–	<5	–	–		–	
Sex																
Male	350	5.56	81	11.54	58	7.86	45	6.48	60	5.77	30	3.81	35	3.29	41	3.22
Female	353	5.86	100	14.92	57	8.18	46	6.96	60	6.07	27	3.57	40	3.91	23	1.87
Ambiguous/Unknown	<5	–	–		<5	–	<5	–	–		–		<5	–	–	
Parity																
1 Live birth	292	5.39	75	14.38	48	6.64	38	5.99	57	6.36	22	3.29	31	3.38	21	1.99
2 or more live births	366	5.45	69	9.59	66	9.26	52	7.22	56	5.11	35	4.02	45	3.87	43	3.00
Unknown	48	–	37	–	<5	–	<5	–	7	–	–		–		–	
Gravidity																
1 Pregnancy	223	4.81	71	14.60	36	5.37	25	3.82	37	5.24	15	2.88	21	2.88	18	2.07
2 or more pregnancies	474	6.35	106	14.04	77	10.06	65	9.28	83	6.47	42	4.13	55	4.08	46	2.87
Unknown	9	–	<5	–	<5	–	<5	–	–		–		–		–	
Plurality																
Singleton	695	5.79	181	13.44	112	7.97	91	6.85	115	5.80	56	3.73	76	3.75	64	2.65
Multiple	11	3.52	–	–	<5	<18.50	<5	<18.44	5	10.81	<5	<12.25	–		–	
Unknown	–		–		–		–		–		–		–		–	

TABLE 8B

SPINA BIFIDA: PERCENTAGE OF CASES BY DESCRIPTIVE CHARACTERISTICS, MACDP, 1968–2003*

Characteristic	Total Cases	Total Percent	1968–1972 Cases	1968–1972 Percent	1973–1978 Cases	1973–1978 Percent	1979–1983 Cases	1979–1983 Percent	1984–1989 Cases	1984–1989 Percent	1990–1993 Cases	1990–1993 Percent	1994–1998 Cases	1994–1998 Percent	1999–2003 Cases	1999–2003 Percent
Birth outcome																
Live birth	588	83.3	144	79.6	98	84.5	86	93.5	107	89.2	47	82.5	53	69.7	53	82.8
Stillbirth	84	11.9	37	20.4	18	15.5	5	5.4	12	10.0	<5	–	6	7.9	<5	–
Elective termination	34	4.8	–	–	–	–	<5	–	<5	–	8	14.0	17	22.4	7	10.9
Unknown	–	–	–	–	–	–	–	–	–	–	–	–	–	–	–	–
Age at diagnosis																
Prenatally or <7 days	678	96.0	180	99.4	115	99.1	89	96.7	114	95.0	55	96.5	68	89.5	57	89.1
8 days–6 months	14	2.0	<5	–	–	–	<5	–	<5	–	<5	–	<5	–	<5	–
6 months–1 year	<5	–	–	–	<5	–	–	–	<5	–	–	–	–	–	<5	–
1–5 years	<5	–	–	–	–	–	–	–	–	–	–	–	–	–	<5	–
>5 years	–	–	–	–	–	–	–	–	–	–	–	–	–	–	–	–
Unknown	11	1.6	–	–	–	–	–	–	<5	–	–	–	5	6.6	5	7.8
Socioeconomic status§																
Upper	117	16.6	–	–	–	29	31.5	45	37.5	16	28.1	22	28.9	5	7.8	–
Middle	114	16.1	–	–	–	–	31	33.7	32	26.7	19	33.3	22	28.9	10	15.6
Lower	129	18.3	–	–	–	–	28	30.4	41	34.2	22	38.6	26	34.2	12	18.8
Unknown	346	49.0	181	100.0	116	100.0	<5	–	<5	–	–	–	6	7.9	37	57.8

* Cells containing fewer than 5 cases are indicated as "<5" Prevalence estimates based on these cells are indicated as less than the prevalence based on 5 cases in Table A. Percentages based on these cells are not provided in Table B. Cells containing zero cases are indicated as "–". Counts are provided, but prevalences are not estimated, for strata with unknown values in Table A. Counts and percentages are provided for strata with unknown values in Table B.

** Prev = Prevalence.

† Data on Hispanic or Latino ethnicity were available beginning in 1990.

‡ The category of All Other Races includes 19 cases of Black or African American race.

§ Information about socioeconomic status was available only for 1979–2001.

TABLE 9A

ENCEPHALOCELE: PREVALENCE (PER 10,000 LIVE BIRTHS) STRATIFIED BY DESCRIPTIVE CHARACTERISTICS, MACDP, 1968–2003*

	Total		1968–1972		1973–1978		1979–1983		1984–1989		1990–1993		1994–1998		1999–2003	
Characteristic	Cases	Prev**	Cases	Prev	Cases	Prev	Cases	Prev	Cases	Prev	Cases	Prev	Cases	Prev	Cases	Prev
Total	**190**	**1.54**	**20**	**1.46**	**31**	**2.16**	**32**	**2.36**	**36**	**1.78**	**21**	**1.36**	**24**	**1.15**	**26**	**1.04**
Maternal age (years)																
<25	82	1.67	9	1.15	17	2.32	15	2.48	18	2.29	6	1.10	9	1.34	8	1.01
25–29	55	1.56	7	1.88	10	2.26	11	2.61	9	1.42	5	1.11	6	1.08	7	1.07
≥30	53	1.37	<5	<2.30	<5	<1.97	6	1.83	9	1.49	10	1.83	9	1.05	11	1.04
Unknown	–	–	–	–	–	–	–	–	–	–	–	–	–	–	–	–
Material race/ethnicity†																
White	98	1.46	16	1.62	25	2.69	12	1.45	21	1.71	6	0.76	11	1.12	7	0.73
Black or African American	74	1.76	–	–	6	1.22	19	3.76	14	1.85	13	2.02	10	1.19	12	1.25
Hispanic or Latino	9	1.38	–	–	–	–	–	–	–	–	–	–	<5	<3.01	6	1.41
All Other Races	9	1.18	<5‡	<1.29	–	–	<5	<26.07	<5	<11.48	<5	<10.58	–	–	<5	<3.27
Unknown	–	–	–	–	–	–	–	–	–	–	–	–	–	–	–	–
Birth weight (grams)																
<2500	78	7.39	8	6.63	11	8.91	13	11.09	15	9.22	11	8.22	11	6.15	9	4.12
≥2500	108	0.96	12	0.96	19	1.47	19	1.54	19	1.02	10	0.71	13	0.68	16	0.70
Unknown	<5	–	–	–	<5	–	–	–	<5	–	–	–	–	–	<5	–
Gestational age (weeks)																
20–36	74	6.47	<5	<4.73	10	8.28	12	9.73	18	9.12	11	6.92	9	4.62	10	4.12
≥37	115	1.09	16	1.38	21	1.74	20	1.77	17	1.02	10	0.77	15	0.81	16	0.72
Unknown	<5	–	–	–	–	–	–	–	<5	–	–	–	–	–	–	–
Sex																
Male	84	1.33	6	0.85	17	2.30	17	2.45	12	1.15	8	1.02	13	1.22	11	0.87
Female	103	1.71	14	2.09	13	1.87	15	2.27	23	2.33	12	1.59	11	1.08	15	1.22
Ambiguous/Unknown	<5	–	–	–	<5	–	<5	–	<5	–	<5	–	–	–	–	–
Parity																
1 Live birth	82	1.51	6	1.15	13	1.80	16	2.52	15	1.67	7	1.05	15	1.63	10	0.95
2 or more live births	101	1.50	9	1.25	18	2.53	15	2.08	20	1.83	14	1.61	9	0.77	16	1.12
Unknown	7	–	5	–	–	–	<5	–	<5	–	–	–	–	–	–	–
Gravidity																
1 Pregnancy	56	1.21	6	1.23	9	1.34	10	1.53	9	1.28	<5	<0.96	10	1.37	8	0.92
2 or more pregnancies	134	1.79	14	1.85	22	2.88	22	3.14	27	2.10	17	1.67	14	1.04	18	1.12
Unknown	–	–	–	–	–	–	–	–	–	–	–	–	–	–	–	–
Plurality																
Singleton	182	1.52	19	1.41	31	2.20	30	2.26	33	1.67	20	1.33	23	1.14	26	1.08
Multiple	8	2.56	<5	<20.05	–	–	<5	<18.44	<5	<10.81	<5	<12.25	<5	<8.05	–	–
Unknown	–	–	–	–	–	–	–	–	–	–	–	–	–	–	–	–

TABLE 9B

ENCEPHALOCELE: PERCENTAGE OF CASES BY DESCRIPTIVE CHARACTERISTICS, MACDP, 1968–2003*

			Period													
	Total		1968–1972		1973–1978		1979–1983		1984–1989		1990–1993		1994–1998		1999–2003	
Characteristic	Cases	Percent	Cases	Percent	Cases	Percent	Cases	Percent	Cases	Percent	Cases	Percent	Cases	Percent	Cases	Percent
Birth outcome																
Live birth	148	77.9	17	85.0	23	74.2	28	87.5	28	77.8	15	71.4	19	79.2	18	69.2
Stillbirth	28	14.7	<5	–	6	19.4	<5	–	7	19.4	<5	–	<5	–	<5	–
Elective termination	14	7.4	–	–	<5	–	–	–	<5	–	<5	–	<5	–	6	23.1
Unknown	–	–	–	–	–	–	–	–	–	–	–	–	–	–	–	–
Age at diagnosis																
Prenatally or <7 days	179	94.2	20	100.0	30	96.8	31	96.9	35	97.2	18	85.7	23	95.8	22	84.6
8 days–6 months	7	3.7	–	–	<5	–	<5	–	<5	–	<5	–	<5	–	<5	–
6 months–1 year	<5	–	–	–	–	–	–	–	–	–	<5	–	–	–	–	–
1–5 years	–	–	–	–	–	–	–	–	–	–	–	–	–	–	–	–
>5 years	–	–	–	–	–	–	–	–	–	–	–	–	–	–	–	–
Unknown	<5	–	–	–	–	–	–	–	–	–	–	–	–	–	<5	–
Socioeconomic status§																
Upper	41	21.6	–	–	–	–	7	21.9	16	44.4	8	38.1	7	29.2	<5	–
Middle	38	20.0	–	–	–	–	11	34.4	9	25.0	7	33.3	5	20.8	6	23.1
Lower	44	23.2	–	–	–	–	14	43.8	11	30.6	6	28.6	11	45.8	<5	–
Unknown	67	35.3	20	100.0	31	100.0	–	–	–	–	–	–	<5	–	15	57.7

* Cells containing fewer than 5 cases are indicated as "<5". Prevalence estimates based on these cells are indicated as less than the prevalence based on 5 cases in Table A. Percentages based on these cells are not provided in Table B. Cells containing zero cases are indicated as "–". Counts are provided, but prevalences are not estimated, for strata with unknown values in Table A. Counts and percentages are provided for strata with unknown values in Table B.
** Prev = Prevalence.
† Data on Hispanic or Latino ethnicity were available beginning in 1990.
‡ The category of All Other Races includes <5 cases of Black or African American race.
§ Information about socioeconomic status was available only for 1979–2001.

TABLE 10A

HYDROCEPHALUS: PREVALENCE (PER 10,000 LIVE BIRTHS) STRATIFIED BY DESCRIPTIVE CHARACTERISTICS, MACDP, 1990–2003*

	Total		1968–1972		1973–1978		1979–1983		1984–1989		1990–1993		1994–1998		1999–2003	
Characteristic	Cases	Prev**	Cases	Prev	Cases	Prev	Cases	Prev	Cases	Prev	Cases	Prev	Cases	Prev	Cases	Prev
Total	296	4.83									67	4.34	104	4.98	125	5.00
Maternal age (years)																
<25	90	4.48									19	3.48	33	4.90	38	4.82
25–29	69	4.16									19	4.22	21	3.80	29	4.43
≥30	137	5.56									29	5.31	50	5.81	58	5.49
Unknown	–	–									–	–	–	–	–	–
Maternal race/ethnicity†																
White	129	4.72									32	4.03	53	5.40	44	4.60
Black or African American	133	5.43									31	4.83	41	4.86	61	6.34
Hispanic or Latino	20	3.08									<5	<8.47	5	3.01	14	3.29
All Other Races	13	4.39									<5	<10.58	5	5.21	5	3.27
Unknown	1	–									–	–	–	–	<5	–
Birth weight (grams)																
<2500	119	22.41									30	22.42	47	26.28	42	19.22
≥2500	169	3.02									37	2.63	56	2.93	76	3.33
Unknown	8	–									–	–	<5	–	7	–
Gestational age (weeks)																
20–36	136	22.30									29	18.24	57	29.28	50	20.59
≥37	155	2.83									36	2.77	45	2.43	74	3.33
Unknown	5	–									<5	–	<5	–	<5	–
Sex																
Male	156	4.99									39	4.95	56	5.26	61	4.80
Female	138	4.59									28	3.71	47	4.59	63	5.13
Ambiguous/Unknown	<5	–									–	–	<5	–	<5	–
Parity																
1 Live birth	128	4.85									20	2.99	47	5.12	61	5.78
2 or more live births	166	4.70									47	5.40	55	4.73	64	4.47
Unknown	2	–									–	–	<5	–	–	–
Gravidity																
1 Pregnancy	94	4.43									11	2.11	37	5.07	46	5.29
2 or more pregnancies	200	5.04									56	5.51	65	4.83	79	4.94
Unknown	2	–									–	–	<5	–	–	–
Plurality																
Singleton	272	4.58									62	4.13	92	4.54	118	4.88
Multiple	24	12.83									5	12.25	12	19.31	7	8.33
Unknown	–	–									–	–	–	–	–	–

TABLE 10B

HYDROCEPHALUS: PERCENTAGE OF CASES BY DESCRIPTIVE CHARACTERISTICS, MACDP, 1990–2003*

	Period															
	Total		1968–1972		1973–1978		1979–1983		1984–1989		1990–1993		1994–1998		1999–2003	
Characteristic	Cases	Percent	Cases	Percent	Cases	Percent	Cases	Percent	Cases	Percent	Cases	Percent	Cases	Percent	Cases	Percent
Birth outcome																
Live birth	258	87.2									55	82.1	91	87.5	112	89.6
Stillbirth	23	7.8									9	13.4	6	5.8	8	6.4
Elective termination	15	5.1									<5	–	7	6.7	5	4.0
Unknown	–	–									–	–	–	–	–	–
Age at diagnosis																
Prenatally or <7 days	208	70.3									58	86.6	73	70.2	77	61.6
8 days–6 months	43	14.5									7	10.4	20	19.2	16	12.8
6 months–1 year	24	8.1									<5	–	5	4.8	17	13.6
1–5 years	4	1.4									–	–	–	–	<5	–
>5 years	–	–									–	–	–	–	–	–
Unknown	17	5.7									–	–	6	5.8	11	8.8
Socioeconomic status§																
Upper	70	23.6									23	34.3	31	29.8	16	12.8
Middle	79	26.7									20	29.9	35	33.7	24	19.2
Lower	83	28.0									23	34.3	32	30.8	28	22.4
Unknown	64	21.6									<5	–	6	5.8	57	45.6

* Numbers of cases and prevalence estimates are not provided for hydrocephalus prior to 1990 because a specific definition for this defect was not applied to all cases prior to that time. Cells containing fewer than 5 cases are indicated as "<5". Prevalence estimates based on these cells are indicated as less than the prevalence based on 5 cases in Table A. Percentages based on these cells are not provided in Table B. Cells containing zero cases are indicated as "–". Cells in years for which no data are provided are left blank. Counts are provided, but prevalences are not estimated, for strata with unknown values in Table A. Counts and percentages are provided for strata with unknown values in Table B.

** Prev = Prevalence.

† Data on Hispanic or Latino ethnicity were available beginning in 1990.

§ Information about socioeconomic status was available only for 1979–2001.

TABLE 11A

CONGENITAL CATARACT: PREVALENCE (PER 10,000 LIVE BIRTHS) STRATIFIED BY DESCRIPTIVE CHARACTERISTICS, MACDP, 1968–2003*

	Total		1968–1972		1973–1978		1979–1983		1984–1989		1990–1993		1994–1998		1999–2003	
Characteristic	Cases	Prev**	Cases	Prev	Cases	Prev	Cases	Prev	Cases	Prev	Cases	Prev	Cases	Prev	Cases	Prev
Total	**265**	**2.15**	**12**	**0.87**	**38**	**2.65**	**41**	**3.02**	**41**	**2.02**	**28**	**1.81**	**44**	**2.11**	**61**	**2.44**
Maternal age (years)																
<25	109	2.22	7	0.89	19	2.60	21	3.47	19	2.42	13	2.38	12	1.78	18	2.28
25–29	64	1.81	<5	<1.34	11	2.48	10	2.38	12	1.89	5	1.11	8	1.45	15	2.29
≥30	92	2.38	<5	<2.30	8	3.15	10	3.04	10	1.65	10	1.83	24	2.79	28	2.65
Unknown	–	–	–	–	–	–	–	–	–	–	–	–	–	–	–	–
Maternal race/ethnicity†																
White	141	2.10	9	0.91	22	2.37	19	2.29	22	1.79	16	2.01	24	2.45	29	3.03
Black or African American	102	2.43	–	–	16	3.26	22	4.35	17	2.24	10	1.56	17	2.02	20	2.08
Hispanic or Latino	15	2.31	–	–	–	–	–	–	–	–	<5	<8.47	<5	<3.01	10	2.35
All Other Races	7	0.92	<5‡	<1.29	–	–	–	–	<5	<11.48	–	–	–	–	<5	<3.27
Unknown	–	–	–	–	–	–	–	–	–	–	–	–	–	–	–	–
Birth weight (grams)																
<2500	68	6.45	5	4.15	13	10.53	13	11.09	6	3.69	5	3.74	11	6.15	15	6.86
≥2500	197	1.75	7	0.56	25	1.93	28	2.26	35	1.88	23	1.63	33	1.73	46	2.02
Unknown	–	–	–	–	–	–	–	–	–	–	–	–	–	–	–	–
Gestational age (weeks)																
20–36	60	5.25	<5	<4.73	7	5.79	11	8.92	6	3.04	6	3.77	10	5.14	16	6.59
≥37	201	1.91	7	0.60	31	2.57	30	2.65	33	1.97	22	1.69	33	1.78	45	2.03
Unknown	<5	–	<5	–	–	–	–	–	<5	–	–	–	<5	–	–	–
Sex																
Male	128	2.03	<5	<0.71	17	2.30	20	2.88	16	1.54	16	2.03	27	2.53	28	2.20
Female	135	2.24	7	1.04	21	3.01	21	3.18	24	2.43	12	1.59	17	1.66	33	2.69
Ambiguous/Unknown	<5	–	<5	–	–	–	–	–	<5	–	–	–	–	–	–	–
Parity																
1 Live birth	107	1.98	5	0.96	12	1.66	12	1.89	13	1.45	11	1.65	23	2.50	31	2.94
2 or more live births	149	2.22	<5	<0.69	25	3.51	27	3.75	26	2.37	17	1.95	21	1.81	30	2.09
Unknown	9	–	<5	–	<5	–	<5	–	<5	–	–	–	–	–	–	–
Gravidity																
1 Pregnancy	81	1.75	<5	<1.03	11	1.64	10	1.53	14	1.98	8	1.54	11	1.51	23	2.64
2 or more pregnancies	183	2.45	8	1.06	26	3.40	31	4.43	27	2.10	20	1.97	33	2.45	38	2.37
Unknown	<5	–	–	–	<5	–	–	–	–	–	–	–	–	–	–	–
Plurality																
Singleton	256	2.13	12	0.89	36	2.56	39	2.94	40	2.02	28	1.86	44	2.17	57	2.36
Multiple	9	2.88	–	–	<5	<18.50	<5	<18.44	<5	<10.81	–	–	–	–	<5	<5.95
Unknown	–	–	–	–	–	–	–	–	–	–	–	–	–	–	–	–

TABLE 11B

CONGENITAL CATARACT: PERCENTAGE OF CASES BY DESCRIPTIVE CHARACTERISTICS, MACDP, 1968–2003*

									Period							
	Total		1968–1972		1973–1978		1979–1983		1984–1989		1990–1993		1994–1998		1999–2003	
Characteristic	Cases	Percent	Cases	Percent	Cases	Percent	Cases	Percent	Cases	Percent	Cases	Percent	Cases	Percent	Cases	Percent
Birth outcome																
Live birth	262	98.9	10	83.3	38	100.0	41	100.0	41	100.0	28	100.0	43	97.7	61	100.0
Stillbirth	<5	–	<5	–	–	–	–	–	–	–	–	–	–	–	–	–
Elective termination	<5	–	–	–	–	–	–	–	–	–	–	–	<5	–	–	–
Unknown	–	–	–	–	–	–	–	–	–	–	–	–	–	–	–	–
Age at diagnosis																
Prenatally or <7 days	162	61.1	11	91.7	24	63.2	27	65.9	26	63.4	19	67.9	26	59.1	29	47.5
8 days–6 months	67	25.3	<5	–	9	23.7	6	14.6	12	29.3	8	28.6	13	29.5	18	29.5
6 months–1 year	19	7.2	–	–	<5	–	8	19.5	<5	–	–	–	<5	–	<5	–
1–5 years	<5	–	–	–	–	–	–	–	–	–	<5	–	<5	–	<5	–
>5 years	<5	–	–	–	–	–	–	–	–	–	–	–	<5	–	–	–
Unknown	13	4.9	–	–	<5	–	–	–	–	–	–	–	<5	–	11	18.0
Socioeconomic status§																
Upper	62	23.4	–	–	–	–	14	34.1	13	31.7	13	46.4	13	29.5	9	14.8
Middle	61	23.0	–	–	–	–	7	17.1	12	29.3	6	21.4	20	45.5	16	26.2
Lower	56	21.1	–	–	–	–	20	48.8	15	36.6	8	28.6	9	20.5	<5	–
Unknown	86	32.5	12	100.0	38	100.0	–	–	<5	–	<5	–	<5	–	32	52.5

* Cells containing fewer than 5 cases are indicated as "<5". Prevalence estimates based on these cells are indicated as less than the prevalence based on 5 cases in Table A. Percentages based on these cells are not provided in Table B. Cells containing zero cases are indicated as "–". Counts are provided, but prevalences are not estimated, for strata with unknown values in Table A. Counts and percentages are provided for strata with unknown values in Table B.

** Prev = Prevalence.

† Data on Hispanic or Latino ethnicity were available beginning in 1990.

‡ The category of All Other Races includes <5 cases of Black or African American race.

§ Information about socioeconomic status was available only for 1979–2001.

TABLE 12A

CONOTRUNCAL HEART DEFECTS: PREVALENCE (PER 10,000 LIVE BIRTHS) STRATIFIED BY DESCRIPTIVE CHARACTERISTICS, MACDP, 1984–2003*

	Total		1968–1972		1973–1978		1979–1983		1984–1989		1990–1993		1994–1998		1999–2003	
Characteristic	Cases	Prev**	Cases	Prev	Cases	Prev	Cases	Prev	Cases	Prev	Cases	Prev	Cases	Prev	Cases	Prev
Total	793	9.72							175	8.63	143	9.27	203	9.72	272	10.88
Maternal age (years)																
<25	262	9.38							60	7.63	49	8.96	73	10.84	80	10.15
25–29	216	9.42							57	8.99	37	8.22	44	7.96	78	11.90
≥30	311	10.13							57	9.41	57	10.44	85	9.87	112	10.61
Unknown	<5	–							<5	–	–		<5	–	<5	–
Maternal race/ethnicity†																
White	398	10.06							113	9.22	75	9.44	106	10.81	104	10.88
Black or African American	295	9.20							58	7.66	55	8.56	75	8.90	107	11.12
Hispanic or Latino	63	9.69							–	–	7	11.85	10	6.03	46	10.83
All Other Race	35	10.31							<5	<11.48	6	12.69	12	12.51	13	8.51
Unknown	<5	–							–		–		–		<5	–
Birth weight (grams)																
<2500	200	28.83							41	25.21	29	21.68	62	34.67	68	31.12
≥2500	592	7.93							134	7.19	114	8.09	141	7.39	203	8.90
Unknown	<5	–							–		–		–		<5	–
Gestational age (weeks)																
20–36	169	21.28							35	17.72	29	18.24	44	22.60	61	25.12
≥37	616	8.74							137	8.19	113	8.68	156	8.42	210	9.45
Unknown	8	–							<5	–	<5	–	<5	–	<5	–
Sex																
Male	442	10.62							90	8.66	81	10.28	112	10.51	159	12.50
Female	351	8.79							85	8.60	62	8.21	91	8.89	113	9.20
Ambiguous/Unknown	–								–		–		–		–	
Parity																
1 Live birth	328	9.27							74	8.26	57	8.53	86	9.36	111	10.53
2 or more live births	458	10.05							96	8.77	86	9.88	116	9.98	160	11.17
Unknown	7	–							5		–		<5		<5	
Gravidity																
1 Pregnancy	211	7.47							53	7.51	31	5.95	49	6.72	78	8.96
2 or more pregnancies	580	11.05							121	9.43	112	11.01	154	11.43	193	12.06
Unknown	<5	–							<5		–		–		<5	
Plurality																
Singleton	759	9.58							168	8.48	140	9.32	190	9.38	261	10.80
Multiple	32	13.72							5	10.81	<5	<12.25	13	20.92	11	13.09
Unknown	<5	–							<5	–	–		–		–	

TABLE 12B

CONOTRUNCAL HEART DEFECTS: PERCENTAGE OF CASES BY DESCRIPTIVE CHARACTERISTICS, MACDP, 1984–2003*

							Period										
	Total		1968–1972		1973–1978		1979–1983		1984–1989		1990–1993		1994–1998		1999–2003	
Characteristic	Cases	Percent	Cases	Percent	Cases	Percent	Cases	Percent	Cases	Percent	Cases	Percent	Cases	Percent	Cases	Percent
Birth outcome																
Live birth	781	98.5							172	98.3	141	98.6	199	98.0	269	98.9
Stillbirth	8	1.0							<5	–	<5	–	<5	–	<5	–
Elective termination	<5	–							–	–	<5	–	<5	–	<5	–
Unknown	–	–							–	–			–	–	–	–
Age at diagnosis																
Prenatally or <7 days	645	81.3							150	85.7	118	82.5	168	82.8	209	76.8
8 days–6 months	90	11.3							20	11.4	21	14.7	22	10.8	27	9.9
6 months–1 year	22	2.8							<5	–	<5	–	9	4.4	5	1.8
1–5 years	9	0.0							<5	–	–	–	–	–	8	2.9
>5 years	<5	–							–	–	–	–	<5	–	–	–
Unknown	26	3.3							–	–	–	–	<5	–	23	8.5
Socioeconomic status§																
Upper	226	28.5							60	34.3	56	39.2	67	33.0	43	15.8
Middle	221	27.9							51	29.1	46	32.2	63	31.0	61	22.4
Lower	201	25.35							63	36	39	27.3	67	33	32	11.8
Unknown	145	18.28							<5	–	<5	–	6	3	136	50

* Numbers of cases and prevalence estimates are not provided for congenital heart defects prior to 1984 because not all of these cases have been reviewed by pediatric cardiologists. Cells containing fewer than 5 cases are indicated as "<5". Prevalence estimates based on these cells are indicated as less than the prevalence based on 5 cases in Table A. Percentages based on these cells are not provided in Table B. Cells containing zero cases are indicated as "–". Cells in years for which no data are provided are left blank. Counts are provided, but prevalences are not estimated, for strata with unknown values in Table A. Counts and percentages are provided for strata with unknown values in Table B.

** Prev = Prevalence.

† Data on Hispanic or Latino ethnicity were available beginning in 1990.

§ Information about socioeconomic status was available only for 1979–2001.

TABLE 13A

DEXTROTRANSPOSITION OF THE GREAT ARTERIES: PREVALENCE (PER 10,000 LIVE BIRTHS) STRATIFIED BY DESCRIPTIVE CHARACTERISTICS, MACDP, 1984–2003*

	Total		1968–1972		1973–1978		1979–1983		1984–1989		1990–1993		1994–1998		1999–2003	
Characteristic	Cases	Prev**	Cases	Prev	Cases	Prev	Cases	Prev	Cases	Prev	Cases	Prev	Cases	Prev	Cases	Prev
Total	**192**	**2.35**							**47**	**2.32**	**34**	**2.20**	**49**	**2.35**	**62**	**2.48**
Maternal age (years)																
<25	61	2.18							15	1.91	12	2.20	14	2.08	20	2.54
25–29	54	2.36							13	2.05	10	2.22	15	2.71	16	2.44
≥30	76	2.46							18	2.97	12	2.20	20	2.32	26	2.46
Unknown	<5	–							<5	–	–	–	–	–	–	–
Maternal race/ethnicity†																
White	105	2.65							34	2.77	8	2.27	30	3.06	23	2.41
Black or African American	61	1.90							12	1.58	14	2.18	15	1.78	20	2.08
Hispanic or Latino	15	2.31							–	–	<5	<8.47	<5	<3.01	13	3.06
All Other Races	10	2.95							<5	<11.48	<5	<10.58	<5	<5.21	5	3.27
Unknown	<5	–							–	–	–	–	–	–	<5	–
Birth weight (grams)																
<2500	23	3.32							8	4.92	<5	<3.74	10	5.59	<5	<2.29
≥2500	169	2.26							39	2.09	32	2.27	39	2.04	59	2.59
Unknown	–	–							–	–	–	–	–	–	–	–
Gestational age (weeks)																
20–36	22	2.77							6	3.04	<5	<3.14	7	3.60	5	2.06
≥37	166	2.36							41	2.45	29	2.23	40	2.16	56	2.52
Unknown	<5	–							–	–	<5	–	<5	–	<5	–
Sex																
Male	116	2.79							23	2.21	23	2.92	31	2.91	39	3.07
Female	76	1.90							24	2.43	11	1.46	18	1.76	23	1.87
Ambiguous/Unknown	–	–							–	–	–	–	–	–	–	–
Parity																
1 Live birth	75	2.12							18	2.01	17	2.54	17	1.85	23	2.18
2 or more live births	115	2.52							28	2.56	17	1.95	31	2.67	39	2.72
Unknown	<5	–							<5	–	–	–	<5	–	–	–
Gravidity																
1 Pregnancy	47	1.66							10	1.42	8	1.54	13	1.78	16	1.84
2 or more pregnancies	144	2.74							36	2.81	26	2.56	36	2.67	46	2.87
Unknown	<5	–							<5	–	–	–	–	–	–	–
Plurality																
Singleton	186	2.35							45	2.27	34	2.26	46	2.27	61	2.52
Multiple	5	2.14							<5	<10.81	–	–	<5	<8.05	<5	<5.95
Unknown	<5	–							<5	–	–	–	–	–	–	–

TABLE 13B

DEXTROTRANSPOSITION OF THE GREAT ARTERIES: PERCENTAGE OF CASES BY DESCRIPTIVE CHARACTERISTICS, MACDP, 1984–2003*

							Period									
	Total		1968–1972		1973–1978		1979–1983		1984–1989		1990–1993		1994–1998		1999–2003	
Characteristic	Cases	Percent	Cases	Percent	Cases	Percent	Cases	Percent	Cases	Percent	Cases	Percent	Cases	Percent	Cases	Percent
Birth outcome																
Live birth	191	99.5							46	97.9	34	100.0	49	100.0	62	100.0
Stillbirth	<5	–							<5	–	–	–	–	–	–	–
Elective termination	–	–							–	–	–	–	–	–	–	–
Age at diagnosis																
Prenatally or <7 days	170	88.5							43	91.5	29	85.3	45	91.8	53	85.5
8 days–6 months	17	8.9							<5	–	<5	–	<5	–	5	8.1
6 months–1 year	<5	0.5							–	–	<5	–	–	–	–	–
1–5 years	–	–							–	–	–	–	–	–	–	–
>5 years	–	–							–	–	–	–	–	–	–	–
Unknown	<5	–							–	–	–	–	–	–	<5	–
Socioeconomic status§																
Upper	61	31.8							20	42.6	14	41.2	15	30.6	12	19.4
Middle	52	27.1							12	25.5	10	29.4	15	30.6	15	24.2
Lower	49	25.5							15	31.9	10	29.4	17	34.7	7	11.3
Unknown	30	15.6							–	–	–	–	<5	–	28	45.2

* Numbers of cases and prevalence estimates are not provided for congenital heart defects prior to 1984 because not all of these cases have been reviewed by pediatric cardiologists. Cells containing fewer than 5 cases are indicated as "<5". Prevalence estimates based on these cells are indicated as less than the prevalence based on 5 cases in Table A. Percentages based on these cells are not provided in Table B. Cells containing zero cases are indicated as "–". Cells in years for which no data are provided are left blank. Counts are provided, but prevalences are not estimated, for strata with unknown values in Table A. Counts and percentages are provided for strata with unknown values in Table B.

** Prev = Prevalence.

† Data on Hispanic or Latino ethnicity were available beginning in 1990.

§ Information about socioeconomic status was available only for 1979–2001.

TABLE 14A

TETRALOGY OF FALLOT: PREVALENCE (PER 10,000 LIVE BIRTHS) STRATIFIED BY DESCRIPTIVE CHARACTERISTICS, MACDP, 1984–2003*

Characteristic	Total		1968–1972		1973–1978		1979–1983		1984–1989		1990–1993		1994–1998		1999–2003	
	Cases	Prev**	Cases	Prev	Cases	Prev	Cases	Prev	Cases	Prev	Cases	Prev	Cases	Prev	Cases	Prev
Total	**376**	**4.61**							**94**	**4.64**	**71**	**4.60**	**93**	**4.45**	**118**	**4.72**
Maternal age (years)																
<25	116	4.15							31	3.94	22	4.02	35	5.20	28	3.55
25–29	108	4.71							35	5.52	21	4.67	15	2.71	37	5.65
≥30	149	4.85							28	4.62	28	5.13	42	4.88	51	4.83
Unknown	<5	–							<5	–	–	–	<5	–	<5	–
Maternal race/ethnicity†																
White	184	4.65							56	4.57	35	4.41	45	4.59	48	5.02
Black or African American	151	4.71							35	4.62	28	4.36	41	4.86	47	4.88
Hispanic or Latino	24	3.69							–	5	<5	8.47	16	3.01	<5	3.77
All Other Races	16	4.71							<5	<11.48	<5	<10.58	<5	<5.21	6	3.93
Unknown	<5	–							–	–	–	–	–	–	<5	–
Birth weight (grams)																
<2500	114	16.43							26	15.99	16	11.96	36	20.13	36	16.47
≥2500	261	3.50							68	3.65	55	3.90	57	2.99	81	3.55
Unknown	<5	–							–	–	–	–	–	<5	–	–
Gestational age (weeks)																
20–36	89	10.96							25	12.66	12	7.55	23	11.82	29	11.94
≥37	283	3.99							66	3.94	59	4.53	69	3.73	89	4.01
Unknown	<5	–							<5	–	–	–	<5	–	–	–
Sex																
Male	204	4.90							45	4.33	36	4.57	50	4.69	73	5.74
Female	172	4.31							49	4.96	35	4.63	43	4.20	45	3.66
Ambiguous/Unknown	–	–							–	–	–	–	–	–	–	–
Parity																
1 Live birth	161	4.55							43	4.80	26	3.89	46	5.01	46	4.36
2 or more live births	212	4.65							49	4.48	45	5.17	47	4.05	71	4.96
Unknown	<5	–							<5	–	–	–	–	–	<5	–
Gravidity																
1 Pregnancy	108	3.82							33	4.68	14	2.69	25	3.43	36	4.14
2 or more pregnancies	267	5.09							61	4.75	57	5.60	68	5.05	81	5.06
Unknown	<5	–							–	–	–	–	–	–	–	–
Plurality																
Singleton	360	4.54							89	4.49	70	4.66	87	4.29	114	4.72
Multiple	15	6.43							<5	<10.81	<5	<12.25	6	9.66	<5	<5.95
Unknown	<5	–							<5	–	–	–	–	–	<5	–

TABLE 14B

TETRALOGY OF FALLOT: PERCENTAGE OF CASES BY DESCRIPTIVE CHARACTERISTICS, MACDP, 1984–2003*

| | \\multicolumn{16}{Period} | | | | | | | | | | | | | | | |
Characteristic	Total Cases	Total Percent	1968–1972 Cases	1968–1972 Percent	1973–1978 Cases	1973–1978 Percent	1979–1983 Cases	1979–1983 Percent	1984–1989 Cases	1984–1989 Percent	1990–1993 Cases	1990–1993 Percent	1994–1998 Cases	1994–1998 Percent	1999–2003 Cases	1999–2003 Percent
Birth outcome																
Live birth	371	98.7							94	100.0	69	97.2	91	97.8	117	99.2
Stillbirth	<5	–							–	–	<5	–	<5	–	<5	–
Elective termination	<5	–							–	–	<5	–	–	–	–	–
Unknown	–	–							–	–	–	–	–	–	–	–
Age at diagnosis																
Prenatally or <7 days	322	85.6							82	87.2	61	85.9	80	86.0	99	83.9
8 days–6 months	35	9.3							8	8.5	9	12.7	9	9.7	9	7.6
6 months–1 year	6	1.6							<5	–	<5	–	<5	–	–	–
1–5 years	<5	–							<5	–	–	–	–	–	–	–
>5 years	–	–							–	–	–	–	–	–	–	–
Unknown	12	3.2							–	–	–	–	<5	–	10	8.5
Socioeconomic status§																
Upper	102	27.1							30	31.9	26	36.6	31	33.3	15	12.7
Middle	109	29.0							27	28.7	24	33.8	30	32.3	28	23.7
Lower	97	25.8							36	38.3	20	28.2	29	31.2	12	10.2
Unknown	68	18.1							<5	–	<5	–	<5	–	63	53.4

* Numbers of cases and prevalence estimates are not provided for congenital heart defects prior to 1984 because not all of these cases have been reviewed by pediatric cardiologists. Cells containing fewer than 5 cases are indicated as "<5". Prevalence estimates based on these cells are indicated as less than the prevalence based on 5 cases in Table A. Percentages based on these cells are not provided in Table B. Cells containing zero cases are indicated as "–". Cells in years for which no data are provided are left blank. Counts are provided, but prevalences are not estimated, for strata with unknown values in Table A. Counts and percentages are provided for strata with unknown values in Table B.
** Prev = Prevalence.
† Data on Hispanic or Latino ethnicity were available beginning in 1990.
§ Information about socioeconomic status was available only for 1979–2001.

TABLE 15A

ATRIOVENTRICULAR SEPTAL DEFECT: PREVALENCE (PER 10,000 LIVE BIRTHS) STRATIFIED BY DESCRIPTIVE CHARACTERISTICS, MACDP, 1984–2003*

Characteristic	Total		1968–1972		1973–1978		1979–1983		1984–1989		1990–1993		1994–1998		1999–2003	
	Cases	Prev**	Cases	Prev	Cases	Prev	Cases	Prev	Cases	Prev	Cases	Prev	Cases	Prev	Cases	Prev
Total	**302**	**3.70**							**71**	**3.50**	**48**	**3.11**	**87**	**4.17**	**96**	**3.84**
Maternal age (years)																
<25	78	2.79							26	3.31	9	1.65	23	3.42	20	2.54
25–29	61	2.66							18	2.84	12	2.67	12	2.17	19	2.90
≥30	161	5.25							26	4.29	27	4.94	51	5.92	57	5.40
Unknown	<5	–							<5	–	–	–	<5	–	–	–
Maternal race ethnicity†																
White	155	3.92							45	3.67	24	3.02	51	5.20	35	3.66
Black or African American	123	3.84							25	3.30	21	3.27	31	3.68	46	4.78
Hispanic or Latino	11	1.69							–	–	–	–	<5	<3.01	10	2.35
All Other Races	12	3.53							<5	<11.48	<5	<10.58	<5	<5.21	5	3.27
Unknown	<5	–							–	–	–	–	<5	–	–	–
Birth weight (grams)																
<2500	93	13.41							19	11.68	15	11.21	25	13.98	34	15.56
≥2500	207	2.77							52	2.79	33	2.34	60	3.14	62	2.72
Unknown	<5	–							–	–	–	–	<5	–	–	–
Gestational age (weeks)																
20–36	85	10.20							17	8.61	13	8.18	25	12.84	30	12.35
≥37	211	2.97							49	2.93	34	2.61	62	3.35	60	2.97
Unknown	6	–							5	–	<5	–	<5	–	–	–
Sex																
Male	129	3.10							32	3.08	24	3.05	36	3.38	37	2.91
Female	172	4.31							39	3.95	24	3.18	51	4.98	58	4.72
Ambiguous/Unknown	<5	–							–	–	–	–	<5	–	<5	–
Parity																
1 Live birth	114	3.22							30	3.35	16	2.39	35	3.81	33	3.13
2 or more live births	184	4.04							38	3.47	32	3.68	52	4.48	62	4.33
Unknown	<5	–							<5	–	<5	–	–	–	–	–
Gravidity																
1 Pregnancy	74	2.62							21	2.98	8	1.54	24	3.29	21	2.41
2 or more pregnancies	226	4.31							49	3.82	40	3.93	63	4.68	74	4.62
Unknown	5	–							<5	–	–	–	–	–	<5	–
Plurality																
Singleton	286	3.61							69	3.48	48	3.19	83	4.10	86	3.56
Multiple	16	6.86							<5	10.81	–	–	<5	<8.05	10	11.90
Unknown	–	–							–	–	–	–	–	–	–	–

TABLE 15B

ATRIOVENTRICULAR SEPTAL DEFECT: PERCENTAGE OF CASES BY DESCRIPTIVE CHARACTERISTICS, MACDP, 1984–2003*

	Total		1968–1972		1973–1978		1979–1983		Period 1984–1989		1990–1993		1994–1998		1999–2003	
Characteristic	Cases	Percent	Cases	Percent	Cases	Percent	Cases	Percent	Cases	Percent	Cases	Percent	Cases	Percent	Cases	Percent
Birth outcome																
Live birth	279	92.4							66	93.0	47	97.9	77	88.5	89	92.7
Stillbirth	11	3.6							<5	–	<5	–	<5	–	<5	–
Elective termination	12	4.0							<5	–	–	–	6	6.9	5	5.2
Unknown	–	–							–	–	–	–	–	–	–	–
Age at diagnosis																
Prenatally or <7 days	246	81.5							60	84.5	40	83.3	72	82.8	74	77.1
8 days–6 months	29	9.6							8	11.3	6	12.5	8	9.2	7	7.3
6 months–1 year	7	2.3							<5	–	<5	–	<5	–	–	–
1–5 years	<5	–							–	–	–	–	<5	–	–	–
>5 years	–	–							–	–	–	–	<5	–	–	–
Unknown	19	6.3							<5	–	–	–	<5	–	15	15.6
Socioeconomic status§																
Upper	98	32.5							33	46.5	19	39.6	31	35.6	15	15.6
Middle	68	22.5							12	16.9	11	22.9	27	31.0	18	18.8
Lower	92	30.5							26	36.6	17	35.4	27	31	22	22.9
Unknown	44	14.6							–	–	<5	–	<5	–	41	42.7

* Numbers of cases and prevalence estimates are not provided for congenital heart defects prior to 1984 because not all of these cases have been reviewed by pediatric cardiologists. Cells containing fewer than 5 cases are indicated as "<5". Prevalence estimates based on these cells are indicated as less than the prevalence based on 5 cases in Table A. Percentages based on these cells are not provided in Table B. Cells containing zero cases are indicated as "–". Cells in years for which no data are provided are left blank. Counts are provided, but prevalences are not estimated, for strata with unknown values in Table A. Counts and percentages are provided for strata with unknown values in Table B.
** Prev = Prevalence.
† Data on Hispanic or Latino ethnicity were available beginning in 1990.
§ Information about socioeconomic status was available only for 1979–2001.

TABLE 16A

COMPLETE ATRIOVENTRICULAR SEPTAL DEFECT: PREVALENCE (PER 10,000 LIVE BIRTHS) STRATIFIED BY DESCRIPTIVE CHARACTERISTICS, MACDP, 1984–2003*

Characteristic	Total Cases	Total Prev**	1968-1972 Cases	1968-1972 Prev	1973-1978 Cases	1973-1978 Prev	1979-1983 Cases	1979-1983 Prev	1984-1989 Cases	1984-1989 Prev	1990-1993 Cases	1990-1993 Prev	1994-1998 Cases	1994-1998 Prev	1999-2003 Cases	1999-2003 Prev
Total	186	2.28							54	2.66	32	2.07	49	2.35	51	2.04
Maternal age (years)																
<25	50	1.79							21	2.67	5	0.91	12	1.78	12	1.52
25–29	31	1.35							15	2.37	8	1.78	<5	<0.90	6	0.92
≥30	104	3.39							18	2.97	19	3.48	34	3.95	33	3.13
Unknown	<5	–							–	–	–	–	<5	–	–	–
Maternal race ethnicity†																
White	90	2.27							29	2.37	17	2.14	27	2.75	17	1.78
Black or African American	77	2.40							24	3.17	12	1.87	19	2.25	22	2.29
Hispanic or Latino	9	1.38							–	–	<5	<8.47	<5	<3.01	7	1.65
All Other Races	9	2.65							<5	<11.48	<5	<10.58	<5	<5.21	5	3.27
Unknown	<5	–							–	–	–	–	<5	–	–	–
Birth weight (grams)																
<2500	59	8.50							17	10.45	9	6.73	14	7.83	19	8.69
≥2500	125	1.67							37	1.99	23	1.63	33	1.73	32	1.40
Unknown	<5	–							–	–	–	–	<5	–	–	–
Gestational age (weeks)																
20–36	53	6.55							15	7.60	9	5.66	12	6.16	17	7.00
≥37	126	1.76							33	1.97	22	1.69	37	2.00	34	1.53
Unknown	7	–							6	–	<5	–	–	–	–	–
Sex																
Male	84	2.02							24	2.31	19	2.41	22	2.07	19	1.49
Female	102	2.55							30	3.03	13	1.72	27	2.64	32	2.61
Ambiguous/Unknown	–	–							–	–	–	–	–	–	–	–
Parity																
1 Live birth	69	1.95							18	2.01	12	1.80	18	1.96	21	1.99
2 or more live births	117	2.57							36	3.29	20	2.30	31	2.67	30	2.09
Unknown	–	–							–	–	–	–	–	–	–	–
Gravidity																
1 Pregnancy	40	1.42							11	1.56	6	1.15	10	1.37	13	1.49
2 or more pregnancies	146	2.78							43	3.35	26	2.56	39	2.90	38	2.37
Unknown	–	–							–	–	–	–	–	–	–	–
Plurality																
Singleton	176	2.22							52	2.62	32	2.13	47	2.32	45	1.86
Multiple	10	4.29							<5	<10.81	–	–	<5	<8.05	6	7.14
Unknown	–	–							–	–	–	–	–	–	–	–

TABLE 16B

COMPLETE ATRIOVENTRICULAR SEPTAL DEFECT: PERCENTAGE OF CASES BY DESCRIPTIVE CHARACTERISTICS, MACDP, 1984–2003*

	Period															
	Total		1968–1972		1973–1978		1979–1983		1984–1989		1990–1993		1994–1998		1999–2003	
Characteristic	Cases	Percent	Cases	Percent	Cases	Percent	Cases	Percent	Cases	Percent	Cases	Percent	Cases	Percent	Cases	Percent
Birth outcome																
Live birth	170	91.4							49	90.7	32	100.0	43	87.8	46	90.2
Stillbirth	9	4.8							<5	–	–	–	<5	–	<5	–
Elective termination	7	3.8							<5	–	–	–	<5	–	<5	–
Unknown	–	–							–	–	–	–	–	–	–	–
Age at diagnosis																
Prenatally or <7 days	157	84.4							47	87.0	30	93.8	41	83.7	39	76.5
8 days–6 months	14	7.5							6	11.1	<5	–	<5	–	<5	–
6 months–1 year	<5	–							<5	–	–	–	<5	–	–	–
1–5 years	–	–							–	–	–	–	–	–	–	–
>5 years	–	–							–	–	–	–	–	–	–	–
Unknown	12	6.5							–	–	–	–	<5	–	10	19.6
Socioeconomic status§																
Upper	65	34.9							19	35.2	16	50.0	21	42.9	9	17.6
Middle	38	20.4							11	20.4	6	18.8	11	22.4	10	19.6
Lower	62	33.3							24	44.4	10	31.3	16	32.7	12	23.5
Unknown	21	11.3							–	–	–	–	<5	–	20	39.2

* Numbers of cases and prevalence estimates are not provided for congenital heart defects prior to 1984 because not all of these cases have been reviewed by pediatric cardiologists. Cells containing fewer than 5 cases are indicated as "<5". Prevalence estimates based on these cells are indicated as less than the prevalence based on 5 cases in Table A. Percentages based on these cells are not provided in Table B. Cells containing zero cases are indicated as "–". Cells in years for which no data are provided are left blank. Counts are provided, but prevalences are not estimated, for strata with unknown values in Table A. Counts and percentages are provided for strata with unknown values in Table B.
** Prev = Prevalence.
† Data on Hispanic or Latino ethnicity were available beginning in 1990.
§ Information about socioeconomic status was available only for 1979–2001.

TABLE 17A

VALVAR PULMONARY STENOSIS: PREVALENCE (PER 10,000 LIVE BIRTHS) STRATIFIED BY DESCRIPTIVE CHARACTERISTICS, MACDP, 1984–2003*

Characteristic	Total		1968–1972		1973–1978		1979–1983		1984–1989		1990–1993		1994–1998		1999–2003	
	Cases	Prev**	Cases	Prev	Cases	Prev	Cases	Prev	Cases	Prev	Cases	Prev	Cases	Prev	Cases	Prev
Total	**346**	**4.24**							**56**	**2.76**	**45**	**2.92**	**116**	**5.55**	**129**	**5.16**
Maternal age (years)																
<25	95	3.40							19	2.42	14	2.56	28	4.16	34	4.31
25–29	101	4.41							19	3.00	11	2.44	31	5.61	40	6.10
≥30	149	4.85							18	2.97	20	3.66	56	6.50	55	5.21
Unknown	<1	–							–	–	–	–	<5	–	–	–
Maternal race/ethnicity†																
White	164	4.14							32	2.61	25	3.15	54	5.51	53	5.54
Black or African American	152	4.74							24	3.17	17	2.65	55	6.52	56	5.82
Hispanic or Latino	21	3.23							–	–	<5	<8.47	<5	<3.01	15	3.53
All Other Races	8	2.36							–	–	–	–	<5	<5.21	5	3.27
Unknown	<1	–							–	–	–	–	<5	–	–	–
Birth weight (grams)																
<2500	107	15.42							15	9.22	10	7.47	32	17.90	50	22.88
≥2500	239	3.20							41	2.20	35	2.48	84	4.40	79	3.46
Unknown	–	–							–	–	–	–	–	–	–	–
Gestational age (weeks)																
20–36	108	13.22							16	8.10	13	8.18	31	15.93	48	19.76
≥37	234	3.26							38	2.27	32	2.46	85	4.59	79	3.56
Unknown	<5	–							<5	–	–	–	–	–	<5	–
Sex																
Male	155	3.72							30	2.89	18	2.28	48	4.51	59	4.64
Female	191	4.78							26	2.63	27	3.57	68	6.65	70	5.70
Ambiguous/Unknown	–	–							–	–	–	–	–	–	–	–
Parity																
1 Live birth	129	3.65							21	2.34	16	2.39	45	4.90	47	4.46
2 or more live births	212	4.65							34	3.11	28	3.22	69	5.94	81	5.66
Unknown	5	–							<5	–	<5	–	<5	–	<5	–
Gravidity																
1 Pregnancy	89	3.15							16	2.27	5	0.96	37	5.07	31	3.56
2 or more pregnancies	254	4.84							40	3.12	40	3.93	77	5.72	97	6.06
Unknown	<5	–							–	–	–	<5	–	<5	–	–
Plurality																
Singleton	317	4.00							54	2.73	41	2.73	105	5.18	117	4.84
Multiple	29	12.43							<5	<10.81	<5	<12.25	11	<17.70	12	14.28
Unknown	–	–							–	–	–	–	–	–	–	–

TABLE 17B

VALVAR PULMONARY STENOSIS: PERCENTAGE OF CASES BY DESCRIPTIVE CHARACTERISTICS, MACDP, 1984–2003*

	Period															
	Total		1968–1972		1973–1978		1979–1983		1984–1989		1990–1993		1994–1998		1999–2003	
Characteristic	Cases	Percent	Cases	Percent	Cases	Percent	Cases	Percent	Cases	Percent	Cases	Percent	Cases	Percent	Cases	Percent
Birth outcome																
Live birth	345	99.7							56	100.0	45	100.00	116	100.0	128	99.2
Stillbirth	—	—							—	—	—	—	—	—	—	—
Elective termination	<5	—							—	—	—	—	—	—	<5	—
Unknown	—	—							—	—	—	—	—	—	—	—
Age at diagnosis																
Prenatally or <7 days	232	67.1							41	73.2	32	71.1	78	67.2	81	62.8
8 days–6 months	89	25.7							15	26.8	10	22.2	32	27.6	32	24.8
6 months–1 year	8	2.3							—	—	<5	—	<5	—	<5	—
1–5 years	7	0.0							—	—	—	—	<5	—	6	4.7
>5 years	—	—							—	—	—	—	—	—	—	—
Unknown	10	2.9							—	—	—	—	<5	—	8	6.2
Socioeconomic status§																
Upper	100	28.9							22	39.3	16	35.6	40	34.5	22	17.1
Middle	94	27.2							16	28.6	16	35.6	37	31.9	25	19.4
Lower	88	25.4							18	32.1	11	24.4	31	26.7	28	21.7
Unknown	64	18.5							—	—	<5	—	8	6.9	54	41.9

* Numbers of cases and prevalence estimates are not provided for congenital heart defects prior to 1984 because not all of these cases have been reviewed by pediatric cardiologists. Cells containing fewer than 5 cases are indicated as "<5". Prevalence estimates based on these cells are indicated as less than the prevalence based on 5 cases in Table A. Percentages based on these cells are not provided in Table B. Cells containing zero cases are indicated as "—". Cells in years for which no data are provided are left blank. Counts are provided, but prevalences are not estimated, for strata with unknown values in Table A. Counts and percentages are provided for strata with unknown values in Table B.

** Prev = Prevalence.

† Data on Hispanic or Latino ethnicity were available beginning in 1990.

§ Information about socioeconomic status was available only for 1979–2001.

TABLE 18A

HYPOPLASTIC LEFT HEART SYNDROME: PREVALENCE (PER 10,000 LIVE BIRTHS) STRATIFIED BY DESCRIPTIVE CHARACTERISTICS, MACDP, 1984–2003*

	Total		1968–1972		1973–1978		1979–1983		1984–1989		1990–1993		1994–1998		1999–2003	
Characteristic	Cases	Prev**	Cases	Prev	Cases	Prev	Cases	Prev	Cases	Prev	Cases	Prev	Cases	Prev	Cases	Prev
Total	204	2.50							45	2.22	45	2.92	56	2.68	58	2.32
Maternal age (years)																
<25	73	2.61							20	2.54	19	3.48	19	2.82	15	1.90
25–29	55	2.40							18	2.84	15	3.33	9	1.63	13	1.98
≥30	76	2.48							7	1.16	11	2.01	28	3.25	30	2.84
Unknown	–	–							–		–		–		–	
Maternal race ethnicity†																
White	95	2.40							26	2.12	21	2.64	27	2.75	21	2.20
Black or African American	83	2.59							19	2.51	20	3.11	18	2.14	26	2.70
Hispanic or Latino	17	2.62							–		<5	<8.47	6	3.62	9	2.12
All Other Races	8	2.36							–		<5	<10.58	5	5.21	<5	<3.27
Unknown	<5	–							–		–		–		<5	–
Birth weight (grams)																
<2500	55	7.93							11	6.76	10	7.47	20	11.18	14	6.41
≥2500	145	1.94							34	1.82	35	2.48	36	1.89	40	1.75
Unknown	<5	–							–		–		–		<5	–
Gestational age (weeks)																
20–36	51	6.42							8	4.05	9	5.66	17	8.73	17	7.00
≥37	153	2.14							37	2.21	36	2.77	39	2.11	41	1.85
Unknown	–	–							–		–		–		–	
Sex																
Male	111	2.67							27	2.60	28	3.55	29	2.72	27	2.12
Female	93	2.33							18	1.82	17	2.25	27	2.64	31	2.52
Ambiguous/Unknown	–	–							–		–		–		–	
Parity																
1 Live birth	81	2.29							24	2.68	21	3.14	15	1.63	21	1.99
2 or more live births	119	2.61							18	1.64	24	2.76	40	3.44	37	2.58
Unknown	<5	–							<5		–		<5		–	
Gravidity																
1 Pregnancy	60	2.12							19	2.69	14	2.69	10	1.37	17	1.95
2 or more pregnancies	143	2.73							26	2.03	31	3.05	45	3.34	41	2.56
Unknown	<5	–							–		–		<5		–	
Plurality																
Singleton	194	2.45							41	2.07	42	2.80	55	2.71	56	2.32
Multiple	10	4.29							<5	<10.81	<5	<12.25	<5	<8.05	<5	<5.95
Unknown	–	–							–		–		–		–	

TABLE 18B

HYPOPLASTIC LEFT HEART SYNDROME: PERCENTAGE OF CASES BY DESCRIPTIVE CHARACTERISTICS, MACDP, 1984–2003*

									Period								
	Total		1968–1972		1973–1978		1979–1983		1984–1989		1990–1993		1994–1998		1999–2003		
Characteristic	Cases	Percent	Cases	Percent	Cases	Percent	Cases	Percent	Cases	Percent	Cases	Percent	Cases	Percent	Cases	Percent	
Birth outcome																	
Live birth	182	89.2							40	88.9	43	95.6	48	85.7	51	87.9	
Stillbirth	12	5.9							5	11.1	<5	–	<5	–	<5	–	
Elective termination	10	4.9							–	–	–	–	7	12.5	<5	–	
Unknown	–	–							–	–	–	–	–	–	–	–	
Age at diagnosis																	
Prenatally or <7 days	183	89.7							42	93.3	40	88.9	54	96.4	47	81.0	
8 days–6 months	11	5.4							<5	–	5	11.1	<5	–	<5	–	
6 months–1 year	–	–							–	–	–	–	–	–	–	–	
1–5 years	–	–							–	–	–	–	–	–	–	–	
>5 years	–	–							–	–	–	–	–	–	–	–	
Unknown	10	4.9							–	–	–	–	–	–	10	17.2	
Socioeconomic status§																	
Upper	55	27.0							16	35.6	14	31.1	19	33.9	6	10.3	
Middle	65	31.9							10	22.2	18	40.0	20	35.7	17	29.3	
Lower	57	27.9							19	42.2	13	28.9	15	26.8	10	17.2	
Unknown	27	13.2							–	–	–	–	<5	–	25	43.1	

* Numbers of cases and prevalence estimates are not provided for congenital heart defects prior to 1984 because not all of these cases have been reviewed by pediatric cardiologists. Cells containing fewer than 5 cases are indicated as "<5". Prevalence estimates based on these cells are indicated as less than the prevalence based on 5 cases in Table A. Percentages based on these cells are not provided in Table B. Cells containing zero cases are indicated as "–". Cells in years for which no data are provided are left blank. Counts are provided, but prevalences are not estimated, for strata with unknown values in Table A. Counts and percentages are provided for strata with unknown values in Table B.
** Prev = Prevalence.
† Data on Hispanic or Latino ethnicity were available beginning in 1990.
§ Information about socioeconomic status was available only for 1979–2001.

TABLE 19A

AORTIC STENOSIS: PREVALENCE (PER 10,000 LIVE BIRTHS) STRATIFIED BY DESCRIPTIVE CHARACTERISTICS, MACDP, 1984–2003*

	Total		1968–1972		1973–1978		1979–1983		1984–1989		1990–1993		1994–1998		1999–2003	
Characteristic	Cases	Prev**	Cases	Prev	Cases	Prev	Cases	Prev	Cases	Prev	Cases	Prev	Cases	Prev	Cases	Prev
Total	90	1.10							26	1.28	13	0.84	19	0.91	32	1.28
Maternal age (years)																
<25	17	0.61							<5	<0.64	<5	<0.91	<5	<0.74	7	0.89
25–29	34	1.48							12	1.89	<5	<1.11	7	1.27	11	1.68
≥30	39	1.27							10	1.65	7	1.28	8	1.14	14	1.33
Unknown	—	—							—	—	—	—	—	—	—	—
Maternal race/ethnicity†																
White	61	1.54							22	1.79	11	1.39	11	1.12	17	1.78
Black or African American	19	0.59							<5	<0.66	<5	<0.78	6	0.71	7	0.73
Hispanic or Latino	9	1.38							—	—	—	—	<5	<3.01	7	1.65
All Other Races	<5	0.29							—	—	—	—	—	<5	<5	<3.27
Unknown	—	—							—	—	—	—	—	—	—	—
Birth weight (grams)																
<2500	23	3.32							<5	<3.07	6	4.48	<5	<2.80	10	4.58
≥2500	67	0.90							23	1.23	7	0.50	15	0.79	22	0.96
Unknown	—	—							—	—	—	—	—	—	—	—
Gestational age (weeks)																
20–36	19	2.39							<5	<2.53	5	3.14	5	2.57	5	2.06
≥37	71	1.01							22	1.31	8	0.61	14	0.76	27	1.22
Unknown	—	—							—	—	—	—	—	—	—	—
Sex																
Male	57	1.37							21	2.02	8	1.02	8	0.75	20	1.57
Female	32	0.80							5	0.51	5	0.66	11	1.08	11	0.90
Ambiguous/Unknown	<5	—						—	—	—	—	—	—	<5	—	—
Parity																
1 Live birth	43	1.22							9	1.00	10	1.50	10	1.09	14	1.33
2 or more live births	47	1.03							17	1.55	<5	<0.57	9	0.77	18	1.26
Unknown	—	—							—	—	—	—	—	—	—	—
Gravidity																
1 Pregnancy	29	1.03							5	0.71	7	1.34	5	0.69	12	1.38
2 or more pregnancies	61	1.16							21	1.64	6	0.59	14	1.04	20	1.25
Unknown	—	—							—	—	—	—	—	—	—	—
Plurality																
Singleton	88	1.11							25	1.26	13	0.87	19	0.94	31	1.28
Multiple	<5	<2.14							—	—	—	—	—	—	<5	<5.95
Unknown	<5	—							<5	—	—	—	—	—	—	—

TABLE 19B

AORTIC STENOSIS: PERCENTAGE OF CASES BY DESCRIPTIVE CHARACTERISTICS, MACDP, 1984–2003*

Characteristic	Total		1968–1972		1973–1978		1979–1983		1984–1989		1990–1993		1994–1998		1999–2003	
	Cases	Percent	Cases	Percent	Cases	Percent	Cases	Percent	Cases	Percent	Cases	Percent	Cases	Percent	Cases	Percent
Birth outcome																
Live birth	87	96.7							26	100.00	13	100.0	17	89.5	31	96.9
Stillbirth	<5	–							–	–	–	–	<5	–	<5	–
Elective termination	<5	–							–	–	–	–	<5	–	–	–
Unknown	–	–							–	–	–	–	–	–	–	–
Age at diagnosis																
Prenatally or <7 days	72	80.0							24	92.3	9	69.2	16	84.2	23	71.9
8 days–6 months	9	10.0							<5	–	<5	–	<5	–	<5	–
6 months–1 year	<5	–							–	–	<5	–	<5	–	<5	–
1–5 years	<5	–							<5	–	–	–	–	–	–	–
>5 years	–	–							–	–	–	–	–	–	–	–
Unknown	5	5.6							–	–	–	–	–	–	5	15.6
Socioeconomic status§																
Upper	33	36.7							13	50.0	5	38.5	6	31.6	9	28.1
Middle	26	28.9							7	26.9	7	53.8	6	31.6	6	18.8
Lower	18	20.0							6	23.1	<5	–	6	31.6	5	15.6
Unknown	13	14.4							–	–	–	–	<5	–	12	37.5

* Numbers of cases and prevalence estimates are not provided for congenital heart defects prior to 1984 because not all of these cases have been reviewed by pediatric cardiologists. Cells containing fewer than 5 cases are indicated as "<5". Prevalence estimates based on these cells are indicated as less than the prevalence based on 5 cases in Table A. Percentages based on these cells are not provided in Table B. Cells containing zero cases are indicated as "_". Cells in years for which no data are provided are left blank. Counts are provided, but prevalences are not estimated, for strata with unknown values in Table A. Counts and percentages are provided for strata with unknown values in Table B.

** Prev = Prevalence.

† Data on Hispanic or Latino ethnicity were available beginning in 1990.

§ Information about socioeconomic status was available only for 1979–2001.

TABLE 20A

COARCTATION OF THE AORTA: PREVALENCE (PER 10,000 LIVE BIRTHS) STRATIFIED BY DESCRIPTIVE CHARACTERISTICS, MACDP, 1984–2003*

Characteristic	Total Cases	Total Prev**	1968–1972 Cases	1968–1972 Prev	1973–1978 Cases	1973–1978 Prev	1979–1983 Cases	1979–1983 Prev	1984–1989 Cases	1984–1989 Prev	1990–1993 Cases	1990–1993 Prev	1994–1998 Cases	1994–1998 Prev	1999–2003 Cases	1999–2003 Prev
Total	317	3.89							81	3.99	43	2.79	92	4.41	101	4.04
Maternal age (years)																
<25	79	2.83							25	3.18	<5	<0.91	21	3.12	29	3.68
25–29	82	3.58							24	3.78	14	3.11	20	3.62	24	3.66
≥30	154	5.02							30	4.95	25	4.58	51	5.92	48	4.55
Unknown	<5	–							<5	–	–	–	–	–	–	–
Maternal race/ethnicity†																
White	180	4.55							56	4.57	25	3.15	54	5.51	45	4.71
Black or African American	102	3.18							24	3.17	14	2.18	31	3.68	33	3.43
Hispanic or Latino	22	3.39							–	–	<5	<8.47	5	3.01	16	3.77
All Other Races	9	2.65							<5	<11.48	<5	<10.58	<5	<5.21	<5	<3.27
Unknown	<5	–							–	–	<5	–	–	–	<5	–
Birth weight (grams)																
<2500	64	9.22							17	10.45	9	6.73	23	12.86	15	6.86
≥2500	253	3.39							64	3.43	34	2.41	69	3.61	86	3.77
Unknown	–	–							–	–	–	–	–	–	–	–
Gestational age (weeks)																
20–36	57	7.18							13	6.58	9	5.66	19	9.76	16	6.59
≥37	255	3.60							66	3.94	34	2.61	73	3.94	82	3.69
Unknown	5	–							<5	–	–	–	–	–	<5	–
Sex																
Male	180	4.32							41	3.95	28	3.55	53	4.98	58	4.56
Female	137	3.43							40	4.05	15	1.99	39	3.81	43	3.50
Ambiguous/Unknown	–	–							–	–	–	–	–	–	–	–
Parity																
1 Live birth	119	3.36							29	3.24	13	1.95	36	3.92	41	3.89
2 or more live births	195	4.28							49	4.48	30	3.45	56	4.82	60	4.19
Unknown	<5	–							<5	–	–	–	–	–	–	–
Gravidity																
1 Pregnancy	76	2.69							24	3.40	7	1.34	22	3.02	23	2.64
2 or more pregnancies	240	4.57							56	4.36	36	3.54	70	5.20	78	4.87
Unknown	<5	–							<5	–	–	–	–	–	–	–
Plurality																
Singleton	295	3.72							75	3.79	41	2.73	85	4.20	94	3.89
Multiple	21	9.00							5	10.81	<5	<12.25	7	11.26	7	8.33
Unknown	<5	–							<5	–	–	–	–	–	–	–

TABLE 20B

COARCTATION OF THE AORTA: PERCENTAGE OF CASES BY DESCRIPTIVE CHARACTERISTICS, MACDP, 1984–2003*

							Period									
	Total		1968–1972		1973–1978		1979–1983		1984–1989		1990–1993		1994–1998		1999–2003	
Characteristic	Cases	Percent	Cases	Percent	Cases	Percent	Cases	Percent	Cases	Percent	Cases	Percent	Cases	Percent	Cases	Percent
Birth outcome																
Live birth	315	99.4							81	100.0	42	97.7	92	100.0	100	99.0
Stillbirth	<5	–							–	–	<5	–	–	–	–	–
Elective termination	<5	–							–	–	–	–	–	–	<5	–
Unknown	–	–							–	–	–	–	–	–	–	–
Age at diagnosis																
Prenatally or <7 days	203	64.0							56	69.1	25	58.1	65	70.7	57	56.4
8 days–6 months	87	27.4							21	25.9	15	34.9	25	27.2	26	25.7
6 months–1 year	7	2.2							<5	–	<5	–	<5	–	<5	–
1–5 years	9	0.0							<5	–	<5	–	<5	–	6	5.9
>5 years	–	–							–	–	–	–	–	–	–	–
Unknown	11	3.5							<5	–	–	–	–	–	10	9.9
Socioeconomic status§																
Upper	110	34.7							37	45.7	16	37.2	35	38.0	22	21.8
Middle	83	26.2							22	27.2	19	44.2	27	29.3	15	14.9
Lower	68	21.5							20	24.7	8	18.6	28	30.4	12	11.9
Unknown	56	17.7							<5	–	–	–	<5	–	52	51.5

* Numbers of cases and prevalence estimates are not provided for congenital heart defects prior to 1984 because not all of these cases have been reviewed by pediatric cardiologists. Cells containing fewer than 5 cases are indicated as "<5". Prevalence estimates based on these cells are indicated as less than the prevalence based on 5 cases in Table A. Percentages based on these cells are not provided in Table B. Cells containing zero cases are indicated as "–". Cells in years for which no data are provided are left blank. Counts are provided, but prevalences are not estimated, for strata with unknown values in Table A. Counts and percentages are provided for strata with unknown values in Table B.

** Prev = Prevalence.

† Data on Hispanic or Latino ethnicity were available beginning in 1990.

§ Information about socioeconomic status was available only for 1979–2001.

TABLE 21A

ATRIAL SEPTAL DEFECT: PREVALENCE (PER 10,000 LIVE BIRTHS) STRATIFIED BY DESCRIPTIVE CHARACTERISTICS, MACDP, 1984–2003*

	Period															
	Total		1968–1972		1973–1978		1979–1983		1984–1989		1990–1993		1994–1998		1999–2003	
Characteristic	Cases	Prev**	Cases	Prev	Cases	Prev	Cases	Prev	Cases	Prev	Cases	Prev	Cases	Prev	Cases	Prev
Total	710	8.70							121	5.97	124	8.03	171	8.19	294	11.76
Maternal age (years)																
<25	208	7.44							36	4.58	35	6.40	48	7.13	89	11.29
25–29	181	7.90							40	6.31	36	8.00	43	7.78	62	9.46
≥30	320	10.43							45	7.43	52	9.52	80	9.29	143	13.54
Unknown	<5	–							–	–	<5	–	–	–	–	–
Maternal race/ethnicity†																
White	320	8.09							81	6.61	60	7.56	83	8.46	96	10.04
Black or African American	288	8.99							36	4.75	54	8.41	74	8.78	124	12.88
Hispanic or Latino	73	11.23							–	–	6	10.16	7	4.22	60	14.12
All Other Races	23	6.77							<5	<11.48	<5	<10.58	<5	5.21	10	6.55
Unknown	6	–							–	–	–	–	<5	–	<5	–
Birth weight (grams)																
<2500	277	39.93							42	25.82	47	35.13	67	37.47	121	55.37
≥2500	433	5.80							79	4.24	77	5.47	104	5.45	173	7.58
Unknown	–	–							–	–	–	–	–	–	–	–
Gestational age (weeks)																
20–36	264	32.87							34	17.22	47	29.56	68	34.93	115	47.35
≥37	437	6.14							83	4.96	77	5.92	100	5.40	177	7.97
Unknown	9	–							<5	–	–	–	<5	–	<5	–
Sex																
Male	297	7.13							47	4.52	54	6.85	81	7.60	115	9.04
Female	413	10.34							74	7.49	70	9.27	90	8.80	179	14.57
Ambiguous/Unknown	–	–							–	–	–	–	–	–	–	–
Parity																
1 Live birth	292	8.26							51	5.69	51	7.63	66	7.19	124	11.76
2 or more live births	410	8.99							64	5.85	73	8.39	105	9.04	168	11.73
Unknown	8	–							6	–	–	–	–	–	<5	–
Gravidity																
1 Pregnancy	198	7.01							38	5.38	32	6.15	40	5.48	88	10.11
2 or more pregnancies	509	9.70							82	6.39	92	9.05	131	9.73	204	12.75
Unknown	<5	–							<5	–	–	–	–	–	<5	–
Plurality																
Singleton	666	8.40							117	5.91	118	7.85	160	7.90	271	11.22
Multiple	44	18.86							<5	<10.81	6	14.70	11	17.70	23	27.37
Unknown	–	–							–	–	–	–	–	–	–	–

TABLE 21B

ATRIAL SEPTAL DEFECT: PERCENTAGE OF CASES BY DESCRIPTIVE CHARACTERISTICS, MACDP, 1984–2003*

Characteristic	Total		1968–1972		1973–1978		1979–1983		1984–1989		1990–1993		1994–1998		1999–2003	
	Cases	Percent	Cases	Percent	Cases	Percent	Cases	Percent	Cases	Percent	Cases	Percent	Cases	Percent	Cases	Percent
Birth outcome																
Live birth	688	96.9							115	95.0	118	95.2	165	96.5	290	98.6
Stillbirth	17	2.4							6	5.0	<5	–	<5	–	<5	–
Elective termination	5	0.7							–	–	<5	–	<5	–	–	–
Unknown	–	–							–	–	–	–	–	–	–	–
Age at diagnosis																
Prenatally or <7 days	455	64.1							88	72.7	78	62.9	107	62.6	182	61.9
8 days–6 months	172	24.2							27	22.3	29	23.4	46	26.9	70	23.8
6 months–1 year	34	4.8							6	5.0	12	9.7	10	5.8	6	2.0
1–5 years	22	0.0							–	–	<5	–	<5	–	14	4.8
>5 years	<5	–							–	–	–	–	–	–	<5	–
Unknown	26	3.7							–	–	<5	–	<5	–	21	7.1
Socioeconomic status§																
Upper	175	24.6							48	39.7	40	32.3	42	24.6	45	15.3
Middle	164	23.1							32	26.4	38	30.6	55	32.2	39	13.3
Lower	190	26.8							40	33.1	45	36.3	61	35.7	44	15
Unknown	181	25.5							<5	–	<5	–	13	7.6	166	56.5

* Numbers of cases and prevalence estimates are not provided for congenital heart defects prior to 1984 because not all of these cases have been reviewed by pediatric cardiologists. Cells containing fewer than 5 cases are indicated as "<5". Prevalence estimates based on these cells are indicated as less than the prevalence based on 5 cases in Table A. Percentages based on these cells are not provided in Table B. Cells containing zero cases are indicated as "–". Cells in years for which no data are provided are left blank. Counts are provided, but prevalences are not estimated, for strata with unknown values in Table A. Counts and percentages are provided for strata with unknown values in Table B.

** Prev = Prevalence.

† Data on Hispanic or Latino ethnicity were available beginning in 1990.

§ Information about socioeconomic status was available only for 1979–2001.

TABLE 22A

SECUNDUM ATRIAL SEPTAL DEFECT: PREVALENCE (PER 10,000 LIVE BIRTHS) STRATIFIED BY DESCRIPTIVE CHARACTERISTICS, MACDP, 1984–2003*

Characteristic	Total		Period						1984–1989		1990–1993		1994–1998		1999–2003	
			1968–1972		1973–1978		1979–1983									
	Cases	Prev**	Cases	Prev	Cases	Prev	Cases	Prev	Cases	Prev	Cases	Prev	Cases	Prev	Cases	Prev
Total	489	5.99							45	2.22	73	4.73	133	6.37	238	9.52
Maternal age (years)																
<25	134	4.80							11	1.40	19	3.48	37	5.49	67	8.50
25–29	121	5.28							17	2.68	20	4.45	32	5.79	52	7.94
≥30	233	7.59							17	2.81	33	6.04	64	7.43	119	11.27
Unknown	<5	–							–	–	<5	–	–	–	–	–
Maternal race/ethnicity†																
White	213	5.38							33	2.69	35	4.41	64	6.53	81	8.47
Black or African American	200	6.24							11	1.45	31	4.83	58	6.88	100	10.39
Hispanic or Latino	55	8.46							–	–	5	8.47	<5	<3.01	46	10.83
All Other Races	16	4.71							<5	<11.48	<5	<10.58	5	5.21	8	5.24
Unknown	5	–							–	–	–	–	<5	–	<5	–
Birth weight (grams)																
<2500	176	25.37							10	6.15	20	14.95	49	27.40	97	44.39
≥2500	313	4.19							35	1.88	53	3.76	84	4.40	141	6.18
Unknown	–	–							–	–	–	–	–	–	–	–
Gestational age (weeks)																
20–36	164	20.53							8	4.05	18	11.32	47	24.15	91	37.47
≥37	318	4.48							35	2.09	55	4.23	83	4.48	145	6.53
Unknown	7	–							<5	–	–	–	<5	–	<5	–
Sex																
Male	201	4.83							14	1.35	35	4.44	63	5.91	89	7.00
Female	288	7.21							31	3.14	38	5.03	70	6.84	149	12.13
Ambiguous/Unknown	–	–							–	–	–	–	–	–	–	–
Parity																
1 Live birth	203	5.74							20	2.23	27	4.04	54	5.88	102	9.67
2 or more live births	281	6.16							22	2.01	46	5.28	79	6.80	134	9.36
Unknown	5	–							<5	–	–	–	–	–	<5	–
Gravidity																
1 Pregnancy	141	4.99							16	2.27	20	3.84	33	4.52	72	8.27
2 or more pregnancies	346	6.59							29	2.26	53	5.21	100	7.42	164	10.25
Unknown	<5	–							–	–	–	–	–	–	<5	–
Plurality																
Singleton	456	5.75							44	2.22	71	4.73	123	6.07	218	9.02
Multiple	33	14.15							<5	<10.81	<5	<12.25	10	16.09	20	23.80
Unknown	–	–							–	–	–	–	–	–	–	–

TABLE 22B

SECUNDUM ATRIAL SEPTAL DEFECT: PERCENTAGE OF CASES BY DESCRIPTIVE CHARACTERISTICS, MACDP, 1984–2003*

Characteristic	Total Cases	Total Percent	1968–1972 Cases	1968–1972 Percent	1973–1978 Cases	1973–1978 Percent	1979–1983 Cases	1979–1983 Percent	1984–1989 Cases	1984–1989 Percent	1990–1993 Cases	1990–1993 Percent	1994–1998 Cases	1994–1998 Percent	1999–2003 Cases	1999–2003 Percent
Birth outcome																
Live birth	482	98.6							44	97.8	72	98.6	131	98.5	235	98.7
Stillbirth	6	1.2							<5	–	<5	–	<5	–	<5	–
Elective termination	<5	–							–	–	–	–	<5	–	–	–
Unknown	–	–							–	–	–	–	–	–	–	–
Age at diagnosis																
Prenatally or <7 days	289	59.1							29	64.4	39	53.4	80	60.2	141	59.2
8 days–6 months	128	26.2							12	26.7	20	27.4	38	28.6	58	24.4
6 months–1 year	29	5.9							<5	–	11	15.1	8	6.0	6	2.5
1–5 years	20	4.1							–	–	<5	–	<5	–	13	5.5
>5 years	<5	–							–	–	–	–	–	–	<5	–
Unknown	22	4.5							–	–	–	–	<5	–	19	8.0
Socioeconomic status§																
Upper	109	22.3							19	42.2	21	28.8	34	25.6	35	14.7
Middle	110	22.5							14	31.1	24	32.9	43	32.3	29	12.2
Lower	116	23.7							11	24.4	27	37	45	33.8	33	13.9
Unknown	154	31.5							<5	–	<5	–	11	8.3	141	59.2

* Numbers of cases and prevalence estimates are not provided for congenital heart defects prior to 1984 because not all of these cases have been reviewed by pediatric cardiologists. Cells containing fewer than 5 cases are indicated as "<5". Prevalence estimates based on these cells are indicated as less than the prevalence based on 5 cases in Table A. Percentages based on these cells are not provided in Table B. Cells containing zero cases are indicated as "—". Cells in years for which no data are provided are left blank. Counts are provided, but prevalences are not estimated, for strata with unknown values in Table A. Counts and percentages are provided for strata with unknown values in Table B.

** Prev = Prevalence.

† Data on Hispanic or Latino ethnicity were available beginning in 1990.

§ Information about socioeconomic status was available only for 1979–2001.

TABLE 23A

VENTRICULAR SEPTAL DEFECT: PREVALENCE (PER 10,000 LIVE BIRTHS) STRATIFIED BY DESCRIPTIVE CHARACTERISTICS, MACDP, 1984–2003*

	Total		1968–1972		1973–1978		1979–1983		1984–1989		1990–1993		1994–1998		1999–2003	
Characteristic	Cases	Prev**	Cases	Prev	Cases	Prev	Cases	Prev	Cases	Prev	Cases	Prev	Cases	Prev	Cases	Prev
Total	**2,416**	**29.61**							**459**	**22.64**	**359**	**23.26**	**627**	**30.02**	**971**	**38.84**
Maternal age (years)																
<25	686	24.55							168	21.37	105	19.21	172	25.54	241	30.57
25–29	673	29.36							142	22.39	110	24.45	167	30.2	254	38.76
≥30	1,053	34.31							149	24.59	143	26.18	288	33.44	473	44.8
Unknown	<5	–							–	–	<5	–	–	–	<5	–
Maternal race/ethnicity[†]																
White	1,282	32.40							294	23.98	205	25.81	337	34.37	446	46.65
Black or African American	776	24.21							155	20.46	128	19.93	210	24.91	283	29.4
Hispanic or Latino	264	40.62							–	–	12	20.32	58	34.97	194	45.66
All Other Races	77	22.68							10	22.96	14	29.61	21	21.88	32	20.95
Unknown	17	–							–	–	–	–	<5	–	16	–
Birth weight (grams)																
<2500	625	90.09							120	73.78	113	84.46	172	96.19	220	100.68
≥2500	1,788	23.96							337	18.08	246	17.46	454	23.78	751	32.92
Unknown	<5	–							<5	–	–	–	<5	–	–	–
Gestational age (weeks)																
20–36	610	75.82							116	58.74	104	65.41	167	85.8	223	91.82
≥37	1,780	24.91							336	26.08	254	19.52	453	24.46	737	33.17
Unknown	26	–							7	–	<5	–	7	–	11	–
Sex																
Male	1,143	27.45							224	21.56	162	20.56	305	28.63	452	35.54
Female	1,271	31.81							235	23.77	196	25.95	322	31.47	518	42.17
Ambiguous/Unknown	<5	–							–	–	<5	–	–	–	<5	–
Parity																
1 Live birth	1,071	30.28							190	21.21	162	24.24	282	30.7	437	41.44
2 or more live births	1,317	28.89							248	22.65	197	22.63	340	29.26	532	37.15
Unknown	28	–							21	–	–	–	5	–	<5	–
Gravidity																
1 Pregnancy	704	24.91							134	18.99	99	19.02	173	23.72	298	34.24
2 or more pregnancies	1,700	32.40							320	24.94	260	25.57	449	33.34	671	41.92
Unknown	12	–							5	–	–	–	5	–	<5	–
Plurality																
Singleton	2,260	28.51							437	22.06	325	21.63	592	29.22	906	37.5
Multiple	156	66.88							22	47.57	34	83.29	35	56.32	65	77.35
Unknown	–	–							–	–	–	–	–	–	–	–

TABLE 23B

VENTRICULAR SEPTAL DEFECT: PERCENTAGE OF CASES BY DESCRIPTIVE CHARACTERISTICS, MACDP, 1984–2003*

| | Period | | | | | | | | | | | | | | | |
Characteristic	Total		1968–1972		1973–1978		1979–1983		1984–1989		1990–1993		1994–1998		1999–2003	
	Cases	Percent	Cases	Percent	Cases	Percent	Cases	Percent	Cases	Percent	Cases	Percent	Cases	Percent	Cases	Percent
Birth outcome																
Live birth	2,373	98.2							451	98.3	349	97.2	613	97.8	960	98.9
Stillbirth	33	1.4							8	1.7	8	2.2	9	1.4	8	0.8
Elective termination	10	0.4							–	–	<5	–	5	0.8	<5	–
Unknown	<5	–							–	–	–	–	–	–	–	–
Age at diagnosis																
Prenatally or <7 days	1,988	82.3							363	79.1	302	84.1	499	79.6	824	84.9
8 days–6 months	330	13.7							80	17.4	48	13.4	105	16.7	97	10.0
6 months–1 year	36	1.5							13	2.8	7	1.9	11	1.8	5	0.5
1–5 years	22	0.0							<5	–	<5	–	8	1.3	11	1.1
>5 years	–	–							–	–	–	–	–	–	–	–
Unknown	40	1.7							<5	–	<5	–	<5	34	3.5	
Socioeconomic status§																
Upper	675	27.9							156	34.0	147	40.9	197	31.4	175	18.0
Middle	642	26.6							145	31.6	120	33.4	212	33.8	165	17.0
Lower	550	22.8							147	32	84	23.4	181	28.9	138	14.2
Unknown	549	22.7							11	2.4	8	2.2	37	5.9	493	50.8

* Numbers of cases and prevalence estimates are not provided for congenital heart defects prior to 1984 because not all of these cases have been reviewed by pediatric cardiologists. Cells containing fewer than 5 cases are indicated as "<5". Prevalence estimates based on these cells are indicated as less than the prevalence based on 5 cases in Table A. Percentages based on these cells are not provided in Table B. Cells containing zero cases are indicated as "—". Cells in years for which no data are provided are left blank. Counts are provided, but prevalences are not estimated, for strata with unknown values in Table A. Counts and percentages are provided for strata with unknown values in Table B.

** Prev = Prevalence.

† Data on Hispanic or Latino ethnicity were available beginning in 1990.

§ Information about socioeconomic status was available only for 1979–2001.

TABLE 24A

PERIMEMBRANOUS VENTRICULAR SEPTAL DEFECT: PREVALENCE (PER 10,000 LIVE BIRTHS) STRATIFIED BY DESCRIPTIVE CHARACTERISTICS, MACDP, 1984–2003*

	Total		1968–1972		1973–1978		1979–1983		1984–1989		1990–1993		1994–1998		1999–2003	
Characteristic	Cases	Prev**	Cases	Prev	Cases	Prev	Cases	Prev	Cases	Prev	Cases	Prev	Cases	Prev	Cases	Prev
Total	684	8.38							96	4.73	102	6.61	208	9.96	278	11.12
Maternal age (years)																
<25	200	7.16							36	4.58	28	5.12	54	8.02	82	10.40
25–29	186	8.11							38	5.99	29	6.45	54	9.76	65	9.92
≥30	298	9.71							22	3.63	45	8.24	100	11.61	131	12.41
Unknown	—	–							—		—		—		—	–
Maternal race/ethnicity§																
White	306	7.73							53	4.32	49	6.17	102	10.40	102	10.67
Black or African American	289	9.02							42	5.54	46	7.16	86	10.20	115	11.95
Hispanic or Latino	53	8.16							—	–	<5	<8.47	12	7.23	38	8.94
All Other Races	29	8.54							<5	<11.48	<5	<10.58	7	7.29	17	11.13
Unknown	7	–							—	–	—	–	<5	–	6	–
Birth weight (grams)																
<2500	195	28.11							22	13.53	34	25.41	60	33.55	79	36.15
≥2500	489	6.55							74	3.97	68	4.83	148	7.75	199	8.72
Unknown	—	–							—	–	—	–	—	–	—	–
Gestational age (weeks)																
20–36	168	21.16							19	9.62	29	18.24	49	25.17	71	29.23
≥37	507	7.09							76	4.54	72	5.53	157	8.48	202	9.09
Unknown	9	–							<5	–	<5	–	<5	–	5	–
Sex																
Male	346	8.31							43	4.14	53	6.73	107	10.05	143	11.25
Female	338	8.46							53	5.36	49	6.49	101	9.87	135	10.99
Ambiguous/Unknown	—	–							—		—		—		—	–
Parity																
1 Live birth	317	8.96							44	4.91	47	7.03	93	10.13	133	12.61
2 or more live births	358	7.85							45	4.11	55	6.32	114	9.81	144	10.05
Unknown	9	–							7		—		<5		<5	–
Gravidity																
1 Pregnancy	196	6.94							32	4.53	34	6.53	44	6.03	86	9.88
2 or more pregnancies	484	9.22							62	4.83	68	6.69	163	12.10	191	11.93
Unknown	<5	–							<5	–	—	–	<5	–	<5	–
Plurality																
Singleton	646	8.15							93	4.69	95	6.32	198	9.77	260	10.76
Multiple	38	16.29							<5	<10.81	7	17.15	10	16.09	18	21.42
Unknown	—	–							—		—		—		—	–

TABLE 24B

PERIMEMBRANOUS VENTRICULAR SEPTAL DEFECT: PERCENTAGE OF CASES BY DESCRIPTIVE CHARACTERISTICS, MACDP, 1984–2003*

	Total		1968–1972		1973–1978		1979–1983		1984–1989		1990–1993		1994–1998		1999–2003	
													Period			
Characteristic	Cases	Percent	Cases	Percent	Cases	Percent	Cases	Percent	Cases	Percent	Cases	Percent	Cases	Percent	Cases	Percent
Birth outcome																
Live birth	672	98.2							94	97.9	100	98.0	201	96.6	277	99.6
Stillbirth	10	1.5							<5	–	<5	–	5	2.4	<5	–
Elective termination	<5	–							–	–	–	–	<5	–	–	–
Unknown	–	–							–	–	–	–	–	–	–	–
Age at diagnosis																
Prenatally or <7 days	478	69.9							62	64.6	75	73.5	133	63.9	208	74.8
8 days–6 months	166	24.3							30	31.3	23	22.5	63	30.3	50	18.0
6 months–1 year	16	2.3							<5	–	<5	–	6	2.9	<5	–
1–5 years	10	1.4							–	–	<5	–	<5	–	6	2.2
>5 years	–	–							–	–	–	–	–	–	–	–
Unknown	14	2.0							–	–	–	–	<5	–	11	4.0
Socioeconomic status§																
Upper	185	27.0							32	33.3	39	38.2	63	30.3	51	18.3
Middle	183	26.8							29	30.2	38	37.3	65	31.3	51	18.3
Lower	172	25.1							32	33.3	23	22.5	68	32.7	49	17.6
Unknown	144	21.1							<5	–	<5	–	12	5.8	127	45.7

* Numbers of cases and prevalence estimates are not provided for congenital heart defects prior to 1984 because not all of these cases have been reviewed by pediatric cardiologists. Cells containing fewer than 5 cases are indicated as "<5". Prevalence estimates based on these cells are indicated as less than the prevalence based on 5 cases in Table A. Percentages based on these cells are not provided in Table B. Cells containing zero cases are indicated as "—". Cells in years for which no data are provided are left blank. Counts are provided, but prevalences are not estimated, for strata with unknown values in Table A. Counts and percentages are provided for strata with unknown values in Table B.
** Prev = Prevalence.
† Data on Hispanic or Latino ethnicity were available beginning in 1990.
§ Information about socioeconomic status was available only for 1979–2001.

TABLE 25A

MUSCULAR VENTRICULAR SEPTAL DEFECT: PREVALENCE (PER 10,000 LIVE BIRTHS) STRATIFIED BY DESCRIPTIVE CHARACTERISTICS, MACDP, 1984–2003*

	Total		1968–1972		1973–1978		1979–1983		1984–1989		1990–1993		1994–1998		1999–2003	
Characteristic	Cases	Prev**	Cases	Prev	Cases	Prev	Cases	Prev	Cases	Prev	Cases	Prev	Cases	Prev	Cases	Prev
Total	1,166	14.29							46	2.27	131	8.49	343	16.42	646	25.48
Maternal age (years)																
<25	298	10.66							15	1.91	43	7.87	96	14.26	144	18.26
25–29	328	14.31							15	2.37	38	8.45	98	17.72	177	27.01
≥30	536	17.46							16	2.64	49	8.97	149	17.30	322	30.50
Unknown	<5	–							–		<5		–		<5	
Maternal race/ethnicity†																
White	658	16.63							34	2.77	82	10.33	203	20.70	339	35.46
Black or African American	288	8.99							11	1.45	41	6.38	97	11.51	139	14.44
Hispanic or Latino	182	28.01							–		<5	<8.47	33	19.90	145	34.12
All Other Races	27	7.95							<5	<11.48	<5	<10.58	10	10.42	12	7.86
Unknown	11	–							–		–		–		11	
Birth weight (grams)																
<2500	246	35.46							7	4.30	39	29.15	87	48.65	113	51.71
≥2500	919	12.31							39	2.09	92	6.53	255	13.36	533	23.37
Unknown	<5	–							–		–		<5		–	
Gestational age (weeks)																
20–36	270	33.38							11	5.57	39	24.53	95	48.81	125	51.47
≥37	884	12.43							34	2.03	92	7.07	244	13.17	514	23.14
Unknown	12	–							<5		–		<5		7	
Sex																
Male	522	12.54							26	2.50	53	6.73	162	15.21	281	22.10
Female	643	16.09							20	2.02	78	10.33	181	17.69	364	29.63
Ambiguous/Unknown	<5	–							–		–		–		<5	
Parity																
1 Live birth	527	14.90							19	2.12	68	10.17	156	16.99	284	26.93
2 or more live births	633	13.88							26	2.37	63	7.24	183	15.75	361	25.21
Unknown	6	–							<5		–		<5		<5	
Gravidity																
1 Pregnancy	355	12.56							14	1.98	40	7.68	105	14.40	196	22.52
2 or more pregnancies	806	15.36							32	2.49	91	8.95	234	17.37	449	28.05
Unknown	5	–							–		–		<5		<5	
Plurality																
Singleton	1,081	13.64							44	2.22	116	7.72	321	15.84	600	24.84
Multiple	85	36.44							<5	<10.81	15	36.75	22	35.40	46	54.74
Unknown	–	–							–		–		–		–	

TABLE 25B

MUSCULAR VENTRICULAR SEPTAL DEFECT: PERCENTAGE OF CASES BY DESCRIPTIVE CHARACTERISTICS, MACDP, 1984–2003*

			Period													
	Total		1968–1972		1973–1978		1979–1983		1984–1989		1990–1993		1994–1998		1999–2003	
Characteristic	Cases	Percent	Cases	Percent	Cases	Percent	Cases	Percent	Cases	Percent	Cases	Percent	Cases	Percent	Cases	Percent
Birth outcome																
Live birth	1,166	100.0							46	100.0	131	100.0	343	100.0	646	100
Stillbirth	—	—							—	—	—	—	—	—	—	—
Elective termination	—	—							—	—	—	—	—	—	—	—
Unknown	—	—							—	—	—	—	—	—	—	—
Age at diagnosis																
Prenatally or <7 days	1,024	87.8							32	69.6	114	87.0	296	86.3	582	90.1
8 days–6 months	104	8.9							11	23.9	12	9.2	40	11.7	41	6.3
6 months–1 year	12	1.0							<5	—	<5	—	<5	—	<5	—
1–5 years	7	0.0							—	—	—	—	<5	—	<5	—
>5 years	—	—							—	—	—	—	—	—	—	—
Unknown	19	1.6							—	—	<5	—	—	—	18	2.8
Socioeconomic status																
Upper	308	26.4							20	43.5	53	40.5	116	33.8	119	18.4
Middle	267	22.9							10	21.7	42	32.1	115	33.5	100	15.5
Lower	218	18.7							14	30.4	32	24.4	91	26.5	81	12.5
Unknown	373	32.0							<5	—	<5	—	21	6.1	346	53.6

* Numbers of cases and prevalence estimates are not provided for congenital heart defects prior to 1984 because not all of these cases have been reviewed by pediatric cardiologists. Cells containing fewer than 5 cases are indicated as "<5". Prevalence estimates based on these cells are indicated as less than the prevalence based on 5 cases in Table A. Percentages based on these cells are not provided in Table B. Cells containing zero cases are indicated as "—". Cells in years for which no data are provided are left blank. Counts are provided, but prevalences are not estimated, for strata with unknown values in Table A. Counts and percentages are provided for strata with unknown values in Table B.

** Prev = Prevalence.

† Data on Hispanic or Latino ethnicity were available beginning in 1990.

§ Information about socioeconomic status was available only for 1979–2001.

TABLE 26A

SINGLE VENTRICLE: PREVALENCE (PER 10,000 LIVE BIRTHS) STRATIFIED BY DESCRIPTIVE CHARACTERISTICS, MACDP, 1984–2003*

Characteristic	Total		1968–1972		1973–1978		1979–1983		1984–1989		1990–1993		1994–1998		1999–2003	
	Cases	Prev**	Cases	Prev	Cases	Prev	Cases	Prev	Cases	Prev	Cases	Prev	Cases	Prev	Cases	Prev
Total	**79**	**0.97**							**18**	**0.89**	**16**	**1.04**	**24**	**1.15**	**21**	**0.84**
Maternal age (years)																
<25	25	0.89							6	0.76	5	0.91	6	0.89	8	1.01
25–29	20	0.87							<5	<0.79	<5	<1.11	6	1.08	6	0.92
≥30	34	1.11							8	1.32	7	1.28	12	1.39	7	0.66
Unknown	–	–							–	–	–	–	–	–	–	–
Maternal race/ethnicity†																
White	45	1.14							14	1.14	8	1.01	1.7	1.73	6	0.63
Black or African American	25	0.78							<5	<0.66	5	0.78	6	0.71	10	1.04
Hispanic or Latino	<5	<0.77							–	–	–	–	–	–	<5	1.18
All Other Races	5	1.47							–	–	<5	<10.58	<5	<5.21	<5	<3.27
Unknown	<5	–							<5	–	–	–	–	–	<5	–
Birth weight (grams)																
<2500	26	3.75							5	3.07	8	5.98	6	3.36	7	3.20
≥2500	52	0.70							13	0.70	7	0.50	18	0.94	14	0.61
Unknown	<5	–							<5	–	<5	–	–	–	–	–
Gestational age (weeks)																
20–36	22	2.77							<5	<2.53	5	3.14	7	3.60	7	2.88
≥37	56	0.79							14	0.84	11	0.85	17	0.92	14	0.63
Unknown	<5	–							<5	–	–	–	–	–	–	–
Sex																
Male	48	1.15							11	1.06	8	1.02	15	1.41	14	1.10
Female	30	0.75							7	0.71	7	0.93	9	0.88	7	0.57
Ambiguous/Unknown	<5	–							7	–	<5	–	–	–	–	–
Parity																
1 Livebirth	31	0.88							<5	<0.56	8	1.20	13	1.42	6	0.57
2 or more live births	47	1.03							13	1.19	8	0.92	11	0.95	15	1.05
Unknown	<5	–							<5	–	–	–	–	–	–	–
Gravidity																
1 Pregnancy	22	0.78							5	0.71	6	1.15	7	0.96	<5	<0.57
2 or more pregnancies	57	1.09							13	1.01	10	0.98	17	1.26	17	1.06
Unknown	–	–							–	–	–	–	–	–	–	–
Plurality																
Singleton	75	0.95							17	0.86	14	0.93	24	1.18	20	0.83
Multiple	<5	2.14							<5	<10.81	<5	<12.25			<5	<5.95
Unknown	–	–							–	–	–	–	–	–	–	–

TABLE 26B

SINGLE VENTRICLE: PERCENTAGE OF CASES BY DESCRIPTIVE CHARACTERISTICS, MACDP, 1984–2003*

| | Period | | | | | | | | | | | | | | | |
| Characteristic | Total | | 1968–1972 | | 1973–1978 | | 1979–1983 | | 1984–1989 | | 1990–1993 | | 1994–1998 | | 1999–2003 | |
	Cases	Percent	Cases	Percent	Cases	Percent	Cases	Percent	Cases	Percent	Cases	Percent	Cases	Percent	Cases	Percent
Birth outcome																
Live birth	69	87.3							18	100.0	13	81.3	19	79.2	19	90.5
Stillbirth	8	10.1							–	–	<5	–	<5	–	<5	–
Elective termination	<5	–							–	–	–	–	<5	–	<5	–
Unknown	–	–							–	–	–	–	–	–	–	–
Age at diagnosis																
Prenatally or <7 days	66	83.5							13	72.2	14	87.5	21	87.5	18	85.7
8 days–6 months	9	11.4							5	27.8	<5	–	<5	–	–	–
6 months–1 year	–	–							–	–	–	–	–	–	–	–
1–5 years	–	–							–	–	–	–	–	–	–	–
>5 years	–	–							–	–	–	–	–	–	–	–
Unknown	<5	–							–	–	–	–	<5	–	<5	–
Socioeconomic status§																
Upper	27	34.2							7	38.9	7	43.8	10	41.7	<5	–
Middle	22	27.8							6	33.3	6	37.5	7	29.2	<5	–
Lower	20	25.3							5	27.8	<5	–	5	20.8	7	33.3
Unknown	10	12.7							–	–	–	–	<5	–	8	38.1

* Numbers of cases and prevalence estimates are not provided for congenital heart defects prior to 1984 because not all of these cases have been reviewed by pediatric cardiologists. Cells containing fewer than 5 cases are indicated as "<5". Prevalence estimates based on these cells are indicated as less than the prevalence based on 5 cases in Table A. Percentages based on these cells are not provided in Table B. Cells containing zero cases are indicated as "–". Cells in years for which no data are provided are left blank. Counts are provided, but prevalences are not estimated, for strata with unknown values in Table A. Counts and percentages are provided for strata with unknown values in Table B.

** Prev = Prevalence.

† Data on Hispanic or Latino ethnicity were available beginning in 1990.

§ Information about socioeconomic status was available only for 1979–2001.

TABLE 27A

PARTIAL AND TOTAL ANOMALOUS PULMONARY VENOUS RETURN: PREVALENCE (PER 10,000 LIVE BIRTHS) STRATIFIED BY DESCRIPTIVE CHARACTERISTICS, MACDP, 1984–2003*

Characteristic	Total Cases	Total Prev**	1968–1972 Cases	1968–1972 Prev	1973–1978 Cases	1973–1978 Prev	1979–1983 Cases	1979–1983 Prev	1984–1989 Cases	1984–1989 Prev	1990–1993 Cases	1990–1993 Prev	1994–1998 Cases	1994–1998 Prev	1999–2003 Cases	1999–2003 Prev
Total	71	0.87							19	0.94	21	1.36	12	0.57	19	0.76
Maternal age (years)																
<25	27	0.97							10	1.27	8	1.46	<5	<0.74	6	0.76
25–29	16	0.70							5	0.79	7	1.56	–	–	<5	<0.76
≥30	28	0.91							<5	<0.83	6	1.10	9	1.05	9	0.85
Unknown	–	–							–	–	–	–	–	–	–	–
Maternal race/ethnicity†																
White	33	0.83							8	0.65	11	1.39	6	0.61	8	0.84
Black or African American	26	0.81							11	1.45	7	1.09	<5	<0.59	<5	<0.52
Hispanic or Latino	10	1.54							–	–	<5	<8.47	<5	<3.01	6	1.41
All Other Races	<5	<1.47							–	–	–	–	<5	<5.21	<5	<3.27
Unknown	–	–							–	–	–	–	–	–	–	–
Birth weight (grams)																
<2500	16	2.31							<5	<3.07	6	4.48	<5	2.80	6	2.75
≥2500	55	0.74							16	0.86	15	1.06	11	0.58	13	0.57
Unknown	–	–							–	–	–	–	–	–	–	–
Gestational age (weeks)																
20–36	16	2.02							6	3.04	5	3.14	<5	<2.57	<5	<2.06
≥37	55	0.78							13	0.78	16	1.23	10	0.54	16	0.72
Unknown	–	–							–	–	–	–	–	–	–	–
Sex																
Male	46	1.10							11	1.06	11	1.40	8	0.75	16	1.26
Female	25	0.63							8	0.81	10	1.32	<5	<0.49	<5	<0.41
Ambiguous/Unknown	–	–							–	–	–	–	–	–	–	–
Parity																
1 Live birth	31	0.88							9	1.00	9	1.35	<5	<0.54	9	0.85
2 or more live births	39	0.86							9	0.82	12	1.38	8	0.69	10	0.70
Unknown	<5	–							<5	–	–	–	–	–	–	–
Gravidity																
1 Pregnancy	28	0.99							8	1.13	8	1.54	<5	<0.69	9	1.03
2 or more pregnancies	43	0.82							11	0.86	13	1.28	9	0.67	10	0.62
Unknown	–	–							–	–	–	–	–	–	–	–
Plurality																
Singleton	67	0.85							19	0.96	20	1.33	11	0.54	17	0.70
Multiple	<5	<2.14							–	–	<5	<12.25	<5	<8.05	<5	<5.95
Unknown	–	–							–	–	–	–	–	–	–	–

TABLE 27B

PARTIAL AND TOTAL ANOMALOUS PULMONARY VENOUS RETURN: PERCENTAGE OF CASES BY DESCRIPTIVE CHARACTERISTICS, MACDP, 1984–2003*

| | | | | | | | | | | Period | | | | | | |
| Characteristic | Total | | 1968–1972 | | 1973–1978 | | 1979–1983 | | 1984–1989 | | 1990–1993 | | 1994–1998 | | 1999–2003 | |
	Cases	Percent	Cases	Percent	Cases	Percent	Cases	Percent	Cases	Percent	Cases	Percent	Cases	Percent	Cases	Percent
Birth outcome																
Live birth	71	100.00							19	100.0	21	100.0	12	100.0	19	100.0
Stillbirth	–	–							–	–	–	–	–	–	–	–
Elective termination	–	–							–	–	–	–	–	–	–	–
Unknown	–	–							–	–	–	–	–	–	–	–
Age at diagnosis																
Prenatally or <7 days	45	63.4							11	57.9	11	52.4	10	83.3	13	68.4
8 days–6 months	21	29.6							6	31.6	9	42.9	<5	–	5	26.3
6 months–1 year	5	7.0							<5	–	<5	–	<5	–	<5	–
1–5 years	–	–							–	–	–	–	–	–	–	–
>5 years	–	–							–	–	–	–	–	–	–	–
Unknown	–	–							–	–	–	–	–	–	–	–
Socioeconomic status§																
Upper	22	31.0							<5	–	11	52.4	<5	–	<5	–
Middle	15	21.1							<5	–	<5	–	<5	–	<5	–
Lower	26	36.6							11	57.9	6	28.6	<5	–	5	26.3
Unknown	8	11.3							–	–	–	–	<5	–	7	36.8

* Numbers of cases and prevalence estimates are not provided for congenital heart defects prior to 1984 because not all of these cases have been reviewed by pediatric cardiologists. Cells containing fewer than 5 cases are indicated as "<5". Prevalence estimates based on these cells are indicated as less than the prevalence based on 5 cases in Table A. Percentages based on these cells are not provided in Table B. Cells containing zero cases are indicated as "–". Cells in years for which no data are provided are left blank. Counts are provided, but prevalences are not estimated, for strata with unknown values in Table A. Counts and percentages are provided for strata with unknown values in Table B.

** Prev = Prevalence.

† Data on Hispanic or Latino ethnicity were available beginning in 1990.

§ Information about socioeconomic status was available only for 1979–2001.

TABLE 28A

CLEFT LIP WITH OR WITHOUT CLEFT PALATE: PREVALENCE (PER 10,000 LIVE BIRTHS) STRATIFIED BY DESCRIPTIVE CHARACTERISTICS, MACDP, 1968–2003*

Characteristic	Total		1968–1972		1973–1978		1979–1983		1984–1989		1990–1993		1994–1998		1999–2003	
	Cases	Prev**	Cases	Prev	Cases	Prev	Cases	Prev	Cases	Prev	Cases	Prev	Cases	Prev	Cases	Prev
Total	1,177	9.55	151	11.01	158	11.01	156	11.51	180	8.88	142	9.20	192	9.19	198	7.92
Maternal age (years)																
<25	512	10.42	88	11.25	78	10.66	81	13.38	75	9.54	44	8.05	71	10.54	75	9.51
25–29	303	8.59	35	9.40	55	12.40	41	9.75	50	7.88	43	9.56	34	6.15	45	6.87
≥30	358	9.25	24	11.04	25	9.85	34	10.34	55	9.08	55	10.07	87	10.10	78	7.39
Unknown	<5	–	<5	–	–	–	–	–	–	–	–	–	–	–	–	–
Maternal race/ethnicity†																
White	764	11.40	126	12.79	125	13.45	104	12.53	124	10.11	81	10.20	107	10.91	97	10.15
Black or African American	279	6.64	–	–	31	6.32	49	9.69	49	6.47	45	7.01	53	6.29	52	5.40
Hispanic or Latino	71	10.93	–	–	–	–	–	–	–	–	7	11.85	22	13.26	42	9.88
All Other Races	62	8.15	25‡	6.46	<5	<33.81	<5	<26.07	7	16.07	9	19.04	10	10.42	6	3.93
Unknown	<5	–	–	–	–	–	–	–	–	–	–	–	–	–	<5	–
Birth weight (grams)																
<2500	276	26.16	28	23.22	30	24.31	40	34.13	44	27.05	40	29.90	39	21.81	55	25.17
≥2500	896	7.97	121	9.72	127	9.81	116	9.38	135	7.24	102	7.24	152	7.96	143	6.27
Unknown	5	–	<5	–	<5	–	–	–	<5	–	–	–	<5	–	–	–
Gestational age (weeks)																
20–36	233	20.37	19	17.96	21	17.38	31	25.14	33	16.71	41	25.79	39	20.04	49	20.18
≥37	933	8.85	132	11.38	137	11.37	124	10.97	143	8.54	98	7.53	152	8.21	147	6.62
Unknown	11	–	–	–	–	–	<5	–	<5	–	<5	–	<5	–	<5	–
Sex																
Male	682	10.83	91	12.96	95	12.87	82	11.81	102	9.82	71	9.01	117	10.98	124	9.75
Female	487	8.09	60	8.95	63	9.04	72	10.89	77	7.79	68	9.00	74	7.23	73	5.94
Ambiguous/Unknown	8	–	–	–	–	–	<5	–	<5	–	<5	–	<5	–	<5	–
Parity																
1 Live birth	523	9.66	63	12.08	83	11.49	63	9.92	70	7.81	59	8.83	86	9.36	99	9.39
2 or more live births	617	9.19	61	8.48	74	10.38	93	12.91	102	9.32	83	9.53	106	9.12	98	6.84
Unknown	37	–	27	–	<5	–	–	–	8	–	–	–	–	–	<5	–
Gravidity																
1 Pregnancy	403	8.69	58	11.93	71	10.59	51	7.79	55	7.79	32	6.15	58	7.95	78	8.96
2 or more pregnancies	772	10.34	93	12.32	87	11.37	105	14.99	124	9.66	110	10.82	134	9.95	119	7.44
Unknown	5	–	–	–	–	–	–	–	<5	–	–	–	–	–	<5	–
Plurality																
Singleton	1,146	9.54	147	10.91	152	10.81	155	11.67	175	8.83	137	9.12	187	9.23	193	7.99
Multiple	31	9.93	<5	<20.05	6	22.21	<5	<18.44	5	10.81	5	12.25	5	8.05	5	5.95
Unknown	–	–	–	–	–	–	–	–	–	–	–	–	–	–	–	–

TABLE 28B

CLEFT LIP WITH OR WITHOUT CLEFT PALATE: PERCENTAGE OF CASES BY DESCRIPTIVE CHARACTERISTICS, MACDP, 1968–2003*

Characteristic	Total		1968–1972		1973–1978		1979–1983		1984–1989		1990–1993		1994–1998		1999–2003	
	Cases	Percent	Cases	Percent	Cases	Percent	Cases	Percent	Cases	Percent	Cases	Percent	Cases	Percent	Cases	Percent
Birth outcome																
Live birth	1,099	93.4	143	94.7	147	93.0	150	96.2	167	92.8	129	90.8	180	93.8	183	92.4
Stillbirth	64	5.4	8	5.3	11	7.0	6	3.8	13	7.2	11	7.7	8	4.2	7	3.5
Elective termination	14	1.2	—	—	—	—	—	—	—	—	<5	—	<5	—	8	4.0
Unknown	—	—	—	—	—	—	—	—	—	—	—	—	—	—	—	—
Age at diagnosis																
Prenatally or <7 days	1,148	97.5	150	99.3	158	100.0	155	99.4	175	97.2	139	97.9	191	99.5	180	90.9
8 days–6 months	8	0.7	<5	—	—	—	<5	—	<5	—	<5	—	—	—	<5	—
6 months–1 year	<5	—	—	—	—	—	—	—	<5	—	<5	—	—	—	—	—
1–5 years	—	—	—	—	—	—	—	—	—	—	—	—	—	—	—	—
>5 years	—	—	—	—	—	—	—	—	—	—	—	—	—	—	—	—
Unknown	19	1.6	—	—	—	—	—	—	<5	—	—	—	<5	—	17	8.6
Socioeconomic status§																
Upper	265	22.5	—	—	—	—	44	28.2	67	37.2	52	36.6	61	31.8	41	20.7
Middle	260	22.1	—	—	—	—	54	34.6	51	28.3	50	35.2	63	32.8	42	21.2
Lower	236	20.1	—	—	—	—	55	35.3	57	31.7	39	27.5	59	30.7	26	13.1
Unknown	416	35.3	151	100.0	158	100.0	<5	—	5	2.8	<5	—	9	4.7	89	44.9

* Cells containing fewer than 5 cases are indicated as "<5". Prevalence estimates based on these cells are indicated as less than the prevalence based on 5 cases in Table A. Percentages based on these cells are not provided in Table B. Cells containing zero cases are indicated as "—". Counts are provided, but prevalences are not estimated, for strata with unknown values in Table A. Counts and percentages are provided for strata with unknown values in Table B.
** Prev = Prevalence.
† Data on Hispanic or Latino ethnicity were available beginning in 1990.
‡ The category of All Other Races includes 25 cases of Black or African American race.
§ Information about socioeconomic status was available only for 1979–2001.

TABLE 29A

CLEFT PALATE ALONE: PREVALENCE (PER 10,000 LIVE BIRTHS) STRATIFIED BY DESCRIPTIVE CHARACTERISTICS, MACDP, 1968–2003*

Characteristic	Total		1968–1972		1973–1978		1979–1983		1984–1989		1990–1993		1994–1998		1999–2003	
	Cases	Prev**	Cases	Prev	Cases	Prev	Cases	Prev	Cases	Prev	Cases	Prev	Cases	Prev	Cases	Prev
Total	**672**	**5.45**	**72**	**5.25**	**99**	**6.90**	**62**	**4.57**	**106**	**5.23**	**75**	**4.86**	**106**	**5.08**	**152**	**6.08**
Maternal age (years)																
<25	258	5.25	41	5.24	53	7.25	32	5.29	33	4.20	19	3.48	40	5.94	40	5.07
25–29	185	5.24	19	5.11	24	5.41	18	4.28	40	6.31	27	6.00	22	3.98	35	5.34
≥30	227	5.87	12	5.52	21	8.27	12	3.65	33	5.45	29	5.31	44	5.11	76	7.20
Unknown	<5	–	–	–	<5	–	–	–	–	–	–	–	–	–	<5	–
Maternal race/ethnicity†																
White	410	6.12	55	5.58	70	7.53	39	4.70	65	5.30	48	6.04	57	5.81	76	7.95
Black or African American	194	4.62	–	–	29	5.91	23	4.55	39	5.15	22	3.43	37	4.39	44	4.57
Hispanic or Latino	29	4.46	–	–	–	–	–	–	–	–	–	–	7	4.22	22	5.18
All Other Races	36	4.73	17‡	4.39	–	–	–	–	<5	<11.48	5	10.58	5	5.21	7	4.58
Unknown	<5	–	–	–	–	–	–	–	–	–	–	–	–	–	<5	–
Birth weight (grams)																
<2500	192	18.20	20	16.59	32	25.93	19	16.21	34	20.91	16	11.96	26	14.54	45	20.59
≥2500	477	4.24	51	4.10	66	5.10	43	3.48	72	3.86	58	4.12	80	4.19	107	4.69
Unknown	<5	–	<5	–	<5	–	–	–	–	–	<5	–	–	–	–	–
Gestational age (weeks)																
20–36	149	13.03	13	12.29	15	12.41	14	11.35	31	15.70	12	7.55	25	12.84	39	16.06
≥37	514	4.87	58	5.00	83	6.89	48	4.25	74	4.42	61	4.69	81	4.37	109	4.91
Unknown	9	–	<5	–	<5	–	–	–	<5	–	<5	–	–	–	<5	–
Sex																
Male	317	5.03	32	4.56	51	6.91	31	4.46	44	4.23	40	5.08	46	4.32	73	5.74
Female	352	5.84	40	5.97	47	6.74	31	4.69	60	6.07	35	4.63	60	5.86	79	6.43
Ambiguous/Unknown	<5	–	–	–	<5	–	–	–	<5	–	–	–	–	–	–	–
Parity																
1 Live birth	284	5.24	32	6.14	41	5.67	33	5.20	35	3.91	27	4.04	53	5.77	63	5.97
2 or more live births	372	5.54	33	4.59	55	7.72	29	4.02	66	6.03	47	5.40	53	4.56	89	6.21
Unknown	16	–	7	–	<5	–	–	–	5	–	<5	–	–	–	–	–
Gravidity																
1 Pregnancy	223	4.81	29	5.96	35	5.22	27	4.12	25	3.54	21	4.03	41	5.62	45	5.17
2 or more pregnancies	446	5.97	43	5.70	62	8.10	35	5.00	81	6.31	53	5.21	65	4.83	107	6.69
Unknown	<5	–	–	–	<5	–	–	–	–	–	<5	–	–	–	–	–
Plurality																
Singleton	652	5.43	70	5.20	97	6.90	61	4.59	104	5.25	73	4.86	101	4.98	146	6.04
Multiple	20	6.40	<5	<20.05	<5	<18.50	<5	<18.44	<5	<10.81	<5	<12.25	5	8.05	6	7.14
Unknown	–	–	–	–	–	–	–	–	–	–	–	–	–	–	–	–

TABLE 29B

CLEFT PALATE ALONE: PERCENTAGE OF CASES BY DESCRIPTIVE CHARACTERISTICS, MACDP, 1968–2003*

Characteristic	Total		1968–1972		1973–1978		1979–1983		1984–1989		1990–1993		1994–1998		1999–2003	
	Cases	Percent	Cases	Percent	Cases	Percent	Cases	Percent	Cases	Percent	Cases	Percent	Cases	Percent	Cases	Percent
Birth outcome																
Live birth	650	96.7	69	95.8	96	97.0	58	93.5	102	96.2	74	98.7	101	95.3	150	98.7
Stillbirth	17	2.5	<5	–	<5	–	<5	–	<5	–	<5	–	<5	–	5	3.3
Elective termination	5	0.7	–	–	–	–	–	–	<5	–	–	–	<5	–	<5	–
Unknown	–	–	–	–	–	–	–	–	–	–	–	–	–	–	–	–
Age at diagnosis																
Prenatally or <7 days	613	91.2	71	98.6	97	98.0	59	95.2	101	95.3	70	93.3	91	85.8	124	81.6
8 days–6 months	19	2.8	<5	–	<5	–	<5	–	<5	–	<5	–	<5	–	5	3.3
6 months–1 year	8	1.2	–	–	<5	–	<5	–	<5	–	–	–	<5	–	<5	–
1–5 years	10	1.5	–	–	–	–	–	–	–	–	<5	–	<5	–	6	3.9
>5 years	<5	–	–	–	–	–	–	–	–	–	–	–	<5	–	–	–
Unknown	20	3.0	–	–	–	–	–	–	–	–	–	–	6	5.7	14	9.2
Socioeconomic status§																
Upper	143	21.3	–	–	–	–	19	30.6	28	26.4	34	45.3	27	25.5	35	23.0
Middle	148	22.0	–	–	–	–	19	30.6	31	29.2	22	29.3	39	36.8	37	24.3
Lower	140	20.8	–	–	–	–	22	35.5	44	41.5	18	24.0	35	33.0	21	13.8
Unknown	241	35.9	72	100.0	99	100.0	<5	–	<5	–	<5	–	5	4.7	59	38.8

* Cells containing fewer than 5 cases are indicated as "<5". Prevalence estimates based on these cells are indicated as less than the prevalence based on 5 cases in Table A. Percentages based on these cells are not provided in Table B. Cells containing zero cases are indicated as "–". Counts are provided, but prevalences are not estimated, for strata with unknown values in Table A. Counts and percentages are provided for strata with unknown values in Table B.

** Prev = Prevalence.

† Data on Hispanic or Latino ethnicity were available beginning in 1990.

‡ The category of All Other Races includes 15 cases of Black or African American race.

§ Information about socioeconomic status was available only for 1979–2001.

TABLE 30A

PYLORIC STENOSIS: PREVALENCE (PER 10,000 LIVE BIRTHS) STRATIFIED BY DESCRIPTIVE CHARACTERISTICS, MACDP, 1968–2003*

Characteristic	Total Cases	Total Prev**	1968–1972 Cases	1968–1972 Prev	1973–1978 Cases	1973–1978 Prev	1979–1983 Cases	1979–1983 Prev	1984–1989 Cases	1984–1989 Prev	1990–1993 Cases	1990–1993 Prev	1994–1998 Cases	1994–1998 Prev	1999–2003 Cases	1999–2003 Prev
Total	1,656	13.44	155	11.30	221	15.40	160	11.80	321	15.83	224	14.51	281	13.46	294	11.76
Maternal age (years)																
<25	629	12.80	78	9.97	102	13.95	67	11.07	110	13.99	71	12.99	95	14.11	106	13.44
25–29	523	14.82	46	12.36	80	18.04	54	12.84	117	18.45	72	16.00	78	14.10	76	11.60
≥30	487	12.59	17	7.82	38	14.97	39	11.86	92	15.18	81	14.83	108	12.54	112	10.61
Unknown	17	–	14	–	<5	–	–	–	<5	–	–	–	–	–	–	–
Maternal race/ethnicity†																
White	1,279	19.09	149	15.13	202	21.73	128	15.42	273	22.27	174	21.91	191	19.48	162	16.95
Black or African American	252	6.00	–	–	18	3.67	32	6.33	43	5.68	41	6.38	58	6.88	60	6.23
Hispanic or Latino	95	14.62	–	–	–	–	–	–	–	–	6	10.16	27	16.28	62	14.59
All Other Races	27	3.55	6‡	1.55	<5	<33.81	–	–	5	11.48	<5	<10.58	<5	<5.21	8	5.24
Unknown	<5	–	–	–	–	–	–	–	–	–	–	–	<5	–	<5	–
Birth weight (grams)																
<2500	111	10.52	9	7.46	8	6.48	12	10.24	16	9.84	17	12.71	18	10.07	31	14.19
≥2500	1,531	13.62	137	11.01	211	16.29	148	11.96	304	16.31	207	14.69	261	13.67	263	11.53
Unknown	14	–	9	–	<5	–	–	–	<5	–	–	–	<5	–	–	–
Gestational age (weeks)																
20–36	151	13.20	11	10.40	12	9.93	16	12.98	15	7.60	24	15.09	19	9.76	54	22.23
≥37	1,492	14.15	144	12.41	208	17.27	144	12.74	303	18.10	199	15.29	259	13.98	235	10.58
Unknown	13	–	–	–	<5	–	–	–	<5	–	<5	–	<5	–	5	–
Sex																
Male	1,377	21.86	128	18.24	183	24.79	132	19.01	263	25.31	184	23.35	238	22.34	249	19.58
Female	279	4.63	27	4.03	38	5.45	28	4.24	58	5.87	40	5.30	43	4.20	45	3.66
Ambiguous/Unknown	–	–	–	–	–	–	–	–	–	–	–	–	–	–	–	–
Parity																
1 Live birth	781	14.42	66	12.66	102	14.12	71	11.19	152	16.97	104	15.56	157	17.09	129	12.23
2 or more live births	825	12.29	66	9.17	118	16.55	86	11.93	153	13.97	119	13.67	121	10.41	162	11.31
Unknown	50	–	23	–	<5	–	<5	–	16	–	<5	–	<5	–	<5	–
Gravidity																
1 Pregnancy	593	12.79	60	12.34	87	12.98	56	8.55	115	16.30	71	13.64	114	15.63	90	10.34
2 or more pregnancies	1,049	14.05	91	12.05	132	17.25	104	14.85	204	15.90	153	15.04	164	12.18	201	12.56
Unknown	14	–	<5	–	<5	–	–	–	<5	–	–	–	<5	–	<5	–
Plurality																
Singleton	1,616	13.46	155	11.51	219	15.58	157	11.82	312	15.75	219	14.58	273	13.47	281	11.63
Multiple	38	12.17	–	–	<5	<18.50	<5	<18.44	7	15.14	5	12.25	8	12.87	13	15.47
Unknown	<5	–	–	–	–	–	–	–	<5	–	–	–	–	–	–	–

TABLE 30B

PYLORIC STENOSIS: PERCENTAGE OF CASES BY DESCRIPTIVE CHARACTERISTICS, MACDP, 1968–2003*

	Total		1968–1972		1973–1978		Period 1979–1983		1984–1989		1990–1993		1994–1998		1999–2003	
Characteristic	Cases	Percent	Cases	Percent	Cases	Percent	Cases	Percent	Cases	Percent	Cases	Percent	Cases	Percent	Cases	Percent
Birth outcome																
Live birth	1,656,	100.0	155	100.0	221	100.0	160	100.0	321	100.00	224	100.00	281	100.0	294	100.0
Stillbirth	–	–	–	–	–	–	–	–	–	–	–	–	–	–	–	–
Elective termination	–	–	–	–	–	–	–	–	–	–	–	–	–	–	–	–
Unknown	–	–	–	–	–	–	–	–	–	–	–	–	–	–	–	–
Age at diagnosis																
Prenatally or <7 days	118	7.1	15	9.7	27	12.2	15	9.4	17	5.3	16	7.1	11	3.9	17	5.8
8 days–6 months	1,525	92.1	140	90.3	194	87.8	142	88.8	301	93.8	208	92.9	269	95.7	271	92.2
6 months–1 year	<5	–	–	–	–	–	<5	–	–	–	–	–	–	–	–	–
1–5 years	<5	–	–	–	–	–	–	–	–	–	–	–	<5	–	–	–
>5 years	–	–	–	–	–	–	–	–	–	–	–	–	–	–	–	–
Unknown	10	0.6	–	–	–	–	<5	–	<5	–	–	–	–	–	6	2.0
Socioeconomic status§																
Upper	475	28.7	–	–	–	–	61	38.1	146	45.5	98	43.8	108	38.4	62	21.1
Middle	403	24.3	–	–	–	–	46	28.8	110	34.3	80	35.7	100	35.6	67	22.8
Lower	255	15.4	–	–	–	–	48	30.0	57	17.8	45	20.1	58	20.6	47	16.0
Unknown	523	31.6	155	100.00	221	100.0	5	3.1	8	2.5	<5	–	15	5.3	118	40.1

* Cells containing fewer than 5 cases are indicated as "<5". Prevalence estimates based on these cells are indicated as less than the prevalence based on 5 cases in Table A. Percentages based on these cells are not provided in Table B. Cells containing zero cases are indicated as "–". Counts are provided, but prevalences are not estimated, for strata with unknown values in Table A. Counts and percentages are provided for strata with unknown values in Table B.
** Prev = Prevalence.
† Data on Hispanic or Latino ethnicity were available beginning in 1990.
‡ The category of All Other Races includes 6 cases of Black or African American race.
§ Information about socioeconomic status was available only for 1979–2001.

TABLE 31A

ESOPHAGEAL ATRESIA OR STENOSIS: PREVALENCE (PER 10,000 LIVE BIRTHS) STRATIFIED BY DESCRIPTIVE CHARACTERISTICS, MACDP, 1968–2003*

	Total		1968–1972		1973–1978		1979–1983		1984–1989		1990–1993		1994–1998		1999–2003	
Characteristic	Cases	Prev**	Cases	Prev	Cases	Prev	Cases	Prev	Cases	Prev	Cases	Prev	Cases	Prev	Cases	Prev
Total	**266**	**2.16**	**27**	**1.97**	**33**	**2.30**	**33**	**2.43**	**49**	**2.42**	**33**	**2.14**	**43**	**2.06**	**48**	**1.92**
Maternal age (years)																
<25	99	2.01	22	2.81	14	1.91	16	2.64	21	2.67	7	1.28	10	1.49	9	1.14
25–29	72	2.04	<5	<1.34	14	3.16	11	2.61	12	1.89	9	2.00	10	1.81	12	1.83
≥30	95	2.46	<5	<2.30	5	1.97	6	1.83	16	2.64	17	3.11	23	2.67	27	2.56
Unknown	–	–	–		–		–		–		–		–		–	
Maternal race/ethnicity†																
White	180	2.69	23	2.34	28	3.01	27	3.25	33	2.69	20	2.52	22	2.24	27	2.82
Black or African American	66	1.57	–		5	1.02	6	1.19	14	1.85	9	1.40	20	2.37	12	1.25
Hispanic or Latino	10	1.54	–		–		–		–		<5	<8.47	<5	<3.01	8	1.88
All Other Races	10	1.31	<5‡	<1.29	–		–		<5	<11.48	<5	<10.58	–		<5	<3.27
Unknown	–		–		–		–		–		–		–		–	
Birth weight (grams)																
<2500	123	11.66	9	7.46	14	11.34	18	15.36	22	13.53	14	10.46	21	11.74	25	11.44
≥2500	142	1.26	18	1.45	19	1.47	15	1.21	26	1.40	19	1.35	22	1.15	23	1.01
Unknown	<5		–		–		–		<5		–		–		–	
Gestational age (weeks)																
20–36	92	8.04	5	4.73	7	5.79	9	7.30	18	9.12	12	7.55	19	9.76	22	9.06
≥37	170	1.61	22	1.90	26	2.16	24	2.12	28	1.67	20	1.54	24	1.30	26	1.17
Unknown	<5		–		–		–		<5		<5		–		–	
Sex																
Male	153	2.43	15	2.14	22	2.98	16	2.30	27	2.60	18	2.28	28	2.63	27	2.12
Female	112	1.86	12	1.79	11	1.58	17	2.57	21	2.12	15	1.99	15	1.47	21	1.71
Ambiguous/Unknown	<5		–		–		–		<5		–		–		–	
Parity																
1 Live birth	135	2.49	14	2.68	15	2.08	18	2.84	26	2.90	12	1.80	23	2.50	27	2.56
2 or more live births	127	1.89	12	1.67	18	2.53	15	2.08	21	1.92	21	2.41	19	1.64	21	1.47
Unknown	<5		<5		–		–		<5		<5		<5		–	
Gravidity																
1 Pregnancy	94	2.03	13	2.67	9	1.34	12	1.83	18	2.55	8	1.54	15	2.06	19	2.18
2 or more pregnancies	170	2.28	14	1.85	24	3.14	21	3.00	30	2.34	25	2.46	27	2.00	29	1.81
Unknown	<5		–		–		–		<5		–		<5		–	
Plurality																
Singleton	254	2.12	27	2.00	32	2.28	33	2.48	46	2.32	32	2.13	41	2.02	43	1.78
Multiple	12	3.84	–		<5	<18.50	–		<5	10.81	<5	12.25	<5	<8.05	5	5.95
Unknown	–		–		–		–		–		–		–		–	

TABLE 31B

ESOPHAGEAL ATRESIA OR STENOSIS: PERCENTAGE OF CASES BY DESCRIPTIVE CHARACTERISTICS, MACDP, 1968–2003*

| | Total | | Period | | | | | | | | | | | | | |
| | | | 1968–1972 | | 1973–1978 | | 1979–1983 | | 1984–1989 | | 1990–1993 | | 1994–1998 | | 1999–2003 | |
Characteristic	Cases	Percent	Cases	Percent	Cases	Percent	Cases	Percent	Cases	Percent	Cases	Percent	Cases	Percent	Cases	Percent
Birth outcome																
Live birth	257	96.6	26	96.3	33	100.0	31	93.9	46	93.9	31	93.9	42	97.7	48	100.0
Stillbirth	9	3.4	<5	–	–	–	<5	–	<5	–	<5	–	<5	–	<5	–
Elective termination	–	–	–	–	–	–	–	–	–	–	–	–	–	–	–	–
Unknown	–	–	–	–	–	–	–	–	–	–	–	–	–	–	–	–
Age at diagnosis																
Prenatally or <7 days	249	93.6	27	100.0	32	97.0	33	100.0	46	93.9	31	93.9	41	95.3	39	81.3
8 days–6 months	8	3.0	–	–	<5	–	–	–	<5	–	<5	–	<5	–	<5	–
6 months–1 year	<5	–	–	–	–	–	–	–	<5	–	–	–	–	–	–	–
1–5 years	–	–	–	–	–	–	–	–	–	–	–	–	–	–	–	–
>5 years	–	–	–	–	–	–	–	–	–	–	–	–	–	–	–	–
Unknown	6	2.3	–	–	–	–	–	–	–	–	–	–	<5	–	5	10.4
Socioeconomic status§																
Upper	74	27.8	–	–	–	–	18	54.5	15	30.6	18	54.5	13	30.2	10	20.8
Middle	55	20.7	–	–	–	–	8	24.2	13	26.5	6	18.2	12	27.9	16	33.3
Lower	57	21.4	–	–	–	–	7	21.2	20	40.8	9	27.3	17	39.5	<5	–
Unknown	80	30.1	27	100.0	33	100.0	–	–	<5	–	–	–	<5	–	18	37.5

* Cells containing fewer than 5 cases are indicated as "<5". Prevalence estimates based on these cells are indicated as less than the prevalence based on 5 cases in Table A. Percentages based on these cells are not provided in Table B. Cells containing zero cases are indicated as "—". Counts are provided, but prevalences are not estimated, for strata with unknown values in Table A. Counts and percentages are provided for strata with unknown values in Table B.
** Prev = Prevalence.
† Data on Hispanic or Latino ethnicity were available beginning in 1990.
‡ The category of All Other Races includes <5 cases of Black or African American race.
§ Information about socioeconomic status was available only for 1979–2001.

TABLE 32A

DUODENAL ATRESIA OR STENOSIS: PREVALENCE (PER 10,000 LIVE BIRTHS) STRATIFIED BY DESCRIPTIVE CHARACTERISTICS, MACDP, 1968–2003*

	Total		1968–1972		1973–1978		1979–1983		1984–1989		1990–1993		1994–1998		1999–2003	
Characteristic	Cases	Prev**	Cases	Prev	Cases	Prev	Cases	Prev	Cases	Prev	Cases	Prev	Cases	Prev	Cases	Prev
Total	**199**	**1.62**	**16**	**1.17**	**21**	**1.46**	**19**	**1.40**	**33**	**1.63**	**24**	**1.56**	**36**	**1.72**	**50**	**2.00**
Maternal age (years)																
<25	72	1.47	8	1.02	7	0.96	10	1.65	17	2.16	7	1.28	10	1.49	13	1.65
25–29	53	1.50	<5	<1.34	13	2.93	6	1.43	7	1.10	6	1.33	8	1.45	10	1.53
≥30	73	1.89	5	2.30	<5	<1.97	<5	<1.52	9	1.49	10	1.83	18	2.09	27	2.56
Unknown	<5	—	—	—	—	—	—	—	—	—	<5	—	—	—	—	—
Material race/ethnicity†																
White	114	1.70	12	1.22	11	1.18	11	1.32	25	2.04	12	1.51	17	1.73	26	2.72
Black or African American	69	1.64	—	—	10	2.04	8	1.58	8	1.06	10	1.56	16	1.90	17	1.77
Hispanic or Latino	10	1.54	—	—	—	—	—	—	—	—	<5	<8.47	<5	<3.01	7	1.65
All Other Races	6	0.79	<5‡	<1.29	—	—	—	—	—	—	—	<5	<10.58	<5	<5.21	—
Unknown	—	—	—	—	—	—	—	—	—	—	—	—	—	—	—	—
Birth weight (grams)																
<2500	98	9.29	10	8.29	9	7.29	10	8.53	17	10.45	7	5.23	21	11.74	24	10.98
≥2500	101	0.90	6	0.48	12	0.93	9	0.73	16	0.86	17	1.21	15	0.79	26	1.14
Unknown	—	—	—	—	—	—	—	—	—	—	—	—	—	—	—	—
Gestational age (weeks)																
20–36	87	7.61	7	6.62	7	5.79	7	5.86	15	7.60	10	6.29	18	9.25	23	9.47
≥37	110	1.04	9	0.78	14	1.16	12	1.06	17	1.02	13	1.00	18	0.97	27	1.22
Unknown	<5	—	—	—	—	—	—	—	<5	—	<5	—	—	—	—	—
Sex																
Male	89	1.41	7	1.00	10	1.35	8	1.15	10	0.96	7	0.89	20	1.88	27	2.12
Female	110	1.83	9	1.34	11	1.58	11	1.66	23	2.33	17	2.25	16	1.56	23	1.87
Ambiguous/Unknown	—	—	—	—	—	—	—	—	—	—	—	—	—	—	—	—
Parity																
1 Live birth	92	1.70	5	0.96	12	1.66	9	1.42	16	1.79	9	1.35	20	2.18	21	1.99
2 or more live births	102	1.52	10	1.39	9	1.26	10	1.39	13	1.19	15	1.72	16	1.38	29	2.02
Unknown	5	—	<5	—	—	—	—	—	<5	—	—	—	—	—	—	—
Gravidity																
1 Pregnancy	67	1.44	6	1.23	9	1.34	6	0.92	13	1.84	7	1.34	13	1.78	13	1.49
2 or more pregnancies	132	1.77	10	1.32	12	1.57	13	1.86	20	1.56	17	1.67	23	1.71	37	2.31
Unknown	—	—	—	—	—	—	—	—	—	—	—	—	—	—	—	—
Plurality																
Singleton	188	1.57	16	1.19	19	1.35	19	1.43	32	1.62	21	1.40	31	1.53	50	2.07
Multiple	11	3.52	—	—	<5	<18.50	—	—	<5	<10.81	<5	<12.25	5	8.05	—	—
Unknown	—	—	—	—	—	—	—	—	—	—	—	—	—	—	—	—

TABLE 32B

DUODENAL ATRESIA OR STENOSIS: PERCENTAGE OF CASES BY DESCRIPTIVE CHARACTERISTICS, MACDP, 1968–2003*

	Total		1968–1972		1973–1978		1979–1983		1984–1989		1990–1993		1994–1998		1999–2003	
Characteristic	Cases	Percent	Cases	Percent	Cases	Percent	Cases	Percent	Cases	Percent	Cases	Percent	Cases	Percent	Cases	Percent
Birth outcome																
Live birth	197	99.0	16	100.0	21	100.0	19	100.0	32	97.0	24	100.0	35	97.2	50	100.0
Stillbirth	<5	–	–	–	–	–	–	–	<5	–	–	–	<5	–	–	–
Elective termination	–	–	–	–	–	–	–	–	–	–	–	–	–	–	–	–
Unknown	–	–	–	–	–	–	–	–	–	–	–	–	–	–	–	–
Age at diagnosis																
Prenatally or <7 days	172	86.4	15	93.8	17	81.0	18	94.7	31	93.9	21	87.5	32	88.9	38	76.0
8 days–6 months	16	8.0	<5	–	<5	–	<5	–	<5	–	<5	–	<5	–	<5	–
6 months–1 year	<5	–	–	–	–	–	–	–	–	–	<5	–	–	–	<5	–
1–5 years	–	–	–	–	–	–	–	–	–	–	–	–	–	–	–	–
>5 years	–	–	–	–	–	–	–	–	–	–	–	–	–	–	–	–
Unknown	9	4.5	–	–	–	–	–	–	–	–	–	–	–	–	9	18.0
Socioeconomic status§																
Upper	40	20.1	–	–	–	–	5	26.3	8	24.2	6	25.0	10	27.8	11	22.0
Middle	57	28.6	–	–	–	–	9	47.4	10	30.3	11	45.8	11	30.6	16	32.0
Lower	43	21.6	–	–	–	–	5	26.3	14	42.4	6	25.0	14	38.9	<5	–
Unknown	59	29.6	16	100.0	21	100.0	–	–	<5	–	–	–	<5	–	19	38.0

* Cells containing fewer than 5 cases are indicated as "<5". Prevalence estimates based on these cells are indicated as less than the prevalence based on 5 cases in Table A. Percentages based on these cells are not provided in Table B. Cells containing zero cases are indicated as "–". Counts are provided, but prevalences are not estimated, for strata with unknown values in Table A. Counts and percentages are provided for strata with unknown values in Table B.
** Prev = Prevalence.
† Data on Hispanic or Latino ethnicity were available beginning in 1990.
‡ The category of All Other Races includes <5 cases of Black or African American race.
§ Information about socioeconomic status was available only for 1979–2001.

TABLE 33A

JEJUNAL AND/OR ILEAL ATRESIA OR STENOSIS: PREVALENCE (PER 10,000 LIVE BIRTHS) STRATIFIED BY DESCRIPTIVE CHARACTERISTICS, MACDP, 1968–2003*

								Period								
	Total		1968–1972		1973–1978		1979–1983		1984–1989		1990–1993		1994–1998		1999–2003	
Characteristic	Cases	Prev**	Cases	Prev	Cases	Prev	Cases	Prev	Cases	Prev	Cases	Prev	Cases	Prev	Cases	Prev
Total	201	1.63	23	1.68	22	1.53	21	1.55	30	1.48	24	1.56	33	1.58	48	1.92
Maternal age (years)																
<25	77	1.57	11	1.41	10	1.37	8	1.32	13	1.65	9	1.65	10	1.49	16	2.03
25–29	60	1.70	8	2.15	7	1.58	8	1.90	8	1.26	<5	<1.11	12	2.17	13	1.98
≥30	64	1.65	<5	<2.30	5	1.97	5	1.52	9	1.49	11	2.01	11	1.28	19	1.80
Unknown	—	—	—	—	—	—	—	—	—	—	—	—	—	—	—	—
Maternal race/ethnicity†																
White	85	1.27	15	1.52	10	1.08	10	1.20	9	0.73	8	1.01	15	1.53	18	1.88
Black or African American	85	2.02	—	—	12	2.44	9	1.78	21	2.77	13	2.02	11	1.30	19	1.97
Hispanic or Latino	19	2.92	—	—	—	—	—	—	—	—	<5	<8.47	6	3.62	10	2.35
All Other Races	12	1.58	8‡	2.07	—	—	<5	<26.07	—	—	—	—	<5	<5.21	<5	<3.27
Unknown	—	—	—	—	—	—	—	—	—	—	—	—	—	—	—	—
Birth weight (grams)																
<2500	94	8.91	15	12.44	12	9.72	10	8.53	15	9.22	7	5.23	12	6.71	23	10.53
≥2500	107	0.95	8	0.64	10	0.77	11	0.89	15	0.80	17	1.21	21	1.10	25	1.10
Unknown	—	—	—	—	—	—	—	—	—	—	—	—	—	—	—	—
Gestational age (weeks)																
20–36	106	9.27	13	12.29	11	9.10	11	8.92	20	10.13	8	5.03	17	8.73	26	10.71
≥37	94	0.89	10	0.86	11	0.91	10	0.88	10	0.60	15	1.15	16	0.86	22	0.99
Unknown	<5	—	—	—	—	—	—	—	—	—	<5	—	—	—	—	—
Sex																
Male	96	1.52	11	1.57	9	1.22	12	1.73	14	1.35	10	1.27	17	1.60	23	1.81
Female	105	1.74	12	1.79	13	1.87	9	1.36	16	1.62	14	1.85	16	1.56	25	2.04
Ambiguous/Unknown	—	—	—	—	—	—	—	—	—	—	—	—	—	—	—	—
Parity																
1 Live birth	90	1.66	15	2.88	11	1.52	11	1.73	14	1.56	13	1.95	12	1.31	14	1.33
2 or more live births	109	1.62	7	0.97	11	1.54	10	1.39	15	1.37	11	1.26	21	1.81	34	2.37
Unknown	<5	—	<5	—	—	—	—	—	<5	—	—	—	—	—	—	—
Gravidity																
1 Pregnancy	70	1.51	15	3.08	10	1.49	8	1.22	13	1.84	8	1.54	7	0.96	9	1.03
2 or more pregnancies	131	1.75	8	1.06	12	1.57	13	1.86	17	1.32	16	1.57	26	1.93	39	2.44
Unknown	—	—	—	—	—	—	—	—	—	—	—	—	—	—	—	—
Plurality																
Singleton	192	1.60	21	1.56	19	1.35	21	1.58	29	1.46	23	1.53	33	1.63	46	1.90
Multiple	9	2.88	<5	<20.05	<5	<18.50	—	—	<5	<10.81	<5	<12.25	—	—	<5	<5.95
Unknown	—	—	—	—	—	—	—	—	—	—	—	—	—	—	—	—

TABLE 33B

JEJUNAL AND/OR ILEAL ATRESIA OR STENOSIS: PERCENTAGE OF CASES BY DESCRIPTIVE CHARACTERISTICS, MACDP, 1968–2003*

| | \multicolumn{16}{c}{Period} | | | | | | | | | | | | | | | |
| Characteristic | Total | | 1968–1972 | | 1973–1978 | | 1979–1983 | | 1984–1989 | | 1990–1993 | | 1994–1998 | | 1999–2003 | |
	Cases	Percent	Cases	Percent	Cases	Percent	Cases	Percent	Cases	Percent	Cases	Percent	Cases	Percent	Cases	Percent
Birth outcome																
Live birth	201	100.0	23	100.0	22	100.0	21	100.0	30	100.0	24	100.0	33	100.0	48	100.0
Stillbirth	–	–	–	–	–	–	–	–	–	–	–	–	–	–	–	–
Elective termination	–	–	–	–	–	–	–	–	–	–	–	–	–	–	–	–
Unknown	–	–	–	–	–	–	–	–	–	–	–	–	–	–	–	–
Age at diagnosis																
Prenatally or <7 days	191	95.0	21	91.3	20	90.9	20	95.2	29	96.7	24	100.0	33	100.0	44	91.7
8 days–6 months	7	3.5	<5	–	<5	–	<5	–	–	–	–	–	<5	–	–	–
6 months–1 year	–	–	–	–	–	–	–	–	–	–	–	–	–	–	–	–
1–5 years	–	–	–	–	–	–	–	–	–	–	–	–	–	–	–	–
>5 years	–	–	–	–	–	–	–	–	–	–	–	–	–	–	–	–
Unknown	<5	–	–	–	–	–	–	–	–	–	–	–	–	–	<5	–
Socioeconomic status§																
Upper	38	18.9	–	–	–	–	8	38.1	<5	–	12	50.0	9	27.3	6	12.5
Middle	43	21.4	–	–	–	–	<5	–	10	33.3	9	37.5	12	36.4	8	16.7
Lower	52	25.9	–	–	–	–	9	42.9	17	56.7	<5	–	9	27.3	14	29.2
Unknown	68	33.8	23	100.0	22	100.0	–	–	–	–	–	–	<5	–	20	41.7

* Cells containing fewer than 5 cases are indicated as "<5". Prevalence estimates based on these cells are indicated as less than the prevalence based on 5 cases in Table A. Percentages based on these cells are not provided in Table B. Cells containing zero cases are indicated as "–". Counts are provided, but prevalences are not estimated, for strata with unknown values in Table A. Counts and percentages are provided for strata with unknown values in Table B.

** Prev = Prevalence.

† Data on Hispanic or Latino ethnicity were available beginning in 1990.

‡ The category of All Other Races includes 8 cases of Black or African American race.

§ Information about socioeconomic status was available only for 1979–2001.

TABLE 34A

ANAL OR RECTAL ATRESIA OR STENOSIS: PREVALENCE (PER 10,000 LIVE BIRTHS) STRATIFIED BY DESCRIPTIVE CHARACTERISTICS, MACDP, 1968–2003*

	Total		1968–1972		1973–1978		1979–1983		1984–1989		1990–1993		1994–1998		1999–2003	
Characteristic	Cases	Prev**	Cases	Prev	Cases	Prev	Cases	Prev	Cases	Prev	Cases	Prev	Cases	Prev	Cases	Prev
Total	457	3.71	58	4.23	61	4.25	49	3.62	82	4.04	54	3.50	76	3.64	77	3.08
Maternal age (years)																
<25	183	3.72	31	3.96	33	4.51	21	3.47	35	4.45	17	3.11	23	3.42	23	2.92
25–29	128	3.63	18	4.84	20	4.51	17	4.04	21	3.31	17	3.78	18	3.25	17	2.59
≥30	146	3.77	9	4.14	8	3.15	11	3.35	26	4.29	20	3.66	35	4.06	37	3.50
Unknown	–	–	–	–	–	–	–	–	–	–	–	–	–	–	–	–
Maternal race/ethnicity†																
White	261	3.89	43	4.37	48	5.16	31	3.73	55	4.49	27	3.40	34	3.47	23	2.41
Black or African American	142	3.38	–	–	13	2.65	17	3.36	23	3.04	25	3.89	34	4.03	30	3.12
Hispanic or Latino	20	3.08	–	–	–	–	–	–	–	–	<5	<8.47	<5	<3.01	15	3.53
All Other Races	31	4.08	15	3.88	–	–	<5	<26.07	<5	<11.48	–	–	5	5.21	6	3.93
Unknown	<5	–	–	–	–	–	–	–	–	–	–	–	–	–	<5	–
Birth weight (grams)																
<2500	173	16.40	20	16.59	20	16.21	26	22.18	30	18.45	20	14.95	34	19.01	23	10.53
≥2500	280	2.49	36	2.89	41	3.17	23	1.86	51	2.74	34	2.41	41	2.15	54	2.37
Unknown	<5	–	<5	–	–	–	–	–	<5	–	–	–	<5	–	–	–
Gestational age (weeks)																
20–36	149	13.03	13	12.29	17	14.07	17	13.39	25	12.66	22	13.84	36	18.49	19	7.82
≥37	299	2.84	45	3.88	44	3.65	31	2.74	54	3.23	31	2.38	38	2.05	56	2.52
Unknown	9	–	–	–	–	–	<5	–	<5	–	<5	–	<5	–	<5	–
Sex																
Male	261	4.14	35	4.99	35	4.74	23	3.31	46	4.43	29	3.68	45	4.22	48	3.77
Female	178	2.96	23	3.43	19	2.73	23	3.48	35	3.54	23	3.05	28	2.74	27	2.20
Ambiguous/Unknown	18	–	–	–	7	–	<5	–	<5	–	<5	–	<5	–	<5	–
Parity																
1 Live birth	211	3.90	28	5.37	24	3.32	23	3.62	37	4.13	29	4.34	34	3.70	36	3.41
2 or more live births	236	3.52	23	3.20	37	5.19	26	3.61	43	3.93	25	2.87	41	3.53	41	2.86
Unknown	10	–	7	–	–	–	–	–	<5	–	–	–	<5	–	–	–
Gravidity																
1 Pregnancy	145	3.13	26	5.35	21	3.13	15	2.29	24	3.40	19	3.65	20	2.74	20	2.30
2 or more pregnancies	311	4.16	32	4.24	40	5.23	34	4.85	58	4.52	35	3.44	55	4.08	57	3.56
Unknown	<5	–	–	–	–	–	–	–	–	–	–	–	<5	–	–	–
Plurality																
Singleton	431	3.59	56	4.16	58	4.13	45	3.39	77	3.89	52	3.46	69	3.41	74	3.06
Multiple	26	8.32	<5	<20.05	<5	<18.50	<5	<18.44	5	10.81	<5	<12.25	7	11.26	<5	<5.95
Unknown	–	–	–	–	–	–	–	–	–	–	–	–	–	–	–	–

TABLE 34B

ANAL OR RECTAL ATRESIA OR STENOSIS: PERCENTAGE OF CASES BY DESCRIPTIVE CHARACTERISTICS, MACDP, 1968–2003*

	Period															
	Total		1968–1972		1973–1978		1979–1983		1984–1989		1990–1993		1994–1998		1999–2003	
Characteristic	Cases	Percent	Cases	Percent	Cases	Percent	Cases	Percent	Cases	Percent	Cases	Percent	Cases	Percent	Cases	Percent
Birth outcome																
Live birth	429	93.9	55	94.8	57	93.4	48	98.0	77	93.9	49	90.7	70	92.1	73	94.8
Stillbirth	22	4.8	<5	–	<5	–	<5	–	5	6.1	<5	–	<5	–	<5	–
Elective termination	6	1.3	–	–	–	–	–	–	–	–	<5	–	<5	–	<5	–
Unknown	–	–	–	–	–	–	–	–	–	–	–	–	–	–	–	–
Age at diagnosis																
Prenatally or <7days	435	95.2	57	98.3	57	93.4	48	98.0	80	97.6	49	90.7	72	94.7	72	93.5
8 days–6 months	15	3.3	<5	–	<5	–	<5	–	<5	–	<5	–	<5	–	<5	–
6 month)–1 year	<5	–	–	–	–	–	–	–	<5	–	<5	–	<5	–	–	–
1–5 years	–	–	–	–	–	–	–	–	–	–	–	–	–	–	–	–
>5 years	–	–	–	–	–	–	–	–	–	–	–	–	–	–	–	–
Unknown	<5	–	–	–	–	–	–	–	<5	–	–	–	<5	–	<5	–
Socioeconomic status§																
Upper	102	22.3	–	–	–	–	17	34.7	26	31.7	20	37.0	24	31.6	15	19.5
Middle	102	22.3	–	–	–	–	14	28.6	30	36.6	14	25.9	25	32.9	19	24.7
Lower	95	20.8	–	–	–	–	17	34.7	25	30.5	20	37.0	23	30.3	10	13.0
Unknown	158	34.6	58	100.0	61	100.0	<5	–	<5	–	–	–	<5	–	33	42.9

* Cells containing fewer than 5 cases are indicated as "<5". Prevalence estimates based on these cells are indicated as less than the prevalence based on 5 cases in Table A. Percentages based on these cells are not provided in Table B. Cells containing zero cases are indicated as "—". Counts are provided, but prevalences are not estimated, for strata with unknown values in Table A. Counts and percentages are provided for strata with unknown values in Table B.

** Prev = Prevalence.

† Data on Hispanic or Latino ethnicity were available beginning in 1990.

‡ The category of All Other Races includes 14 cases of Black or African American race.

§ Information about socioeconomic status was available only for 1979–2001.

TABLE 35A

HIRSCHSPRUNG DISEASE: PREVALENCE (PER 10,000 LIVE BIRTHS) STRATIFIED BY DESCRIPTIVE CHARACTERISTICS, MACDP, 1968–2003*

	Total		1968–1972		1973–1978		1979–1983		1984–1989		1990–1993		1994–1998		1999–2003	
Characteristic	Cases	Prev**	Cases	Prev	Cases	Prev	Cases	Prev	Cases	Prev	Cases	Prev	Cases	Prev	Cases	Prev
Total	227	1.84	10	0.73	23	1.60	25	1.84	31	1.53	39	2.53	43	2.06	56	2.24
Maternal age (years)																
<25	72	1.47	<5	<0.64	12	1.64	8	1.32	8	1.02	13	2.38	10	1.49	18	2.28
25–29	69	1.96	<5	<1.34	9	2.03	9	2.14	10	1.58	14	3.11	15	2.71	8	1.27
≥30	83	2.15	<5	<2.30	<5	<1.97	8	2.43	13	2.15	12	2.20	17	1.97	29	2.75
Unknown	<5	–	<5	–	–	–	–	–	–	–	–	–	<5	–	<5	–
Maternal race/ethnicity†																
White	108	1.61	8	0.81	15	1.61	16	1.93	19	1.55	13	1.64	18	1.84	19	1.99
Black or African American	97	2.31	–	–	8	1.63	9	1.78	9	1.19	23	3.58	19	2.25	29	3.01
Hispanic or Latino	9	1.38	–	–	–	–	–	–	–	–	<5	<8.47	<5	<3.01	7	1.65
All Other Races	12	1.58	<5‡	<129	–	–	–	–	<5	<11.48	<5	<10.58	<5	<5.21	<5	<3.27
Unknown	<5	–	–	–	–	–	–	–	–	–	–	–	<5	–	–	–
Birth weight (grams)																
<2500	29	2.75	<5	<4.15	<5	<4.05	<5	<4.27	<5	<3.07	5	3.74	6	3.36	11	5.03
≥2500	194	1.73	6	0.48	22	1.70	23	1.86	29	1.56	34	2.41	36	1.89	44	1.93
Unknown	<5	–	<5	–	–	–	–	–	–	–	–	–	<5	–	<5	–
Gestational age (weeks)																
20–36	33	2.88	<5	<4.73	<5	<4.14	<5	<4.05	5	2.53	<5	<3.14	10	5.14	9	3.71
≥37	193	1.83	9	0.78	21	1.74	22	1.95	26	1.55	36	2.77	32	1.73	47	2.12
Unknown	<5	–	–	–	–	–	–	–	–	–	–	–	<5	–	–	–
Sex																
Male	172	2.73	7	1.00	19	2.57	18	2.59	22	2.12	28	3.55	36	3.38	42	3.30
Female	55	0.91	<5	<0.75	<5	<0.72	7	1.06	9	0.91	11	1.46	7	0.68	14	1.14
Ambiguous/Unknown	–	–	–	–	–	–	–	–	–	–	–	–	–	–	–	–
Parity																
1 Live birth	87	1.61	<5	<0.96	8	1.11	8	1.26	11	1.23	17	2.54	18	1.96	23	2.18
2 or more live births	133	1.98	<5	<0.69	15	2.10	16	2.22	20	1.83	22	2.53	24	2.07	32	2.23
Unknown	7	–	<5	–	–	–	<5	–	–	–	–	–	<5	–	<5	–
Gravidity																
1 Pregnancy	55	1.19	<5	<1.03	7	1.04	6	0.92	5	0.71	12	2.31	10	1.37	13	1.49
2 or more pregnancies	169	2.26	7	0.93	16	2.09	19	2.71	26	2.03	27	2.65	32	2.38	42	2.62
Unknown	<5	–	<5	–	–	–	–	–	–	–	–	–	<5	–	<5	–
Plurality																
Singleton	216	1.80	10	0.74	23	1.64	23	1.73	30	1.51	37	2.46	40	1.97	53	2.19
Multiple	11	3.52	–	–	–	–	<5	<18.44	<5	<10.81	<5	<12.25	<5	<8.05	<5	<5.95
Unknown	–	–	–	–	–	–	–	–	–	–	–	–	–	–	–	–

TABLE 35B

HIRSCHSPRUNG DISEASE: PERCENTAGE OF CASES BY DESCRIPTIVE CHARACTERISTICS, MACDP, 1968–2003*

Characteristic	Total		1968–1972		1973–1978		1979–1983		1984–1989		1990–1993		1994–1998		1999–2003	
	Cases	Percent	Cases	Percent	Cases	Percent	Cases	Percent	Cases	Percent	Cases	Percent	Cases	Percent	Cases	Percent
Birth outcome																
Live birth	227	100.0	10	100.0	23	100.0	25	100.0	31	100.0	39	100.0	43	100.0	56	100.0
Stillbirth	–	–	–	–	–	–	–	–	–	–	–	–	–	–	–	–
Elective termination	–	–	–	–	–	–	–	–	–	–	–	–	–	–	–	–
Unknown	–	–	–	–	–	–	–	–	–	–	–	–	–	–	–	–
Age at diagnosis																
Prenatally or <7 days	144	63.4	7	70.0	12	52.2	16	64.0	22	71.0	18	46.2	27	62.8	42	75.0
8 days–6 months	72	31.7	<5	–	11	47.8	7	28.0	7	22.6	19	48.7	11	25.6	14	25.0
6 months–1 year	9	4.0	–	–	–	–	<5	–	<5	–	<5	–	<5	–	–	–
1–5 years	<5	–	–	–	–	–	–	–	–	–	<5	–	<5	–	–	–
>5 years	–	–	–	–	–	–	–	–	–	–	–	–	–	–	–	–
Unknown	–	–	–	–	–	–	–	–	–	–	–	–	–	–	–	–
Socioeconomic status§																
Upper	49	21.6	–	–	–	–	5	20.0	10	32.3	11	28.2	14	32.6	9	16.1
Middle	63	27.8	–	–	–	–	8	32.0	13	41.9	11	28.2	18	41.9	13	23.2
Lower	53	23.3	–	–	–	–	11	44.0	7	22.6	16	41.0	11	25.6	8	14.3
Unknown	62	27.3	10	100.0	23	100.0	<5	–	<5	–	<5	–	–	–	26	46.4

* Cells containing fewer than 5 cases are indicated as "<5". Prevalence estimates based on these cells are indicated as less than the prevalence based on 5 cases in Table A. Percentages based on these cells are not provided in Table B. Cells containing zero cases are indicated as "–". Counts are provided, but prevalences are not estimated, for strata with unknown values in Table A. Counts and percentages are provided for strata with unknown values in Table B.

** Prev = Prevalence.

† Data on Hispanic or Latino ethnicity were available beginning in 1990.

‡ The category of All Other Races includes <5 cases of Black or African American race.

§ Information about socioeconomic status was available only for 1979–2001.

TABLE 36A

HYPOSPADIAS: PREVALENCE (PER 10,000 LIVE BIRTHS) STRATIFIED BY DESCRIPTIVE CHARACTERISTICS, MACDP, 1968–2003*

Characteristic	Total		1968–1972		1973–1978		1979–1983		1984–1989		1990–1993		1994–1998		1999–2003	
	Cases	Prev**	Cases	Prev	Cases	Prev	Cases	Prev	Cases	Prev	Cases	Prev	Cases	Prev	Cases	Prev
Total	3,730	30.27	271	19.75	429	29.89	367	27.08	682	33.64	483	31.30	705	33.76	793	31.72
Maternal age (years)																
<25	1,313	26.72	152	19.43	219	29.94	165	27.36	240	30.53	163	29.82	197	29.26	177	22.45
25–29	1,048	29.70	78	20.96	133	29.99	106	25.20	233	36.74	128	28.45	177	32.01	193	29.45
≥30	1,359	35.12	38	17.48	76	29.94	96	29.21	209	34.49	191	34.97	328	38.09	421	39.88
Unknown	10	–	<5	–	<5	–	–	–	–	–	<5	–	<5	–	<5	–
Maternal race/ethnicity†																
White	2,332	34.80	229	23.25	329	35.39	243	29.27	459	37.44	284	35.76	391	39.87	397	41.53
Black or African American	1,195	28.44	–	–	98	19.96	122	24.13	213	28.11	182	28.34	273	32.39	307	31.90
Hispanic or Latino	85	13.08	–	–	<5	–	–	–	–	–	11	18.63	16	9.65	58	13.65
All Other Races	103	13.54	42‡	10.85	<5	<33.81	–	–	10	22.96	6	12.69	20	20.84	23	15.06
Unknown	15	–	–	–	<5	–	<5	–	–	.	–	–	5	–	8	–
Birth weight (grams)																
<2500	809	76.68	52	43.12	61	49.43	83	70.81	115	70.71	101	75.49	189	105.69	208	95.19
≥2500	2,914	25.93	217	17.44	367	28.34	284	22.96	567	30.42	382	27.12	514	26.92	583	25.56
Unknown	7	–	<5	–	<5	–	–	–	–	–	–	–	<5	–	<5	–
Gestational age (weeks)																
20–36	725	63.38	42	39.71	45	37.24	66	53.52	101	51.15	84	52.83	179	91.96	208	85.64
≥37	2,973	28.20	229	19.74	383	31.79	301	26.62	571	34.12	396	30.44	521	28.13	572	25.75
Unknown	32	–	–	–	<5	–	–	–	10	–	<5	–	5	–	13	–
Sex																
Male	3,725	59.14	271	38.61	429	58.11	365	52.36	682	65.64	482	61.17	704	66.09	792	62.28
Female	–	–	–	–	–	–	–	–	–	–	–	–	–	–	–	–
Ambiguous/Unknown	5	–	–	–	–	–	<5	–	–	–	<5	–	<5	–	<5	–
Parity																
1 Live birth	1,830	33.97	112	21.48	207	28.65	194	30.56	336	37.51	244	36.51	356	38.76	391	37.08
2 or more live births	1,803	26.86	112	15.56	221	31.01	169	23.45	319	29.14	238	27.34	344	29.61	400	27.93
Unknown	87	–	47	–	<5	–	<5	–	27	–	<5	–	5	–	<5	–
Gravidity																
1 Pregnancy	1,333	28.75	99	20.36	179	26.71	153	23.36	242	34.29	159	30.54	224	30.71	277	31.83
2 or more pregnancies	2,382	31.90	170	22.52	249	32.55	211	30.12	438	34.13	323	31.76	477	35.42	514	32.11
Unknown	15	–	<5	–	<5	–	<5	–	<5	–	<5	–	<5	–	<5	–
Plurality																
Singleton	3,549	29.56	261	19.38	410	29.16	354	26.65	655	33.06	465	30.95	668	32.97	736	30.46
Multiple	178	56.99	10	40.10	19	70.32	12	44.25	25	54.05	18	44.10	37	59.54	57	67.83
Unknown	<5	–	–	–	–	–	<5	–	<5	–	–	–	–	–	–	–

TABLE 36B

HYPOSPADIAS: PERCENTAGE OF CASES BY DESCRIPTIVE CHARACTERISTICS, MACDP, 1968–2003*

Characteristic	Total		1968–1972		1973–1978		1979–1983		1984–1989		1990–1993		1994–1998		1999–2003	
	Cases	Percent	Cases	Percent	Cases	Percent	Cases	Percent	Cases	Percent	Cases	Percent	Cases	Percent	Cases	Percent
Birth outcome																
Live birth	3,715	99.6	268	98.9	426	99.3	363	98.9	681	99.9	482	99.8	704	99.9	791	99.7
Stillbirth	11	0.3	<5	–	<5	–	<5	–	<5	–	–	–	<5	–	–	–
Elective termination	<5	–	–	–	–	–	–	–	–	–	<5	–	–	–	<5	–
Unknown	<5	–	–	0.2	–	–	<5	–	–	–	–	–	–	–	–	–
Age at diagnosis																
Prenatally or <7 days	3,522	94.4	269	99.3	423	98.6	348	94.8	655	96.0	466	96.5	652	92.5	709	89.4
8 days–6 months	63	1.7	<5	–	5	1.2	6	1.6	17	2.5	7	1.4	11	1.6	16	2.0
6 months–1 year	73	2.0	<5	–	<5	–	13	3.5	10	1.5	6	1.2	23	3.3	19	2.4
1–5 years	26	0.7	–	–	–	–	–	–	–	–	–	–	10	1.4	16	2.0
>5 years	<5	–	–	–	–	–	–	–	–	–	<5	–	–	–	–	–
Unknown	45	1.2	–	–	–	–	–	–	–	–	<5	–	9	1.3	33	4.2
Socioeconomic status§																
Upper	992	26.6	–	–	–	–	133	36.2	254	37.2	189	39.1	255	36.2	161	20.3
Middle	901	24.2	–	–	–	–	107	29.2	229	33.6	161	33.3	255	36.2	149	18.8
Lower	706	18.9	–	–	–	–	120	32.7	192	28.2	122	25.3	170	24.1	102	12.9
Unknown	1,131	30.3	271	100.0	429	100.0	7	1.9	7	1.0	11	2.3	25	3.5	381	48.0

* Cells containing fewer than 5 cases are indicated as "<5." Prevalence estimates based on these cells are indicated as less than the prevalence based on 5 cases in Table A. Percentages based on these cells are not provided in Table B. Cells containing zero cases are indicated as "–". Counts are provided, but prevalences are not estimated, for strata with unknown values in Table A. Counts and percentages are provided for strata with unknown values in Table B.
** Prev = Prevalence.
† Data on Hispanic or Latino ethnicity were available beginning in 1990.
‡ The category of All Other Races includes 42 cases of Black or African American race.
§ Information about socioeconomic status was available only for 1979–2001.

TABLE 37A

BILATERAL RENAL AGENESIS OR DYSGENESIS: PREVALENCE (PER 10,000 LIVE BIRTHS) STRATIFIED BY DESCRIPTIVE CHARACTERISTICS, MACDP, 1968–2003*

	Total		1968–1972		1973–1978		1979–1983		1984–1989		1990–1993		1994–1998		1999–2003	
Characteristic	Cases	Prev**	Cases	Prev	Cases	Prev	Cases	Prev	Cases	Prev	Cases	Prev	Cases	Prev	Cases	Prev
Total	**169**	**1.37**	**12**	**0.87**	**26**	**1.81**	**26**	**1.92**	**26**	**1.28**	**23**	**1.49**	**31**	**1.48**	**25**	**1.00**
Maternal age (years)																
<25	73	1.49	5	0.64	14	1.91	16	2.64	13	1.65	6	1.10	11	1.63	8	1.01
25–29	44	1.25	<5	<1.34	5	1.13	<5	<1.19	7	1.10	8	1.78	10	1.81	6	0.92
≥30	51	1.32	<5	<2.30	7	2.76	6	1.83	6	0.99	9	1.65	10	1.16	11	1.04
Unknown	<5	–	<5	–	–	–	–	–	–	–	–	–	–	–	–	–
Maternal race/ethnicity†																
White	97	1.45	10	1.02	18	1.94	18	2.17	18	1.47	10	1.26	12	1.22	11	1.15
Black or African American	62	1.48	–	–	8	1.63	8	1.58	8	1.06	12	1.87	17	2.02	9	0.94
Hispanic or Latino	<5	<0.77	–	–	–	–	–	–	–	–	–	–	–	–	<5	<1.18
All Other Races	6	0.79	<5‡	<1.29	–	–	–	–	–	–	<5	<10.58	<5	<5.21	<5	<3.27
Unknown	<5	–	–	–	–	–	–	–	–	–	–	–	<5	–	–	–
Birth weight (grams)																
<2500	132	12.51	10	8.29	21	17.02	20	17.06	20	12.30	19	14.20	22	12.30	20	9.15
≥2500	36	0.32	<5	<0.40	5	0.39	6	0.49	5	0.27	<5	<0.35	9	0.47	5	0.22
Unknown	<5	–	–	–	–	–	–	–	<5	–	–	–	–	–	–	–
Gestational age (weeks)																
20–36	104	9.09	<5	<4.73	8	6.62	15	12.16	14	7.09	19	11.95	24	12.33	20	8.23
≥37	64	0.61	8	0.69	18	1.49	11	0.97	12	0.72	<5	<0.38	7	0.38	<5	<0.23
Unknown	<5	–	–	–	–	–	<5	–	–	–	–	–	–	–	<5	–
Sex																
Male	104	1.65	10	1.42	20	2.71	12	1.73	15	1.44	16	2.03	15	1.41	16	1.26
Female	61	1.01	<5	<0.75	6	0.86	13	1.97	11	1.11	6	0.79	15	1.47	8	0.65
Ambiguous/Unknown	<5	–	–	–	–	–	<5	–	–	–	<5	–	<5	–	<5	–
Parity																
1 Live birth	72	1.33	6	1.15	15	2.08	12	1.89	10	1.12	10	1.50	10	1.09	9	0.85
2 or more live births	95	1.42	6	0.83	11	1.54	14	1.94	14	1.28	13	1.49	21	1.81	16	1.12
Unknown	<5	–	–	–	–	–	<5	–	<5	–	–	–	<5	–	–	–
Gravidity																
1 Pregnancy	54	1.16	5	1.03	12	1.79	9	1.37	8	1.13	5	0.96	6	0.82	9	1.03
2 or more pregnancies	115	1.54	7	0.93	14	1.83	17	2.43	18	1.40	18	1.77	25	1.86	16	1.00
Unknown	–	–	–	–	–	–	–	–	–	–	–	–	–	–	–	–
Plurality																
Singleton	163	1.36	12	0.89	25	1.78	24	1.81	26	1.31	23	1.53	30	1.48	23	0.95
Multiple	6	1.92	–	–	<5	<18.50	<5	<18.44	–	–	–	–	<5	<8.05	<5	<5.95
Unknown	–	–	–	–	–	–	–	–	–	–	–	–	–	–	–	–

TABLE 37B

BILATERAL RENAL AGENESIS OR DYSGENESIS: PERCENTAGE OF CASES BY DESCRIPTIVE CHARACTERISTICS, MACDP, 1968–2003*

	Total		1968–1972		1973–1978		1979–1983		1984–1989		1990–1993		1994–1998		1999–2003	
Characteristic	Cases	Percent	Cases	Percent	Cases	Percent	Cases	Percent	Cases	Percent	Cases	Percent	Cases	Percent	Cases	Percent
Birth outcome																
Live birth	132	78.1	10	83.3	23	88.5	24	92.3	21	80.8	17	73.9	23	74.2	14	56.0
Stillbirth	22	13.0	<5	–	<5	–	<5	–	5	19.2	<5	–	<5	–	5	20.0
Elective termination	15	8.9	–	–	–	–	–	–	–	–	<5	–	6	19.4	6	24.0
Unknown	–	–	–	–	–	–	–	–	–	–	–	–	–	–	–	–
Age at diagnosis																
Prenatally or <7 days	159	94.1	12	100.0	25	96.2	25	96.2	24	92.3	23	100.0	29	93.5	21	84.0
8 days–6 months	7	4.1	–	–	<5	–	<5	–	<5	–	–	–	<5	–	<5	–
6 months–1 year	<5	–	–	–	–	–	–	–	–	–	–	–	–	–	–	–
1–5 years	–	–	–	–	–	–	–	–	–	–	–	–	–	–	<5	–
>5 years	–	–	–	–	–	–	–	–	–	–	–	–	–	–	–	–
Unknown	<5	–	–	–	–	–	–	–	–	–	–	–	<5	–	<5	–
Socioeconomic status§																
Upper	48	28.4	–	–	–	–	11	42.3	13	50.0	5	21.7	12	38.7	7	28.0
Middle	34	20.1	–	–	–	–	6	23.1	5	19.2	14	60.9	7	22.6	<5	–
Lower	36	21.3	–	–	–	–	9	34.6	8	30.8	<5	–	12	38.7	<5	–
Unknown	51	30.2	12	100.0	26	100.0	–	–	–	–	–	–	<5	–	13	52.0

* Cells containing fewer than 5 cases are indicated as "<5". Prevalence estimates based on these cells are indicated as less than the prevalence based on 5 cases in Table A. Percentages based on these cells are not provided in Table B. Cells containing zero cases are indicated as "–". Counts are provided, but prevalences are not estimated, for strata with unknown values in Table A. Counts and percentages are provided for strata with unknown values in Table B.

** Prev = Prevalence.

† Data on Hispanic or Latino ethnicity were available beginning in 1990.

‡ The category of All Other Races includes <5 cases of Black or African American race.

§ Information about socioeconomic status was available only for 1979–2001.

TABLE 38A

ANY CYSTIC KIDNEY DISEASE: PREVALENCE (PER 10,000 LIVE BIRTHS) STRATIFIED BY DESCRIPTIVE CHARACTERISTICS, MACDP, 1968–2003*

	Total		1968–1972		1973–1978		1979–1983		1984–1989		1990–1993		1994–1998		1999–2003	
Characteristic	Cases	Prev**	Cases	Prev	Cases	Prev	Cases	Prev	Cases	Prev	Cases	Prev	Cases	Prev	Cases	Prev
Total	**507**	**4.11**	**32**	**2.33**	**32**	**2.23**	**37**	**2.73**	**86**	**4.24**	**75**	**4.86**	**107**	**5.12**	**138**	**5.52**
Maternal age (years)																
<25	205	4.17	16	2.05	16	2.19	20	3.30	44	5.60	24	4.39	40	5.94	45	5.71
25–29	140	3.97	9	2.42	11	2.48	12	2.85	26	4.10	18	4.00	27	4.88	37	5.65
≥30	162	4.19	7	3.22	5	1.97	5	1.52	16	2.64	33	6.04	40	4.64	56	5.30
Unknown	–	–	–	–	–	–	–	–	–	–	–	–	–	–	–	–
Maternal race/ethnicity†																
White	225	3.36	23	2.34	19	2.04	24	2.89	45	3.67	34	4.28	38	3.88	42	4.39
Black or African American	228	5.43	–	–	13	2.65	13	2.57	39	5.15	38	5.92	56	6.64	69	7.17
Hispanic or Latino	29	4.46	–	–	–	–	–	–	–	–	<5	<8.47	8	4.82	19	4.47
All Other Races	24	3.16	9‡	2.33	–	–	–	–	<5	<11.48	<5	<10.58	5	5.21	7	4.58
Unknown	<5	–	–	–	–	–	–	–	–	–	–	–	–	–	<5	–
Birth weight (grams)																
<2500	194	18.39	18	14.93	15	12.15	18	15.36	35	21.52	34	25.41	37	20.69	37	16.93
≥2500	308	2.74	13	1.04	17	1.31	19	1.54	50	2.68	39	2.77	70	3.67	100	4.38
Unknown	5	–	<5	–	–	–	–	–	<5	–	<5	–	–	–	<5	–
Gestational age (weeks)																
20–36	214	18.71	18	17.02	17	14.07	18	14.60	35	17.72	38	23.90	41	21.06	47	19.35
≥37	286	2.71	14	1.21	15	1.25	18	1.59	49	2.93	35	2.69	66	3.56	89	4.01
Unknown	7	–	–	–	<5	–	<5	–	<5	–	<5	–	–	–	<5	–
Sex																
Male	292	4.64	22	3.13	23	3.12	18	2.59	49	4.72	40	5.08	64	6.01	76	5.98
Female	207	3.44	9	1.34	8	1.15	19	2.87	35	3.54	35	4.63	41	4.01	60	4.88
Ambiguous/Unknown	8	–	<5	–	<5	–	–	–	<5	–	–	–	<5	–	<5	–
Parity																
1 Live birth	211	3.90	8	1.53	14	1.94	19	2.99	33	3.68	33	4.94	46	5.01	58	5.50
2 or more live births	285	4.25	19	2.64	18	2.53	18	2.50	49	4.48	42	4.82	59	5.08	80	5.59
Unknown	11	–	5	–	–	–	<5	–	<5	–	<5	–	<5	–	–	–
Gravidity																
1 Pregnancy	143	3.08	6	1.23	13	1.94	12	1.83	19	2.69	22	4.23	26	3.57	45	5.17
2 or more pregnancies	362	4.85	26	3.44	19	2.48	25	3.57	67	5.22	53	5.21	79	5.87	93	5.81
Unknown	<5	–	–	–	–	–	–	–	–	–	–	–	<5	–	–	–
Plurality																
Singleton	492	4.10	32	2.38	31	2.20	37	2.79	85	4.29	74	4.93	102	5.03	131	5.42
Multiple	14	4.48	–	–	<5	<18.50	–	–	–	–	<5	<12.25	5	8.05	7	8.33
Unknown	<5	–	–	–	–	–	–	–	<5	–	–	–	–	–	–	–

TABLE 38B

ANY CYSTIC KIDNEY DISEASE: PERCENTAGE OF CASES BY DESCRIPTIVE CHARACTERISTICS, MACDP, 1968–2003*

| | Total | | 1968–1972 | | 1973–1978 | | 1979–1983 | | 1984–1989 | | 1990–1993 | | 1994–1998 | | 1999–2003 | |
| | | | | | | | | Period | | | | | | | | |
Characteristic	Cases	Percent	Cases	Percent	Cases	Percent	Cases	Percent	Cases	Percent	Cases	Percent	Cases	Percent	Cases	Percent
Birth outcome																
Live birth	467	92.1	28	87.5	30	93.8	36	97.3	81	94.2	63	84.0	99	92.5	130	94.2
Stillbirth	20	3.9	<5	–	<5	–	<5	–	<5	–	5	6.7	<5	–	<5	–
Elective termination	20	3.9	–	–	–	–	–	–	<5	–	7	9.3	7	6.5	5	3.6
Unknown	–	–	–	–	–	–	–	–	–	–	–	–	–	–	–	–
Age at diagnosis																
Prenatally or <7 days	444	87.6	31	96.9	31	96.9	29	78.4	83	96.5	74	98.7	91	85.0	105	76.1
8 days–6 months	22	4.3	<5	–	<5	–	8	21.6	<5	–	<5	–	7	6.5	<5	–
6 months–1 year	<5	–	–	–	–	–	–	–	–	–	–	–	<5	–	–	–
1–5 years	<5	–	–	–	–	–	–	–	–	–	–	–	–	–	<5	–
>5 years																
Unknown	37	7.3	–	–	–	–	–	–	–	–	–	–	6	5.6	31	22.5
Socioeconomic status§																
Upper	109	21.5	–	–	–	–	8	21.6	24	27.9	25	33.3	31	29.0	21	15.2
Middle	130	25.6	–	–	–	–	10	27.0	26	30.2	28	37.3	37	34.6	29	21.0
Lower	144	28.4	–	–	–	–	19	51.4	35	40.7	22	29.3	39	36.4	29	21.0
Unknown	124	24.5	32	100.0	32	100.0	–	–	<5	–	–	–	–	–	59	42.8

* Cells containing fewer than 5 cases are indicated as "<5". Prevalence estimates based on these cells are indicated as less than the prevalence based on 5 cases in Table A. Percentages based on these cells are not provided in Table B. Cells containing zero cases are indicated as "—". Counts are provided, but prevalences are not estimated, for strata with unknown values in Table A. Counts and percentages are provided for strata with unknown values in Table B.

** Prev = Prevalence.

† Data on Hispanic or Latino ethnicity were available beginning in 1990.

‡ The category of All Other Races includes 9 cases of Black or African American race.

§ Information about socioeconomic status was available only for 1979–2001.

TABLE 39A

CONGENITAL DISLOCATION OR DYSPLASIA OF THE HIP: PREVALENCE (PER 10,000 LIVE BIRTHS) STRATIFIED BY DESCRIPTIVE CHARACTERISTICS, MACDP, 1968–2003*

Characteristic	Total Cases	Total Prev**	1968–1972 Cases	Prev	1973–1978 Cases	Prev	1979–1983 Cases	Prev	1984–1989 Cases	Prev	1990–1993 Cases	Prev	1994–1998 Cases	Prev	1999–2003 Cases	Prev
Total	**959**	**7.78**	**97**	**7.97**	**154**	**10.73**	**98**	**7.23**	**163**	**8.04**	**161**	**10.43**	**140**	**6.70**	**146**	**5.84**
Maternal age (years)																
<25	340	6.92	57	7.29	72	9.84	47	7.76	51	6.49	43	7.87	31	4.60	39	4.95
25–29	296	8.39	28	7.52	60	13.53	32	7.61	51	8.04	47	10.45	39	7.05	39	5.95
≥30	321	8.30	11	5.06	22	8.67	19	5.78	61	10.07	71	13.00	69	8.01	68	6.44
Unknown	<5	–	<5	–	–	–	–	–	–	–	–	–	<5	–	–	–
Maternal race/ethnicity†																
White	737	11.00	84	8.53	135	14.52	71	8.55	139	11.34	119	14.98	105	10.71	84	8.79
Black or African American	130	3.09	–	–	18	3.67	26	5.14	21	2.77	30	4.67	21	2.49	14	1.45
Hispanic or Latino	58	8.93	–	–	–	–	–	–	–	–	10	16.93	11	6.63	37	8.71
All Other Races	28	3.68	13‡	3.36	–	–	<5	<26.07	<5	<11.48	<5	<10.58	<5	<5.21	6	3.93
Unknown	6	–	–	–	<5	–	–	–	–	–	–	–	–	–	5	–
Birth weight (grams)																
<2500	118	11.19	15	12.44	19	15.40	20	17.06	18	11.07	15	11.21	17	9.51	14	6.41
≥2500	839	7.46	80	6.43	135	10.43	78	6.31	145	7.78	146	10.36	123	6.44	132	5.79
Unknown	<5	–	<5	–	–	–	–	–	–	–	–	–	–	–	–	–
Gestational age (weeks)																
20–36	111	9.70	11	10.40	13	10.76	11	8.92	16	8.10	19	11.95	17	8.75	24	9.88
≥37	839	7.96	86	7.41	141	11.70	87	7.69	146	8.72	140	10.76	119	6.42	120	5.40
Unknown	9	–	–	–	–	–	–	–	<5	–	<5	–	<5	–	<5	–
Sex																
Male	243	3.86	32	4.56	40	5.42	26	3.74	38	3.66	31	3.93	37	3.47	39	3.07
Female	714	11.85	64	9.55	113	16.22	72	10.89	125	12.65	130	17.21	103	10.07	107	8.71
Ambiguous/Unknown	<5	–	<5	–	<5	–	–	–	–	–	–	–	–	–	–	–
Parity																
1 Live birth	567	10.47	55	10.55	87	12.04	57	8.98	92	10.27	107	16.01	79	8.60	90	8.53
2 or more live births	365	5.44	25	3.47	66	9.26	40	5.55	64	5.85	54	6.20	60	5.16	56	3.91
Unknown	27	–	17	–	<5	–	<5	–	7	–	–	–	<5	–	–	–
Gravidity																
1 Pregnancy	426	9.19	53	10.90	68	10.15	48	7.33	61	8.64	76	14.60	60	8.23	60	6.89
2 or more pregnancies	529	7.08	43	5.70	84	10.98	50	7.14	102	7.95	85	8.36	79	5.87	86	5.37
Unknown	<5	–	<5	–	<5	–	–	–	–	–	–	–	<5	–	–	–
Plurality																
Singleton	947	7.89	95	7.05	149	10.60	98	7.38	162	8.18	159	10.58	139	6.86	145	6.00
Multiple	12	3.84	<5	<20.05	5	18.50	–	–	<5	<10.81	<5	<12.25	<5	<8.05	<5	<5.95
Unknown	–	–	–	–	–	–	–	–	–	–	–	–	–	–	–	–

TABLE 39B

CONGENITAL DISLOCATION OR DYSPLASIA OF THE HIP: PERCENTAGE OF CASES BY DESCRIPTIVE CHARACTERISTICS, MACDP, 1968–2003*

	Total		1968–1972		1973–1978		1979–1983		1984–1989		1990–1993		1994–1998		1999–2003	
Characteristic	Cases	Percent	Cases	Percent	Cases	Percent	Cases	Percent	Cases	Percent	Cases	Percent	Cases	Percent	Cases	Percent
Birth outcome																
Live birth	953	99.4	94	96.9	151	98.1	98	100.0	163	100.0	161	100.0	140	100.0	146	100.0
Stillbirth	6	0.6	<5	—	<5	—	—	—	—	—	—	—	—	—	—	—
Elective termination	—	—	—	—	—	—	—	—	—	—	—	—	—	—	—	—
Unknown	—	—	—	—	—	—	—	—	—	—	—	—	—	—	—	—
Age at diagnosis																
Prenatally or <7 days	844	88.0	91	93.8	128	83.1	82	83.7	146	89.6	152	94.4	118	84.3	127	87.0
8 days–6 months	57	5.9	5	5.2	19	12.3	7	7.1	9	5.5	6	3.7	6	4.3	5	3.4
6months–1 year	36	3.8	<5	—	7	4.5	9	9.2	6	3.7	<5	—	6	4.3	5	3.4
1–5 years	13	1.4	—	—	—	—	—	—	<5	—	—	—	10	7.1	<5	—
>5 years	—	—	—	—	—	—	—	—	—	—	—	—	—	—	—	—
Unknown	9	0.9	—	—	—	—	—	—	<5	—	<5	—	—	—	7	4.8
Socioeconomic status§																
Upper	254	26.5	—	—	—	—	33	33.7	76	46.6	67	41.6	54	38.6	24	16.4
Middle	211	22.0	—	—	—	—	40	40.8	49	30.1	51	31.7	48	34.3	23	15.8
Lower	150	15.6	—	—	—	—	23	23.5	34	20.9	37	23.0	33	23.6	23	15.8
Unknown	344	35.9	97	100.0	154	100.0	<5	—	<5	—	6	3.7	5	3.6	76	52.1

* Cells containing fewer than 5 cases are indicated as "<5". Prevalence estimates based on these cells are indicated as less than the prevalence based on 5 cases in Table A. Percentages based on these cells are not provided in Table B. Cells containing zero cases are indicated as "—". Counts are provided, but prevalences are not estimated, for strata with unknown values in Table A. Counts and percentages are provided for strata with unknown values in Table B.
** Prev = Prevalence.
† Data on Hispanic or Latino ethnicity were available beginning in 1990.
‡ The category of All Other Races includes 13 cases of Black or African American race.
§ Information about socioeconomic status was available only for 1979–2001.

TABLE 40A

CLUBFOOT WITHOUT A NEURAL TUBE DEFECT: PREVALENCE (PER 10,000 LIVE BIRTHS) STRATIFIED BY DESCRIPTIVE CHARACTERISTICS, MACDP, 1968–2003*

	Total		1968–1972		1973–1978		1979–1983		1984–1989		1990–1993		1994–1998		1999–2003	
Characteristic	Cases	Prev**	Cases	Prev	Cases	Prev	Cases	Prev	Cases	Prev	Cases	Prev	Cases	Prev	Cases	Prev
Total	2,099	17.03	344	25.07	401	27.94	265	19.55	304	14.99	202	13.09	305	14.61	278	11.12
Maternal age (years)																
<25	943	19.19	197	25.18	226	30.90	148	24.45	126	16.03	74	13.54	85	12.62	87	11.03
25–29	604	17.12	100	26.87	111	25.03	78	18.54	94	14.82	58	12.89	89	16.09	74	11.29
≥30	549	14.19	44	20.24	64	25.21	39	11.86	84	13.86	70	12.82	131	15.21	117	11.08
Unknown	<5	–	<5	–	–	–	<5	–	–	–	–	–	–	–	–	–
Maternal race/ethnicity‡																
White	1,386	20.68	283	28.73	308	33.13	185	22.28	204	16.64	116	14.61	155	15.81	135	14.12
Black or African American	539	12.83	–	–	88	17.93	79	15.62	95	12.54	75	11.68	118	14.09	84	8.73
Hispanic or Latino	69	10.62	–	–	–	–	–	–	–	–	7	11.85	16	9.65	46	10.83
All Other Races	98	12.88	61‡	15.76	<5	<33.81	–	–	5	11.48	<5	<10.58	14	14.59	10	6.55
Unknown	7	–	–	–	<5	–	<5	–	–	–	–	–	<5	–	<5	–
Birth weight (grams)																
<2500	442	41.90	59	48.93	70	56.72	61	52.04	60	36.89	51	38.12	77	43.06	64	29.29
≥2500	1,645	14.64	281	22.58	329	25.41	204	16.49	243	13.04	150	10.65	227	11.89	211	9.25
Unknown	12	–	<5	–	<5	–	–	–	<5	–	<5	<10.58	<5	–	<5	–
Gestational age (weeks)																
20–36	390	34.09	43	40.65	63	52.14	54	43.79	45	22.79	55	34.59	73	37.50	57	23.47
≥37	1,696	16.09	301	25.95	337	27.97	211	18.66	255	15.24	144	11.07	231	12.47	217	9.77
Unknown	13	–	–	–	<5	–	–	–	<5	–	<5	–	<5	–	<5	–
Sex																
Male	1,275	20.24	198	28.21	239	32.37	150	21.60	194	18.67	123	15.61	191	17.93	180	14.15
Female	818	13.58	146	21.79	159	22.82	115	17.40	110	11.13	79	10.46	113	11.04	96	7.82
Ambiguous/Unknown	6	–	–	–	<5	–	–	–	–	–	–	–	<5	–	<5	–
Parity																
1 Live birth	1,070	19.76	173	33.18	215	29.76	141	22.21	137	15.29	108	16.16	151	16.44	145	13.75
2 or more live births	958	14.27	118	16.40	186	26.10	123	17.07	151	13.79	94	10.80	153	13.17	133	9.29
Unknown	71	–	53	–	–	–	<5	–	16	–	–	–	<5	–	–	–
Gravidity																
1 Pregnancy	833	17.96	161	33.11	182	27.15	103	15.73	106	15.02	66	12.68	105	14.40	110	12.64
2 or more pregnancies	1,260	16.87	183	24.24	218	28.49	161	22.98	195	15.19	136	13.37	199	14.78	168	10.50
Unknown	6	–	–	–	<5	–	<5	–	<5	–	–	–	<5	–	–	–
Plurality																
Singleton	2,045	17.03	339	25.17	393	27.95	254	19.12	294	14.84	198	13.18	299	14.76	268	11.09
Multiple	53	16.97	5	20.05	8	29.61	11	40.56	10	21.62	<5	<12.25	6	9.66	9	10.71
Unknown	<5	–	–	–	–	–	–	–	–	–	–	–	–	–	<5	–

TABLE 40B

CLUBFOOT WITHOUT A NEURAL TUBE DEFECT: PERCENTAGE OF CASES BY DESCRIPTIVE CHARACTERISTICS, MACDP, 1968–2003*

									Period							
	Total		1968–1972		1973–1978		1979–1983		1984–1989		1990–1993		1994–1998		1999–2003	
Characteristic	Cases	Percent	Cases	Percent	Cases	Percent	Cases	Percent	Cases	Percent	Cases	Percent	Cases	Percent	Cases	Percent
Birth outcome																
Live birth	2,033	96.9	337	98.0	392	97.8	258	97.4	296	97.4	191	94.6	290	95.1	269	96.8
Stillbirth	54	2.6	7	2.0	9	2.2	7	2.6	8	2.6	7	3.5	11	3.6	5	1.8
Elective termination	12	0.6	—	—	—	—	—	—	—	—	<5	—	<5	—	<5	—
Unknown	—	—	—	—	—	—	—	—	—	—	—	—	—	—	—	—
Age at diagnosis																
Prenatally or <7 days	2,041	97.2	341	99.1	394	98.3	264	99.6	292	96.1	197	97.5	295	96.7	258	92.8
8 days–6 months	28	1.3	<5	—	7	1.7	<5	—	7	2.3	<5	—	<5	—	<5	—
6 months–1 year	10	0.5	—	—	—	—	—	—	5	1.6	<5	—	<5	—	<5	—
1–5 years	<5	—	—	—	—	—	—	—	—	—	—	—	<5	—	<5	—
>5 years	—	—	—	—	—	—	—	—	—	—	—	—	—	—	—	—
Unknown	18	0.9	—	—	—	—	—	—	—	—	—	—	<5	—	14	5.0
Socioeconomic status§																
Upper	399	19.0	—	—	—	—	74	27.9	114	37.5	72	35.6	95	31.1	44	15.8
Middle	437	20.8	—	—	—	—	88	33.2	88	28.9	72	35.6	123	40.3	66	23.7
Lower	356	17.0	—	—	—	—	95	35.8	95	31.3	53	26.2	74	24.3	39	14.0
Unknown	907	43.2	344	100.0	401	100.0	8	3.0	7	2.3	5	2.5	13	4.3	129	46.4

* Cells containing fewer than 5 cases are indicated as "<5". Prevalence estimates based on these cells are indicated as less than the prevalence based on 5 cases in Table A. Percentages based on these cells are not provided in Table B. Cells containing zero cases are indicated as "—". Counts are provided, but prevalences are not estimated, for strata with unknown values in Table A. Counts and percentages are provided for strata with unknown values in Table B.

** Prev = Prevalence.

† Data on Hispanic or Latino ethnicity were available beginning in 1990.

‡ The category of All Other Races includes 58 cases of Black or African American race.

§ Information about socioeconomic status was available only for 1979–2001.

TABLE 41A

POLYDACTYLY: PREVALENCE (PER 10,000 LIVE BIRTHS) STRATIFIED BY DESCRIPTIVE CHARACTERISTICS, MACDP, 1968–2003*

	Total		Period 1968–1972		1973–1978		1979–1983		1984–1989		1990–1993		1994–1998		1999–2003	
Characteristic	Cases	Prev**	Cases	Prev	Cases	Prev	Cases	Prev	Cases	Prev	Cases	Prev	Cases	Prev	Cases	Prev
Total	1,913	15.53	155	11.30	199	13.24	474	34.97	285	14.06	167	10.82	294	14.08	348	13.92
Maternal age (years)																
<25	884	17.99	80	10.23	110	15.04	268	44.27	132	16.79	62	11.34	107	15.89	125	15.85
25–29	516	14.62	43	11.55	48	10.82	127	30.19	76	11.98	46	10.22	76	13.74	100	15.26
≥30	509	13.16	31	14.26	32	12.61	79	24.03	76	12.54	59	10.80	110	12.77	122	11.56
Unknown	<5	–	<5	–	–	–	–	–	<5	–	–	–	<5	–	<5	–
Maternal race/ethnicity†																
White	778	11.61	119	12.08	118	12.69	98	11.80	139	11.34	88	11.08	117	11.93	99	10.36
Black or African American	974	23.18	–	–	71	14.46	373	73.76	143	18.87	61	9.50	146	17.32	180	18.70
Hispanic or Latino	79	12.16	–	–	–	–	–	–	–	–	7	11.85	20	12.06	52	12.24
All Other Races	76	9.99	36‡	9.30	<5	<33.81	<5	<26.07	<5	<11.48	10	21.15	10	10.42	15	9.82
Unknown	6	–	–	–	–	–	<5	–	<5	–	<5	–	<5	–	<5	–
Birth weight (grams)																
<2500	339	32.13	29	24.05	31	25.12	70	59.72	55	33.82	35	26.16	50	27.96	69	31.58
≥<2500	1,570	13.97	124	9.96	158	12.20	404	32.66	229	12.29	132	9.37	244	12.78	279	12.23
Unknown	<5	–	<5	–	<5	–	–	–	<5	–	–	–	–	–	–	–
Gestational age (weeks)																
20–36	319	27.89	23	21.75	30	24.83	73	59.20	50	25.32	30	18.87	43	22.09	70	28.82
≥37	1,569	14.88	132	11.38	160	13.28	399	35.29	231	13.80	134	10.30	246	13.28	267	12.02
Unknown	25	–	–	–	<5	–	<5	–	<5	–	<5	–	<5	–	11	–
Sex																
Male	1,118	17.75	92	13.11	107	14.49	268	38.59	171	16.46	99	12.56	173	16.24	208	16.36
Female	792	13.15	62	9.25	83	11.91	206	31.17	114	11.53	66	8.74	121	11.83	140	11.40
Ambiguous/Unknown	<5	–	<5	–	–	–	–	–	<5	–	<5	–	–	–	–	–
Parity																
1 Live birth	814	15.03	66	12.66	89	12.32	219	34.50	112	12.50	72	10.77	119	12.96	137	12.99
2 or more live births	1,051	15.66	61	8.48	100	14.03	255	35.39	155	14.16	95	10.91	175	15.06	210	14.66
Unknown	48	–	28	–	<5	–	–	–	18	–	–	–	–	–	<5	–
Gravidity																
1 Pregnancy	606	13.07	61	12.54	73	10.89	154	23.52	94	13.32	51	9.80	78	10.70	95	10.92
2 or more pregnancies	1,301	17.42	93	12.32	117	15.29	317	45.25	190	14.81	116	11.41	216	16.04	252	15.74
Unknown	6	–	<5	–	–	–	<5	–	<5	–	–	–	–	–	<5	–
Plurality																
Singleton	1,588	15.47	152	11.28	186	13.23	462	34.78	277	13.98	159	10.58	286	14.12	336	13.91
Multiple	55	17.61	<5	<20.05	<5	<18.50	12	44.25	8	17.30	8	19.60	8	12.87	12	14.28
Unknown	–	–	–	–	–	–	–	–	–	–	–	–	–	–	–	–

TABLE 41B

POLYDACTYLY: PERCENTAGE OF CASES BY DESCRIPTIVE CHARACTERISTICS, MACDP, 1968–2003*

	Total		1968–1972		1973–1978		1979–1983		1984–1989		1990–1993		1994–1998		1999–2003	
Characteristic	Cases	Percent	Cases	Percent	Cases	Percent	Cases	Percent	Cases	Percent	Cases	Percent	Cases	Percent	Cases	Percent
Birth outcome																
Live birth	1,856	97.0	150	96.8	185	97.4	467	98.5	276	96.8	160	95.8	283	96.3	335	96.3
Stillbirth	40	2.1	5	3.2	5	2.6	7	1.5	8	2.8	5	3.0	6	2.0	<5	–
Elective termination	17	0.9	–	–	–	–	–	–	<5	–	<5	–	5	1.7	9	2.6
Unknown	–	–	–	–	–	–	–	–	–	–	–	–	–	–	–	–
Age at diagnosis																
Prenatally or <7 days	1,856	97.0	154	99.4	186	97.9	469	98.9	279	97.9	162	97.0	276	93.9	330	94.8
8 days–6 months	33	1.7	<5	–	<5	–	<5	–	5	1.8	<5	–	7	2.4	8	2.3
6 months–1 year	6	0.3	–	–	–	–	<5	–	<5	–	<5	–	<5	–	<5	–
1–5 years	<5	–	–	–	–	–	–	–	–	–	–	–	<5	–	–	–
>5 years	<5	–	–	–	–	–	–	–	–	–	–	–	<5	–	–	–
Unknown	15	0.8	–	–	–	–	–	–	–	–	–	–	7	2.4	8	2.3
Socioeconomic status§																
Upper	347	18.1	–	–	–	–	65	13.7	87	30.5	59	35.3	89	30.3	47	13.5
Middle	425	22.2	–	–	–	–	111	23.4	72	25.3	57	34.1	97	33.0	88	25.3
Lower	603	31.5	–	–	–	–	294	62.0	121	42.5	48	28.7	92	31.3	48	13.8
Unknown	536	28.1	155	100.0	190	100.0	<5	–	5	1.8	<5	–	16	5.4	165	47.4

* Cells containing fewer than 5 cases are indicated as "<5". Prevalence estimates based on these cells are indicated as less than the prevalence based on 5 cases in Table A. Percentages based on these cells are not provided in Table B. Cells containing zero cases are indicated as "–". Counts are provided, but prevalences are not estimated, for strata with unknown values in Table A. Counts and percentages are provided for strata with unknown values in Table B.
** Prev = Prevalence.
† Data on Hispanic or Latino ethnicity were available beginning in 1990.
‡ The category of All Other Races includes 36 cases of Black or African American race.
§ Information about socioeconomic status was available only for 1979–2001.

TABLE 42A

TRANSVERSE LIMB DEFICIENCY: PREVALENCE (PER 10,000 LIVE BIRTHS) STRATIFIED BY DESCRIPTIVE CHARACTERISTICS, MACDP, 1968–2003*

	Total		1968–1972		1973–1978		1979–1983		1984–1989		1990–1993		1994–1998		1999–2003	
Characteristic	Cases	Prev**	Cases	Prev	Cases	Prev	Cases	Prev	Cases	Prev	Cases	Prev	Cases	Prev	Cases	Prev
Total	**377**	**3.06**	**54**	**3.94**	**55**	**3.83**	**38**	**2.80**	**52**	**2.56**	**48**	**3.11**	**67**	**3.21**	**63**	**2.52**
Maternal age (years)																
<25	173	3.52	25	3.20	31	4.24	25	4.13	24	3.05	20	3.66	25	4.16	20	2.54
25–29	105	2.98	19	5.11	17	3.83	7	1.66	13	2.05	17	3.78	23	4.16	9	1.37
≥30	98	2.53	9	4.14	7	2.76	6	1.83	15	2.48	11	2.01	16	1.86	34	3.22
Unknown	<5	–	<5	–	–	–	–	–	–	–	–	–	–	–	–	–
Maternal race/ethnicity†																
White	212	3.16	37	3.76	38	4.09	21	2.53	36	2.94	23	2.90	35	3.57	22	2.30
Black or African American	121	2.88	–	–	17	3.46	17	3.36	14	1.85	24	3.74	24	2.85	25	2.60
Hispanic or Latino	7	2.62	–	–	–	–	–	–	–	–	–	–	5	3.01	12	2.82
All Other Races	26	3.42	17‡	4.39	–	–	–	–	<5	<11.48	<5	<10.58	<5	<5.21	<5	<3.27
Unknown	<5	–	<5	–	–	–	<5	–	–	–	–	–	<5	–	–	–
Birth weight (grams)																
<2500	138	13.08	22	18.24	16	12.96	13	11.09	19	11.68	16	11.96	29	16.22	23	10.53
≥2500	235	2.09	31	2.49	39	3.01	24	1.94	31	1.66	32	2.27	38	1.99	40	1.75
Unknown	<5	–	<5	–	–	–	<5	–	<5	–	–	–	–	–	–	–
Gestational age (weeks)																
20–36	118	10.32	11	10.40	17	14.07	7	5.68	17	8.61	15	9.43	29	14.90	22	9.06
≥37	255	2.42	42	3.62	38	3.15	31	2.74	32	1.91	33	2.54	38	2.05	41	1.85
Unknown	<5	–	<5	–	–	–	–	–	<5	–	–	–	–	–	–	–
Sex																
Male	208	3.30	32	4.56	28	3.79	22	3.17	22	2.12	30	3.81	37	3.47	37	2.91
Female	164	2.72	22	3.28	27	3.87	16	2.42	27	2.73	17	2.25	29	2.83	26	2.12
Ambiguous/Unknown	5	–	–	–	–	–	<5	–	<5	–	<5	–	<5	–	–	–
Parity																
1 Live birth	196	3.62	23	4.41	31	4.29	21	3.31	26	2.90	28	4.19	39	4.25	28	2.66
2 or more live births	170	2.53	23	3.20	24	3.37	17	2.36	23	2.10	20	2.30	28	2.41	35	2.44
Unknown	11	–	8	–	–	–	–	–	<5	–	–	–	–	–	–	–
Gravidity																
1 Pregnancy	162	3.49	18	3.70	30	4.48	18	2.75	22	3.12	23	4.42	29	3.98	22	2.53
2 or more pregnancies	215	2.88	36	4.77	25	3.27	20	2.85	30	2.34	25	2.46	38	2.82	41	2.56
Unknown	–	–	–	–	–	–	–	–	–	–	–	–	–	–	–	–
Plurality																
Singleton	361	3.01	53	3.93	55	3.91	36	2.71	47	2.37	46	3.06	63	3.11	61	2.52
Multiple	16	5.12	<5	<20.05	–	–	<5	<18.44	5	10.81	<5	<12.25	<5	<8.05	<5	<5.95
Unknown	–	–	–	–	–	–	–	–	–	–	–	–	–	–	–	–

TABLE 42B

TRANSVERSE LIMB DEFICIENCY: PERCENTAGE OF CASES BY DESCRIPTIVE CHARACTERISTICS, MACDP, 1968–2003*

	Total		Period 1968–1972		1973–1978		1979–1983		1984–1989		1990–1993		1994–1998		1999–2003	
Characteristic	Cases	Percent	Cases	Percent	Cases	Percent	Cases	Percent	Cases	Percent	Cases	Percent	Cases	Percent	Cases	Percent
Birth outcome																
Live birth	344	91.2	52	96.3	52	94.5	34	89.5	47	90.4	43	89.6	60	89.6	56	88.9
Stillbirth	25	6.6	<5	–	<5	–	<5	–	5	9.6	<5	–	<5	–	<5	–
Elective termination	8	2.1	–	–	–	–	–	–	–	–	<5	–	<5	–	<5	–
Unknown	–	–	–	–	–	–	–	–	–	–	–	–	–	–	–	–
Age at diagnosis																
Prenatally or <7days	375	99.5	54	100.0	55	100.0	38	100.0	51	98.1	48	100.0	67	100.0	62	98.4
8 days–6 months	<5	–	–	–	–	–	–	–	<5	–	–	–	–	–	–	–
6 months–1 year	–	–	–	–	–	–	–	–	–	–	–	–	–	–	–	–
1–5 years	–	–	–	–	–	–	–	–	–	–	–	–	–	–	–	–
>5 years	–	–	–	–	–	–	–	–	–	–	–	–	–	–	–	–
Unknown	<5	–	–	–	–	–	–	–	–	–	–	–	–	–	<5	–
Socioeconomic status§																
Upper	68	18.0	–	–	–	–	8	21.1	15	28.8	14	29.2	19	28.4	12	19.0
Middle	81	21.5	–	–	–	–	11	28.9	14	26.9	15	31.3	27	40.3	14	22.2
Lower	88	23.3	–	–	–	–	16	42.1	22	42.3	19	39.6	19	28.4	12	19.0
Unknown	140	37.1	54	100.0	55	100.0	<5	–	<5	–	–	–	<5	–	25	39.7

* Cells containing fewer than 5 cases are indicated as "<5". Prevalence estimates based on these cells are indicated as less than the prevalence based on 5 cases in Table A. Percentages based on these cells are not provided in Table B. Cells containing zero cases are indicated as "–". Counts are provided, but prevalences are not estimated, for strata with unknown values in Table A. Counts and percentages are provided for strata with unknown values in Table B.
** Prev = Prevalence.
† Data on Hispanic or Latino ethnicity were available beginning in 1990.
‡ The category of All Other Races includes 16 cases of Black or African American race.
§ Information about socioeconomic status was available only for 1979–2001.

TABLE 43A

CRANIOSYNOSTOSIS: PREVALENCE (PER 10,000 LIVE BIRTHS) STRATIFIED BY DESCRIPTIVE CHARACTERISTICS, MACDP, 1968–2003*

Characteristic	Total Cases	Prev**	1968–1972 Cases	Prev	1973–1978 Cases	Prev	1979–1983 Cases	Prev	1984–1989 Cases	Prev	1990–1993 Cases	Prev	1994–1998 Cases	Prev	1999–2003 Cases	Prev
Total	**481**	**3.90**	**30**	**2.19**	**56**	**3.90**	**44**	**3.25**	**69**	**3.40**	**93**	**6.03**	**88**	**4.21**	**101**	**4.04**
Maternal age (years)																
<25	129	2.63	13	1.66	23	3.14	13	2.15	21	2.67	23	4.21	19	2.82	17	2.16
25–29	136	3.85	8	2.15	19	4.28	11	2.61	16	2.52	30	6.67	28	5.06	24	3.66
≥30	215	5.56	8	3.68	14	5.52	20	6.08	32	5.28	40	7.32	41	4.76	60	5.68
Unknown	<5	–	<5	–	–	–	–	–	–	–	–	–	–	–	–	–
Maternal race/ethnicity†																
White	353	5.27	25	2.54	46	4.95	42	5.06	61	4.98	74	9.32	52	5.30	53	5.54
Black or African American	82	1.95	–	–	9	1.83	<5	<0.99	7	0.92	17	2.65	25	2.97	22	2.29
Hispanic or Latino	30	4.62	–	–	–	–	–	–	–	–	–	–	9	5.43	21	4.94
All Other Races	14	1.84	5‡	1.29	<5	<33.81	–	–	–	–	<5	<10.58	<5	<5.21	<5	3.27
Unknown	<5	–	–	–	–	–	–	–	<5	–	<5	–	–	–	–	–
Birth weight (grams)																
<2500	78	7.39	<5	<4.15	10	8.10	5	4.27	12	7.38	16	11.96	13	7.27	19	8.69
≥2500	401	3.57	26	2.09	46	3.55	39	3.15	57	3.06	77	5.47	75	3.93	81	3.55
Unknown	<5	–	<5	–	–	–	–	–	–	–	–	–	–	–	<5	–
Gestational age (weeks)																
20–36	83	7.26	<5	<4.73	7	5.79	<5	<4.05	13	6.58	17	10.69	16	8.22	23	9.47
≥37	394	3.74	27	2.33	49	4.07	40	3.54	54	3.23	76	5.84	71	3.83	77	3.47
Unknown	<5	–	–	–	–	–	–	–	<5	–	–	–	<5	–	<5	–
Sex																
Male	322	5.11	22	3.13	33	4.47	34	4.90	47	4.52	57	7.23	65	6.10	64	5.03
Female	159	2.64	8	1.19	23	3.30	10	1.51	22	2.23	36	4.77	23	2.25	37	3.01
Ambiguous/Unknown	–	–	–	–	–	–	–	–	–	–	–	–	–	–	–	–
Parity																
1 Live birth	213	3.93	14	2.68	21	2.91	18	2.84	36	4.02	48	7.18	37	4.03	39	3.70
2 or more live births	263	3.92	13	1.81	35	4.91	26	3.61	32	2.92	45	5.17	50	4.30	62	4.33
Unknown	<5	–	<5	–	–	–	–	–	<5	–	–	–	<5	–	–	–
Gravidity																
1 Pregnancy	132	2.85	10	2.06	19	2.83	14	2.14	22	3.12	24	4.61	20	2.74	23	2.64
2 or more pregnancies	345	4.62	18	2.38	37	4.84	30	4.28	46	3.58	69	6.78	67	4.97	78	4.87
Unknown	<5	–	<5	–	–	–	–	–	<5	–	–	–	<5	–	–	–
Plurality																
Singleton	452	3.76	28	2.08	55	3.91	43	3.24	65	3.28	85	5.66	80	3.95	96	3.97
Multiple	28	8.97	<5	<20.05	<5	<18.50	<5	<18.44	<5	<10.81	8	19.60	8	12.87	5	5.95
Unknown	<5	–	–	–	–	–	–	–	<5	–	–	–	–	–	–	–

TABLE 43B

CRANIOSYNOSTOSIS: PERCENTAGE OF CASES BY DESCRIPTIVE CHARACTERISTICS, MACDP, 1968–2003*

																Period
	Total		1968–1972		1973–1978		1979–1983		1984–1989		1990–1993		1994–1998		1999–2003	
Characteristic	Cases	Percent	Cases	Percent	Cases	Percent	Cases	Percent	Cases	Percent	Cases	Percent	Cases	Percent	Cases	Percent
Birth outcome																
Live birth	480	99.8	30	100.0	56	100.0	44	100.0	69	100.0	93	100.0	88	100.0	100	99.0
Stillbirth	<5	–	–	–	–	–	–	–	–	–	–	–	–	–	<5	–
Elective termination	–	–	–	–	–	–	–	–	–	–	–	–	–	–	–	–
Unknown	–	–	–	–	–	–	–	–	–	–	–	–	–	–	–	–
Age at diagnosis																
Prenatally or <7 days	176	36.6	13	43.3	29	51.8	28	63.6	27	39.1	33	35.5	21	23.9	25	24.8
8 days–6 months	191	39.7	16	53.3	24	42.9	13	29.5	26	37.7	40	43.0	42	47.7	30	29.7
6 months–1 year	73	15.2	<5	–	<5	–	<5	–	14	20.3	17	18.3	14	15.9	22	21.8
1–5 years	18	3.7	–	–	–	–	–	–	–	–	<5	–	8	9.1	9	8.9
>5 years	<5	–	–	–	–	–	–	–	–	–	–	–	<5	–	–	–
Unknown	22	4.6	–	–	–	–	<5	–	<5	–	<5	–	<5	–	15	14.9
Socioeconomic status§																
Upper	175	36.4	–	–	–	–	19	43.2	36	52.2	60	64.5	36	40.9	24	23.8
Middle	76	15.8	–	–	–	–	12	27.3	16	23.2	14	15.1	22	25.0	12	11.9
Lower	66	13.7	–	–	–	–	<5	–	13	18.8	19	20.4	23	26.1	7	6.9
Unknown	164	34.1	30	100.0	56	100.0	9	20.5	<5	–	–	–	7	8.0	58	57.4

* Cells containing fewer than 5 cases are indicated as "<5". Prevalence estimates based on these cells are indicated as less than the prevalence based on 5 cases in Table A. Percentages based on these cells are not provided in Table B. Cells containing zero cases are indicated as "–". Counts are provided, but prevalences are not estimated, for strata with unknown values in Table A. Counts and percentages are provided for strata with unknown values in Table B.

** Prev = Prevalence.

† Data on Hispanic or Latino ethnicity were available beginning in 1990.

‡ The category of All Other Races includes 5 cases of Black or African American race.

§ Information about socioeconomic status was available only for 1979–2001.

TABLE 44A

SKELETAL DYSPLASIA: PREVALENCE (PER 10,000 LIVE BIRTHS) STRATIFIED BY DESCRIPTIVE CHARACTERISTICS, MACDP, 1968–2003*

Characteristic	Total Cases	Total Prev**	1968–1972 Cases	1968–1972 Prev	1973–1978 Cases	1973–1978 Prev	1979–1983 Cases	1979–1983 Prev	1984–1989 Cases	1984–1989 Prev	1990–1993 Cases	1990–1993 Prev	1994–1998 Cases	1994–1998 Prev	1999–2003 Cases	1999–2003 Prev
Total	**226**	**1.83**	**19**	**1.38**	**17**	**1.18**	**26**	**1.92**	**38**	**1.87**	**38**	**2.46**	**47**	**2.25**	**41**	**1.64**
Maternal age (years)																
<25	75	1.53	10	1.28	6	0.82	9	1.49	10	1.27	16	2.93	14	2.08	10	1.27
25–29	71	2.01	6	1.61	8	1.80	11	2.61	12	1.89	13	2.89	14	2.53	7	1.07
≥30	80	2.07	<5	<2.30	<5	<1.97	6	1.83	16	2.64	9	1.65	19	2.21	24	2.27
Unknown	–	–	–	–	–	–	–	–	–	–	–	–	–	–	–	–
Maternal race/ethnicity†																
White	122	1.82	9	0.91	14	1.51	12	1.45	20	1.63	17	2.14	30	3.06	20	2.09
Black or African American	79	1.88	–	–	<5	<1.02	13	2.57	18	2.38	19	2.96	13	1.54	13	1.35
Hispanic or Latino	12	1.85	–	–	–	–	–	–	–	–	<5	<8.47	<5	<3.01	6	1.41
All Other Races	12	1.58	10‡	2.58	–	–	<5	<26.07	–	–	–	–	–	–	<5	<3.27
Unknown	<5	–	–	–	–	–	–	–	<5	–	–	–	–	–	<5	–
Birth weight (grams)																
<2500	95	9.00	7	5.80	6	4.86	12	10.24	17	10.45	13	9.72	24	13.42	16	7.32
≥2500	130	1.16	12	0.96	11	0.85	14	1.13	21	1.13	25	1.77	22	1.15	25	1.10
Unknown	<5	–	–	–	–	–	–	–	–	–	–	–	<5	–	–	–
Gestational age (weeks)																
20–36	80	6.99	6	5.67	<5	<4.14	7	5.68	13	6.58	16	10.06	22	11.30	12	4.94
≥37	143	1.36	13	1.12	13	1.08	19	1.68	23	1.37	22	1.69	25	1.35	28	1.26
Unknown	<5	–	–	–	–	–	–	–	<5	–	–	–	–	–	<5	–
Sex																
Male	103	1.64	10	1.42	7	0.95	13	1.87	12	1.15	21	2.67	23	2.16	17	1.34
Female	122	2.03	9	1.34	10	1.44	13	1.97	26	2.63	17	2.25	23	2.25	24	1.95
Ambiguous/Unknown	<5	–	–	–	–	–	–	–	–	–	–	–	<5	–	–	–
Parity																
1 Live birth	89	1.64	9	1.73	10	1.38	8	1.26	14	1.56	17	2.54	18	1.96	13	1.23
2 or more live births	133	1.98	8	1.11	7	0.98	18	2.50	22	2.01	21	2.41	29	2.50	28	1.96
Unknown	<5	–	<5	–	–	–	–	–	<5	–	–	–	–	–	–	–
Gravidity																
1 Pregnancy	58	1.25	8	1.65	7	1.04	<5	<0.76	8	1.13	11	2.11	13	1.78	7	0.80
2 or more pregnancies	167	2.24	11	1.46	10	1.31	22	3.14	29	2.26	27	2.65	34	2.52	34	2.12
Unknown	<5	–	–	–	–	–	–	–	<5	–	–	–	–	–	–	–
Plurality																
Singleton	219	1.82	19	1.41	17	1.21	25	1.88	36	1.82	37	2.46	45	2.22	40	1.66
Multiple	6	1.92	–	–	–	–	<5	<18.44	<5	<10.81	<5	<12.25	<5	<8.05	<5	<5.95
Unknown	<5	–	–	–	–	–	–	–	<5	–	–	–	–	–	–	–

TABLE 44B

SKELETAL DYSPLASIA: PERCENTAGE OF CASES BY DESCRIPTIVE CHARACTERISTICS, MACDP, 1968–2003*

Characteristic	Total		1968–1972		1973–1978		1979–1983		1984–1989		1990–1993		1994–1998		1999–2003	
	Cases	Percent	Cases	Percent	Cases	Percent	Cases	Percent	Cases	Percent	Cases	Percent	Cases	Percent	Cases	Percent
Birth outcome																
Live birth	193	85.4	18	94.7	16	94.1	23	88.5	32	84.2	32	84.2	37	78.7	35	85.4
Stillbirth	16	7.1	<5	–	<5	–	<5	–	5	13.2	<5	–	<5	–	<5	–
Elective termination	17	7.5	–	–	–	–	–	–	<5	–	<5	–	7	14.9	5	12.2
Unknown																
Age at diagnosis																
Prenatally or <7 days	191	84.5	18	94.7	16	94.1	25	96.2	36	94.7	29	76.3	36	76.6	31	75.6
8 days–6 months	11	4.9	<5	–	–	–	<5	–	<5	–	<5	–	<5	–	–	–
6 months–1 year	9	4.0	<5	–	<5	–	–	–	–	–	<5	–	<5	–	<5	–
1–5 years	<5	–	–	–	–	–	–	–	–	–	–	–	–	–	<5	–
>5 years	–	–	–	–	–	–	–	–	–	–	–	–	–	–	–	–
Unknown	13	5.8	–	–	–	–	–	–	–	–	<5	–	5	10.6	6	14.6
Socioeconomic status§																
Upper	50	22.1	–	–	–	–	7	26.9	10	26.3	9	23.7	19	40.4	5	12.2
Middle	51	22.6	–	–	–	–	9	34.6	12	31.6	13	34.2	12	25.5	5	12.2
Lower	58	25.7	–	–	–	–	9	34.6	16	42.1	14	36.8	11	23.4	8	19.5
Unknown	67	29.6	19	100.0	17	100.0	<5	–	–		<5	–	5	10.6	23	56.1

*Cells containing fewer than 5 cases are indicated as "<5". Prevalence estimates based on these cells are indicated as less than the prevalence based on 5 cases in Table A. Percentages based on these cells are not provided in Table B. Cells containing zero cases are indicated as "–". Counts are provided, but prevalences are not estimated, for strata with unknown values in Table A. Counts and percentages are provided for strata with unknown values in Table B.

** Prev = Prevalence.

† Data on Hispanic or Latino ethnicity were available beginning in 1990.

‡ The category of All Other Races includes 10 cases of Black or African American race.

§ Information about socioeconomic status was available only for 1979–2001.

TABLE 45A

DIAPHRAGMATIC HERNIA: PREVALENCE (PER 10,000 LIVE BIRTHS) STRATIFIED BY DESCRIPTIVE CHARACTERISTICS, MACDP, 1968–2003*

Characteristic	Total Cases	Prev**	1968–1972 Cases	Prev	1973–1978 Cases	Prev	1979–1983 Cases	Prev	1984–1989 Cases	Prev	1990–1993 Cases	Prev	1994–1998 Cases	Prev	1999–2003 Cases	Prev
Total	280	2.27	27	1.97	34	2.37	24	1.77	47	2.32	38	2.46	40	1.92	70	2.80
Maternal age (years)																
<25	104	2.12	10	1.28	19	2.60	12	1.98	16	2.04	11	2.01	12	1.78	24	3.04
25–29	73	2.07	10	2.69	10	2.26	5	1.19	11	1.73	11	2.44	12	2.17	14	2.14
≥30	101	2.61	6	2.76	5	1.97	7	2.13	19	3.14	16	2.93	16	1.86	32	3.03
Unknown	<5	–	<5	–	–	–	–	–	<5	–	–	–	–	–	–	–
Maternal race/ethnicity†																
White	158	2.36	19	1.93	21	2.26	17	2.05	32	2.61	19	2.39	17	1.73	33	3.45
Black or African American	90	2.14	–	–	13	2.65	6	1.19	15	1.98	18	2.80	14	1.66	24	2.49
Hispanic or Latino	19	2.92	–	–	–	–	–	–	–	–	–	–	8	4.82	11	2.59
All Other Races	12	1.58	8‡	2.07	–	–	<5	<26.07	–	–	<5	<10.58	<5	<5.21	<5	<3.27
Unknown	<5	–	–	–	–	–	–	–	–	–	–	–	–	–	<5	–
Birth weight (grams)																
<2500	76	7.20	8	6.63	9	7.29	5	4.27	12	7.38	15	11.21	14	7.83	13	5.95
≥2500	198	1.76	17	1.37	24	1.85	17	1.37	35	1.88	23	1.63	26	1.36	56	2.45
Unknown	6	–	<5	–	<5	–	<5	–	–	–	–	–	–	–	<5	–
Gestational age (weeks)																
20–36	78	6.82	6	5.67	8	6.62	5	4.05	13	6.58	14	8.81	14	7.19	18	7.41
≥37	200	1.90	21	1.81	26	2.16	19	1.68	32	1.91	24	1.84	26	1.40	52	2.34
Unknown	<5	–	–	–	–	–	<5	–	<5	–	–	–	–	–	–	–
Sex																
Male	159	2.52	19	2.71	17	2.30	16	2.30	31	2.98	22	2.79	22	2.07	32	2.52
Female	121	2.01	8	1.19	17	2.44	8	1.21	16	1.62	16	2.12	18	1.76	38	3.09
Ambiguous/Unknown	–	–	–	–	–	–	–	–	–	–	–	–	–	–	–	–
Parity																
1 Live birth	126	2.33	10	1.92	17	2.35	14	2.21	18	2.01	17	2.54	19	2.07	31	2.94
2 or more live births	145	2.16	11	1.53	17	2.39	10	1.39	26	2.37	21	2.41	21	1.81	39	2.72
Unknown	9	–	6	–	–	–	–	–	<5	–	–	–	–	–	–	–
Gravidity																
1 Pregnancy	92	1.98	10	2.06	12	1.79	13	1.99	15	2.13	8	1.54	14	1.92	20	2.30
2 or more pregnancies	156	2.49	17	2.25	22	2.88	11	1.57	30	2.34	30	2.95	26	1.93	50	3.12
Unknown	<5	–	–	–	–	–	–	–	<5	–	–	–	–	–	–	–
Plurality																
Singleton	273	2.27	26	1.93	34	2.42	23	1.73	46	2.32	36	2.40	40	1.97	68	2.81
Multiple	7	2.24	<5	<20.05	–	–	<5	<18.44	<5	<10.81	<5	<12.25	–	–	<5	<5.95
Unknown	–	–	–	–	–	–	–	–	–	–	–	–	–	–	–	–

Period

TABLE 45B

DIAPHRAGMATIC HERNIA: PERCENTAGE OF CASES BY DESCRIPTIVE CHARACTERISTICS, MACDP, 1968–2003*

	Period															
	Total		1968–1972		1973–1978		1979–1983		1984–1989		1990–1993		1994–1998		1999–2003	
Characteristic	Cases	Percent	Cases	Percent	Cases	Percent	Cases	Percent	Cases	Percent	Cases	Percent	Cases	Percent	Cases	Percent
Birth outcome																
Live birth	262	93.6	26	96.3	33	97.1	23	95.8	45	95.7	35	92.1	34	85.0	66	94.3
Stillbirth	9	3.2	<5	–	<5	–	<5	–	<5	–	<5	–	<5	–	<5	–
Elective termination	9	3.2	–	–	–	–	–	–	–	–	<5	–	5	12.5	<5	–
Unknown																
Age at diagnosis																
Prenatally or <7 days	252	90.0	26	96.3	30	88.2	23	95.8	44	93.6	37	97.4	36	90.0	56	80.0
8 days–6 months	12	4.3	<5	–	<5	–	–	–	<5	–	<5	–	<5	–	<5	–
6 months–1 year	6	2.1	–	–	<5	–	<5	–	<5	–	–	–	<5	–	<5	–
1–5 years	<5	–	–	–	–	–	–	–	–	–	–	–	<5	–	<5	–
>5 years	–	–	–	–	–	–	–	–	–	–	–	–	–	–	–	–
Unknown	8	2.9	–	–	–	–	–	–	–	–	–	–	<5	–	7	10.0
Socioeconomic status§																
Upper	72	25.7	–	–	–	–	10	41.7	21	44.7	18	47.4	13	32.5	10	14.3
Middle	55	19.6	–	–	–	–	7	29.2	14	29.8	9	23.7	10	25.0	15	21.4
Lower	52	18.6	–	–	–	–	7	29.2	11	23.4	10	26.3	14	35.0	10	14.3
Unknown	101	36.1	27	100.0	34	100.0	–	–	<5	–	<5	–	<5	–	35	50.0

* Cells containing fewer than 5 cases are indicated as "<5". Prevalence estimates based on these cells are indicated as less than the prevalence based on 5 cases in Table A. Percentages based on these cells are not provided in Table B. Cells containing zero cases are indicated as "–". Counts are provided, but prevalences are not estimated, for strata with unknown values in Table A. Counts and percentages are provided for strata with unknown values in Table B.
** Prev = Prevalence.
† Data on Hispanic or Latino ethnicity were available beginning in 1990.
‡ The category of All Other Races includes 8 cases of Black or African American race.
§ Information about socioeconomic status was available only for 1979–2001.

TABLE 46A

OMPHALOCELE: PREVALENCE (PER 10,000 LIVE BIRTHS) STRATIFIED BY DESCRIPTIVE CHARACTERISTICS. MACDP, 1968–2003*

Characteristic	Total Cases	Total Prev**	1968–1972 Cases	Prev	1973–1978 Cases	Prev	1979–1983 Cases	Prev	1984–1989 Cases	Prev	1990–1993 Cases	Prev	1994–1998 Cases	Prev	1999–2003 Cases	Prev
Total	337	2.73	48	3.50	57	3.97	47	3.47	54	2.66	33	2.14	51	2.44	47	1.88
Maternal age (years)																
<25	148	3.01	27	3.45	35	4.79	19	3.14	25	3.1	11	2.01	16	2.38	15	1.90
25–29	88	2.49	15	4.03	14	3.16	12	2.85	16	2.52	13	2.89	10	1.81	8	1.22
≥30	101	2.61	6	2.76	8	3.15	16	4.87	13	2.15	9	1.65	25	2.90	24	2.27
Unknown	–	–	–	–	–	–	–	–	–	–	–	–	–	–	–	–
Maternal race/ethnicity†																
White	198	2.95	37	3.76	38	4.09	37	4.46	29	2.37	15	1.89	23	2.35	19	1.99
Black or African American	110	2.62	–	–	19	3.87	10	1.98	24	3.17	16	2.49	22	2.61	19	1.97
Hispanic or Latino	10	1.54	–	–	–	–	–	–	–	–	<5	<8.47	<5	<3.01	5	1.18
All Other Races	16	2.10	11‡	2.84	–	–	–	–	–	–	–	–	<5	<5.21	<5	<3.27
Unknown	<5	–	<5	–	–	–	–	–	<5	–	–	–	–	–	<5	–
Birth weight (grams)																
<2500	171	16.21	28	23.22	33	26.74	20	17.06	25	15.37	18	13.45	27	15.10	20	9.15
≥2500	149	1.33	17	1.37	21	1.62	23	1.86	26	1.40	14	0.99	23	1.20	25	1.10
Unknown	17	–	<5	–	<5	–	<5	–	<5	–	<5	–	<5	–	<5	–
Gestational age (weeks)																
20–36	167	14.60	26	24.58	30	24.83	15	12.16	22	11.14	20	12.58	29	14.90	25	10.29
≥37	167	1.58	21	1.81	27	2.24	32	2.83	30	1.79	13	1.00	22	1.19	22	0.99
Unknown	<5	–	<5	–	–	–	–	–	<5	–	–	–	–	–	–	–
Sex																
Male	171	2.71	21	2.99	25	3.39	30	4.32	22	2.12	18	2.28	27	2.53	28	2.20
Female	157	2.61	27	4.03	27	3.87	17	2.57	30	3.03	14	1.85	24	2.35	18	1.47
Ambiguous/Unknown	9	–	–	–	5	–	–	–	<5	–	<5	–	–	–	<5	–
Parity																
1 Live birth	190	3.51	24	4.60	38	5.26	29	4.57	25	2.79	22	3.29	28	3.05	24	2.28
2 or more live births	136	2.03	16	2.22	19	2.67	18	2.50	26	2.37	11	1.26	23	1.98	23	1.61
Unknown	11	–	8	–	–	–	–	–	<5	–	–	–	–	–	–	–
Gravidity																
1 Pregnancy	134	2.89	20	4.11	32	4.77	18	2.75	16	2.27	17	3.27	14	1.92	17	1.95
2 or more pregnancies	203	2.72	28	3.71	25	3.27	29	4.14	38	2.96	16	1.57	37	2.75	30	1.87
Unknown	–	–	–	–	–	–	–	–	–	–	–	–	–	–	–	–
Plurality																
Singleton	312	2.60	45	3.34	53	3.77	44	3.31	49	2.47	29	1.93	48	2.37	44	1.82
Multiple	25	8.00	<5	<20.05	<5	<18.50	<5	<18.44	5	10.81	<5	<12.25	<5	<8.05	<5	<5.95
Unknown	–	–	–	–	–	–	–	–	–	–	–	–	–	–	–	–

TABLE 46B

OMPHALOCELE: PERCENTAGE OF CASES BY DESCRIPTIVE CHARACTERISTICS, MACDP, 1968–2003*

									Period							
	Total		1968–1972		1973–1978		1979–1983		1984–1989		1990–1993		1994–1998		1999–2003	
Characteristic	Cases	Percent	Cases	Percent	Cases	Percent	Cases	Percent	Cases	Percent	Cases	Percent	Cases	Percent	Cases	Percent
Birth outcome																
Live birth	246	73.0	34	70.8	36	63.2	36	76.6	41	75.9	25	75.8	36	70.6	38	80.9
Stillbirth	80	23.7	14	29.2	20	35.1	11	23.4	13	24.1	6	18.2	10	19.6	6	12.8
Elective termination	11	3.3	–	–	<5	–	–	–	–	–	<5	–	5	9.8	<5	–
Unknown	–	–	–	–	–	–	–	–	–	–	–	–	–	–	–	–
Age at diagnosis																
Prenatally or <7 days	325	96.4	48	100.0	57	100.0	47	100.0	54	100.0	33	100.0	47	92.2	39	83.0
8 days–6 months	<5	–	–	–	–	–	–	–	–	–	–	–	<5	–	–	–
6 months–1 year	–	–	–	–	–	–	–	–	–	–	–	–	–	–	–	–
1–5 years	–	–	–	–	–	–	–	–	–	–	–	–	–	–	–	–
>5 years	–	–	–	–	–	–	–	–	–	–	–	–	–	–	–	–
Unknown	11	3.3	–	–	–	–	–	–	–	–	–	–	<5	–	8	17.0
Socioeconomic status§																
Upper	75	22.3	–	–	–	–	17	36.2	18	33.3	13	39.4	18	35.3	9	19.1
Middle	71	21.1	–	–	–	–	20	42.6	14	25.9	10	30.3	14	27.5	13	27.7
Lower	63	18.7	–	–	–	–	9	19.1	21	38.9	9	27.3	17	33.3	7	14.9
Unknown	128	38.0	48	100.0	57	100.0	<5	–	<5	–	<5	–	<5	–	18	38.3

* Cells containing fewer than 5 cases are indicated as "<5". Prevalence estimates based on these cells are indicated as less than the prevalence based on 5 cases in Table A. Percentages based on these cells are not provided in Table B. Cells containing zero cases are indicated as "–". Counts are provided, but prevalences are not estimated, for strata with unknown values in Table A. Counts and percentages are provided for strata with unknown values in Table B.

** Prev = Prevalence.

† Data on Hispanic or Latino ethnicity were available beginning in 1990.

‡ The category of All Other Races includes 10 cases of Black or African American race.

§ Information about socioeconomic status was available only for 1979–2001.

TABLE 47A

GASTROSCHISIS: PREVALENCE (PER 10,000 LIVE BIRTHS) STRATIFIED BY DESCRIPTIVE CHARACTERISTICS, MACDP, 1968–2003*

Characteristic	Total		1968–1972		1973–1978		1979–1983		1984–1989		1990–1993		1994–1998		1999–2003	
	Cases	Prev**	Cases	Prev	Cases	Prev	Cases	Prev	Cases	Prev	Cases	Prev	Cases	Prev	Cases	Prev
Total	**244**	**1.98**	**12**	**0.87**	**19**	**1.32**	**27**	**1.99**	**41**	**2.02**	**42**	**2.72**	**38**	**1.82**	**65**	**2.60**
Maternal age (years)																
<25	175	3.56	9	1.15	4	1.91	20	3.30	29	3.69	30	5.49	25	3.71	48	6.09
25–29	40	1.13	–	–	<5	<1.13	6	1.43	5	0.79	7	1.56	6	1.08	13	1.98
≥30	28	0.72	<5	<2.30	<5	<1.97	<5	<1.52	7	1.16	5	0.92	7	0.81	<5	<0.47
Unknown	<5	–	<5	–	–	–	–	–	–	–	–	–	–	–	–	–
Maternal race/ethnicity[†]																
White	128	1.91	11	1.12	16	1.72	17	2.05	29	2.37	19	2.39	17	1.73	19	1.99
Black or African American	85	2.02	–	–	<5	<1.02	10	1.98	11	1.45	21	3.27	18	2.14	22	2.29
Hispanic or Latino	25	3.85	–	–	–	–	–	–	–	–	<5	<8.47	<5	<3.01	22	5.18
All Other Races	6	0.79	<5[‡]	<1.29	–	–	–	–	<5	<11.48	–	–	<5	<5.21	<5	<3.27
Unknown	–	–	–	–	–	–	–	–	–	–	–	–	–	–	–	–
Birth weight (grams)																
<2500	152	14.41	9	7.46	15	12.15	19	16.21	19	11.68	24	17.94	24	13.42	42	19.22
≥2500	89	0.79	<5	<0.40	<5	<0.39	8	0.65	21	1.13	18	1.28	13	0.68	22	0.96
Unknown	<5	–	–	–	–	–	–	–	<5	–	–	–	<5	–	<5	–
Gestational age (weeks)																
20–36	141	12.33	6	5.67	9	7.45	14	11.35	20	10.13	25	15.72	23	11.82	44	18.12
≥37	97	0.92	6	0.52	10	0.83	13	1.15	18	1.08	17	1.31	13	0.70	20	0.90
Unknown	6	–	–	–	–	–	–	–	<5	–	–	–	<5	–	<5	–
Sex																
Male	111	1.76	9	1.28	13	1.76	10	1.44	15	1.44	16	2.03	17	1.60	31	2.44
Female	133	2.21	<5	<0.75	6	0.86	17	2.57	26	2.63	26	3.44	21	2.05	34	2.77
Ambiguous/Unknown	–	–	–	–	–	–	–	–	–	–	–	–	–	–	–	–
Parity																
1 Live birth	158	2.92	10	1.92	13	1.80	19	2.99	24	2.68	26	3.89	24	2.61	42	3.98
2 or more live births	84	1.25	<5	<0.69	6	0.84	8	1.11	17	1.55	16	1.84	13	1.12	23	1.61
Unknown	<5	–	<5	–	–	–	–	–	–	–	–	–	<5	–	–	–
Gravidity																
1 Pregnancy	114	2.46	9	1.85	9	1.34	8	1.22	15	2.13	18	3.46	21	2.88	34	3.91
2 or more pregnancies	129	1.73	<5	<0.66	10	1.31	19	2.71	26	2.03	24	2.36	16	1.19	31	1.94
Unknown	<5	–	–	–	–	–	–	–	–	–	–	–	<5	–	–	–
Plurality																
Singleton	236	1.97	11	0.82	18	1.28	26	1.96	40	2.02	39	2.60	38	1.88	64	2.65
Multiple	8	2.56	<5	<20.05	<5	<18.50	<5	<18.44	<5	<10.81	<5	<12.25	–	–	<5	<5.95
Unknown	–	–	–	–	–	–	–	–	–	–	–	–	–	–	–	–

TABLE 47B

GASTROSCHISIS: PERCENTAGE OF CASES BY DESCRIPTIVE CHARACTERISTICS, MACDP, 1968–2003*

| | Total | | 1968–1972 | | 1973–1978 | | 1979–1983 | | 1984–1989 | | 1990–1993 | | 1994–1998 | | 1999–2003 | |
Characteristic	Cases	Percent	Cases	Percent	Cases	Percent	Cases	Percent	Cases	Percent	Cases	Percent	Cases	Percent	Cases	Percent
Birth outcome																
Live birth	214	87.7	9	75.0	17	89.5	24	88.9	38	92.7	37	88.1	30	78.9	59	90.8
Stillbirth	28	11.5	<5	–	<5	–	<5	–	<5	–	5	11.9	8	21.1	5	7.7
Elective termination	<5	–	–	<5	–	–	–	–	<5	–	–	–	–	–	<5	–
Unknown	–	–	–	–	–	–	–	–	–	–	–	–	–	–	–	–
Age at diagnosis																
Prenatally or <7 days	235	96.3	12	100.0	19	100.0	27	100.0	40	97.6	42	100.0	38	100.0	57	87.7
8 days–6 months	–	–	–	–	–	–	–	–	–	–	–	–	–	–	–	–
6 months–1 year	–	–	–	–	–	–	–	–	–	–	–	–	–	–	–	–
1–5 years	–	–	–	–	–	–	–	–	–	–	–	–	–	–	–	–
>5 years	–	–	–	–	–	–	–	–	–	–	–	–	–	–	–	–
Unknown	9	3.7	–	–	–	–	–	–	<5	–	–	–	–	–	8	12.3
Socioeconomic status§																
Upper	42	17.2	–	–	–	–	<5	–	11	26.8	11	26.2	10	26.3	6	9.2
Middle	63	25.8	–	–	–	–	12	44.4	16	39.0	12	28.6	10	26.3	13	20.0
Lower	67	27.5	–	–	–	–	10	37.0	12	29.3	17	40.5	16	42.1	12	18.5
Unknown	72	29.5	12	100.0	19	100.0	<5	–	<5	–	<5	–	<5	–	34	52.3

* Cells containing fewer than 5 cases are indicated as "<5". Prevalence estimates based on these cells are indicated as less than the prevalence based on 5 cases in Table A. Percentages based on these cells are not provided in Table B. Cells containing zero cases are indicated as "–". Counts are provided, but prevalences are not estimated, for strata with unknown values in Table A. Counts and percentages are provided for strata with unknown values in Table B.
** Prev = Prevalence.
† Data on Hispanic or Latino ethnicity were available beginning in 1990.
‡ The category of All Other Races includes <5 cases of Black or African American race.
§ Information about socioeconomic status was available only for 1979–2001.

TABLE 48A

DOWN SYNDROME, MATERNAL AGE 35 YEARS OR OLDER: PREVALENCE (PER 10,000 LIVE BIRTHS) STRATIFIED BY DESCRIPTIVE CHARACTERISTICS, MACDP, 1968–2003*

															Period
	Total		1968–1972		1973–1978		1979–1983		1984–1989		1990–1993		1994–1998		1999–2003	
Characteristic	Cases	Prev**	Cases	Prev	Cases	Prev	Cases	Prev	Cases	Prev	Cases	Prev	Cases	Prev	Cases	Prev
Total	**419**	**3.40**	**31**	**2.26**	**26**	**1.81**	**19**	**1.40**	**43**	**2.12**	**43**	**2.79**	**95**	**4.55**	**162**	**6.48**
Maternal age (years)																
<25	–	–	–	–	–	–	–	–	–	–	–	–	–	–	–	–
25–29	–	–	–	–	–	–	–	–	–	–	–	–	–	–	–	–
≥30	419	10.83	31	14.26	26	10.24	19	5.78	43	7.10	43	7.87	95	11.03	162	15.34
Unknown	–	–	–	–	–	–	–	–	–	–	–	–	–	–	–	–
Maternal race/ethnicity†																
White	235	3.51	22	2.23	6	1.72	13	1.57	25	2.04	26	3.27	56	5.71	77	8.05
Black or African American	141	3.36	–	–	10	2.04	6	1.19	16	2.11	17	2.65	30	3.56	62	6.44
Hispanic or Latino	21	3.23	–	–	–	–	–	–	–	–	–	–	<5	<3.01	17	4.00
All Other Races	22	2.89	9‡	2.33	–	–	–	–	<5	<11.48	–	–	5	5.21	6	3.93
Unknown	–	–	–	–	–	–	–	–	–	–	–	–	–	–	–	–
Birth weight (grams)																
<2500	119	11.28	9	7.46	5	4.05	<5	<4.27	10	6.15	17	12.71	28	15.66	46	21.05
≥2500	298	2.65	22	1.77	21	1.62	15	1.21	32	1.72	26	1.85	66	3.46	116	5.09
Unknown	<5	–	–	–	–	–	–	–	<5	–	–	–	<5	–	–	–
Gestational age (weeks)																
20–36	127	11.10	<5	<4.73	<5	<4.14	<5	<4.05	16	8.10	18	11.32	31	15.93	52	21.41
≥37	288	2.73	28	2.41	22	1.83	16	1.42	25	1.49	25	1.92	63	3.40	109	4.91
Unknown	<5	–	–	–	–	–	–	–	<5	–	–	–	<5	–	<5	–
Sex																
Male	232	3.68	16	2.28	12	1.63	9	1.30	24	2.31	30	3.81	52	4.88	89	7.00
Female	187	3.10	15	2.24	14	2.01	10	1.51	19	1.92	13	1.72	43	4.20	73	5.94
Ambiguous/Unknown	–	–	–	–	–	–	–	–	–	–	–	–	–	–	–	–
Parity																
1 Live birth	72	1.33	<5	<0.96	<5	<0.69	<5	<0.79	5	0.56	7	1.05	25	2.72	29	2.75
2 or more live births	335	4.99	20	2.78	23	3.23	16	2.22	38	3.47	36	4.14	69	5.94	133	9.29
Unknown	12	–	10	–	<5	–	–	–	–	–	–	–	<5	–	–	–
Gravidity																
1 Pregnancy	40	0.86	<5	<1.03	<5	<0.75	<5	<0.76	<5	<0.71	5	0.96	11	1.51	16	1.84
2 or more pregnancies	375	5.02	28	3.71	23	3.01	17	2.43	40	3.12	38	3.74	83	6.16	146	9.12
Unknown	<5	–	<5	–	<5	–	–	–	–	–	–	–	<5	–	–	–
Plurality																
Singleton	401	3.34	30	2.23	25	1.78	19	1.43	41	2.07	42	2.80	92	4.54	152	6.29
Multiple	18	5.76	<5	<20.05	<5	<18.50	–	–	<5	<10.81	<5	<12.25	<5	<8.05	10	11.90
Unknown	–	–	–	–	–	–	–	–	–	–	–	–	–	–	–	–

TABLE 48B

DOWN SYNDROME, MATERNAL AGE 35 YEARS OR OLDER: PERCENTAGE OF CASES BY DESCRIPTIVE CHARACTERISTICS, MACDP, 1968–2003*

	Total		1968–1972		1973–1978		1979–1983		1984–1989		1990–1993		1994–1998		1999–2003	
Characteristic	Cases	Percent	Cases	Percent	Cases	Percent	Cases	Percent	Cases	Percent	Cases	Percent	Cases	Percent	Cases	Percent
Birth outcome																
Live birth	382	91.2	31	100.0	25	96.2	17	89.5	36	83.7	38	88.4	86	90.5	149	92.0
Stillbirth	14	3.3	–	–	<5	–	<5	–	5	11.6	–	–	<5	–	<5	–
Elective termination	23	5.5	–	–	–	–	–	–	<5	–	5	11.6	6	6.3	10	6.2
Unknown	–	–	–	–	–	–	–	–	–	–	–	–	–	–	–	–
Age at diagnosis																
Prenatally or <7 days	397	94.7	30	96.8	26	100.0	17	89.5	42	97.7	43	100.0	92	96.8	147	90.7
8 days–6 months	9	2.1	<5	–	–	–	<5	–	<5	–	–	–	<5	–	<5	–
6 months–1 year	<5	–	–	–	–	–	–	–	–	–	–	–	–	–	<5	–
1–5 years	<5	–	–	–	–	–	–	–	–	–	–	–	–	–	<5	–
>5 years	–	–	–	–	–	–	–	–	–	–	–	–	–	–	–	–
Unknown	11	2.6	–	–	–	–	–	–	–	–	–	–	<5	–	9	5.6
Socioeconomic status§																
Upper	115	27.4	–	–	–	–	8	42.1	15	34.9	19	44.2	43	45.3	30	18.5
Middle	94	22.4	–	–	–	–	6	31.6	16	37.2	18	41.9	23	24.2	31	19.1
Lower	71	16.9	–	–	–	–	5	26.3	12	27.9	6	14.0	28	29.5	20	12.3
Unknown	139	33.2	31	100.0	26	100.0	–	–	–	–	–	–	<5	–	81	50.0

* Cells containing fewer than 5 cases are indicated as "<5". Prevalence estimates based on these cells are indicated as less than the prevalence based on 5 cases in Table A. Percentages based on these cells are not provided in Table B. Cells containing zero cases are indicated as "–". Counts are provided, but prevalences are not estimated, for strata with unknown values in Table A. Counts and percentages are provided for strata with unknown values in Table B.

** Prev = Prevalence.

† Data on Hispanic or Latino ethnicity were available beginning in 1990.

‡ The category of All Other Races includes 9 cases of Black or African American race.

§ Information about socioeconomic status was available only for 1979–2001.

TABLE 49A

DOWN SYNDROME, MATERNAL AGE YOUNGER THAN 35 YEARS: PREVALENCE (PER 10,000 LIVE BIRTHS) STRATIFIED BY DESCRIPTIVE CHARACTERISTICS, MACDP, 1968–2003*

Characteristic	Total		1968–1972		1973–1978		1979–1983		1984–1989		1990–1993		1994–1998		1999–2003	
	Cases	Prev**	Cases	Prev	Cases	Prev	Cases	Prev	Cases	Prev	Cases	Prev	Cases	Prev	Cases	Prev
Total	874	7.09	87	6.34	92	6.41	115	8.48	150	7.40	101	6.54	154	7.37	175	7.00
Maternal age (years)																
<25	314	6.39	42	5.37	44	6.02	40	6.61	52	6.61	34	6.22	50	7.43	52	6.60
25–29	246	6.97	27	7.25	26	5.86	31	7.37	44	6.94	31	6.89	39	7.05	48	7.33
≥30	314	8.12	18	8.28	22	8.67	44	13.39	54	8.91	36	6.59	65	7.55	75	7.10
Unknown	–	–	–	–	–	–	–	–	–	–	–	–	–	–	–	–
Maternal race/ethnicity†																
White	479	7.15	60	6.09	63	6.78	68	8.19	101	8.24	54	6.80	67	6.83	66	6.90
Black or African American	278	6.62	–	–	28	5.70	45	8.90	47	6.20	38	5.92	59	7.00	61	6.34
Hispanic or Latino	57	8.77	–	–	–	–	–	–	–	–	<5	<8.47	16	9.65	40	9.41
All Other Races	50	7.36	27‡	6.98	<5	<33.81	<5	<26.07	<5	<11.48	8	16.92	9	9.38	7	4.58
Unknown	<5	–	–	–	–	–	–	–	–	–	–	–	<5	–	<5	–
Birth weight (grams)																
<2500	221	20.95	19	15.76	20	16.21	29	24.74	30	18.45	22	16.44	50	27.96	51	23.34
≥2500	644	5.73	67	5.38	70	5.41	86	6.95	120	6.44	79	5.61	101	5.29	121	5.30
Unknown	9	–	<5	–	<5	–	–	–	–	–	–	–	<5	–	<5	–
Gestational age (weeks)																
20–36	185	16.17	10	9.45	15	12.41	16	12.98	23	11.65	20	12.58	45	23.12	56	23.06
≥37	683	6.48	77	6.64	77	6.39	99	8.76	125	7.47	78	5.99	109	5.88	118	5.31
Unknown	6	–	–	–	–	–	–	–	<5	–	<5	–	–	–	<5	–
Sex																
Male	477	7.57	51	7.27	48	6.50	71	10.22	68	6.54	60	7.61	85	7.98	94	7.39
Female	397	6.59	36	5.37	44	6.31	44	6.66	82	8.30	41	5.43	69	6.74	81	6.59
Ambiguous/Unknown	–	–	–	–	–	–	–	–	–	–	–	–	–	–	–	–
Parity																
1 Live birth	366	6.76	36	6.90	35	4.84	45	7.09	57	6.36	45	6.73	65	7.08	83	7.87
2 or more live births	489	7.28	39	5.42	56	7.86	70	9.71	89	8.13	56	6.43	89	7.66	90	6.28
Unknown	19	–	12	–	<5	–	–	–	<5	–	<5	–	–	–	<5	–
Gravidity																
1 Pregnancy	268	5.78	35	7.20	28	4.18	35	5.34	42	5.95	31	5.95	43	5.90	54	6.20
2 or more pregnancies	603	8.07	51	6.76	64	8.37	80	11.42	107	8.34	70	6.88	111	8.24	120	7.50
Unknown	<5	–	<5	–	–	–	–	–	<5	–	–	–	–	–	<5	–
Plurality																
Singleton	855	7.12	86	6.38	89	6.33	113	8.51	148	7.47	99	6.59	148	7.30	172	7.12
Multiple	18	5.76	<5	<20.05	<5	<18.50	<5	<18.44	<5	<10.81	<5	<12.25	6	9.66	<5	<5.95
Unknown	<5	–	–	–	–	–	–	–	<5	–	–	–	–	–	–	–

TABLE 49B

DOWN SYNDROME, MATERNAL AGE YOUNGER THAN 35 YEARS: PERCENTAGE OF CASES BY DESCRIPTIVE CHARACTERISTICS, MACDP, 1968–2003*

| | Total | | Period | | | | | | | | | | | | | |
| | | | 1968–1972 | | 1973–1978 | | 1979–1983 | | 1984–1989 | | 1990–1993 | | 1994–1998 | | 1999–2003 | |
Characteristic	Cases	Percent	Cases	Percent	Cases	Percent	Cases	Percent	Cases	Percent	Cases	Percent	Cases	Percent	Cases	Percent
Birth outcome																
Live birth	836	95.7	86	98.9	92	100.0	115	100.0	147	98.0	98	97.0	141	91.6	157	89.7
Stillbirth	13	1.5	<5	–	–	–	–	–	<5	–	<5	–	<5	–	5	2.9
Elective termination	25	2.9	–	–	–	–	–	–	–	–	<5	–	10	6.5	13	7.4
Unknown	–	–	–	–	–	–	–	–	–	–	–	–	–	–	–	–
Age at diagnosis																
Prenatally or <7 days	813	93.0	81	93.1	83	90.2	109	94.8	145	96.7	95	94.1	143	92.9	157	89.7
8 days–6 months	37	4.2	5	5.7	7	7.6	5	4.3	<5	–	<5	–	8	5.2	<5	–
6 months–1 year	8	0.9	<5	–	<5	–	<5	–	<5	–	<5	–	<5	–	–	–
1–5 years	–	–	–	–	–	–	–	–	–	–	–	–	–	–	–	–
>5 years	–	–	–	–	–	–	–	–	–	–	–	–	–	–	–	–
Unknown	16	1.8	–	–	–	–	–	–	–	–	–	–	<5	–	14	8.0
Socioeconomic status§																
Upper	199	22.8	–	–	–	–	35	30.4	55	36.7	43	42.6	40	26.0	26	14.9
Middle	213	24.3	–	–	–	–	32	27.8	56	37.3	31	30.7	53	34.4	41	23.4
Lower	197	22.5	–	–	–	–	47	40.9	39	26.0	25	24.8	57	37.0	29	16.6
Unknown	265	30.3	87	100.0	92	100.0	<5	–	–	–	<5	–	<5	–	79	45.1

* Cells containing fewer than 5 cases are indicated as "<5". Prevalence estimates based on these cells are indicated as less than the prevalence based on 5 cases in Table A. Percentages based on these cells are not provided in Table B. Cells containing zero cases are indicated as "—". Counts are provided, but prevalences are not estimated, for strata with unknown values in Table A. Counts and percentages are provided for strata with unknown values in Table B.

** Prev = Prevalence.

† Data on Hispanic or Latino ethnicity were available beginning in 1990.

‡ The category of All Other Races includes 26 cases of Black or African American race.

§ Information about socioeconomic status was available only for 1979–2001.

TABLE 50A

ANY AUTOSOMAL TRISOMY, MATERNAL AGE 35 YEARS OR OLDER: PREVALENCE (PER 10,000 LIVE BIRTHS) STRATIFIED BY DESCRIPTIVE CHARACTERISTICS, MACDP, 1968–2003*

Characteristic	Total		Period 1968–1972		1973–1978		1979–1983		1984–1989		1990–1993		1994–1998		1999–2003	
	Cases	Prev**	Cases	Prev	Cases	Prev	Cases	Prev	Cases	Prev	Cases	Prev	Cases	Prev	Cases	Prev
Total	528	4.29	34	2.48	32	2.23	24	1.77	53	2.61	59	3.82	122	5.84	204	8.16
Maternal age (years)																
<25	—	—	—	—	—	—	—	—	—	—	—	—	—	—	—	—
25–29	—	—	—	—	—	—	—	—	—	—	—	—	—	—	—	—
≥30	525	13.65	34	15.64	32	12.61	24	7.30	53	8.75	59	10.80	122	14.17	204	19.32
Unknown	—	—	—	—	—	—	—	—	—	—	—	—	—	—	—	—
Maternal race/ethnicity†																
White	286	4.27	24	2.44	18	1.94	17	2.05	30	2.45	32	4.03	71	7.24	94	9.83
Black or African American	189	4.50	—	—	14	2.85	7	1.38	21	2.77	26	4.05	38	4.51	83	8.62
Hispanic or Latino	26	4.00	—	—	—	—	—	—	—	—	—	—	6	3.62	20	4.71
All Other Races	27	3.55	10‡	2.58	—	—	—	—	<5	<11.48	<5	<10.58	7	7.29	7	4.58
Unknown	—	—	—	—	—	—	—	—	—	—	—	—	—	—	—	—
Birth weight (grams)																
<2500	199	18.86	10	8.29	9	7.29	6	5.12	15	9.22	30	22.42	50	27.96	79	36.15
≥2500	320	2.85	24	1.93	22	1.70	17	1.37	36	1.93	29	2.06	69	3.61	123	5.39
Unknown	9	—	—	—	<5	—	<5	—	<5	—	—	—	<5	—	<5	—
Gestational age (weeks)																
20–36	191	16.70	<5	<4.73	7	5.79	7	5.68	23	11.65	27	16.98	46	23.63	78	32.12
≥37	330	3.13	31	2.67	25	2.08	17	1.50	28	1.67	30	2.31	74	4.00	125	5.63
Unknown	7	—	—	—	—	—	—	—	<5	—	<5	—	<5	—	<5	—
Sex																
Male	275	4.37	18	2.56	13	1.76	10	1.44	27	2.60	39	4.95	63	5.91	105	8.26
Female	253	4.20	16	2.39	19	2.73	14	2.12	26	2.63	20	2.65	59	5.77	99	8.06
Ambiguous/Unknown	—	—	—	—	—	—	—	—	—	—	—	—	—	—	—	—
Parity																
1 Live birth	88	1.62	<5	<0.96	<5	<0.69	<5	<0.79	5	0.56	11	1.65	31	3.38	35	3.32
2 or more live births	426	6.35	22	3.06	29	4.07	21	2.91	47	4.29	48	5.51	90	7.75	169	11.80
Unknown	14	—	11	—	<5	—	—	—	<5	—	—	—	<5	—	—	—
Gravidity																
1 Pregnancy	48	1.04	<5	<1.03	<5	<0.75	<5	<0.76	<5	<0.71	7	1.34	14	1.92	19	2.18
2 or more pregnancies	476	6.37	31	4.11	29	3.79	22	3.14	50	3.90	52	5.11	107	7.94	185	11.56
Unknown	<5	—	<5	—	—	—	—	—	—	—	—	—	<5	—	—	—
Plurality																
Singleton	505	4.21	33	2.45	31	2.20	24	1.81	51	2.57	57	3.79	118	5.82	191	7.91
Multiple	23	7.36	<5	<20.05	<5	<18.50	—	—	<5	<10.81	<5	<12.25	<5	<8.05	13	15.47
Unknown	—	—	—	—	—	—	—	—	—	—	—	—	—	—	—	—

TABLE 50B

ANY AUTOSOMAL TRISOMY, MATERNAL AGE 35 YEARS OR OLDER: PERCENTAGE OF CASES BY DESCRIPTIVE CHARACTERISTICS, MACDP, 1968–2003*

									Period							
	Total		1968–1972		1973–1978		1979–1983		1984–1989		1990–1993		1994–1998		1999–2003	
Characteristic	Cases	Percent	Cases	Percent	Cases	Percent	Cases	Percent	Cases	Percent	Cases	Percent	Cases	Percent	Cases	Percent
Birth outcome																
Live birth	450	85.2	34	100.0	30	93.8	19	79.2	44	83.0	47	79.7	99	81.1	177	86.8
Stillbirth	40	7.6	–	–	<5	–	5	20.8	7	13.2	5	8.5	10	8.2	11	5.4
Elective termination	38	7.2	–	–	–	–	–	–	<5	–	7	11.9	13	10.7	16	7.8
Unknown	–	–	–	–	–	–	–	–	–	–	–	–	–	–	–	–
Age at diagnosis																
Prenatally or <7 days	498	94.3	33	97.1	32	100.0	22	91.7	52	98.1	58	98.3	118	96.7	183	89.7
8 days–6 months	9	1.7	<5	–	–	–	<5	–	<5	–	–	–	<5	–	<5	–
6 months–1 year	<5	–	–	–	–	–	–	–	–	–	<5	–	<5	–	<5	–
1–5 years	<5	–	–	–	–	–	–	–	–	–	–	–	–	–	<5	–
>5 years	–	–	–	–	–	–	–	–	–	–	–	–	–	–	–	–
Unknown	17	3.2	–	–	–	–	–	–	–	–	–	–	<5	–	15	7.4
Socioeconomic status§																
Upper	148	28.0	–		–		12	50.0	19	35.8	23	39.0	54	44.3	40	19.6
Middle	116	22.0	–		–		6	25.0	18	34.0	24	40.7	29	23.8	39	19.1
Lower	97	18.4	–		–		6	25.0	16	30.2	11	18.6	38	31.1	26	12.7
Unknown	167	31.6	34	100.0	32	100.0	–	–	–	–	<5	–	<5	–	99	48.5

* Cells containing fewer than 5 cases are indicated as "<5". Prevalence estimates based on these cells are indicated as less than the prevalence based on 5 cases in Table A. Percentages based on these cells are not provided in Table B. Cells containing zero cases are indicated as "–". Counts are provided, but prevalences are not estimated, for strata with unknown values in Table A. Counts and percentages are provided for strata with unknown values in Table B.

** Prev = Prevalence.

† Data on Hispanic or Latino ethnicity were available beginning in 1990.

‡ The category of All Other Races includes 10 cases of Black or African American race.

§ Information about socioeconomic status was available only for 1979–2001.

TABLE 51A

ANY AUTOSOMAL TRISOMY, MATERNAL AGE YOUNGER THAN 35 YEARS: PREVALENCE (PER 10,000 LIVE BIRTHS) STRATIFIED BY DESCRIPTIVE CHARACTERISTICS, MACDP, 1968–2003*

Characteristic	Total		1968–1972		1973–1978		1979–1983		1984–1989		1990–1993		1994–1998		1999–2003	
	Cases	Prev**	Cases	Prev	Cases	Prev	Cases	Prev	Cases	Prev	Cases	Prev	Cases	Prev	Cases	Prev
Total	1,156	9.38	104	7.58	109	7.59	141	10.40	206	10.16	142	9.20	216	10.34	238	9.52
Maternal age (years)																
<25	426	8.67	55	7.03	53	7.25	53	8.76	75	9.54	46	8.42	72	10.69	72	9.13
25–29	331	9.38	30	8.06	32	7.22	40	9.51	55	8.67	47	10.45	53	9.58	74	11.29
≥30	399	10.31	19	8.74	24	9.46	48	14.60	76	12.54	49	8.97	91	10.57	92	8.71
Unknown	–	–	–	–	–	–	–	–	–	–	–	–	–	–	–	–
Maternal race/ethnicity†																
White	611	9.12	72	7.31	73	7.85	85	10.24	131	10.69	70	8.81	95	9.69	85	8.89
Black or African American	397	9.45	–	–	35	7.13	54	10.68	73	9.64	59	9.19	87	10.32	89	9.25
Hispanic or Latino	80	12.31	–	–	–	–	–	–	–	–	<5	<8.47	22	13.26	54	12.71
All Other Races	64	8.41	32‡	8.27	<5	<33.81	<5	<26.07	<5	<11.48	9	19.04	9	9.38	9	5.89
Unknown	<5	–	–	–	–	–	–	–	–	–	–	–	<5	–	–	–
Birth weight (grams)																
<2500	434	41.14	30	24.88	27	21.88	50	42.66	72	44.27	52	38.87	104	58.16	99	45.30
≥2500	704	6.26	72	5.79	79	6.10	91	7.36	134	7.19	90	6.39	107	5.60	131	5.74
Unknown	18	–	<5	–	<5	–	–	–	–	–	–	–	5	–	8	–
Gestational age (weeks)																
20–36	311	27.19	12	11.35	17	14.07	25	20.27	46	23.29	44	27.67	78	40.07	89	36.65
≥37	835	7.92	91	7.84	91	7.55	116	10.26	157	9.38	95	7.30	137	7.40	148	6.66
Unknown	10	–	<5	–	<5	–	–	–	<5	–	<5	–	<5	–	<5	–
Sex																
Male	607	9.64	55	7.84	57	7.72	83	11.95	93	8.95	81	10.28	115	10.80	123	9.67
Female	548	9.10	49	7.31	52	7.46	58	8.78	112	11.33	61	8.08	101	9.87	115	9.36
Ambiguous/Unknown	<5	–	–	–	–	–	–	–	<5	–	–	–	–	–	–	–
Parity																
1 Live birth	467	8.62	45	8.63	42	5.81	55	8.66	76	8.48	55	8.23	82	8.93	112	10.62
2 or more live births	661	9.85	43	5.97	65	9.12	86	11.93	122	11.14	87	9.99	134	11.53	124	8.66
Unknown	28	–	16	–	<5	–	–	–	8	–	–	–	<5	–	<5	–
Gravidity																
1 Pregnancy	344	7.42	44	9.05	35	5.22	44	6.72	54	7.65	37	7.11	54	7.40	76	8.73
2 or more pregnancies	807	10.81	59	7.82	73	9.54	97	13.85	150	11.69	105	10.32	162	12.03	161	10.06
Unknown	5	–	<5	–	<5	–	–	–	<5	–	–	–	–	–	<5	–
Plurality																
Singleton	1,132	9.43	103	7.65	106	7.54	138	10.39	204	10.30	139	9.25	208	10.27	234	9.69
Multiple	23	7.36	<5	<20.05	<5	<18.50	<5	<18.44	<5	<10.81	<5	<12.25	8	12.87	<5	<5.95
Unknown	<5	–	–	–	–	–	–	–	<5	–	–	–	–	–	–	–

TABLE 51B

ANY AUTOSOMAL TRISOMY, MATERNAL AGE YOUNGER THAN 35 YEARS: PERCENTAGE OF CASES BY DESCRIPTIVE CHARACTERISTICS, MACDP, 1968–2003*

	Period															
	Total		1968–1972		1973–1978		1979–1983		1984–1989		1990–1993		1994–1998		1999–2003	
Characteristic	Cases	Percent	Cases	Percent	Cases	Percent	Cases	Percent	Cases	Percent	Cases	Percent	Cases	Percent	Cases	Percent
Birth outcome																
Live birth	1,052	91.0	100	96.2	109	100.0	141	100.0	200	97.1	132	93.0	177	81.9	193	81.1
Stillbirth	49	4.2	<5	–	–	–	–	–	5	2.4	<5	–	16	7.4	20	8.4
Elective termination	55	4.8	–	–	–	–	–	–	<5	–	6	4.2	23	10.6	25	10.5
Unknown	–	–	–	–	–	–	–	–	–	–	–	–	–	–	–	–
Age at diagnosis																
Prenatally or <7 days	1,083	9.37	97	93.3	99	90.8	135	95.7	200	97.1	135	95.1	202	93.5	215	90.3
8 days–6 months	41	3.5	6	5.8	8	7.3	5	3.5	5	2.4	5	3.5	8	3.7	<5	–
6 months–1 year	8	0.7	<5	–	<5	–	<5	–	<5	–	<5	–	<5	–	–	–
1–5 years	–	–	–	–	–	–	–	–	–	–	–	–	–	–	–	–
>5 years	–	–	–	–	–	–	–	–	1	–	–	–	–	–	–	–
Unknown	24	2.1	–	–	–	–	–	–	–	–	–	–	5	2.3	19	8.0
Socioeconomic status§																
Upper	276	23.9	–	–	–	–	47	33.3	78	37.9	58	40.8	58	26.9	35	14.7
Middle	272	23.5	–	–	–	–	36	25.5	68	33.0	44	31.0	71	32.9	53	22.3
Lower	277	24.0	–	–	–	–	56	39.7	60	29.1	38	26.8	81	37.5	42	17.6
Unknown	331	28.6	104	100.0	109	100.0	<5	–	–	–	<5	–	6	2.8	108	45.4

* Cells containing fewer than 5 cases are indicated as "<5". Prevalence estimates based on these cells are indicated as less than the prevalence based on 5 cases in Table A. Percentages based on these cells are not provided in Table B. Cells containing zero cases are indicated as "–". Counts are provided, but prevalences are not estimated, for strata with unknown values in Table A. Counts and percentages are provided for strata with unknown values in Table B.
** Prev = Prevalence.
† Data on Hispanic or Latino ethnicity were available beginning in 1990.
‡ The category of All Other Races includes 31 cases of Black or African American race.
§ Information about socioeconomic status was available only for 1979–2001.

TABLE 52A

SELECTED DEFECTS: TOTAL PREVALENCE (PER 10,000 LIVE BIRTHS) STRATIFIED BY DESCRIPTIVE CHARACTERISTICS, MACDP, 1968–2003*

Characteristic	Anophthalmia		Truncus arteriosus		Pulmonary atresia		Levo transposition of the great arteries		Vascular ring		Ebstein anomaly		Choanal atresia or stenosis		Large intestinal atresia or stenosis	
	Cases	Prev**	Cases	Prev	Cases	Prev	Cases	Prev	Cases	Prev	Cases	Prev	Cases	Prev	Cases	Prev
Total	62	0.50	44	0.54	37	0.45	27	0.33	86	1.05	45	0.55	152	1.23	25	0.20
Maternal age (years)																
<25	35	0.71	21	0.75	15	0.54	9	0.32	26	0.93	15	0.54	49	1.00	9	0.18
25–29	15	0.43	6	0.26	7	0.31	6	0.26	21	0.92	15	0.65	46	1.30	5	0.14
≥30	12	0.31	17	0.55	15	0.49	12	0.39	39	1.27	15	0.49	57	1.47	11	0.28
Unknown	–	–	–	–	–	–	–	–	–	–	–	–	–	–	–	–
Maternal race/ethnicity†																
White	41	0.61	23	0.58	15	0.38	12	0.30	49	1.24	28	0.71	93	1.39	16	0.24
Black or African American	14	0.33	12	0.37	17	0.53	11	0.34	27	0.84	10	0.31	44	1.05	7	0.17
Hispanic or Latino	<5	<0.77	6	0.92	<5	<0.77	<5	<0.77	7	1.08	<5	<0.77	7	1.08	–	–
All Other Races	<5	<0.66	<5	<1.47	<5	<1.47	<5	<1.47	<5	<1.47	<5	<1.47	8	1.05	<5	<0.66
Unknown	–	–	–	–	<5	–	–	–	–	–	–	–	–	–	–	–
Birth weight (grams)																
<2500	38	3.60	17	2.45	9	1.30	<5	<0.72	17	2.45	7	1.01	42	3.98	9	0.85
≥2500	24	0.21	27	0.36	28	0.38	25	0.33	69	0.92	38	0.51	110	0.98	16	0.14
Unknown	–	–	–	–	–	–	–	–	–	–	–	–	–	–	–	–
Gestational age (weeks)																
20–36	26	2.27	13	1.64	5	0.63	<5	<0.63	15	1.89	11	1.39	47	4.11	10	0.87
≥37	36	0.34	31	0.44	30	0.43	22	0.31	71	1.01	34	0.48	102	0.97	15	0.14
Unknown	–	–	–	–	<5	–	<5	–	–	–	–	–	<5	–	–	–
Sex																
Male	24	0.38	22	0.53	23	0.55	22	0.53	56	1.34	20	0.48	74	1.17	18	0.29
Female	37	0.61	22	0.55	14	0.35	5	0.13	30	0.75	25	0.63	78	1.30	7	0.12
Ambiguous/Unknown	<5	–	–	–	–	–	–	–	–	–	–	–	–	–	–	–
Parity																
1 Live birth	28	0.52	15	0.42	17	0.48	12	0.34	40	1.13	18	0.51	65	1.20	15	0.28
2 or more live births	33	0.49	29	0.64	19	0.42	14	0.31	45	0.99	26	0.57	87	1.30	10	0.15
Unknown	<5	–	–	–	<5	–	<5	–	<5	–	<5	–	–	–	–	–
Gravidity																
1 Pregnancy	18	0.39	9	0.32	14	0.50	8	0.28	26	0.92	12	0.42	47	1.01	11	0.24
2 or more pregnancies	44	0.59	35	0.67	23	0.44	18	0.34	60	1.14	32	0.61	105	1.41	14	0.19
Unknown	–	–	–	–	–	–	<5	–	–	–	<5	–	–	–	–	–
Plurality																
Singleton	59	0.49	40	0.50	35	0.44	27	0.34	80	1.01	44	0.56	143	1.19	25	0.21
Multiple	<5	<1.60	<5	<2.14	<5	–	–	–	6	2.57	<5	<2.14	9	2.88	–	–
Unknown	–	–	–	–	–	–	–	–	–	–	–	–	–	–	–	–

TABLE 52B
SELECTED DEFECTS: PERCENTAGE OF CASES BY DESCRIPTIVE CHARACTERISTICS, MACDP, 1968–2003*

Defects

Characteristic	Anophthalmia		Truncus arteriosus		Pulmonary atresia		Levo transposition of the great arteries		Vascular ring		Ebstein anomaly		Choanal atresia or stenosis		Large intestinal atresia or stenosis	
	Cases	Percent	Cases	Percent	Cases	Percent	Cases	Percent	Cases	Percent	Cases	Percent	Cases	Percent	Cases	Percent
Birth outcome																
1 Live birth	49	79.0	41	93.2	36	97.3	27	100.0	86	100.0	40	88.9	150	98.7	24	96.0
Stillbirth	12	19.4	<5	–	–	–	–	–	–	–	5	11.1	<5	–	<5	–
Elective termination	<5	–	<5	–	<5	–	–	–	–	–	–	–	–	–	–	–
Unknown	–	–	–	–	–	–	–	–	–	–	–	–	–	–	–	–
Age at diagnosis																
Prenatally or <7 days	57	91.9	38	86.4	35	94.6	22	81.5	36	41.9	40	88.9	133	87.5	24	96.0
8 days–6 months	<5	–	<5	–	<5	–	<5	–	24	27.9	<5	–	11	7.2	–	–
6 months–1 year	<5	–	–	–	–	–	–	–	13	15.1	–	–	<5	–	–	–
1–5 years	–	–	–	–	–	–	–	–	8	0.0	–	–	<5	–	–	–
>5 years	–	–	–	–	–	–	–	–	<5	–	–	–	<5	–	–	–
Unknown	<5	–	<5	–	<5	–	<5	–	<5	–	<5	–	<5	–	<5	–
Socioeconomic status§																
Upper	17	27.4	14	31.8	9	24.3	<5	–	27	31.4	15	33.3	48	31.6	5	20.0
Middle	8	0.0	10	22.7	13	35.1	7	25.9	26	30.2	17	37.8	40	26.3	9	36.0
Lower	5	24.2	11	25.0	9	24.3	10	37.0	15	17.4	5	11.1	22	14.5	<5	–
Unknown	22	35.5	9	20.5	6	16.2	6	22.2	18	20.9	8	17.8	42	27.6	7	28.0

* Cells containing fewer than 5 cases are indicated as "<5". Prevalence estimates based on these cells are indicated as less than the prevalence based on 5 cases in Table A. Percentages based on these cells are not provided in Table B. Cells containing zero cases are indicated as "–". Counts are provided, but prevalences are not estimated, for strata with unknown values in Table A. Counts and percentages are provided for strata with unknown values in Table B.

** Prev = Prevalence.

† Data on Hispanic or Latino ethnicity were available beginning in 1990.

§ Information about socioeconomic status was available only for 1979–2001.

TABLE 53A

SELECTED DEFECTS: TOTAL PREVALENCE (PER 10,000 LIVE BIRTHS) STRATIFIED BY DESCRIPTIVE CHARACTERISTICS, MACDP, 1968–2003*

| | Birth Defects | | | | | | | | | | | | | | | |
| | Biliary atresia | | Exstrophy of the bladder | | Posterior urethral valves | | Intercalary limb deficiency | | Longitudinal limb deficiency | | Split-hand and/or split-foot malformation | | Other and unspecified limb deficiency | | Urethral obstruction sequence | |
Characteristic	Cases	Prev**	Cases	Prev	Cases	Prev	Cases	Prev	Cases	Prev	Cases	Prev	Cases	Prev	Cases	Prev
Total	**98**	**0.80**	**19**	**0.15**	**137**	**1.11**	**40**	**0.32**	**176**	**1.43**	**49**	**0.40**	**26**	**0.21**	**50**	**0.41**
Maternal age (years)																
<25	46	0.94	8	0.16	59	1.20	15	0.31	83	1.69	18	0.37	11	0.22	22	0.45
25–29	27	0.77	8	0.23	33	0.94	14	0.40	36	1.02	12	0.34	<5	<0.14	14	0.40
≥30	25	0.65	<5	<0.13	44	1.14	11	0.28	57	1.47	19	0.49	11	0.28	14	0.36
Unknown	–	–	–	–	<5	–	–	–	–	–	–	–	–	–	–	–
Maternal race/ethnicity†																
White	42	0.63	15	0.22	52	0.78	27	0.40	93	1.39	27	0.40	14	0.21	26	0.39
Black or African American	44	1.05	<5	<0.12	75	1.78	9	0.21	61	1.45	18	0.43	10	–	18	0.43
Hispanic or Latino	<5	<0.77	–	–	<5	<0.77	–	–	12	1.85	<5	<0.77	<5	<0.77	<5	<0.77
All Other Races	9	1.18	<5	<0.66	6	0.79	<5	<0.66	10	1.31	–	–	–	–	5	0.66
Unknown	–	–	–	–	<5	–	–	–	–	–	<5	–	<5	–	–	–
Birth weight (grams)																
<2500	23	2.18	<5	<0.47	38	3.60	24	2.27	72	6.82	20	1.90	13	1.23	22	2.09
≥2500	73	0.65	16	0.14	98	0.87	15	0.13	102	0.91	29	0.26	13	0.12	28	0.25
Unknown	<5	–	–	–	<5	–	<5	–	<5	–	–	–	–	–	–	–
Gestational age (weeks)																
20–36	20	1.75	<5	<0.44	48	4.20	16	1.40	58	5.07	16	1.40	11	0.96	24	2.10
≥37	75	0.71	16	0.15	89	0.84	21	0.20	116	1.10	33	0.31	14	0.13	26	0.25
Unknown	<5	–	–	–	–	–	<5	–	<5	–	–	–	<5	–	–	–
Sex																
Male	51	0.81	10	0.16	137	2.18	21	0.33	97	1.54	23	0.37	14	0.22	45	0.71
Female	47	0.78	8	0.13	–	–	19	0.32	74	1.23	25	0.42	12	0.20	5	0.08
Ambiguous/Unknown	–	–	<5	–	–	–	–	–	5	–	<5	–	–	–	–	–
Parity																
1 Live birth	48	0.89	5	0.09	58	1.07	13	0.24	80	1.48	22	0.41	11	0.20	23	0.42
2 or more live births	47	0.70	13	0.19	75	1.12	24	0.36	90	1.34	25	0.37	15	0.22	27	0.40
Unknown	<5	–	<5	–	<5	–	<5	–	6	–	<5	–	–	–	–	–
Gravidity																
1 Pregnancy	37	0.80	<5	<0.11	40	0.86	9	0.19	55	1.19	13	0.28	10	0.22	16	0.35
2 or more pregnancies	60	0.80	15	0.20	95	1.27	30	0.40	121	1.62	36	0.48	16	0.21	34	0.46
Unknown	<5	–	–	–	<5	–	<5	–	–	–	–	–	–	–	–	–
Plurality																
Singleton	97	0.81	18	0.15	130	1.08	39	0.32	174	1.45	48	0.40	24	0.20	43	0.36
Multiple	<5	<1.60	<5	<1.60	7	2.24	<5	<1.60	<5	<1.60	<5	<1.60	<5	<1.60	7	2.24
Unknown	–	–	–	–	–	–	–	–	–	–	–	–	–	–	–	–

TABLE 53B

SELECTED DEFECTS: PERCENTAGE OF CASES BY DESCRIPTIVE CHARACTERISTICS, MACDP, 1968–2003*

Birth Defects

Characteristic	Biliary atresia		Exstrophy of the bladder		Posterior urethral valves		Intercalary limb deficiency		Longitudinal limb deficiency		Split-hand and/or split-foot malformation		Other and unspecified limb deficiency		Urethral obstruction sequence	
	Cases	Percent	Cases	Percent	Cases	Percent	Cases	Percent	Cases	Percent	Cases	Percent	Cases	Percent	Cases	Percent
Birth outcome																
Live birth	96	98.0	17	89.5	132	96.4	34	85.0	160	90.9	47	95.9	19	73.1	46	92.0
Stillbirth	<5	–	<5	–	<5	–	<5	–	12	6.8	<5	–	<5	–	<5	–
Elective termination	–	–	–	–	<5	–	<5	–	<5	–	–	–	<5	–	<5	–
Unknown	–	–	–	–	–	–	–	–	–	–	–	–	–	–	–	–
Age at diagnosis																
Prenatally or <7 days	21	21.4	19	100.0	94	68.6	39	97.5	172	97.7	47	95.9	23	88.5	47	94.0
8 days–6 months	73	74.5	–	–	26	19.0	<5	–	–	–	<5	–	<5	–	<5	–
6 months–1 year	<5	–	–	–	<5	–	–	–	–	–	–	–	<5	–	–	–
1–5 years	–	–	–	–	<5	–	–	–	–	–	–	–	–	–	–	–
>5 Years	–	–	–	–	–	–	–	–	<5	–	–	–	<5	–	–	–
Unknown	<5	–	–	–	10	7.3	–	–	–	–	–	–	–	–	<5	–
Socioeconomic status§																
Upper	19	19.4	<5	–	19	13.9	5	12.5	36	20.5	9	18.4	<5	–	9	18.0
Middle	20	20.4	<5	–	36	26.3	12	30.0	31	17.6	7	14.3	<5	–	16	32.0
Lower	24	24.5	<5	–	42	30.7	5	12.5	45	25.6	16	32.7	<5	–	9	18.0
Unknown	35	35.7	9	47.4	40	29.2	18	45.0	64	36.4	17	34.7	16	61.5	16	32.0

* Cells containing fewer than 5 cases are indicated as "<5". Prevalence estimates based on these cells are indicated as less than the prevalence based on 5 cases in Table A. Percentages based on these cells are not provided in Table B. Cells containing zero cases are indicated as "–". Counts are provided, but prevalences are not estimated, for strata with unknown values in Table A. Counts and percentages are provided for strata with unknown values in Table B.
** Prev = Prevalence.
† Data on Hispanic or Latino ethnicity were available beginning in 1990.
§ Information about socioeconomic status was available only for 1979–2001.

TABLE 54A

SELECTED DEFECTS: TOTAL PREVALENCE (PER 10,000 LIVE BIRTHS) STRATIFIED BY DESCRIPTIVE CHARACTERISTICS, MACDP, 1968–2003*

	Birth Defects											
	Trisomy 13, maternal age 35 years or older		Trisomy 13, maternal age younger than 35 years		Trisomy 18, maternal age 35 years or older		Trisomy 18, maternal age younger than 35 years		Turner syndrome		Conjoined twins	
Characteristic	Cases	Prev**	Cases	Prev	Cases	Prev	Cases	Prev	Cases	Prev	Cases	Prev
Total	**27**	**0.22**	**104**	**0.84**	**71**	**0.58**	**150**	**1.22**	**110**	**0.89**	**15**	**0.12**
Maternal age (years)												
<25	–	–	42	0.85	–	–	59	1.20	36	0.73	5	0.10
25–29	–	–	33	0.94	–	–	43	1.22	31	0.88	8	0.23
≥30	27	0.70	29	0.75	71	1.84	48	1.24	43	1.11	<5	<0.13
Unknown	–	–	–	–	–	–	–	–	–	–	–	–
Maternal race/ethnicity†												
White	18	0.27	46	0.69	26	0.39	73	1.09	66	0.98	13	0.19
Black or African American	7	0.17	47	1.12	38	0.90	59	1.40	28	0.67	<5	<0.12
Hispanic or Latino	<5	<0.77	8	1.23	<5	<0.77	13	2.00	11	1.69	–	–
All Other Races	–	–	<5	<0.66	<5	<0.66	5	0.66	<5	<0.66	<5	<0.66
Unknown	–	–	–	–	–	–	–	–	<5	–	–	–
Birth weight (grams)												
<2500	17	1.61	60	5.69	56	5.31	136	12.89	41	3.89	<5	<0.47
≥2500	8	0.07	40	0.36	10	0.09	11	0.10	67	0.60	11	0.10
Unknown	<5	–	<5	–	5	–	<5	–	<5	–	–	–
Gestational age (weeks)												
20–36	18	1.57	44	3.85	40	3.50	66	5.77	46	4.02	8	0.70
≥37	8	0.08	57	0.54	29	0.28	83	0.79	63	0.60	7	0.07
Unknown	<5	–	<5	–	<5	–	<5	–	<5	–	–	–
Sex												
Male	9	0.14	56	0.89	28	0.44	63	1.00	5	0.08	6	0.10
Female	18	0.30	47	0.78	43	0.71	87	1.44	103	1.71	9	0.15
Ambiguous/Unknown	–	–	<5	–	–	–	–	–	<5	–	–	–
Parity												
1 Live birth	<5	<0.09	38	0.70	9	0.17	52	0.96	54	1.00	<5	<0.09
2 or more live births	23	0.34	63	0.94	60	0.89	93	1.39	55	0.82	10	0.15
Unknown	–	–	<5	–	<5	–	5	–	<5	–	<5	–
Gravidity												
1 Pregnancy	<5	<0.11	26	0.56	<5	<0.11	44	0.95	39	0.84	<5	<0.11
2 or more pregnancies	24	0.32	77	1.03	67	0.90	105	1.41	71	0.95	11	0.15
Unknown	–	–	<5	–	–	–	<5	–	–	–	–	–
Plurality												
Singleton	26	0.22	103	0.86	67	0.56	146	1.22	107	0.89	<5	<0.04
Multiple	<5	<1.60	<5	<1.60	<5	<1.60	<5	<1.60	<5	<1.60	14	4.48
Unknown	–	–	–	–	–	–	–	–	<5	–	–	–

TABLE 54B

SELECTED DEFECTS: PERCENTAGE OF CASES BY DESCRIPTIVE CHARACTERISTICS, MACDP, 1968–2003*

Birth Defects

Characteristic	Trisomy 13, maternal age 35 years or older		Trisomy 13, maternal age younger than 35 years		Trisomy 18, maternal age 35 years or older		Trisomy 18, maternal age younger than 35 years		Turner syndrome		Conjoined twins	
	Cases	Percent	Cases	Percent	Cases	Percent	Cases	Percent	Cases	Percent	Cases	Percent
Birth outcome												
Live birth	18	66.7	83	79.8	43	60.6	109	72.7	74	67.3	13	86.7
Stillbirth	5	18.5	9	8.7	20	28.2	25	16.7	23	20.9	<5	–
Elective termination	<5	–	12	11.5	8	11.3	16	10.7	13	11.8	<5	–
Unknown	–	–	–	–	–	–	–	–	–	–	–	–
Age at diagnosis												
Prenatally or <7 days	26	96.3	97	93.3	66	93.0	147	98.0	101	91.8	15	100.0
8 days–6 months	–	–	<5	–	<5	–	–	–	5	4.5	–	–
6 months–1 year	–	–	–	–	–	–	–	–	<5	–	–	–
1–5 years	–	–	–	–	–	–	–	–	<5	–	–	–
>5 years	–	–	–	–	–	–	–	–	–	–	–	–
Unknown	<5	–	5	4.8	<5	–	<5	–	<5	–	–	–
Socioeconomic status§												
Upper	9	33.3	26	25.0	19	26.8	46	30.7	34	30.9	–	–
Middle	8	29.6	26	25.0	12	16.9	27	18.0	31	28.2	<5	–
Lower	6	22.2	26	25.0	18	25.3	42	28.0	22	20.0	<5	–
Unknown	<5	–	26	25.0	22	31.0	35	23.3	23	20.9	10	66.7

* Cells containing fewer than 5 cases are indicated as "<5." Prevalence estimates based on these cells are indicated as less than the prevalence based on 5 cases in Table A. Percentages based on these cells are not provided in Table B. Cells containing zero cases are indicated as "–". Counts are provided, but prevalences are not estimated, for strata with unknown values in Table A. Counts and percentages are provided for strata with unknown values in Table B.
** Prev = Prevalence.
† Data on Hispanic or Latino ethnicity were available beginning in 1990.
§ Information about socioeconomic status was available only for 1979–2001.

APPENDIX II
INFANT MORTALITY STATISTICS

The data in Appendix II is drawn from the Linked Birth and Infant Death Data Set from the National Vital Statistics System, administered by the Centers for Disease Control's National Center for Health Statistics. In the Linked Birth and Infant Death Data Set, information from the death certificate is linked to the birth certificate for each infant under one year of age who dies in the United States, Puerto Rico, the Virgin Islands, and Guam. Information available in the birth certificate is then used to conduct more detailed analyses of infant mortality patterns.

AVERAGE LIFETIME COST PER CHILD WITH SELECTED BIRTH DEFECTS, 2001

Birth Defects	Estimated Cost
Genetic Defects	
Down Syndrome	$647,200
Heart Defects	
Truncus arteriosus	$724,692
Transposition of the great vessels	$383,154
Tetralogy of Fallot	$375,979
Limb Defects	
Reduction defect-lower limbs	$285,572
Reduction defect-upper limbs	$142,068
Muscle Defects	
Diaphragmatic hernia	$358,759
Esophageal atresia/tracheoesophageal fistula	$208,080
Colon, rectal or anal atresia	$176,509
Gastroschisis	$156,419
Neural Tube Defects	
Spina bifida	$421,900
Oral-Facial Defects	
Cleft lip or palate	$144,938

Note: Figures are based on lifetime cost estimates for the 1988 California birth cohort (adjusted for differences in costs and numbers of births between California and the nation and for cost inflation between 1988 and 1992; 1992 cost figures were adjusted for inflation and are presented in 2001 dollars).

Source: Trust for America's Health.

Infant, Neonatal, and Postneonatal Mortality Rates: United States, 1950–2002

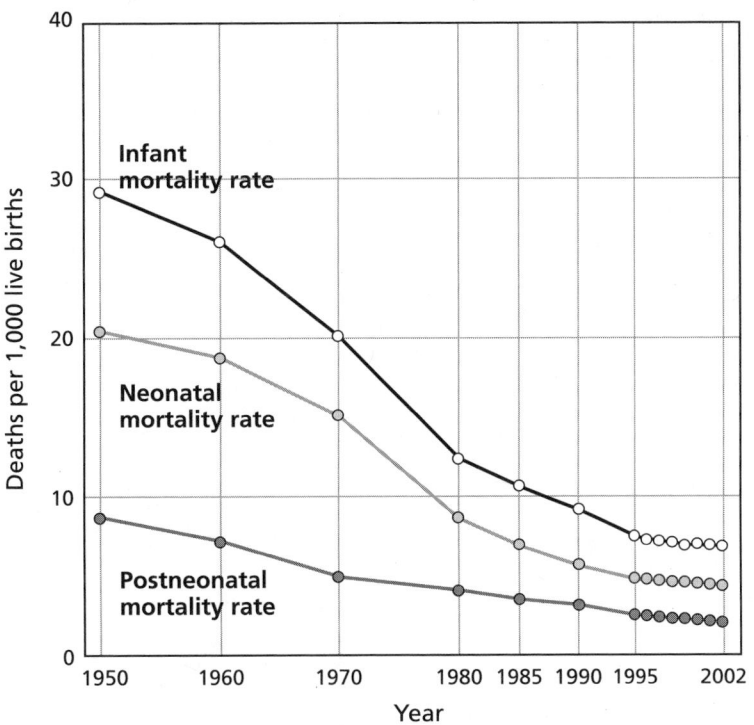

Year	Infant	Neonatal	Postneonatal
	Deaths per 1,000 live births		
1950	29.2	20.5	8.7
1960	26.0	18.7	7.3
1970	20.0	15.1	4.9
1980	12.6	8.5	4.1
1985	10.6	7.0	3.7
1990	9.2	5.8	3.4
1995	7.6	4.9	2.7
1996	7.3	4.8	2.5
1997	7.2	4.8	2.5
1998	7.2	4.8	2.4
1999	7.1	4.7	2.3
2000	6.9	4.6	2.3
2001	6.8	4.5	2.3
2002	7.0	4.7	2.3

Notes: "Infant" is defined as under 1 year of age, "neonatal" as under 28 days of age, and "postneonatal" as between 28 days and 1 year of age. See Data Table for data points graphed and additional notes.

Source: Centers for Disease Control and Prevention, National Center for Health Statistics, National Vital Statistics System.

© Infobase Publishing

INFANT MORTALITY RATES BY DETAILED RACE AND ORIGIN OF MOTHER: UNITED STATES, 2000–2002

Race and origin of mother	Infant deaths per 1,000 live birth
White, not Hispanic or Latino	5.7
Black or African American, not Hispanic or Latino	13.6
Hispanic or Latino	5.5
Puerto Rican	8.3
Other and unknown Hispanic or Latino	6.7
Mexican	5.4
Central and South American	4.9
Cuban	4.2
Asian or Pacific Islander	4.8
Hawaiian	8.7
Filipino	5.7
Other Asian or Pacific Islander	4.8
Japanese	4.5
Chinese	3.2
American Indian or Alaska Native	8.9

NOTES: Infant is defined as under 1 year of age. Persons of Hispanic origin may be of any race. Asian or Pacific Islander and American Indian or Alaska Native races include persons of Hispanic and non-Hispanic origin.

SOURCE: Centers for Disease Control and Prevention, National Center for Health Statistics, National Vital Statistics System, National Linked Birth/Infant Death Data Sets.

INFANT, NEONATAL, AND POSTNEONATAL DEATHS AND MORTALITY RATES BY SPECIFIED RACE OR NATIONAL ORIGIN OF MOTHER: UNITED STATES, 2002

Race of mother	Live births	Number of deaths			Mortality rate per 1,000 live births		
		Infant	Neonatal	Postneonatal	Infant	Neonatal	Postneonatal
All races	4,021,825	27,970	18,791	9,179	7.0	4.7	2.3
White	3,174,807	18,395	12,352	6,044	5.8	3.9	1.9
Black	593,743	8,201	5,533	2,668	13.8	9.3	4.5
American Indian[1]	42,367	366	195	171	8.6	4.6	4.0
Asian or Pacific Islander	210,908	1,006	710	296	4.8	3.4	1.4
Chinese	33,673	101	79	22	3.0	2.4	0.7
Japanese	9,264	45	34	11	4.9	3.7	*
Hawaiian	6,772	65	38	27	9.6	5.6	4.0
Filipino	33,016	190	134	55	5.7	4.1	1.7
Other Asian or Pacific Islander	128,183	605	424	181	4.7	3.3	1.4

* Figure does not meet standard of reliability or precision: based on fewer than 20 deaths in the numerator.
[1]Includes Aleuts and Eskimos.

NOTES: Infant deaths are weighted so numbers may not exactly add to totals due to rounding. Neonatal is less than 28 days, and postneonatal is 28 days to under 1 year.

INFANT, NEONATAL, AND POSTNEONATAL DEATHS AND MORTALITY RATES BY HISPANIC ORIGIN OF MOTHER AND BY RACE OF MOTHER FOR MOTHERS OF NON-HISPANIC ORIGIN: UNITED STATES, 2002

Hispanic origin and race of mother	Live births	Number of deaths			Mortality rate per 1,000 live births		
		Infant	Neonatal	Postneonatal	Infant	Neonatal	Postneonatal
All origins[1]	4,021,825	27,970	18,791	9,179	7.0	4.7	2.3
Total Hispanic	876,654	4,927	3,360	1,567	5.6	3.8	1.8
Mexican	627,510	3,399	2,283	1,116	5.4	3.6	1.8
Puerto Rican	57,469	471	334	137	8.2	5.8	2.4
Cuban	14,232	53	46	7	3.7	3.2	*
Central and South American	125,984	637	435	202	5.1	3.5	1.6
Other and unknown Hispanic	51,459	368	263	105	7.1	5.1	2.0
Non-Hispanic total[2]	3,119,987	22,647	15,109	7,538	7.3	4.8	2.4
Non-Hispanic white	2,298,168	13,327	8,853	4,474	5.8	3.9	1.9
Non-Hispanic black	578,366	8,031	5,399	2,632	13.9	9.3	4.6
Not stated	25,184	395	322	74	. . .	. . .	. . .

* Figure does not meet standard of reliability or precision; based on fewer than 20 deaths in the numerator.
. . . Category not applicable.
[1]Origin of mother not stated included in "All origins" but not distributed among origins.
[2]Includes races other than white or black.

NOTES: Infant deaths are weighted so numbers may not exactly add to totals due to rounding. Neonatal is less than 28 days, and postneonatal is 28 days to under 1 year.

INFANT, NEONATAL, AND POSTNEONATAL DEATHS AND MORTALITY RATES BY RACE OR NATIONAL ORIGIN OF MOTHER: TOTAL OF 11 STATES, 2002

Race of mother	Live births	Number of deaths			Mortality rate per 1,000 live births		
		Infant	Neonatal	Postneonatal	Infant	Neonatal	Postneonatal
All races	1,808,792	11,232	7,501	3,731	6.2	4.1	2.1
Total Asian or Pacific Islander	147,907	674	453	221	4.6	3.1	1.5
Chinese	26,727	83	63	20	3.1	2.4	0.8
Japanese	7,251	35	24	11	4.9	3.4	*
Filipino	26,982	158	111	46	5.8	4.1	1.7
Vietnamese	16,211	60	47	13	3.7	2.9	*
Asian Indian	28,532	105	71	34	3.7	2.5	1.2
Korean	10,430	38	23	15	3.7	2.2	*
Hawaiian	5,931	55	34	21	9.3	5.7	3.5
Samoan	1,616	11	5	6	*	*	*
Guamanian	529	8	2	6	*	*	*
Remaining Asian or Pacific Islander	23,698	119	71	48	5.0	3.0	2.0
White	1,433,745	7,687	5,155	2,532	5.4	3.6	1.8
Black	218,206	2,789	1,855	934	12.8	8.5	4.3
American Indian[1]	8,934	82	37	44	9.1	4.2	4.9

* Figure does not meet standard of reliability or precision; based on fewer than 20 deaths in the numerator.
[1]Includes Aleuts and Eskimos.

NOTES: Infant deaths are weighted so numbers may not exactly add to totals due to rounding. States included are California, Hawaii, Illinois, Minnesota, Missouri, New Jersey, New York, Texas, Virginia, Washington, and West Virginia. Neonatal is less than 28 days, and postneonatal is 28 days to under 1 year.

INFANT MORTALITY RATES BY RACE AND ORIGIN OF MOTHER: UNITED STATES, 1995–2002

Race and Hispanic origin of mother	1995	1996	1997	1998	1999	2000	2001	2002	Percent change 1995 to 2002	Percent change 2001 to 2002
All races	7.6	7.3	7.2	7.2	7.0	6.9	6.8	7.0	−7.9	2.9
White	6.3	6.1	6.0	6.0	5.8	5.7	5.7	5.8	− 7.9	1.8**
Black	14.6	14.1	13.7	13.8	14.0	13.5	13.3	13.8	− 5.5	3.8
American Indian[1]	9.0	10.0	8.7	9.3	9.3	8.3	9.7	8.6	−4.4**	−11.3**
Asian or Pacific Islander	5.3	5.2	5.0	5.5	4.8	4.9	4.7	4.8	−9.4	2.1**
Chinese	3.8	3.2	3.1	4.0	2.9	3.5	3.2	3.0	−21.1**	−6.3**
Japanese	5.3	4.2	5.3	3.5	3.4	4.5	4.0	4.9	−7.5**	22.5**
Hawaiian	6.6	5.6	9.0	10.0	7.1	9.0	7.3	9.6	45. 5**	31.5**
Filipino	5.6	5.8	5.8	6.2	5.8	5.7	5.5	5.7	1.8 **	3.6**
Hispanic	6.3	6.1	6.0	5.8	5.7	5.6	5.4	5.6	− 11.1	3.7**
Mexican	6.0	5.8	5.8	5.6	5.5	5.4	5.2	5.4	−10.0	3.8**
Puerto Rican	8.9	8.6	7.9	7.8	8.3	8.2	8.5	8.2	−79**	−3.5**
Cuban	5.3	5.1	5.5	3.6	4.7	4.6	4.2	3.7	− 30.2**	−11.9**
Central and South American	5.5	5.0	5.5	5.3	4.7	4.6	5.0	5.1	−7.3**	2.0**
Non-Hispanic white	6.3	6.0	6.0	6.0	5.8	5.7	5.7	5.8	−7.9	1.8**
Non-Hispanic black	14.7	14.2	13.7	13.9	14.1	13.6	13.5	13.9	−5.4	3.0**

** Not significant at p<.05.
[1]Includes Aleuts and Eskimos.

INFANT MORTALITY RATES, LIVE BIRTHS, AND INFANT DEATHS, BY SELECTED CHARACTERISTICS AND SPECIFIED RACE OF MOTHER: UNITED STATES, 2002

	infant mortality rate per 1,000 live births in specified group				
		Race of mother			
Characteristics	All races	White	Black	American Indian[1]	Asian or Pacific Islander
Total	7.0	5.8	13.8	8.6	4.8
Age at death:					
Total neonatal	4.7	3.9	9.3	4.6	3.4
Early neonatal (less than 7 days)	3.7	3.1	7.6	3.2	2.7
Late neonatal (7–27 days)	0.9	0.8	1.7	1.4	0.7
Postneonatal	2.3	1.9	4.5	4.0	1.4
Sex:					
Male	7.6	6.4	14.8	9.7	5.1
Female	6.3	5.1	12.8	7.6	4.4
Plurality:					
Single births	6.1	5.0	12.3	7.9	4.3
Plural births	32.3	28.0	55.9	38.4	23.5
Birth weight:					
Less than 2,500 grams	59.5	54.7	76.5	64.2	41.0
Less than 1,500 grams	250.8	242.1	272.1	249.1	218.4
1,500–2,499 grams	15.1	15.3	15.4	24.0	10.7
2,500 grams or more	2.4	2.2	3.9	4.3	1.6
Period of gestation:					
Less than 32 weeks	186.4	175.8	212.9	158.6	163.4
32–36 weeks	9.2	8.7	11.1	13.1	7.3
37–41 weeks	2.5	2.2	4.0	4.3	1.7
42 weeks or more	3.1	2.8	4.7	5.9	2.5
Trimester of pregnancy prenatal care began:					
First trimester	6.2	5.2	12.8	7.9	4.4
After first trimester or no care	9.0	7.6	14.3	9.5	5.3
Second trimester	7.3	6.5	10.5	8.9	4.3
Third trimester	6.0	4.9	9.3	*	4.5
No prenatal care	38.4	29.9	58.0	*	30.5
Age of mother:					
Under 20 years	10.4	8.8	15.2	9.1	9.2
20–24 years	7.8	6.4	13.9	9.4	5.2
25–29 years	6.0	5.1	12.4	7.6	3.9
30–34 years	5.6	4.7	13.4	7.6	4.3
35–39 years	6.5	5.5	14.5	8.5	5.4
40–54 years	8.5	7.3	16.1	*	8.2
Educational attainment of mother:					
0–8 years	6.6	6.1	14.7	*	4.0
9–11 years	9.6	8.0	15.8	8.3	5.9
12 years	7.8	6.5	13.4	9.1	5.6
13–15 years	6.0	4.9	11.7	8.6	4.7
16 years and over	4.2	3.7	9.9	*	3.7

| | | infant mortality rate per 1,000 live births in specified group | | | |
| | | Race of mother | | | |
Characteristics	All races	White	Black	American Indian[1]	Asian or Pacific Islander
Live-birth order:					
1	7.0	5.9	14.2	9.1	4.7
2	6.1	5.2	12.3	8.4	4.0
3	6.6	5.6	12.2	6.8	5.2
4	8.3	6.7	15.1	7.9	7.8
5 or more	11.1	8.7	18.7	11.2	7.7
Marital status:					
Married	5.4	5.0	11.8	7.2	4.4
Unmarried	9.9	7.9	14.8	9.6	7.1
Mother's place of birth:					
Born in the 50 States and DC	7.3	5.9	14.2	8.7	6.6
Born elsewhere	5.1	4.9	8.8	*	4.3
Maternal smoking during pregnancy:[2]					
Smoker	11.1	9.8	20.0	12.1	11.6
Nonsmoker	6.6	5.3	13.1	7.7	4.7
			Live births		
Total	4,021,825	3,174,807	593,743	42,367	210,908
Sex:					
Male	2,058,037	1,626,328	301,530	21,423	108,756
Female	1,963,788	1,548,479	292,213	20,944	102,152
Plurality:					
Single births	3,889,276	3,069,960	572,699	41,362	205,255
Plural births	132,549	104,847	21,044	1,005	5,653
Birth weight:					
Less than 2,500 grams	315,028	216,373	79,137	3,072	16,446
Less than 1,500 grams	59,361	37,569	18,841	549	2,402
1,500–2,499 grams	255,667	178,804	60,296	2,523	14,044
2,500 grams or more	3,705,556	2,957,532	514,367	39286	194,371
Not stated	1,241	902	239	9	91
Period of gestation:					
Less than 32 weeks	77,877	50,326	23,660	868	3,023
32–36 weeks	402,972	299,956	79,801	4,625	18,590
37–41 weeks	3,231,562	2,577,101	448,002	32,923	173,536
42 weeks or more	268,096	214,606	37,956	3,557	11,977
Not stated	41,318	32,818	4,324	394	3,782
Trimester of pregnancy prenatal care began:					
First trimester	3,301,213	2,664,128	434,099	28,833	174,153
After first trimester or no care	641,456	454,505	143,167	12,460	31,324
Second trimester	499,014	357,575	107,393	9,158	24,888
Third trimester	103,325	71,673	23,757	2,548	5,347
No prenatal care	39,117	25,257	12,017	754	1,089
Not stated	79,156	56,174	16,477	1,074	5,431
Age of mother:					
Under 20 years	432,825	309,879	106,993	7,840	8,113
20–24 years	1,022,132	783,010	194,719	14,343	30,060
25–29 years	1,060,420	851,159	136,604	10,138	62,519
30–34 years	951,229	779,538	95,013	6,338	70,340
35–39 years	453,939	369,840	48,393	2,976	32,730
40–54 years	101,280	81,381	12,021	732	7,146
Educational attainment of mother:					
0–8 years	239,622	216,932	13,913	1,705	7,072
9–11 years	614,968	461,280	128,424	11,153	14,111
12 years	1,234,741	937,997	231,845	16,446	48,453
13–15 years	851,738	664,946	135,547	8,828	42,417
16 years and over	1,026,820	854,863	73,837	3,639	94,481
Not stated	53,936	38,789	10,177	596	4,374
Live-birth order:					
1	1,594,949	1,258,506	222,845	14,837	98,761
2	1,306,795	1,049,590	173,145	11,784	72,276
3	675,278	536,537	105,569	7,568	25,604
4	264,268	202,695	49,309	4,087	8,177
5 or more	170,266	119,760	41,063	3,962	5,481
Not stated	10,269	7,719	1,812	129	609
Marital status:					
Married	2,655,815	2,270,333	188,848	17,070	179,564
Unmarried	1,366,010	904,474	404,895	25,297	31,344
Mother's place of birth:					
Born in the 50 States and DC	3,079,253	2,489,080	514,714	39,931	35,528
Born elsewhere	933,408	679,913	76,574	2,362	174,559
Not stated	9,164	5,814	2,455	74	821

See footnotes at end of table.

(table continues)

Characteristics	All races	infant mortality rate per 1,000 live births in specified group — Race of mother			
		White	Black	American Indian[1]	Asian or Pacific Islander
Maternal smoking during pregnancy:[2]					
Smoker	397,199	337,313	48,579	7,672	3,635
Nonsmoker	3,077,208	2,394,749	509,900	31,273	141,286
Not stated	18,046	14,185	2,607	389	865
			Infant deaths		
Total	27,970	18,395	8,201	366	1,006
Age at death:					
Total neonatal	18,791	12,352	5,533	195	710
Early neonatal (less than 7 days)	15,020	9,804	4,506	137	573
Late neonatal (7–27 days)	3,771	2,548	1,027	58	138
Postneonatal	9,179	6,044	2,668	171	296
Sex:					
Male	15,690	10,459	4,467	208	556
Female	12,279	7,936	3,734	158	450
Plurality:					
Single births	23,691	15,465	7,025	328	874
Plural births	4,278	2,931	1,176	39	133
Birthweight:					
Less than 2,500 grams	18,758	11,830	6,056	197	675
Less than 1,500 grams	14,885	9,097	5,127	137	525
1,500–2,499 grams	3,873	2,733	929	61	150
2,500 grams or more	8,840	6,366	1,993	168	313
Not stated	371	199	152	1	19
Period of gestation:					
Less than 32 weeks	14,515	8,845	5,038	138	494
32–36 weeks	3,692	2,612	884	61	135
37–41 weeks	8,001	5,761	1,801	141	298
42 weeks or more	824	594	179	21	29
Not stated	937	582	299	6	50
Trimester of pregnancy prenatal care began:					
First trimester	20,521	13,957	5,569	227	769
After first trimester or no care	5,758	3,433	2,042	118	165
Second trimester	3,637	2,324	1,124	81	108
Third trimester	618	354	222	18	24
No prenatal care	1,503	755	697	18	33
Not stated	1,690	1,005	591	21	73
Age of mother:					
Under 20 years	4,496	2,724	1,626	72	75
20–24 years	8,016	5,014	2,711	135	156
25–29 years	6,352	4,334	1,700	77	241
30–34 years	5,312	3,695	1,269	48	299
35–39 years	2,934	2,031	701	25	176
40–54 years	858	597	194	9	59
Educational attainment of mother:					
0–8 years	1,581	1,332	205	15	28
9–11 years	5,875	3,671	2,027	93	84
12 years	9,641	6,107	3,114	150	270
13–15 years	5,099	3,236	1,587	76	200
16 years and over	4,290	3,192	731	17	349
Not stated	1,484	857	536	16	75
Live-birth order:					
1	11,139	7,383	3,155	134	467
2	7,927	5,410	2,131	99	287
3	4,481	3,008	1,289	51	133
4	2,194	1,352	746	32	64
5 or more	1,898	1,043	769	44	42
Not stated	330	199	112	5	13
Marital status:					
Married	14,404	11,277	2,220	124	783
Unmarried	13,566	7,118	5,981	243	224
Mother's place of birth:					
Born in the 50 States and DC	22,581	14,706	7,293	346	236
Born elsewhere	4,777	3,338	676	16	747
Not stated	612	352	232	4	24
Maternal smoking during pregnancy:[2]					
Smoker	4,406	3,298	973	93	42
Nonsmoker	20,255	12,653	6,693	239	671
Not stated	436	268	146	10	11

* Figure does not meet standard of reliability or precision; based on fewer than 20 deaths in the numerator.
[1] Includes Aleuts and Eskimos.
[2] Excludes data for California, which does not report tobacco use on the birth certificate.

NOTES: Infant deaths are weighted so numbers may not exactly add to totals due to rounding. Not stated responses were included in totals but not distributed among groups for rate computations.

INFANT MORTALITY RATES, LIVE BIRTHS, AND INFANT DEATHS, BY SELECTED CHARACTERISTICS AND ORIGIN OF MOTHER AND BY RACE OF MOTHER: UNITED STATES, 2002

	Infant mortality rates per 1,000 live births in specified group									
		Hispanic						Non-Hispanic		
Characteristics	All origins[1]	Total	Mexican	Puerto Rican	Cuban	Central and South American	Other and unknown Hispanic	Total[2]	White	Black
Total	7.0	5.6	5.4	8.2	3.7	5.1	7.1	7.3	5.8	13.9
Age at death:										
Total neonatal	4.7	3.8	3.6	5.8	3.2	3.5	5.1	4.8	3.9	9.3
Early neonatal (less than 7 days)	3.7	3.0	2.9	4.9	2.7	2.7	4.3	3.9	3.0	7.6
Late neonatal (7–27 days)	0.9	0.8	0.8	0.9	*	0.8	0.9	1.0	0.8	1.8
Postneonatal	2.3	1.8	1.8	2.4	*	1.6	2.0	2.4	1.9	4.6
Sex:										
Male	7.6	6.0	5.9	8.7	4.5	4.9	8.0	8.0	6.5	14.9
Female	6.3	5.2	4.9	7.7	2.9	5.3	6.2	6.5	5.1	12.8
Plurality:										
Single births	6.1	5.1	4.9	7.1	3.2	4.5	6.4	6.3	5.0	12.3
Plural births	32.3	31.1	30.0	42.9	*	27.6	37.7	32.3	27.1	55.9
Birthweight:										
Less than 2,500 grams	59.5	56.7	57.0	59.2	46.6	52.0	62.2	59.7	53.4	76.5
Less than 1,500 grams	250.8	241.8	247.7	234.4	188.6	213.7	268.1	250.9	239.5	272.1
1,500–2,499 grams	15.1	16.1	16.6	14.1	*	15.2	15.3	14.9	14.9	15.4
2,500 grams or more	2.4	2.0	2.0	2.6	*	1.7	2.3	2.5	2.2	3.9
Period of gestation:										
Less than 32 weeks	186.4	160.9	159.3	182.2	144.5	147.6	176.7	191.1	179.9	212.9
32–36 weeks	9.2	8.0	7.8	8.9	*	7.7	10.2	9.4	8.9	11.1
37–41 weeks	2.5	2.1	2.1	2.7	*	1.9	2.3	2.6	2.3	4.1
42 weeks or more	3.1	2.5	2.6	*	*	*	*	3.3	2.9	4.9
Trimester of pregnancy prenatal care began:										
First trimester	6.2	5.3	5.1	7.5	3.4	4.8	6.1	6.4	5.2	12.9
After first trimester or no care	9.0	6.0	5.7	9.7	*	5.5	7.7	10.2	8.6	14.4
Second trimester	7.3	5.2	5.0	7.9	*	4.6	6.5	8.2	7.4	10.5
Third trimester	6.0	3.4	3.3	*	*	*	*	7.1	6.1	9.5
No prenatal care	38.4	23.0	19.7	49.2	*	29.3	36.5	45.5	36.4	57.9
Age of mother:										
Under 20 years	10.4	7.3	6.8	10.6	*	6.8	10.9	11.6	9.7	15.2
20–24 years	7.8	5.3	5.0	8.2	*	4.8	6.5	8.7	6.9	14.0
25–29 years	6.0	5.1	4.8	7.4	*	4.9	6.8	6.2	5.1	12.5
30–34 years	5.6	5.0	5.1	7.2	*	4.4	4.4	5.6	4.6	13.4
35–39 years	6.5	6.2	6.3	7.6	*	5.1	7.3	6.4	5.3	14.6
40–54 years	8.5	8.9	9.2	*	*	8.2	*	8.3	6.8	16.3
Educational attainment of mother:										
0–8 years	6.6	5.3	5.1	11.5	*	5.8	7.6	10.4	9.9	15.2
9–11 years	9.6	6.1	5.7	9.7	*	6.0	7.4	11.7	9.9	15.9
12 years	7.8	5.6	5.3	8.8	*	4.7	7.4	8.4	6.9	13.6
13–15 years	6.0	4.9	5.0	6.0	*	4.3	5.3	6.1	4.8	11.9
16 years and over	4.2	4.0	4.1	3.9	*	4.4	*	4.2	3.7	10.0
Live-birth order:										
1	7.0	5.8	5.7	8.2	3.8	4.9	8.2	7.2	5.8	14.3
2	6.1	5.0	5.0	7.6	*	4.4	5.4	6.3	5.1	12.4
3	6.6	5.3	5.0	7.6	*	5.4	6.2	7.0	5.7	12.2
4	8.3	5.6	5.0	7.8		6.4	9.8	9.4	7.3	15.3
5 or more	11.1	7.9	7.4	13.8	*	7.7	*	12.3	9.1	18.8
Marital status:										
Married	5.4	5.0	5.0	6.9	3.0	4.4	5.8	5.5	4.9	11.8
Unmarried	9.9	6.4	6.0	9.1	5.4	5.9	8.9	11.2	8.8	14.8
Mother's place of birth:										
Born in the 50 States and DC	7.3	6.6	6.3	8.2	3.9	5.5	7.5	7.4	5.8	14.2
Born elsewhere	5.1	5.0	4.8	7.9	3.6	5.0	4.7	5.3	4.6	9.1
Maternal smoking during pregnancy:[3]										
Smoker	11.1	10.7	9.8	12.4	*	*	10.7	11.1	9.7	20.1
Nonsmoker	6.6	5.6	5.4	7.9	3.5	4.9	6.8	6.8	5.2	13.2

See footnotes at end of table.   *(table continues)*

		Live births								
		Hispanic						Non-Hispanic			
Characteristics	All origins[1]	Total	Mexican	Puerto Rican	Cuban	Central and South American	Other and unknown Hispanic	Total[2]	White	Black	Not stated
Total	4,021,825	876,654	627,510	57,469	14,232	125,98 4	51,459	3,119,987	2,298,168	578,366	25,184
Sex:											
Male	2,058,037	447,036	319,627	29,582	7,309	64,395	26,123	1,598,106	1,179,142	293,771	12,895
Female	1,963,788	429,618	307,883	27,887	6,923	61,589	25,336	1,521,881	1,1 19,026	284,595	12,289
Plurality:											
Single births	3,889,276	857,787	615,022	55,709	13,795	123,073	50,188	3,007,230	2,212,465	557,702	24,259
Plural births	132,549	18,867	12,488	1,760	437	2,911	1,271	112,757	85,703	20,664	925
Birthweight:											
Less than 2,500 grams	315,028	57,541	38,728	5,581	926	8,242	4,064	255,406	159,001	77,690	2,081
Less than 1,500 grams	59,361	10,359	6,771	1,143	165	1,526	754	48,494	27,225	18,485	508
1,500–2,499 grams	255,667	47,182	31,957	4,438	761	6,716	3,310	206,912	131,776	59,205	1,573
2,500 grams or more	3,705,556	818,987	588,705	51,874	13,304	117,728	47,376	2,863,735	2,138,60	500,481	22,834
Not stated	1,241	126	77	14	2	14	19	846	562	195	269
Period of gestation:											
Less than 32 weeks	77,877	14,737	9,880	1,471	222	2,133	1,031	62,573	35,662	23,244	567
32–36 weeks	402,972	84,780	59,761	6,538	1,262	11,744	5,475	315,868	215,479	78,199	2,324
37–41 weeks	3,231,562	692,314	493,514	45,212	11,808	101,253	40,527	2,520,020	1,885,188	435,923	19,228
42 weeks or more	268,096	64,998	47,247	4,016	882	8,997	3,856	201,650	149,898	36,896	1,448
Not stated	41,318	19,825	17,108	232	58	1,857	570	19,876	11,941	4,104	1,617
Trimester of pregnancy prenatal care began:											
First trimester	3,301,213	657,244	464,446	44,363	13,004	97,144	38,287	2,625,196	2,006,374	423,026	18,773
After first trimester or no care	641,456	199,151	148,970	11,155	1,134	26,287	11,605	438,624	257,102	139,867	3,681
Second trimester	499,014	152,459	113,453	8,872	944	20,236	8,954	343,841	206,536	104,923	2,714
Third trimester	103,325	34,096	25,378	1,730	149	4,910	1,929	68,609	37,993	23,085	620
No prenatal care	39,117	12,596	10,139	553	41	1,141	722	26,174	12,573	11,859	347
Not stated	79,156	20,259	14,094	1,951	94	2,553	1,567	56,167	34,692	15,473	2,730
Age of mother:											
Under 20 years	432,825	130,322	99,593	10,212	1,159	10,750	8,608	300,084	181,008	104,631	2,419
20–24 years	1,022,132	265,239	196,866	18,725	2,410	31,548	15,690	750,968	519,154	190,251	5,925
25–29 years	1,060,420	236,146	170,148	13,842	4,025	35,429	12,702	817,980	614,912	132,833	6,294
30–34 years	951,229	157,887	106,177	9,415	3,881	29,222	9,192	787,081	620,175	92,157	6,261
35–39 years	453,939	71,481	45,129	4,386	2,283	15,366	4,317	379,118	297,438	46,834	3,340
40–54 years	101,280	15,579	9,597	889	474	3,669	950	84,756	65,481	11,660	945
Educational attainment of mother:											
0–8 years	239,622	180,514	150,043	2,276	192	23,609	4,394	58,406	37,288	12,999	702
9–11 years	614,968	233,255	184,000	15,648	1,475	20,647	11,485	379,286	230,460	125,346	2,427
12 years	1,234,741	260,239	179,483	19,515	5,082	38,473	17,686	968,554	680,852	226,230	5,948
13–15 years	851,738	115,398	68,074	12,688	3,104	21,650	9,882	732,297	550,547	132,333	4,043
16 years and over	1,026,820	71,041	34,149	6,730	4,321	19,216	6,625	950,500	781,618	72,045	5,279
Not stated	53,936	16,207	11,761	612	58	2,389	1,387	30,944	17,403	9,413	6,785
Live-birth order:											
1	1,594,949	320,585	221,759	22,370	6,554	49,915	19, 987	1,264,645	938,381	216,536	9,719
2	1,306,795	268,911	189,759	17,742	5,103	40,242	16, 065	1,030,619	780,783	168,586	7,265
3	675,278	166,130	122,873	10,270	1,866	21,981	9,1 40	505,265	370,717	102,964	3,883
4	264,268	72,829	55,841	4,145	486	8,619	3,738	189,82 9	130,048	48,266	1,610
5 or more.	170,266	46,249	35,919	2,839	209	4,978	2,304	122,734	73,547	40,367	1,283
Not stated	10,269	1,950	1,359	103	14	249	225	6,895	4,692	1,647	1,424
Marital status:											
Married	2,655,815	495,181	363,544	23,506	9,984	69, 544	28,603	2,143,669	1,769,630	182,807	16,965
Unmarried	1,366,010	381,473	263,966	33,963	4,248	56, 440	22,856	976,318	528,538	395,559	8,219
Mother's place of birth:											
Born in the 50 States and DC	3,079,253	321,261	226,150	37,713	6,396	14,455	36,547	2,737,913	2,161,864	507,205	20,079
Born elsewhere	933,408	553,846	400,550	19,586	7,832	111,420	14,458	375,391	132,638	68,953	4,171
Not stated	9,164	1,547	810	170	4	109	454	6,683	3,666	2,208	934
Maternal smoking during pregnancy:[3]											
Smoker	397,199	18,488	8,879	4,964	378	1,265	3,002	375 ,981	317,666	47,852	2,730
Nonsmoker	3,077,208	592,561	386,433	50,317	13,142	99,626	43,043	2,467,722	1,805,185	496,605	16,925
Not stated	18,046	2,536	1,807	158	13	248	310	14,243	10,667	2,455	1,267

See footnotes at end of table.

(table continues)

Characteristics	All origins[1]	Total	Mexican	Puerto Rican	Cuban	Central and South American	Other and unknown Hispanic	Total[2]	White	Black	Not stated
			Infant deaths — Hispanic					**Non-Hispanic**			
Total	27,970	4,927	3,399	471	53	637	368	22,647	13,327	8,031	395
Age at death:											
Total neonatal	18,791	3,360	2,283	334	46	435	263	15,109	8,853	5,399	322
Early neonatal (less than 7 days)	15,020	2,673	1,794	282	38	339	219	12,056	7,002	4,386	291
Late neonatal (7–27 days)	3,771	687	489	51	8	95	44	3,053	1,851	1,014	31
Postneonatal	9,179	1,567	1,116	137	7	202	105	7,538	4,474	2,632	74
Sex:											
Male	15,690	2,699	1,886	256	33	314	210	12,760	7,665	4,3 77	231
Female	12,279	2,228	1,512	215	20	323	158	9,887	5,661	3,654	164
Plurality:											
Single births	23,691	4,340	3,024	395	44	557	320	19,006	11,003	6,876	345
Plural births	4,278	587	374	76	9	80	48	3,641	2,323	1,155	51
Birthweight:											
Less than 2,500 grams	18,758	3,263	2,209	330	43	428	253	15,245	8,487	5,943	250
Less than 1,500 grams	14,885	2,504	1,677	268	31	326	202	12,169	6,519	5,029	212
1,500–2,499 grams	3,873	759	532	62	12	102	51	3,075	1,968	913	38
2,500 grams or more	8,840	1,621	1,163	135	9	205	109	7,141	4,723	1,962	79
Not stated	371	43	26	5	1	4	6	262	116	126	67
Period of gestation:											
Less than 32 weeks	14,515	2,371	1,574	268	32	315	182	11,958	6,415	4,949	187
32–36 weeks	3,692	680	466	58	9	91	56	2,976	1,928	867	36
37–41 weeks	8,001	1,450	1,035	122	10	190	93	6,495	4,307	1,771	56
42 weeks or more	824	161	123	12	–	17	8	655	428	179	8
Not stated	937	266	201	10	2	25	29	563	249	264	108
Trimester of pregnancy prenatal care began:											
First trimester	20,521	3,459	2,382	334	44	464	235	16,879	10,462	5,474	184
After first trimester or no care	5,758	1,203	851	108	9	145	89	4,495	2,221	2,011	61
Second trimester	3,637	796	567	70	6	94	58	2,815	1,532	1,105	26
Third trimester	618	117	84	10	–	18	5	488	232	219	12
No prenatal care	1,503	290	200	27	3	33	26	1,191	458	687	22
Not stated	1,690	266	165	29	–	27	44	1,273	644	547	151
Age of mother:											
Under 20 years	4,496	956	673	108	7	74	94	3,477	1,765	1,588	64
20–24 years	8,016	1,399	984	154	7	152	102	6,534	3,589	2,668	83
25–29 years	6,352	1,199	824	102	12	174	86	5,075	3,108	1,666	78
30–34 years	5,312	796	544	67	15	128	41	4,422	2,855	1,235	94
35–39 years	2,934	440	285	33	11	79	32	2,438	1,566	684	56
40–54 years	858	138	88	6	1	30	13	700	444	190	20
Educational attainment of mother:											
0–8 years	1,581	961	765	26	–	136	34	606	371	198	13
9–11 years	5,875	1,422	1,049	152	12	123	85	4,432	2,274	1,998	21
12 years	9,641	1,455	952	171	19	181	131	8,131	4,674	3,066	56
13–15 years	5,099	569	340	76	9	92	53	4,502	2,668	1,571	28
16 years and over	4,290	283	141	26	13	84	19	3,988	2,906	718	19
Not stated	1,484	237	151	19	–	20	46	988	433	480	258
Live-birth order:											
1	11,139	1,873	1,257	183	25	243	164	9,124	5,470	3,087	143
2	7,927	1,356	944	135	12	178	87	6,483	4,016	2,096	88
3	4,481	883	620	78	11	118	57	3,558	2,122	1,260	40
4	2,194	405	280	32	2	55	37	1,776	954	738	13
5 or more	1,898	366	267	39	3	38	18	1,511	670	761	21
Not stated	330	43	31	3	–	4	5	197	95	90	90
Marital status:											
Married	14,404	2,477	1,812	163	30	306	166	11,690	8,661	2,164	237
Unmarried	13,566	2,450	1,587	308	23	330	202	10,957	4,665	5,867	159
			Infant deaths								
Mother's place of birth:											
Born in the 50 States and DC	22,581	2,118	1,431	309	25	80	273	20,241	12,511	7,207	222
Born elsewhere	4,777	2,744	1,939	154	28	555	68	1,975	604	627	58
Not stated	612	65	29	7	–	2	27	431	212	197	115
Maternal smoking during pregnancy:[3]											
Smoker	4,406	198	87	62	3	14	32	4,165	3,078	961	43
Nonsmoker	20,255	3,322	2,100	396	46	486	294	16,756	9,316	6,579	177
Not stated	436	44	29	4	–	5	5	292	153	119	100

*Figure does not meet standard of reliability or precision; based on fewer than 20 deaths in the numerator.
– Quantity zero.
[1]Includes origin not stated.
[2]Includes races other than black or white.
[3]Exctudes data for California, which does not report tobacco use on the birth certificate.

NOTES: Infant deaths are weighted so numbers may not exactly add to totals due to rounding. Not stated responses were included in totals but not distributed among groups for rate computations.

INFANT MORTALITY RATES BY RACE AND ORIGIN OF MOTHER: UNITED STATES AND EACH STATE, PUERTO RICO, VIRGIN ISLANDS, AND GUAM, 2000–2002 [By place of residence]

		Infant mortality rates per 1,000 live births in specified group						
		Race of mother				Hispanic origin of mother		
State	Total	White	Black	American Indian[1]	Asian or Pacific Islander	Hispanic	Non-Hispanic white	Non-Hispanic black
United States[2]	6.9	5.7	13.5	8.9	4.8	5.5	5.7	13.6
Alabama	9.3	6.8	14.8	*	*	7.0	6.8	14.7
Alaska	6.8	5.4	*	11.2	*	*	5.1	*
Arizona	6.7	6.3	14.4	9.4	5.3	6.0	6.5	14.4
Arkansas	8.3	7.2	12.8	*	*	4.5	7.5	12.8
California	5.4	5.0	11.4	7.6	4.5	5.1	4.7	11.4
Colorado	6.0	5.5	13.8	11.8	6.2	6.2	5.2	13.7
Connecticut	6.4	5.4	14.2	*	3.7	7.1	4.9	14.3
Delaware	9.6	7.9	14.8	*	*	7.9	7.9	14.9
District of Columbia	11.4	4.8	15.2	*	*	7.5	*	15.3
Florida	7.2	5.6	12.9	5.8	5.1	5.2	5.7	13.0
Georgia	8.7	6.3	13.4	*	6.8	6.0	6.3	13.4
Hawaii	7.2	6.6	*	*	7.3	6.0	6.3	*
Idaho	6.6	6.6	*	*	*	8.8	6.2	*
Illinois	7.8	6.1	15.8	*	6.5	6.4	5.9	15.8
Indiana	7.7	6.9	13.9	*	*	6.4	7.0	13.9
Iowa	5.8	5.6	11.7	*	*	6.7	5.5	11.4
Kansas	7.0	6.5	14.6	*	*	7.1	6.4	14.7
Kentucky	6.7	6.3	10.7	*	*	4.8	6.4	10.8
Louisiana	9.8	6.8	13.8	*	8.1	6.0	6.9	13.7
Maine	5.1	5.1	*	*	*	*	5.0	*
Maryland	7.7	5.3	12.6	*	4.5	5.7	5.3	12.7
Massachusetts	4.8	4.3	9.6	*	3.7	6.0	4.0	10.5
Michigan	8.1	6.3	16.9	*	4.9	6.7	6.0	16.9
Minnesota	5.5	4.9	10.8	10.3	6.1	6.5	4.7	10.8
Mississippi	10.5	7.0	14.8	*	*	*	7.0	14.7
Missouri	7.7	6.3	15.6	*	4.5	7.2	6.3	15.6
Montana	6.9	6.5	*	9.9	*	*	6.4	*
Nebraska	7.0	6.3	14.8	15.8	*	7.2	6.2	15.0
Nevada	6.0	5.3	13.6	*	4.7	5.1	5.1	13.7
New Hampshire	4.9	4.9	*	*	*	*	4.5	*
New Jersey	6.1	4.8	13.1	*	3.3	6.3	4.0	13.6
New Mexico	6.4	6.2	15.6	6.8	*	6.3	6.0	15.8
New York	6.1	5.0	10.7	*	3.4	5.5	4.8	11.2
North Carolina	8.4	6.3	15.0	10.6	5.9	5.6	6.4	15.1
North Dakota	7.8	7.2	*	13.4	*	*	6.8	*
Ohio	7.7	6.4	15.5	*	4.8	7.6	6.3	15.3
Oklahoma	8.0	7.3	14.6	7.6	*	5.7	7.4	14.5
Oregon	5.5	5.5	10.3	*	3.7	5.1	5.6	10.4
Pennsylvania	7.3	6.2	14.6	*	4.0	8.6	5.9	14.4
Rhode Island	6.7	6.2	11.9	*	*	8.0	5.3	12.6
South Carolina	9.0	5.9	15.0	*	*	4.6	6.0	14.9
South Dakota	6.4	5.5	*	11.6	*	*	5.4	*
Tennessee	9.0	7.0	17.0	*	*	6.2	7.0	17.0
Texas	5.9	5.3	11.1	*	4.0	5.1	5.5	11.1
Utah	5.3	5.2	*	*	8.4	6.5	5.0	*
Vermont	5.5	5.6	*	*	*	*	5.5	*
Virginia	7.2	5.4	13.7	*	4.6	4.8	5.5	13.6
Washington	5.5	5.3	9.5	10.6	4.8	5.1	5.2	9.5
West Virginia	7.9	7.8	12.1	*	*	*	7.7	11.7
Wisconsin	6.9	5.6	17.9	11.5	5.2	6.2	5.6	17.9
Wyoming	6.5	6.6	*	*	*	*	6.3	*
Puerto Rico	9.4	9.4	10.4	. . .	. . .	. . .	. . .	. . .
Virgin Islands	7.0	*	6.0	*	*	*	*	*
Guam	7.3	*	*	*	7.7	*	*	*

* Figure does not meet standard of reliability or precision; based on fewer than 20 deaths in the numerator.
. . . Data not available.
[1]Includes Aleuts and Eskimos.
[2]Excludes data for Puerto Rico, Virgin Islands, and Guam.

PERCENT OF LIVE BIRTHS WITH SELECTED MATERNAL AND INFANT CHARACTERISTICS BY SPECIFIED RACE OF MOTHER: UNITED STATES, 2002

Characteristic	All races	White	Black	American Indian[1]	Asian or Pacific Islander Total	Chinese	Japanese	Hawaiian	Fillipino	Other
Birthweight:										
Less than 1,500 grams	1.5	1.2	3.2	1.3	1.1	0.7	1.0	1.6	1.3	1.2
Less than 2,500 grams	7.8	6.8	13.3	7.3	7.8	5.5	7.6	8.2	8.6	8.2
Preterm births[2]	12.1	11.1	17.6	13.1	10.4	7.7	9.2	13.5	12.7	10.5
Prenatal care beginning in the first trimester	83.7	85.4	75.2	69.8	84.8	87.2	90.5	78.1	85.4	83.9
Births to mothers under 20 years	10.8	9.8	18.0	18.5	3.8	0.9	1.7	14.6	4.5	4.0
Fourth and higher order births	10.8	10.2	15.3	19.1	6.5	2.1	3.9	16.3	7.3	7.1
Births to unmarried mothers	34.0	28.5	68.2	59.7	14.9	9.0	10.3	50.4	20.0	13.5
Mothers completing 12 or more years of school	78.5	78.4	75.6	69.2	89.7	88.7	97.8	85.7	94.7	88.4
Mothers born in the 50 States and DC	76.7	78.5	87.0	94.4	16.9	10.0	40.4	97.4	21.5	11.6
Mother smoked during pregnancy[3]	11.4	12.3	8.7	19.7	2.5	0.5	4.0	13.7	2.9	2.1

[1]Includes births to Aleuts and Eskimos.
[2]Born prior to 37 completed weeks of gestation.
[3]Excludes data for California, which does not report tobacco use on the birth certificate.

PERCENT OF LIVE BIRTHS WITH SELECTED MATERNAL AND INFANT CHARACTERISTICS BY ORIGIN OF MOTHER AND RACE OF MOTHER: UNITED STATES, 2002

Characteristic	All origins[1]	Hispanic Total	Mexican	Puerto Rican	Cuban	Central and South American	Other and unknown Hispanic	Non-Hispanic Total[2]	White	Black
Birthweight:										
Less than 1,500 grams	1.5	1.2	1.1	2.0	1.2	1.2	1.5	1.6	1.2	3.2
Less than 2,500 grams	7.8	6.6	6.2	9.7	6.5	6.5	7.9	8.2	6.9	13.4
Preterm births[3]	12.1	11.6	11.4	14.0	10.5	11.2	12.8	12.2	11.0	17.7
Prenatal care beginning in the first trimester	83.7	76.7	75.7	79.9	92.0	78.7	76.7	85.7	88.6	75.2
Births to mothers under 20 years	10.8	14.9	15.9	17.8	8.1	8.5	16.7	9.6	7.9	18.1
Fourth and higher order births	10.8	13.6	14.7	12.2	4.9	10.8	11.8	10.0	8.9	15.4
Births to unmarried mothers	34.0	43.5	42.1	59.1	29.8	44.8	44.4	31.3	23.0	68.4
Mothers completing 12 or more years of school	78.5	51.9	45.8	68.5	88.2	64.2	68.3	85.8	88.3	75.7
Mothers born in the 50 States and DC	76.7	36.7	36.1	65.8	45.0	11.5	71.7	87.9	94.2	88.0
Mother smoked during pregnancy[4]	11.4	3.0	2.2	9.0	2.8	1.3	6.5	13.2	15.0	8.8

[1]Includes origin not stated.
[2]Includes races other than black or white.
[3]Born prior to 37 completed weeks of gestation.
[4]Excludes data for California, which does not report tobacco use on the birth certificate.

LIVE BIRTHS, INFANT, NEONATAL, AND POSTNEONATAL DEATHS AND MORTALITY RATES, BY RACE AND ORIGIN OF MOTHER AND BIRTHWEIGHT: UNITED STATES, 2002 LINKED FILE, AND PERCENT CHANGE IN BIRTHWEIGHT-SPECIFIC INFANT MORTALITY, 1995–2002

Race and birthweight	Number in 2002				Mortality rate per 1,000 live births in 2002			Percent change in infant mortality rate 1995–2002
	Live births	Infant deaths	Neonatal deaths	Postneonatal deaths	Infant	Neonatal	Postneonatal	
All races[1]	4,021,825	27,970	18,791	9,179	7.0	4.7	2.3	-7.9
Less than 2,500 grams	315,028	18,758	15,324	3,434	59.5	48.6	10.9	-7.9
Less than 1,500 grams	59,361	14,885	13,078	1,807	250.8	220.3	30.4	-6.6
Less than 500 grams	6,780	5,844	5,688	156	861.9	838.9	23.0	-4.6**
500–749 grams	11,290	5,528	4,792	736	489.6	424.4	65.2	-7.3
750–999 grams	11,803	1,831	1,374	458	155.1	116.4	38.8	-14.8
1,000–1,249 grams	13,599	956	712	243	70.3	52.4	17.9	-17.8
1,250–1,499 grams	15,889	726	512	214	45.7	32.2	13.5	-16.3
1,500–1,999 grams	61,705	1,636	1,067	569	26.5	17.3	9.2	-20.2
2,000–2,499 grams	193,962	2,237	1,180	1,057	11.5	6.1	5.4	-14.8
2,500 grams or more	3,705,556	8,840	3,103	5,737	2.4	0.8	1.5	-20.0
2,500–2,999 grams	688,845	3,082	1,208	1,874	4.5	1.8	2.7	-16.7
3,000–3,499 grams	1,522,223	3,435	1,107	2,328	2.3	0.7	1.5	-20.7
3,500–3,999 grams	1,126,215	1,771	560	1,211	1.6	0.5	1.1	-20.0
4,000–4,499 grams	314,255	427	164	264	1.4	0.5	0.8	-22.2
4,500–4,999 grams	48,621	98	46	52	2.0	0.9	1.1	-9.1**
5,000 grams or more	5,397	27	18	9	5.0	*	*	-40.5**
Not stated	1,241	371	363	8	...	...	...	...
White	3,174,807	18,395	12,352	6,044	5.8	3.9	1.9	-7.9
Less than 2,500 grams	216,373	11,830	9,787	2,043	54.7	45.2	9.4	-8.4
Less than 1,500 grams	37,569	9,097	8,104	992	242.1	215.7	26.4	-7.1
Less than 500 grams	3,873	3,368	3,277	91	869.6	846.1	23.5	-4.6**
500–749 grams	6,690	3,382	3,003	379	505.5	448.9	56.7	-7.5
750–999 grams	7,370	1,201	936	265	163.0	127.0	36.0	-15.5
1,000–1,249 grams	8,937	652	516	136	73.0	57.7	15.2	-19.7
1,250–1,499 grams	10,699	492	371	121	46.0	34.7	11.3	-17.1
1,500–1,999 grams	43,113	1,142	792	350	26.5	18.4	8.1	-20.2
2,000–2,499 grams	135,691	1,591	890	701	11.7	6.6	5.2	-14.6
2,500 grams or more	2,957,532	6,366	2,370	3,996	2.2	0.8	1.4	-18.5
2,500–2,999 grams	495,210	2,133	900	1,233	4.3	1.8	2.5	-18.9
3,000–3,499 grams	1,191,645	2,463	848	1,615	2.1	0.7	1.4	-22.2
3,500–3,999 grams	948,175	1,354	444	910	1.4	0.5	1.0	-22.2
4,000–4,499 grams	275,107	321	129	191	1.2	0.5	0.7	-25.0
4,500–4,999 grams	42,764	74	34	39	1.7	0.8	0.9	-15.0**
5,000 grams or more	4,631	21	13	8	4.5	*	*	-41.6**
Not stated	902	199	195	4	...	...		
Black	593,743	8,201	5,533	2,668	13.8	9.3	4.5	-5.5
Less than 2,500 grams	79,137	6,056	4,830	1,226	76.5	61.0	15.5	-3.4**
Less than 1,500 grams	18,841	5,127	4,397	731	272.1	233.4	38.8	-4.7
Less than 500 grams	2,617	2,231	2,173	58	852.5	830.3	22.2	-4.7**
500–749 grams	4,095	1,907	1,584	323	465.7	386.8	78.9	-6.7**
750–999 grams	3,827	541	371	170	141.4	96.9	44.4	-13.3
1,000–1,249 grams	3,970	258	160	98	65.0	40.3	24.7	-12.8**
1,250–1,499 grams	4,332	190	109	82	43.9	25.2	18.9	-9.7**
1,500–1,999 grams	15,156	409	216	193	27.0	14.3	12.7	-16.7
2,000–2,499 grams	45,140	520	218	302	11.5	4.8	6.7	-14.8
2,500 grams or more	514,367	1,993	554	1,439	3.9	1.1	2.8	-13.3
2,500–2,999 grams	140,541	798	239	558	5.7	1.7	4.0	-8.1**
3,000–3,499 grams	226,502	774	192	582	3.4	0.8	2.6	-17.1
3,500–3,999 grams	117,810	322	88	234	2.7	0.7	2.0	-22.9
4,000–4,499 grams	25,298	79	23	55	3.1	0.9	2.2	-27.9**
4,500–4,999 grams	3,741	16	7	9	*	*	*	*
5,000 grams or more	475	5	5	–	*	*	*	*
Not stated	239	152	149	3	...	...	...	...

See footnotes at end of table.

(table continues)

Race and birthweight	Number in 2002				Mortality rate per 1,000 live births in 2002			Percent change in infant mortality rate 1995–2002
	Live births	Infant deaths	Neonatal deaths	Postneonatal deaths	Infant	Neonatal	Postneonatal	
American Indian[2]	42,367	366	195	171	8.6	4.6	4.0	-4.4**
Less than 2,500 grams	3,072	197	146	51	64.1	47.5	16.6	11.3**
Less than 1,500 grams	549	137	113	24	249.5	205.8	43.7	5.4**
Less than 500 grams	57	50	47	3	877.2	824.6	*	-1.3**
500–749 grams	103	42	37	5	407.8	359.2	*	-33.1**
750–999 grams	113	14	10	4	*	*	*	*
1,000–1,249 grams	124	14	9	5	*	*	*	*
1,250–1,499 grams	152	16	9	7	*	*	*	*
1,500–1,999 grams	591	19	15	4	*	*	*	*
2,000–2,499 grams	1,932	41	18	23	21.2	*	11.9	10.4**
2,500 grams or more	39,286	168	49	119	4.3	1.2	3.0	-18.9**
2,500–2,999 grams	6,746	45	17	28	6.7	*	4.2	-36.8**
3,000–3,499 grams	15,490	74	18	56	4.8	*	3.6	0.0**
3,500–3,999 grams	12,304	33	9	24	2.7	*	2.0	-34.1**
4,000–4,499 grams	3,870	10	3	7	*	*	*	*
4,500–4,999 grams	769	4	2	2	*	*	*	*
5,000 grams or more	107	1	–	1	*	*	*	*
Not stated	9	1	–	1	...	...	...	...
Asian or Pacific Islander	210,908	1,006	710	296	4.8	3.4	1.4	-9.4
Less than 2,500 grams	16,446	675	561	113	41.0	34.1	6.9	-11.4
Less than 1,500 grams	2,402	525	464	60	218.6	193.2	25.0	-8.8**
Less than 500 grams	233	195	192	3	836.9	824.0	*	-7.5**
500–749 grams	402	197	167	29	490.0	415.4	72.1	-5.1**
750–999 grams	493	75	57	18	152.1	115.6	*	-20.4**
1,000–1,249 grams	568	31	26	5	54.6	45.8	*	-39.9**
1,250–1,499 grams	706	27	22	5	38.2	31.2	*	-48.4**
1,500–1,999 grams	2,845	66	44	22	23.2	15.5	7.7	-43.7
2,000–2,499 grams	11,199	85	54	31	7.6	4.8	2.8	-26.9**
2,500 grams or more	194,371	313	130	183	1.6	0.7	0.9	-27.3
2,500–2,999 grams	46,348	106	52	54	2.3	1.1	1.2	-34.3
3,000–3,499 grams	88,586	123	49	74	1.4	0.6	0.8	-26.3
3,500–3,999 grams	47,926	61	19	42	1.3	*	0.9	-7.1**
4,000–4,499 grams	9,980	18	8	10	*	*	*	*
4,500–4,999 grams	1,347	4	2	2	*	*	*	*
5,000 grams or more	184	–	–	–	*	*	*	*
Not stated	91	19	19	–	...			
Hispanic	876,654	4,927	3,360	1,567	5.6	3.8	1.8	-11.1
Less than 2,500 grams	57,541	3,263	2,695	569	56.7	46.8	9.9	-7.5
Less than 1,500 grams	10,359	2,504	2,203	301	241.7	212.7	29.1	-8.2
Less than 500 grams	1,070	875	848	27	817.8	792.5	25.2	-6.4**
500–749 grams	1,951	985	863	123	504.9	442.3	63.0	-6.7**
750–999 grams	2,085	328	247	81	157.3	118.5	38.8	-17.0
1,000–1,249 grams	2,390	172	140	32	72.0	58.6	13.4	-15.6**
1,250–1,499 grams	2,863	144	105	38	50.3	36.7	13.3	-7.5**
1,500–1,999 grams	10,952	321	230	90	29.3	21.0	8.2	-13.3**
2,000–2,499 grams	36,230	438	261	177	12.1	7.2	4.9	-6.9**
2,500 grams or more	818,987	1,621	624	997	2.0	0.8	1.2	-20.0
2,500–2,999 grams	149,252	552	255	297	3.7	1.7	2.0	-17.8
3,000–3,499 grams	349,880	615	204	411	1.8	0.6	1.2	-21.7
3,500–3,999 grams	245,269	354	116	238	1.4	0.5	1.0	-22.2
4,000–4,499 grams	63,677	69	30	39	1.1	0.5	0.6	-26.7**
4,500–4,999 grams	9,692	23	14	9	2.4	*	*	-20.0**
5,000 grams or more	1,217	8	5	3	*	*	*	*
Not stated	126	43	42	1	...	...		

See footnotes at end of table.

(table continues)

Race and birthweight	Number in 2002				Mortality rate per 1,000 live births in 2002			Percent change in infant mortality rate 1995–2002
	Live births	Infant deaths	Neonatal deaths	Postneonatal deaths	Infant	Neonatal	Postneonatal	
Non-Hispanic white	2,298,168	13,327	8,853	4,474	5.8	3.9	1.9	-7.9
Less than 2,500 grams	159,001	8,487	7,008	1,480	53.4	44.1	9.3	-9.2
Less than 1,500 grams	27,225	6,519	5,819	700	239.4	213.7	25.7	-7.2
Less than 500 grams	2,745	2,437	2,373	64	887.8	864.5	23.3	-3.7**
500–749 grams	4,733	2,383	2,120	262	503.5	447.9	55.4	-8.1
750–999 grams	5,316	875	691	184	164.6	130.0	34.6	-14.0
1,000–1,249 grams	6,554	478	374	104	72.9	57.1	15.9	-20.8
1,250–1,499 grams	7,877	346	260	86	43.9	33.0	10.9	-21.0
1,500–1,999 grams	32,175	817	559	258	25.4	17.4	8.0	-23.0
2,000–2,499 grams	99,601	1,151	630	521	11.6	6.3	5.2	-16.5
2,500 grams or more	2,138,605	4,723	1,730	2,993	2.2	0.8	1.4	-18.5
2,500–2,999 grams	346,644	1,575	637	939	4.5	1.8	2.7	-18.2
3,000–3,499 grams	842,563	1,840	641	1,199	2.2	0.8	1.4	-21.4
3,500–3,999 grams	702,068	992	324	669	1.4	0.5	1.0	-22.2
4,000–4,499 grams	210,936	252	100	152	1.2	0.5	0.7	-25.0
4,500–4,999 grams	33,000	50	20	30	1.5	0.6	0.9	-21.1**
5,000 grams or more	3,394	13	8	5	*	*	*	*
Not stated	562	116	115	1	...	...	...	...
Non-Hispanic black	578,366	8,031	5,399	2,632	13.9	9.3	4.6	-5.4
Less than 2,500 grams	77,690	5,943	4,733	1,209	76.5	60.9	15.6	-3.2**
Less than 1,500 grams	18,485	5,029	4,311	719	272.1	233.2	38.9	-4.6
Less than 500 grams	2,561	2,185	2,127	57	853.2	830.5	22.3	-4.7**
500–749 grams	4,030	1,878	1,558	320	466.0	386.6	79.4	-6.3**
750–999 grams	3,760	527	360	166	140.2	95.7	44.1	-14.3
1,000–1,249 grams	3,898	255	157	98	65.4	40.3	25.1	-12.0**
1,250–1,499 grams	4,236	184	107	78	43.4	25.3	18.4	-10.0**
1,500–1,999 grams	14,890	402	211	191	27.0	14.2	12.8	-16.4
2,000–2,499 grams	44,315	512	212	300	11.6	4.8	6.8	-13.4
2,500 grams or more	500,481	1,962	542	1,420	3.9	1.1	2.8	-15.2
2,500–2,999 grams	137,618	783	233	549	5.7	1.7	4.0	-8.1**
3,000–3,499 grams	220,512	761	187	574	3.5	0.8	2.6	-14.6
3,500–3,999 grams	113,987	321	88	233	2.8	0.8	2.0	-20.0
4,000–4,499 grams	24,313	77	22	54	3.2	0.9	2.2	-27.3**
4,500–4,999 grams	3,589	16	7	9	*	*	*	*
5,000 grams or more	462	5	5	–	*	*	*	*
Not stated	195	126	124	2	...	...	...	...

** Not significant at $p<.05$.
* Figure does not meet standard of reliability or precision; based on fewer than 20 deaths in the numerator.
... Category not applicable.
– Quantity zero.
[1]Includes races other than white or black.
[2]Includes Aleuts and Eskimos.
NOTES: Infant deaths are weighted so numbers may not exactly add to totals due to rounding. Neonatal is less than 28 days, and postneonatal is 28 days to under 1 year.

INFANT DEATHS AND MORTALITY RATES FOR THE FIVE LEADING CAUSES OF INFANT DEATH, BY RACE AND ORIGIN OF MOTHER: UNITED STATES, 2002

[Rates per 100,000 live births in specified group]

Cause of death (Based on the *International Classification of Diseases, Tenth Revision*, 1992)	All races			Non-Hispanic white			Non-Hispanic black[1]			American Indian[2,3]			Asian or Pacific Islander[4]		
	Rank	Number	Rate	Rank	Number	Rate	Rank	Number	Rate	Rank	Number	Rate	Rank	Number	Rate
All causes	...	27,970	695.4	...	13,327	579.9	...	8,031	1,388.6	...	366	864.8	...	1,006	477.2
Congenital malformations, deformations and chromosomal abnormalities (Q00–Q99)	1	5,630	140.0	1	2,999	130.5	2	987	170.6	1	80	188.1	1	225	106.8
Disorders related to short gestation and low birthweight, not elsewhere classified (P07)	2	4,636	115.3	2	1,769	77.0	1	1,828	316.0	3	46	108.0	2	161	76.4
Sudden infant death syndrome (R95)	3	2,295	57.1	3	1,269	55.2	3	642	110.9	2	52	123.3	4	51	24.3
Newborn affected by maternal complications of pregnancy (P01)[5]	4	1,704	42.4	4	797	34.7	4	548	94.8	4	22	52.6	3	68	32.1
Newborn affected by complications of placenta, cord and membranes (P02)	5	1,013	25.2	5	491	21.3	6	308	53.2	9	7	*	6	32	15.0

Cause of death (Based on the *International Classification of Diseases, Tenth Revision*, 1992)	Total Hispanic			Mexican			Puerto Rican[6]			Central and South American[7]		
	Rank	Number	Rate	Rank	Number	Rate	Rank	Number	Rate	Rank	Number	Rate
All causes	...	4,927	562.0	...	3,399	541.6	...	471	818.9	...	637	505.6
Congenital malformations, deformations and chromosomal abnormalities (Q00–Q99)	1	1,277	145.6	1	914	145.6	2	96	166.6	1	172	136.4
Disorders related to short gestation and low birthweight, not elsewhere classified (P07)	2	759	86.6	2	503	80.1	1	97	168.6	2	93	74.1
Sudden infant death syndrome (R95)	3	260	29.7	3	181	28.8	3	31	54.3	5	26	20.8
Newborn affected by maternal complications of pregnancy (P01)[5]	4	241	27.5	4	149	23.8	4	28	48.9	4	27	21.1
Newborn affected by complications of placenta, cord and membranes (P02)	5	158	18.0	5	112	17.8	6	18	*	9	12	*

... Category not applicable.

* Figure does not meet standard of reliability or precision; based on fewer than 20 deaths in the numerator.

[1] For non-Hispanic blacks, Respiratory distress of newborn was the fifth leading cause of death, with 319 deaths and a rate of 55.1.

[2] Includes Aleuts and Eskimos.

[3] For American Indians, Accidents (unintentional injuries) was the fifth leading cause of death; however, with only 16 deaths, a reliable infant mortality rate could not be computed.

[4] For Asian or Pacific Islanders, Diseases of the circulatory system was the fifth leading cause of death, with 34 deaths and a rate of 16.2.

[5] Cause-of-death coding changes may affect comparability with the previous year's data for this cause; see "Technical Notes."

[6] For Puerto Ricans, Respiratory distress of newborn was the fifth leading cause of death, with 20 deaths and a rate of 35.1.

[7] For Central and South Americans, Respiratory distress of newborn was the third leading cause of death, with 32 deaths and a rate of 25.1.

NOTE: Reliable cause-specific infant mortality rates cannot be computed for Cubans because of the small number of infant deaths (53).

NEONATAL MORTALITY RATES, ACCORDING TO RACE, ORIGIN, GEOGRAPHIC DIVISION, AND STATE: UNITED STATES, AVERAGE ANNUAL 1989–91, 1997–99, AND 2000–2002

| | All races | | | Not Hispanic or Latino | | | | | |
| | | | | White | | | Black or African American | | |
Geographic division and State	1989–91[1]	1997–99[2]	2000–2002[2]	1989–91[1]	1997–99[2]	2000–2002[2]	1989–91[1]	1997–99[2]	2000–2002[2]
				Neonatal[3] deaths per 1,000 live births					
United States	5.7	4.8	4.6	4.6	3.9	3.8	11.1	9.4	9.2
New England[4]	5.1	4.4	4.0	4.2	3.6	3.3	11.0	8.8	9.0
Connecticut	5.7	5.1	4.8	4.2	3.7	3.8	12.5	10.0	10.1
Maine	4.5	3.9	3.8	4.2	3.9	3.7	*	*	*
Massachusetts	4.9	4.0	3.7	4.1	3.4	3.0	10.4	8.3	8.0
New Hampshire[4]	4.3	3.6	3.4	4.4	3.4	3.1	*	*	*
Rhode Island	6.4	5.0	5.1	5.3	3.9	3.8	*9.8	*	*10.2
Vermont	4.1	4.4	3.5	3.9	4.4	3.6	*	*	*
Middle Atlantic	6.3	4.7	4.5	4.6	3.5	3.6	12.3	9.2	8.6
New Jersey	5.8	4.6	4.3	4.5	3.2	2.9	11.4	9.6	9.3
New York	6.5	4.5	4.3	4.3	3.2	3.4	12.6	8.2	7.8
Pennsylvania	6.2	5.1	5.2	4.9	4.0	4.3	12.5	11.1	9.6
East North Central	6.3	5.4	5.3	4.9	4.3	4.2	12.1	10.6	10.4
Illinois	7.0	5.7	5.3	5.1	4.3	4.2	12.7	11.1	10.0
Indiana	6.0	5.2	5.1	5.2	4.6	4.6	11.5	10.3	8.6
Michigan	6.9	5.5	5.6	4.9	4.0	4.2	14.0	11.0	11.4
Ohio	5.5	5.3	5.3	4.8	4.6	4.2	9.8	9.4	10.4
Wisconsin	5.1	4.6	4.6	4.6	3.7	3.9	9.1	10.5	11.3
West North Central	5.0	4.5	4.3	4.5	4.0	3.7	10.2	10.0	9.6
Iowa	4.8	4.0	3.7	4.5	3.7	3.5	*10.5	*11.3	*8.4
Kansas	4.9	4.8	4.6	4.6	4.7	4.0	8.3	8.1	10.3
Minnesota	4.3	3.9	3.6	3.9	3.6	3.2	10.7	8.1	6.4
Missouri	6.0	4.9	5.1	5.0	3.9	4.1	10.6	10.8	10.7
Nebraska	4.5	4.9	4.8	4.2	4.3	4.3	*9.8	*11.6	*10.9
North Dakota	5.0	4.4	5.1	4.7	4.5	4.5	*	*	*
South Dakota	5.1	4.6	3.4	4.5	4.2	3.4	*	*	*
South Atlantic	6.9	5.7	5.5	4.9	4.1	4.0	11.7	10.0	9.6
Delaware	7.5	5.9	7.0	5.8	3.8	5.8	12.4	12.8	11.1
District of Columbia	14.1	9.8	8.3	*5.2	*	*	16.7	12.4	10.9
Florida	6.2	4.8	4.8	4.7	3.9	3.6	10.5	8.3	8.7
Georgia	7.9	5.8	5.8	5.5	4.0	4.1	12.0	9.4	9.2
Maryland	5.9	6.2	5.6	3.9	3.8	3.8	10.2	10.8	9.2
North Carolina	7.3	6.5	5.9	5.3	4.8	4.4	11.9	11.5	11.0
South Carolina	7.7	6.9	6.2	5.4	4.3	3.9	11.3	11.6	10.6
Virginia	6.8	5.3	4.9	4.8	3.9	3.6	13.0	9.8	9.6
West Virginia	5.8	5.3	5.1	5.6	5.2	5.0	*9.7	*8.1	*9.8
East South Central	6.6	5.6	5.6	5.0	4.2	4.2	10.6	9.5	9.8
Alabama	7.5	6.3	5.9	5.7	4.6	4.2	11.1	9.9	9.4
Kentucky	5.0	4.7	4.2	4.6	4.4	4.0	8.9	7.6	6.3
Mississippi	7.1	6.2	6.6	4.9	3.9	4.2	9.5	9.0	9.5
Tennessee	6.5	5.2	5.8	4.9	3.9	4.3	11.8	9.9	11.4
West South Central[4]	5.0	4.4	4.2	4.2	3.9	3.7	8.4	7.6	7.7
Arkansas	5.4	5.1	4.9	4.5	4.4	4.2	8.5	7.5	8.1
Louisiana[4]	6.3	6.0	6.3	4.8	4.1	4. 3	8.5	8.9	8.9
Oklahoma[4]	4.4	5.0	4.8	4.1	4.9	4. 6	6.3	8.1	8.5
Texas	4.7	3.9	3.6	4.1	3.5	3.3	8.5	6.7	6.7
Mountain	4.8	4.2	4.1	4.4	3.9	3.7	10.1	8.2	8.9
Arizona	5.3	4.6	4.3	4.9	4.3	4.2	11.0	9.0	9.6
Colorado	5.0	4.5	4.2	4.7	4.0	3.5	10.9	9.8	10.5
Idaho	5.3	4.4	4.5	5.2	4.3	4.1	*	*	*
Montana	4.6	3.7	4.5	4.2	3.2	4.3	*	*	*
Nevada	4.3	3.8	3.6	3.8	3.5	2.9	*8.3	*	7.4
New Mexico	5.0	3.9	4.0	4.8	4.3	3.5	*	*	*
Utah	3.7	3.5	3.5	3.6	3.3	3.4	*	*	*
Wyoming	3.9	3.8	4.3	3.8	3.5	4.3	*	*	*
Pacific	4.6	3.7	3.6	4.0	3.3	3.2	9.2	7.5	7.2
Alaska	4.1	3.1	3.1	3.7	2.9	*2.9	*	*	*
California	4.6	3.8	3.6	4.1	3.3	3.1	9.2	7.7	7.5
Hawaii	4.3	4.7	5.0	3.5	*3.9	5.3	*	*	*
Oregon	4.4	3.6	3.6	4.0	3.4	3.6	*11.6	*	*
Washington	4.3	3.4	3.5	3.8	3.0	3.3	9.7	7.1	6.0

See footnotes at end of table.

(table continues)

Geographic division and State	Hispanic or Latino[5]			American Indian or Alaska Native[6]			Asian or Pacific Islander[6]		
	1989–91[1]	1997–99[2]	2000–2002[2]	1989–91[1]	1997–99[2]	2000–2002[2]	1989–91[1]	1997–99[2]	2000–2002[2]
	Neonatal[3] deaths per 1,000 live births								
United States	4.8	3.9	3.8	5.9	4.8	4.4	3.9	3.4	3.3
New England[7]	5.5	5.7	4.9	*	*	*	4.4	*2.6	3.1
Connecticut	5.3	6.5	5.3	*	*	*	*	*	*
Maine	*	*	*	*	*	*	*	*	*
Massachusetts	5.8	5.1	4.6	*	*	*	*3.9	*2.5	*2.7
New Hampshire[7]	- - -	*	*	*	*	*	*	*	*
Rhode Island	*4.9	*5.4	*6.0	*	*	*	*	*	*
Vermont	*	*	*	*	*	*	*	*	*
Middle Atlantic	6.2	4.5	4.2	*	*	*	4.1	3.0	2.3
New Jersey	5.1	4.6	4.3	*	*	*	*3.4	3.1	2.2
New York	6.4	4.2	3.9	*	*	*	4.1	2.9	2.3
Pennsylvania	7.3	5.5	5.8	*	*	*	*5.2	*3.4	*2.7
East North Central	5.9	5.1	4.5	*6.2	*5.3	*5.0	3.6	4.1	4.3
Illinois	6.4	4.8	4.4	*	*	*	3.9	4.4	4.8
Indiana	*4.7	5.2	4.8	*	*	*	*	*	*
Michigan	5.2	4.8	4.7	*	*	*	*	*3.9	*3.8
Ohio	*5.4	6.7	5.3	*	*	*	*	*3.0	*4.0
Wisconsin	*3.9	7.3	4.4	*	*	*	*	*4.2	*3.8
West North Central	5.3	4.5	4.9	6.1	5.3	5.3	4.6	4.5	3.9
Iowa	*	*3.9	*4.9	*	*	*	*	*	*
Kansas	*5.4	*3.7	4.9	*	*	*	*	*	*
Minnesota	*	*4.7	4.6	*4.9	*	*	*3.2	*4.5	*4.2
Missouri	*	*4.6	*5.2	*	*	*	*	*	*
Nebraska	*	*6.5	*4.6	*	*	*	*	*	*
North Dakota	*	*	*	*	*	*	*	*	*
South Dakota	*	*	*	*8.2	*6.1	*4.7	*	*	*
South Atlantic	5.2	3.6	3.7	7.4	8.0	5.8	4.6	3.5	4.0
Delaware	*	*	*	*	*	*	*	*	*
District of Columbia	*	*	*	*	*	*	*	*	*
Florida	5.1	3.2	3.6	*	*	*	*4.4	*2.9	3.8
Georgia	*5.7	3.3	4.0	*	*	*	*5.3	*3.2	5.4
Maryland	*4.7	*4.4	4.2	*	*	*	*4.5	*4.0	*3.6
North Carolina	*5.5	4.8	3.8	*7.7	11.2	*8.1	*	*3.6	*4.4
South Carolina	*	*5.5	*3.6	*	*	*	*	*	*
Virginia	*4.8	3.8	3.5	*	*	*	*4.1	4.0	3.2
West Virginia	*	*	*	*	*	*	*	*	*
East South Central	*	4.3	3.9	*	*	*	*	*4.7	*3.6
Alabama	*	*	*4.6	*	*	*	*	*	*
Kentucky	*	*	*	*	*	*	*	*	*
Mississippi	*	*	*	*	*	*	*	*	*
Tennessee	*	*4.9	*3.8	*	*	*	*	*	*
West South Central[7]	4.2	3.5	3.2	4.3	4.4	3.7	4.1	2.7	2.9
Arkansas	*	*4.1	*3.1	*	*	*	*	*	*
Louisiana[7]	- - -	*	*	*	*	*	*	*	*7.1
Oklahoma[7]	- - -	*3.1	*3.3	*3.7	4.5	3.9	*	*	*
Texas	4.2	3.5	3.2	*	*	*	4.0	2.8	2.5
Mountain	4.7	4.3	4.2	5.8	4.4	4.3	4.6	3.6	3.7
Arizona	5.0	4.6	4.1	5.4	4.4	4.4	*	*	*
Colorado	4.4	4.8	4.6	*	*	*	*	*	*47
Idaho	*	*4.3	6.8	*	*	*	*	*	*
Montana	*	*	*	7.6	*5.3	*5.9	*	*	*
Nevada	*4.1	3.4	3.3	*	*	*	*	*	*
New Mexico	4.9	3.6	4.3	4.9	*3.6	*3.5	*	*	*
Utah	*3.6	4.0	4.1	*	*	*	*	*	*5.0
Wyoming	*	*	*	*	*	*	*	*	*
Pacific	4.5	3.6	3.5	6.5	4.3	4.1	3.7	3.4	3.3
Alaska	*	*	*	*5.7	*3.3	*3.9	*	*	*
California	4.4	3.6	3.5	6.3	*4.6	*4.0	3.6	3.1	3.0
Hawaii	*6.6	*4.3	*3.8	*	*	*	4.2	5.0	4.9
Oregon	6.5	4.7	3.6	*	*	*	*5.3	*3.8	*
Washington	4.9	3.4	3.2	*8.5	*5.6	*4.1	*2.7	3.1	3.2

* Estimates are considered unreliable. Rates preceded by an asterisk are based on fewer than 50 deaths. Rates not shown are based on fewer than 20 deaths.
- - - Data not available.
[1]Rates based on unweighted birth cohort data.
[2]Rates based on period file using weighted data. See Appendix I, National Vital Statistics System, Linked Birth/Infant Death Data Set.
[3]Infants under 28 days of age.
[4]Rates for white and black are substituted for non-Hispanic white and non-Hispanic black for Louisiana 1989, Oklahoma 1989–90, and New Hampshire 1989–91.
[5]Persons of Hispanic origin may be of any race.
[6]Includes persons of Hispanic origin.
[7]Rates for Hispanic origin exclude data from States not reporting Hispanic origin on the birth certificate for 1 or more years in a 3-year period.
NOTE: National linked files do not exist for 1992–94.

SOURCE: Centers for Disease Control and Prevention, National Center for Health Statistics, National Vital Statistics System, Linked Birth/Infant Death Data Set.

INFANT MORTALITY RATES AND INTERNATIONAL RANKINGS: SELECTED COUNTRIES, SELECTED YEARS 1960–2002

[Data are based on reporting by countries]

Country[2]	1960	1970	1980	1990	2000	2001	2002	International rankings[1]	
								1960	2002
	Infant[3] deaths per 1,000 live births								
Australia	20.2	17.9	10.7	8.2	5.2	5.3	5.0	5	17
Austria	37.5	25.9	14.3	7.8	4.8	4.8	4.1	24	8
Belgium	31.2	21.1	12.1	8.0	4.8	4.5	4.9	20	16
Bulgaria	45.1	27.3	20.2	14.8	13.3	14.4	13.3	30	36
Canada	27.3	18.8	10.4	6.8	5.3	5.2	5.4	14	23
Chile	120.3	82.2	33.0	16.0	11.7	8.3	7.8	36	32
Costa Rica	67.8	65.4	20.3	15.3	10.2	10.8	11.2	33	34
Cuba	37.3	38.7	19.6	10.7	7.2	6.2	6.5	23	27
Czech Republic	20.0	20.2	16.9	10.8	4.1	4.0	4.2	4	10
Denmark	21.5	14.2	8.4	7.5	5.3	4.9	4.4	8	12
England and Wales	22.4	18.5	12.1	7.9	5.6	5.5	5.2	9	21
Finland	21.0	13.2	7.6	5.6	3.8	3.2	3.0	6	4
France	27.5	18.2	10.0	7.3	4.6	4.5	4.1	15	8
Germany[4]	35.0	22.5	12.4	7.0	4.4	4. 3	4.3	22	11
Greece	40.1	29.6	17.9	9.7	6.1	5.1	5.9	25	25
Hong Kong	41.5	19.2	11.2	6.2	3.0	2.6	2.3	26	1
Hungary	47.6	35.9	23.2	14.8	9.2	8.1	7.2	31	29
Ireland	29.3	19.5	11.1	8.2	6.2	5.7	5.1	17	20
Israel[5]	31.0	18.9	15.6	9.9	5.4	5.1	5.4	19	23
Italy	43.9	29.6	14.6	8.2	4.5	4.7	4.7	29	14
Japan	30.7	13.1	7.5	4.6	3.2	3.1	3.0	18	4
Netherlands	17.9	12.7	8.6	7.1	5.1	5.4	5.0	2	17
New Zealand	22.6	16.7	13.0	8.4	6.3	5.6	6.2	10	26
Northern Ireland	27.2	22.9	13.4	7.5	5.1	6.1	4.7	13	14
Norway	18.9	12.7	8.1	7.0	3.8	3.9	3.5	3	7
Poland	54.8	36.7	25.5	19.3	8.1	7.7	7.5	32	30
Portugal	77.5	55.5	24.3	11.0	5.5	5.0	5.0	35	17
Puerto Rico	43.3	27.9	18.5	13.4	9.9	9.2	9.8	27	33
Romania	75.7	49.4	29.3	26.9	18.6	18.4	17.3	34	37
Russian Federation[6]	- - -	- - -	22.0	17.6	15.2	14.6	13.2	- - -	35
Scotland	26.4	19.6	12.1	7.7	5.7	5.5	5.3	12	22
Singapore	34.8	21.4	11.7	6.7	2.5	2.2	2.9	21	3
Slovakia	28.6	25.7	20.9	12.0	8.6	6.2	7.6	16	31
Spain	43.7	28.1	12.3	7.6	3.9	3.5	3.4	28	6
Sweden	16.6	11.0	6.9	6.0	3.4	3.7	2.8	1	2
Switzerland	21.1	15.1	9.1	6.8	4.9	5.0	4.5	7	13
United States	26.0	20.0	12.6	9.2	6.9	6.8	7.0	11	28

- - - Data not available.

[1]Rankings are from lowest to highest infant mortality rates (IMR). Countries with the same IMR receive the same rank. The country with the next highest IMR is assigned the rank it would have received had the lower-ranked countries not been tied, i.e., skip a rank. Some of the variation in IMRs is due to differences among countries in distinguishing between fetal and infant deaths.

[2]Refers to countries, territories, cities, or geographic areas with at least 1 million population and with "complete" counts of live births and infant deaths as indicated in the United Nations Demographic Yearbook.

[3]Under 1 year of age.

[4]Rates for 1990 and earlier years were calculated by combining information from the Federal Republic of Germany and the German Democratic Republic.

[5]Includes data for East Jerusalem and Israeli residents in certain other territories under occupation by Israeli military forces since June 1967.

[6]Excludes infants born alive after less than 28 weeks' gestation, of less than 1,000 grams in weight and 35 centimeters in length, who die within 7 days of birth.

NOTE: Some rates for selected countries and selected years were revised and differ from the previous edition of Health, United States.

SOURCES: Organization for Economic Cooperation and Development (OECD): OECD Health Data 2004 3rd edition, A Comparative Analysis of 30 Countries, www.oecd.org/els/health/; United Nations: 2000 Demographic Yearbook, United Nations Publication, Sales No. E/F.02.XIII.1, New York, 2002; World Health Organization Statistical Information System (WHOSIS), www3.who.int/whosis/; United States and Puerto Rico: Centers for Disease Control and Prevention, National Center for Health Statistics. Vital Statistics of the United States, vol. II, mortality part A (selected years). Public Health Service. Washington; Sweden: Statistics Sweden; Costa Rica: Dirección General de Estadísticas y Censos. Elaboración y estimación, Centro Centroamericano de Población, Universidad de Costa Rica, populi.eest.ucr.ac.cr/observa/index1.htm; Russian Federation: Goskomstat, www.gks.ru/eng/. Israel: Central Bureau Statistics of Israel, www.cbs.gov.il/engindex.htm.

INFANT, NEONATAL, AND POSTNEONATAL MORTALITY RATES, ACCORDING TO DETAILED RACE AND ORIGIN OF MOTHER: UNITED STATES, SELECTED YEARS 1983–2002

Race and origin of mother	1983[1]	1985[1]	1990[1]	1995[2]	1998[2]	1999[2]	2000[2]	2001[2]	2002[2]
	Infant[3] deaths per 1,000 live births								
All mothers	10.9	10.4	8.9	7.6	7.2	7.0	6.9	6.8	7.0
White	9.3	8.9	7.3	6.3	6.0	5.8	5.7	5.7	5.8
Black or African American	19.2	18.6	16.9	14.6	13.8	14.0	13.5	13.3	13.8
American Indian or Alaska Native	15.2	13.1	13.1	9.0	9.3	9.3	8.3	9.7	8.6
Asian or Pacific Islander	8.3	7.8	6.6	5.3	5.5	4.8	4.9	4.7	4.8
Chinese	9.5	5.8	4.3	3.8	4.0	2.9	3.5	3.2	3.0
Japanese	*5.6	*6.0	*5.5	*5.3	*3.4	*3.5	*4.5	*4.0	*4.9
Filipino	8.4	7.7	6.0	5.6	6.2	5.8	5.7	5.5	5.7
Hawaiian	11.2	*9.9	*8.0	*6.5	9.9	*7.0	9.0	*7.3	9.6
Other Asian or Pacific Islander	8.1	8.5	7.4	5.5	5.7	5.1	4.8	4.8	4.7
Hispanic or Latino[4,5]	9.5	8.8	7.5	6.3	5.8	5.7	5.6	5.4	5.6
Mexican	9.1	8.5	7.2	6.0	5.6	5.5	5.4	5.2	5.4
Puerto Rican	12.9	11.2	9.9	8.9	7.8	8.3	8.2	8.5	8.2
Cuban	7.5	8.5	7.2	5.3	*3.7	4.6	4.6	4.2	3.7
Central and South American	8.5	8.0	6.8	5.5	5.3	4.7	4.6	5.0	5.1
Other and unknown Hispanic or Latino	10.6	9.5	8.0	7.4	6.5	7.2	6.9	6.0	7.1
Not Hispanic or Latino:									
White[5]	9.2	8.6	7.2	6.3	6.0	5.8	5.7	5.7	5.8
Black or African American[5]	19.1	18.3	16.9	14.7	13.9	14.1	13.6	13.5	13.9
	Neonatal[3] deaths per 1,000 live births								
All mothers	7.1	6.8	5.7	4.9	4.8	4.7	4.6	4.5	4.7
White	6.1	5.8	4.6	4.1	4.0	3.9	3.8	3.8	3.9
Black or African American	12.5	12.3	11.1	9.6	9.4	9.5	9.1	8.9	9.3
American Indian or Alaska Native	7.5	6.1	6.1	4.0	5.0	5.0	4.4	4.2	4.6
Asian or Pacific Islander	5.2	4.8	3.9	3.4	3.9	3.2	3.4	3.1	3.4
Chinese	5.5	3.3	2.3	2.3	2.7	1.8	2.5	1.9	2.4
Japanese	*3.7	*3.1	*3.5	*3.3	*2.5	*2.8	*2.6	*2.5	*3.7
Filipino	5.6	5.1	3.5	3.4	4.6	3.9	4.1	4.0	4.1
Hawaiian	*7.0	*5.7	*4.3	*4.0	*7.2	*4.9	*6.2	*3.6	*5.6
Other Asian or Pacific Islander	5.0	5.4	4.4	3.7	3.9	3.3	3.4	3.2	3.3
Hispanic or Latino[4,5]	6.2	5.7	4.8	4.1	3.9	3.9	3.8	3.6	3.8
Mexican	5.9	5.4	4.5	3.9	3.7	3.7	3.6	3.5	3.6
Puerto Rican	8.7	7.6	6.9	6.1	5.2	5.9	5.8	6.0	5.8
Cuban	*5.0	6.2	5.3	*3.6	*2.7	*3.5	*3.2	*2.5	*3.2
Central and South American	5.8	5.6	4.4	3.7	3.6	3.3	3.3	3.4	3.5
Other and unknown Hispanic or Latino	6.4	5.6	5.0	4.8	4.5	4.8	4.6	3.9	5.1
Not Hispanic or Latino:									
White[5]	5.9	5.6	4.5	4.0	3.9	3.8	3.8	3.8	3.9
Black or African American[5]	12.0	11.9	11.0	9.6	9.4	9.6	9.2	9.0	9.3
	Postneonatal[3] deaths per 1,000 live births								
All mothers	3.8	3.6	3.2	2.6	2.4	2.3	2.3	2.3	2.3
White	3.2	3.1	2.7	2.2	2.0	1.9	1.9	1.9	1.9
Black or African American	6.7	6.3	5.9	5.0	4.4	4.5	4.3	4.4	4.5
American Indian or Alaska Native	7.7	7.0	7.0	5.1	4.4	4.3	3.9	5.4	4.0
Asian or Pacific Islander	3.1	2.9	2.7	1.9	1.7	1.7	1.4	1.6	1.4
Chinese	4.0	*2.5	*2.0	*1.5	*1.3	*1.2	*1.0	*1.3	*0.7
Japanese	*	*2.9	*	*	*	*	*	*	*
Filipino	*2.8	2.7	2.5	2.2	1.6	1.9	1.6	*1.5	1.7
Hawaiian	*4.2	*4.3	*3.8	*	*	*	*	*3.7	*4.0
Other Asian or Pacific Islander	3.0	3.0	3.0	1.9	1.8	1.8	1.4	1.6	1.4
Hispanic or Latino[4,5]	3.3	3.2	2.7	2.1	1.9	1.8	1.8	1.8	1.8
Mexican	3.2	3.2	2.7	2.1	1.9	1.8	1.8	1.7	1.8
Puerto Rican	4.2	3.5	3.0	2.8	2.6	2.4	2.4	2.5	2.4
Cuban	*2.5	*2.3	*1.9	*1.7	*	*	*	*1.7	*
Central and South American	2.6	2.4	2.4	1.9	1.7	1.4	1.4	1.6	1.6
Other and unknown Hispanic or Latino	4.2	3.9	3.0	2.6	2.0	2.5	2.3	2.1	2.0
Not Hispanic or Latino:									
White[5]	3.2	3.0	2.7	2.2	2.0	1.9	1.9	1.9	1.9
Black or African American[5]	7.0	6.4	5.9	5.0	4.5	4.6	4.4	4.5	4.6

See footnotes at end of table.

(table continues)

(Table continued)

Race and origin of mother	1983–85[1,6]	1986–88[1,6]	1989–91[1,6]	1996–98[2,6]	1997–99[2,6]	2000–2002[2,6]
			Infant[3] deaths per 1,000 live births			
All mothers	10.6	9.8	9.0	7.2	7.1	6.9
White	9.0	8.2	7.4	6.0	5.9	5.7
Black or African American	18.7	17.9	17.1	13.9	13.8	13.5
American Indian or Alaska Native	13.9	13.2	12.6	9.3	9.1	8.9
Asian or Pacific Islander	8.3	7.3	6.6	5.2	5.1	4.8
Chinese	7.4	5.8	5.1	3.4	3.3	3.2
Japanese	6.0	6.9	5.3	4.3	4.1	4.5
Filipino	8.2	6.9	6.4	5.9	6.0	5.7
Hawaiian	11.3	11.1	9.0	8.2	8.6	8.7
Other Asian or Pacific Islander	8.6	7.6	7.0	5.5	5.2	4.8
Hispanic or Latino[4,5]	9.2	8.3	7.5	5.9	5.8	5.5
Mexican	8.8	7.9	7.2	5.8	5.6	5.4
Puerto Rican	12.3	11.1	10.4	8.1	8.0	8.3
Cuban	8.0	7.3	6.2	4.7	4.6	4.2
Central and South American	8.2	7.5	6.6	5.2	5.1	4.9
Other and unknown Hispanic or Latino	9.8	9.0	8.2	6.8	6.7	6.7
Not Hispanic or Latino:						
White[5]	8.8	8.1	7.3	6.0	5.9	5.7
Black or African American[5]	18.5	17.9	17.2	13.9	13.9	13.6
			Neonatal[3] deaths per 1,000 live births			
All mothers	6.9	6.3	5.7	4.8	4.8	4.6
White	5.9	5.2	4.7	4.0	3.9	3.8
Black or African American	12.2	11.7	11.1	9.3	9.4	9.1
American Indian or Alaska Native	6.7	5.9	5.9	4.7	4.8	4.4
Asian or Pacific Islander	5.2	4.5	3.9	3.5	3.4	3.3
Chinese	4.3	3.3	2.7	2.3	2.2	2.3
Japanese	3.4	4.4	3.0	2.6	2.8	2.9
Filipino	5.3	4.5	4.0	4.1	4.0	4.1
Hawaiian	7.4	7.1	4.8	5.6	6.1	5.2
Other Asian or Pacific Islander	5.5	4.7	4.2	3.6	3.5	3.3
Hispanic or Latino[4,5]	6.0	5.3	4.8	3.9	3.9	3.8
Mexican	5.7	5.0	4.5	3.8	3.8	3.6
Puerto Rican	8.3	7.2	7.0	5.4	5.5	5.9
Cuban	5.9	5.3	4.6	3.5	3.4	3.0
Central and South American	5.7	4.9	4.4	3.6	3.6	3.4
Other and unknown Hispanic or Latino	6.1	5.8	5.2	4.5	4.3	4.5
Not Hispanic or Latino:						
White[5]	5.7	5.1	4.6	3.9	3.9	3.8
Black or African American[5]	11.8	11.4	11.1	9.3	9.4	9.2
			Postneonatal[3] deaths per 1,000 live births			
All mothers	3.7	3.5	3.3	2.5	2.4	2.3
White	3.1	3.0	2.7	2.1	2.0	1.9
Black or African American	6.4	6.2	6.0	4.6	4.5	4.4
American Indian or Alaska Native	7.2	7.3	6.7	4.6	4.3	4.5
Asian or Pacific Islander	3.1	2.8	2.6	1.8	1.7	1.5
Chinese	3.1	2.5	2.4	1.2	1.1	1.0
Japanese	2.6	2.5	2.2	*1.7	*1.3	*1.6
Filipino	2.9	2.4	2.3	1.9	1.9	1.6
Hawaiian	3.9	4.0	4.1	*2.6	*2.5	3.5
Other Asian or Pacific Islander	3.1	2.9	2.8	1.8	1.8	1.5
Hispanic or Latino[4,5]	3.2	3.0	2.7	2.0	1.9	1.8
Mexican	3.2	2.9	2.7	2.0	1.9	1.8
Puerto Rican	4.0	3.9	3.4	2.7	2.5	2.4
Cuban	2.2	2.0	1.6	*1.3	*1.2	*1.2
Central and South American	2.5	2.6	2.2	1.6	1.5	1.5
Other and unknown Hispanic or Latino	3.7	3.2	3.0	2.3	2.3	2.1
Not Hispanic or Latino:						
White[5]	3.1	3.0	2.7	2.1	2.0	1.9
Black or African American[5]	6.7	6.5	6.1	4.6	4.5	4.5

* Estimates are considered unreliable. Rates preceded by an asterisk are based on fewer than 50 deaths in the numerator. Rates not shown are based on fewer than 20 deaths in the numerator.
[1] Rates based on unweighted birth cohort data.
[2] Rates based on a period file using weighted data. See Appendix I, National Vital Statistics System, Linked Birth/Infant Death Data Set.
[3] Infant (under 1 year of age), neonatal (under 28 days), and postneonatal (28 days–11 months).
[4] Persons of Hispanic origin may be of any race.
[5] Prior to 1995, data shown only for States with an Hispanic-origin item on their birth certificates. See Appendix II, Hispanic origin.
[6] Average annual mortality rate.
NOTES: The race groups white, black, American Indian or Alaska Native, and Asian or Pacific Islander include persons of Hispanic and non-Hispanic origin. National linked files do not exist for 1992–94. Data for additional years are available. See Appendix III.

SOURCE: Centers for Disease Control and Prevention, National Center for Health Statistics, National Vital Statistics System, Linked Birth/Infant Death Data Set.

INFANT MORTALITY BY CAUSE: US, 2000–2002 (SOURCE: NVSS)

[Rate per 100,000 live births]

Race/Ethnicity	All	White	Black	American Indian/ Alaska Native	Asian or Pacific Islanders	Non-Hispanic White	Non-Hispanic Black	Hispanic
Cause								
All causes	689.3	573.3	1,353.9	887.0	479.1	573.7	1,364.1	555.0
Congenital malformations, deformations and chromosomal abnormalities	139.8	136.1	166.7	163.0	112.2	131.5	167.2	145.5
Disorders related to short gestation and low birthweight, not elsewhere classified	111.1	77.6	300.3	95.4	72.0	74.6	302.9	81.3
Sudden infant death syndrome	58.3	48.6	115.3	129.8	24.1	55.2	116.7	30.4
Newborn affected by maternal complications of pregnancy	38.0	29.5	86.6	34.0	25.5	31.2	87.4	23.0
Newborn affected by complications of placenta, cord and membranes	25.3	21.7	48.2	25.7	14.8	22.4	48.2	17.9
Accidents (unintentional injuries)	23.0	19.2	44.5	61.8	11.4	20.7	45.3	14.7
Respiratory distress of newborn	24.6	19.4	55.7	19.4	14.1	19.1	55.8	19.8
Bacterial sepsis of newborn	18.4	14.7	40.1	17.0	10.3	14.5	40.5	15.5
Diseases of the circulatory system	16.0	13.5	28.9	19.2	15.2	13.8	29.1	12.8
Intrauterine hypoxia and birth asphyxia	14.4	13.0	22.3	19.4	11.3	13.5	22.5	11.2
Septicemia	7.3	5.7	16.6	*	4.8	5.2	16.9	6.8
Chronic respiratory disease originating in the perinatal period	7.6	5.5	20.2	*	3.8	6.0	20.5	3.9
Birth trauma	4.3	3.8	7.4	*	*	3.7	7.5	4.0

* Unreliable data

APPENDIX III

BIRTH DEFECTS DATA FROM SELECTED STATES AND THE DEPARTMENT OF DEFENSE

The following tables present rates and counts for birth defects reported by the Department of Defense, Puerto Rico, and the following states:

Alabama
Alaska
Arizona
Arkansas
California
Colorado
Delaware
Florida
Georgia
Hawaii
Illinois
Iowa
Kentucky
Massachusetts

Michigan
Mississippi
Missouri
Montana
New Jersey
New Mexico
New York
North Carolina
North Dakota
Oklahoma
Rhode Island
South Carolina
Tennessee
Texas
Utah
Virginia
West Virginia
Wisconsin

Alabama

BIRTH DEFECTS COUNTS AND RATES 1998–2001

(Rates per 10,000 Live Births)

Defect	Non-Hispanic White	Non-Hispanic Black or African	Hispanic	Asian or Pacific Islander	American Indian or Alaskan Native	Other/ Unknown	Total	Notes
Amniotic bands	3	0	1	0	0	0	4	
	1.17	0.00	15.38	0.00	0.00		0.95	
Anencephalus	5	3	1	0	0	0	9	
	1.96	1.94	15.38	0.00	0.00		2.13	
Aniridia	2	1	0	0	0	0	3	
	0.78	0.65	0.00	0.00	0.00		0.71	
Anophthalmia / microphthalmia	7	8	0	0	0	0	15	
	2.74	5.17	0.00	0.00	0.00		3.55	
Anotia/microtia	1	2	0	1	0	0	4	
	0.39	1.29	0.00	29.24	0.00		0.95	
Aortic valve stenosis	7	2	0	1	0	0	10	
	2.74	1.29	0.00	29.24	0.00		2.37	
Atrial septal defect	46	24	1	1	0	0	72	isolated cases not reported
	18.00	15.52	15.38	29.24	0.00		17.03	
Biliary atresia	2	2	0	0	0	0	4	
	0.78	1.29	0.00	0.00	0.00		0.95	
Bladder exstrophy	2	1	0	0	0	0	3	
	0.78	0.65	0.00	0.00	0.00		0.71	
Choanal atresia	3	3	0	0	0	0	6	
	1.17	1.94	0.00	0.00	0.00		1.42	
Cleft lip with and without cleft palate	34	9	0	1	0	0	44	
	13.31	5.82	0.00	29.24	0.00		10.41	
Cleft palate without cleft lip	31	9	0	1	0	0	41	
	12.13	5.82	0.00	29.24	0.00		9.70	
Coarctation of aorta	11	9	0	0	0	0	20	
	4.31	5.82	0.00	0.00	0.00		4.73	
Common truncus		1	3	0	0	0	4	
	0.39	1.94	0.00	0.00	0.00		0.95	
Congenital cataract	4	3	0	0	0	0	7	
	1.57	1.94	0.00	0.00	0.00		1.66	
Congenital hip dislocation	2	3	0	0	0	0	5	isolated cases not reported
	0.78	1.94	0.00	0.00	0.00		1.18	
Diaphragmatic hernia	9	7	0	0	0	0	16	
	3.52	4.53	0.00	0.00	0.00		3.79	
Down syndrome	31	21	1	0	0	0	53	
	12.13	13.58	15.38	0.00	0.00		12.54	
Ebstein's anomaly	3	2	0	0	0	0	5	
	1.17	1.29	0.00	0.00	0.00		1.18	
Encephalocele	2	1	1	0	1	0	5	
	0.78	0.65	15.38	0.00	45.25		1.18	
Endocardial cushion defect	8	11	1	0	0	0	20	
	3.13	7.11	15.38	0.00	0.00		4.73	
Esophageal atresia / tracheoesophageal fistula	5	2	0	0	0	0	7	
	1.96	1.29	0.00	0.00	0.00		1.66	
Fetal alcohol syndrome	0	7	0	0	0	0	7	
	0.00	4.53	0.00	0.00	0.00		1.66	
Gastroschisis	10	2	0	3	0	0	15	
	3.91	1.29	0.00	87.72	0.00		3.55	
Hirschsprung's disease (congenital megacolon)	5	4	0	0	0	0	9	
	1.96	2.59	0.00	0.00	0.00		2.13	
Hydrocephalus without Spina Bifida	26	12	1	0	0	0	39	
	10.18	7.76	15.38	0.00	0.00		9.23	

(Table continues)

(Table continued)

Defect	Race/Ethnicity							Notes
	Non-Hispanic White	Non-Hispanic Black or African	Hispanic	Asian or Pacific Islander	American Indian or Alaskan Native	Other/ Unknown	Total	
Hypoplastic left heart syndrome	5 *1.96*	3 *1.94*	0 *0.00*	0 *0.00*	0 *0.00*	0	8 *1.89*	
Hypospadias and Epispadias	39 *15.26*	23 *14.87*	0 *0.00*	1 *29.24*	0 *0.00*	0	63 *14.91*	isolated 1st degree hypospadias not reported
Microcephalus	15 *5.87*	18 *11.64*	0 *0.00*	1 *29.24*	0 *0.00*	0	34 *8.04*	
Obstructive genitourinary defect	67 *26.22*	46 *29.74*	1 *15.38*	0 *0.00*	0 *0.00*	0	114 *26.97*	
Omphalocele	8 *3.13*	4 *2.59*	0 *0.00*	0 *0.00*	0 *0.00*	0	12 *2.84*	
Pulmonary valve atresia and stenosis	11 *4.31*	6 *3.88*	0 *0.00*	0 *0.00*	0 *0.00*	0	17 *4.02*	
Pyloric stenosis	59 *23.09*	13 *8.40*	0 *0.00*	0 *0.00*	0 *0.00*	0	72 *17.03*	
Rectal and large intestinal atresia/stenosis	11 *4.31*	10 *6.47*	0 *0.00*	1 *29.24*	0 *0.00*	0	22 *5.21*	
Reduction deformity, lower limbs	1 *0.39*	3 *1.94*	0 *0.00*	1 *29.24*	0 *0.00*	0	5 *1.18*	
Reduction deformity, upper limbs	14 *5.48*	1 *0.65*	1 *15.38*	1 *29.24*	0 *0.00*	0	17 *4.02*	
Renal agenesis/hypoplasia	25 *9.78*	18 *11.64*	0 *0.00*	1 *29.24*	0 *0.00*	0	44 *10.41*	
Spina bifida without anencephalus	10 *3.91*	8 *5.17*	1 *15.38*	1 *29.24*	0 *0.00*	0	20 *4.73*	
Tetralogy of Fallot	12 *4.70*	9 *5.82*	0 *0.00*	0 *0.00*	0 *0.00*	0	21 *4.97*	
Transposition of great arteries	13 *5.09*	3 *1.94*	1 *15.38*	0 *0.00*	0 *0.00*	0	17 *4.02*	
Tricuspid valve atresia and stenosis	4 *1.57*	1 *0.65*	0 *0.00*	0 *0.00*	0 *0.00*	0	5 *1.18*	
Trisomy 13	10 *3.91*	2 *1.29*	0 *0.00*	0 *0.00*	0 *0.00*	0	12 *2.84*	
Trisomy 18	9 *3.52*	5 *3.23*	0 *0.00*	0 *0.00*	0 *0.00*	0	14 *3.31*	
Ventricular septal defect	37 *14.48*	20 *12.93*	2 *30.77*	0 *0.00*	0 *0.00*	0	59 *13.96*	isolated cases not reported
Total Live Births	25,551	15,467	650	342	221		42,267	

TRISOMY COUNTS AND RATES BY MATERNAL AGE 1998–2001
(Rates per 10,000 Live Births)

Defect	Age		
	<35	35 and >	Total*
Down syndrome	32 *8.32*	21 *55.02*	53 *12.54*
Trisomy 13	8 *2.08*	4 *10.48*	12 *2.84*
Trisomy 18	7 *1.82*	7 *18.34*	14 *3.31*
Total Live Births	38,444	3,817	42,267

*Total includes unknown age.

Alaska

BIRTH DEFECTS COUNTS AND RATES 1997–2001

(Rates per 10,000 Live Births)

Defect	Non-Hispanic White	Non-Hispanic Black or African	Hispanic	Asian or Pacific Islander	American Indian or Alaskan Native	Other/ Unknown	Total	Notes
Amniotic bands							0	Live births only
							0.00	
Anencephalus							8	
							1.60	
Aniridia							1	
							0.20	
Anophthalmia / microphthalmia							18	
							3.61	
Anotia/microtia							23	
							4.61	
Aortic valve stenosis							15	
							3.00	
Atrial septal defect							429	
							86.08	
Biliary atresia							11	
							2.20	
Bladder exstrophy							4	
							0.80	
Choanal artesia							15	
							3.00	
Cleft lip with and without cleft palate							88	
							17.65	
Cleft palate without cleft lip							57	
							11.43	
Coarctation of aorta							25	
							5.01	
Common truncus							9	
							1.80	
Congenital cataract							24	
							4.81	
Congenital hip dislocation							137	
							27.49	
Diaphragmatic hernia							28	
							5.61	
Down syndrome							67	
							13.44	
Ebstein's anomaly							4	
							0.80	
Encephalocele							15	
							3.00	
Endocardial cushion defect							27	
							5.41	
Esophageal atresia / tracheoesophageal fistula							15	
							3.00	
Hirschsprung's disease (congenital megacolon)							64	
							12.84	
Hydrocephalus without Spina Bifida							65	
							13.04	
Hypoplastic left heart syndrome							12	
							2.40	
Hypospadias and Epispadias							191	
							38.32	

(Table continues)

(Table continued)

Defect	Race/Ethnicity						Total	Notes
	Non-Hispanic White	Non-Hispanic Black or African	Hispanic	Asian or Pacific Islander	American Indian or Alaskan Native	Other/Unknown		
Microcephalus							150 *30.09*	
Obstructive genitourinary defect							141 *28.29*	
Patent ductus arteriosus							285 *57.18*	include birth weight ≥2500 grams only
Pulmonary valve atresia and stenosis							32 *6.42*	Adjusted for over-reporting, based on medical chart review
Pyloric stenosis							149 *29.89*	
Rectal and large intestinal atresia/stenosis							48 *9.63*	
Reduction deformity, lower limbs							41 *8.22*	
Reduction deformity, upper limbs							20 *4.01*	
Renal agenesis/hypoplasia							26 *5.21*	
Spina bifida without anencephalus							21 *4.21*	Live births only
Tetralogy of Fallot							42 *8.42*	
Transposition of great arteries							23 *4.61*	
Tricuspid valve atresia and stenosis							13 *2.60*	
Trisomy 13							9 *1.80*	
Trisomy 18							9 *1.80*	
Ventricular septal defect							384 *77.05*	
Total Live Births							49,835	

Notes:
1. Alaska conducts surveillance for FAS using FASSNET methodology. ICD-9 case counts do not accurately reflect FAS prevalence. Contact the program for data on FAS.

TRISOMY COUNTS AND RATES BY MATERNAL AGE 1997–2001
(Rates per 10,000 Live Births)

Defect	Age		
	<35	35 and >	Total*
Down syndrome	40 *13.44*	27 *9.30*	67 *39.67*
Trisomy 13	5 *1.16*	4 *5.88*	9 *1.81*
Trisomy 18	4 *0.92*	4 *5.88*	9 *1.81*
Total Live Births	43,017	6,806	49,835

*Total includes unknown age.

Arizona

BIRTH DEFECTS COUNTS AND RATES 1997

(Rates per 10,000 Live Births)

Defect	Non-Hispanic White	Non-Hispanic Black or African	Hispanic	Asian or Pacific Islander	American Indian or Alaskan Native	Other/Unknown	Total	Notes
Amniotic bands	8	0	3	0	1	0	12	
	2.11	*0.00*	*1.07*	*0.00*	*1.90*		*1.59*	
Anencephalus	9	0	13	0	1	1	24	
	2.38	*0.00*	*4.65*	*0.00*	*1.90*		*3.18*	
Aniridia	0	0	2	0	0	0	2	
	0.00	*0.00*	*0.72*	*0.00*	*0.00*		*0.26*	
Anophthalmia / microphthalmia	9	1	4	0	5	0	19	
	2.38	*4.02*	*1.43*	*0.00*	*9.49*		*2.51*	
Anotia/microtia	11	0	10	2	8	0	31	
	2.90	*0.00*	*3.58*	*12.48*	*15.18*		*4.10*	
Aortic valve stenosis	14	0	12	0	1	0	27	
	3.70	*0.00*	*4.29*	*0.00*	*1.90*		*3.57*	
Atrial septal defect	42	4	33	1	18	1	99	
	11.09	*16.10*	*11.81*	*6.24*	*34.15*		*13.10*	
Biliary atresia	2	0	0	0	0	0	2	
	0.53	*0.00*	*0.00*	*0.00*	*0.00*		*0.26*	
Bladder exstrophy	1	0	0	0	0	0	1	
	0.26	*0.00*	*0.00*	*0.00*	*0.00*		*0.13*	
Choanal atresia	8	2	1	0	0	0	11	
	2.11	*8.05*	*0.36*	*0.00*	*0.00*		*1.46*	
Cleft lip with and without cleft palate	52	1	22	2	22	3	102	
	13.73	*4.02*	*7.87*	*12.48*	*41.74*		*13.50*	
Cleft palate without cleft lip	21	0	17	0	3	3	44	
	5.55	*0.00*	*6.08*	*0.00*	*5.69*		*5.82*	
Coarctation of aorta	22	0	15	0	1	0	38	
	5.81	*0.00*	*5.37*	*0.00*	*1.90*		*5.03*	
Common truncus		7	1	2	1	0	11	
	1.85	*4.02*	*0.72*	*6.24*	*0.00*		*1.46*	
Congenital cataract	5	0	6	0	1	1	13	
	1.32	*0.00*	*2.15*	*0.00*	*1.90*		*1.72*	
Congenital hip dislocation	26	1	20	0	8	0	55	
	6.87	*4.02*	*7.16*	*0.00*	*15.18*		*7.28*	
Diaphragmatic hernia	8	0	5	0	1	1	15	
	2.11	*0.00*	*1.79*	*0.00*	*1.90*		*1.99*	
Down syndrome	45	5	35	1	12	2	100	
	11.88	*20.12*	*12.53*	*6.24*	*22.77*		*13.23*	
Ebstein's anomaly	4	0	4	0	1	0	9	
	1.06	*0.00*	*1.43*	*0.00*	*1.90*		*1.19*	
Encephalocele	1	1	6	0	1	0	9	
	0.26	*4.02*	*2.15*	*0.00*	*1.90*		*1.19*	
Endocardial cushion defect	15	0	12	0	0	1	28	
	3.96	*0.00*	*4.29*	*0.00*	*0.00*		*3.71*	
Esophageal atresia / tracheoesophageal fistula	15	0	6	0	1	0	22	
	3.96	*0.00*	*2.15*	*0.00*	*1.90*		*2.91*	
Fetal alcohol syndrome	1	0	0	0	6	1	8	
	0.26	*0.00*	*0.00*	*0.00*	*11.38*		*1.06*	
Gastroschisis	10	5	19	0	2	0	36	
	2.64	*20.12*	*6.80*	*0.00*	*3.79*		*4.76*	
Hirschsprung's disease (congenital megacolon)	6	0	2	0	0	0	8	
	1.58	*0.00*	*0.72*	*0.00*	*0.00*		*1.06*	
Hydrocephalus without Spina Bifida	18	0	10	0	3	0	31	
	4.75	*0.00*	*3.58*	*0.00*	*5.69*		*4.10*	

(Table continues)

(Table continued)

Defect	Race/Ethnicity							
	Non-Hispanic White	Non-Hispanic Black or African	Hispanic	Asian or Pacific Islander	American Indian or Alaskan Native	Other/ Unknown	Total	Notes
Hypoplastic left heart syndrome	9 *2.38*	0 *0.00*	3 *1.07*	0 *0.00*	0 *0.00*	0	12 *1.59*	
Hypospadias and Epispadias	134 *35.39*	10 *40.24*	42 *15.03*	7 *43.70*	6 *11.38*	2	201 *26.60*	
Microcephalus	22 *5.81*	3 *12.07*	32 *11.45*	1 *6.24*	8 *15.18*	3	69 *9.13*	
Obstructive genitourinary defect	52 *13.73*	1 *4.02*	47 *16.82*	3 *18.73*	8 *15.18*	1	112 *14.82*	
Omphalocele	6 *1.58*	0 *0.00*	3 *1.07*	0 *0.00*	1 *1.90*	0	10 *1.32*	
Pulmonary valve atresia and stenosis	33 *8.71*	3 *12.07*	22 *7.87*	2 *12.48*	7 *13.28*	0	67 *8.87*	
Pyloric stenosis	86 *22.71*	4 *16.10*	43 *15.39*	0 *0.00*	12 *22.77*	7	152 *20.12*	
Rectal and large intestinal atresia/stenosis	12 *3.17*	1 *4.02*	7 *2.51*	0 *0.00*	0 *0.00*	0	20 *2.65*	
Reduction deformity, lower limbs	14 *3.70*	0 *0.00*	1 *0.36*	0 *0.00*	2 *3.79*	0	17 *2.25*	
Reduction deformity, upper limbs	17 *4.49*	0 *0.00*	7 *2.51*	0 *0.00*	2 *3.79*	0	26 *3.44*	
Renal agenesis/hypoplasia	15 *3.96*	1 *4.02*	12 *4.29*	3 *18.73*	2 *3.79*	0	33 *4.37*	
Spina bifida without anencephalus	16 *4.23*	0 *0.00*	12 *4.29*	0 *0.00*	2 *3.79*	2	32 *4.23*	
Tetralogy of Fallot	18 *4.75*	2 *8.05*	7 *2.51*	1 *6.24*	5 *9.49*	0	33 *4.37*	
Transposition of great arteries	17 *4.49*	2 *8.05*	15 *5.37*	1 *6.24*	3 *5.69*	1	39 *5.16*	
Tricuspid valve atresia and stenosis	4 *1.06*	0 *0.00*	4 *1.43*	0 *0.00*	0 *0.00*	0	8 *1.06*	
Trisomy 13	1 *0.26*	0 *0.00*	3 *1.07*	0 *0.00*	0 *0.00*	1	5 *0.66*	
Trisomy 18	7 *1.85*	1 *4.02*	5 *1.79*	0 *0.00*	2 *3.79*	0	15 *1.99*	
Ventricular septal defect	66 *17.43*	5 *20.12*	53 *18.97*	2 *12.48*	18 *34.15*	1	145 *19.19*	
Total Live Births	37,869	2,485	27,941	1,602	5,271		75,563	

TRISOMY COUNTS AND RATES BY MATERNAL AGE 1997

(Rates per 10,000 Live Births)

Defect	Age		
	<35	35 and >	Total*
Down syndrome	63 *9.49*	37 *40.31*	100 *13.23*
Trisomy 13	3 *0.45*	2 *2.18*	5 *0.66*
Trisomy 18	13 *1.96*	2 *2.18*	15 *1.99*
Total Live Births	66,362	9,179	75,563

*Total includes unknown age.

Arkansas

BIRTH DEFECTS COUNTS AND RATES 1997–2001

(Rates per 10,000 Live Births)

Defect	Non-Hispanic White	Non-Hispanic Black or African	Hispanic	Asian or Pacific Islander	American Indian or Alaskan Native	Other/ Unknown	Total	Notes
Amniotic bands	28	10	1	0	0	2	41	
	2.12	2.58	0.98	0.00	0.00		2.22	
Anencephalus	54	11	6	1	0	3	75	
	4.08	2.84	5.89	4.86	0.00		4.06	
Aniridia	0	0	0	0	0	0	0	
	0.00	0.00	0.00	0.00	0.00		0.00	
Anophthalmia / microphthalmia	42	7	1	0	0	0	50	
	3.18	1.81	0.98	0.00	0.00		2.71	
Anotia/microtia	27	3	2	0	0	0	31	
	2.04	0.77	0.98	0.00	0.00		1.68	
Aortic valve stenosis	51	14	2	2	0	0	69	
	3.86	3.61	1.96	9.73	0.00		3.74	
Atrial septal defect	465	143	31	2	0	9	650	
	35.17	36.91	30.42	9.73	0.00		35.19	
Biliary atresia	5	5	2	1	0	0	13	
	0.38	1.29	1.96	4.86	0.00		0.70	
Bladder exstrophy	5	0	0	0	0	0	5	
	0.38	0.00	0.00	0.00	0.00		0.27	
Choanal artesia	15	3	2	0	0	0	20	
	1.13	0.77	1.96	0.00	0.00		1.08	
Cleft lip with and without cleft palate	168	27	10	1	2	3	211	
	12.71	6.97	9.81	4.86	18.81		11.42	
Cleft palate without cleft lip	107	18	3	1	0	1	130	
	8.09	4.65	2.94	4.86	0.00		7.04	
Coarctation of aorta	76	12	6	0	0	0	94	
	5.75	3.10	5.89	0.00	0.00		5.09	
Common truncus	11	1	1	0	0	0	13	
	0.83	0.26	0.98	0.00	0.00		0.70	
Congenital cataract	36	18	2	0	0	1	57	
	2.72	4.65	1.96	0.00	0.00		3.09	
Congenital hip dislocation	82	8	14	0	1	1	106	inclusion criteria altered after 1998
	6.20	2.06	13.74	0.00	9.41		5.74	
Diaphragmatic hernia	67	8	2	0	0	0	77	
	5.07	2.06	1.96	0.00	0.00		4.17	
Down syndrome	155	42	19	1	0	3	220	
	11.72	10.84	18.64	4.86	0.00		11.91	
Ebstein's anomaly	15	0	1	0	0	0	16	
	1.13	0.00	0.98	0.00	0.00		0.87	
Encephalocele	19	7	0	0	0	0	26	
	1.44	1.81	0.00	0.00	0.00		1.41	
Endocardial cushion defect	61	19	2	0	0	1	83	
	4.61	4.90	1.96	0.00	0.00		4.49	
Esophageal atresia / tracheoesophageal fistula	35	7	3	1	1	0	47	
	2.65	1.81	2.94	4.86	9.41		2.54	
Fetal alcohol syndrome	5	26	0	0	0	0	31	
	0.38	6.71	0.00	0.00	0.00		1.68	
Gastroschisis	71	13	5	0	0	3	92	
	5.37	3.36	4.91	0.00	0.00		4.98	
Hirschsprung's disease (congenital megacolon)	15	6	0	0	0	0	21	
	1.13	1.55	0.00	0.00	0.00		1.14	
Hydrocephalus without Spina Bifida	154	62	7	1	0	4	228	inclusion criteria altered in 1998
	11.65	16.00	6.87	4.86	0.00		12.34	
Hypoplastic left heart syndrome	51	5	2	0	0	0	58	
	3.86	1.29	1.96	0.00	0.00		3.14	

(Table continues)

(Table continued)

Defect	Race/Ethnicity						Total	Notes
	Non-Hispanic White	Non-Hispanic Black or African	Hispanic	Asian or Pacific Islander	American Indian or Alaskan Native	Other/ Unknown		
Hypospadias and	512	86	13	0	1	5	617	
Epispadias	*38.73*	*22.20*	*12.76*	*0.00*	*9.41*		*33.40*	
Microcephalus	88	40	4	1	1	1	135	inclusion criteria
	6.66	*10.32*	*3.93*	*4.86*	*9.41*		*7.31*	altered in 1998
Obstructive genitourinary	205	47	18	3	0	1	274	
defect	*15.51*	*12.13*	*17.66*	*14.59*	*0.00*		*14.83*	
Omphalocele	30	12	4	0	0	1	47	
	2.27	*3.10*	*3.93*	*0.00*	*0.00*		*2.54*	
Patent ductus arteriosus	378	127	32	3	0	3	543	only if weight ≥2500
	28.59	*32.78*	*31.40*	*14.59*	*0.00*		*29.39*	grams; inclusion criteria altered in 2001
Pulmonary valve atresia	136	41	8	0	0	4	189	
and stenosis	*10.29*	*10.58*	*7.85*	*0.00*	*0.00*		*10.23*	
Pyloric stenosis	201	20	12	0	0	3	236	inclusion criteria
	15.20	*5.16*	*11.78*	*0.00*	*0.00*		*12.78*	altered after 1998
Rectal and large intestinal	82	18	4	0	0	1	105	
atresia/stenosis	*6.20*	*4.65*	*3.93*	*0.00*	*0.00*		*5.68*	
Reduction deformity,	20	10	2	0	0	0	32	
lower limbs	*1.51*	*2.58*	*1.96*	*0.00*	*0.00*		*1.73*	
Reduction deformity,	51	14	3	0	0	1	69	
upper limbs	*3.86*	*3.61*	*2.94*	*0.00*	*0.00*		*3.74*	
Renal agenesis/hypoplasia	65	15	8	0	0	1	89	
	4.92	*3.87*	*7.85*	*0.00*	*0.00*		*4.82*	
Spina bifida without	76	16	4	0	0	2	98	
anencephalus	*5.75*	*4.13*	*3.93*	*0.00*	*0.00*		*5.31*	
Tetralogy of Fallot	45	18	7	1	0	2	73	
	3.40	*4.65*	*6.87*	*4.86*	*0.00*		*3.95*	
Transposition of great	66	12	6	1	0	0	85	
arteries	*4.99*	*3.10*	*5.89*	*4.86*	*0.00*		*4.60*	
Tricuspid valve atresia	17	4	1	0	0	0	22	
and stenosis	*1.29*	*1.03*	*0.98*	*0.00*	*0.00*		*0.92*	
Trisomy 13	14	3	0	0	0	0	17	
	1.06	*0.77*	*0.00*	*0.00*	*0.00*		*0.92*	
Trisomy 18	23	6	1	0	0	0	30	
	1.74	*1.55*	*0.98*	*0.00*	*0.00*		*1.62*	
Ventricular septal defect	506	149	44	7	2	10	718	
	38.28	*38.46*	*43.18*	*34.05*	*18.81*		*38.87*	
Total Live Births	132,199	38,744	10,191	2,056	1,063		184,731	

TRISOMY COUNTS AND RATES BY MATERNAL AGE 1997–2001
(Rates per 10,000 Live Births)

Defect	Age		
	<35	35 and >	Total*
Down syndrome	136	78	220
	7.94	*58.63*	*11.91*
Trisomy 13	15	2	17
	0.88	*1.50*	*0.92*
Trisomy 18	18	12	30
	1.05	*9.02*	*1.62*
Total Live Births	171,380	13,304	184,731

*Total includes unknown age.
Notes:
1. All data for 2001 are provisional.

California

BIRTH DEFECTS COUNTS AND RATES 1997–2001

(Rates per 10,000 Live Births)

Defect	Non-Hispanic White	Non-Hispanic Black or African	Hispanic	Asian or Pacific Islander	American Indian or Alaskan Native	Other/Unknown	Total	Notes
Amniotic bands	12	<5	27	9	<5	0	51	
	1.28		*1.75*	*7.20*			*1.80*	
Anencephalus	26	<5	35	10	<5	22	95	
	2.78		*2.27*	*8.00*			*3.36*	
Anophthalmia / microphthalmia	12	0	13	0	0	0	25	
	1.28	*0.00*	*0.84*	*0.00*	*0.00*		*0.88*	
Anotia/microtia	13	<5	64	6	0	<5	86	
	1.39		*4.15*	*4.80*	*0.00*		*3.04*	
Aortic valve stenosis	24	<5	12	<5	<5	0	43	
	2.57		*0.78*				*1.52*	
Atrial septal defect	161	25	289	26	5	12	518	
	17.21	*18.68*	*18.75*	*20.80*	*22.37*		*18.30*	
Biliary atresia	6	5	10	0	0	0	21	
	0.64	*3.74*	*0.65*	*0.00*	*0.00*		*0.74*	
Bladder exstrophy	<5	0	0	0	0	0	<5	
		0.00	*0.00*	*0.00*	*0.00*			
Choanal artesia	6	0	<5	<5	0	0	11	
	0.64	*0.00*			*0.00*		*0.39*	
Cleft lip with and without cleft palate	106	10	145	9	<5	9	281	
	11.33	*7.47*	*9.41*	*7.20*			*9.93*	
Cleft palate without cleft lip	49	7	51	7	<5	9	126	
	5.24	*5.23*	*3.31*	*5.60*			*4.45*	
Coarctation of aorta	40	5	55	6	<5	<5	110	
	4.28	*3.74*	*3.57*	*4.80*			*3.89*	
Common truncus	5	0	6	0	0	0	11	
	0.53	*0.00*	*0.39*	*0.00*	*0.00*		*0.39*	
Diaphragmatic hernia	19	<5	38	<5	0	<5	66	
	2.03		*2.47*		*0.00*		*2.33*	
Down syndrome	100	11	224	11	<5	6	354	
	10.69	*8.22*	*14.54*	*8.80*			*12.51*	
Ebstein's anomaly	<5	0	<5	0	0	<5	8	
		0.00		*0.00*	*0.00*		*0.28*	
Encephalocele	5	<5	10	<5	<5	<5	20	
	0.53		*0.65*				*0.71*	
Endocardial cushion defect	40	<5	63	5	<5	5	117	
	4.28		*4.09*	*4.00*			*4.13*	
Esophageal atresia / tracheoesophageal fistula	11	<5	19	<5	0	0	34	
	1.18		*1.23*		*0.00*		*1.20*	
Fetal alcohol syndrome	5	<5	6	<5	0	<5	17	
	0.53		*0.39*		*0.00*		*0.60*	
Gastroschisis	38	<5	58	7	0	<5	110	
	4.06		*3.76*	*5.60*	*0.00*		*3.89*	
Hydrocephalus without Spina Bifida	26	5	40	6	0	<5	780	
	2.78	*3.74*	*2.60*	*4.80*	*0.00*		*2.76*	
Hypoplastic left heart syndrome	24	<5	31	<5	<5	0	63	
	2.57		*2.01*				*2.23*	
Hypospadias and Epispadias	23	5	32	<5	<5	<5	67	
	2.46	*3.74*	*2.08*				*2.37*	
Omphalocele	13	<5	11	<5	0	0	27	
	1.39		*0.71*		*0.00*		*0.95*	
Pulmonary valve atresia and stenosis	9	<5	19	0	0	<5	31	
	0.96		*1.23*	*0.00*	*0.00*		*1.10*	

(Table continues)

(Table continued)

Defect	Race/Ethnicity							Notes
	Non-Hispanic White	Non-Hispanic Black or African	Hispanic	Asian or Pacific Islander	American Indian or Alaskan Native	Other/Unknown	Total	
Rectal and large intestinal atresia/stenosis	26 *2.78*	<5	43 *2.79*	6 *4.80*	0 *0.00*	<5	77 *2.72*	
Reduction deformity, lower limbs	13 *1.39*	<5	23 *1.49*	<5	0 *0.00*	<5	45 *1.59*	
Reduction deformity, upper limbs	27 *2.89*	<5	60 *3.89*	5 *4.00*	0 *0.00*	<5	99 *3.50*	
Renal agenesis/hypoplasia	<5	0 *0.00*	10 *0.65*	<5	<5	<5	16 *0.57*	
Spina bifida without anencephalus	39 *4.17*	<5	63 *4.09*	<5	0 *0.00*	8	116 *4.10*	
Tetralogy of Fallot	31 *3.31*	<5	57 *3.70*	6 *4.80*	<5	5	104 *3.67*	
Transposition of great arteries	41 *4.38*	7 *5.23*	60 *3.89*	5 *4.00*	<5	<5	116 *4.10*	
Tricuspid valve atresia and stenosis	<5	<5 *1.17*	18	<5 *0.00*	0	0	25 *0.88*	
Trisomy 13	5 *0.53*	<5	17 *1.10*	<5	0 *0.00*	0	26 *0.92*	
Trisomy 18	12 *1.28*	<5	24 *1.56*	6 *4.80*	0 *0.00*	<5	50 *1.77*	
Ventricular septal defect	143 *15.29*	18 *13.45*	254 *16.48*	17 *13.60*	<5	8	443 *15.65*	
Total Live Births	93,528	13,383	154,101	12,497	2,235		283,066	

TRISOMY COUNTS AND RATES BY MATERNAL AGE 1997–2001
(Rates per 10,000 Live Births)

Defect	Age		Total*
	<35	35 and >	
Down syndrome	217 *8.56*	133 *45.10*	354 *12.51*
Trisomy 13	20 *0.79*	6 *2.03*	26 *0.92*
Trisomy 18	26 *1.03*	20 *6.78*	50 *1.77*
Total Live Births	253,564	29,491	283,066

*Total includes unknown age.

Notes:
1. Anophthalmia/microphthalmia—Bilateral confirmed by geneticist (14), pathologist (25), ophthalmologist (22) or neurologist (19).
2. Anotia/microtia—Exclude any case with Downs (758.000); 744.214—Diagnosis confirmed by geneticist (14), ENT (24) or pathologist (25).
3. Cardiovascular defects—Diagnosis confirmed by cardiac surgeon (8), cardiologist (9), pathologist (25) or by autopsy (18), echo (5), catheterization (16), or surgery (15).
4. ASD and VSD—A) Reportable in isolation only with positive catheterization, CHF, diuretics, medication or surgery. Prior to 1/1/00 were reportable in combination only. B) If the ASD and/or VSD is a component of another major heart malformation, it is not counted. C) The only chromosomal abnormalities included in this dataset are Trisomy 13, 18, 21. If the baby had ASD and /or VSD and a chromosome anomaly that was not Trisomy 13, 18, 21, the ASD and/or VSD was excluded. D) ASD and/or VSD not confirmed to echo, cardiac catherization, surgery, or baby did not have congestive heart failure or was not taking diuretics was excluded. E) ASD and/or VSD were excluded if physician review determined the baby did not have the defect.
5. Hypospadias and Epispadias—No epispadias in registry; 2nd and 3rd degree hypospadias only.
6. Pulmonary valve atresia and stenosis—No stenosis in registry.
7. Rectal and large intestinal atresia/stenosis—Diagnosis confirmed by autopsy (18), CT scan (3), scope (11), surgery (15) or X-ray (6).
8. Trisomy 13, Down syndrome, and trisomy 18—Diagnosis confirmed by cytogeneticist (19, 119).
9. CBDPMP does not report rates based on <5 cases.

Colorado

BIRTH DEFECTS COUNTS AND RATES 1997–2001

(Rates per 10,000 Live Births)

Defect	Race/Ethnicity							
	Non-Hispanic White	Non-Hispanic Black or African	Hispanic	Asian or Pacific Islander	American Indian or Alaskan Native	Other/Unknown	Total	Notes
Anencephalus	18	1	12	1	1	8	41	live births/fetal deaths—
	0.89	*0.73*	*1.46*	*1.08*	*4.05*		*1.32*	any gestational age
Aniridia	2	0	1	2	0	0	5	
	0.10	*0.00*	*0.12*	*2.16*	*0.00*		*0.16*	
Anophthalmia / microphthalmia	23	0	14	0	0	2	39	
	1.13	*0.00*	*1.71*	*0.00*	*0.00*		*1.26*	
Anotia/microtia	29	0	25	2	0	1	57	
	1.43	*0.00*	*3.05*	*2.16*	*0.00*		*1.83*	
Aortic valve stenosis	74	3	26	3	1	5	112	
	3.65	*2.18*	*3.17*	*3.24*	*4.05*		*3.61*	
Atrial septal defect	1,031	69	394	52	15	4	1,565	
	50.79	*50.12*	*48.00*	*56.22*	*60.78*		*50.38*	
Biliary atresia	27	4	13	2	0	0	46	
	1.33	*2.91*	*1.58*	*2.16*	*0.00*		*1.48*	
Bladder exstrophy	6	0	5	0	0	3	14	
	0.30	*0.00*	*0.61*	*0.00*	*0.00*		*0.45*	
Choanal artesia	31	1	8	1	0	2	43	
	1.53	*0.73*	*0.97*	*1.08*	*0.00*		*1.38*	
Cleft lip with and without cleft palate	241	14	102	12	4	12	385	
	11.87	*10.17*	*12.43*	*12.97*	*16.21*		*12.39*	
Cleft palate without cleft lip	171	6	47	4	1	5	234	
	8.42	*4.36*	*5.73*	*4.32*	*4.05*		*7.53*	
Coarctation of aorta	203	3	53	7	1	6	273	
	10.00	*2.18*	*6.46*	*7.57*	*4.05*		*8.79*	
Common truncus	21	2	6	0	2	1	32	
	1.03	*1.45*	*0.73*	*0.00*	*8.10*		*1.03*	
Congenital cataract	55	4	26	3	0	0	88	
	2.71	*2.91*	*3.17*	*3.24*	*0.00*		*2.83*	
Congenital hip dislocation	374	7	143	15	3	2	544	
	18.43	*5.08*	*17.42*	*16.22*	*12.16*		*17.51*	
Diaphragmatic hernia	81	9	41	4	0	11	146	
	3.99	*6.54*	*4.99*	*4.32*	*0.00*		*4.70*	
Down syndrome	258	15	92	10	2	186	563	
	12.71	*10.89*	*11.21*	*10.81*	*8.10*		*18.12*	
Ebstein's anomaly	24	0	8	0	0	2	34	
	1.18	*0.00*	*0.97*	*0.00*	*0.00*		*1.09*	
Encephalocele	17	0	10	0	0	6	33	
	0.84	*0.00*	*1.22*	*0.00*	*0.00*		*1.06*	
Endocardial cushion defect	71	5	29	4	0	10	119	
	3.50	*3.63*	*3.53*	*4.32*	*0.00*		*3.83*	
Esophageal atresia / tracheoesophageal fistula	106	5	25	4	0	5	145	
	5.22	*3.63*	*3.05*	*4.32*	*0.00*		*4.67*	
Gastroschisis	58	3	46	5	0	4	116	medical record review
	2.86	*2.18*	*5.60*	*5.41*	*0.00*		*3.73*	
Hirschsprung's disease (congenital megacolon)	46	7	20	2	1	1	77	
	2.27	*5.08*	*2.44*	*2.16*	*4.05*		*2.48*	
Hydrocephalus without Spina Bifida	168	9	70	9	3	26	285	
	8.28	*6.54*	*8.53*	*9.73*	*12.16*		*9.17*	
Hypoplastic left heart syndrome	57	1	17	2	0	6	83	
	2.81	*0.73*	*2.07*	*2.16*	*0.00*		*2.67*	
Hypospadias and Epispadias	1,118	75	187	24	6	6	1,416	
	55.08	*54.47*	*22.78*	*25.95*	*24.31*		*45.58*	

(Table continues)

(Table continued)

Defect	Race/Ethnicity							Notes
	Non-Hispanic White	Non-Hispanic Black or African	Hispanic	Asian or Pacific Islander	American Indian or Alaskan Native	Other/ Unknown	Total	
Microcephalus	86	12	53	6	1	1	159	
	4.24	*8.72*	*6.46*	*6.49*	*4.05*		*5.12*	
Obstructive genitourinary defect	602	36	232	35	5	13	923	
	29.66	*26.15*	*28.26*	*37.84*	*20.26*		*29.71*	
Omphalocele	56	1	21	2	0	8	88	medical record review
	2.76	*0.73*	*2.56*	*2.16*	*0.00*		*2.83*	
Patent ductus arteriosus	825	62	301	38	10	0	1,236	cases w/ birth weight
	40.65	*45.03*	*36.67*	*41.08*	*40.52*		*39.79*	of ≥2500 grams
Pulmonary valve atresia and stenosis	213	24	82	9	2	3	333	
	10.49	*17.43*	*9.99*	*9.73*	*8.10*		*10.72*	
Pyloric stenosis	386	6	152	6	1	0	551	
	19.02	*4.36*	*18.52*	*6.49*	*4.05*		*17.74*	
Rectal and large intestinal atresia/stenosis	116	6	47	4	0	5	178	
	5.71	*4.36*	*5.73*	*4.32*	*0.00*		*5.73*	
Reduction deformity, lower limbs	34	4	19	2	0	5	64	
	1.68	*2.91*	*2.31*	*2.16*	*0.00*		*2.06*	
Reduction deformity, upper limbs	77	7	29	4	0	7	124	
	3.79	*5.08*	*3.53*	*4.32*	*0.00*		*3.99*	
Renal agenesis/hypoplasia	90	8	38	5	1	11	153	
	4.43	*5.81*	*4.63*	*5.41*	*4.05*		*4.93*	
Spina bifida without anencephalus	62	0	20	0	0	14	96	live births/fetal deaths—
	3.05	*0.00*	*2.44*	*0.00*	*0.00*		*3.09*	any gestational age
Tetralogy of Fallot	85	8	24	3	0	2	122	
	4.19	*5.81*	*2.92*	*3.24*	*0.00*		*3.93*	
Transposition of great arteries	88	4	27	2	1	1	123	
	4.34	*2.91*	*3.29*	*2.16*	*4.05*		*3.96*	
Tricuspid valve atresia and stenosis	27	2	16	2	1	0	48	
	1.33	*1.45*	*1.95*	*2.16*	*4.05*		*1.55*	
Trisomy 13	22	2	17	0	1	35	77	
	1.08	*1.45*	*2.07*	*0.00*	*4.05*		*2.48*	
Trisomy 18	57	7	20	4	0	68	156	
	2.81	*5.08*	*2.44*	*4.32*	*0.00*		*5.02*	
Ventricular septal defect	819	57	354	34	12	13	1,289	includes probable cases
	40.35	*41.40*	*43.12*	*36.76*	*48.62*		*41.50*	
Total Live Births	**202,976**	**13,768**	**82,090**	**9,250**	**2,468**		**310,632**	

TRISOMY COUNTS AND RATES BY MATERNAL AGE 1997–2001
(Rates per 10,000 Live Births)

Defect	Age		
	<35	35 and >	Total*
Down syndrome	286	274	·563
	10.73	*62.39*	*18.12*
Trisomy 13	48	29	77
	1.80	*6.60*	*2.48*
Trisomy 18	79	75	156
	2.96	*17.08*	*5.02*
Total Live Births	**266,567**	**43,919**	**310,632**

*Total includes unknown age.

Notes:
1. Data for fetal alcohol syndrome are available through the FAS Surveillance Network. Contact CRCSN at crcsn@state.co.us for these data.
2. See pregnancy outcome section of Colorado's program description for detailed pregnancy outcome collected for all birth defects.
3. Colorado residency rule has changed from previous years. Please contact CRCSN for further information.

Delaware

BIRTH DEFECTS COUNTS AND RATES 1997–2000

(Rates per 10,000 Live Births)

Defect	Race/Ethnicity						Total	Notes
	Non-Hispanic White	Non-Hispanic Black or African	Hispanic	Asian or Pacific Islander	American Indian or Alaskan Native	Other/ Unknown		
Anencephalus	0	0	0	0	0	0	0	Live births only
	0.00	*0.00*	*0.00*	*0.00*	*0.00*		*0.00*	
Aniridia	0	0	0	0	0	0	0	
	0.00	*0.00*	*0.00*	*0.00*	*0.00*		*0.00*	
Anophthalmia / microphthalmia	51	25	4	0	0	3	83	
	18.44	*24.25*	*12.13*	*0.00*	*0.00*		*19.51*	
Anotia/microtia	0	0	0	0	0	0	0	
	0.00	*0.00*	*0.00*	*0.00*	*0.00*		*0.00*	
Aortic valve stenosis	7	1	0	0	0	0	8	
	2.53	*0.97*	*0.00*	*0.00*	*0.00*		*1.88*	
Atrial septal defect	121	56	10	6	0	7	200	
	43.75	*54.33*	*30.33*	*54.89*	*0.00*		*47.02*	
Biliary atresia	1	3	0	0	0	0	4	
	0.36	*2.91*	*0.00*	*0.00*	*0.00*		*0.94*	
Bladder exstrophy	1	0	1	0	0	0	2	
	0.36	*0.00*	*3.03*	*0.00*	*0.00*		*0.47*	
Choanal atresia	5	2	0	0	0	0	7	
	1.81	*1.94*	*0.00*	*0.00*	*0.00*		*1.65*	
Cleft lip with and without cleft palate	22	7	1	0	0	0	30	
	7.95	*6.79*	*3.03*	*0.00*	*0.00*		*7.05*	
Cleft palate without cleft lip	17	5	1	0	0	1	24	
	6.15	*4.85*	*3.03*	*0.00*	*0.00*		*5.64*	
Coarctation of aorta	15	2	0	1	0	1	19	
	5.42	*1.94*	*0.00*	*9.15*	*0.00*		*4.47*	
Common truncus	1	1	0	0	0	0	2	
	0.36	*0.97*	*0.00*	*0.00*	*0.00*		*0.47*	
Congenital cataract	2	3	1	0	0	0	6	
	0.72	*2.91*	*3.03*	*0.00*	*0.00*		*1.41*	
Congenital hip dislocation	54	5	8	4	0	2	71	
	19.52	*3.88*	*21.23*	*36.60*	*0.00*		*16.69*	
Diaphragmatic hernia	6	3	0	0	0	1	10	
	2.17	*2.91*	*0.00*	*0.00*	*0.00*		*2.35*	
Down syndrome	30	8	5	3	0	1	47	
	10.85	*7.76*	*15.17*	*27.45*	*0.00*		*11.05*	
Ebstein's anomaly	2	0	0	0	0	0	2	
	0.72	*0.00*	*0.00*	*0.00*	*0.00*		*0.47*	
Encephalocele	1	2	1	0	0	1	5	
	0.36	*1.94*	*3.03*	*0.00*	*0.00*		*1.18*	
Endocardial cushion defect	13	4	3	2	0	0	22	
	4.70	*3.88*	*9.10*	*18.30*	*0.00*		*5.17*	
Esophageal atresia / tracheoesophageal fistula	8	1	1	0	0	0	10	
	2.89	*0.97*	*3.03*	*0.00*	*0.00*		*2.35*	
Fetal alcohol syndrome	4	7	1	0	0	0	12	
	1.45	*6.79*	*3.03*	*0.00*	*0.00*		*2.82*	
Hirschsprung's disease (congenital megacolon)	6	2	0	1	0	2	11	
	2.17	*1.94*	*0.00*	*9.15*	*0.00*		*2.59*	
Hydrocephalus without Spina Bifida	9	11	0	1	0	4	25	
	3.25	*10.67*	*0.00*	*9.15*	*0.00*		*5.88*	
Hypoplastic left heart syndrome	8	4	0	0	0	1	13	
	2.89	*3.88*	*0.00*	*0.00*	*0.00*		*3.06*	
Hypospadias and Epispadias	106	40	7	4	0	2	159	
	38.32	*38.80*	*21.23*	*36.60*	*0.00*		*37.38*	

(Table continues)

(Table continued)

Defect	Race/Ethnicity							Notes
	Non-Hispanic White	Non-Hispanic Black or African	Hispanic	Asian or Pacific Islander	American Indian or Alaskan Native	Other/ Unknown	Total	
Microcephalus	1	1	2	0	0	1	5	
	0.36	*0.97*	*6.07*	*0.00*	*0.00*		*1.18*	
Obstructive genitourinary defect	100	23	13	3	0	13	152	
	36.15	*22.31*	*39.43*	*27.45*	*0.00*		*35.74*	
Omphalocele	6	0	0	0	0	1	7	
	8.57	*0.00*	*0.00*	*0.00*	*0.00*		*6.34*	
Patent ductus arteriosus	133	70	8	4	0	9	224	1997–1999 cases with birth weight of ≥2500 grams
	48.09	*67.91*	*24.26*	*36.60*	*0.00*		*52.66*	
Pulmonary valve atresia and stenosis	7	8	1	0	0	1	17	
	2.53	*7.76*	*3.03*	*0.00*	*0.00*		*4.00*	
Pyloric stenosis	63	17	4	0	0	16	100	
	22.78	*16.49*	*12.13*	*0.00*	*0.00*		*23.51*	
Rectal and large intestinal atresia/stenosis	1	5	0	1	0	0	7	
	0.36	*4.85*	*0.00*	*9.15*	*0.00*		*1.65*	
Reduction deformity, lower limbs	1	1	0	1	0	0	3	
	0.36	*0.97*	*0.00*	*9.15*	*0.00*		*0.71*	
Reduction deformity, upper limbs	8	2	0	0	0	0	10	
	2.89	*1.94*	*0.00*	*0.00*	*0.00*		*2.35*	
Renal agenesis/hypoplasia	12	3	3	0	0	1	19	
	4.34	*2.91*	*9.10*	*0.00*	*0.00*		*4.47*	
Spina bifida without anencephalus	6	2	7	0	0	0	15	Live births only
	2.17	*1.94*	*21.23*	*0.00*	*0.00*		*3.53*	
Tetralogy of Fallot	16	8	1	0	0	0	25	
	5.78	*7.76*	*3.03*	*0.00*	*0.00*		*5.88*	
Transposition of great arteries	7	3	0	0	0	2	12	
	2.53	*2.91*	*0.00*	*0.00*	*0.00*		*2.82*	
Tricuspid valve atresia and stenosis	2	1	0	0	0	0	3	
	0.72	*0.97*	*0.00*	*0.00*	*0.00*		*0.71*	
Trisomy 13	3	1	0	0	0	0	4	
	1.08	*0.97*	*0.00*	*0.00*	*0.00*		*0.94*	
Trisomy 18	0	2	2	0	0	0	4	
	0.00	*1.94*	*6.07*	*0.00*	*0.00*		*0.94*	
Ventricular septal defect	108	39	15	3	1	9	175	do not include probable cases
	39.05	*37.83*	*45.50*	*27.45*	*89.29*		*41.14*	
Total Live Births	27,659	10,308	3,297	1,093	112		42,533	

TRISOMY COUNTS AND RATES BY MATERNAL AGE 1997–2000
(Rates per 10,000 Live Births)

Defect	Age		
	<35	35 and >	Total*
Down syndrome	29	17	47
	7.79	*32.06*	*11.05*
Trisomy 13	2	2	4
	0.54	*3.77*	*0.94*
Trisomy 18	2	2	4
	0.54	*3.77*	*0.94*
Total Live Births	37,231	5,302	42,533

*Total includes unknown age.

Florida

BIRTH DEFECTS COUNTS AND RATES 1997–2000

(Rates per 10,000 Live Births)

Defect	Non-Hispanic White	Non-Hispanic Black or African	Hispanic	Asian or Pacific Islander	American Indian or Alaskan Native	Other/ Unknown	Total	Notes
Anencephalus	18	4	13	0	0	0	35	
	0.44	*0.24*	*0.70*	*0.00*	*0.00*		*0.44*	
Aniridia	5	4	3	0	0	0	12	
	0.12	*0.24*	*0.16*	*0.00*	*0.00*		*0.15*	
Anophthalmia / microphthalmia	39	22	15	3	0	0	79	
	0.94	*1.34*	*0.81*	*1.57*	*0.00*		*1.00*	
Anotia/microtia	26	7	20	0	0	0	53	
	0.63	*0.43*	*1.07*	*0.00*	*0.00*		*0.67*	
Aortic valve stenosis	82	12	19	2	0	0	115	
	1.98	*0.73*	*1.02*	*1.05*	*0.00*		*1.46*	
Atrial septal defect	2,727	1,298	1,608	113	19	7	5,772	
	65.99	*78.95*	*86.35*	*59.10*	*52.50*		*73.27*	
Biliary atresia	44	31	17	1	1	0	94	
	1.06	*1.89*	*0.91*	*0.52*	*2.76*		*1.19*	
Bladder exstrophy	17	6	4	0	0	0	27	
	0.41	*0.36*	*0.21*	*0.00*	*0.00*		*0.34*	
Choanal atresia	75	32	25	1	2	0	135	
	1.81	*1.95*	*1.34*	*0.52*	*5.53*		*1.71*	
Cleft lip with and without cleft palate	445	107	151	16	6	1	726	
	10.77	*6.51*	*8.11*	*8.37*	*16.58*		*9.22*	
Cleft palate without cleft lip	244	68	57	4	4	0	377	
	5.90	*4.14*	*3.06*	*2.09*	*11.05*		*4.79*	
Coarctation of aorta	202	79	79	3	2	1	366	
	4.89	*4.80*	*4.24*	*1.57*	*5.53*		*4.65*	
Common truncus	45	17	17	0	1	0	80	
	1.09	*1.03*	*0.91*	*0.00*	*2.76*		*1.02*	
Congenital cataract	46	33	23	1	0	1	104	
	1.11	*2.01*	*1.24*	*0.52*	*0.00*		*1.32*	
Congenital hip dislocation	628	89	266	25	4	1	1,013	
	15.20	*5.41*	*14.28*	*13.08*	*11.05*		*12.86*	
Diaphragmatic hernia	119	38	59	4	1	1	222	
	2.88	*2.31*	*3.17*	*2.09*	*2.76*		*2.82*	
Down syndrome	518	172	268	22	2	0	982	
	12.53	*10.46*	*14.39*	*11.51*	*5.53*		*12.47*	
Ebstein's anomaly	29	4	12	2	1	0	48	
	0.70	*0.24*	*0.64*	*1.05*	*2.76*		*0.61*	
Encephalocele	37	18	11	1	1	0	68	
	0.90	*1.09*	*0.59*	*0.52*	*2.76*		*0.86*	
Endocardial cushion defect	161	62	60	6	1	0	290	
	3.90	*3.77*	*3.22*	*3.14*	*2.76*		*3.68*	
Esophageal atresia / tracheoesophageal fistula	124	29	44	5	1	0	203	
	3.00	*1.76*	*2.36*	*2.62*	*2.76*		*2.58*	
Fetal alcohol syndrome	146	123	17	4	1	0	291	
	3.53	*7.48*	*0.91*	*2.09*	*2.76*		*3.69*	
Hirschsprung's disease (congenital megacolon)	84	47	42	2	2	0	177	
	2.03	*2.86*	*2.26*	*1.05*	*5.53*		*2.25*	
Hydrocephalus without Spina Bifida	279	201	127	11	2	0	620	
	6.75	*12.23*	*6.82*	*5.75*	*5.53*		*7.87*	
Hypoplastic left heart syndrome	101	48	37	3	2	0	191	
	2.44	*2.92*	*1.99*	*1.57*	*5.53*		*2.42*	
Hypospadias and Epispadias	1,648	469	427	39	12	2	2,597	
	39.88	*28.53*	*22.93*	*20.40*	*33.16*		*32.97*	

(Table continues)

(Table continued)

Defect	Race/Ethnicity							Notes
	Non-Hispanic White	Non-Hispanic Black or African	Hispanic	Asian or Pacific Islander	American Indian or Alaskan Native	Other/ Unknown	Total	
Microcephalus	252	193	143	11	3	1	603	
	6.10	*11.74*	*7.68*	*5.75*	*8.29*		*7.65*	
Obstructive genitourinary defect	998	289	491	50	10	3	1,841	
	24.15	*17.58*	*26.37*	*26.15*	*27.63*		*23.37*	
Patent ductus arteriosus	2,841	1,486	1,429	140	19	13	5,928	
	68.74	*90.38*	*76.74*	*73.22*	*52.50*		*75.25*	
Pulmonary valve atresia and stenosis	374	255	187	16	2	3	837	
	9.05	*15.51*	*10.04*	*8.37*	*5.53*		*10.62*	
Pyloric stenosis	928	197	274	15	8	1	1,423	
	22.46	*11.98*	*14.71*	*7.85*	*22.11*		*18.06*	
Rectal and large intestinal atresia/stenosis	149	72	73	4	2	1	301	
	3.61	*4.38*	*3.92*	*2.09*	*5.53*		*3.82*	
Reduction deformity, lower limbs	63	33	21	2	0	0	119	
	1.52	*2.01*	*1.13*	*1.05*	*0.00*		*1.51*	
Reduction deformity, upper limbs	86	44	33	2	0	0	165	
	2.08	*2.68*	*1.77*	*1.05*	*0.00*		*2.09*	
Renal agenesis/hypoplasia	137	56	72	5	2	1	273	
	3.32	*3.41*	*3.87*	*2.62*	*5.53*		*3.47*	
Spina bifida without anencephalus	168	62	73	4	2	0	309	
	4.07	*3.77*	*3.92*	*2.09*	*5.53*		*3.92*	
Tetralogy of Fallot	222	106	88	4	0	1	421	
	5.37	*6.45*	*4.73*	*2.09*	*0.00*		*5.34*	
Transposition of great arteries	176	64	68	4	2	0	314	
	4.26	*3.89*	*3.65*	*2.09*	*5.53*		*3.99*	
Tricuspid valve atresia and stenosis	56	30	30	1	0	0	117	
	1.36	*1.82*	*1.61*	*0.52*	*0.00*		*1.49*	
Trisomy 13	47	27	24	2	0	1	101	
	1.14	*1.64*	*1.29*	*1.05*	*0.00*		*1.28*	
Trisomy 18	46	20	39	3	1	1	110	
	1.11	*1.22*	*2.09*	*1.57*	*2.76*		*1.40*	
Ventricular septal defect	2,006	685	912	60	18	4	6,685	
	48.54	*41.66*	*48.97*	*31.38*	*49.74*		*46.78*	
Total Live Births	**413,270**	**164,413**	**186,225**	**19,120**	**3,619**		**787,769**	

TRISOMY COUNTS AND RATES BY MATERNAL AGE 1997–2000
(Rates per 10,000 Live Births)

Defect	Age		
	<35	35 and >	Total*
Down syndrome	599	383	982
	8.81	*35.52*	*12.47*
Trisomy 13	72	29	101
	1.06	*2.69*	*1.28*
Trisomy 18	70	40	110
	1.03	*3.71*	*1.40*
Total Live Births	**679,761**	**107,825**	**787,769**

*Total includes unknown age.

Georgia

BIRTH DEFECTS COUNTS AND RATES 1997–2001

(Rates per 10,000 Live Births)

Defect	Non-Hispanic White	Non-Hispanic Black or African	Hispanic	Asian or Pacific Islander	American Indian or Alaskan Native	Other/ Unknown	Total	Notes
Amniotic bands	14	15	6	0	0	0	35	
	1.44	*1.60*	*1.94*	*0.00*	*0.00*		*1.49*	
Anencephalus	34	29	10	4	0	3	80	Includes terminations
	3.49	*3.09*	*3.23*	*3.66*	*0.00*		*3.40*	
Aniridia	2	1	0	1	0	0	4	
	0.21	*0.11*	*0.00*	*0.91*	*0.00*		*0.17*	
Anophthalmia / microphthalmia	35	24	4	2	0	0	65	
	3.59	*2.55*	*1.29*	*1.83*	*0.00*		*2.76*	
Anotia/microtia	13	7	9	5	0	1	35	
	1.33	*0.74*	*2.91*	*4.57*	*0.00*		*1.49*	
Aortic valve stenosis	28	12	7	2	0	0	49	
	2.87	*1.28*	*2.26*	*1.83*	*0.00*		*2.08*	
Atrial septal defect	224	269	70	21	1	11	596	
	22.98	*28.62*	*22.62*	*19.19*	*22.78*		*25.30*	
Biliary atresia	7	10	0	1	0	0	18	
	0.72	*1.06*	*0.00*	*0.91*	*0.00*		*0.76*	
Bladder exstrophy	2	1	0	0	0	0	3	
	0.21	*0.11*	*0.00*	*0.00*	*0.00*		*0.13*	
Choanal atresia	17	15	4	0	0	0	36	
	1.74	*1.60*	*1.29*	*0.00*	*0.00*		*1.53*	
Cleft lip with and without cleft palate	104	56	28	9	0	1	198	
	10.67	*5.96*	*9.05*	*8.22*	*0.00*		*8.40*	
Cleft palate without cleft lip	93	49	16	7	0	2	167	
	9.54	*5.21*	*5.17*	*6.40*	*0.00*		*7.09*	
Coarctation of aorta	61	48	15	4	0	1	129	
	6.26	*5.11*	*4.85*	*3.66*	*0.00*		*5.48*	
Common truncus	8	8	1	1	0	0	18	
	0.82	*0.85*	*0.32*	*0.91*	*0.00*		*0.76*	
Congenital cataract	30	16	4	1	0	0	51	
	3.08	*1.70*	*1.29*	*0.91*	*0.00*		*2.16*	
Congenital hip dislocation	95	19	27	6	0	4	151	
	9.75	*2.02*	*8.73*	*5.48*	*0.00*		*6.41*	
Diaphragmatic hernia	24	20	8	2	0	0	54	
	2.46	*2.13*	*2.59*	*1.83*	*0.00*		*2.29*	
Down syndrome	146	104	36	19	0	2	307	
	14.98	*11.06*	*11.63*	*17.36*	*0.00*		*13.03*	
Ebstein's anomaly	2	5	3	0	0	0	10	
	0.21	*0.53*	*0.97*	*0.00*	*0.00*		*0.42*	
Encephalocele	13	13	4	0	0	2	32	Includes terminations
	1.33	*1.38*	*1.29*	*0.00*	*0.00*		*1.36*	
Endocardial cushion defect	42	50	5	7	0	0	104	
	4.31	*5.32*	*1.62*	*6.40*	*0.00*		*4.41*	
Esophageal atresia / tracheoesophageal fistula	32	16	7	1	0	0	56	
	3.28	*1.70*	*2.26*	*0.91*	*0.00*		*2.38*	
Fetal alcohol syndrome	5	27	0	0	0	0	32	
	0.51	*2.87*	*0.00*	*0.00*	*0.00*		*1.36*	
Gastroschisis	17	19	14	1	0	0	51	
	1.74	*2.02*	*4.52*	*0.91*	*0.00*		*2.16*	
Hirschsprung's disease (congenital megacolon)	16	27	6	5	0	1	55	
	1.64	*2.87*	*1.94*	*4.57*	*0.00*		*2.33*	
Hydrocephalus without Spina Bifida	77	85	22	8	0	0	192	
	7.90	*9.04*	*7.11*	*7.31*	*0.00*		*8.15*	

(Table continues)

(Table continued)

Defect	Race/Ethnicity						Total	Notes
	Non-Hispanic White	Non-Hispanic Black or African	Hispanic	Asian or Pacific Islander	American Indian or Alaskan Native	Other/ Unknown		
Hypoplastic left heart syndrome	33	26	8	3	0	2	72	
	3.39	*2.77*	*2.59*	*2.74*	*0.00*		*3.06*	
Hypospadias and Epispadias	392	317	36	19	0	6	770	
	40.21	*33.72*	*11.63*	*17.36*	*0.00*		*32.68*	
Microcephalus	45	108	22	11	0	1	187	
	4.62	*11.49*	*7.11*	*10.05*	*0.00*		*7.94*	
Obstructive genitourinary defect	241	180	82	33	0	7	543	
	24.72	*19.15*	*26.50*	*30.16*	*0.00*		*23.05*	
Omphalocele	25	25	4	4	0	1	59	
	2.56	*2.66*	*1.29*	*3.66*	*0.00*		*2.50*	
Patent ductus arteriosus	311	255	96	38	1	10	711	
	31.90	*27.13*	*31.02*	*34.73*	*22.78*		*30.18*	
Pulmonary valve atresia and stenosis	69	71	19	4	0	2	165	
	7.08	*7.55*	*6.14*	*3.66*	*0.00*		*7.00*	
Pyloric stenosis	198	62	46	8	0	2	316	
	20.31	*6.60*	*14.87*	*7.31*	*0.00*		*13.41*	
Rectal and large intestinal atresia/stenosis	36	39	12	5	1	2	95	
	3.69	*4.15*	*3.88*	*4.57*	*22.78*		*4.03*	
Reduction deformity, lower limbs	13	21	6	1	0	0	41	
	1.33	*2.23*	*1.94*	*0.91*	*0.00*		*1.74*	
Reduction deformity, upper limbs	43	31	16	2	0	3	95	
	4.41	*3.30*	*5.17*	*1.83*	*0.00*		*4.03*	
Renal agenesis/hypoplasia	47	45	7	3	0	1	103	
	4.82	*4.79*	*2.26*	*2.74*	*0.00*		*4.37*	
Spina bifida without anencephalus	40	30	11	0	0	3	84	Includes terminations
	4.10	*3.19*	*3.55*	*0.00*	*0.00*		*3.57*	
Tetralogy of Fallot	38	40	8	2	0	0	88	
	3.90	*4.26*	*2.59*	*1.83*	*0.00*		*3.73*	
Transposition of great arteries	51	48	16	10	0	1	126	
	5.23	*5.11*	*5.17*	*9.14*	*0.00*		*5.35*	
Tricuspid valve atresia and stenosis	18	17	4	0	0	0	39	
	1.85	*1.81*	*1.29*	*0.00*	*0.00*		*1.66*	
Trisomy 13	16	14	4	0	0	0	34	
	1.64	*1.49*	*1.29*	*0.00*	*0.00*		*1.44*	
Trisomy 18	21	32	5	2	0	0	60	
	2.15	*3.40*	*1.62*	*1.83*	*0.00*		*2.55*	
Ventricular septal defect	432	307	150	39	1	10	939	
	44.32	*32.66*	*48.47*	*35.64*	*22.78*		*39.85*	
Total Live Births	97,481	93,996	30,945	10,943	439		235,616	

TRISOMY COUNTS AND RATES BY MATERNAL AGE 1997–2001
(Rates per 10,000 Live Births)

Defect	Age		Total*
	<35	35 and >	
Down syndrome	165	141	307
	8.29	*38.63*	*13.03*
Trisomy 13	23	11	34
	1.16	*3.01*	*1.44*
Trisomy 18	38	22	60
	1.91	*6.03*	*2.55*
Total Live Births	199,054	36,504	235,616

*Total includes unknown age.

Hawaii

BIRTH DEFECTS COUNTS AND RATES 1997–2001

(Rates per 10,000 Live Births)

Defect	Non-Hispanic White	Non-Hispanic Black or African	Hispanic	Asian or Pacific Islander	American Indian or Alaskan Native	Other/ Unknown	Total	Notes
Amniotic bands	3	1	0	13	0	1	18	
	1.69	*3.45*	*0.00*	*2.17*	*0.00*		*2.08*	
Anencephalus	7	0	2	19	0	4	32	
	3.95	*0.00*	*12.15*	*3.17*	*0.00*		*3.69*	Includes stillbirths/ terminations
Aniridia	0	0	0	2	0	0	2	
	0.00	*0.00*	*0.00*	*0.33*	*0.00*		*0.23*	
Anophthalmia / microphthalmia	5	0	0	15	0	0	20	
	2.82	*0.00*	*0.00*	*2.51*	*0.00*		*2.31*	
Anotia/microtia	1	0	2	20	3	0	26	
	0.56	*0.00*	*12.15*	*3.34*	*30.30*		*3.00*	
Aortic valve stenosis	0	0	0	6	0	1	7	
	0.00	*0.00*	*0.00*	*1.00*	*0.00*		*0.81*	
Atrial septal defect	37	5	7	144	2	1	196	
	20.90	*17.26*	*42.53*	*24.06*	*20.20*		*22.60*	
Biliary atresia	0	0	0	5	0	0	5	
	0.00	*0.00*	*0.00*	*0.84*	*0.00*		*0.58*	
Bladder exstrophy	1	0	0	2	1	0	4	
	0.56	*0.00*	*0.00*	*0.33*	*10.10*		*0.46*	
Choanal atresia	1	0	1	5	0	0	7	
	0.56	*0.00*	*6.08*	*0.84*	*0.00*		*0.81*	
Cleft lip with and without cleft palate	13	3	5	84	2	3	110	
	7.34	*10.36*	*30.38*	*14.03*	*20.20*		*12.68*	
Cleft palate without cleft lip	15	0	2	37	0	0	54	
	8.47	*0.00*	*12.15*	*6.18*	*0.00*		*6.23*	
Coarctation of aorta	8	0	1	10	0	1	20	
	4.52	*0.00*	*6.08*	*1.67*	*0.00*		*2.31*	
Common truncus	2	0	0	4	0	0	6	
	1.13	*0.00*	*0.00*	*0.67*	*0.00*		*0.69*	
Congenital cataract	3	0	2	3	0	0	8	
	1.69	*0.00*	*12.15*	*0.50*	*0.00*		*0.92*	
Congenital hip dislocation	8	0	0	36	0	0	44	
	4.52	*0.00*	*0.00*	*6.01*	*0.00*		*5.07*	
Diaphragmatic hernia	5	0	0	11	0	1	17	
	2.82	*0.00*	*0.00*	*1.84*	*0.00*		*1.96*	
Down syndrome	26	2	0	84	3	13	128	
	14.68	*6.90*	*0.00*	*14.03*	*30.30*		*14.76*	
Ebstein's anomaly	3	0	0	2	0	1	6	
	1.69	*0.00*	*0.00*	*0.33*	*0.00*		*0.69*	
Encephalocele	2	0	1	9	0	0	12	
	1.13	*0.00*	*6.08*	*1.50*	*0.00*		*1.38*	
Endocardial cushion defect	2	0	1	11	0	0	14	
	1.13	*0.00*	*6.08*	*1.84*	*0.00*		*1.61*	
Esophageal atresia / tracheoesophageal fistula	6	1	0	6	0	0	13	
	3.39	*3.45*	*0.00*	*1.00*	*0.00*		*1.50*	
Fetal alcohol syndrome	3	0	0	4	1	0	8	
	1.69	*0.00*	*0.00*	*0.67*	*10.10*		*0.92*	
Gastroschisis	6	1	2	21	0	1	31	
	3.39	*3.45*	*12.15*	*3.51*	*0.00*		*3.57*	
Hirschsprung's disease (congenital megacolon)	2	1	0	15	1	0	19	
	1.13	*3.45*	*0.00*	*2.51*	*10.10*		*2.19*	
Hydrocephalus without Spina Bifida	13	0	2	46	1	7	69	
	7.34	*0.00*	*12.15*	*7.68*	*10.10*		*7.95*	

(Table continues)

(Table continued)

Defect	Race/Ethnicity							
	Non-Hispanic White	Non-Hispanic Black or African	Hispanic	Asian or Pacific Islander	American Indian or Alaskan Native	Other/ Unknown	Total	Notes
Hypoplastic left heart syndrome	1	0	1	8	0	1	11	
	0.56	*0.00*	*6.08*	*1.34*	*0.00*		*1.27*	
Hypospadias and Epispadias	48	6	8	170	2	2	236	
	27.11	*20.71*	*48.60*	*28.40*	*20.20*		*27.21*	
Microcephalus	9	2	0	50	2	1	64	
	5.08	*6.90*	*0.00*	*8.35*	*20.20*		*7.38*	
Obstructive genitourinary defect	33	3	5	84	1	2	128	
	18.64	*10.36*	*30.38*	*14.03*	*10.10*		*14.76*	
Omphalocele	5	0	0	16	0	3	24	
	2.82	*0.00*	*0.00*	*2.67*	*0.00*		*2.77*	
Patent ductus arteriosus	144	20	29	694	8	12	907	
	81.32	*69.04*	*176.18*	*115.94*	*80.81*		*104.56*	
Pulmonary valve atresia and stenosis	3	0	1	18	0	0	22	
	1.69	*0.00*	*6.08*	*3.01*	*0.00*		*2.54*	
Pyloric stenosis	17	1	3	23	0	0	44	
	9.60	*3.45*	*18.23*	*3.84*	*0.00*		*5.07*	
Rectal and large intestinal atresia/stenosis	8	2	1	26	0	2	39	
	4.52	*6.90*	*6.08*	*4.34*	*0.00*		*4.50*	
Reduction deformity, lower limbs	2	1	0	11	0	0	14	
	1.13	*3.45*	*0.00*	*1.84*	*0.00*		*1.61*	
Reduction deformity, upper limbs	3	1	0	20	0	0	24	
	1.69	*3.45*	*0.00*	*3.34*	*0.00*		*2.77*	
Renal agenesis/hypoplasia	7	4	0	22	0	4	37	
	3.95	*13.81*	*0.00*	*3.68*	*0.00*		*4.27*	
Spina bifida without anencephalus	7	1	1	20	0	3	32	Includes stillbirths/ terminations
	3.95	*3.45*	*6.08*	*3.34*	*0.00*		*3.69*	
Tetralogy of Fallot	5	1	0	19	0	0	25	
	2.82	*3.45*	*0.00*	*3.17*	*0.00*		*2.88*	
Transposition of great arteries	7	0	0	26	1	2	36	
	3.95	*0.00*	*0.00*	*4.34*	*10.10*		*4.15*	
Tricuspid valve atresia and stenosis	3	0	0	11	0	1	15	
	1.69	*0.00*	*0.00*	*1.84*	*0.00*		*1.73*	
Trisomy 13	6	0	1	12	0	3	22	
	3.39	*0.00*	*6.08*	*2.00*	*0.00*		*2.54*	
Trisomy 18	10	0	0	20	1	8	39	
	5.65	*0.00*	*0.00*	*3.34*	*10.10*		*4.50*	
Ventricular septal defect	65	6	8	252	5	5	341	
	36.71	*20.71*	*48.60*	*42.10*	*50.51*		*39.31*	
Total Live Births	17,707	2,897	1,646	59,860	990		86,743	

TRISOMY COUNTS AND RATES BY MATERNAL AGE 1997–2001
(Rates per 10,000 Live Births)

Defect	Age		
	<35	35 and >	Total*
Down syndrome	54	74	128
	7.43	*52.47*	*14.76*
Trisomy 13	10	11	22
	1.38	*7.80*	*2.54*
Trisomy 18	20	19	39
	2.75	*13.47*	*4.50*
Total Live Births	72,631	14,103	86,743

*Total includes unknown age.

Illinois

BIRTH DEFECTS COUNTS AND RATES 1997–2001

(Rates per 10,000 Live Births)

Defect	Non-Hispanic White	Non-Hispanic Black or African	Hispanic	Asian or Pacific Islander	American Indian or Alaskan Native	Other/ Unknown	Total	Notes
Anencephalus	84	21	47	4	3	1	159	Live births and
	1.62	*1.22*	*2.54*	*1.09*	*17.11*		*1.74*	stillbirths only
Aniridia	0	1	0	0	0	0	1	
	0.00	*0.06*	*0.00*	*0.00*	*0.00*		*0.01*	
Anophthalmia / microphthalmia	47	10	11	0	0	1	69	
	0.91	*0.58*	*0.59*	*0.00*	*0.00*		*0.75*	
Anotia/microtia	22	2	12	2	0	0	38	
	0.42	*0.12*	*0.65*	*0.55*	*0.00*		*0.42*	
Aortic valve stenosis	64	5	9	0	0	1	79	
	1.24	*0.29*	*0.49*	*0.00*	*0.00*		*0.86*	
Atrial septal defect	1,263	387	350	58	3	44	2,105	
	24.40	*22.57*	*18.91*	*15.82*	*25.66*		*23.03*	
Biliary atresia	17	12	7	1	0	6	43	
	0.33	*0.70*	*0.38*	*0.27*	*0.00*		*0.47*	
Bladder exstrophy	28	4	1	1	0	0	34	
	0.54	*0.23*	*0.05*	*0.27*	*0.00*		*0.37*	
Choanal atresia	67	9	18	5	1	1	101	
	1.29	*0.52*	*0.97*	*1.36*	*8.55*		*1.10*	
Cleft lip with and without cleft palate	346	77	121	19	2	5	570	
	6.68	*4.49*	*6.54*	*5.18*	*17.11*		*6.23*	
Cleft palate without cleft lip	223	4	52	10	1	1	328	
	4.31	*2.39*	*2.81*	*2.73*	*8.55*		*3.59*	
Coarctation of aorta	127	29	37	7	0	1	201	
	2.45	*1.69*	*2.00*	*1.91*	*0.00*		*2.20*	
Common truncus	19	10	6	2	0	0	37	
	0.37	*0.58*	*0.32*	*0.55*	*0.00*		*0.40*	
Congenital cataract	33	7	7	0	0	0	47	
	0.64	*0.41*	*0.38*	*0.00*	*0.00*		*0.51*	
Congenital hip dislocation	101	15	34	4	0	1	155	
	1.95	*0.87*	*1.84*	*1.09*	*0.00*		*1.70*	
Diaphragmatic hernia	151	38	49	10	0	0	248	
	2.92	*2.22*	*2.65*	*2.73*	*0.00*		*2.71*	
Down syndrome	617	160	225	37	2	19	1,060	
	11.92	*9.33*	*12.16*	*10.09*	*17.11*		*11.59*	
Ebstein's anomaly	33	1	6	0	0	1	41	
	0.64	*0.06*	*0.32*	*0.00*	*0.00*		*0.45*	
Encephalocele	32	17	10	2	0	1	62	
	0.62	*0.99*	*0.54*	*0.55*	*0.00*		*0.68*	
Endocardial cushion defect	146	34	29	6	0	2	217	
	2.82	*1.98*	*1.57*	*1.64*	*0.00*		*2.37*	
Esophageal atresia / tracheoesophageal fistula	144	31	22	10	0	1	208	
	2.78	*1.81*	*1.19*	*2.73*	*0.00*		*2.28*	
Fetal alcohol syndrome	39	115	8	2	1	3	168	
	0.75	*6.71*	*0.43*	*0.55*	*8.55*		*1.84*	
Hirschsprung's disease (congenital megacolon)	81	57	24	6	0	5	173	
	1.56	*3.32*	*1.30*	*1.64*	*0.00*		*1.89*	
Hydrocephalus without Spina Bifida	275	184	100	15	2	10	586	
	5.31	*10.73*	*5.40*	*4.09*	*17.11*		*6.41*	
Hypoplastic left heart syndrome	93	20	25	5	0	1	144	
	1.80	*1.17*	*1.35*	*1.36*	*0.00*		*1.58*	
Hypospadias and Epispadias	571	115	78	15	2	1	782	
	11.03	*6.71*	*4.22*	*4.09*	*17.11*		*8.55*	
Lung agenesis/hypoplasia	140	49	34	7	1	4	235	
	3.36	*3.54*	*2.36*	*2.45*	*10.66*		*3.22*	
Microcephalus	113	144	57	5	0	10	329	
	2.18	*8.40*	*3.08*	*1.36*	*0.00*		*3.60*	

(Table continues)

(Table continued)

Defect	Race/Ethnicity							Notes
	Non-Hispanic White	Non-Hispanic Black or African	Hispanic	Asian or Pacific Islander	American Indian or Alaskan Native	Other/Unknown	Total	
Obstructive genitourinary defect	595 *11.49*	139 *8.11*	161 *8.70*	36 *9.82*	3 *25.66*	4	938 *10.26*	
Patent ductus arteriosus	1,139 *22.00*	295 *17.20*	253 *13.67*	61 *16.64*	5 *34.22*	18	1,770 *19.36*	only birthweight ≥2500 grams
Pulmonary valve atresia and stenosis	197 *3.81*	54 *3.15*	55 *2.97*	12 *3.27*	0 *0.00*	13	331 *3.62*	
Pyloric stenosis	194 *3.75*	48 *2.80*	96 *5.19*	5 *1.36*	0 *0.00*	22	365 *3.99*	
Rectal and large intestinal atresia/stenosis	175 *3.38*	47 *2.74*	44 *2.38*	10 *2.73*	0 *0.00*	5	281 *3.07*	
Reduction deformity, lower limbs	42 *0.81*	14 *0.82*	10 *0.54*	2 *0.55*	0 *0.00*	1	69 *0.75*	
Reduction deformity, upper limbs	81 *1.56*	24 *1.40*	26 *1.41*	2 *0.55*	2 *17.11*	3	138 *1.51*	
Renal agenesis/hypoplasia	103 *1.99*	29 *1.69*	23 *1.24*	1 *0.27*	0 *0.00*	5	161 *1.76*	
Spina bifida without anencephalus	153 *2.96*	47 *2.74*	63 *3.40*	6 *1.64*	0 *0.00*	8	277 *3.03*	Live births and still births only
Tetralogy of Fallot	154 *2.97*	59 *3.44*	22 *1.19*	7 *1.91*	1 *8.55*	10	253 *2.77*	
Transposition of great arteries	148 *2.86*	37 *2.16*	37 *2.00*	4 *1.09*	0 *0.00*	3	229 *2.50*	
Tricuspid valve atresia and stenosis	19 *0.37*	9 *0.52*	10 *0.54*	0 *0.00*	0 *0.00*	0	38 *0.42*	
Trisomy 13	51 *0.99*	18 *1.05*	8 *0.43*	0 *0.00*	1 *8.55*	2	80 *0.88*	
Trisomy 18	109 *2.11*	36 *2.10*	33 *1.78*	5 *1.36*	2 *17.11*	2	187 *2.05*	
Ventricular septal defect	1,196 *23.10*	323 *18.84*	362 *19.56*	67 *18.27*	7 *59.88*	44	1,999 *21.87*	Includes probable cases
Total Live Births	517,719	171,476	185,053	36,663	1,169		914,204	

TRISOMY COUNTS AND RATES BY MATERNAL AGE 1997–2001

(Rates per 10,000 Live Births)

Defect	Age		Total*
	<35	35 and >	
Down syndrome	525 *6.66*	407 *32.37*	1,060 *11.59*
Trisomy 13	52 *0.66*	26 *2.07*	80 *0.88*
Trisomy 18	102 *1.29*	72 *5.73*	187 *2.05*
Total Live Births	788,409	125,729	914,204

*Total includes unknown age.

Notes:

1. Illinois used primarily passive newborn reporting during 1997–2001. However, a number of projects were undertaken to enhance case identification during this time period:

a. In each year except 1998, some active case finding was undertaken. APORS staff reviewed hospital charts to identify children with major birth defects. The targeted hospitals and conditions varied from year to year. Birth defects identified through these projects may not have been diagnosed during the newborn period.

b. In 2000 and 2001, APORS staff matched records with birth certificate information. Facilities were asked to provide birth defect information about very low birth-weight previously unreported to APORS.

c. In 2000 and 2001, APORS staff matched some hospital discharge records with APORS records to obtain more complete case ascertainment. The facilities that provided most of the hospital discharge records were Level III facilities.

d. In 2000, APORS staff undertook a reabstraction study. For a sample of reported cases, hospital charts were reviewed to determine the accuracy of hospital reporting.

2. ICD-9 codes were used to define the birth defect groups.

3. The data include fetal deaths >20 weeks, or if death certificate issued. It does not include terminations.

4. Probable/possible diagnoses are included in Illinois cases.

Iowa

BIRTH DEFECTS COUNTS AND RATES 1997–2001

(Rates per 10,000 Live Births)

Defect	Non-Hispanic White	Non-Hispanic Black or African	Hispanic	Asian or Pacific Islander	American Indian or Alaskan Native	Other/ Unknown	Total	Notes
Amniotic bands	27	2	1	0	0	0	30	
	1.63	*3.57*	*0.90*	*0.00*	*0.00*		*1.60*	
Anencephalus	44	3	3	1	0	7	58	
	2.66	*5.36*	*2.70*	*2.55*	*0.00*		*3.10*	
Aniridia	1	1	0	0	0	3	5	
	0.06	*1.79*	*0.00*	*0.00*	*0.00*		*0.27*	
Anophthalmia / microphthalmia	34	2	3	0	0	2	41	
	2.06	*3.57*	*2.70*	*0.00*	*0.00*		*2.19*	
Anotia/microtia	99	4	8	1	0	2	114	
	5.98	*7.15*	*7.20*	*2.55*	*0.00*		*6.09*	
Aortic valve stenosis	72	3	1	0	0	1	77	
	4.35	*5.36*	*0.90*	*0.00*	*0.00*		*4.11*	
Atrial septal defect	413	23	13	9	2	16	476	
	24.97	*41.10*	*11.70*	*22.99*	*21.25*		*25.41*	
Biliary atresia	14	0	1	0	0	0	15	
	0.85	*0.00*	*0.90*	*0.00*	*0.00*		*0.80*	
Bladder exstrophy	8	1	2	0	0	0	11	
	0.48	*1.79*	*1.80*	*0.00*	*0.00*		*0.59*	
Choanal atresia	46	1	0	1	0	2	50	
	2.78	*1.79*	*0.00*	*2.55*	*0.00*		*2.67*	
Cleft lip with and without cleft palate	207	6	12	4	1	5	235	
	12.51	*10.72*	*10.80*	*10.22*	*10.63*		*12.55*	
Cleft palate without cleft lip	124	3	4	2	0	11	144	
	7.50	*5.36*	*3.60*	*5.11*	*0.00*		*7.69*	
Coarctation of aorta	123	6	3	0	0	7	139	
	7.44	*10.72*	*2.70*	*0.00*	*0.00*		*7.42*	
Common truncus		23	0	1	2	0	228	
	1.39	*0.00*	*0.90*	*5.11*	*0.00*		*1.49*	
Congenital cataract	50	3	3	0	1	1	58	
	3.02	*5.36*	*2.70*	*0.00*	*10.63*		*3.10*	
Congenital hip dislocation	143	1	13	0	1	10	168	
	8.64	*1.79*	*11.70*	*0.00*	*10.63*		*8.97*	
Diaphragmatic hernia	36	1	1	1	1	2	42	
	2.18	*1.79*	*0.90*	*2.55*	*10.63*		*2.24*	
Down syndrome	231	7	12	1	0	20	271	
	13.96	*12.51*	*10.80*	*2.55*	*0.00*		*14.47*	
Ebstein's anomaly	15	0	1	0	0	0	16	
	0.91	*0.00*	*0.90*	*0.00*	*0.00*		*0.85*	
Encephalocele	18	2	2	0	0	1	23	
	1.09	*3.57*	*1.80*	*0.00*	*0.00*		*1.23*	
Endocardial cushion defect	88	7	0	4	0	4	103	
	5.32	*12.51*	*0.00*	*10.22*	*0.00*		*5.50*	
Esophageal atresia / tracheoesophageal fistula	51	0	0	1	0	3	55	
	3.08	*0.00*	*0.00*	*2.55*	*0.00*		*2.94*	
Fetal alcohol syndrome	6	0	0	0	1	2	9	
	0.36	*0.00*	*0.00*	*0.00*	*10.63*		*0.48*	
Gastroschisis	62	6	2	3	1	4	78	
	3.75	*10.72*	*1.80*	*7.66*	*10.63*		*4.16*	
Hirschsprung's disease (congenital megacolon)	37	2	0	2	0	4	45	
	2.24	*3.57*	*0.00*	*5.11*	*0.00*		*2.40*	
Hydrocephalus without Spina Bifida	178	4	12	3	1	6	204	
	10.76	*7.15*	*10.80*	*7.66*	*10.63*		*10.89*	
Hypoplastic left heart syndrome	63	4	0	0	0	0	67	
	3.81	*7.15*	*0.00*	*0.00*	*0.00*		*3.58*	

(Table continues)

(Table continued)

Defect	Race/Ethnicity							Notes
	Non-Hispanic White	Non-Hispanic Black or African	Hispanic	Asian or Pacific Islander	American Indian or Alaskan Native	Other/ Unknown	Total	
Hypospadias and	587	13	16	5	1	15	637	
Epispadias	*35.49*	*23.23*	*14.40*	*12.77*	*10.63*		*34.01*	
Microcephalus	138	14	11	2	2	13	180	
	8.34	*25.02*	*9.90*	*5.11*	*21.25*		*9.61*	
Obstructive genitourinary	387	16	20	2	3	23	451	
defect	*23.39*	*28.59*	*18.00*	*5.11*	*31.88*		*24.08*	
Omphalocele	44	0	3	2	1	3	53	
	2.66	*0.00*	*2.70*	*5.11*	*10.63*		*2.83*	
Patent ductus arteriosus	479	31	23	4	2	5	544	
	28.96	*55.40*	*20.69*	*10.22*	*21.25*		*29.04*	
Pulmonary valve atresia	190	8	8	5	0	11	222	
and stenosis	*11.49*	*14.30*	*7.20*	*12.77*	*0.00*		*11.85*	
Pyloric stenosis	522	6	31	1	2	28	590	
	31.56	*10.72*	*27.89*	*2.55*	*21.25*		*31.50*	
Rectal and large intestinal	82	3	5	0	0	4	94	
atresia/stenosis	*4.96*	*5.36*	*4.50*	*0.00*	*0.00*		*5.02*	
Reduction deformity,	53	4	0	0	0	2	59	
lower limbs	*3.20*	*7.15*	*0.00*	*0.00*	*0.00*		*3.15*	
Reduction deformity,	97	2	0	2	0	4	105	
upper limbs	*5.86*	*3.57*	*0.00*	*5.11*	*0.00*		*5.61*	
Renal agenesis/hypoplasia	96	2	4	0	0	5	107	
	5.80	*3.57*	*3.60*	*0.00*	*0.00*		*5.71*	
Spina bifida without	100	2	8	0	1	2	113	
anencephalus	*6.05*	*3.57*	*7.20*	*0.00*	*10.63*		*6.03*	
Tetralogy of Fallot	66	2	1	1	0	1	71	
	3.99	*3.57*	*0.90*	*2.55*	*0.00*		*3.79*	
Transposition of great	89	3	6	3	0	3	104	
arteries	*5.38*	*5.36*	*5.40*	*7.66*	*0.00*		*5.55*	
Tricuspid valve atresia	16	0	4	2	0	0	22	
and stenosis	*0.97*	*0.00*	*3.60*	*5.11*	*0.00*		*1.17*	
Trisomy 13	24	0	2	0	1	1	28	
	1.45	*0.00*	*1.80*	*0.00*	*10.63*		*1.49*	
Trisomy 18	29	2	5	3	0	6	45	
	1.75	*3.57*	*4.50*	*7.66*	*0.00*		*2.40*	
Ventricular septal defect	718	34	41	11	1	28	833	
	43.40	*60.76*	*36.89*	*28.10*	*10.63*		*44.47*	
Total Live Births	**165,422**	**5,596**	**11,114**	**3,914**	**941**		**187,312**	

TRISOMY COUNTS AND RATES BY MATERNAL AGE 1997–2001
(Rates per 10,000 Live Births)

Defect	Age		
	<35	35 and >	Total*
Down syndrome	170	100	271
	10.16	*49.93*	*14.47*
Trisomy 13	18	10	28
	1.08	*4.99*	*1.49*
Trisomy 18	26	19	45
	1.55	*9.49*	*2.40*
Total Live Births	**167,264**	**20,029**	**187,312**

*Total includes unknown age.

Kentucky

BIRTH DEFECTS COUNTS AND RATES 1997–2001

(Rates per 10,000 Live Births)

Defect	Non-Hispanic White	Non-Hispanic Black or African	Hispanic	Asian or Pacific Islander	American Indian or Alaskan Native	Other/ Unknown	Total	Notes
Amniotic bands	22	6	1	0	0	0	29	
	1.15	*3.02*	*2.37*	*0.00*	*0.00*		*1.32*	
Anencephalus	76	4	2	0	0	0	82	1997–2001 data
	3.20	*1.63*	*4.05*	*0.00*	*0.00*		*3.00*	
Aniridia	6	3	0	0	0	0	9	
	0.31	*1.51*	*0.00*	*0.00*	*0.00*		*0.41*	
Anophthalmia / microphthalmia	35	2	0	1	0	1	39	
	1.82	*1.01*	*0.00*	*4.48*	*0.00*		*1.77*	
Anotia/microtia	26	1	1	2	0	0	30	
	1.36	*0.50*	*2.37*	*8.96*	*0.00*		*1.36*	
Aortic valve stenosis	62	4	0	0	0	0	66	
	3.23	*2.01*	*0.00*	*0.00*	*0.00*		*3.00*	
Atrial septal defect	1,194	263	19	10	2	14	1,502	
	62.26	*132.42*	*44.99*	*44.78*	*59.00*		*68.23*	
Biliary atresia	13	2	0	0	0	0	15	
	0.68	*1.01*	*0.00*	*0.00*	*0.00*		*0.68*	
Bladder exstrophy	10	1	0	0	0	1	12	
	0.52	*0.50*	*0.00*	*0.00*	*0.00*		*0.55*	
Choanal atresia	32	2	0	0	0	0	34	
	1.67	*1.01*	*0.00*	*0.00*	*0.00*		*1.54*	
Cleft lip with and without cleft palate	215	7	2	4	0	1	229	
	11.21	*3.52*	*4.74*	*17.91*	*0.00*		*10.40*	
Cleft palate without cleft lip	160	6	2	3	1	0	172	
	8.34	*3.02*	*4.74*	*13.43*	*29.50*		*7.81*	
Coarctation of aorta	119	10	5	1	0	1	136	
	6.20	*5.03*	*11.84*	*4.48*	*0.00*		*6.18*	
Common truncus	12	3	2	0	0	0	17	
	0.63	*1.51*	*4.74*	*0.00*	*0.00*		*0.77*	
Congenital cataract	21	4	1	0	0	0	26	
	1.09	*2.01*	*2.37*	*0.00*	*0.00*		*1.18*	
Congenital hip dislocation	232	9	2	4	1	0	248	
	12.10	*4.53*	*4.74*	*17.91*	*29.50*		*11.26*	
Diaphragmatic hernia	68	4	0	1	0	1	74	
	3.55	*2.01*	*0.00*	*4.48*	*0.00*		*3.36*	
Down syndrome	210	16	3	4	0	1	234	
	10.95	*8.06*	*7.10*	*17.91*	*0.00*		*10.63*	
Ebstein's anomaly	13	1	0	0	0	0	14	
	0.68	*0.50*	*0.00*	*0.00*	*0.00*		*0.64*	
Encephalocele	19	2	1	0	0	0	22	1997–2001 data
	0.80	*0.82*	*2.02*	*0.00*	*0.00*		*0.80*	
Endocardial cushion defect	80	9	0	0	0	0	89	
	4.17	*4.53*	*0.00*	*0.00*	*0.00*		*4.04*	
Esophageal atresia / tracheoesophageal fistula	66	7	0	1	0	0	74	
	3.44	*3.52*	*0.00*	*4.48*	*0.00*		*3.36*	
Fetal alcohol syndrome	14	10	0	0	0	1	25	
	0.73	*5.03*	*0.00*	*0.00*	*0.00*		*1.14*	
Gastroschisis	83	6	5	1	0	0	95	756.72
	4.33	*3.02*	*11.84*	*4.48*	*0.00*		*4.32*	
Hirschsprung's disease (congenital megacolon)	48	7	0	1	0	0	56	
	2.50	*3.52*	*0.00*	*4.48*	*0.00*		*2.54*	
Hydrocephalus without Spina Bifida	174	29	1	0	0	0	204	
	9.07	*14.60*	*2.37*	*0.00*	*0.00*		*9.27*	
Hypoplastic left heart syndrome	53	4	3	0	1	0	61	
	2.76	*2.01*	*7.10*	*0.00*	*29.50*		*2.77*	

(Table continues)

(Table continued)

Defect	Race/Ethnicity							Notes
	Non-Hispanic White	Non-Hispanic Black or African	Hispanic	Asian or Pacific Islander	American Indian or Alaskan Native	Other/ Unknown	Total	
Hypospadias and Epispadias	711 *37.07*	74 *37.26*	7 *16.58*	2 *8.96*	2 *59.00*	3	799 *36.29*	
Microcephalus	133 *6.93*	14 *7.05*	5 *11.84*	3 *13.43*	0 *0.00*	1	156 *7.09*	
Obstructive genitourinary defect	355 *18.51*	30 *15.10*	6 *14.21*	7 *31.35*	1 *29.50*	0	399 *18.12*	
Omphalocele	30 *1.56*	6 *3.02*	0 *0.00*	2 *8.96*	0 *0.00*	1	39 *1.77*	756.73
Patent ductus arteriosus	909 *47.40*	174 *87.61*	16 *37.89*	8 *35.83*	2 *59.00*	3	1,112 *50.51*	>2500 gms only
Pulmonary valve atresia and stenosis	216 *11.26*	23 *11.58*	7 *16.58*	0 *0.00*	0 *0.00*	0	246 *11.17*	
Pyloric stenosis	516 *26.91*	25 *12.59*	2 *4.74*	1 *4.48*	1 *29.50*	0	545 *24.76*	
Rectal and large intestinal atresia/stenosis	99 *5.16*	8 *4.03*	2 *4.74*	0 *0.00*	0 *0.00*	2	111 *5.04*	
Reduction deformity, lower limbs	40 *2.09*	6 *3.02*	0 *0.00*	1 *4.48*	0 *0.00*	0	47 *2.13*	
Reduction deformity, upper limbs	66 *3.44*	9 *4.53*	1 *2.37*	0 *0.00*	0 *0.00*	0	76 *3.45*	
Renal agenesis/hypoplasia	57 *2.97*	4 *2.01*	1 *2.37*	1 *4.48*	0 *0.00*	1	64 *2.91*	
Spina bifida without anencephalus	90 *3.78*	2 *0.82*	2 *4.05*	0 *0.00*	0 *0.00*	1	95 *3.48*	1997–2001 data
Tetralogy of Fallot	82 *4.28*	11 *5.54*	0 *0.00*	0 *0.00*	0 *0.00*	2	95 *4.32*	
Transposition of great arteries	92 *4.80*	6 *3.02*	2 *4.74*	1 *4.48*	0 *0.00*	0	101 *4.59*	
Tricuspid valve atresia and stenosis	18 *0.94*	3 *1.51*	0 *0.00*	0 *0.00*	1 *29.50*	0	22 *1.00*	
Trisomy 13	22 *1.15*	2 *1.01*	0 *0.00*	1 *4.48*	0 *0.00*	0	25 *1.14*	
Trisomy 18	56 *2.92*	8 *4.03*	2 *4.74*	0 *0.00*	0 *0.00*	0	66 *3.00*	
Ventricular septal defect	963 *50.21*	114 *57.40*	34 *80.51*	4 *17.91*	1 *29.50*	8	1,124 *51.06*	
Total Live Births	**191,783**	**19,861**	**4,223**	**2,233**	**339**		**220,151**	

TRISOMY COUNTS AND RATES BY MATERNAL AGE 1998–2001
(Rates per 10,000 Live Births)

Defect	Age		
	<35	35 and >	Total*
Down syndrome	142 *7.07*	92 *47.64*	234 *10.63*
Trisomy 13	18 *0.90*	6 *3.11*	25 *1.14*
Trisomy 18	47 *2.34*	19 *9.84*	66 *3.00*
Total Live Births	**200,737**	**19,313**	**220,151**

*Total includes unknown age.
Notes:
1. Births covered include live births and fetal deaths.
2. Unknown race category includes unknowns for Hispanic origin or an unknown race.
3. Heart defects include probable diagnoses.
4. Neural tube defect data is available from 1997 through 2001. The remaining codes are available for 1998 through 2001 only.

Maryland

BIRTH DEFECTS COUNTS AND RATES 1997–2001

(Rates per 10,000 Live Births)

Defect	Non-Hispanic White	Non-Hispanic Black or African	Hispanic	Asian or Pacific Islander	American Indian or Alaskan Native	Other/ Unknown	Total	Notes
			Race/Ethnicity					
Anencephalus	51	25				16	92	
	2.56	*2.48*					*2.71*	
Cleft lip with and without cleft palate	189	65				31	285	
	9.49	*6.45*					*8.40*	
Cleft palate without cleft lip	116	31				17	164	
	5.83	*3.08*					*4.83*	
Congenital hip dislocation	74	10				12	96	
	3.72	*0.99*					*2.83*	
Down syndrome	252	103				52	407	
	12.66	*10.23*					*12.00*	
Esophageal atresia / tracheoesophageal fistula	33	17				6	56	
	1.66	*1.69*					*1.65*	
Hydrocephalus without Spina Bifida	72	46				14	132	
	3.62	*4.57*					*3.89*	
Hypospadias and Epispadias	548	189				42	779	
	27.52	*18.76*					*22.97*	
Rectal and large intestinal atresia/stenosis	62	22				9	93	
	3.11	*2.18*					*2.74*	
Reduction deformity, lower limbs	50	31				3	84	
	2.51	*3.08*					*2.48*	
Reduction deformity, upper limbs	72	27				8	106	
	3.62	*2.68*					*3.12*	
Spina bifida without anencephalus	91	19				8	118	
	4.57	*1.89*					*3.48*	
Total Live Births	**199,115**	**100,723**					**339,205**	

TRISOMY COUNTS AND RATES BY MATERNAL AGE 1997–2001

(Rates per 10,000 Live Births)

Defect	<35	35 and >	Total*
		Age	
Down syndrome	233	174	407
	8.24	*30.79*	*12.00*
Total Live Births	**282,621**	**56,515**	**339,205**

*Total includes unknown age.

Massachusetts

BIRTH DEFECTS COUNTS AND RATES 1999–2001

Defect	Non-Hispanic White	Non-Hispanic Black or African	Hispanic	Asian or Pacific Islander	American Indian or Alaskan Native	Other/ Unknown	Total	Notes
Amniotic bands	7	1	1	0	0	1	10	
	0.39	0.57	0.36	0.00	0.00		0.41	
Anencephalus	10	2	1	0	0	2	15	
	0.56	1.15	0.36	0.00	0.00		0.62	
Aniridia	9	0	0	0	0	0	9	
	0.50	0.00	0.00	0.00	0.00		0.37	
Anophthalmia / microphthalmia	15	2	1	3	0	0	21	
	0.84	1.15	0.36	2.21	0.00		0.86	
Anotia/microtia	19	0	7	3	0	2	31	
	1.06	0.00	2.55	2.21	0.00		1.27	
Aortic valve stenosis	27	2	3	1	0	0	33	
	1.50	1.15	1.09	0.74	0.00		1.36	
Atrial septal defect	280	33	48	20	0	13	394	
	15.59	18.90	17.47	14.72	0.00		16.18	
Biliary atresia	6	2	2	0	0	0	10	
	0.33	1.15	0.73	0.00	0.00		0.41	
Bladder exstrophy	5	1	1	0	0	0	7	
	0.28	0.57	0.36	0.00	0.00		0.29	
Choanal artesia	8	0	1	0	0	0	9	
	0.45	0.00	0.36	0.00	0.00		0.37	
Cleft lip with and without cleft palate	136	5	33	18	0	7	199	
	7.57	2.86	12.01	13.25	0.00		8.17	
Cleft palate without cleft lip	107	2	18	6	1	4	138	
	5.96	1.15	6.55	4.42	25.71		5.67	
Coarctation of aorta	65	10	9	2	0	5	91	
	3.62	5.73	3.28	1.47	0.00		3.74	
Common truncus	8	1	0	0	0	0	9	
	0.45	0.57	0.00	0.00	0.00		0.37	
Congenital cataract	18	2	4	2	0	0	26	
	1.00	1.15	1.46	1.47	0.00		1.07	
Diaphragmatic hernia	40	1	5	1	0	1	48	
	2.23	0.57	1.82	0.74	0.00		1.97	
Down syndrome	192	20	34	2	1	9	258	
	10.69	11.45	12.38	1.47	25.71		10.60	
Ebstein's anomaly	7	1	3	0	0	1	12	
	0.39	0.57	1.09	0.00	0.00		0.49	
Encephalocele	5	3	1	1	0	1	11	
	0.28	1.72	0.36	0.74	0.00		0.45	
Endocardial cushion defect	68	10	8	2	0	4	92	
	3.79	5.73	2.91	1.47	0.00		3.78	
Esophageal atresia / tracheoesophageal fistula	41	3	8	3	0	4	59	
	2.28	1.72	2.91	2.21	0.00		2.42	
Gastroschisis	34	0	11	2	0	1	48	
	1.89	0.00	4.00	1.47	0.00		1.97	
Hirschsprung's disease (congenital megacolon)	27	3	6	2	0	1	39	
	1.50	1.72	2.18	1.47	0.00		1.60	
Hydrocephalus without Spina Bifida	39	6	12	5	1	2	65	
	2.17	3.44	4.37	3.68	25.71		2.67	
Hypoplastic left heart syndrome	24	4	6	0	0	1	35	
	1.34	2.29	2.18	0.00	0.00		1.44	
Hypospadias and Epispadias	136	16	24	12	0	4	192	Excludes 1st degree hypospadias and epispadias
	7.57	9.16	8.74	8.83	0.00		7.89	
Microcephalus	41	6	14	2	0	0	63	Defined as head circumference 2 std below normal
	2.28	3.44	5.10	1.47	0.00		2.59	
Obstructive genitourinary defect	137	11	25	7	0	2	182	Excludes isolated diagnosis without surgical intervention and secondary diagnosis without postnatal confirmation
	7.63	6.30	9.10	5.15	0.00		7.48	

(Table continued)

Defect	Race/Ethnicity							Notes
	Non-Hispanic White	Non-Hispanic Black or African	Hispanic	Asian or Pacific Islander	American Indian or Alaskan Native	Other/ Unknown	Total	
Omphalocele	23	5	5	2	0	1	36	
	1.28	*2.86*	*1.82*	*1.47*	*0.00*		*1.48*	
Patent ductus arteriosus	263	39	40	17	0	10	369	Excludes GA 35 weeks and persists 5 days. For 2001: If >35 weeks: ligated surgically, catheter, with codable defect
	14.65	*22.34*	*14.56*	*12.51*	*0.00*		*15.16*	
Pulmonary valve atresia and stenosis	87	13	11	3	0	5	119	
	4.84	*7.45*	*4.00*	*2.21*	*0.00*		*4.89*	
Rectal and large intestinal atresia/stenosis	57	4	14	4	0	3	82	
	3.17	*2.29*	*5.10*	*2.94*	*0.00*		*3.37*	
Reduction deformity, lower limbs	22	3	5	0	0	3	33	
	1.23	*1.72*	*1.82*	*0.00*	*0.00*		*1.36*	
Reduction deformity, upper limbs	43	5	10	3	0	3	64	
	2.39	*2.86*	*3.64*	*2.21*	*0.00*		*2.63*	
Renal agenesis/hypoplasia	5	1	2	0	0	1	9	Excludes isolated cases
	0.28	*0.57*	*0.73*	*0.00*	*0.00*		*0.37*	
Spina bifida without anencephalus	29	3	4	4	0	0	40	
	1.61	*1.72*	*1.46*	*2.94*	*0.00*		*1.64*	
Tetralogy of Fallot	72	10	12	8	0	0	102	
	4.01	*5.73*	*4.37*	*5.89*	*0.00*		*4.19*	
Transposition of great arteries	48	4	9	3	0	3	67	
	2.67	*2.29*	*3.28*	*2.21*	*0.00*		*2.75*	
Tricuspid valve atresia and stenosis	11	1	4	0	0	1	17	
	0.61	*0.57*	*1.46*	*0.00*	*0.00*		*0.70*	
Trisomy 13	9	1	2	1	0	0	13	
	0.50	*0.57*	*0.73*	*0.74*	*0.00*		*0.53*	
Trisomy 18	23	3	3	1	0	2	32	
	1.28	*1.72*	*1.09*	*0.74*	*0.00*		*1.31*	
Ventricular septal defect	261	35	43	11	1	8	359	Excludes isolated muscular VSDs
	14.53	20.04	15.65	8.09	25.71		14.75	
Total Live Births	**179,568**	**17,461**	**27,472**	**13,589**	**389**		**243,462**	

TRISOMY COUNTS AND RATES BY MATERNAL AGE 1999–2001
(Rates per 10,000 Live Births)

Defect	Age		
	<35	35 and >	Total*
Down syndrome	117	141	258
	6.12	*26.96*	*10.60*
Trisomy 13	7	6	13
	0.37	*1.15*	*0.53*
Trisomy 18	15	18	33
	0.78	*3.44*	*1.36*
Total Live Births	**191,156**	**52,300**	**243,462**

*Total includes unknown age.

Notes:
1. Stillbirths are included. Terminations are not included.
2. Coding system is CDC/BPA.
3. CHANGE: Previous years submission have included possible/probable cases. This year submissions for all years (1999–2001) exclude possible/probable cases.
4. CHANGE: Tetralogy of Fallot, included the code 746030 (defined as "Pulmonary atresia/VSD not TOF/PA") in past submissions. Clinical decision was made that this was an error and the code should be "Pulmonary valve atresia and stenosis." Submissions for 1999–2001 include this change.

Michigan

BIRTH DEFECTS COUNTS AND RATES 1997–2001

(Rates per 10,000 Live Births)

Defect	Non-Hispanic White	Non-Hispanic Black or African	Hispanic	Asian or Pacific Islander	American Indian or Alaskan Native	Other/ Unknown	Total	Notes
Anencephalus	54	7	1	0	8	72		
	1.09	*0.59*	*0.32*	*1.17*	*0.00*		*1.07*	
Aniridia	7	1	2	0	1	2	13	
	0.14	*0.08*	*0.64*	*0.00*	*2.86*		*0.19*	
Anophthalmia/ microphthalmia	67	18	6	6	1	4	102	
	1.35	*1.50*	*1.91*	*3.52*	*2.86*		*1.52*	
Anotia/microtia	40	6	5	4	0	3	58	
	0.81	*0.50*	*1.59*	*2.35*	*0.00*		*0.87*	
Aortic valve stenosis	128	8	5	0	2	8	151	
	2.59	*0.67*	*1.59*	*0.00*	*5.72*		*2.25*	
Atrial septal defect	2,428	642	136	62	20	65	3,353	
	49.07	*53.67*	*43.29*	*36.40*	*57.22*		*50.02*	
Biliary atresia	46	22	2	3	0	3	76	
	0.93	*1.84*	*0.64*	*1.76*	*0.00*		*1.13*	
Bladder exstrophy	17	3	0	0	1	0	21	
	0.34	*0.25*	*0.00*	*0.00*	*2.86*		*0.31*	
Choanal atresia	78	12	3	2	0	4	99	
	1.58	*1.00*	*0.95*	*1.17*	*0.00*		*1.48*	
Cleft lip with and without cleft palate	511	54	31	17	6	30	649	
	10.33	*4.51*	*9.87*	*9.98*	*17.17*		*9.68*	
Cleft palate without cleft lip	259	50	12	8	3	21	353	
	5.23	*4.18*	*3.82*	*4.70*	*8.58*		*5.27*	
Coarctation of aorta	278	44	16	4	4	8	354	
	5.62	*3.68*	*5.09*	*2.35*	*11.44*		*5.28*	
Common truncus	58	12	2	0	1	6	79	
	1.17	*1.00*	*0.64*	*0.00*	*2.86*		*1.18*	
Congenital cataract	90	23	3	4	2	4	126	
	1.82	*1.92*	*0.95*	*2.35*	*5.72*		*1.88*	
Congenital hip dislocation	686	57	24	29	3	20	819	
	13.86	*4.77*	*7.64*	*17.03*	*8.58*		*12.22*	
Diaphragmatic hernia	133	35	5	8	1	9	191	
	2.69	*2.93*	*1.59*	*4.70*	*2.86*		*2.85*	
Down syndrome	524	90	36	22	2	31	714	
	10.59	*8.28*	*11.46*	*12.92*	*5.72*		*10.65*	
Ebstein's anomaly	103	6	2	3	1	11	126	
	2.08	*0.50*	*0.64*	*1.76*	*2.86*		*1.88*	
Encephalocele	30	13	3	0	0	1	47	
	0.61	*1.09*	*0.95*	*0.00*	*0.00*		*0.70*	
Endocardial cushion defect	177	43	7	4	0	15	246	
	3.58	*3.59*	*2.23*	*2.35*	*0.00*		*3.67*	
Esophageal atresia/ tracheoesophageal fistula	133	32	6	1	3	5	180	
	2.69	*2.68*	*1.91*	*0.59*	*8.58*		*2.69*	
Fetal alcohol syndrome	55	40	3	1	0	2	101	
	1.11	*3.34*	*0.95*	*0.59*	*0.00*		*1.51*	
Hirschsprung's disease (congenital megacolon)	136	47	8	6	1	9	207	
	2.75	*3.93*	*2.55*	*3.52*	*2.86*		*3.09*	
Hydrocephalus without Spina Bifida	360	125	17	9	4	18	533	
	7.28	*10.45*	*5.41*	*5.28*	*11.44*		*7.95*	
Hypoplastic left heart syndrome	191	28	10	4	1	28	262	
	3.86	*2.34*	*3.18*	*2.35*	*2.86*		*3.91*	

(Table continued)

Defect	Race/Ethnicity							
	Non-Hispanic White	Non-Hispanic Black or African	Hispanic	Asian or Pacific Islander	American Indian or Alaskan Native	Other/Unknown	Total	Notes
Hypospadias and Epispadias	1,360 *27.48*	224 *18.73*	43 *13.69*	17 *9.98*	7 *20.03*	66	1,717 *25.61*	
Microcephalus	268 *5.42*	108 *9.03*	13 *4.14*	11 *6.46*	3 *8.58*	13	416 *6.21*	
Obstructive genitourinary defect	795 *16.07*	156 *13.04*	62 *19.74*	21 *12.33*	6 *17.17*	35	1,075 *16.04*	
Patent ductus arteriosus	1,171 *23.66*	306 *25.58*	67 *21.33*	34 *19.96*	10 *28.61*	8	1,596 *23.81*	
Pulmonary valve atresia and stenosis	444 *8.97*	144 *12.04*	29 *9.23*	18 *10.57*	4 *11.44*	22	661 *9.86*	
Pyloric stenosis	944 *19.08*	108 *9.03*	59 *18.78*	8 *4.70*	7 *20.03*	24	1,150 *17.15*	
Rectal and large intestinal atresia/stenosis	221 *4.47*	50 *4.18*	9 *2.86*	8 *4.70*	1 *2.86*	14	303 *4.52*	
Reduction deformity, lower limbs	59 *1.19*	17 *1.42*	3 *0.95*	2 *1.17*	0 *0.00*	3	84 *1.25*	
Reduction deformity, upper limbs	107 *2.16*	29 *2.42*	2 *0.64*	2 *1.17*	0 *0.00*	5	145 *2.16*	
Renal agenesis/hypoplasia	256 *5.17*	46 *3.85*	16 *5.09*	10 *5.87*	1 *2.86*	12	341 *5.09*	
Spina bifida without anencephalus	188 *3.80*	40 *3.34*	11 *3.50*	4 *2.35*	3 *8.58*	13	259 *3.86*	
Tetralogy of Fallot	238 *4.81*	44 *3.68*	20 *6.37*	11 *6.46*	2 *5.72*	18	333 *4.97*	
Transposition of great arteries	227 *4.59*	33 *2.76*	12 *3.82*	6 *3.52*	1 *2.86*	23	302 *4.51*	
Tricuspid valve atresia and stenosis	49 *0.99*	21 *1.76*	6 *1.91*	2 *1.17*	0 *0.00*	2	80 *1.19*	
Trisomy 13	39 *0.79*	11 *0.92*	4 *1.27*	3 *1.76*	0 *0.00*	8	65 *0.97*	
Trisomy 18	62 *1.25*	10 *0.84*	3 *0.95*	3 *1.76*	1 *2.86*	9	88 *1.31*	
Ventricular septal defect	1,813 *36.64*	299 *25.00*	85 *27.06*	70 *41.10*	15 *42.92*	96	2,378 *35.47*	
Total Live Births	494,839	119,613	31,415	17,031	3,495		670,359	

TRISOMY COUNTS AND RATES BY MATERNAL AGE 1997–2001

(Rates per 10,000 Live Births)

Defect	Age		
	<35	35 and >	Total*
Down syndrome	403 *6.85*	285 *34.70*	714 *10.65*
Trisomy 13	46 *0.78*	11 *1.34*	65 *0.97*
Trisomy 18	48 *0.82*	32 *3.90*	88 *1.31*
Total Live Births	588,034	82,126	670,254

*Total includes unknown age.

Mississippi

BIRTH DEFECTS COUNTS AND RATES 2000–2001

(Rates per 10,000 Live Births)

Defect	Non-Hispanic White	Non-Hispanic Black or African	Hispanic	Asian or Pacific Islander	American Indian or Alaskan Native	Other/ Unknown	Total	Notes
Anencephalus	4	5	0	0	0	1	10	live births only
	0.89	*1.29*	*0.00*	*0.00*	*0.00*		*1.16*	
Aniridia	1	1	0	0	0	0	2	
	0.22	*0.26*	*0.00*	*0.00*	*0.00*		*0.23*	
Anophthalmia/ microphthalmia	4	6	0	0	0	0	10	
	0.89	*1.55*	*0.00*	*0.00*	*0.00*		*1.16*	
Anotia/microtia	3	3	0	0	1	0	7	
	0.67	*0.78*	*0.00*	*0.00*	*19.65*		*0.81*	
Aortic valve stenosis	4	1	0	0	0	0	5	
	0.89	*0.26*	*0.00*	*0.00*	*0.00*		*0.58*	
Atrial septal defect	82	115	4	1	2	0	204	
	18.19	*29.71*	*31.27*	*12.80*	*39.29*		*23.62*	
Biliary atresia	2	3	0	0	0	0	5	
	0.44	*0.78*	*0.00*	*0.00*	*0.00*		*0.58*	
Bladder exstrophy	2	1	0	0	0	0	3	
	0.44	*0.26*	*0.00*	*0.00*	*0.00*		*0.35*	
Choanal atresia	2	1	0	0	0	0	3	
	0.44	*0.26*	*0.00*	*0.00*	*0.00*		*0.35*	
Cleft lip with and without cleft palate	34	24	0	0	1	0	59	
	7.54	*6.20*	*0.00*	*0.00*	*19.65*		*6.83*	
Cleft palate without cleft lip	26	18	1	0	1	0	46	
	5.77	*4.65*	*7.82*	*0.00*	*19.65*		*5.33*	
Coarctation of aorta	15	9	0	0	1	0	25	
	3.33	*2.33*	*0.00*	*0.00*	*19.65*		*2.90*	
Common truncus	5	3	0	0	0	0	8	
	1.11	*0.78*	*0.00*	*0.00*	*0.00*		*0.93*	
Congenital cataract	7	4	0	0	0	0	11	
	1.55	*1.03*	*0.00*	*0.00*	*0.00*		*1.27*	
Congenital hip dislocation	17	12	1	1	1	1	33	
	3.77	*3.10*	*7.82*	*12.80*	*19.65*		*3.82*	
Diaphragmatic hernia	7	17	1	0	1	1	27	
	1.55	*4.39*	*7.82*	*0.00*	*19.65*		*3.13*	
Down syndrome	44	21	1	0	1	0	67	
	9.76	*5.43*	*7.82*	*0.00*	*19.65*		*7.76*	
Ebstein's anomaly	2	2	0	0	0	0	4	
	0.44	*0.52*	*0.00*	*0.00*	*0.00*		*0.46*	
Encephalocele	7	4	0	0	0	0	11	
	1.55	*1.03*	*0.00*	*0.00*	*0.00*		*1.27*	
Endocardial cushion defect	10	8	0	0	0	0	18	
	2.22	*2.07*	*0.00*	*0.00*	*0.00*		*2.08*	
Esophageal atresia/ tracheoesophageal fistula	9	11	0	0	0	0	20	
	2.00	*2.84*	*0.00*	*0.00*	*0.00*		*2.32*	
Fetal alcohol syndrome	2	3	0	0	2	0	7	
	0.44	*0.78*	*0.00*	*0.00*	*39.29*		*0.81*	
Hirschsprung's disease (congenital megacolon)	7	14	0	0	0	1	22	
	1.55	*3.62*	*0.00*	*0.00*	*0.00*		*2.55*	
Hydrocephalus without Spina Bifida	21	34	0	0	2	0	57	
	4.66	*8.78*	*0.00*	*0.00*	*39.29*		*6.60*	
Hypoplastic left heart syndrome	12	6	1	0	1	3	23	
	2.66	*1.55*	*7.82*	*0.00*	*19.65*		*2.66*	
Hypospadias and Epispadias	62	64	0	0	1	0	127	
	13.75	*16.54*	*0.00*	*0.00*	*19.65*		*14.71*	

(Table continued)

Defect	Race/Ethnicity							Notes
	Non-Hispanic White	Non-Hispanic Black or African	Hispanic	Asian or Pacific Islander	American Indian or Alaskan Native	Other/ Unknown	Total	
Microcephalus	18	48	1	1	3	3	74	
	3.99	*12.40*	*7.82*	*12.80*	*58.94*		*8.57*	
Obstructive genitourinary defect	64	45	0	0	1	2	112	
	14.20	*11.63*	*0.00*	*0.00*	*19.65*		*12.97*	
Patent ductus arteriosus	70	94	1	0	1	0	166	Only >2500 g Birth Weights are included. 75 cases did not have a birth weight available.
	15.53	*24.29*	*7.82*	*0.00*	*19.65*		*19.22*	
Pulmonary valve atresia and stenosis	12	29	0	0	1	0	42	
	2.66	*7.49*	*0.00*	*0.00*	*19.65*		*4.86*	
Pyloric stenosis	84	22	1	0	1	1	109	
	18.64	*5.68*	*7.82*	*0.00*	*19.65*		*12.62*	
Rectal and large intestinal atresia/stenosis	9	10	0	0	0	1	20	
	2.00	*2.58*	*0.00*	*0.00*	*0.00*		*2.32*	
Reduction deformity, lower limbs	2	5	0	0	0	1	8	
	0.44	*1.29*	*0.00*	*0.00*	*0.00*		*0.93*	
Reduction deformity, upper limbs	4	10	0	0	1	0	15	
	0.89	*2.58*	*0.00*	*0.00*	*19.65*		*1.74*	
Renal agenesis/hypoplasia	10	18	0	0	0	1	29	
	2.22	*4.65*	*0.00*	*0.00*	*0.00*		*3.36*	
Spina bifida without anencephalus	15	12	2	0	1	1	31	
	3.33	*3.10*	*15.64*	*0.00*	*19.65*		*3.59*	
Tetralogy of Fallot	12	13	0	0	0	0	25	
	2.66	*3.36*	*0.00*	*0.00*	*0.00*		*2.90*	
Transposition of great arteries	20	13	0	0	0	1	34	
	4.44	*3.36*	*0.00*	*0.00*	*0.00*		*3.94*	
Tricuspid valve atresia and stenosis	1	5	0	0	0	0	6	
	0.22	*1.29*	*0.00*	*0.00*	*0.00*		*0.69*	
Trisomy 13	2	4	0	0	0	0	6	
	0.44	*1.03*	*0.00*	*0.00*	*0.00*		*0.69*	
Trisomy 18	4	8	0	0	0	0	12	
	0.89	*2.07*	*0.00*	*0.00*	*0.00*		*1.39*	
Ventricular septal defect	116	129	0	1	2	2	250	MSDH does not indicate probable causes.
	25.73	*33.33*	*0.00*	*12.80*	*39.29*		*28.95*	
Total Live Births	45,075	38,704	1,279	781	509		86,352	

TRISOMY COUNTS AND RATES BY MATERNAL AGE 2000–2001

(Rates per 10,000 Live Births)

Defect	Age		
	<35	35 and >	Total*
Down syndrome	43	24	67
	5.38	*37.13*	*7.76*
Trisomy 13	5	1	6
	0.63	*1.55*	*0.69*
Trisomy 18	6	6	12
	0.75	*9.28*	*1.39*
Total Live Births	79,882	6,464	86,352

*Total includes unknown age.

Missouri

BIRTH DEFECTS COUNTS AND RATES 1997–2001

(Rates per 10,000 Live Births)

Defect	Non-Hispanic White	Non-Hispanic Black or African	Hispanic	Asian or Pacific Islander	American Indian or Alaskan Native	Other/ Unknown	Total	Notes
Anencephalus	52	8	5	2	0	0	67	
	2.16	*1.79*	*5.54*	*3.99*	*0.00*		*2.23*	
Aniridia	12	2	0	0	0	0	14	
	0.50	*0.45*	*0.00*	*0.00*	*0.00*		*0.47*	
Anophthalmia/ microphthalmia	47	13	3	0	0	0	63	
	1.95	*2.91*	*3.32*	*0.00*	*0.00*		*2.09*	
Anotia/microtia	11	5	2	0	0	0	18	
	0.46	*1.12*	*2.22*	*0.00*	*0.00*		*0.60*	
Aortic valve stenosis	55	9	2	0	0	0	66	
	2.29	*2.01*	*2.22*	*0.00*	*0.00*		*2.19*	
Atrial septal defect	1,518	458	68	25	7	5	2,081	
	63.11	*102.40*	*75.36*	*49.92*	*62.33*		*69.16*	
Biliary atresia	23	6	0	0	0	0	29	
	0.96	*1.34*	*0.00*	*0.00*	*0.00*		*0.96*	
Bladder exstrophy	15	1	0	0	0	0	16	
	0.62	*0.22*	*0.00*	*0.00*	*0.00*		*0.53*	
Choanal atresia	61	10	1	2	0	0	74	
	2.54	*2.24*	*1.11*	*3.99*	*0.00*		*2.46*	
Cleft lip with and without cleft palate	301	20	12	5	0	0	338	
	12.51	*4.47*	*13.30*	*9.98*	*0.00*		*11.23*	
Cleft palate without cleft lip	159	26	6	1	1	1	194	
	6.61	*5.81*	*6.65*	*2.00*	*8.90*		*6.45*	
Coarctation of aorta	162	22	2	5	0	0	191	
	6.74	*4.92*	*2.22*	*9.98*	*0.00*		*6.35*	
Common truncus	25	2	0	0	0	0	27	
	1.04	*0.45*	*0.00*	*0.00*	*0.00*		*0.90*	
Congenital cataract	64	10	3	0	0	0	77	
	2.66	*2.24*	*3.32*	*0.00*	*0.00*		*2.56*	
Congenital hip dislocation	369	22	10	1	2	0	404	
	15.34	*4.92*	*11.08*	*2.00*	*17.81*		*13.43*	
Diaphragmatic hernia	103	23	4	6	0	0	136	
	4.28	*5.14*	*4.43*	*11.98*	*0.00*		*4.52*	
Down syndrome	353	56	15	6	0	1	432	
	14.68	*12.52*	*16.62*	*11.98*	*0.00*		*14.36*	
Ebstein's anomaly	20	1	0	0	0	1	22	
	0.83	*0.22*	*0.00*	*0.00*	*0.00*		*0.73*	
Encephalocele	30	2	2	1	0	0	35	
	1.25	*0.45*	*2.22*	*2.00*	*0.00*		*1.16*	
Endocardial cushion defect	126	19	2	2	0	0	149	
	5.24	*4.25*	*2.22*	*3.99*	*0.00*		*4.95*	
Esophageal atresia/ tracheoesophageal fistula	75	10	4	0	0	0	89	
	3.12	*2.24*	*4.43*	*0.00*	*0.00*		*2.96*	
Fetal alcohol syndrome	26	15	0	1	0	0	42	
	1.08	*3.35*	*0.00*	*2.00*	*0.00*		*1.40*	
Hirschsprung's disease (congenital megacolon)	85	18	3	2	0	0	108	
	3.53	*4.02*	*3.32*	*3.99*	*0.00*		*3.59*	
Hydrocephalus without Spina Bifida	221	62	5	4	0	2	294	
	9.19	*13.86*	*5.54*	*7.99*	*0.00*		*9.77*	
Hypoplastic left heart syndrome	85	20	2	1	0	0	108	
	3.53	*4.47*	*2.22*	*2.00*	*0.00*		*3.59*	
Hypospadias and Epispadias	1,087	183	26	11	1	5	1,313	
	45.19	*40.92*	*28.82*	*21.96*	*8.90*		*43.64*	

(Table continued)

Defect	Race/Ethnicity						Total	Notes
	Non-Hispanic White	Non-Hispanic Black or African	Hispanic	Asian or Pacific Islander	American Indian or Alaskan Native	Other/ Unknown		
Microcephalus	138	49	3	1	1	0	192	
	5.74	*10.96*	*3.32*	*2.00*	*8.90*		*6.38*	
Obstructive genitourinary defect	524	84	11	12	3	2	636	
	21.79	*18.78*	*12.19*	*23.96*	*26.71*		*21.14*	
Patent ductus arteriosus	1,214	311	43	26	2	4	1,600	
	50.48	*69.53*	*47.66*	*51.92*	*17.81*		*53.18*	
Pulmonary valve atresia and stenosis	285	90	8	6	0	2	391	
	11.85	*20.12*	*8.87*	*11.98*	*0.00*		*13.00*	
Pyloric stenosis	838	72	16	5	5	0	936	
	34.84	*16.10*	*17.73*	*9.98*	*44.52*		*31.11*	
Rectal and large intestinal atresia/stenosis	135	11	6	1	0	0	153	
	5.61	*2.46*	*6.65*	*2.00*	*0.00*		*5.09*	
Reduction deformity, lower limbs	45	12	2	0	1	0	60	
	1.87	*2.68*	*2.22*	*0.00*	*8.90*		*1.99*	
Reduction deformity, upper limbs	67	17	2	2	1	0	89	
	2.79	*3.80*	*2.22*	*3.99*	*8.90*		*2.96*	
Renal agenesis/hypoplasia	122	17	5	1	0	0	145	
	5.07	*3.80*	*5.54*	*2.00*	*0.00*		*4.82*	
Spina bifida without anencephalus	122	14	9	0	0	0	145	
	5.07	*3.13*	*9.97*	*0.00*	*0.00*		*4.82*	
Tetralogy of Fallot	141	28	9	3	1	0	182	
	5.86	*6.26*	*9.97*	*5.99*	*8.90*		*6.05*	
Transposition of great arteries	118	21	0	2	0	0	141	
	4.91	*4.70*	*0.00*	*3.99*	*0.00*		*4.69*	
Tricuspid valve atresia and stenosis	37	10	1	0	0	0	48	
	1.54	*2.24*	*1.11*	*0.00*	*0.00*		*1.60*	
Trisomy 13	20	8	0	1	0	0	29	
	0.83	*1.79*	*0.00*	*2.00*	*0.00*		*0.96*	
Trisomy 18	51	13	2	1	0	0	67	
	2.12	*2.91*	*2.22*	*2.00*	*0.00*		*2.23*	
Ventricular septal defect	1,057	204	33	14	3	4	1,315	
	43.95	*45.61*	*36.57*	*27.96*	*26.71*		*43.71*	
Total Live Births	**240,514**	**44,726**	**9,023**	**5,008**	**1,123**		**300,876**	

TRISOMY COUNTS AND RATES BY MATERNAL AGE 1997–2001
(Rates per 10,000 Live Births)

Defect	Age		
	<35	35 and >	Total*
Down syndrome	354	178	432
	9.47	*54.80*	*14.36*
Trisomy 13	22	7	29
	0.82	*2.15*	*0.96*
Trisomy 18	47	20	67
	1.75	*6.16*	*2.23*
Total Live Births	**268,352**	**32,483**	**300,876**

*Total includes unknown age.

Montana

BIRTH DEFECTS COUNTS AND RATES 2000–2001

(Rates per 10,000 Live Births)

| Defect | Race/Ethnicity | | | | | | | Notes |
	Non-Hispanic White	Non-Hispanic Black or African	Hispanic	Asian or Pacific Islander	American Indian or Alaskan Native	Other/Unknown	Total	
Amniotic bands	0	0	0	0	0	0	0	
	0.00	*0.00*	*0.00*	*0.00*	*0.00*		*1.83*	
Anencephalus	1	0	0	0	0	1	2	
	0.55	*0.00*	*0.00*	*0.00*	*0.00*		*0.91*	
Aniridia	0	0	0	0	0	0	0	
	0.00	*0.00*	*0.00*	*0.00*	*0.00*		*0.00*	
Anophthalmia/ microphthalmia	0	0	0	1	0	0	1	
	0.00	*0.00*	*0.00*	*55.87*	*0.00*		*0.46*	
Anotia/microtia	0	0	0	0	0	0	0	
	0.00	*0.00*	*0.00*	*0.00*	*0.00*		*0.00*	
Aortic valve stenosis	2	0	0	0	0	3	5	
	1.10	*0.00*	*0.00*	*0.00*	*0.00*		*2.28*	
Atrial septal defect	24	0	0	1	5	32	62	
	13.19	*0.00*	*0.00*	*55.87*	*18.89*		*28.32*	
Biliary atresia	0	0	0	0	0	0	0	
	0.00	*0.00*	*0.00*	*0.00*	*0.00*		*0.00*	
Bladder exstrophy	0	0	0	0	0	0	0	
	0.00	*0.00*	*0.00*	*0.00*	*0.00*		*0.00*	
Choanal atresia	0	0	0	0	0	0	0	
	0.00	*0.00*	*0.00*	*0.00*	*0.00*		*0.00*	
Cleft lip with and without cleft palate	8	1	0	0	7	8	24	
	4.40	*129.87*	*0.00*	*0.00*	*26.45*		*10.96*	
Cleft palate without cleft lip	9	0	0	0	2	6	17	
	4.95	*0.00*	*0.00*	*0.00*	*7.56*		*7.77*	
Coarctation of aorta	4	0	0	0	0	0	4	
	2.20	*0.00*	*0.00*	*0.00*	*0.00*		*1.83*	
Common truncus	0	0	0	0	0	1	1	
	0.00	*0.00*	*0.00*	*0.00*	*0.00*		*0.46*	
Congenital cataract	2	0	0	0	0	0	2	
	1.10	*0.00*	*0.00*	*0.00*	*0.00*		*0.91*	
Congenital hip dislocation	0	0	0	0	0	0	0	
	0.00	*0.00*	*0.00*	*0.00*	*0.00*		*0.00*	
Diaphragmatic hernia	1	0	0	0	0	1	2	
	0.55	*0.00*	*0.00*	*0.00*	*0.00*		*0.91*	
Down syndrome	26	0	0	0	2	22	50	
	14.29	*0.00*	*0.00*	*0.00*	*7.56*		*22.84*	
Ebstein's anomaly	2	0	0	0	0	1	3	
	1.10	*0.00*	*0.00*	*0.00*	*0.00*		*1.37*	
Encephalocele	0	0	0	0	0	0	0	
	0.00	*0.00*	*0.00*	*0.00*	*0.00*		*0.00*	
Endocardial cushion defect	2	0	0	0	1	5	8	
	1.10	*0.00*	*0.00*	*0.00*	*3.78*		*3.65*	
Esophageal atresia/ tracheoesophageal fistula	0	0	0	1	0	1	2	
	0.00	*0.00*	*0.00*	*55.87*	*0.00*		*0.91*	
Gastroschisis	4	0	0	0	0	1	5	
	2.20	*0.00*	*0.00*	*0.00*	*0.00*		*2.28*	
Hirschsprung's disease (congenital megacolon)	0	0	0	0	0	1	1	
	0.00	*0.00*	*0.00*	*0.00*	*0.00*		*0.46*	
Hydrocephalus without Spina Bifida	3	0	0	0	0	2	5	
	1.65	*0.00*	*0.00*	*0.00*	*0.00*		*2.28*	
Hypoplastic left heart syndrome	2	0	0	0	0	1	3	
	1.10	*0.00*	*0.00*	*0.00*	*0.00*		*1.37*	

(Table continued)

Defect	Race/Ethnicity							Notes
	Non-Hispanic White	Non-Hispanic Black or African	Hispanic	Asian or Pacific Islander	American Indian or Alaskan Native	Other/ Unknown	Total	
Hypospadias and Epispadias	8 *4.40*	0 *0.00*	0 *0.00*	0 *0.00*	0 *0.00*	2	10 *4.57*	
Microcephalus	13 *7.15*	0 *0.00*	0 *0.00*	0 *0.00*	1 *3.78*	10	24 *10.96*	
Obstructive genitourinary defect	5 *2.75*	0 *0.00*	0 *0.00*	0 *0.00*	1 *3.78*	3	9 *4.11*	
Omphalocele	1 *0.55*	0 *0.00*	0 *0.00*	0 *0.00*	0 *0.00*	0	1 *0.46*	
Patent ductus arteriosus	14 *7.70*	0 *0.00*	0 *0.00*	1 *55.87*	2 *7.56*	25	42 *19.18*	>2500 gms
Pulmonary valve atresia and stenosis	2 *1.10*	0 *0.00*	0 *0.00*	0 *0.00*	0 *0.00*	10	12 *5.48*	
Pyloric stenosis	1 *0.55*	0 *0.00*	0 *0.00*	0 *0.00*	0 *0.00*	0	1 *0.46*	
Rectal and large intestinal atresia/stenosis	0 *0.00*	0 *0.00*	0 *0.00*	0 *0.00*	0 *0.00*	1	1 *0.46*	
Reduction deformity, lower limbs	2 *1.10*	0 *0.00*	0 *0.00*	0 *0.00*	0 *0.00*	0	2 *0.91*	
Reduction deformity, upper limbs	2 *1.10*	0 *0.00*	0 *0.00*	0 *0.00*	0 *0.00*	0	2 *0.91*	
Renal agenesis/hypoplasia	0 *0.00*	0 *0.00*	0 *0.00*	0 *0.00*	0 *0.00*	1	1 *0.46*	
Spina bifida without anencephalus	3 *1.65*	0 *0.00*	0 *0.00*	0 *0.00*	1 *3.78*	0	4 *1.83*	Live Births
Tetralogy of Fallot	2 *1.10*	0 *0.00*	0 *0.00*	0 *0.00*	1 *3.78*	5	8 *3.65*	
Transposition of great arteries	2 *1.10*	0 *0.00*	0 *0.00*	0 *0.00*	1 *3.78*	1	4 *1.83*	
Tricuspid valve atresia and stenosis	0 *0.00*	0 *0.00*	0 *0.00*	0 *0.00*	0 *0.00*	0	0 *0.00*	
Trisomy 13	3 *1.65*	0 *0.00*	0 *0.00*	0 *0.00*	1 *3.78*	1	5 *2.28*	
Trisomy 18	4 *2.20*	0 *0.00*	0 *0.00*	0 *0.00*	0 *0.00*	1	5 *2.28*	
Ventricular septal defect	26 *14.29*	0 *0.00*	0 *0.00*	0 *0.00*	1 *3.78*	48	75 *34.26*	
Total Live Births	**18,190**	**77**	**704**	**179**	**2,647**		**21,893**	

TRISOMY COUNTS AND RATES BY MATERNAL AGE 2000–2001
(Rates per 10,000 Live Births)

Defect	Age		
	<35	35 and >	Total*
Down syndrome	21 *10.94*	19 *70.90*	50 *22.84*
Trisomy 13	2 *1.04*	3 *11.19*	5 *2.28*
Trisomy 18	2 *1.04*	1 *3.73*	5 *2.28*
Total Live Births	**19,204**	**2,680**	**21,893**

*Total includes unknown age.

New Jersey

BIRTH DEFECTS COUNTS AND RATES 1997–2001

(Rates per 10,000 Live Births)

Defect	Race/Ethnicity						Total	Notes
	Non-Hispanic White	Non-Hispanic Black or African	Hispanic	Asian or Pacific Islander	American Indian or Alaskan Native	Other/ Unknown		
Amniotic bands	12	9	7	0	0	0	28	
	0.38	0.96	0.66	0.00	0.00		0.49	
Anencephalus	8	3	11	1	0	0	23	
	0.25	0.32	1.04	0.25	0.00		0.40	
Aniridia	2	0	0	0	0	0	2	
	0.06	0.00	0.00	0.00	0.00		0.03	
Anophthalmia/ microphthalmia	27	11	11	2	0	0	51	
	0.85	1.18	1.04	0.49	0.00		0.89	
Anotia/microtia	33	1	29	2	0	1	66	
	1.04	0.11	2.75	0.49	0.00		1.15	
Aortic valve stenosis	47	7	10	6	0	1	71	
	1.49	0.75	0.95	1.48	0.00		1.24	
Atrial septal defect	2,472	1,143	848	281	11	50	4,805	
	78.15	122.18	80.28	69.24	139.95		84.03	
Biliary atresia	10	1	3	3	0	0	17	
	0.32	0.11	0.28	0.74	0.00		0.30	
Bladder exstrophy	9	1	3	1	0	0	14	
	0.28	0.11	0.28	0.25	0.00		0.24	
Choanal atresia	53	17	7	2	0	0	79	
	1.68	1.82	0.66	0.49	0.00		1.38	
Cleft lip with and without cleft palate	239	51	94	46	0	7	437	
	7.56	5.45	8.90	11.34	0.00		7.64	
Cleft palate without cleft lip	186	50	51	19	0	4	310	
	5.88	5.34	4.83	4.68	0.00		5.42	
Coarctation of aorta	111	25	32	10	1	1	180	
	3.51	2.67	3.03	2.46	12.72		3.15	
Common truncus	27	4	5	0	0	0	36	
	0.85	0.43	0.47	0.00	0.00		0.63	
Congenital cataract	41	15	15	3	0	0	74	
	1.30	1.60	1.42	0.74	0.00		1.29	
Congenital hip dislocation	338	34	104	31	0	2	509	
	10.69	3.63	9.85	7.64	0.00		8.90	
Diaphragmatic hernia	63	21	19	13	0	3	119	
	1.99	2.24	1.80	3.20	0.00		2.08	
Down syndrome	366	117	122	27	1	9	642	
	11.57	12.51	11.55	6.65	12.72		11.23	
Ebstein's anomaly	17	1	3	3	0	0	24	
	0.54	0.11	0.28	0.74	0.00		0.42	
Encephalocele	8	6	7	2	0	0	23	
	0.25	0.64	0.66	0.49	0.00		0.40	
Endocardial cushion defect	85	40	27	7	0	2	161	
	2.69	4.28	2.56	1.72	0.00		2.82	
Esophageal atresia/ tracheoesophageal fistula	83	18	23	8	0	1	133	
	2.62	1.92	2.18	1.97	0.00		2.33	
Fetal alcohol syndrome	10	9	1	0	0	0	20	
	0.32	0.96	0.09	0.00	0.00		0.35	
Gastroschisis	41	24	32	3	1	3	104	
	1.30	2.57	3.03	0.74	12.72		1.82	
Hirschsprung's disease (congenital megacolon)	51	27	15	6	0	4	103	
	1.61	2.89	1.42	1.48	0.00		1.80	
Hydrocephalus without Spina Bifida	92	69	51	11	0	5	228	
	2.91	7.38	4.83	2.71	0.00		3.99	

(Table continued)

Defect	Race/Ethnicity							Notes
	Non-Hispanic White	Non-Hispanic Black or African	Hispanic	Asian or Pacific Islander	American Indian or Alaskan Native	Other/ Unknown	Total	
Hypoplastic left heart syndrome	63 *1.99*	25 *2.67*	20 *1.89*	11 *2.71*	1 *12.72*	2	122 *2.13*	
Hypospadias and Epispadias	1,396 *44.13*	304 *32.50*	238 *22.53*	109 *26.86*	3 *38.17*	32	2,082 *36.41*	
Microcephalus	106 *3.35*	102 *10.90*	68 *6.44*	12 *2.96*	0 *0.00*	6	294 *5.14*	
Obstructive genitourinary defect	826 *26.11*	161 *17.21*	255 *24.14*	116 *28.58*	2 *25.45*	14	1,374 *24.03*	
Omphalocele	36 *1.14*	21 *2.24*	16 *1.51*	1 *0.25*	0 *0.00*	0	74 *1.29*	
Patent ductus arteriosus	1,832 *57.92*	640 *68.41*	496 *46.95*	196 *48.30*	5 *63.61*	21	3,190 *55.78*	
Pulmonary valve atresia and stenosis	365 *11.54*	282 *30.14*	127 *12.02*	35 *8.62*	1 *12.72*	9	819 *14.32*	
Pyloric stenosis	615 *19.44*	114 *12.19*	252 *23.86*	23 *5.67*	2 *25.45*	14	1,020 *17.84*	
Rectal and large intestinal atresia/stenosis	106 *3.35*	33 *3.53*	40 *3.79*	17 *4.19*	0 *0.00*	2	198 *3.46*	
Reduction deformity, lower limbs	48 *1.52*	24 *2.57*	17 *1.61*	2 *0.49*	1 *12.72*	1	93 *1.63*	
Reduction deformity, upper limbs	87 *2.75*	34 *3.63*	39 *3.69*	12 *2.96*	0 *0.00*	2	174 *3.04*	
Renal agenesis/hypoplasia	112 *3.54*	22 *2.35*	37 *3.50*	12 *2.96*	1 *12.72*	4	188 *3.29*	
Spina bifida without anencephalus	55 *1.74*	19 *2.03*	26 *2.46*	5 *1.23*	0 *0.00*	1	106 *1.85*	
Tetralogy of Fallot	125 *3.95*	42 *4.49*	39 *3.69*	13 *3.20*	1 *12.72*	3	223 *3.90*	
Transposition of great arteries	117 *3.70*	34 *3.63*	40 *3.79*	15 *3.70*	1 *12.72*	5	212 *3.71*	
Tricuspid valve atresia and stenosis	23 *0.73*	15 *1.60*	5 *0.47*	4 *0.99*	0 *0.00*	1	48 *0.84*	
Trisomy 13	21 *0.66*	8 *0.86*	8 *0.76*	0 *0.00*	0 *0.00*	0	37 *0.65*	
Trisomy 18	28 *0.89*	9 *0.96*	14 *1.33*	4 *0.99*	0 *0.00*	0	55 *0.96*	
Ventricular septal defect	1,761 *55.67*	448 *47.89*	528 *49.98*	171 *42.14*	5 *63.61*	27	2,940 *51.41*	
Total Live Births	**316,311**	**93,551**	**105,634**	**786**	**40,582**		**571,846**	

TRISOMY COUNTS AND RATES BY MATERNAL AGE 1997–2001
(Rates per 10,000 Live Births)

Defect	Age		
	<35	35 and >	Total*
Down syndrome	338 *7.38*	290 *25.55*	642 *11.23*
Trisomy 13	25 *0.55*	12 *1.06*	37 *0.65*
Trisomy 18	31 *0.68*	23 *2.03*	55 *0.96*
Total Live Births	**458,242**	**113,503**	**571,846**

*Total includes unknown age.

New Mexico

BIRTH DEFECTS COUNTS AND RATES 1997–2001

(Rates per 10,000 Live Births)

Defect	Non-Hispanic White	Non-Hispanic Black or African	Hispanic	Asian or Pacific Islander	American Indian or Alaskan Native	Other/Unknown	Total	Notes
Amniotic bands	0	0	0	0	0	0	0	
	0.00	*0.00*	*0.00*	*0.00*		*0.00*		
Anencephalus	5	0	13	4	4		26	1997–1999: Includes 740; 1998–2000: Includes prenatally diagnosed
	1.35	*0.00*	*2.39*	*3.96*			*2.40*	
Aniridia	0	0	1	0	0		1	
	0.00	*0.00*	*0.18*	*0.00*			*0.09*	
Anophthalmia/ microphthalmia	4	0	3	0	0		7	
	1.08	*0.00*	*0.55*	*0.00*			*0.65*	
Anotia/microtia	4	4	5	5	0		18	
	1.08	*19.98*	*0.92*	*4.95*			*1.66*	
Aortic valve stenosis	3	0	2	1	0		6	
	0.81	*0.00*	*0.37*	*0.99*			*0.55*	
Atrial septal defect	82	2	102	42	3		231	
	22.10	*9.99*	*18.79*	*41.58*			*21.30*	
Biliary atresia	1	0	1	2	1		5	
	0.27	*0.00*	*0.18*	*1.98*			*0.46*	
Bladder exstrophy	3	0	1	0	0		4	
	0.81	*0.00*	*0.18*	*0.00*			*0.37*	
Choanal atresia	1	1	0	0	0		2	
	0.27	*5.00*	*0.00*	*0.00*			*0.18*	
Cleft lip with and without cleft palate	65	0	87	45	6		203	1998–2000: Includes 749
	17.52	*0.00*	*16.02*	*44.55*			*18.71*	
Cleft palate without cleft lip	6	1	17	5	0		29	
	1.62	*5.00*	*3.13*	*4.95*			*2.67*	
Coarctation of aorta	3	0	2	0	0		5	
	0.81	*0.00*	*0.37*	*0.00*			*0.46*	
Common truncus	0	0	0	0	0		0	
	0.00	*0.00*	*0.00*	*0.00*			*0.00*	
Congenital cataract	4	0	4	3	0		11	
	1.08	*0.00*	*0.74*	*2.97*			*1.01*	
Congenital hip dislocation	114	3	159	71	5		352	1997–1998: Includes 754.3
	30.73	*14.99*	*29.29*	*70.30*			*32.45*	
Diaphragmatic hernia	8	0	23	9	1		41	
	2.16	*0.00*	*4.24*	*8.91*			*3.78*	
Down syndrome	36	0	53	14	0		103	
	9.70	*0.00*	*9.76*	*13.86*			*9.50*	
Ebstein's anomaly	3	0	3	1	0		3	
	0.81	*0.00*	*0.55*	*0.99*			*0.28*	
Encephalocele	1	0	1	1	1		4	
	0.27	*0.00*	*0.18*	*0.99*			*0.37*	
Endocardial cushion defect	3	1	5	0	0		9	
	0.81	*5.00*	*0.92*	*0.00*			*0.83*	
Esophageal atresia/ tracheoesophageal fistula	3	0	9	2	0		14	
	0.81	*0.00*	*1.66*	*1.98*			*1.29*	
Fetal alcohol syndrome	2	0	7	1	0		10	
	0.54	*0.00*	*1.29*	*0.99*			*0.92*	
Hirschsprung's disease (congenital megacolon)	8	0	4	0	0		12	
	2.16	*0.00*	*0.74*	*0.00*			*1.11*	
Hydrocephalus without Spina Bifida	22	1	31	12	0		66	
	5.93	*5.00*	*5.71*	*11.88*			*6.08*	

(Table continued)

Defect	Non-Hispanic White	Non-Hispanic Black or African	Hispanic	Asian or Pacific Islander	American Indian or Alaskan Native	Other/ Unknown	Total	Notes
Hypoplastic left heart syndrome	6	0	4		1	0	11	
	1.62	*0.00*	*0.74*		*0.99*		*1.01*	
Hypospadias and Epispadias	46	3	39		7	1	96	
	12.40	*14.99*	*7.18*		*6.93*		*8.85*	
Microcephalus	29	0	42		5	1	77	
	7.82	*0.00*	*7.74*		*4.95*		*7.10*	
Obstructive genitourinary defect	18	2	19		4	0	43	
	4.85	*9.99*	*3.50*		*3.96*		*3.96*	
Patent ductus arteriosus	51	4	71		24	2	152	1997–1998 data only
	26.95	*39.53*	*26.54*		*36.05*		*28.08*	
Pulmonary valve atresia and stenosis	9	0	19		2	0	30	
	2.43	*0.00*	*3.50*		*1.98*		*2.77*	
Pyloric stenosis	12	0	36		8	0	56	
	3.23	*0.00*	*6.63*		*7.92*		*5.16*	
Rectal and large intestinal atresia/stenosis	16	0	22		9	0	47	
	4.31	*0.00*	*4.05*		*8.91*		*4.33*	
Reduction deformity, lower limbs	7	1	12		5	1	26	
	1.89	*5.00*	*2.21*		*4.95*		*2.40*	
Reduction deformity, upper limbs	10	0	16		4	1	31	
	2.70	*0.00*	*2.95*		*3.96*		*2.86*	
Renal agenesis/hypoplasia	7	2	3		1	0	13	
	1.89	*9.99*	*0.55*		*0.99*		*1.20*	
Spina bifida without anencephalus	23	0	36		3	3	65	1997–2000: Includes 741; 1998–2000: Includes prenatally diagnosed
	6.20	*0.00*	*6.63*		*2.97*		*5.99*	
Tetralogy of Fallot	9	1	24		7	0	41	
	2.43	*5.00*	*4.42*		*6.93*		*3.78*	
Transposition of great arteries	8	0	9		3	0	20	
	2.16	*0.00*	*1.66*		*2.97*		*1.84*	
Tricuspid valve atresia and stenosis	4	0	6		1	0	11	
	1.08	*0.00*	*1.11*		*0.99*		*1.01*	
Trisomy 13	3	0	6		1	0	10	
	0.81	*0.00*	*1.11*		*0.99*		*0.92*	
Trisomy 18	3	0	5		3	0	11	
	0.81	*0.00*	*0.92*		*2.97*		*1.01*	
Ventricular septal defect	151	4	206		79	6	446	
	40.70	*19.98*	*37.94*		*78.22*		*41.12*	
Total Live Births	**37,101**	**2,002**	**54,291**		**10,100**		**108,476**	

Notes:
1. Patent ductus arteriosus data for 1999–2000 not available.

New York

BIRTH DEFECTS COUNTS AND RATES 1997–2001

(Rates per 10,000 Live Births)

Defect	Race/Ethnicity						Total	Notes
	Non-Hispanic White	Non-Hispanic Black or African	Hispanic	Asian or Pacific Islander	American Indian or Alaskan Native	Other/ Unknown		
Amniotic bands	16	3	3	1	0	0	23	
	0.23	*0.13*	*0.11*	*0.12*	*0.00*		*0.18*	
Anencephalus	28	9	10	3	0	1	51	
	0.41	*0.38*	*0.38*	*0.35*	*0.00*		*0.40*	
Aniridia	7	2	1	1	0	0	11	
	0.13	*0.08*	*0.04*	*0.12*	*0.00*		*0.09*	
Anophthalmia/ microphthalmia	48	22	19	6	0	0	95	
	0.70	*0.92*	*0.72*	*0.70*	*0.00*		*0.74*	
Anotia/microtia	48	5	19	6	1	2	81	
	0.70	*0.21*	*0.72*	*0.70*	*3.14*		*0.63*	
Aortic valve stenosis	131	13	24	5	0	2	175	
	1.92	*0.54*	*0.91*	*0.58*	*0.00*		*1.37*	
Atrial septal defect	1,583	1,136	696	211	7	27	3,660	
	23.24	*47.52*	*26.44*	*24.58*	*21.96*		*28.56*	
Biliary atresia	49	39	18	12	1	2	121	
	0.72	*1.63*	*0.68*	*1.40*	*3.14*		*0.94*	
Bladder exstrophy	26	2	2	0	0	0	30	
	0.38	*0.08*	*0.08*	*0.00*	*0.00*		*0.23*	
Choanal atresia	116	20	45	6	0	1	188	
	1.70	*0.84*	*1.71*	*0.70*	*0.00*		*1.47*	
Cleft lip with and without cleft palate	551	113	166	70	2	11	913	
	8.09	*4.73*	*6.31*	*8.15*	*6.27*		*7.12*	
Cleft palate without cleft lip	461	88	148	45	1	5	748	
	6.77	*3.68*	*5.62*	*5.24*	*3.14*		*5.84*	
Coarctation of aorta	299	74	78	31	5	5	492	
	4.39	*3.10*	*2.96*	*3.61*	*15.68*		*3.84*	
Common truncus	42	19	14	3	0	0	78	
	0.62	*0.79*	*0.53*	*0.35*	*0.00*		*0.61*	
Congenital cataract	97	26	23	7	1	0	154	
	1.42	*1.09*	*0.87*	*0.82*	*3.14*		*1.20*	
Congenital hip dislocation	886	122	295	115	4	3	1,425	
	13.01	*5.10*	*11.21*	*13.39*	*12.55*		*11.12*	
Diaphragmatic hernia	88	29	25	9	1	0	152	
	1.29	*1.21*	*0.95*	*1.05*	*3.14*		*1.19*	
Down syndrome	796	220	262	69	2	13	1,362	
	11.69	*9.20*	*9.95*	*8.04*	*6.27*		*10.63*	
Ebstein's anomaly	43	8	15	5	0	0	71	
	0.63	*0.33*	*0.57*	*0.58*	*0.00*		*0.55*	
Encephalocele	35	19	24	4	2	0	84	
	0.51	*0.79*	*0.91*	*0.47*	*6.27*		*0.66*	
Endocardial cushion defect	201	75	41	13	0	0	330	
	2.95	*3.14*	*1.56*	*1.51*	*0.00*		*2.57*	
Esophageal atresia/ tracheoesophageal fistula	192	32	53	5	1	0	283	
	2.82	*1.34*	*2.01*	*0.58*	*3.14*		*2.21*	
Fetal alcohol syndrome	29	96	14	1	0	4	144	
	0.43	*4.02*	*0.53*	*0.12*	*0.00*		*1.12*	
Gastroschisis	82	32	32	2	0	0	148	
	1.20	*1.34*	*1.22*	*0.23*	*0.00*		*1.15*	
Hirschsprung's disease (congenital megacolon)	131	56	44	20	1	1	253	
	1.92	*2.34*	*1.67*	*2.33*	*3.14*		*1.97*	
Hydrocephalus without Spina Bifida	413	251	199	53	1	7	924	
	6.06	*10.50*	*7.56*	*6.17*	*3.14*		*7.21*	
Hypoplastic left heart syndrome	124	48	57	5	0	2	236	
	1.82	*2.01*	*2.17*	*0.58*	*0.00*		*1.84*	

(Table continued)

Defect	Race/Ethnicity							Notes
	Non-Hispanic White	Non-Hispanic Black or African	Hispanic	Asian or Pacific Islander	American Indian or Alaskan Native	Other/ Unknown	Total	
Hypospadias and	2,791	719	499	197	11	24	4,241	
Epispadias	*40.98*	*30.08*	*18.95*	*22.95*	*34.50*		*33.09*	
Microcephalus	224	190	131	45	2	1	593	
	3.29	*7.95*	*4.98*	*5.24*	*6.27*		*4.63*	
Obstructive genitourinary	1,769	427	649	225	5	16	3,091	
defect	*25.97*	*17.86*	*24.65*	*26.21*	*15.68*		*24.12*	
Omphalocele	69	34	24	7	1	2	137	
	1.01	*1.42*	*0.91*	*0.82*	*3.14*		*1.07*	
Patent ductus arteriosus	377	221	135	35	2	9	779	
	5.54	*9.24*	*5.13*	*4.08*	*6.27*		*6.08*	
Pulmonary valve atresia	517	295	184	43	1	10	1,050	
and stenosis	*7.59*	*12.34*	*6.99*	*5.01*	*3.14*		*8.19*	
Pyloric stenosis	1,357	227	533	64	3	4	2,188	
	19.93	*9.50*	*20.25*	*7.45*	*9.41*		*17.07*	
Rectal and large intestinal	279	73	103	37	1	2	495	
atresia/stenosis	*4.10*	*3.05*	*3.91*	*4.31*	*3.14*		*3.86*	
Reduction deformity,	84	29	28	7	1	1	150	
lower limbs	*1.23*	*1.21*	*1.06*	*0.82*	*3.14*		*1.17*	
Reduction deformity,	130	34	42	8	0	2	216	
upper limbs	*1.91*	*1.42*	*1.60*	*0.93*	*0.00*		*1.69*	
Renal agenesis/hypoplasia	220	65	66	15	2	4	372	
	3.23	*2.72*	*2.51*	*1.75*	*6.27*		*2.90*	
Spina bifida without	133	60	80	16	0	2	291	
anencephalus	*1.95*	*2.51*	*3.04*	*1.86*	*0.00*		*2.27*	
Tetralogy of Fallot	274	108	106	51	0	6	545	
	4.02	*4.52*	*4.03*	*5.94*	*0.00*		*4.25*	
Transposition of great	280	69	76	32	2	5	464	
arteries	*4.11*	*2.89*	*2.89*	*3.73*	*6.27*		*3.62*	
Tricuspid valve atresia	52	29	23	5	1	0	110	
and stenosis	*0.76*	*1.21*	*0.87*	*0.58*	*3.14*		*0.86*	
Trisomy 13	48	22	25	5	0	1	101	
	0.70	*0.92*	*0.95*	*0.58*	*0.00*		*0.79*	
Trisomy 18	5	9	5	0	0	0	19	
	0.07	*0.38*	*0.19*	*0.00*	*0.00*		*0.15*	
Ventricular septal defect	2,511	761	844	282	13	20	4,431	
	36.87	*31.83*	*32.06*	*32.85*	*40.78*		*34.57*	
Total Live Births	**681,042**	**239,059**	**263,266**	**85,854**	**3,188**		**1,281,686**	

TRISOMY COUNTS AND RATES BY MATERNAL AGE 1997–2001

(Rates per 10,000 Live Births)

Defect	Age		
	<35	35 and >	Total*
Down syndrome	715	646	1,362
	6.80	*28.13*	*10.63*
Trisomy 13	71	30	101
	0.68	*1.31*	*0.79*
Trisomy 18	14	5	19
	0.13	*0.22*	*0.15*
Total Live Births	**1,051,809**	**229,668**	**1,281,686**

*Total includes unknown age.
Notes:
1. The New York State data for 2001 are incomplete. The live birth files have not been finalized and we are currently auditing some hospitals for case reports to the Congenital Malformations Registry.

North Carolina

BIRTH DEFECTS COUNTS AND RATES 1997–2000

(Rates per 10,000 Live Births)

Defect	Non-Hispanic White	Non-Hispanic Black or African	Hispanic	Asian or Pacific Islander	American Indian or Alaskan Native	Other/ Unknown	Total	Notes
Anencephalus	45	16	19	2	1	6	89	
	1.57	*1.42*	*5.12*	*2.07*	*1.49*		*1.97*	
Aniridia	31	15	5	1	1	0	53	
	1.08	*1.33*	*1.35*	*1.03*	*1.49*		*1.17*	
Anophthalmia/ microphthalmia	46	12	5	1	2	0	66	
	1.61	*1.06*	*1.35*	*1.03*	*2.97*		*1.46*	
Anotia/microtia	133	82	38	7	3	0	263	
	4.65	*7.26*	*10.24*	*7.24*	*4.46*		*5.81*	
Aortic valve stenosis	65	22	5	0	0	0	92	
	2.27	*1.95*	*1.35*	*0.00*	*0.00*		*2.03*	
Atrial septal defect	1,024	542	174	29	28	1	1,798	
	35.82	*47.98*	*46.90*	*30.01*	*41.59*		*39.73*	
Biliary atresia	57	27	7	2	3	1	97	
	1.99	*2.39*	*1.89*	*2.07*	*4.46*		*2.14*	
Bladder exstrophy	17	7	1	1	1	0	27	
	0.59	*0.62*	*0.27*	*1.03*	*1.49*		*0.60*	
Choanal atresia	53	26	8	0	1	0	88	
	1.85	*2.30*	*2.16*	*0.00*	*1.49*		*1.94*	
Cleft lip with and without cleft palate	301	68	35	17	10	3	434	
	10.53	*6.02*	*9.43*	*17.59*	*14.85*		*9.59*	
Cleft palate without cleft lip	199	52	27	3	6	0	287	
	6.96	*4.60*	*7.28*	*3.10*	*8.91*		*6.34*	
Coarctation of aorta	170	64	21	1	2	0	258	
	5.95	*5.67*	*5.66*	*1.03*	*2.97*		*5.70*	
Common truncus	31	11	5	0	0	0	47	
	1.08	*0.97*	*1.35*	*0.00*	*0.00*		*1.04*	
Congenital cataract	50	23	4	3	3	0	83	
	1.75	*2.04*	*1.08*	*3.10*	*4.46*		*1.83*	
Congenital hip dislocation	486	68	77	9	11	0	651	
	17.00	*6.02*	*20.76*	*9.31*	*16.34*		*14.38*	
Diaphragmatic hernia	88	41	17	4	4	0	154	
	3.08	*3.63*	*4.58*	*4.14*	*5.94*		*3.40*	
Down syndrome	341	133	70	12	4	2	562	
	11.93	*11.77*	*18.87*	*12.42*	*5.94*		*12.42*	
Ebstein's anomaly	20	2	1	0	0	0	23	
	0.70	*0.18*	*0.27*	*0.00*	*0.00*		*0.51*	
Encephalocele	29	19	9	2	0	2	61	
	1.01	*1.68*	*2.43*	*2.07*	*0.00*		*1.35*	
Endocardial cushion defect	106	55	19	4	2	1	187	
	3.71	*4.87*	*5.12*	*4.14*	*2.97*		*4.73*	
Esophageal atresia/ tracheoesophageal fistula	102	34	11	2	4	1	154	
	3.57	*3.01*	*2.97*	*2.07*	*5.94*		*3.40*	
Gastroschisis	67	17	10	0	3	1	98	1999–2000 data
	4.60	*2.96*	*4.49*	*0.00*	*8.78*		*4.19*	
Hirschsprung's disease (congenital megacolon)	91	46	6	4	0	0	147	
	3.18	*4.07*	*1.62*	*4.14*	*0.00*		*3.25*	
Hydrocephalus without Spina Bifida	288	159	30	13	7	1	498	
	10.07	*14.07*	*8.09*	*13.45*	*10.40*		*11.00*	
Hypoplastic left heart syndrome	86	36	11	1	1	2	137	
	3.01	*3.19*	*2.97*	*1.03*	*1.49*		*3.03*	
Hypospadias and Epispadias	1,541	603	116	57	45	1	2,363	
	53.91	*53.38*	*31.27*	*58.99*	*66.84*		*52.21*	

(Table continued)

Defect	Race/Ethnicity						Total	Notes
	Non-Hispanic White	Non-Hispanic Black or African	Hispanic	Asian or Pacific Islander	American Indian or Alaskan Native	Other/Unknown		
Microcephalus	147	108	34	7	4	1	301	
	5.14	*9.56*	*9.16*	*7,24*	*5.94*		*6.65*	
Obstructive genitourinary defect	591	224	74	18	14	1	922	
	20.67	*19.83*	*19.95*	*18.63*	*20.80*		*20.37*	
Omphalocele	19	15	2	1	1	1	39	1999–2000 data
	1.31	*2.61*	*0.90*	*1.92*	*2.93*		*1.67*	
Patent ductus arteriosus	962	526	145	25	20	0	1,678	
	33.65	*46.56*	*39.08*	*25.87*	*29.71*		*37.08*	
Pulmonary valve atresia and stenosis	329	169	52	11	6	0	567	
	11.51	*14.96*	*14.02*	*11.38*	*8.91*		*12.53*	
Pyloric stenosis	736	132	61	1	10	0	940	
	25.75	*11.68*	*16.44*	*1.03*	*14.85*		*20.77*	
Rectal and large intestinal atresia/stenosis	151	63	22	4	7	0	247	
	5.28	*5.58*	*5.93*	*4.14*	*10.40*		*5.46*	
Reduction deformity, lower limbs	53	22	6	3	3	0	87	
	1.85	*1.95*	*1.62*	*3.10*	*4.46*		*1.92*	
Reduction deformity, upper limbs	80	41	9	3	2	2	137	
	2.80	*3.63*	*2.43*	*3.10*	*2.97*		*3.03*	
Renal agenesis/hypoplasia	146	50	14	2	2	2	216	
	5.11	*4.43*	*3.77*	*2.07*	*2.97*		*4.77*	
Spina bifida without anencephalus	140	40	34	3	1	6	224	
	4.90	*3.54*	*9.16*	*3.10*	*1.49*		*4.95*	
Tetralogy of Fallot	148	76	10	4	4	1	243	
	5.18	*6.73*	*2.70*	*4.14*	*5.94*		*5.37*	
Transposition of great arteries	135	50	22	4	2	1	214	
	4.72	*4.43*	*5.93*	*4.14*	*2.97*		*4.73*	
Tricuspid valve atresia and stenosis	34	14	3	0	0	1	52	
	1.19	*1.24*	*0.81*	*0.00*	*0.00*		*1.15*	
Trisomy 13	39	27	11	2	0	5	84	
	1.36	*2.39*	*2.97*	*2.07*	*0.00*		*1.86*	
Trisomy 18	65	26	10	2	0	2	105	
	2.27	*2.30*	*2.70*	*2.07*	*0.00*		*2.32*	
Ventricular septal defect	1,155	454	200	31	28	1	1,869	
	40.40	*40.19*	*53.91*	*32.08*	*41.59*		*41.30*	
Total Live Births	**285,864**	**112,972**	**37,099**	**9,663**	**6,732**		**452,582**	

TRISOMY COUNTS AND RATES BY MATERNAL AGE 1997–2000

(Rates per 10,000 Live Births)

Defect	Age		Total*
	<35	35 and >	
Down syndrome	368	194	562
	9.09	*40.54*	*12.42*
Trisomy 13	61	19	84
	1.51	*3.97*	*1.86*
Trisomy 18	77	27	105
	1.90	*5.64*	*2.32*
Total Live Births	**404,713**	**47,855**	**452,582**

*Total includes unknown age.

North Dakota

BIRTH DEFECTS COUNTS AND RATES 1997–2001

(Rates per 10,000 Live Births)

Defect	Race/Ethnicity						Total	Notes
	Non-Hispanic White	Non-Hispanic Black or African	Hispanic	Asian or Pacific Islander	American Indian or Alaskan Native	Other/Unknown		
Anencephalus							10 *2.55*	
Aortic valve stenosis							16 *4.08*	
Atrial septal defect							173 *44.06*	
Cleft lip with and without cleft palate							56 *14.26*	
Cleft palate without cleft lip							28 *7.13*	
Coarctation of aorta							23 *5.85*	
Common truncus							8 *2.03*	
Down syndrome							41 *10.44*	
Ebstein's anomaly							3 *0.76*	
Endocardial cushion defect							13 *3.31*	
Fetus or newborn affected by maternal alcohol use							29 *7.38*	
Hydrocephalus without Spina Bifida							53 *13.50*	
Hypoplastic left heart syndrome							15 *3.82*	
Microcephalus							53 *13.50*	
Patent ductus arteriosus							80 *20.38*	
Pulmonary valve atresia and stenosis							53 *13.50*	
Spina bifida without anencephalus							27 *6.88*	
Tetralogy of Fallot							22 *5.60*	
Transposition of great arteries							14 *3.56*	
Tricuspid valve atresia and stenosis							2 *0.50*	
Trisomy 13							7 *1.78*	
Trisomy 18							9 *2.29*	
Ventricular septal defect							181 *46.10*	
Total Live Births							39,263	

Oklahoma

BIRTH DEFECTS COUNTS AND RATES 1997–2001

(Rates per 10,000 Live Births)

Defect	Non-Hispanic White	Non-Hispanic Black or African	Hispanic	Asian or Pacific Islander	American Indian or Alaskan Native	Other/ Unknown	Total	Notes
Amniotic bands	21	3	3	0	3	0	30	
	1.21	*1.29*	*1.50*	*0.00*	*1.22*		*1.22*	
Anencephalus	42	5	5	0	7	0	59	
	2.43	*2.15*	*2.49*	*0.00*	*2.85*		*2.40*	
Aniridia	4	0	0	0	1	0	5	
	0.23	*0.00*	*0.00*	*0.00*	*0.41*		*0.20*	
Anophthalmia/ microphthalmia	30	0	3	0	5	0	38	
	1.73	*0.00*	*1.50*	*0.00*	*2.03*		*1.54*	
Anotia/microtia	19	2	3	1	4	1	30	
	1.10	*0.86*	*1.50*	*2.23*	*1.63*		*1.22*	
Aortic valve stenosis	79	4	6	0	5	0	94	
	4.57	*1.72*	*2.99*	*0.00*	*2.03*		*3.82*	
Atrial septal defect	830	111	70	9	141	12	1,173	
	48.00	*47.73*	*34.90*	*20.09*	*57.38*		*47.65*	
Biliary atresia	15	1	1	1	1	0	19	
	0.87	*0.43*	*0.50*	*2.23*	*0.41*		*0.77*	
Bladder exstrophy	8	1	0	0	0	0	9	
	0.46	*0.43*	*0.00*	*0.00*	*0.00*		*0.37*	
Choanal atresia	32	3	3	0	6	1	45	
	1.85	*1.29*	*1.50*	*0.00*	*2.44*		*1.83*	
Cleft lip with and without cleft palate	235	14	16	6	32	0	303	
	13.59	*6.02*	*7.98*	*13.40*	*13.02*		*12.31*	
Cleft palate without cleft lip	135	7	11	2	15	0	170	
	7.81	*3.01*	*5.48*	*4.47*	*6.10*		*6.91*	
Coarctation of aorta	85	8	3	4	5	3	108	
	4.92	*3.44*	*1.50*	*8.93*	*2.03*		*4.39*	
Common truncus	15	1	1	0	2	0	19	
	0.87	*0.43*	*0.50*	*0.00*	*0.81*		*0.77*	
Congenital cataract	38	5	3	1	6	2	55	
	2.20	*2.15*	*1.50*	*2.23*	*2.44*		*2.23*	
Congenital hip dislocation	133	3	7	2	15	1	161	
	7.69	*1.29*	*3.49*	*4.47*	*6.10*		*6.54*	
Diaphragmatic hernia	75	3	6	1	11	0	96	
	4.34	*1.29*	*2.99*	*2.23*	*4.48*		*3.90*	
Down syndrome	233	24	31	9	26	5	328	
	13.47	*10.32*	*15.46*	*20.09*	*10.58*		*13.32*	
Ebstein's anomaly	12	0	2	1	0	0	15	
	0.69	*0.00*	*1.00*	*2.23*	*0.00*		*0.61*	
Encephalocele	20	2	2	0	1	0	25	
	1.16	*0.86*	*1.00*	*0.00*	*0.41*		*1.02*	
Endocardial cushion defect	80	14	4	0	12	1	111	
	4.63	*6.02*	*1.99*	*0.00*	*4.88*		*4.51*	
Esophageal atresia/ tracheoesophageal fistula	55	5	3	0	6	0	69	
	3.18	*2.15*	*1.50*	*0.00*	*2.44*		*2.80*	
Fetal alcohol syndrome	5	1	0	0	3	0	9	
	0.29	*0.43*	*0.00*	*0.00*	*1.22*		*0.37*	
Gastroschisis	91	4	4	0	9	1	109	
	5.26	*1.72*	*1.99*	*0.00*	*3.66*		*4.43*	
Hirschsprung's disease (congenital megacolon)	38	10	1	1	3	0	53	
	2.20	*4.30*	*0.50*	*2.23*	*1.22*		*2.15*	
Hydrocephalus without Spina Bifida	145	14	10	1	14	0	184	
	8.39	*6.02*	*4.99*	*2.23*	*5.70*		*7.47*	

(Table continues)

(Table continued)

Defect	Race/Ethnicity							Notes
	Non-Hispanic White	Non-Hispanic Black or African	Hispanic	Asian or Pacific Islander	American Indian or Alaskan Native	Other/ Unknown	Total	
Hypoplastic left heart syndrome	38	4	3	0	6	0	51	
	2.20	*1.72*	*1.50*	*0.00*	*2.44*		*2.07*	
Hypospadias and Epispadias	547	60	28	3	41	5	684	
	31.63	*25.80*	*13.96*	*6.70*	*16.68*		*27.79*	
Microcephalus	162	22	16	3	30	3	236	
	9.37	*9.46*	*7.98*	*6.70*	*12.21*		*9.59*	
Obstructive genitourinary defect	404	33	59	16	52	4	568	
	23.36	*14.19*	*29.42*	*35.72*	*21.16*		*23.07*	
Omphalocele	39	8	1	1	7	1	57	
	2.26	*3.44*	*0.50*	*2.23*	*2.85*		*2.32*	
Pulmonary valve atresia and stenosis	119	9	13	3	27	1	172	
	6.88	*3.87*	*6.48*	*6.70*	*10.99*		*6.99*	
Pyloric stenosis	464	20	32	0	50	1	567	
	26.83	*8.60*	*15.95*	*0.00*	*20.35*		*23.03*	
Rectal and large intestinal atresia/stenosis	140	9	10	2	27	3	191	
	8.10	*3.87*	*4.99*	*4.47*	*10.99*		*7.76*	
Reduction deformity, lower limbs	24	2	4	1	3	1	35	
	1.39	*0.86*	*1.99*	*2.23*	*1.22*		*1.42*	
Reduction deformity, upper limbs	56	11	11	2	5	1	86	
	3.24	*4.73*	*5.48*	*4.47*	*2.03*		*3.49*	
Renal agenesis/hypoplasia	88	6	6	1	8	0	109	
	5.09	*2.58*	*2.99*	*2.23*	*3.26*		*4.43*	
Spina bifida without anencephalus	77	5	10	2	9	0	103	
	4.45	*2.15*	*4.99*	*4.47*	*3.66*		*4.18*	
Tetralogy of Fallot	81	6	8	3	12	0	110	
	4.68	*2.58*	*3.99*	*6.70*	*4.88*		*4.47*	
Transposition of great arteries	82	4	11	1	10	2	110	
	4.74	*1.72*	*5.48*	*2.23*	*4.07*		*4.47*	
Tricuspid valve atresia and stenosis	10	0	4	0	0	0	14	
	0.58	*0.00*	*1.99*	*0.00*	*0.00*		*0.57*	
Trisomy 13	32	1	3	1	1	0	38	
	1.85	*0.43*	*1.50*	*2.23*	*0.41*		*1.54*	
Trisomy 18	46	7	2	1	2	0	58	
	2.66	*3.01*	*1.00*	*2.23*	*0.81*		*2.36*	
Ventricular septal defect	767	73	97	17	100	10	1,064	
	44.36	*31.39*	*48.36*	*37.95*	*40.70*		*43.22*	
Total Live Births	172,916	23,257	20,057	4,479	24,573		246,168	

TRISOMY COUNTS AND RATES BY MATERNAL AGE 1997–2001
(Rates per 10,000 Live Births)

Defect	Age		
	<35	35 and >	Total*
Down syndrome	203	125	328
	9.00	*62.07*	*13.32*
Trisomy 13	31	7	38
	1.37	*3.48*	*1.54*
Trisomy 18	38	20	58
	1.68	*9.93*	*2.36*
Total Live Births	225,543	20,138	246,168

*Total includes unknown age.

Puerto Rico

BIRTH DEFECTS COUNTS AND RATES 1997–2001
(Rates per 10,000 Live Births)

Defect	Non-Hispanic White	Non-Hispanic Black or African	Hispanic	Asian or Pacific Islander	American Indian or Alaskan Native	Other/ Unknown	Total	Notes
Anencephalus	0	0	99 *3.30*	0	0	0	99 *3.30*	
Cleft lip with and without cleft palate	0	0	118 *3.94*	0	0	0	118 *3.94*	
Cleft palate without cleft lip	0	0	67 *2.23*	0	0	0	67 *2.23*	
Down syndrome	0	0	34 *6.07*	0	0	0	34 *6.07*	2001 data only
Encephalocele	0	0	25 *0.83*	0	0	0	25 *0.83*	
Spina bifida without anencephalus	0	0	178 *5.94*	0	0	0	178 *5.94*	
Total Live Births			299,859				299,859	

TRISOMY COUNTS AND RATES BY MATERNAL AGE 2001
(Rates per 10,000 Live Births)

Defect	<35	35 and >	Total*
Down syndrome	20 **3.87**	14 **32.57**	34 **6.07**
Total Live Births	**277,208**	**22,475**	**299,859**

*Total includes unknown age.

Rhode Island

BIRTH DEFECTS COUNTS AND RATES 1997–2001

(Rates per 10,000 Live Births)

Defect	Non-Hispanic White	Non-Hispanic Black or African	Hispanic	Asian or Pacific Islander	American Indian or Alaskan Native	Other/ Unknown	Total	Notes
Anencephalus	1	0	0	0	0	1	2	
	0.24	0.00	0.00	0.00	0.00		0.34	
Aniridia	0	0	0	0	0	1	1	
	0.00	0.00	0.00	0.00	0.00		0.21	
Anophthalmia/ microphthalmia	2	1	0	1	0	2	4	
	0.47	2.24	0.00	5.87	0.00		0.67	
Anotia/microtia	2	1	1	0	0	0	4	
	0.47	2.24	1.27	0.00	0.00		0.67	
Aortic valve stenosis	5	1	1	0	0	0	7	
	1.19	2.24	1.27	0.00	0.00		1.18	
Atrial septal defect	246	36	47	11	1	13	354	
	58.31	80.79	59.92	64.52	133.33		59.57	
Biliary atresia	0	0	1	0	0	0	1	
	0.00	0.00	1.27	0.00	0.00		0.17	
Bladder exstrophy	2	0	0	0	0	0	2	
	0.47	0.00	0.00	0.00	0.00		0.34	
Choanal atresia	5	0	2	0	0	0	7	
	1.19	0.00	2.55	0.00	0.00		1.18	
Cleft lip with and without cleft palate	26	3	3	1	0	3	44	
	6.16	6.73	3.82	5.87	0.00		7.40	
Cleft palate without cleft lip	16	2	0	1	0	0	19	
	3.79	4.49	0.00	5.87	0.00		3.20	
Coarctation of aorta	11	0	1	0	0	0	12	
	2.61	0.00	1.27	0.00	0.00		2.02	
Congenital cataract	6	0	2	0	0	2	10	
	1.42	0.00	2.55	0.00	0.00		1.68	
Congenital hip dislocation	57	4	8	1	0	5	75	
	13.51	8.98	10.20	5.87	0.00		12.62	
Diaphragmatic hernia	6	0	2	0	0	1	9	
	1.42	0.00	2.55	0.00	0.00		1.51	
Down syndrome	46	6	13	1	0	6	73	
	10.90	13.46	16.57	5.87	0.00		12.29	
Ebstein's anomaly	2	0	0	0	0	0	2	
	0.47	0.00	0.00	0.00	0.00		0.34	
Encephalocele	1	0	0	0	0	2	3	
	0.24	0.00	0.00	0.00	0.00		0.50	
Endocardial cushion defect	5	0	0	0	0	1	6	
	1.19	0.00	0.00	0.00	0.00		1.01	
Esophageal atresia/ tracheoesophageal fistula	11	1	1	0	0	0	13	
	2.61	2.24	1.27	0.00	0.00		2.19	
Fetal alcohol syndrome	2	1	0	0	1	0	4	
	0.60	2.87	0.00	0.00	175.44		0.85	
Hirschsprung's disease (congenital megacolon)	5	1	2	0	0	1	9	
	1.19	2.24	2.55	0.00	0.00		1.51	
Hydrocephalus without Spina Bifida	13	4	4	1	0	0	22	
	3.08	8.98	5.10	5.87	0.00		3.70	
Hypoplastic left heart syndrome	3	0	1	0	0	1	5	
	0.71	0.00	1.27	0.00	0.00		0.84	
Hypospadias and Epispadias	173	12	12	2	1	16	216	
	41.01	26.93	15.30	11.73	133.33		36.35	
Microcephalus	9	1	2	2	0	1	15	
	2.13	2.24	2.55	11.73	0.00		2.52	

(Table continued)

Defect	Race/Ethnicity							Notes
	Non-Hispanic White	Non-Hispanic Black or African	Hispanic	Asian or Pacific Islander	American Indian or Alaskan Native	Other/ Unknown	Total	
Obstructive genitourinary defect	102	7	23	4	1	2	139	
	24.18	*15.71*	*29.32*	*23.46*	*133.33*		*23.39*	
Patent ductus arteriosus	209	30	42	12	0	10	303	1997: Unable to exclude birth weights = 2500 grams; 2001: ≥2500 grams
	49.54	*67.32*	*53.54*	*70.38*	*0.00*		*50.99*	
Pulmonary valve atresia and stenosis	59	15	7	2	0	1	84	
	13.99	*33.66*	*8.92*	*11.73*	*0.00*		*14.14*	
Pyloric stenosis	5	0	3	0	0	0	8	
	1.19	*0.00*	*3.82*	*0.00*	*0.00*		*1.35*	
Rectal and large intestinal atresia/stenosis	15	3	6	0	0	2	26	
	3.56	*6.73*	*7.65*	*0.00*	*0.00*		*4.38*	
Reduction deformity, lower limbs	3	1	0	0	0	0	4	
	0.71	*2.24*	*0.00*	*0.00*	*0.00*		*0.67*	
Reduction deformity, upper limbs	7	2	2	0	0	0	11	
	1.66	*4.49*	*2.55*	*0.00*	*0.00*		*1.85*	
Renal agenesis/hypoplasia	6	1	0	0	0	1	8	
	1.42	*2.24*	*0.00*	*0.00*	*0.00*		*1.35*	
Spina bifida without anencephalus	11	0	3	0	0	2	16	
	2.61	*0.00*	*3.82*	*0.00*	*0.00*		*2.69*	
Tetralogy of Fallot	9	3	4	2	0	0	18	
	2.13	*6.73*	*5.10*	*11.73*	*0.00*		*3.03*	
Transposition of great arteries	4	1	1	0	0	1	7	
	0.95	*2.24*	*1.27*	*0.00*	*0.00*		*1.18*	
Tricuspid valve atresia and stenosis	7	0	1	0	0	0	8	
	1.66	*0.00*	*1.27*	*0.00*	*0.00*		*1.35*	
Trisomy 13	1	0	1	0	0	0	2	
	0.24	*0.00*	*1.27*	*0.00*	*0.00*		*0.34*	
Trisomy 18	4	1	0	1	0	0	6	
	0.95	*2.24*	*0.00*	*5.87*	*0.00*		*1.01*	
Ventricular septal defect	201	18	31	8	1	17	276	
	47.65	*40.39*	*39.52*	*46.92*	*133.33*		*46.45*	
Total Live Births	42,185	4,456	7,844	1,705	75		59,422	

TRISOMY COUNTS AND RATES BY MATERNAL AGE 1998–2001
(Rates per 10,000 Live Births)

Defect	Age		
	<35	35 and >	Total*
Down syndrome	27	32	62
	6.71	*38.91*	*12.79*
Trisomy 13	2	2	2
	0.00	*2.43*	*0.41*
Trisomy 18	2	2	6
	0.50	*2.43*	*1.24*
Total Live Births	40,213	8,225	48,460

*Total includes unknown age.

Notes:
1. One RI Hospital failed to code approximately 500 births/year for years '97 & '98.
2. Total live birth data are provided from Vital Statistics. Hospital Discharge Database does not link infant & mother's record.

South Carolina

BIRTH DEFECTS COUNTS AND RATES 1997–2001

(Rates per 10,000 Live Births)

Defect	Race/Ethnicity						Total	Notes
	Non-Hispanic White	Non-Hispanic Black or African	Hispanic	Asian or Pacific Islander	American Indian or Alaskan Native	Other/ Unknown		
Anencephalus	77	32	6	2	1	1	119	
	4.69	*3.23*	*6.32*				*4.36*	
Encephalocele	29	9	0	0	0	0	38	
	1.76	*0.90*	*0.00*				*1.39*	
Spina bifida without anencephalus	67	31	4	0	1	1	104	
	4.08	*3.13*	*4.21*				*3.81*	
Total Live Births	**164,166**	**98,940**	**9,486**				**272,592**	

Tennessee

BIRTH DEFECTS COUNTS AND RATES 2000–2001

(Rates per 10,000 Live Births)

Defect	Non-Hispanic White	Non-Hispanic Black or African	Hispanic	Asian or Pacific Islander	American Indian or Alaskan Native	Other/ Unknown	Total	Notes
				Race/Ethnicity				
Anencephalus	10	2	3	0	0	0	15	
	0.91	0.56	3.34	0.00	0.00		0.95	
Aniridia	2	0	0	0	0	0	2	
	0.18	0.00	0.00	0.00	0.00		0.13	
Anophthalmia/ microphthalmia	8	2	1	1	0	1	13	
	0.73	0.56	1.11	3.51	0.00		0.82	
Anotia/microtia	1	1	1	1	0	0	4	
	0.09	0.28	1.11	3.51	0.00		0.25	
Aortic valve stenosis	22	2	1	1	0	0	26	
	2.01	0.56	1.11	3.51	0.00		1.65	
Atrial septal defect	407	124	19	7	0	17	574	
	37.23	34.43	21.16	24.56	0.00		36.36	
Biliary atresia	6	2	0	0	0	0	8	
	0.55	0.56	0.00	0.00	0.00		0.51	
Bladder exstrophy	5	0	0	0	0	0	5	
	0.46	0.00	0.00	0.00	0.00		0.32	
Choanal atresia	23	4	0	0	0	0	27	
	2.10	1.11	0.00	0.00	0.00		1.71	
Cleft lip with and without cleft palate	145	29	10	4	0	0	188	
	13.26	8.05	11.14	14.04	0.00		11.91	
Cleft palate without cleft lip	122	25	9	2	0	1	159	
	11.16	6.94	10.02	7.02	0.00		10.07	
Coarctation of aorta	64	17	4	4	0	0	89	
	5.85	4.72	4.45	14.04	0.00		5.64	
Common truncus	5	5	2	0	0	1	13	
	0.46	1.39	2.23	0.00	0.00		0.82	
Congenital cataract	18	8	2	1	0	0	29	
	1.65	2.22	2.23	3.51	0.00		1.84	
Congenital hip dislocation	102	10	4	0	0	8	124	
	9.33	2.78	4,45	0.00	0.00		7.86	
Diaphragmatic hernia	31	13	1	3	2	1	51	
	2.84	3.61	1.11	10.53	38.99		3.23	
Down syndrome	143	42	10	4	0	1	200	
	13.08	11.66	11.14	14.04	0.00		12.67	
Ebstein's anomaly	14	2	2	1	0	1	20	
	1.28	0.56	2.23	3.51	0.00		1.27	
Encephalocele	13	6	0	1	0	1	21	
	1.19	1.67	0.00	3.51	0.00		1.33	
Endocardial cushion defect	31	8	1	1	0	1	42	
	2.84	2.22	1.11	3.51	0.00		2.66	
Esophageal atresia/ tracheoesophageal fistula	29	14	1	0	0	0	44	
	2.65	3.89	1.11	0.00	0.00		2.79	
Fetal alcohol syndrome	24	24	0	0	0	2	50	
	2.20	6.66	0.00	0.00	0.00		3.17	
Hirschsprung's disease (congenital megacolon)	39	11	1	1	0	1	53	
	3.57	3.05	1.11	3.51	0.00		3.36	
Hydrocephalus without Spina Bifida	89	39	8	2	0	2	140	
	8.14	10.83	8.91	7.02	0.00		8.87	
Hypoplastic left heart syndrome	52	14	5	1	0	1	73	
	4.76	3.89	5.57	3.51	0.00		4.62	
Hypospadias and Epispadias	495	150	18	7	2	29	701	
	45.28	41.65	20.05	24.56	38.99		44.41	

(Table continues)

(Table continued)

Defect	Race/Ethnicity							Notes
	Non-Hispanic White	Non-Hispanic Black or African	Hispanic	Asian or Pacific Islander	American Indian or Alaskan Native	Other/Unknown	Total	
Microcephalus	46	30	4	0	0	0	80	
	4.21	*8.33*	*4.45*	*0.00*	*0.00*		*5.07*	
Obstructive genitourinary	25	10	2	2	0	0	39	
defect	*2.29*	*2.78*	*2.23*	*7.02*	*0.00*		*2.47*	
Patent ductus arteriosus	336	122	23	11	1	0	493	birthweight ≥2500
	30.74	*33.88*	*25.62*	*38.60*	*19.49*		*31.23*	
Pulmonary valve atresia	57	26	5	2	0	3	93	
and stenosis	*5.21*	*7.22*	*5.57*	*7.02*	*0.00*		*5.89*	
Pyloric stenosis	340	35	15	3	2	6	401	
	31.10	*9.72*	*16.71*	*10.53*	*38.99*		*25.40*	
Rectal and large intestinal	66	33	3	0	0	1	103	
atresia/stenosis	*6.04*	*9.16*	*3.34*	*0.00*	*0.00*		*6.52*	
Reduction deformity,	17	4	1	1	0	0	23	
lower limbs	*1.56*	*1.11*	*1.11*	*3.51*	*0.00*		*1.46*	
Reduction deformity,	22	7	2	1	0	1	33	
upper limbs	*2.01*	*1.94*	*2.23*	*3.51*	*0.00*		*2.09*	
Renal agenesis/hypoplasia	45	14	7	0	0	1	67	
	4.12	*3.89*	*7.80*	*0.00*	*0.00*		*4.24*	
Spina bifida without	46	10	2	1	0	1	60	
anencephalus	*4.21*	*2.78*	*2.23*	*3.51*	*0.00*		*3.80*	
Tetralogy of Fallot	60	26	3	1	0	0	90	
	5.49	*7.22*	*3.34*	*3.51*	*0.00*		*5.70*	
Transposition of great	51	16	5	0	0	1	73	
arteries	*4.67*	*4.44*	*5.57*	*0.00*	*0.00*		*4.62*	
Tricuspid valve atresia	18	5	0	0	0	1	24	
and stenosis	*1.65*	*1.39*	*0.00*	*0.00*	*0.00*		*1.52*	
Trisomy 13	9	4	0	0	0	0	13	
	0.82	*1.11*	*0.00*	*0.00*	*0.00*		*0.82*	
Trisomy 18	19	11	1	0	0	2	33	
	1.74	*3.05*	*1.11*	*0.00*	*0.00*		*2.09*	
Ventricular septal defect	450	108	33	8	0	20	619	
	41.17	*29.99*	*36.75*	*28.07*	*0.00*		*39.21*	
Total Live Births	**109,312**	**36,011**	**8,979**	**2,850**	**513**		**157,857**	

TRISOMY COUNTS AND RATES BY MATERNAL AGE 2000–2001
(Rates per 10,000 Live Births)

Defect	Age		
	<35	35 and >	Total*
Down syndrome	110	73	200
	7.76	*46.08*	*12.67*
Trisomy 13	12	1	13
	0.85	*0.63*	*0.82*
Trisomy 18	21	8	33
	1.48	*5.05*	*2.09*
Total Live Births	**141,751**	**15,843**	**157,857**

*Total includes unknown age.
Notes:
1. Total live births, birth weight, and maternal age are from Vital Statistics birth certificate files; diagnoses are from Hospital Discharge (UB-92 data).
2. Data are for live births only.

Texas

BIRTH DEFECTS COUNTS AND RATES 1997–2001

(Rates per 10,000 Live Births)

Defect	Non-Hispanic White	Non-Hispanic Black or African	Hispanic	Asian or Pacific Islander	American Indian or Alaskan Native	Other/ Unknown	Total	Notes
Amniotic bands	35	17	66	4	1	2	125	
	0.58	*1.02*	*0.90*	*0.88*	*3.10*		*0.80*	
Anencephalus	151	32	270	9	0	9	471	
	2.48	*1.92*	*3.70*	*1.99*	*0.00*		*3.03*	
Aniridia	8	2	8	0	0	0	18	
	0.13	*0.12*	*0.11*	*0.00*	*0.00*		*0.12*	
Anophthalmia/ microphthalmia	164	43	26	8	3	0	444	
	2.70	*2.58*	*3.10*	*1.77*	*9.31*		*2.85*	
Anotia/microtia	105	19	301	5	1	0	431	
	1.73	*1.14*	*4.13*	*1.10*	*3.10*		*2.77*	
Aortic valve stenosis	173	17	165	10	1	0	366	
	2.84	*1.02*	*2.26*	*2.21*	*3.10*		*2.35*	
Atrial septal defect	2,350	640	3,056	140	15	9	6,210	
	38.62	*38.39*	*41.88*	*30.91*	*46.57*		*39.91*	
Biliary atresia	26	17	52	7	0	0	102	
	0.43	*1.02*	*0.71*	*1.55*	*0.00*		*0.66*	
Bladder exstrophy	17	3	11	0	0	0	31	
	0.28	*0.18*	*0.15*	*0.00*	*0.00*		*0.20*	
Choanal atresia	77	15	99	2	0	0	193	
	1.27	*0.90*	*1.36*	*0.44*	*0.00*		*1.24*	
Cleft lip with and without cleft palate	660	130	879	50	12	1	1,732	
	10.85	*7.80*	*12.05*	*11.04*	*37.26*		*11.13*	
Cleft palate without cleft lip	439	74	404	24	4	2	947	
	7.21	*4.44*	*5.54*	*5.30*	*12.42*		*6.09*	
Coarctation of aorta	315	47	306	18	0	0	686	
	5.18	*2.82*	*4.19*	*3.97*	*0.00*		*4.41*	
Common truncus	47	13	68	5	0	0	133	
	0.77	*0.78*	*0.93*	*1.10*	*0.00*		*0.85*	
Congenital cataract	78	26	106	1	0	0	211	
	1.28	*1.56*	*1.45*	*0.22*	*0.00*		*1.36*	
Congenital hip dislocation	343	47	372	13	1	0	776	
	5.64	*2.82*	*5.10*	*2.87*	*3.10*		*4.99*	
Diaphragmatic hernia	147	34	202	11	0	1	395	
	2.42	*2.04*	*2.77*	*2.43*	*0.00*		*2.54*	
Down syndrome	725	127	970	49	2	17	1,890	
	11.91	*7.62*	*13.29*	*10.82*	*6.21*		*12.15*	
Ebstein's anomaly	34	5	58	4	0	0	101	
	0.56	*0.30*	*0.79*	*0.88*	*0.00*		*0.65*	
Encephalocele	47	13	83	8	0	2	153	
	0.77	*0.78*	*1.14*	*1.77*	*0.00*		*0.98*	
Endocardial cushion defect	241	74	259	14	1	3	592	
	3.96	*4.44*	*3.55*	*3.09*	*3.10*		*3.80*	
Esophageal atresia/ tracheoesophageal fistula	150	25	150	4	1	0	330	
	2.47	*1.50*	*2.06*	*0.88*	*3.10*		*2.12*	
Fetal alcohol syndrome	17	9	12	0	0	0	38	
	0.28	*0.54*	*0.16*	*0.00*	*0.00*		*0.24*	
Gastroschisis	229	40	334	11	4	2	620	
	3.76	*2.40*	*4.58*	*2.43*	*12.42*		*3.98*	
Hirschsprung's disease (congenital megacolon)	94	44	51	3	1	0	193	
	1.54	*2.64*	*0.70*	*0.66*	*3.10*		*1.24*	
Hydrocephalus without Spina Bifida	426	160	546	20	1	6	1,159	
	7.00	*9.60*	*7.48*	*4.42*	*3.10*		*7.45*	
Hypoplastic left heart syndrome	142	28	140	7	0	2	319	
	2.33	*1.68*	*1.92*	*1.55*	*0.00*		*2.05*	

(Table continues)

(Table continued)

Defect	Race/Ethnicity							
	Non-Hispanic White	Non-Hispanic Black or African	Hispanic	Asian or Pacific Islander	American Indian or Alaskan Native	Other/ Unknown	Total	Notes
Hypospadias and	2,352	564	1,281	111	4	8	4,320	
Epispadias	*38.65*	*33.83*	*17.56*	*24.50*	*12.42*		*27.76*	
Microcephalus	324	163	487	31	3	2	1,010	
	5.32	*9.78*	*6.67*	*6.84*	*9.31*		*6.49*	
Obstructive genitourinary	1,290	289	1,411	77	10	7	3,084	
defect	*21.20*	*17.33*	*19.34*	*17.00*	*31.05*		*19.82*	
Omphalocele	140	47	153	9	4	7	360	
	2.30	*2.82*	*2.10*	*1.99*	*12.42*		*2.31*	
Patent ductus arteriosus	2,481	667	3,643	169	13	7	6,980	
	40.77	*40.01*	*49.93*	*37.31*	*40.36*		*44.86*	
Pulmonary valve atresia	376	115	466	29	6	3	995	
and stenosis	*6.18*	*6.90*	*6.39*	*6.40*	*18.63*		*6.39*	
Pyloric stenosis	1,322	131	1,519	20	3	3	2,998	
	21.73	*7.86*	*20.82*	*4.42*	*9.31*		*19.27*	
Rectal and large intestinal	264	82	386	15	1	3	751	
atresia/stenosis	*4.34*	*4.92*	*5.29*	*3.31*	*3.10*		*4.83*	
Reduction deformity,	98	44	143	10	1	2	298	
lower limbs	*1.61*	*2.64*	*1.96*	*2.21*	*3.10*		*1.92*	
Reduction deformity,	230	67	329	16	2	2	646	
upper limbs	*3.78*	*4.02*	*4.51*	*3.53*	*6.21*		*4.15*	
Renal agenesis/hypoplasia	298	93	391	17	1	3	803	
	4.90	*5.58*	*5.36*	*3.75*	*3.10*		*5.16*	
Spina bifida without	215	49	343	7	2	6	622	
anencephalus	*3.53*	*2.94*	*4.70*	*1.55*	*6.21*		*4.00*	
Tetralogy of Fallot	185	54	226	18	0	0	483	
	3.04	*3.24*	*3.10*	*3.97*	*0.00*		*3.10*	
Transposition of great	316	58	357	24	3	1	759	
arteries	*5.19*	*3.48*	*4.89*	*5.30*	*9.31*		*4.88*	
Tricuspid valve atresia	144	49	187	16	1	1	398	
and stenosis	*2.37*	*2.94*	*2.56*	*3.53*	*3.10*		*2.56*	
Trisomy 13	66	25	87	9	0	4	191	
	1.08	*1.50*	*1.19*	*1.99*	*0.00*		*1.23*	
Trisomy 18	141	36	147	17	1	10	352	
	2.32	*2.16*	*2.01*	*3.75*	*3.10*		*2.26*	
Ventricular septal defect	2,316	500	3,614	127	8	11	6,576	
	38.06	*29.99*	*49.53*	*28.04*	*24.84*		*42.26*	
Total Live Births	**608,482**	**166,725**	**729,626**	**45,300**	**3,221**		**1,556,101**	

TRISOMY COUNTS AND RATES BY MATERNAL AGE 1997–2001
(Rates per 10,000 Live Births)

Defect	Age		
	<35	35 and >	Total*
Down syndrome	1,121	769	1,890
	8.02	*48.57*	*12.15*
Trisomy 13	133	58	191
	0.9	*366*	*1.23*
Trisomy 18	191	161	352
	1.37	*10.17*	*2.26*
Total Live Births	**1,397,553**	**158,315**	**1,556,101**

*Total includes unknown age.
Notes:
1. Data are provisional. They do not include possible/probable diagnoses. They do include cases from all pregnancy outcomes.

Utah

BIRTH DEFECTS COUNTS AND RATES 1997–2001

(Rates per 10,000 Live Births)

Defect	Non-Hispanic White	Non-Hispanic Black or African	Hispanic	Asian or Pacific Islander	American Indian or Alaskan Native	Other/ Unknown	Total	Notes
Amniotic bands	11	0	3	0	0	0	14	'91–'01 data
	0.95	*0.00*	*1.67*	*0.00*	*0.00*		*0.98*	
Anencephalus	40	0	9	0	1	4	54	
	2.11	*0.00*	*3.31*	*0.00*	*3.04*		*2.35*	
Aniridia	1	0	0	0	0	0	1	'99–'01 data
	0.09	*0.00*	*0.00*	*0.00*	*0.00*		*0.07*	
Anophthalmia/ microphthalmia	25	0	7	1	0	0	33	'99–'01 data
	2.16	*0.00*	*3.89*	*2.38*	*0.00*		*2.33*	
Anotia/microtia	44	0	4	3	3	1	52	'99–'01 data
	3.81	*0.00*	*2.22*	*7.13*	*15.15*		*3.68*	
Aortic valve stenosis	60	0	7	1	1	0	69	
	3.17	*0.00*	*2.58*	*1.50*	*3.04*		*3.00*	
Atrial septal defect	197	5	43	4	8	4	261	'99–'01 data
	17.06	*56.37*	*23.88*	*9.51*	*40.40*		*18.45*	
Biliary atresia	7	1	1	0	0	0	9	'99–'01 data
	0.61	*11.27*	*0.56*	*0.00*	*0.00*		*0.64*	
Bladder exstrophy	4	0	0	0	0	0	4	'99–'01 data
	0.35	*0.00*	*0.00*	*0.00*	*0.00*		*0.28*	
Choanal atresia	20	1	3	0	0	1	25	'99–'01 data
	1.73	*11.27*	*1.67*	*0.00*	*0.00*		*1.77*	
Cleft lip with and without cleft palate	268	1	44	7	6	6	332	Includes 4 NOS
	14.14	*7.19*	*16.19*	*10.47*	*18.26*		*14.46*	
Cleft palate without cleft lip	152	1	17	7	4	2	183	
	8.02	*7.19*	*6.26*	*10.47*	*20.00*		*7.97*	
Coarctation of aorta	168	0	15	1	0	2	186	
	8.86	*0.00*	*5.52*	*1.50*	*0.00*		*8.10*	
Common truncus	22	0	2	0	0	0	24	
	1.16	*0.00*	*0.74*	*0.00*	*0.00*		*1.05*	
Congenital cataract	25	1	3	0	0	0	29	'99–'01 data
	2.16	*11.27*	*1.67*	*0.00*	*0.00*		*2.05*	
Diaphragmatic hernia	34	1	8	0	0	2	45	'99–'01 data
	2.94	*11.27*	*4.44*	*0.00*	*0.00*		*3.18*	
Down syndrome	263	2	45	12	4	13	339	
	13.88	*14.38*	*16.56*	*17.95*	*12.17*		*14.76*	
Ebstein's anomaly	9	0	0	0	0	0	9	'99–'01 data
	0.78	*0.00*	*0.00*	*0.00*	*0.00*		*0.63*	
Encephalocele	17	0	16	1	0	1	94	
	0.90	*0.00*	*8.89*	*2.38*	*0.00*		*6.64*	
Endocardial cushion defect	74	0	18	3	2	2	127	'99–'01 data
	6.41	*0.00*	*10.00*	*7.13*	*10.10*		*8.98*	
Esophageal atresia/ tracheoesophageal fistula	29	0	7	1	2	0	39	'99–'01 data
	2.51	*0.00*	*3.89*	*2.38*	*10.10*		*2.75*	
Gastroschisis	70	3	13	3	2	2	93	Excludes those with limb body wall complex
	3.69	*21.54*	*4.78*	*4.49*	*6.09*		*4.05*	
Hirschsprung's disease (congenital megacolon)	21	1	5	2	0	0	29	'99–'01 data
	1.82	*11.27*	*2.78*	*4.76*	*0.00*		*2.05*	
Hydrocephalus without Spina Bifida	55	0	9	3	0	1	68	'99–'01 data
	4.76	*0.00*	*5.00*	*7.13*	*0.00*		*4.81*	
Hypoplastic left heart syndrome	63	0	11	2	0	6	82	
	3.32	*0.00*	*4.05*	*2.99*	*0.00*		*3.57*	
Hypospadias and Epispadias	359	2	21	10	3	4	399	'99–'01 data
	31.08	*22.55*	*11.66*	*23.78*	*15.15*		*28.20*	

(Table continues)

(Table continued)

Defect	Race/Ethnicity						Total	Notes
	Non-Hispanic White	Non-Hispanic Black or African	Hispanic	Asian or Pacific Islander	American Indian or Alaskan Native	Other/Unknown		
Microcephalus	27	0	5	0	0	1	33	'99–'01 data
	2.34	*0.00*	*2.78*	*0.00*	*0.00*		*2.33*	
Obstructive genitourinary defect	247	1	28	10	5	1	292	'99–'01 data
	21.39	*11.27*	*15.55*	*23.78*	*25.25*		*20.64*	
Omphalocele	46	0	8	3	0	1	58	
	2.43	*0.00*	*2.94*	*4.49*	*0.00*		*2.53*	
Pulmonary valve atresia and stenosis	128	1	18	2	1	1	151	'99–'01 data
	11.08	*7.19*	*6.62*	*4.76*	*3.04*		*10.67*	
Pyloric stenosis	155	0	28	1	0	2	186	'99–'01 data
	13.42	*0.00*	*15.55*	*2.38*	*0.00*		*13.15*	
Rectal and large intestinal atresia/stenosis	40	0	6	0	0	1	47	'99–'01 data
	3.46	*0.00*	*3.33*	*0.00*	*0.00*		*3.32*	
Reduction deformity, lower limbs	34	0	4	0	0	0	38	
	1.79	*0.00*	*1.47*	*0.00*	*0.00*		*1.65*	
Reduction deformity, upper limbs	110	0	18	2	1	8	139	
	5.80	*0.00*	*6.62*	*2.99*	*3.04*		*6.05*	
Renal agenesis/hypoplasia	43	0	2	2	1	1	49	'99–'01 data
	3.72	*0.00*	*1.11*	*4.76*	*5.05*		*3.46*	
Spina bifida without anencephalus	68	0	10	3	3	0	84	
	3.59	*0.00*	*3.68*	*4.49*	*9.13*		*3.66*	
Tetralogy of Fallot	71	1	7	2	0	2	82	
	3.75	*7.19*	*2.58*	*2.99*	*0.00*		*3.57*	
Transposition of great arteries	93	2	16	3	2	1	117	
	4.91	*14.38*	*5.89*	*4.49*	*6.09*		*5.10*	
Tricuspid valve atresia and stenosis	15	1	2	1	0	0	19	'99–'01 data
	1.30	*11.27*	*1.11*	*2.38*	*0.00*		*1.34*	
Trisomy 13	25	0	1	1	1	2	29	
	2.16	*0.00*	*0.37*	*1.50*	*3.04*		*1.26*	
Trisomy 18	62	0	9	4	0	3	78	
	3.27	*0.00*	*3.31*	*5.98*	*0.00*		*3.40*	
Total Live Births	**189,519**	**1,391**	**27,170**	**6,684**	**3,286**		**229,626**	

TRISOMY COUNTS AND RATES BY MATERNAL AGE 1997–2001
(Rates per 10,000 Live Births)

Defect	Age		Total*
	<35	35 and >	
Down syndrome	187	141	339
	8.95	*68.04*	*14.76*
Trisomy 13	24	3	29
	1.15	*1.45*	*1.26*
Trisomy 18	43	33	78
	2.06	*15.93*	*3.40*
Total Live Births	**208,856**	**20,722**	**229,626**

*Total includes unknown age.

Virginia

BIRTH DEFECTS COUNTS AND RATES 1997–2001

(Rates per 10,000 Live Births)

Defect	Non-Hispanic White	Non-Hispanic Black or African	Hispanic	Asian or Pacific Islander	American Indian or Alaskan Native	Other/Unknown	Total	Notes
Anencephalus	22	6	2	1	0	0	31	
	0.90	*0.70*	*0.80*	*0.58*	*0.00*		*0.83*	
Aniridia	2	0	0	0	0	0	2	
	0.08	*0.00*	*0.00*	*0.00*	*0.00*		*0.05*	
Anophthalmia/ microphthalmia	14	5	2	0	0	0	21	
	0.57	*0.58*	*0.80*	*0.00*	*0.00*		*0.56*	
Anotia/microtia	9	4	1	1	0	0	15	
	0.37	*0.46*	*0.40*	*0.58*	*0.00*		*0.40*	
Aortic valve stenosis	23	6	1	3	0	0	33	
	0.94	*0.70*	*0.40*	*1.73*	*0.00*		*0.88*	
Atrial septal defect	679	199	100	55	2	7	1,042	
	27.84	*23.09*	*39.90*	*31.63*	*31.70*		*27.77*	
Biliary atresia	9	4	1	2	0	0	16	
	0.37	*0.46*	*0.40*	*1.15*	*0.00*		*0.43*	
Bladder exstrophy	9	0	0	0	0	0	9	
	0.37	*0.00*	*0.00*	*0.00*	*0.00*		*0.24*	
Choanal atresia	26	8	2	0	0	0	36	
	1.07	*0.93*	*0.80*	*0.00*	*0.00*		*0.96*	
Cleft lip with and without cleft palate	220	42	24	12	0	0	298	
	9.02	*4.87*	*9.58*	*6.90*	*0.00*		*7.94*	
Cleft palate without cleft lip	100	29	6	7	0	1	143	
	4.10	*3.36*	*2.39*	*4.03*	*0.00*		*3.81*	
Coarctation of aorta	104	21	5	5	0	1	136	
	4.26	*2.44*	*2.00*	*2.88*	*0.00*		*3.62*	
Common truncus	18	5	1	1	0	0	25	
	0.74	*0.58*	*0.40*	*0.58*	*0.00*		*0.67*	
Congenital cataract	21	4	1	0	0	0	26	
	0.86	*0.46*	*0.40*	*0.00*	*0.00*		*0.69*	
Congenital hip dislocation	299	27	19	11	0	4	360	
	12.26	*3.13*	*7.58*	*6.33*	*0.00*		*9.59*	
Diaphragmatic hernia	59	14	6	7	0	1	87	
	2.42	*1.62*	*2.39*	*4.03*	*0.00*		*2.32*	
Down syndrome	219	57	31	13	1	1	322	
	8.98	*6.61*	*12.37*	*7.48*	*15.85*		*8.58*	
Ebstein's anomaly	9	0	0	1	0	0	10	
	0.37	*0.00*	*0.00*	*0.58*	*0.00*		*0.27*	
Encephalocele	5	8	0	0	0	0	13	
	0.20	*0.93*	*0.00*	*0.00*	*0.00*		*0.35*	
Endocardial cushion defect	49	12	4	0	0	2	67	
	2.01	*1.39*	*1.60*	*0.00*	*0.00*		*1.79*	
Esophageal atresia/ tracheoesophageal fistula	61	11	5	0	0	1	78	
	2.50	*1.28*	*2.00*	*0.00*	*0.00*		*2.08*	
Fetal alcohol syndrome	22	29	3	0	1	1	56	
	0.90	*3.36*	*1.20*	*0.00*	*15.85*		*1.49*	
Hirschsprung's disease (congenital megacolon)	34	22	4	0	0	0	60	
	1.39	*2.55*	*1.60*	*0.00*	*0.00*		*1.60*	
Hydrocephalus without Spina Bifida	85	58	14	3	0	0	160	
	3.48	*6.73*	*5.59*	*1.73*	*0.00*		*4.26*	
Hypoplastic left heart syndrome	42	9	0	1	0	0	52	
	1.72	*1.04*	*0.00*	*0.58*	*0.00*		*1.39*	
Hypospadias and Epispadias	313	110	17	6	2	1	449	
	12.83	*12.76*	*6.78*	*3.45*	*31.70*		*11.96*	

(Table continues)

(Table continued)

Defect	Race/Ethnicity							Notes
	Non-Hispanic White	Non-Hispanic Black or African	Hispanic	Asian or Pacific Islander	American Indian or Alaskan Native	Other/Unknown	Total	
Microcephalus	61	40	8.	6	0	0	115	
	2.50	*4.64*	*3.19*	*3.45*	*0.00*		*3.06*	
Obstructive genitourinary defect	144	52	10	8	0	1	215	
	5.90	*6.03*	*3.99*	*4.60*	*0.00*		*5.73*	
Patent ductus arteriosus	1,072	546	140	80	5	10	1,853	
	43.95	*63.34*	*55.87*	*46.00*	*79.24*		*49.38*	
Pulmonary valve atresia and stenosis	168	97	17	17	1	3	303	
	6.89	*11.25*	*6.78*	*9.78*	*15.85*		*8.07*	
Pyloric stenosis	238	31	10	7	1	2	289	
	9.76	*3.60*	*3.99*	*4.03*	*15.85*		*7.70*	
Rectal and large intestinal atresia/stenosis	88	32	5	7	0	0	132	
	3.61	*3.71*	*2.00*	*4.03*	*0.00*		*3.52*	
Reduction deformity, lower limbs	23	11	3	0	0	0	37	
	0.94	*1.28*	*1.20*	*0.00*	*0.00*		*0.99*	
Reduction deformity, upper limbs	43	14	2	0	0	0	59	
	1.76	*1.62*	*0.80*	*0.00*	*0.00*		*1.57*	
Renal agenesis/hypoplasia	81	23	9	3	0	0	116	
	3.32	*2.67*	*3.59*	*1.73*	*0.00*		*3.09*	
Spina bifida without anencephalus	95	25	14	3	0	0	137	
	3.89	*2.90*	*5.59*	*1.73*	*0.00*		*3.65*	
Tetralogy of Fallot	92	23	9	6	0	2	132	
	3.77	*2.67*	*3.59*	*3.45*	*0.00*		*3.52*	
Transposition of great arteries	78	12	8	0	0	0	98	
	3.20	*1.39*	*3.19*	*0.00*	*0.00*		*2.61*	
Tricuspid valve atresia and stenosis	13	13	0	2	0	2	30	
	0.53	*1.51*	*0.00*	*1.15*	*0.00*		*0.80*	
Trisomy 13	9	6	2	0	0	0	17	
	0.37	*0.70*	*0.80*	*0.00*	*0.00*		*0.45*	
Trisomy 18	22	7	1	0	0	0	30	
	0.90	*0.81*	*0.40*	*0.00*	*0.00*		*0.80*	
Ventricular septal defect	610	161	70	30	1	9	881	
	25.01	*18.68*	*27.93*	*77.25*	*15.85*		*23.48*	
Total Live Birth	243,925	86,203	25,060	17,390	631		375,277	

TRISOMY COUNTS AND RATES BY MATERNAL AGE 1997–2000
(Rates per 10,000 Live Births)

Defect	Age		
	<35	35 and >	Total*
Down syndrome	173	148	322
	5.43	*26.60*	*8.58*
Trisomy 13	14	3	17
	0.44	*0.54*	*0.45*
Trisomy 18	18	12	30
	0.56	*2.16*	*0.80*
Total Live Births	318,737	55,639	375,277

*Total includes unknown age.
Notes:
1. Only live births are included in the report.
2. Only children who were born to VA residents are included in the report.
3. Race is the mother's race reported on the birth certificate.
4. Data for 2000 may not be completed.
5. ICD9 codes were used to define birth defects.

West Virginia

BIRTH DEFECTS COUNTS AND RATES 1997–2001

(Rates per 10,000 Live Births)

Defect	Non-Hispanic White	Non-Hispanic Black or African	Hispanic	Asian or Pacific Islander	American Indian or Alaskan Native	Other/ Unknown	Total	Notes
Amniotic bands	0	0	0	0	0	0	0	
	0.00	*0.00*	*0.00*	*0.00*			*0.00*	
Anencephalus	5	0	1	0	0	0	6	
	0.51	*0.00*	*23.31*	*0.00*			*0.58*	
Aniridia	9	0	0	0	0	0	9	
	0.91	*0.00*	*0.00*	*0.00*			*0.87*	
Anophthalmia/ microphthalmia	10	0	0	0	0	0	10	
	1.02	*0.00*	*0.00*	*0.00*			*0.97*	
Anotia/microtia	7	0	0	0	0	1	8	
	0.71	*0.00*	*0.00*	*0.00*			*0.77*	
Aortic valve stenosis	16	1	0	0	0	0	17	
	1.62	*2.70*	*0.00*	*0.00*			*1.64*	
Atrial septal defect	459	16	0	0	0	10	485	
	46.61	*43.15*	*0.00*	*0.00*			*46.87*	
Biliary atresia	6	0	0	0	0	0	6	
	0.61	*0.00*	*0.00*	*0.00*			*0.58*	
Bladder exstrophy	2	0	0	0	0	0	2	
	0.20	*0.00*	*0.00*	*0.00*			*0.19*	
Choanal atresia	8	0	0	0	0	0	8	
	0.81	*0.00*	*0.00*	*0.00*			*0.77*	
Cleft lip with and without cleft palate	51	2	0	0	0		53	Provisional data
	5.18	*5.39*	*0.00*	*0.00*			*5.12*	
Cleft palate without cleft lip	40	0	0	0	0	1	41	Provisional data
	4.06	*0.00*	*0.00*	*0.00*			*3.96*	
Coarctation of aorta	48	3	0	0	0	0	51	
	4.87	*8.09*	*0.00*	*0.00*			*4.93*	
Common truncus	8	0	0	0	0	0	8	
	0.81	*0.00*	*0.00*	*0.00*			*0.77*	
Congenital cataract	10	0	0	0	0	0	10	
	1.02	*0.00*	*0.00*	*0.00*			*0.97*	
Congenital hip dislocation	31	0	0	0	0	0	31	
	3.15	*0.00*	*0.00*	*0.00*			*3.00*	
Diaphragmatic hernia	15	1	0	0	0	0	16	
	1.52	*2.70*	*0.00*	*0.00*			*1.55*	
Down syndrome	63	5	0	0	0	3	71	
	6.40	*13.48*	*0.00*	*0.00*			*6.86*	
Ebstein's anomaly	7	0	0	0	0	0	7	
	0.71	*0.00*	*0.00*	*0.00*			*0.68*	
Encephalocele	1	0	0	0	0	0	1	
	0.10	*0.00*	*0.00*	*0.00*			*0.10*	
Endocardial cushion defect	31	4	0	0	0	0	35	
	3.15	*10.79*	*0.00*	*0.00*			*3.38*	
Esophageal atresia/ tracheoesophageal fistula	13	1	0	0	0	0	14	
	1.32	*2.70*	*0.00*	*0.00*			*1.35*	
Fetus or newborn affected by maternal alcohol use	40	5	0	0	0	1	46	
	4.06	*13.48*	*0.00*	*0.00*			*4.45*	
Gastroschisis	15	0	0	0	0	0	15	
	1.52	*0.00*	*0.00*	*0.00*			*1.45*	
Hirschsprung's disease (congenital megacolon)	11	0	0	0	0	0	11	
	1.12	*0.00*	*0.00*	*0.00*			*1.06*	
Hydrocephalus without Spina Bifida	41	0	0	0	0	1	42	
	4.16	*0.00*	*0.00*	*0.00*			*4.06*	

(Table continues)

(Table continued)

Defect	Race/Ethnicity						Total	Notes
	Non-Hispanic White	Non-Hispanic Black or African	Hispanic	Asian or Pacific Islander	American Indian or Alaskan Native	Other/ Unknown		
Hypoplastic left heart syndrome	25	3	0	0	0	0	28	
	2.54	*8.09*	*0.00*	*0.00*			*2.71*	
Hypospadias and Epispadias	123	5	0	0	0	3	131	
	12.49	*13.48*	*0.00*	*0.00*			*12.66*	
Microcephalus	42	2	0	0	0	1	45	
	4.27	*5.39*	*0.00*	*0.00*			*4.35*	
Obstructive genitourinary defect	93	2	0	0	0	1	96	
	9.44	*5.39*	*0.00*	*0.00*			*9.28*	
Omphalocele	0	0	0	0	0	0	0	
	0.00	*0.00*	*0.00*	*0.00*			*0.00*	
Patent ductus arteriosus	458	11	0	0	0	7	476	
	46.51	*29.67*	*0.00*	*0.00*			*46.00*	
Pulmonary valve atresia and stenosis	83	1	0	0	0	1	85	
	8.43	*2.70*	*0.00*	*0.00*			*8.21*	
Pyloric stenosis	29	1	0	0	0	2	32	
	2.94	*2.70*	*0.00*	*0.00*			*3.09*	
Rectal and large intestinal atresia/stenosis	21	0	0	0	0	0	21	
	2.13	*0.00*	*0.00*	*0.00*	*0.00*		*2.03*	
Reduction deformity, lower limbs	10	1	0	0	0	0	11	
	1.02	*2.70*	*0.00*	*0.00*			*1.06*	
Reduction deformity, upper limbs	10	0	0	0	0	0	10	
	1.02	*0.00*	*0.00*	*0.00*			*0.97*	
Renal agenesis/hypoplasia	16	1	0	0	0	0	17	
	1.62	*2.70*	*0.00*	*0.00*			*1.64*	
Spina bifida without anencephalus	14	0	0	2	0	0	16	
	1.42	*0.00*	*0.00*	*33.50*			*1.55*	
Tetralogy of Fallot	33	2	0	0	0	1	36	
	3.35	*5.39*	*0.00*	*0.00*			*3.48*	
Transposition of great arteries	37	1	0	0	0	0	38	
	3.76	*2.70*	*0.00*	*0.00*			*3.67*	
Tricuspid valve atresia and stenosis	11	0	0	0	0	0	11	
	1.12	*0.00*	*0.00*	*0.00*			*1.06*	
Trisomy 13	3	0	0	0	0	0	3	
	0.30	*0.00*	*0.00*	*0.00*			*0.29*	
Trisomy 18	5	0	0	0	0	0	5	
	0.51	*0.00*	*0.00*	*0.00*			*0.48*	
Ventricular septal defect	202	8	0	0	0	7	217	
	20.51	*21.57*	*0.00*	*0.00*			*20.97*	
Total Live Births	**3,708**	**429**	**597**	**0**			**103,485**	

TRISOMY COUNTS AND RATES BY MATERNAL AGE 1997–2001
(Rates per 10,000 Live Births)

Defect	Age		Total*
	<35	35 and >	
Down syndrome	48	20	71
	5.07	*23.99*	*6.86*
Trisomy 13	2	1	3
	0.21	*1.20*	*0.29*
Trisomy 18	4	1	5
	0.42	*1.20*	*0.48*
Total Live Births	**94,688**	**8,338**	**103,485**

*Total includes unknown age.

Wisconsin

BIRTH DEFECTS COUNTS AND RATES 1997–2001

(Rates per 10,000 Live Births)

Defect	Non-Hispanic White	Non-Hispanic Black or African	Hispanic	Asian or Pacific Islander	American Indian or Alaskan Native	Other/ Unknown	Total	Notes
Anencephalus	39	2	5	2	1	0	49	includes stillbirths
	1.42	*0.62*	*2.43*	*1.95*	*2.29*		*1.43*	
Aniridia	0	1	0	0	0	0	1	
	0.00	*0.31*	*0.00*	*0.00*	*0.00*		*0.02*	
Anophthalmia/ microphthalmia	10	0	1	0	0	0	11	
	0.36	*0.00*	*0.48*	*0.00*	*0.00*		*0.32*	
Anotia/microtia	7	0	2	0	0	0	9	
	0.25	*0.00*	*0.97*	*0.00*	*0.00*		*0.26*	
Aortic valve stenosis	16	0	0	0	2	0	18	
	0.58	*0.00*	*0.00*	*0.00*	*4.58*		*0.52*	
Atrial septal defect	609	60	28	17	17	0	731	
	22.30	*18.63*	*13.65*	*16.63*	*38.98*		*21.47*	
Biliary atresia	2	0	0	0	0	0	2	
	0.07	*0.00*	*0.00*	*0.00*	*0.00*		*0.05*	
Bladder exstrophy	17	1	0	0	0	0	18	
	0.62	*0.31*	*0.00*	*0.00*	*0.00*		*0.52*	
Choanal atresia	41	2	5	1	1	0	50	
	1.50	*0.62*	*2.43*	*0.97*	*2.29*		*1.46*	
Cleft lip with and without cleft palate	245	10	12	8	5	0	280	
	8.97	*3.10*	*5.85*	*7.82*	*11.46*		*8.22*	
Cleft palate without cleft lip	171	7	9	12	4	0	203	
	6.26	*2.17*	*4.38*	*11.73*	*9.17*		*5.96*	
Coarctation of aorta	37	3	1	0	0	0	41	
	1.35	*0.93*	*0.48*	*0.00*	*0.00*		*1.20*	
Common truncus	6	2	2	0	0	0	10	
	0.21	*0.62*	*0.97*	*0.00*	*0.00*		*0.29*	
Congenital cataract	28	3	2	1	1	0	35	
	1.02	*0.93*	*0.97*	*0.97*	*2.29*		*1.02*	
Congenital hip dislocation	328	18	19	11	7	0	383	
	12.01	*5.59*	*9.26*	*10.76*	*16.05*		*11.25*	
Diaphragmatic hernia	63	7	3	1	1	0	75	
	2.30	*2.17*	*1.46*	*0.97*	*2.29*		*2.20*	
Down syndrome	264	22	34	14	3	0	337	
	9.67	*6.83*	*16.58*	*13.69*	*6.87*		*9.90*	
Ebstein's anomaly	6	2	1	0	0	0	9	
	0.21	*0.62*	*0.48*	*0.00*	*0.00*		*0.26*	
Encephalocele	15	0	4	1	1	0	21	
	0.54	*0.00*	*1.95*	*0.97*	*2.29*		*0.61*	
Endocardial cushion defect	47	1	1	0	0	0	49	
	1.72	*0.31*	*0.48*	*0.00*	*0.00*		*1.43*	
Esophageal atresia/ tracheoesophageal fistula	46	2	4	1	2	0	55	
	1.68	*0.62*	*1.95*	*0.97*	*4.58*		*1.61*	
Fetus or newborn affected by maternal alcohol use	25	32	1	0	8	0	66	
	0.91	*9.93*	*0.48*	*0.00*	*18.34*		*1.93*	
Gastroschisis	106	18	11	5	1	0	141	
	3.88	*5.59*	*5.36*	*4.89*	*2.29*		*4.14*	
Hirschsprung's disease (congenital megacolon)	13	5	0	0	0	0	18	
	0.47	*1.55*	*0.00*	*0.00*	*0.00*		*0.52*	
Hydrocephalus without Spina Bifida	84	26	11	2	1	0	124	
	3.07	*8.07*	*5.36*	*1.95*	*2.29*		*3.64*	
Hypoplastic left heart syndrome	37	5	0	0	2	0	44	
	1.35	*1.55*	*0.00*	*0.00*	*4.58*		*1.29*	

(Table continues)

(Table continued)

Defect	Race/Ethnicity							
	Non-Hispanic White	Non-Hispanic Black or African	Hispanic	Asian or Pacific Islander	American Indian or Alaskan Native	Other/Unknown	Total	Notes
Hypospadias and Epispadias	920	94	40	12	14	0	1,080	
	33.69	*29.19*	*19.50*	*11.73*	*32.10*		*31.73*	
Microcephalus	35	16	4	3	0	0	58	
	1.28	*4.96*	*1.95*	*2.93*	*0.00*		*1.70*	
Obstructive genitourinary defect	344	39	24	12	3	0	422	
	12.60	*12.11*	*11.70*	*11.73*	*6.87*		*12.39*	
Patent ductus arteriosus	658	46	42	20	15	0	781	Excl bthwt
	24.10	*14.28*	*20.48*	*19.56*	*34.39*		*22.94*	
Pulmonary valve atresia and stenosis	119	43	16	1	4	0	183	
	4.35	*13.35*	*7.80*	*0.97*	*9.17*		*5.37*	
Pyloric stenosis	4	0	0	0	0	0	4	
	0.14	*0.00*	*0.00*	*0.00*	*0.00*		*0.11*	
Rectal and large intestinal atresia/stenosis	93	15	5	8	1	0	122	
	3.40	*4.65*	*2.43*	*7.82*	*2.29*		*3.58*	
Reduction deformity, lower limbs	42	3	1	1	1	0	48	
	1.53	*0.93*	*0.48*	*0.97*	*2.29*		*1.41*	
Reduction deformity, upper limbs	72	7	2	3	2	0	86	
	2.63	*2.17*	*0.97*	*2.93*	*4.58*		*2.52*	
Renal agenesis/hypoplasia	77	7	5	1	3	0	93	
	2.82	*2.17*	*2.43*	*0.97*	*6.87*		*2.73*	
Spina bifida without anencephalus	77	12	9	0	0	0	98	Includes stillbirths
	2.82	*3.72*	*4.38*	*0.00*	*0.00*		*2.87*	
Tetralogy of Fallot	40	5	5	5	0	0	55	
	1.46	*1.55*	*2.43*	*4.89*	*0.00*		*1.61*	
Transposition of great arteries	48	5	2	0	0	0	55	
	1.75	*1.55*	*0.97*	*0.00*	*0.00*		*1.61*	
Tricuspid valve atresia and stenosis	9	3	0	0	1	0	13	
	0.32	*0.93*	*0.00*	*0.00*	*2.29*		*0.38*	
Trisomy 13	17	3	1	1	1	0	23	
	0.62	*0.93*	*0.48*	*0.97*	*2.29*		*0.67*	
Trisomy 18	27	4	2	2	0	0	35	
	0.98	*1.24*	*0.97*	*1.95*	*0.00*		*1.02*	
Ventricular septal defect	554	47	48	27	14	0	690	
	20.29	*14.59*	*23.41*	*26.41*	*32.10*		*20.27*	
Total Live Births	**273,000**	**32,194**	**20,504**	**10,222**	**4,361**		**340,351**	

TRISOMY COUNTS AND RATES BY MATERNAL AGE 1997–2001
(Rates per 10,000 Live Births)

Defect	Age		
	<35	35 and >	Total*
Down syndrome	187	150	337
	6.32	*33.91*	*9.90*
Trisomy 13	18	5	23
	0.61	*1.13*	*0.68*
Trisomy 18	19	16	35
	0.64	*3.62*	*1.03*
Total Live Births	**296,096**	**44,232**	**340,351**

Department of Defense

BIRTH DEFECTS COUNTS AND RATES 1998–2001

(Rates per 10,000 Live Births)

Defect	Non-Hispanic White	Non-Hispanic Black or African	Hispanic	Asian or Pacific Islander	American Indian or Alaskan Native	Other/ Unknown	Total	Notes
			Race/Ethnicity					
Anencephalus	42	12	3	3		3	63	
	1.69	*1.76*	*0.97*	*2.46*			*1.66*	
Aniridia	12	1	0	0		0	13	
	0.48	*0.15*	*0.00*	*0.00*			*0.34*	
Anophthalmia/ microphthalmia	76	14	7	1		4	102	
	3.06	*2.06*	*2.26*	*0.82*			*2.68*	
Anotia/microtia	48	6	13	4		5	76	
	1.93	*0.88*	*4.20*	*3.28*			*2.00*	
Aortic valve stenosis	126	14	12	3		9	164	
	5.08	*2.06*	*3.88*	*2.46*			*4.31*	
Atrial septal defect	2,458	782	320	106		193	3,859	
	99.06	*114.89*	*103.34*	*87.00*			*101.50*	
Biliary atresia	42	8	2	3		6	61	
	1.69	*1.18*	*0.65*	*2.46*			*1.60*	
Bladder exstrophy	6	2	1	0		1	10	
	0.24	*0.29*	*0.32*	*0.00*			*0.26*	
Choanal atresia	82	30	8	1		4	125	
	3.30	*4.41*	*2.58*	*0.82*			*3.29*	
Cleft lip with and without cleft palate	363	55	43	21		19	501	
	14.63	*8.08*	*13.89*	*17.24*			*13.18*	
Cleft palate without cleft lip	358	66	37	19		18	498	
	14.43	*9.70*	*11.95*	*15.59*			*13.10*	
Coarctation of aorta	228	38	33	8		16	323	
	9.19	*5.58*	*10.66*	*6.57*			*8.50*	
Common truncus	68	14	8	5		5	100	
	2.74	*2.06*	*2.58*	*4.10*			*2.63*	
Congenital cataract	97	44	14	4		4	163	
	3.91	*6.46*	*4.52*	*3.28*			*4.29*	
Congenital hip dislocation	1,103	156	108	50		85	1,502	
	44.45	*22.92*	*34.88*	*41.04*			*39.51*	
Diaphragmatic hernia	118	38	14	3		6	179	
	4.76	*5.58*	*4.52*	*2.46*			*4.71*	
Down syndrome	393	89	46	24		37	589	
	15.84	*13.08*	*14.86*	*19.70*			*15.49*	
Ebstein's anomaly	62	2	4	3		3	74	
	2.50	*0.29*	*1.29*	*2.46*			*1.95*	
Encephalocele	49	20	10	2		7	88	
	1.97	*2,94*	*3.23*	*1.64*			*2.31*	
Endocardial cushion defect	183	39	15	5		11	253	
	7.37	*5.73*	*4.84*	*4.10*			*6.65*	
Esophageal atresia/ tracheoesophageal fistula	95	20	12	3		3	133	
	3.83	*2.94*	*3.88*	*2.46*			*3.50*	
Fetus or newborn affected by maternal alcohol use	15	4	0	0		3	22	
	0.60	*0.59*	*0.00*	*0.00*			*0.58*	
Gastroschisis	248	90	35	15		14	402	
	9.99	*13.22*	*11.30*	*12.31*			*10.57*	
Hirschsprung's disease (congenital megacolon)	145	62	19	7		11	244	
	5.84	*9.11*	*6.14*	*5.75*			*6.42*	
Hydrocephalus without Spina Bifida	391	121	48	13		25	598	
	15.76	*17.78*	*15.50*	*10.67*			*15.73*	
Hypoplastic left heart syndrome	98	34	14	6		7	159	
	3.95	*5.00*	*4.52*	*4.92*			*4.18*	

(Table continues)

(Table continued)

Defect	Race/Ethnicity							Notes
	Non-Hispanic White	Non-Hispanic Black or African	Hispanic	Asian or Pacific Islander	American Indian or Alaskan Native	Other/Unknown	Total	
Hypospadias and	1,435	326	115	50		93	2,019	
Epispadias	*57.83*	*47.89*	*37.14*	*41.04*			*53.10*	
Microcephalus	360	110	51	15		23	559	
	14.51	*16.16*	*16.47*	*12.31*			*14.70*	
Obstructive genitourinary	854	175	99	37		57	1,222	
defect	*34.42*	*25.71*	*31.97*	*30.37*			*32.14*	
Pulmonary valve atresia	602	266	77	37		44	1,026	
and stenosis	*24.26*	*39.08*	*24.87*	*30.37*			*26.99*	
Pyloric stenosis	864	120	90	9		52	1,135	
	34.82	*17.63*	*29.07*	*7.39*			*29.85*	
Rectal and large intestinal	188	49	17	6		12	272	
atresia/stenosis	*7.58*	*7.20*	*5.49*	*4.92*			*7.15*	
Reduction deformity,	90	34	12	6		8	150	
lower limbs	*3.63*	*5.00*	*3.88*	*4.92*			*3.95*	
Reduction deformity, upper limbs	83	23	9	4		4	123	
	3.34	*3.38*	*2.91*	*3.28*			*3.24*	
Renal agenesis/hypoplasia	138	39	16	6		9	208	
	5.56	*5.73*	*5.17*	*4.92*			*5.47*	
Spina bifida without	200	27	28	6		15	276	
anencephalus	*8.06*	*3.97*	*9.04*	*4.92*			*7.26*	
Tetralogy of Fallot	209	61	15	7		9	301	
	8.42	*8.96*	*4.84*	*5.75*			*7.92*	
Transposition of great	165	27	14	9		14	229	
arteries	*6.65*	*3.97*	*4.52*	*7.39*			*6.02*	
Tricuspid valve atresia	53	14	4	3		4	78	
and stenosis	*2.14*	*2.06*	*1.29*	*2.46*			*2.05*	
Trisomy 13	25	14	4	3		2	48	
	1.01	*2.06*	*1.29*	*2.46*			*1.26*	
Trisomy 18	59	16	9	6		2	92	
	2.38	*2.35*	*2.91*	*4.92*			*2.42*	
Ventricular septal defect	1,953	478	244	69		114	2,858	
	78.71	*70.22*	*78.80*	*56.63*			*75.17*	
Total Live Births	248,136	68,068	30,965	12,184			380,201	

TRISOMY COUNTS AND RATES BY MATERNAL AGE 1998–2001
(Rates per 10,000 Live Births)

Defect	Age		
	<35	35 and >	Total*
Down syndrome	378	159	589
	11.63	*54.15*	*15.49*
Trisomy 13	33	10	48
	1.02	*3.41*	*1.26*
Trisomy 18	61	17	92
	1.88	*5.79*	*2.42*
Total Live Births	324,932	29,362	380,201

*Total includes unknown age.
Notes:
1. DoD Registry data unable to distinguish "American Indian or Alaskan Native" race/ethnicity category.

APPENDIX IV
STATE AGENCIES AND BIRTH DEFECT SURVEILLANCE PROGRAMS

Alabama

Alabama Birth Defects Surveillance and Prevention Program (ABDSPP)
CCCB, Room 214
307 University Boulevard
Mobile, AL 36688
(251) 460-7505
(251) 461-1591 (fax)
http://www.usouthal.edu/genetics

Alaska

Alaska Birth Defects Registry (ABDR)
MCH Epidemiology Unit; Section of Epidemiology
3601 C Street
Suite 934
P.O. Box 240249
Anchorage, AK 99524-0249
(907) 269-3442
(907) 269-3493
http://www.akepi.org/mchepi/ABDR

Arizona

Arizona Birth Defects Monitoring Program (ABDMP)
Arizona Department of Health Services
150 North 18th Avenue
Suite 550
Phoenix, AZ 85007
(602) 542-7331
(602) 364-0082 (fax)
http://www.hs.state.az.us/phs/phstats/bdr/index.htm

Arkansas

Arkansas Reproductive Health Monitoring System (ARHMS)
Arkansas Center for Birth Defects and Research Prevention
11219 Financial Center Parkway
Financial Park Place
Suite 250
Little Rock, AR 72211
(501) 364-8951
(501) 364-5107
http://www.ARbirthdefectsresearch.uams.edu

California

California Birth Defects Monitoring Program (CBDMP)
1917 Fifth Street
Berkeley, CA 94710-1916
(209) 384-8388
(510) 549-4175 (fax)
http://www.cbdmp.org

Colorado

Colorado Responds to Children with Special Needs: Colorado (CRCSN)
4300 Cherry Creek Drive
Denver, CO 80246-1530
(303) 692-2636
(303) 782-0904 (fax)
http://www.cdphe.state.co.us/dc/crcsn/crcsnhome.asp

Connecticut

Connecticut Birth Defects Registry (CTBDR)
Family Health Division
410 Capitol Avenue, MS #11FHD
Hartford, CT 06134
(860) 509-8066
(860) 509-7720

Delaware

Delaware Birth Defects Surveillance Project
DE Division of Public Health
P.O. Box 637
Dover, DE 19903
(302) 744-4554
(302) 739-6653 (fax)

District of Columbia

District of Columbia Birth Defects Surveillance
and Prevention Program (DC BDSPP)
DC Department of Health, Maternal and
Family Health Administration
825 N. Capitol Street NE, Room 3181
· Washington, DC 20002
(202) 442-9343
(202) 442-4828 (fax)

Florida

Florida Birth Defects Registry (FBDR)
Florida Department of Health
4052 Bald Cypress Way, Bin A08
Tallahassee, FL 32399-1712
(850) 245-4444, ext. 2198
(850) 922-8473 (fax)
http://flbdr.hsc.usf.edu

Georgia

Centers for Disease Control and Prevention,
Metropolitan Atlanta Congenital Defects
Program (MACDP)
Centers for Disease Control and Prevention
1600 Clifton Road, MS E-86
Atlanta, GA 30333
(404) 498-3808

(404) 498-3040 (fax)
http://www.cdc.gov/ncbddd/bd

Georgia Birth Defects Reporting and
Information System (GBDRIS)
GA Division of Public Health, MCH
Epidemiology Section
2 Peachtree Street NW
Suite 14-04
Atlanta, GA 30303
(404) 651-5131
(404) 657-7517
http://health.state.ga.us/epi/mch/publications.
shtml

Hawaii

Hawaii Birth Defects Program (HBDP)
76 North King Street, #208
Honolulu, HI 96817-5157
(808) 587-4120
(808) 587-4130 (fax)
http://www.members.aol.com/entropynot/hbdp.
html

Idaho

Idaho Bureau of Clinical and Preventive
Services
450 W. State Street
Boise, ID 83720
(208) 334-0670
(208) 332-7307
http://www.healthandwelfare.idaho.gov/
site/3367/default.aspx

Illinois

Adverse Pregnancy Outcomes Reporting
System (APORS)
Illinois Department of Public Health
605 W. Jefferson Street
Springfield, IL 62761
(217) 785-7133
(217) 557-5152 (fax)
http://www.idph.state.il.us/about/epi/aporsrpt.
htm

Indiana

Indiana Birth Defects and Problems Registry (IBDPR)
Indiana State Department of Health
2 North Meridian Street
Indianapolis, IN 46204
(317) 233-7827
(317) 233-1300 (fax)
http://www.in.gov/isdh/programs/idbpr

Iowa

Iowa Birth Defects Registry (IBDR)
University of Iowa, C21-E GH
200 Hawkins Drive
Iowa City, IA 52242
(319) 384-5012
(319) 353-8711 (fax)
http://www.public-health.uiowa.edu/birthdefects

Kansas

Birth Defects Reporting System
Kansas Department of Health and Environment
1000 SW Jackson
Suite 220
Topeka, KS 66612-1274
(785) 291-3363
(785) 291-3493

Kentucky

Kentucky Birth Surveillance Registry (KBSR)
Kentucky Department for Public Health
275 East Main Street, HS 2GW-A
Frankfort, KY 40621
(502) 564-2154
(502) 564-8389 (fax)
http://publichealth.state.ky.us/kbsr.htm

Louisiana

Louisiana Birth Defects Monitoring Network (LBDMN)
DHH/Office of Public Health
325 Loyola Avenue
Suite 607
New Orleans, LA 70112

(504) 568-5055
(504) 568-7529 (fax)
http://oph.dhh.state.la.us/childrensspecial/
birthdefect/index.html

Maine

Maine Birth Defects Program (MBDP)
Maine Bureau of Health
11 State House Station
286 Water Street, 7th Floor
Augusta, ME 04333
(207) 287-4623
(207) 287-4743

Maryland

Maryland Birth Defects Reporting and Information System (BDRIS)
Maryland Department of Health and Mental Hygiene
201 W. Preston Street, Room 421A
Baltimore, MD 21201
(410) 767-6730
(410) 333-5047 (fax)
http://fha.state.md.us/genetics

Massachusetts

Massachusetts Center for Birth Defects Research and Prevention, Birth Defect Monitoring Program (MCBDRP)
Massachusetts Department of Public Health
250 Washington Street, 5th Floor
Boston, MA 02108-4619
(617) 624-5507
(617) 624-5574 (fax)

Michigan

Michigan Birth Defects Registry (MBDR)
3423 N. Logan
Lansing, MI 48909
(517) 335-8677
(517) 335-9513 (fax)
http://www.michigan.gov/mdch/0,1607,7-132-
2944_4670-,00.html

Minnesota

Minnesota Department of Health
121 E 7th Place
Suite 220
St. Paul, MN 55164
(651) 215-0877
(651) 215-0975 (fax)
http://www.health.state.mn.us

Mississippi

Mississippi Birth Defects Registry (MBDR)
Mississippi State Department of Health
P.O. Box 1700
Jackson, MS 39215-1700
(601) 576-7619
(601) 576-7498 (fax)

Missouri

Missouri Birth Defects Registry
Missouri Department of Health, Health Data
** Analysis**
P.O. Box 570, 920 Wildwood
Jefferson City, MO 65102
(573) 751-6278
(573) 526-4102

Montana

Montana Birth Outcomes Monitoring System
** (MBOMS)**
FCHB/DPHHS
P.O. Box 202951
Helena, MT 59620-2951
(406) 444-4119
(406) 444-2606 (fax)

Nebraska

Nebraska Birth Defects Registry
Nebraska Health and Human Services System
301 Centennial Mall South
P.O. Box 95007
Lincoln, NE 68509-5007

(402) 471-3575
(402) 471-9728 (fax)

Nevada

Nevada Birth Defects Registry
Bureau of Family Health Services—State
** Health Division**
3427 Goni Road
Suite 108
Carson City, NV 89706
(775) 684-4285
(775) 684-4245 (fax)

New Hampshire

New Hampshire Birth Conditions Program
** (NHBCP)**
Division of Genetics and Child Development
Department of Pediatrics
Dartmouth Hitchcock Medical Center
1 Medical Center Drive
Lebanon, NH 03756
(603) 653-6053
(603) 650-8268 (fax)

New Jersey

Special Child Health Services Registry (SCHS
** REGISTRY)**
New Jersey Department of Health and
** Senior Services**
P.O. Box 364
Trenton, NJ 08625-0364
(609) 292-5676
(609) 633-7820 (fax)
http://www.state.nj.us/health/fhs/scregis.htm

New Mexico

New Mexico Birth Defects Prevention and
** Surveillance System (NM BDPASS)**
New Mexico Department of Human Health
2040 S. Pacheco
Santa Fe, NM 87505
(505) 476-8889
(505) 476-8898 (fax)
http://www.health.state.nm.us

New York

**New York State Congenital Malformations
    Registry (CMR)**
New York Department of Health
Flanigan Square, Room 200
547 River Street
Troy, NY 12180
(518) 402-7990
(518) 402-7959 (fax)
http://www.health.state.ny.us/nysdoh/cmr/
    cmrhome.htm

North Carolina

**North Carolina Birth Defects Monitoring
    Program (NCBDMP)**
North Carolina Center for Health Statistics
1908 Mail Service Center
Raleigh, NC 27699-1908
(919) 715-4476
(919) 733-8485
http://www.schs.state.nc.us.SCHS

North Dakota

**North Dakota Birth Defects Monitoring
    System (NDBDMS)**
**Children's Special Health Services Division
    ND**
Department of Human Services
600 East Boulevard Avenue, Department 301
Bismarck, ND 58505-0200
(701) 328-4963
(701) 328-1412 (fax)
http://www.health.state.nd.us/ndhd/admin/vital/

Ohio

**Ohio Connection for Children with Special
    Needs (OCCSN)**
Ohio Department of Health
246 N. High Street
Columbus, OH 43216-0118
(614) 466-1663
(614) 728-9163

Oklahoma

Oklahoma Birth Defects Registry (OBDR)
**Oklahoma State Screening Department of
    Health, Screening**
Special Services, and SoonerStart
1000 NE 10th Street, Room 710
Oklahoma City, OK 73117-1299
(405) 271-9444
(405) 271-4892 (fax)

Pennsylvania

**Pennsylvania Follow-Up, Outreach, Referral,
    and Education for Families (PA FORE
    FAMILIES)**
Pennsylvania Department of Health
P.O. Box 90, 7th Floor, East Wing, Health and
    Welfare Building
Harrisburg, PA 17108
(717) 783-8143
(717) 772-0323 (fax)

Puerto Rico

**Puerto Rico Folic Acid Campaign and
    Birth Defects Surveillance System
    (PRFAC/BDSS)**
Puerto Rico Department of Health
P.O. Box 70814
San Juan, PR 00936
(787) 751-3654
(787) 764-4259 (fax)
http://www.salud.gov.pr/AF/Afindex.htm

Rhode Island

**Rhode Island Birth Defects Surveillance
    Program**
Rhode Island Department of Health
3 Capitol Hill, Room 302
Providence, RI 02908-5097
(401) 222-5935
(401) 222-1442

South Carolina

**South Carolina Birth Defects Surveillance
    and Prevention Program**
Greenwood Genetic Center
1 Gregor Mendel Circle
Greenwood, SC 29646
(864) 941-8146
(864) 388-1707
http://www.ggc.org

South Dakota

Sioux Valley Children's Specialty Clinic
1305 W 18th Street
Sioux Falls, SD 57117
(605) 333-4298
(605) 333-1585

Tennessee

Tennessee Birth Defects Registry (TBDR)
Tennessee Department of Health—PPA
425 Fifth Avenue, North, 4th Floor
Nashville, TN 37247
(615) 253-4702
(615) 253-1688 (fax)

Texas

**Texas Birth Defects Monitoring Division
    (TBDMD)**
1100 West 49th Street
Austin, TX 78756-3180
(512) 458-7232
(512) 458-7330 (fax)
http://www.tdh.state.tx.us/tbdmd/index.htm

U.S. Department of Defense

**United States Department of Defense (DoD)
    Birth and Infant Health Registry**
**DoD Department for Deployment Health
    Research, Code 25, Naval Research
    Center**
P.O. Box 85122

San Diego, CA 92186-5122
(619) 553-8097
(619) 553-7601 (fax)
http://www.nhrc.navy.mil/rsch/code25/projects/
    birthdefects.htm

Utah

Utah Birth Defects Network (UBDN)
44 North Medical Drive
P.O. Box 144697
Salt Lake City, UT 84114-4697
http://www.health.utah.gov/birthdefect

Vermont

Birth Information Network
Vermont Department of Health
P.O. Box 70
108 Cherry Street
Burlington, VT 05402
(802) 863-7298
(802) 865-7701

Virginia

**Virginia Congenital Anomalies Reporting
    and Education System (VACARES)**
Virginia Department of Health
109 Governor Street, 8th Floor
Richmond, VA 23219
(804) 864-7712
(804) 864-7721 (fax)
http://www.vahealth.org/genetics

Washington

**Washington State Birth Defects Surveillance
    System (BDSS)**
Washington Department of Health
Maternal and Child Health
P.O. Box 47835
Olympia, WA 98504-7835
(360) 236-3553
(360) 236-2323 (fax)

West Virginia

**West Virginia Congenital Abnormalities
    Registry, Education, and Surveillance
    System (WVCARESS)**
OMCFH
350 Capitol Street
Charleston, WV 25301
(304) 558-71717
(304) 558-3510 (fax)
http://www.wvdhhr.org

Wisconsin

Wisconsin Birth Defects Registry (WBDR)
Division of Public Health
Department of Health and Family Services
1 West Wilson

P.O. Box 2659
Madison, WI 53701
(608) 261-9304
(608) 267-3824
http://www.dhfs.state.wi.us/dph_bfch/cshcn
http://www.wbdr.han.wisc.edu

Wyoming

**Wyoming Department of Health,
    Community, and Family**
Health Division
4020 House Avenue
Cheyenne, WY 82002
(307) 777-5413
(307) 777-7215 (fax)

APPENDIX V
RESOURCES

A

AARSKOG SYNDROME
Aarskog Syndrome Support Group
62 Robin Hill Lane
Levittown, PA 19055-1411
(215) 943-7131
shannonfaith49@msn.com

Dagfinn Aarskog, M.D.
Department of Pediatrics
N-5021 Bergen
Newline, Norway

ABETALIPOTPROTEINEMIA
See TAY-SACHS DISEASE

ABORTION
Center for Reproductive Law and Policy
1146 19th Street NW
Washington, D.C. 20036
(202) 530-2975
http://www.crlp.org

Planned Parenthood Federation of America
1108 16th Street NW
Washington, D.C. 20036
(800) 230-7526
(202) 347-8500 or (202) 783-3219
http://plannedparenthood.org

ACANTHOSIS NIGRICANS
See ARTHRITIS

ACHONDROPLASIA
See SHORT STATURE

ADOPTION
C.A.S.E.
The Center for Adoption Support and Education, Inc.

Maryland office:
11120 New Hampshire Avenue
Suite 205
Silver Spring, MD 20904
(301) 593-9200
(301) 593-9203
http://www.adoptionsupport.org
caseadopt@adoptionsupport.org

Virginia office:
King's Park Professional Building
8996 Burke Lake Road
Suite 201
Burke, VA 22015
(703) 425-3703
(703) 425-3704
http://www.adoptionsupport.org
caseadopt@adoptionsupport.org

National Adoption Center
1500 Walnut Street
Suite 701
Philadelphia, PA 19102
(800) TO-ADOPT
http://www.adopt.org/

ADRENOGENITAL SYNDROMES
Androgen Insensitivity Syndrome Support Network
4203 Genesee Avenue, #103-436
San Diego, CA 92117-4950
(619) 569-5254
http://www.medhelp.org/www/ais/

CARES Foundation, Inc.
189 Main Street
2nd Floor
Millburn, NJ 7041
(973) 912-3895
(973) 912-3894
http://www.caresfoundation.org
kelly@caresfoundation.org

**Congenital Adrenal Hyperplasia
  Support Association, Inc.**
801 Country Road, #3
Wrenshall, MN 55797
(218) 384-3863
http://www.childhealthinfo.com/a/
  adrenal-hyperplasia.htm

Intersex Society of North America
979 Golf Course Drive, #282
Rohnert Park, CA 94928
http://www.isna.org
info@isna.org

The MAGIC Foundation
6645 W. North Avenue
Oak Park, IL 60302
(800) 3-MAGIC-3
http://www.magicfoundation.org

National Adrenal Diseases Foundation
505 Northern Boulevard
Great Neck, NY 11021
(516) 487-4992
http://www.medhelp.org/nadf/
nadfmail@aol.com

ADRENOLEUKODYSTROPHY
United Leukodystrophy Foundation
2304 Highland Drive
Sycamore, IL 60178
(800) 728-5483
(815) 895-2432
http://www.ulf.org/
office@ulf.org

AICARDI SYNDROME
**Aicardi Syndrome Awareness and Support
  Network**
29 Delavan Avenue
Toronto, Ontario M5P 1T2

(416) 481-4095
asasn@sympatico.ca

**Aicardi Syndrome Foundation
Aicardi Syndrome Newsletter**
1510 Polo Fields Court
Louisville, KY 40245
(502) 244-9152
(502) 244-9152
newsletter@aicardisyndrome.org

Aicardi Syndrome Foundation
PO Box 3202
St. Charles, IL 60174
(800) 374-8518
http://www.aicardisyndrome.org/
aicardi@aol.com

AIDS
**CDC National AIDS Hotline
American Social Health Association**
PO Box 13827
Research Triangle Park, NC 27709
(919) 361-8400
(919) 361-8425
http://www.ashastd.org/

ALAGILLE SYNDROME
Alagille Syndrome Alliance
10500 SW Starr Drive
Tualatin, OR 97062
(503) 885-0455
http://www.alagille.org
alagille@alagille.org

American Liver Foundation
75 Maiden Lane
Suite 603
New York, NY 10038
(212) 668-1000
(973) 256-3214
http://www.liverfoundation.org
webmail@liverfoundation.org

Children's Liver Alliance
3835 Richmond Avenue
Box 190
Staten Island, NY 10312
(718) 987-6200
http://www.liverkids.org.au/
livers4kids@earthlink.net

ALBINISM

Albinism Fellowship
PO Box 77, Burnley
GB BB11 5GN, Lancashire
(+44)-01282-771900
http://www.albinism.org/
m.sanderson@virgin.net

Hermansky-Pudlak Syndrome Network, Inc.
One South Road
Oyster Bay, NY 11771-1905
(800) 789-9477
(516) 922-3440 or 4022
http://www.medhelp.org/web/hpsn.htm
appell@worldnet.att.net

International Albinism Center
Box 485 UMHC
The University of Minnesota Hospital and Clinic
420 Delaware Street, X.E.
Minneapolis, MN 55455
http://albinism.med.umn.edu/

National Organization for Albinism & Hypopigmentation
PO Box 959
East Hampstead, NH 03826
(603) 887-2310
(800) 648-2310
http://www.albinism.org/
info@albinism.org

ALBRIGHT HEREDITARY OSTEODYSTROPHY

See McCune-Albright syndrome

ALCOHOLISM

National Council on Alcoholism
22 Cortlandt Street
Suite 801
New York, NY 10007-3128
(212) 269-7797
(212) 269-7510
800-NCA-CALL (HOPELINE/24-hour affiliate referral)
http://www.ncadd.org
national@ncadd.org

SAMHSA's National Clearinghouse for Alcohol and Drug Information
PO Box 2345
Rockville, MD 20847-2345
(800) 729-6686
(301) 468-6433
http://www.health.org/govpubs/MS498/

ALKAPTONURIA

The Alkaptonuria Society
12 High Beeches
Childwall
Liverpool, L16 3GA
United Kingdom
(+44) 0151 737 1862
http://www.alkaptonuria.info
manager@alkaptonuria.info

ALLERGY

Allergy/Asthma Information Association AAIA National Office
Box 100
Toronto, Ontario M9W 5K9
(416) 679-9521
(800) 611-7011
(416) 679-9524 (fax)
http://www.aaia.ca/ENGLISH/Main_Pages/Welcomepg.htm

American Academy of Allergy, Asthma & Immunology
555 East Wells Street
Suite 1100
Milwaukee, WI 53202-3823
(414) 272-6071
http://www.aaaai.org/patients/contact.stm
info@aaaai.org

American Allergy Association
PO Box 7273
Menlo Park, CA 94025
(415) 322-1663

National Institute of Allergy and Infectious Diseases (NIAID)
Building 31
Room 7A32
9000 Rockville Pike
Bethesda, MD 20892

(301) 496-5717
(301) 402-0120 (fax)

ALOPECIA

Bald Headed Men of America
3725 Bridges Street
Morehead City, NC 28557
(252) 726-1855
(252) 726-6061 (fax)
http://www.members.aol.com/baldusa/
jcapps4102@aol.com

National Alopecia Areata Foundation
14 Mitchell Boulevard
San Rafael, CA 94903
(415) 472-3780
(415) 472-5343 (fax)
http://www.naaf.org
vicki@naaf.org

ALPHA-1-ANTRITRYPSIN DEFICIENCY

Alpha-1 Advocacy Alliance
PO Box 182
103 Rapidan Church Lane
Wolftown, VA 22748
(540) 948-6777
(540) 948-6763
http://http://www.alpha1advocacy.org
alpha1advocacyalliance@yahoo.com

Alpha-1 Association
815 Connecticut Avenue
Suite 1200
Washington, D.C. 20006-4004
(202) 887-1900
(202) 857-9799 (fax)
http://www.alpha1.org
info@alpha1.org

Alpha-1 Canadian Registry
Toronto Hospital Western Division
Edith Cavell Wing
Suite 4-011
399 Bathurst Street
Toronto, Ontario M5T 2S8
(416) 603-5020
(800) 352-8186

Alpha-1 Foundation
2937 SW 27 Avenue
Suite 302
Miami, FL 33133
(305) 567-9888
(305) 567-1317
http://www.alphaone.org
mmcguire@alphaone.org

American Liver Foundation
75 Maiden Lane
Suite 603
New York, NY 10038
(212) 668-1000
(973) 256-3214
http://www.liverfoundation.org
webmail@liverfoundation.org

ALSTROM SYNDROME

Alstrom Syndrome International
14 Whitney Farm Road
Mt. Desert, ME 4660
(207) 244-7043
(207) 288-6078
(800) 371-3628
http://www.jax.org/alstrom/
jdm@jax.org

**National Association for Parents of the
    Visually Impaired**
PO Box 317
Watertown, MA 2471
(617) 972-7441
(617) 972-7444
napvi@perkins.pvt.k12.ma.us

ALZHEIMER DISEASE

Alzheimer's Association
919 North Michigan Avenue
Suite 1100
Chicago, IL 60611-1676
(312) 335-8700
(312) 335-1110
(312) 335-8882 (TDD)
http://www.alz.org
info@alz.org

Alzheimer's Disease Education & Referral Center
PO Box 8250
Silver Spring, MD 20907-8250
(301) 495-3334 (fax)
http://www.alzheimers.org/
adear@alzheimers.org

Canadian Association for Alzheimer's Disease
http://www.alzheimer.ca/

National Endowment for Alzheimer's Disease
3741 Walnut Street
Suite 101
Philadelphia, PA 19104
(856) 757-9773
(856) 757-9647
http://http://www.memorymatters.org
janson@memorymatters.org

AMBIGUOUS GENITALIA

Ambiguous Genitalia Support Network
PO Box 313
Clements, CA 95227
(209) 727-0313
(209) 727-0313
http://www.jps.net/agsn/
agsn@jps.net

Intersex Society of North America
PO Box 3070
Ann Arbor, MI 48106-3070
(734) 994-7369
(734) 994-7379
http://www.isna.org
info@isna.org

AMYLOIDOSIS

Amyloidosis Support Network, Inc.
1490 Herndon Lane
Marietta, GA 30062
info@amyloidosis.org
http://www.amyloidosis.org/AboutUs.asp

AMYOTROPHIC LATERAL SCLEROSIS

ALS Society of Canada
265 Yorkland Boulevard
Suite 300
Toronto, Ontario M2J 1S5
(800) 267-4ALS

(416) 497-1256 (fax)
http://www.als.ca/

Amyotrophic Lateral Sclerosis Association
27001 Agoura Road
Suite 150
Calabasas Hills, CA 91301
(818) 880-9006 or 9007
(818) 340-7573 (TDD)
http://www.alsa.org
alsinfo@alsa-national.org

Les Turner ALS Foundation
8142 N. Lawndale Avenue
Skokie, IL 60076
(847) 679-3311
(847) 679-9109
http://www.lesturnerals.org
info@lesturnerals.org

ANEMIA

Aplastic Anemia and Myelodysplasia Association of Canada
23 Hamills Crescent
Richmond Hill, Ontario L4S 1C1
(905) 780-0698
(888) 840-0039
(905) 780-1648
http://www.aamac.ca/
lori.lockwood@aamac.ca

Cooley's Anemia Foundation
National Office
129-09 26th Avenue, #203
Flushing, NY 11354
(800) 522-7222
(718) 321-CURE (2873)
(718) 321-3340 (fax)
http://www.thalassemia.org/

Fanconi Anemia Research Fund, Inc.
1801 Willamette Street
Suite 200
Eugene, OR 97401
(541) 687-4658
(541) 687-0548
http://www.fanconi.org
info@fanconi.org

Iron Disorders Institute
PO Box 2031
Greenville, SC 20602
(864) 292-1175
(864) 292-1878 (fax)
http://www.irondisorders.org
publications@irondisorders.org

ANGELMAN SYNDROME

Angelman Syndrome Foundation
414 Plaza Drive
Suite 209
Westmont, IL 60559
(630) 734-9267
(630) 655-0391
http://www.angelman.org
info@angelman.org

Canadian Angelman Syndrome Society
PO Box 37
Priddis, Alberta T0L 1W0
(403) 931-2415
(403) 931-4237 (fax)
info@AngelmanCanada.org

ANKYLOSING SPONDYLITIS

Kickas.org
http://www.kickas.org
kickas@kickas.org

Spondylitis Association of America
PO Box 5872
Sherman Oaks, CA 91413
(800) 777-8189
(818) 981-1616
info@spondylitis.org
http://www.spondylitis.org/

APERT SYNDROME

AboutFace International
123 Edward Street
Suite 1003
CA M5G 1E2 Toronto, Ontario
(416) 597-2229
(416) 597-8494 (fax)
http://www.aboutfaceinternational.org
info@aboutfaceinternational.org

AboutFace USA
PO Box 93
Limekiln, PA 19535
http://http://www.aboutfaceusa.org/
abtface@interlog.com

AboutFace USA/CleftAdvocate
PO Box 969
Batavia, IL 60510-0969
(888) 486-1209
(630) 761-2985 (fax)
http://www.aboutfaceusa.org
http://www.cleftadvocate.org
AboutFaceUSA@comcast.net
debbie@cleftadvocate.org

**Apert Support and Information Network
Don & Cathie Sears**
PO Box 2571
Columbia, SC 29202
(803) 732-2372
http://www.apert.org/
catndon@apert.org

Apert Syndrome Pen Pals
PO Box 115
Providence, RI 2901
(401) 454-4849

Children's Craniofacial Association (CCA)
13140 Coit Road
Suite 307
Dallas, TX 75240
(800) 535-3643
(214) 570-8811
contactCCA@ccakids.com

ARTHRITIS

**National Institute of Arthritis and
   Musculoskeletal and Skin Diseases
   Information Clearinghouse**
National Institutes of Health
1 AMS Circle
Bethesda, MD 20892-3675
(301) 495-4484
(877) 22-NIAMS (226-4267)
(301) 565-2966 (TTY)
(301) 718-6366 (fax)
http://www.niams.nih.gov/hi/index.htm
NIAMSinfo@mail.nih.gov

ARTHRYGRYPOSIS MULTIPLEX CONGENITA

National Support Group for Arthrogryposis
PO Box 5192
Sonora, CA 95370
(209)-928-3688
http://http://www.sonnet.com/avenues
avenues@sonnet.com

ASTHMA

Asthma & Allergy Foundation of American National Headquarters
1233 20th Street NW
Suite 402
Washington, D.C. 20036
(202) 466-7643
(202) 466-8940 (fax)
http://www.aafa.org
info@aafa.org

Asthma Society of Canada
130 Bridgeland Avenue
Suite 425
Toronto, Ontario M6A 1Z4
(866) 787-4050
(416) 787-4050
(416) 787-5807 (fax)
info@asthma.ca
http://www.asthma.ca/adults/

ATAXIA

A-T Children's Project
668 S. Military Trail
Deerfield Beach, FL 33442-3023
(954) 481-6611
(954) 725-1153
(800) 5-HELP-A-T
info@atcp.org
http://www.atcp.org/

Connaitre les Syndromes Cerbelleux
3, allee Xavier Bichat
FR 77420 Champs sur Marne 77420
01-64-68-70-36

National Ataxia Foundation
2600 Fernbrook Lane
Suite 119
Minneapolis, MN 55447-4730

(763) 553-0020
(763) 553-0167 (fax)
http://www.ataxia.org
naf@ataxia.org

ATTENTION DEFICIT HYPERACTIVITY DISORDER

The ADHD Challenge
PO Box 488
West Peabody, MA 01985-7277
(800) 233-2322
(978) 535-3276

Attention Deficit Information Network (AD-IN)
475 Hillside Avenue
Needham, MA 02194
(617) 455-9895
(781) 444-5466 (fax)
http://www.infonetwork.com

Autism Treatment Services of Canada
404 - 94th Avenue SE
Calgary, Alberta T2J 0E8
atsc@autism.ca
(403) 253-6961
http://www.autism.ca/

Children and Adults with Attention Deficit Disorders (CHADD)
499 NW 70th Avenue
Suite 101
Plantation, FL 33317
(800) 233-4050
(305) 587-3700
(305) 587-4599 (fax)
http://www.chadd.org

National ADD Association
PO Box 972
Mentor, OH 44061
(800) 487-2282
(440) 350-9595
(440) 350-0223 (fax)
http://www.add.org

National Center for Learning Disabilities
381 Park Avenue South
Suite 1401
New York, NY 10016
(212) 545-7510

(212) 545-9665 (fax)
http://www.ncld.org

National Mental Health Association
1021 Prince Street
Alexandria, VA 22314
(703) 684-7722
(800) 433-5959
(703) 684-5968 (fax)
http://www.nmha.org

Parent to Parent of NYS
45 Mall Drive
Commack, NY 11725
(631) 493-1716
http://www.parenttoparentnys.org/longisland.htm
rr815@aol.com

AZOREAN DISEASE

International Joseph Diseases Foundation
PO Box 994268
Redding, CA 96099
(530) 246-4722
http://69.10.163.110/bastiana/
mjd@ijdf.net

B

BARDET-BIEDL SYNDROME

Laurence Moon Bardet-Beidl Syndrome E-mail Group
124 Lincoln Avenue
Purchase, NY 10577
(914) 251-1163
hawkfan5@ozramp.net.au

BASAL CELL CARCINOMA

See CANCER

BATTEN DISEASE

Batten Disease Support and Research Association
120 Humphries Drive
Suite 2
Reynoldsburg, OH 43068
(740) 927-4298
http://www.bdsra.org/
BDSRA1@bdsra.org

Batten Disease Support and Research Association
c/o Bev Martin
17 Bell Street
Regina, Saskatchewan S4S 4B7
(306) 789-9047
(800) 448-4570
gmaxim@cableregina.com
http://www.bdsra.org

National Batten Disease Registry
New York Institute for Basic Research in
   Developmental Disabilities
1050 Forest Hill Road
Staten Island, NY 10314
(718) 494-5201
(800) 952-9628
(718) 982-6346 (fax)
battenkw@aol.com

BECKWITH WIEDEMANN SYNDROME

Beckwith-Wiedemann Support Network
2711 Colony Road
Ann Arbor, MI 48104
(734) 973-0263
(734) 973-9721
http://www.beckwith-wiedemann.org
a800bwsn@aol.com

BILARY ATRESIA

See LIVER DISORDERS

BIRTH DEFECTS

Association of Birth Defect Children (ABDC)
930 Woodcock Road
Suite 225
Orlando, FL 32803
http://www.birthdefects.org/default.htm
staff@birthdefects.org

Birth Defect Research for Children, Inc.
930 Woodcock Road
Suite 225
Orlando, FL 32803
(407) 895-0802
(407) 895-0824 (fax)
http://www.birthdefects.org

March of Dimes
1275 Mamaroneck Avenue

White Plains, NY 10605
(914) 428-7100
http://www.marchofdimes.com/

National Center for Education in Maternal and Child Health
2115 Wisconsin Avenue NW
Suite 601
Washington, D.C. 20007-2292
(202) 784-9770
(202) 784-9777
http://www.ncemch.org/
mchlibrary@ncemch.org

National Easter Seal Society
230 West Monroe Street
Suite 1800
Chicago, IL 60606
(312) 726-6200
(312) 726-4258
(800) 221-6827
(312) 726-1494 (fax)
http://www.easterseals.com/site/PageServer

National Institute of Child Health and Human Development
PO Box 3006
Rockville, MD 20847
(800) 370-2943
(888) 320-6942
(301) 984-1473 (fax)
http://www.nichd.nih.gov/
nichdinformationresourcecenter@mail.nih.gov

BLEPHAROPHIMOSIS

Blepharophimosis, Ptosis, Epicanthus Inversus Family Network
820 SE Meadow Vale Drive
Pullman, WA 99163
(509) 332-6628
lschauble@gocougs.wsu.edu

BLOOM SYNDROME

Bloom Syndrome Registry
c/o James L German III, M.D.
Department of Pediatrics
Box 103
Weill Medical College of Cornell University
1300 York Avenue
New York, NY 10021

(212) 746-3956
(212) 746-0300 (fax)
jlg2003@med.cornell.edu

Chicago Center for Jewish Genetic Disorders
One South Franklin Street
Suite 2910
Chicago, IL 60606
(312) 357-4717
(312) 855-3295
http://www.jewishgeneticscenter.org
jewishgeneticsctr@juf.org

BREAST CANCER

See CANCER

C

CANAVAN DISEASE

See LEUKODYSTROPHY

CANCER

American Cancer Society
15999 Clifton Road NE
Atlanta, GA 303329-4251
(800) 227-2345
(404) 320-3333
(404) 329-5787 (fax)
http://www.cancer.org/

Canadian Cancer Society National Office
10 Alcorn Avenue
Suite 200
Toronto, Ontario M4V 3B1
(416) 961-7223
(416) 961-4189 (fax)
ccs@cancer.ca

Cancer Information & Support Network
2792 Sanderling Way
Pleasanton, CA 94566
(925) 462-4963
(925) 461-8463 (fax)

Candlelighters Childhood Cancer Foundation
3910 Warner Street
Kensington, MD 20895
(301) 962-3520

(301) 962-3521 (fax)
http://www.candlelighters.org
info@candlelighters.org

Childhood Cancer Foundation Candlelighters Canada

55 Eglinton Avenue East
Suite 401
Toronto, Ontario M4P 1G8
(416) 489-6440
(800) 363-1062
(416) 489-9812 (fax)
staff@childhoodcancer.ca
http://www.childhoodcancer.ca

David G. Jagelman Cancer Registry

Department of Medical Genetics
T-10 Cleveland Clinic Foundation
805 15th Street NW
Room 500
Washington, D.C. 20005
(205) 496-4070
http://www.clevelandclinic.org/registries/registry/
david.htm

Gilda Radner Familial Ovarian Cancer Registry
Roswell Park Cancer Institute

Elm and Carlton Streets
Buffalo, NY 14263-0001
(716) 845-4503
(716) 845-8266 (fax)
http://www.ovariancancer.com
cathy.fahey@roswellpark.org

Hereditary Colon Cancer Newsletter and Webpage

Department of Behavioral Sciences
243, 1515 Holcombe Boulevard
Houston, TX 77030
(713) 745-2385
(713) 794-4730 (fax)
http://www.epigenetic.org/~pjs/homepage.html
wsternit@mdanderson.org

Intestinal Multiple Polyposis and Colorectal Cancer Foundation

PO Box 11
Conyngham, PA 18219
(570) 788-3712

(717) 788-1818 (fax)
impacc@epix.net

National Alliance of Breast Cancer Organizations

9 East 37th Street
10th Floor
New York, NY 10016
(212) 889-0606
(212) 689-1213 (fax)
http://www.nabco.org
nabcoinfo@aol.com

National Breast Cancer Coalition

1707 L Street NW
Suite 1060
Washington, D.C. 20036
(202) 296-7477
(202) 265-6854 (fax)
http://www.natlbcc.org

National Cancer Institute

805 15th Street NW
Room 500
Washington, D.C. 20005
(800) 4-CANCER
(800) 332-8615
http://www.cancer.gov
cancergovstaff@mail.nih.gov

National Coalition for Cancer Survivorship

1010 Wayne Avenue
Suite 770
Silver Spring, MD 20910
(301) 565-9670 (fax)
http://www.cansearch.org
info@cansearch.org

National Ovarian Cancer Coalition, Inc.

500 NE Spanish River Boulevard
Suite 14
Boca Raton, FL 33431
(561) 393-0005
(561) 393-7275 (fax)
http://www.ovarian.org
nocc@ovarian.org

Ovarian Cancer National Alliance

910 17th Street NW
Suite 413
Washington, D.C. 20006
(202) 331-1332

(202) 331-2292 (fax)
http://www.ovariancancer.org
ovarian@aol.com

Susan G. Komen Breast Cancer Foundation
5005 LBJ Freeway
Suite 370
Dallas, TX 75244
(972) 855-1600
(800) IM-AWARE
(972) 855-1605 (fax)
http://www.breastcancerinfo.com
helpline@komen.org

**The University of Texas M. D. Anderson
    Cancer Center**
1515 Holcombe Boulevard
Houston, TX 77030
(800) 392-1611
http://www.mdanderson.org/

Y-ME National Breast Cancer Organization
212 W. Van Buren
Suite 1000
Chicago, IL 60640
(312) 986-8338
(312) 294-8597 (fax)
http://www.y-me.org
contact@y-me.org

CARDIAC ANOMALIES

**Adult Congenital Heart Association, Inc.
    (ACHA)**
1500 Sunday Drive
Suite 102
Raleigh, NC 27607-5151
(919) 861-4547
http://www.achaheart.org/
info@achaheart.org

**American Heart Association
National Center**
7272 Greenville Avenue
Dallas, TX 75231
AHA: (800) AHA-USA-1
or (800) 242-8721
ASA: (888) 4-STROKE
or (888) 478-7653
http://www.americanheart.org

**Cardiac Arrhythmias Research and
    Education Foundation, Inc**
C.A.R.E. Foundation, Inc.
26425 NE Allen Street
Suite 103
P.O. Box 369
Duvall, Washington 98019
(800) 404-9500
(425) 788-1987
(425) 788-1927 (fax)
care@longqt.org
http://www.longqt.org/

Children's Cardiomyopathy Foundation
PO Box 547
Tenafly, NJ 07670
(201) 227-8852
(201) 227-7016 (fax)
http://www.childrenscardiomyopathy.org
info@childrenscardiomyopathy.org

**Children's Heart Association for Support and
    Education**
CHASE – Hospital for Sick Children
c/o Cardiology Department
5555 University Avenue
Toronto, Ontario M5G 1X8
(416) 410-2427
http://www.chasekids.org/

**Congenital Heart Anomalies Support,
    Education, & Resources, Inc.**
CHASER News
2112 North Wilkins Road
Swanton, OH 43558
(419) 825-5575
(419) 825-2880 (fax)
http://www.csun.edu/~hcmth011/chaser/
    chaser-news.html
myer106w@wonder.em.cdc.gov
chaser@compuserve.com

Coronary Club, Inc.
9500 Euclid Avenue
Suite EE37
Cleveland, OH 44195
(800) 478-4255
(216) 444-3690
(216) 444-9385 (fax)

International Bundle Branch Block Association
6631 W. 83rd Street
Los Angeles, CA 90045-2875
(310) 670-9132

Kids with Heart National Association for Children's Heart Disorders
1578 Careful Drive
Green Bay, WI 54304-2941
(920) 498-0058
(800) 538-5390 (fax) (U.S. only)
http://www.kidswithheart.org

Mended Hearts
7272 Greenville Avenue
Dallas, TX 75231
(888) 432-7899
(214) 706-5245 (fax)
http://www.mendedhearts.org
info@mendedhearts.org

Montgomery Heart Foundation for Cardiomyopathy
1419 Mt. Carmel Road
Parkton, MD 21120
(410) 357-8401
http://www.med.jhu.edu/cardiomyopathy
rmonty@jhmi.edu

CARNITINE DEFICIENCY

See MITOCHONDRIAL DISORDERS

CARPENTER SYNDROME

Carpenter Syndrome Network
Box 4215-48
26661 Bear Valley Road
Tehachapi, CA 93561
(805) 821-1313

CELL BANK

Human Genetic Mutant Cell Repository Coriell Institute
401 Haddon Avenue
Camden, NJ 08103
(800) 752-3805
(856) 757-4848
(856) 757-9737 (fax)
ccr@coriell.org

CEREBRAL PALSY

Ontario Foundation for Cerebral Palsy
104-1630 Lawrence Avenue West
Toronto, Ontario M6L 1C5
(416) 244-9686
(877) 244-9686
(416) 244-6543 (fax)
http://www.ofcp.on.ca/med.html
info@ofcp.on.ca

United Cerebral Palsy Association, Inc.
1660 L Street NW
Suite 700
Washington, D.C. 20036-5602
(202) 776-0406
(202) 973-7197
(202) 776-0414 (fax)
http://www.ucpa.org

CESAREAN BIRTHS

American College of Obstetricians and Gynecologists
409 12th Street, SW
PO Box 96920
Washington, D.C. 20090-6920
(202) 638-5577
http://www.acog.org/

CHARCOT-MARIE-TOOTH SYNDROME

Charcot-Marie-Tooth Association
2700 Chestnut Street
Chester, PA 19013
(610) 499-9264
(810) 499-9267
http://www.charcot-marie-tooth.org
cmtassoc@aol.com

Charcot-Marie-Tooth International
1 Springbank Drive
St. Catharines, Ontario CA L2S 2K1
(905) 687-3630
(905) 687-8753 (fax)
http://www.cmtint.org
cmtint@vaxxine.com

CHARGE

CHARGE Syndrome Foundation, Inc.
2004 Parkade Boulevard
Columbia, MO 65202

(573) 499-4694
(573) 499-4694 (fax)
http://www.chargesyndrome.org
meg@chargesyndrome.org

CHOLESTEROL ESTER STORAGE DISEASE

See TAY-SACHS DISEASE

CHONDRODYSPLASIA PUNCTATA

See SHORT STATURE

CHROMOSOME ABNORMALITIES

4p- Support Group (Wolf Hirschhorn Syndrome)
2585 Taylor
Longview, WA 98632
(360) 577-9033
http://www.4p-supportgroup.org
fourpminus@4p-supportgroup.org

5p- Society (Cri-du-Chat)
11609 Oakmont
Overland Park, KS 66210
(913) 469-8900
http://www.fivepminus.org/
fivepminus@aol.com

8p Duplication Support Group
c/o Faith Callif-Daley
Genetics Center, Children's Medical Center
1 Children's Plaza
Dayton, OH 45404
(937) 641-5645
(937) 641-5325 (fax)
callif-daleyf@childrensdayton.org

11q Research and Resource Group
6123 A. Duncan Road
Petersburg, VA 23803
(804) 863-2114
(804) 828-5383 (fax)
http://www.11q.net
mspace@vcu.edu

22q and You Center
Clinical Genetics Center
The Children's Hospital of Philadelphia
34th Street and Civic Center Boulevard
Philadelphia, PA 19104-4399
(215) 590-2920

http://www.chop.edu/consumer/jsp/division/
    service.jsp?id=74652
mcginn@email.chop.edu

49, XXXXY Information
Klinefelter Syndrome Organization
10001 N E 74th Street
Vancouver, WA 98662-3801
(360) 892-7547
kimbj@juno.com

Associazione Internazionale Ring14
34 - 42100 Reggio Emilia, Italy
39 0522/322607
39 0522/324835 (fax)
http://www.ring14.com
info@ring14.com

Chromosome 7 Information
The Hospital for Sick Children
Department of Genetics Room 9102
555 University Avenue, Toronto, Ontario M5G 1X8
http://www.genet.sickkids.on.ca/chromosome7/

Chromosome 9p Network (merger of Support Group for Monosomy 9p- and Support Group for 9p-)
393 N. Grass Valley Road
Pine Valley, UT 84781
(435) 574-1121
(435) 574-2000 (fax)
http://www.9pminus.org
beverly.udell@9pminus.org

Chromosome 11 Deletion/WAGR Syndrome Support Group
2063 Regina
Lincoln Park, MI 48146
TheMooZoo@aol.com

Chromosome 18 Registry & Research Society
6302 Fox Head
San Antonio, TX 78247
(210) 657-4968
(210) 657-4968 (fax)
http://www.chromosome18.org/
cody@uthscsa.edu

Chromosome 22 Central
237 Kent Avenue
Timmins, Ontario P4N 3C2
(705) 268-3099

(705) 267-3370 (fax)
http://www.c22c.org
a815@c22c.org

Chromosome Deletion Outreach
PO Box 724
Boca Raton, FL 33429-0724
(888) 236-6880
http://www.chromodisorder.org/
info@chromodisorder.org

Cri Du Chat Support Group of Australia, Inc.
5 Connal Drive
Frankston, VIC 3199
http://www.vicnet.net.au/~criduch/
maggiecdc@bigfoot.com

European Chromosome 11q Network
Annet van Betuw
Else Mauhsstraat 7
6708 NJ Wageningen, Netherlands
http://www.11q.org (http://home01.wxs.
    nl/~avbetuw/home.htm)
avbetuw@wxs.nl
Materials in Dutch, English, German, Italian, and
    "Scandinavian" (for Norwegian, Swedish and
    Danish families)

International 11; 22 Translocation Network
Stephanie St-Pierre
232 Kent Avenue
Timmins, Ontario P4N 3C3
(705) 268-3099
http://www.nt.net/~a815/index.html
mum2_1@hotmail.com

International 22q 1 1.2 Deletion Syndrome Foundation
PO Box 872
Lansdale, PA 19446
(215) 453-1819
http://www.22q.org
mabissi@comcast.net

Isodicentric 15 Exchange, Advocacy, and Support (IDEAS)
416 Big Mount Road
Thomasville, PA 17364-9768
(717) 225-5229
(610) 891-2062 (fax)
http://www.idic15.org
ideas@craftech.com

Parents & Researchers Interested in Smith Magenis Syndrome (PRISMS)
11875 Fawn Ridge Lane
Reston, VA 22094
(703) 709-0568
acmsmith@nchgr.nih.gov
http://www.kumc.edu/gec/support/smith-ma.html

SOFT (Support Organization for Trisomy 18, 13, Other)
Support Organization for Trisomy 18, 13 and
    Related Disorders
2982S Union Street
Rochester, NY 14624
(716) 594-4621
http://www.trisomy.org/

SOFT (Support Organization for Trisomy 18, 13, Other) - for Families with Child with Trisomy 18, 13 or Other Chromosome Disorders - Annual Conferences, Literature, Newsletter, and Other
http://www.trisomy.org/

S.O.F.T. Australia
198 Oak Road
Kirrawee NSW 2232 Australia
02 9521 6039
http://www.challengenet.com/~SOFT/index.htm
karens@tig.com.au

Support Organization for Trisomy 18, 13 and Related Disorders
2982S Union Street
Rochester, NY 14624
(716) 594-4621

Tetrasomy X/Pentasomy X Support Group
1402 Governor House Circle
Wilmington, DE 19809
(302) 764-3924
cyndibradley@hotmail.com

UNIQUE: Rare Chromosome Disorder Support Group
PO Box 2189
Caterham Surrey, England CR3 5GN
44 (0)1883 330766
http://www.rarechromo.org
info@rarechromo.org

Velo-Cardio-Facial Syndrome Educational Foundation, Inc.
PO Box 874
Milltown, NJ 08850
(732) 238-8803
(866) VCF-SEF5
http://www.vcfsef.org/
info@vcfsef.org

CLEFT LIP, PALATE

AboutFace International
123 Edward Street
Suite 1003
CA M5G 1E2 Toronto, Ontario M5G 1E2
(416) 597-2229
(416) 597-8494 (fax)
http://www.aboutfaceinternational.org
info@aboutfaceinternational.org

AboutFace USA
PO Box 93
Limekiln, PA 19535
http://www.aboutfaceusa.org/
abtface@interlog.com

AboutFace USA/CleftAdvocate
PO Box 969
Batavia, IL 60510-0969
(888) 486-1209
(630) 761-2985 (fax)
http://www.aboutfaceusa.org, http://www.
    cleftadvocate.org
aboutfaceusa@comcast.net, debbie@cleftadvocate.
    org

American Cleft Palate-Craniofacial Association/Cleft Palate Foundation
1504 East Franklin Street
Suite 102
Chapel Hill, NC 27514-2820
(919) 933-9044
http://www.cleftline.org/#
info@cleftline.org

Birth Defect Research for Children, Inc.
930 Woodcock Road
Suite 225
Orlando, FL 32803
(407) 895-0802

(407) 895-0824 (fax)
http://www.birthdefects.org

CleftAdvocate
5201 Sequin Drive
Las Vegas, NV 89130
(702) 228-8662
(702) 341-5351 (fax)
http://www.cleftadvocate.org
debbie@cleftadvocate.org

COCKAYNE SYNDROME

Share and Care Cockayne Syndrome Network, Inc.
PO Box 570618
Dallas, TX 75357
(972) 613-6273
(972) 613-4590 (fax)
http://www.cockayne-syndrome.com
J93082@aol.com

COFFIN-LOWRY SYNDROME

Coffin-Lowry Syndrome Foundation
3045 255th Avenue, SE
Sammamish, WA 98075
(425) 427-0939
http://www.clsf.info
clsfoundation@yahoo.com

COFFIN-SIRIS SYNDROME

Coffin-Siris Syndrome Support Group
1524 Marshall Street
Antioch, CA 94509
(925) 754-6568
http://members.aol.com/CoffinSiri/index.html
jxgarris@aol.com

Congenital Lactic Acidosis Family Support Group
1620 Marble Avenue
Denver, CO 80229
(303) 287-4953

COLORECTAL CANCER

See CANCER; FAMILIAL POLYPOSIS/POLYCYSTIC KIDNEY DISEASE

CONGENITAL GLAUCOMA

See OCULAR DISORDERS

CONJOINED TWINS

Twin Hope
2592 West 14th Street
Cleveland, OH 44113
(502) 243-2110
http://www.twinhope.com
twinhope@twinhope.com

CORNELIA DE LANGE SYNDROME

Cornelia de Lange Syndrome Canada
http://www.cdlscanada.com/
questions@cdlscanada.com

Cornelia de Lange Syndrome Foundation, Inc.
302 West Main Street
Suite 100
Avon, CT 6001
(860) 676-8166
(860) 676-8337
http://www.cdlsusa.org
info@cdlsusa.org

CRANIOFACIAL DISORDERS

AboutFace International
123 Edward Street
Suite 1003
CA M5G 1E2, Toronto, Ontario M5G 1E2
(416) 597-2229
(416) 597-8494 (fax)
http://www.aboutfaceinternational.org
info@aboutfaceinternational.org

AboutFace USA
PO Box 93
Limekiln, PA 19535
http://www.aboutfaceusa.org/
abtface@interlog.com

AboutFace USA/CleftAdvocate
PO Box 969
Batavia, IL 60510-0969
(888) 486-1209
(630) 761-2985 (fax)
http://www.aboutfaceusa.org, http://www.
   cleftadvocate.org
aboutfaceusa@comcast.net, debbie@cleftadvocate.
   org

The Center for Craniofacial Disorders
Montefiore Medical Center
Albert Einstein College of Medicine
111 East 210th Street
Bronx, NY 10467-2490
Medical Director:
Alan Shanske, MD (Genetics)
(718) 920-4300
Surgical Director:
David A. Staffenberg, MD (Plastic Surgery)
(718) 920-4462
dstaffen@montefiore.org

Children's Craniofacial Association
13140 Coit Road
Suite 307
Dallas, TX 75240
(214) 570-8811
(972) 240-7607 (fax)
http://www.masterlink.com/children
char_smith@prodigy.net

CleftAdvocate
5201 Sequin Drive
Las Vegas, NV 89130
(702) 228-8662
(702) 341-5351 (fax)
http://www.cleftadvocate.org
debbie@cleftadvocate.org

Craniofacial Foundation of America
975 East Third Street
Chattanooga, TN 37403
(423) 778-9192
(423) 778-8172 (fax)
http://www.erlanger.org/cranio
farmertm@erlanger.org

FACES, The National Craniofacial Association
PO Box 11082
Chattanooga, TN 37401
(423) 266-1632
(423) 267-3124 (fax)
http://www.faces-cranio.org
faces@mindspring.com

Forward Face
317 East 34th Street
Suite 901A

New York, NY 10016
(212) 684-5860
(212) 684-5864 (fax)
http://www.forwardface.org
info@forwardface.org

Let's Face It USA
PO Box 29972
Bellingham, WA 98228
(360) 676-7325
http://www.faceit.org
letsfaceit@faceit.org

National Foundation for Facial Reconstruction
317 East 34th Street
Room 901
New York, NY 10016
(212) 263-6656
(212) 263-7534 (fax)
info@nffr.org

CRI-DU-CHAT SYNDROME

See CHROMOSOME ABNORMALITIES

CRANIOSYNOSTOSIS

See CRANIOFACIAL DISORDERS

CROHN'S DISEASE AND COLITIS

American Autoimmune Related Diseases Association, Inc.
22100 Gratiot Avenue
East Detroit, MI 48021
(810) 776-3900
(810) 776-3903 (fax)
http://www.aarda.org
aarda@aol.com

Crohn's & Colitis Foundation of America, Inc.
386 Park Avenue South
17th Floor
New York, NY 10016
(212) 685-3440
(212) 779-4098 (fax)
http://www.ccfa.org
info@ccfa.org

Crohn's and Colitis Foundation of Canada
60 St. Clair Avenue East
Suite 600
Toronto, Ontario M4T 1N5
(416) 920-5035

(800) 387-1479
(416) 929-0364 (fax)
http://www.ccfc.ca/english/index.html
ccfc@ccfc.ca

Pediatric Crohn's & Colitis Association, Inc.
PO Box 188
Newton, MA 02468
(617) 489-5854
http://pcca.hypermart.net/

CROUZON SYNDROME

Crouzon/Meniere's Parent Support Network
c/o Kathleen Handsaker
3757 N. Catherine Drive
Prescott Valley, AZ 86314-8320
(520) 772-1784
(800) 842-4681
http://www.crouzon.org/
katy@northlink.com

CUTIS LAXA

See MARFAN SYNDROME

CYSTIC FIBROSIS

Canadian Cystic Fibrosis Foundation
2221 Yonge Street
Suite 601
Toronto, Ontario M4S 2B4
(416) 485-9149
(800) 378-2233 (toll-free from Canada only)
(416) 485-5707
(416) 485-0960 (fax)
info@cysticfibrosis.ca
http://www.ccff.ca/home.asp

Cystic Fibrosis Foundation
6931 Arlington Road
Bethesda, MD 20814
(301) 907-2548
(301) 951-6378 (fax)
http://www.cff.org
spattee@cff.org

Cystic Fibrosis Research, Inc.
2672 Bayshore Parkway
Suite 520
Mountain View, CA 94043
(650) 404-9975
(650) 404-9981 (fax)

http://www.cfri.org
cfri@cfri.org

Cystic Fibrosis World Wide
210 Park Ave, #267
Worcester, MA 01609
(508) 733-6120
http://www.cfww.org/
cnoke@cfww.org

CYSTINOSIS

Cystinosis Foundation, Inc.
604 Vernon Street
Oakland, CA 94610
(559) 222-7997
http://www.cystinosisfoundation.org
jean.cystinosis@sbcglobal.net

Cystinosis Research Network
8 Sylvester Road
Burlington, MA 1803
(781) 229-6182
(781) 229-6030 (fax)
http://www.cystinosis.org
crn@cystinosis.org

CYSTINURIA

Cystinuria Support Network
21001 NE 36th Street
Sammamish, WA 98074
(425) 868-2996
(425) 897-0675 (fax)
http://www.cystinuria.com
cystinuria@aol.com

D

DANDY-WALKER SYNDROME

Dandy-Walker Syndrome Network
5030 142nd Path W
Apple Valley, MN 55124
(952) 423-4008

DES

DES Action USA
158 S. Stanwood Road
Columbus, OH 43209
(800) DES-9288

http://www.desaction.org/
desaction@columbus.rr.com

DIABETES

American Diabetes Association
ATTN: National Call Center
1701 North Beauregard Street
Alexandria, VA 22311
(800) DIABETES
http://www.diabetes.org/home.jsp

Canadian Diabetes Association
National Life Building
1400-522 University Avenue
Toronto, Ontario M5G 2R5
(800) 226-8464
info@diabetes.ca
http://www.diabetes.ca/section_main/welcome.
    asp

Diabetes Action, Research, and Education Foundation
426 C Street NE
Washington, D.C. 20002
(202) 333-4520
http://www.daref.org
daref@diabetesaction.org

Juvenile Diabetes Research Foundation International
120 Wall Street
New York, NY 10005-4001
(800) 533-CURE
(212) 785-9595 (fax)
feedback@jdrf.org
info@jdrf.org

London Diabetes and Lipid Centre
168 Lavender Hill
Room 101 Limited, Shakespeare House
GB SW11 5TF, London SW11 5TF
08707-300-004
08707-300-005 (fax)
http://www.room101.co.uk/

DIGEORGE SYNDROME (VELO-CARDIO-FACIAL SYNDROME)

See CHROMOSOME ABNORMALITIES - 22

DISABILITIES

American Self-Help Group Clearinghouse
100 Hanover Avenue
Room 202
Cedar Knolls, NJ 07927-2020
(973) 326-6789
(973) 326-9467 (fax)
http://www.selfhelpgroups.org
ed@selfhelpgroups.org

Canadian Organization for Rare Disorders
PO Box 814
Coaldale, Alberta T1M 1M7
(403) 345-4544
(403) 345-3948 (fax)
http://www.cord.ca
office@cord.ca

Council for Exceptional Children
1920 Association Drive
Reston, VA 22091
(703) 620-3660
http://www.cec.sped.org

Developmental Disabilites Nurses Association
1733 H Street
Suite 330, PMB 1214
Blaine, WA 98230
(800) 888-6733
(360) 332-2280 (fax)
ddnahq@aol.com
http://ddna.bluestep.net

Eunice Kennedy Shriver Center
200 Trapelo Road
Waltham, MA 2462
(781) 642-0001
(781) 893-5340
http://www.shriver.org
preilly@shriver.org

Families of Children Under Stress (FOCUS)
3050 Presidential Drive
Suite 114
Atlanta, GA 30340
(770) 234-9111
(770) 234-9131 (fax)
http://focus-ga.org/
focus-ga@mindspring.com

Family Center on Technology and Disability (FCTD)
Academy for Educational Development (AED)
1825 Connecticut Avenue NW
7th Floor
Washington, D.C. 20009-5721
(202) 884-8068
(202) 884-8441 (fax)
http://www.fctd.info/contact.php
fctd@aed.org

Family Resource Center on Disabilities
20 East Jackson
Room 900
Chicago, IL 60604
(312) 939-3513
(312) 939-3519
(312) 939-7297 (fax)

Institute on Disability
1640 West Roosevelt Road
Chicago, IL 60608
(312) 413-1504

International Patient Advocacy Association
800 Bellevue Way
MGM Building
Suite 400
Bellevue, WA 98004
(425) 462-4037
(425) 646-3768
(425) 462-9532 (fax)
http://gaucher.mgh.harvard.edu/ipaa.html

National Council on Independent Living
1916 Wilson Boulevard
Suite 209
Arlington, VA 22201
(703) 525-3406
(703) 525-4153
(877) 525-3400
(703) 525-3409 (fax)
ncil@ncil.org
http://www.ncil.org/

National Information Center for Children and Youth With Disabilities
PO Box 1492
Washington, D.C. 20013-1492
(202) 884-8200

(202) 884-8200
(202) 884-8441 (fax)
http://www.NICHCY.org
nichcy@aed.org

DOWN SYNDROME

Apoyo al Niño Down
Department of Genetics
111 Michigan Avenue NW
Washington, D.C. 20010
(202) 884-5480
(202) 884-2390 (fax)
curuburo@cnmc.org

Association for Children with Down Syndrome, Inc.
4 Fern Place
Plainview, NY 11803-4725
(516) 933-4700
(516) 933-9524 (fax)
http://www.acds.org
acds_lyal@hotmail.com

Foundation for Children with Down Syndrome
17646 N. Cave Creek Road
Suite 152
Phoenix, AZ 85032
(602) 493-7688
(602) 265-8216 (fax)
http://www.ffcwds.org

International Mosaic Down Syndrome Association
PO Box 1052
Franklin, TX 77856
(979) 828-1868
(775) 295-9373
http://www.imdsa.com
imdsapresident@imdsa.com

Massachusetts Down Syndrome Congress
PO Box 866
Melrose, MA 02176-0005
(508) 278-7769
http://www.mdsc.org
mdsc@mdsc.org

National Down Syndrome Congress
1370 Center Drive, #102
Atlanta, GA 30338

(770) 604-9500
(770) 604-9898
http://www.ndsccenter.org
info@ndsccenter.com

National Down Syndrome Society
666 Broadway
8th floor
New York, NY 10012-2317
(212) 460-9330
(212) 979-2873 (fax)
http://www.ndss.org
info@ndss.org

Parent Assistance Committee on Down Syndrome
12 Justine Court
Briarcliff Manor, NY 10510-2534
(914) 739-4085

DRUG ABUSE

National Association for Perinatal Addiction Research and Education
11 E. Hubbard Street
Suite 200
Chicago, IL 60611
(312) 329-2512

National Clearinghouse for Alcohol and Drug Information (NCADI)
PO Box 2345
Rockville, MD 20852
(800) 729-6686
http://www.health.org

DUBOWITZ SYNDROME

NE Dubowitz Syndrome Family Support
106 Verndale Street
Warwick, RI 2889
(401) 737-3138
flamingo@netzero.net

DWARFISM

See SHORT STATURE

DYSAUTONOMIA

Dysautonomia Foundation
315 West 39th Street
Suite 701
New York, NY 10018

(212) 279-1066
http://www.familialdysautonomia.org/
info@familialdysautonomia.org

Dysautonomia Foundation, Inc., Toronto Chapter
343 Clark Avenue West
Suite 1103
Thornhill, Ontario L4J 7K5
(905) 882-7725
(905) 764-7752 (fax)

Dysautonomia Treatment and Evaluation Center
New York University Medical Center
530 First Avenue
Suite 9Q
New York, NY 10016
(212) 263-7225
(212) 263-7041 (fax)
http://www.med.nyu.edu/fd/fdcenter.html
Felicia.Axelrod@med.nyu.edu

Familial Dysautonomia Hope Foundation
1170 Green Knolls Drive
Buffalo Grove, IL 60089
(847) 913-0455
(847) 913-8589 (fax)
http://www.fdhope.org
fdhope@comcast.net

National Dysautonomia Research Foundation
1407 West 4th Street
Suite 160
Red Wing, MN 55066-2108
(651) 267-0525
(651) 267-0524 (fax)
http://www.ndrf.org
ndrf@ndrf.org

DYSKERATOSIS CONGENITA

See ECTODERMAL DYSPLASIA

DYSLEXIA

Dyslexia Research Institute (DRI)
4745 Centerville Road
Tallahassee, FL 32308-2899
(850) 893-2216
(850) 893-2440 (fax)
http://www.dyslexia-add.org/

International Dyslexia Association
8600 LaSalle Road
Chester Building
Suite 382
Baltimore, MD 21286-2044
(410) 296-0232
(410) 321-5069 (fax)
http://www.interdys.org
info@interdys.org

National Center for Learning Disabilities
381 Park Avenue South
Suite 1401
New York, NY 10016
(212) 545-7510
(212) 545-9665 (fax)
http://www.ncld.org

DYSPASTIC NEVUS SYNDROME

See CANCER; NEVUS

E

EBSTEIN ANOMALY

See CARDIAC ANOMALIES

ECTODERMAL DYSPLASIA

Canadian Society for Ectodermal Dysplasias (Eastern Canada)
250 The East Mall
Suite 1770
Toronto, Ontario M9B 6L3
(416) 622-2874
info@edscanada.org

Canadian Society for Ectodermal Dysplasia (Western Canada)
304 Hawkwood Boulevard NW
Calgary, Alberta T3G 2Y5
(416) 664-6121

Coalition for Heritable Disorders of Connective Tissue
4301 Connecticut Avenue
Suite 404
Washington, D.C. 20008-2304
(781) 784-3817
(781) 784-6672

http://www.chdct.org
chdct@pxe.org

National Foundation for Ectodermal Dysplasias
410 E. Main
PO Box 114
Mascoutah, IL 62258-0114
(618) 566-2020
(618) 566-4718
http://www.nfed.org
info@nfed.org

EDWARD SYNDROME
See CHROMOSOME ABNORMALITIES

EHLERS DANLOS SYNDROME
Coalition for Heritable Disorders of Connective Tissue
4301 Connecticut Avenue
Suite 404
Washington, D.C. 20008-2304
(781) 784-3817
(781) 784-6672
http://www.chdct.org
chdct@pxe.org

EDS Today
PO Box 88814
Seattle, WA 98138
(253) 835-1735
(253) 835-1735
http://www.edstoday.org
info@edstoday.org

Ehlers Danlos Foundation of New Zealand
Craggy Range Road, RD 12
Havelock North, Hawkes Bay, 4230
64-6-874-7799
64-6-874-7799 (fax)
http://www.edfnz.org.nz
flopsy@ihug.co.nz

Ehlers-Danlos National Foundation
6399 Wilshire Boulevard
Suite 200
Los Angeles, CA 90048
(323) 651-3038
(323) 651-1366 (fax)

http://www.ednf.org
loosejoint@aol.com

Ehlers-Danlos Support Group
P.O. Box 337
Aldershot GU12 6WZ
01252 690940
http://www.ehlers-danlos.org/

Hypermobility & Fibromyalgia Website & Mailing List
http://anaiis.tripod.com/hmedfm/index.html
hm-ed-fm@hotmail.com

ELLIS-VAN CREVALD SYNDROME
See ECTODERMAL DYSLPASIA; SHORT STATURE

ENCEPHALY
Fighters for Encephaly Defects Support (FEDS)
3032 Brereton Street
Pittsburgh, PA 15219
(412) 687-6437

EPIDERMAL NEVUS SYNDROME
See NEVUS; ICHTHYOSIS

EPIDERMOLYSIS BULLOSA
Dystrophic Epidermolysis Bullosa Research Association
5 West 36th Street
Suite 404
New York, NY 10018
(212) 868-1573
(212) 868-9296
http://www.debra.org
jwolf@debra.org

EPIDERMOLYTIC HYPERKERATOSIS
See ARTHRITIS; ICHTHYOSIS

EPILEPSY
American Epilepsy Society
638 Prospect Avenue
Hartford, CT 06105-4240
(860) 586-7505
(860) 586-7550 (fax)
http://www.aesnet.org/

EPILEPSY CANADA
National Office
1470 Peel Street
Suite 745
Montreal, Quebec H3A 1T1
(514) 845-7855
(877) SEIZURE
(514) 845-7866
http://www.epilepsy.ca/eng/mainSet.html
epilepsy@epilepsy.ca

Epilepsy Foundation
4351 Garden City Drive
Landover, MD 20785-2267
(301) 459-3700
(301) 577-4941
http://www.epilepsyfoundation.org
postmaster@efa.org

ETHICS

Hastings Center, the
21 Malcolm Gordon Road
Garrison, NY 10524-5555
(845) 424-4040
(845) 424-4545 (fax)
http://www.thehastingscenter.org/
mail@thehastingscenter.org

Kennedy Institute of Ethics
Georgetown University
Box 571212
Washington, D.C. 20057-1212
(202) 687-3885
(800) MED-ETHX
(202) 687-6770 (fax)
medethx@gunet.georgetown.edu

EXSTROPHY

National Support Group for Exstrophy
5075 Medhurst Street
Solon, OH 44139
(216) 248-6851

F

FABRY DISEASE

Fabry Support & Information Group
PO Box 569
Concordia, MO 64020-0569

(660) 463-1355
(660) 463-1356
http://www.fabry.org
jack@fabry.org

International Center for Fabry Disease
Department of Human Genetics
Mount Sinai School of Medicine
Box 1498
Fifth Avenue at 100th Street
New York, NY 10029
(866) FABRY-MD (866-322-7963)
http://www.mssm.edu/genetics/fabry/
fabry.disease@mssm.edu

FAMILIAL DYSAUTONOMIA

Chicago Center for Jewish Genetic Disorders
One South Franklin Street
Suite 2910
Chicago, IL 60606
(312) 357-4717
(312) 855-3295 (fax)
http://www.jewishgeneticscenter.org
jewishgeneticsctr@juf.org

Dysautonomia Foundation
315 West 39th Street
Suite 701
New York, NY 10018
(212) 279-1066
http://www.familialdysautonomia.org/
info@familialdysautonomia.org

Dysautonomia Treatment and Evaluation Center
New York University Medical Center
530 First Avenue
Suite 9Q
New York, NY 10016
(212) 263-7225
(212) 263-7041 (fax)
http://www.med.nyu.edu/fd/fdcenter.html
Felicia.Axelrod@med.nyu.edu

Mount Sinai School of Medicine
One Gustave L. Levy Place, Box 1497
New York, NY 10029
(212) 659-6774 (Main)
(212) 241-6947 (Consultation/Screening)
http://www.mssm.edu/jewish_genetics/

FAMILIAL DYSTONIA

Dystonia Medical Research Foundation
One E. Wacker Drive
Suite 2430
Chicago, IL 60601-1905
(312) 755-0198
(312) 803-0138 (fax)
http://www.dystonia-foundation.org
dystonia@dystonia-foundation.org

National Dysautonomia Research Foundation
PO Box 301
Red Wing, MN 55066-0301
(651) 267-0525
(651) 267-0524 (fax)
http://www.ndrf.org

FAMILIAL POLYPOSIS/POLYCYSTIC KIDNEY DISEASE

American Kidney Fund
6110 Executive Boulevard
Suite 1010
Rockville, MD 20852
(800) 638-8299
http://www.kidneyfund.org/
webmaster@kidneyfund.org

Autosomal Recessive Polycystic Kidney
Disease Family Support Group
PO Box 70
Kirkwood, PA 17536
(717) 529-5555
(717) 529-5500
info@arpkd.org

Familial GI Cancer Registry
Mount Sinai Hospital, #1157
600 University Avenue
Toronto, Ontario M5G 1X5
(416) 596-4200
(416) 586-8555 (fax)

National Kidney Foundation
30 East 33rd Street
New York, NY 10016
(800) 622-9010
(212) 889-2210
(212) 689-9261 (fax)
http://www.kidney.org/

Polycystic Kidney Disease Foundation
4901 Main Street
Suite 200
Kansas City, MO 64112-2634
(816) 931-2600
(816) 931-8655 (fax)
http://www.pkdcure.org
pkdcure@pkdcure.org

FANCONI'S ANEMIA

Fanconi Anemia Research Fund, Inc.
1801 Willamette Street
Suite 200
Eugene, OR 97401
(541) 687-4658
(541) 687-0548 (fax)
http://www.fanconi.org
info@fanconi.org

Fanconi Canada
PO Box 38157
Toronto, Ontario M5N 3A9
(416) 489-6393
admin@fanconicanada.org

FETAL ALCOHOL SYNDROME

Bergen County Council on Alcoholism & Drug
10 East Broadway
Hackensack, NJ 07601-6820
(201) 261-2183
(201) 261-0807 (fax)
http://www.acbr.com/fas/
info@faslink.org

Family Empowerment Network
610 Langdon Street
Room 519
Madison, WI 53703
(608) 262-6590
(608) 265-3352 (fax)
gwilton@berbee.com

Fetal Alcohol Education Program (FAEP)
Boston University School of Medicine
1975 Main Street
Concord, MA 01742
(978) 369-7713
Fax: 978-287-4993 (fax)

Fetal Alcohol Support Network
2266 Homelands Drive
Mississauga, Ontario L5K 1G6
(905) 822-0733
http://www.acbr.com/fas

Fetal Alcohol Syndrome Family Resource Institute (FAS*FRI)
PO Box 2525
Lynnwood, WA 98036
(253) 531-2878
(253) 640-9155 (fax)
vicfas@hotmail.com

National Center for Education in Maternal & Child Health
Georgetown University
Box 571272
Washington, D.C. 20057-1272
(202) 784-9770
(202) 784-9777 (fax)
mchlibrary@ncemch.org

National Organization on Fetal Alcohol Syndrome
900 17th Street NW
Suite 910
Washington, D.C. 20006
(202) 785-4585
(202) 466-6456 (fax)
http://www.nofas.org
information@nofas.org

Support and Education Network for FAS
Parents and Caregivers
PO Box 626
Paramus, NJ 07653
(201) 261-2183
(201)-261-0807 (fax)

FETAL SURGERY

International Fetal Medicine and Surgery Society
3rd and Parnassus Avenue
San Francisco, CA 94143-0510
(415) 476-4086

FG SYNDROME

FG Syndrome Family Alliance, Inc.
946 NW Circle Boulevard, #290
Corvallis, OR 97330

(617) 577-9050
http://www.fg-syndrome.org/

FG Syndrome Support Group
66 Ford Road
Dagenhamk, Essex RM 10 9JR

FIBRODYSPLASIS OSSIFICANS PROGRESSIVA

International FOP Association
PO Box 196217
Winter Springs, FL 32719-6217
(407) 365-4194
http://www.ifopa.org
jlpfop@aol.com

FRAGILE X SYNDROME

FRAXA Research Foundation, Inc.
45 Pleasant Street
Newburyport, MA 01950
(978) 462-1866
(978) 463-9985 (fax)
http://www.fraxa.org
kclapp@fraxa.org

National Fragile X Foundation
PO Box 190488
San Francisco, CA 94119-0488
(925) 938-9300
(925) 938-9315 (fax)
http://www.FragileX.org
NATLFX@FragileX.org

FRIEDREICH'S ATAXIA

Friedreich's Ataxia Group in America, Inc.
POI Box 11116
Oakland, CA 94611
(415) 658-7014

Friedreich's Ataxia Research Alliance
2001 Jefferson Davis Highway, #209
Arlington, VA 22202
(703) 413-4468
(703) 413-4467 (fax)
http://http://www.frda.org
fara@frda.org

National Ataxia Foundation
2600 Fernbrook Lane
Suite 119
Minneapolis, MN 55447-4730

(763) 553-0020
(763) 553-0167 (fax)
http://www.ataxia.org
naf@ataxia.org

G

GALACTOSEMIA
American Liver Foundation
75 Maiden Lane
Suite 603
New York, NY 10038
(212) 668-1000
(973) 256-3214
http://www.liverfoundation.org
webmail@liverfoundation.org

Association for Neuro-Metabolic Disorders
PO Box 0202/L3220
1500 Medical Center Drive
Ann Arbor, MI 48109
(313) 763-4697
(313) 764-7502 (fax)

Children's Liver Alliance
3835 Richmond Avenue
Box 190
Staten Island, NY 10312
(718) 987-6200
(718) 987-6200 (fax)
http://livertx.org
livers4kids@earthlink.net

Metabolic Information Network
PO Box 670847
Dallas, TX 75367-0847
(214) 696-2188
(800) 955-3258
(214) 696-3258 (fax)
mizeg@ix.netcom.com

Parents of Galactosemic Children, Inc.
1519 Magnolia Bluff
Gautier, MS 39553
(228) 497-5886
(228) 497-5886 (fax)
http://www.galactosemia.org
president@galactosemia.org

GAUCHER DISEASE
Chicago Center for Jewish Genetic Disorders
One South Franklin Street
Suite 2910
Chicago, IL 60606
(312) 357-4717
(312) 855-3295 (fax)
http://www.jewishgeneticscenter.org
jewishgeneticsctr@juf.org

National Gaucher Foundation
5410 Edson Lane
Suite 260
Rockville, MD 20852
(301) 816-1515
(301) 816-1516 (fax)
http://www.gaucherdisease.org
ngf@gaucherdisease.org

GENETIC COUNSELING
American Society of Human Genetics
9650 Rockville Pike
Bethesda, MD 20814
(866) HUM-GENE
(301) 634-7300
http://genetics.faseb.org/genetics/ashg/ashgmenu.
    htm
society@ashg.org

Canadian Association of Genetic Counsellors
http://www.cagc-accg.ca/

**National Society of Genetic Counselors
Executive Office**
233 Canterbury Drive
Wallingford, PA 19086-6617
(610) 872-7608
http://www.nsgc.org/
FYI@nsgc.org

GENETIC DISORDERS
American Society of Human Genetics
9650 Rockville Pike
Bethesda, MD 20814
(866) HUM-GENE
(301) 634-7300
http://genetics.faseb.org/genetics/ashg/ashgmenu.
    htm
society@ashg.org

Association of Genetic Support/Australia (AGSA)
66 Albion Street
Surry Hills, New South Wales, Australia 2010
+61 2 9211 1462
+61 2 9211 8077 (fax)
agsa@ozemail.com.au

Genetic Alliance, Inc.
4301 Connecticut Avenue NW
Suite 404
Washington, D.C. 20008-2369
(202) 966-5557
(202) 966-8553 (fax)
info@geneticalliance.org

Hereditary Disease Foundation
1303 Pico Boulevard
Santa Monica, CA 90405
(310) 450-9913
(310) 450-9532 (fax)
http://www.hdfoundation.org/

National Organization for Rare Disorders
55 Kenosia Avenue
PO Box 1968
Danbury, CT 06813-1968
(203) 744-0100
(800) 999-6673 (voicemail only)
(203) 797-9590
(203) 798-2291 (fax)
http://http://www.rarediseases.org/
orphan@rarediseases.org

GLUTARIC ACIDURIA

International Organization for Glutaric Aciduria, Type I
c/o Mike Metil and Cay Welch
RD 3, Box 167A
Jersey Shore, PA 17740
(717) 321-6487

GLUTEN INDUCED ENTEROPATHY

Gluten Intolerance Group
15110 10th Avenue SW
Suite A
Seattle, WA 98166
(206) 246-6652

(206) 246-6531 (fax)
http://www.gluten.net
info@gluten.net

Canadian Celiac Association
5170 Dixie Road
Suite 204
Mississauga, Ontario L4W 1E3
(905) 507-6208
(800) 363-7296
(905) 507-4673 (fax)
info@celiac.ca
http://www.celiac.ca/englishcca.html

Celiac Sprue Association USA, Inc.
PO Box 31700
Omaha, NE 68131-0700
(402) 558-0600
(402) 558-1347 (fax)
http://www.csaceliacs.org
celiacs@csaceliacs.org

GLYCOGEN STORAGE DISEASE

Association for Glycogen Storage Disease
PO Box 896
Durant, IA 52747
(563) 785-6038
(563) 785-6038 (fax)
http://www.agsdus.org

GOLDENHAR SYNDROME

Goldenhar Syndrome Research & Information Fund
PO Box 61643
St. Petersburg, FL 33714
(813) 522-5772
gsrif@tampabay.rr.com

Goldenhar Syndrome Support Network Society
9325 163 Street
Edmonton, Alberta T5R 2P4
http://www.goldenharsyndrome.org
support@goldenharsyndrome.org

GREBE CHONDRODYSPLASIA

See SHORT STATURE

GRIEF

AMEND (Aiding Mothers and Fathers Experiencing Neonatal Death)
PO Box 20260
Wichita, KS 67208-1260
(316) 268-8441
info@amendinc.com
webmaster@amendinc.com

Center for Loss in Multiple Birth, Inc. (CLIMB)
PO Box 1064
Palmer, AK 99654
(907) 745-2706

Compassionate Friends, Inc., the
PO Box 3696
Oak Brook, IL 60522-3696
s(877) 969-0010
(630) 990-0010
(630) 990-0246 (fax)
http://www.compassionatefriends.org/

National Share Office
St. Joseph Health Center
300 First Capitol Drive
St. Charles, MO 63301-2893
(800) 821-6819
(636) 947-6164
(636) 947-7486 (fax)
http://www.nationalshareoffice.com/index.shtml
share@nationalshareoffice.com

H

HALLERMANN-STREIFF SYNDROME

National Hallermann-Streiff Support
1367 Beulah Park Drive
Lexington, KY 40517
(606) 273-6928

HANDICAP

See BIRTH DEFECTS; DISABILITIES; GENETIC DISORDERS

HEARING IMPAIRMENT

American Society for Deaf Children
PO Box 3355
Gettysburg, PA 17325

(717) 334-7922 (Business V/TTY)
(800) 942-ASDC (Parent Hotline)
(717) 334-8808 (fax)
http://www.deafchildren.org
asdc@deafchildren.com

American Speech Language Hearing Association
10801 Rockville Pike
Rockville, MD 20852
(800) 498-2071
(301) 897-5700
(800) 638-8255
(301) 571-0457 (fax)
http://www.asha.org/default.htm

Better Hearing Institute
515 King Street
Suite 420
Alexandria, VA 22314
(703) 684-3391
http://www.betterhearing.org/
mail@betterhearing.org

DELTA: Deaf Education through Listening and Talking
PO Box 20
Haverhill, Suffolk CB9 7BD
01440 783 689 (phone/fax)
http://www.deafeducation.org.uk
enquiries@deafeducation.org.uk

Hear Now
745 E. Hampden Avenue, #300
Denver, CO 80231
(303) 695-7797
(800) 648-HEAR

National Deaf Education Network & Clearinghouse
Galludet University
800 Florida Avenue NE
KDES PAS-6
Washington, D.C. 20002-3695
(202) 651-5051
(202) 651-5052
(202) 651-5044 (fax)
http://clerccenter.gallaudet.edu
clearinghouse.Infotogo@gallaudet.edu

National Fraternal Society of the Deaf
1118 South Sixth Street
Springfield, IL 62703
(217) 789-7429
(217) 789-7438
(217) 789-7489 (fax)
http://www.nfsd.com/
thefrat@nfsd.com

Research Registry for Hereditary Hearing Loss
555 N. 30th Street
Omaha, NE 68131
(800) 320-1171
(402) 498-6331 (fax)
http://www.boystownhospital.org/Hearing/info/
    genetics/syndromes/bor.asp

Self Help for Hard of Hearing People
7910 Woodmont Avenue
Suite 1200
Bethesda, MD 20814
(301) 657-2248
(301) 657-2249
(301) 913-9413 (fax)
http://www.shhh.org
national@shhh.org

Usher Family Support
4918 42nd Avenue, S
Minneapolis, MN 55417
(612) 724-6982
kadbmn@aol.com

HEMANGIOMA

Cindy Dougan
8400 Rohl Road
North East, PA 16428
(814) 898-1054
(814) 899-5962 (fax)
http://members.tripod.com/~michelle_g/indexh.
    html
cdouganhh@aol.com

HEMOCHROMATOSIS

American Hemochromatosis Society, Inc. (AHS)
Sandra Thomas, President/Founder
4044 W. Lake Mary Boulevard
Unit #104, PMB 416

Lake Mary, FL 32746-2012
(407) 829-4488
(407) 333-1284 (fax)
http://www.americanhs.org
mail@americanhs.org

Hemochromatosis Foundation, Inc.
164 Colonial Avenue
Albany, NY 12208
(518) 489-0972
(518) 489-0227 (fax)
http://www.hemochromatosis.org

Iron Disorders Institute
PO Box 2031
Greenville, SC 20602
(864) 292-1175
(864) 292-1878 (fax)
http://www.irondisorders.org
publications@irondisorders.org

Iron Overload Diseases Association, Inc.
433 Westwind Drive
N. Palm Beach, FL 33408
(561) 840-8512
(561) 840-8513
(561) 842-9881 (fax)
http://www.ironoverload.org
iod@ironoverload.org

HEMOPHILIA

Canadian Hemophilia Society
National Office
625 Avenue Président Kennedy
Suite 505
Montréal, Québec H3A 1K2
(514) 848-0503
(800) 668-2686
(514) 848-9661 (fax)
http://www.hemophilia.ca
chs@hemophilia.ca

Hemophilia Federation of America
102 B Westmark Boulevard
Lafayette, LA 70506
(337) 991-0067
(337) 991-0087 (fax)
http://www.hemophiliafed.org
j.hamilton@cox-internet.com

National Hemophilia Foundation
116 West 32nd Street
11th Floor
New York, NY 10001
(212) 328-3700
(212) 328-3777 (fax)
http://www.hemophilia.org
info@hemophilia.org

HIRSCHSPRUNG'S DISEASE

American Pseudo-obstruction and Hirschsprung's Disease Society, Inc. (APHS)
158 Pleasant Street
North Andover, MA 01845-2797
(508) 685-4477
(508) 685-4488 (fax)
aphs@mail.tiac.net

Hirschsprung's & Motility Disorders Support Network
Washington
http://www.hirschsprungs.info
lisa@hirschsprungs.info

International Foundation for Functional Gastrointestinal Disorders
PO Box 170864
Milwaukee, WI 53217
(414) 964-1799
(414) 964-7176 (fax)
http://www.iffgd.org
iffgd@iffgd.org

Pull-thru Network, Inc.
2312 Savoy Street
Hoover, AL 35226-1528
(205) 978-2930
http://www.pullthrough.org
info@pullthrough.org

HUNTINGTON DISEASE

Donald J. Allen Memorial Huntington's Disease Clinic Association
2721 Boulevard Plaza
Wichita, KS 67211
(800) 759-0135
(316) 684-3443

Foundation for the Care and Cure of Huntington Disease
82682 Overseas Highway
PO Box 1084
Islamorada, FL 33036
(305) 243-6767
http://medgen.med.miami.edu/service/clinics.
   asp#huntinton

Huntington's Disease Society of America
158 West 29th Street
7th Floor
New York, NY 10001-5300
(212) 242-1968
(212) 239-3430 (fax)
http://www.hdsa.org
hdsainfo@hdsa.org

Huntington's Disease Society of America— MA Chapter
6 Courthouse Lane
Chelmsford, MA 01824
(978) 454-8102
(867) 454-8101 (fax)
http://www.hdsa-ne.org

Huntington's Disease Society of America— Michigan Chapter
5400 Mason Street
Midland, MI 48642-3239
(989) 835-9933
(989) 835-1891
http://www.hdsa.org
RRLent@concentric.net

Huntington's Disease Society of America— Western PA Chapter
PO Box 110223
Pittsburgh, PA 15232
(412) 833-8180
(412) 624-8524 (fax)
http://www.hdsawpa.org
pegpolito@aol.com

Huntington Society of Canada (la société Huntington du Canada)
13 Water Street North
Box 1269
Cambridge, Ontario N1R 7G6

(519) 622-1002
(519) 622-7370 (fax)
http://www.hsc-ca.org
info@hsc-ca.org

HYDROCEPHALUS

**Association for Spina Bifida &
    Hydrocephalus**
ASBAH House
42 Park Road
GB PE124Q Peterborough
01 733 555988
01 733 555985 (fax)
http://www.asbah.demon.co.uk
postmaster@asbah.demon.co.uk

**Guardians of Hydrocephalus Research
    Foundation**
2618 Avenue Z
Brooklyn, NY 11235-2023
(800) 458-8655
(718) 743-4476
(718) 743-1171 (fax)

Hydrocephalus Association
870 Market Street
Suite 705
San Francisco, CA 94102
(415) 732-7040
(415) 732-7044 (fax)
http://www.hydroassoc.org
info@hydroassoc.org

Hydrocephalus Research Foundation
1670 Green Oak Circle
Lawrenceville, GA 30243
(770) 995-9570
(770) 995-8982 (fax)
ann_liakos@atlmug.org

Hydrocephalus Support Group, Inc.
PO Box 4236
Chesterfield, MO 63006-4236
(636) 532-8228
(314) 995-4108 (fax)
hydro@inlink.com

National Hydrocephalus Foundation
12313 Centralia Road
Lakewood, CA 9015-1623

HYPOCHONDROPLASIA
See SHORT STATURE

I

ICHTHYOSIS

**Foundation for Ichthyosis and Related Skin
    Types, Inc.**
650 North Cannon Avenue
Suite 17
Lansdale, PA 19446
(215) 631-1411
(215) 631-1413
http://www.scalyskin.org
info@scalyskin.org

Immune Deficiencies
Immune Deficiency Foundation
40 W. Chesapeake Avenue
Suite 308
Towson, MD 21204
(800) 296-4433
(410) 461-5292
http://www.primaryimmune.org/
idf@primaryimmune.org

Jeffrey Modell Foundation
747 Third Avenue
New York, NY 10017
(212) 819-0200
(212) 764-4180
http://www.jmfworld.com
info@jmfworld.org

INCONTINENTIA PIGMENTI

**Incontinentia Pigmenti International
    Foundation**
30 East 72nd Street
Suite 16
New York, NY 10021
(212) 452-1231
(212) 452-1406 (fax)
http://imgen.bcm.tmc.edu/ipif
ipif@ipif.org

INFANTILE AUTISM

Autism Research Institute
4182 Adams Avenue
San Diego, CA 92116

(619) 281-7165
(619) 563-6840 (fax)
http://www.autismwebsite.com/ari/index.htm

Autism Society of America
7910 Woodmont Avenue
Suite 300
Bethesda, MD 20814-3015
(301) 657-0881
(301) 657-0869 (fax)
http://www.autism-society.org
rlbeck@autism-society.org

Autism Treatment Services of Canada
404 94th Avenue, SE
Calgary, Alberta T2J 0E8
(403) 253-6961
http://www.autism.ca/
atsc@autism.ca

National Alliance for Autism Research (NAAR)
Research Park
99 Wall Street
Princeton, NJ 08540
(888) 777-NAAR
(609) 430-9163 (fax)

National Autism Hotline/Autism Services Center
605 Ninth Street
Prichard Building
PO Box 507
Huntington, WV 25710-0507
(304) 525-8014
(304) 525-8026 (fax)

INTRAUTERINE GROWTH RETARDATION
See SHORT STATURE

J

JACKSON-WEISS SYNDROME
See CRANIOFACIAL DISORDERS

JERVELL AND LANGE-NIELSEN SYNDROME
See HEARING IMPAIRMENT

JEWISH GENETIC DISEASE

Center for Jewish Genetic Diseases
Mount Sinai School of Medicine
One Gustave L. Levy Place
Box 1497
New York, NY 10029
(212) 659-6774 (Main)
(212) 241-6947 (Consultation/Screening)
http://www.mssm.edu/jewish_genetics/

Chicago Center for Jewish Genetic Disorders
One South Franklin Street
Suite 2910
Chicago, IL 60606
(312) 357-4717
(312) 855-3295 (fax)
http://www.jewishgeneticscenter.org
jewishgeneticsctr@juf.org

JOUBERT SYNDROME

Joubert Syndrome Foundation
6931 South Carlinda Avenue
Columbia, MD 21046
(410) 997-8084
(410) 992-9184 (fax)
http://www.joubertsyndrome.org
joubertduquette@comcast.net

K

KLINEFELTER SYNDROME

American Association for Klinefelter Syndrome Information & Support (AAKSIS)
c/o Roberta Rappaport
2945 W. Farwell Avenue
Chicago, IL 60645-2925
(888) 466-KSIS
http://www.aaksis.org/
ksinfo@aaksis.org

Canada Klinefelter Support Group
2867 Young Street, Apartment 3
Toronto, Ontario M4N 2J5
(416) 481-3171

Klinefelter Syndrome & Associates, Inc.
PO Box 119
Roseville, CA 95678

(916) 660-1899 (fax)
http://www.genetic.org/ks/
ks47xxy@ix.netcom.com

Klinefelter's Syndrome Association of America
N5879 30th Road
Pine River, WI 54965
(920) 987-5782

KLIPPEL-TRENAUNAY SYNDROME

Klippel-Trenaunay Support Group
5404 Dundee Road
Edina, MN 55436
(952) 925-2596
(952) 925-4708 (fax)
http://www.k-t.org
jvessey@worldnet.att.net

Klippel-Trenaunay Support Group (K-T Support Group) of Canada
c/o Denise Westlake
3265 Turner Road
Windsor, Ontario N8W 3M
(519) 966-0604
deewestlake@aol.com

KNIEST DYSPLASIA

See SHORT STATURE

KNIEST SYNDROME

Kniest Syndrome Group
4956 Queen Avenue South
Minneapolis, MN 55410
(612) 922-6184
(612) 922-8732 (fax)
sondrols@aol.com

KRABBE DISEASE

See LEUKODYSTROPHY

L

LESCH-NYHAN SYNDROME

International Lesch-Nyhan Disease Association
11402 Ferndale Street
Philadelphia, PA 19116
(215) 677-4206

Lesch-Nyhan Registry
NYU School of Medicine Dept of Psychiatry
550 First Avenue
New York, NY 10016
(212) 263-6458
lta1@is2.nyu.edu

LEUKODYSTROPHY

Fight ALD
PO Box 3318
Vista, CA 92085
(760) 212-5731
http://www.fightald.org
janis@fightald.org

MLD (Metachromatic Leukodystrophy) Foundation
21345 Miles Drive
West Linn, OR 97068
(503) 656-4808
(800) 617-8387
(503) 212-0159 (fax)
http://www.MLDfoundation.org
info@mldfoundation.org

United Leukodystrophy Foundation, Inc.
2304 Highland Drive
Sycamore, IL 60178
(815) 895-3211
(815) 895-2432 (fax)
http://www.ulf.org
paula@tbcnet.com

LISSENCEPHALY

Lissencephaly Network
c/o Debbie Bloor
1549 Regent Street
Regina, Saskatchewan S4N 1S1
(306) 569-0146

Lissencephaly Network, Inc.
c/o Dianna Fitzgerald
716 Autumn Ridge
Fort Wayne, IN 46804-6402
(219) 432-4310
(219) 749-6337 (fax)
http://www.lissencephaly.org
lissnet@lissencephaly.org or pjoliver@ghg.net

LIVER DISORDERS

American Liver Foundation
75 Maiden Lane
Suite 603
New York, NY 10038
(212) 668-1000
(973) 256-3214
http://www.liverfoundation.org
webmail@liverfoundation.org

Children's Liver Alliance
3835 Richmond Avenue
Box 190
Staten Island, NY 10312
(718) 987-6200
718.987.6200 (fax) (call first)
http://livertx.org
livers4kids@earthlink.net

Children's Liver Foundation
155 Maplewood Avenue
Maplewood, NJ 07040
(201) 761-1111

LOWE SYNDROME

Lowe Syndrome Association
222 Lincoln Street
West Lafayette, IN 47906
(765) 743-3634
http://www.lowesyndrome.org
info@lowesyndrome.org

LUPUS

Lupus Canada
590 Alden Road
Suite 211
Markham, Ontario L3R 8N2
(800) 661-1468
(905) 513-0004
(905) 513-9516 (fax)
http://www.lupuscanada.org/en/index.html
lupuscanada@bellnet.ca

Lupus Foundation of America
1300 Piccard Drive
Suite 200
Rockville, MD 20850-4303
(301) 670-9292
(301) 670-9486 (fax)

http://www.lupus.org
lupusinfo@lupus.org

S.L.E. Lupus Foundation
149 Madison Avenue
Suite 205
New York, NY 10016
(212) 685-4118
(800) 74-LUPUS
(212) 545-1843 (fax)
lupus@lupusny.org
http://www.lupusny.org/

M

MALE PATTERN BALDNESS

See ALOPECIA

MALIGNANT HYPERTHERMIA

Malignant Hyperthermia Association of Canada, the
200 Elizabeth Street
Room ES3-403
Toronto, Ontario M5G 2C4
(416) 340-3128
(416) 340-4960 (fax)
http://www.mhacanada.org
nancy.bueler@uhn.on.ca

Malignant Hyperthermia Association of the United States
PO Box 1069
11 East State Street
Sherburne, NY 13460
(607) 674-7901
(607) 674-7910 (fax)
http://www.mhaus.org
dianne@mhaus.org

North American Malignant Hyperthermia Registry of the Hyperthermia Association of the United States Department of Anesthesia
Penn State University
Hershy, PA 17033
(888) 274-7899
http://www.mhreg.org
bwb+@pitt.edu

MANIC DEPRESSION

Depression and Bipolar Support Alliance
730 N. Franklin Street
Suite 501
Chicago, IL 60610-7224
(800) 826-3632
(312) 642-7243 (fax)
http://www.dbsalliance.org
questions@dbsalliance.org

**Depression and Related Affective Disorders
  Association**
2330 West Joppa Road
Suite 100
Lutherville, MD 21093
(410) 583-2919
http://www.drada.org

National Alliance for the Mentally Ill
Colonial Place Three
2107 Wilson Boulevard
Suite 300
Arlington, VA 22201-3042
(703) 524-7600
(703) 516-7227
(703) 524-9094 (fax)
http://www.nami.org

MAPLE SYRUP URINE DISEASE

Association of Neuro-Metabolic Disorders
5223 Brookfield Lane
Sylvania, OH 43560-1809
(419) 885-1809

Families with Maple Syrup Urine Disease
24806 SR 119
Goshen, IN 46526
(219) 862-2922

MARFAN SYNDROME

Canadian Marfan Association
Centre Plaza Postal Outlet
128 Queen Street South
PO Box 42257
Mississauga, Ontario L5M 4Z0
(866) 722-1722
(905) 826-3223
(905) 826-2125 (fax)

http://www.marfan.ca
info@marfan.ca

**Coalition for Heritable Disorders of
  Connective Tissue**
4301 Connecticut Avenue
Suite 404
Washington, D.C. 20008-2304
(781) 784-3817
(781) 784-6672 (fax)
http://www.chdct.org
chdct@pxe.org

National Marfan Foundation
22 Manhasset Avenue
Port Washington, NY 11050
(516) 883-8712
(516) 883-8040 (fax)
http://www.marfan.org
staff@marfan.org

McCUNE-ALBRIGHT SYNDROME

MAGIC Foundation
6645 West North Avenue
Oak Park, IL 60302
(708) 383-0808
(708) 383-0899 (fax)
http://www.magicfoundation.org
mary@magicfoundation.org

MENKE'S DISEASE

Corporation for Menke's Disease
5720 Buckfield Court
Fort Wayne, IN 46814
(219) 436-0137

MENTAL RETARDATION

American Association on Mental Retardation
444 North Capitol Street NW
Suite #846
Washington, D.C. 20001
(202) 387-1968
(202) 387-2193 (fax)
http://www.aamr.org
dcroser@aamr.org

Arc of the United States
Professional & Family Services
1010 Wayne Avenue
Suite 650

Silver Spring, MD 20910
(301) 565-5478
(301) 565-3843 (fax)
http://thearc.org
davis@thearc.org

Mental Retardation Association of America, Inc.
211 East 300 South
Suite 212
Salt Lake City, UT 84111
(801) 328-1575

National Center for Learning Disabilities
381 Park Avenue South
Suite 1401
New York, NY 10016
888-575-7373
(212) 545-7510
(212) 545-9665 (fax)
http://www.ncld.org

Voice of the Retarded
5005 Newport Drive
Suite 108
Rolling Meadows, IL 60008
(847) 253-6020
(847) 253-6054 (fax)
http://www.vor.net
vor@compuserve.com

MESOMELIC DYSPLASIA

See SHORT STATURE

METACHROMATIC LEUKODYSTROPHY

See LEUKODYSTROPHY

METAPHYSEAL CHONDRODYSPLASIA

See SHORT STATURE

METATROPIC DYSPLASIA

See SHORT STATURE

MITOCHONDRIAL DISEASES

Association for Neurometabolic Disorders
5223 Brookfield Lane
Sylvania, OH 43560
(419) 885-1497

FOD (Fatty Oxidation Disorders) Family Support Group
1559 New Garden Road, 2E
Greensboro, NC 27410
(336) 547-8682
http://www.fodsupport.org
deb@fodsupport.org

United Mitochondrial Disease Foundation
8085 Saltsburg Road
Suite 201
Pittsburgh, PA 15239
(412) 793-8077
(412) 793-6477 (fax)
http://www.umdf.org
info@umdf.org

MOEBIUS SYNDROME

Moebius Syndrome Foundation
PO Box 147
Pilot Grove, MO 65276
(660) 834-3406
(660) 834-3407 (fax)
http://www.moebiussyndrome.com
vickimc@iland.net

Moving Forward
2934 Glenmore Avenue
Kettering, OH 45409
(937) 293-0409
movingforward@aol.com

MUCOLIPIDOSIS

Mucolipidosis IV Foundation
719 East 17th Street
Brooklyn, NY 11230
(718) 434-5067
http://www.ml4.org
www@ml4.org

MUCOPOLYSACCHARIDOSIS

Canadian Society for Mucopolysaccharide and Related Diseases Inc.
PO Box 30034
RPO Parkgate, North Vancouver, BC V7H 2Y8
(604) 924-5130
(604) 924-5131 (fax)
http://www.mpssociety.ca
kirsten@mpssociety.ca

National MPS Society
PO Box 736
Bangor, ME 04402-0736
(207) 947-1445
(207) 990-3074 (fax)
http://www.mpssociety.org
info@mpssociety.org

MULTIPLE EPIPHYSEAL DYSPLASIA

See SHORT STATURE

MULTIPLE EXOSTOSES

The MHE Coalition
8838 Holly Lane
Olmsted Falls, OH 44138-2701
(440) 235-0325
(440) 427-9032 (fax)
http://www.mhecoalition.com
chelez1@aol.com

MULTIPLE SCLEROSIS

Multiple Sclerosis Society of Canada
175 Bloor Street East
Suite 700, North Tower
Toronto, Ontario M4W 3R8
(800) 268-7582
(416) 922-6065
(416) 922-7538 (fax)
http://www.mssociety.ca
info@mssociety.ca

National Multiple Sclerosis Society
733 Third Avenue
New York, NY 10017
(212) 476-0435
(212) 986-7981 (fax)
http://www.nmss.org
sara.collins@nmss.org

**Organization for Myelin Disorders Research
    and Support**
PO Box 54759
Cincinnati, OH 45254-0759
(513) 734-6338
(513) 734-6378 (fax)
myelinrs@dot-net.net

MUSCULAR DYSTROPHY

FSH Society, Inc.
3 Westwood Road
Lexington, MA 02420
(781) 860-0501
(781) 862-8422
(781) 860-0599 (fax)
http://www.fshsociety.org/

Muscular Dystrophy Association
3300 East Sunrise Drive
Tucson, AZ 85718-3208
(520) 529-2000
(520) 529-5300 (fax)
http://www.mdausa.org
mda@mdausa.org

Muscular Dystrophy Canada
2345 Yonge Street
Suite 900
Toronto, Ontario M4P 2E5
(866) MUSCLE-8
(416) 488-7523 (fax)
http://www.muscle.ca
info@muscle.ca

Parent Project Muscular Dystrophy
158 Linwood Plaza
Ft. Lee, NJ 07024
(201) 944-9985
(201) 944-9987 (fax)
http://www.parentprojectmd.org
pat@parentprojectmd.org

**Society for Muscular Dystrophy Information
    International**
PO Box 479
Bridgewater, NS B4V 2X6
(902) 685-3961
(902) 685-3962 (fax)
http://users.auracom.com/smdi/
smdi@auracom.com

MYASTHENIA GRAVIS

Myastenia Gravis Foundation of America, Inc.
1821 University Avenue, W
Suite S256
St. Paul, MN 55104
(651) 917-6256

(651) 917-1835 (fax)
http://www.myasthenia.org
mgfa@myasthenia.org

MYOCLONUS

Moving Forward
2934 Glenmore Avenue
Kettering, OH 45409
(937) 293-0409
movingforward@aol.com

Myoclonus Families United
1564 E. 24th Street
Brooklyn, NY 11234
(718) 252-2133

N

NAGER AND MILLER SYNDROMES

Foundation for Nager and Miller Syndromes
13210 SE 342nd Street
Auburn, WA 98092-8505
(253) 333-1483
(253) 288-7679 (fax)
http://www.fnms.net
ddfnms@aol.com

NAIL-PATELLA SYNDROME

Nail Patella Syndrome Worldwide
25826 Norrington Square
South Riding, VA 20152
(703) 391-0690
(703) 391-0690 (fax)
http://www.nailpatella.com
medical@nailpatella.org

NARCOLEPSY

Narcolepsy and Cataplexy Foundation of America
445 East 68th Street
Suite 12L
New York, NY 10021
(212) 570-5506

Narcolepsy Network, Inc.
631B Ten Rod Road
North Kingstown, RI 02852
(401) 667-2523
(401) 633-6567 (fax)

http://www.narcolepsynetwork.org
narnet@narcolepsynetwork.org

NEIMANN-PICK SYNDROME

Canadian Society for Mucopolysaccharide & Related Disease Inc.
PO Box 30034
RPO Parkgate
North Vancouver, British Columbia V7H 2Y8
(800) 667-1846
(604) 924-5130
(604) 924-5131(fax)
http://www.mpssociety.ca

National Niemann-Pick Disease Foundation, Inc.
415 Madison Avenue
PO Box 49
Fort Atkinson, WI 53538-0049
(920) 563-0930
(920) 563-0931 (fax)
http://www.nnpdf.org
nnpdf@idcnet.com

National Vascular Malformations Foundation
8230 Nightingale Street
Dearborn Heights, MI 48127
(313) 274-1243
(313) 274-1393 (fax)

NEUROFIBROMATOSIS

Children's Tumor Foundation (formerly the National Neurofibromatosis Foundation), the
95 Pine Street
16th Floor
New York, NY 10005
(800) 323-7938
(212) 344-NNFF
(212) 747-0004 (fax)
http://www.ctf.org
nnff@aol.com

Neurofibromatosis, Inc.
9320 Annapolis Road
Suite 300
Lanham, MD 20706-2924
(301) 918-4600
(301) 918-0009 (fax)
http://www.nfinc.org

Neurofibromatosis Institute, Inc., the
5415 Briggs Avenue
La Crescenta, CA 91214
(818) 957-3508
(818) 957-4926 (fax)
riccardi@medconsumer.com

Neurofibromatosis Society of Ontario
180 Circle Lake Road
North Bay, Ontario P1A 3T2
(866) THE-NFSO
(705) 685-1409
info@nfon.com

NEVUS

Congenital Nevus Support Group, the
PO Box 305
West Salem, OH 44287
(419) 853-4525
http://www.nevusnetwork.org
info@nevusnetwork.org

Nevoid Basal Cell Carcinoma Syndrome Support Network
162 Clover Hill Street
Marlboro, MA 01752
(508) 485-4873
(301) 847-2012 (fax)
souldansur@aol.com

Nevus Network, the
PO Box 1981
Woodbridge, VA 22193
(703) 492-0253
http://www.nevusnetwork.org

Skin Cancer Foundation, the
245 5th Avenue
Suite 1403
New York, NY 10016
(800) SKIN-490
(212) 725-5751 (fax)
http://www.skincancer.org
info@skincancer.org

NOONAN SYNDROME

Noonan Syndrome Support Group
PO Box 145
Upperco, MD 21155
(410) 374-5245
(509) 272-2360 (fax)

http://www.noonansyndrome.org
wandar@bellatlantic.net

NORRIE DISEASE

Norrie Disease Association
Massachusetts General Hospital
149 13th Street
E # 6217
Charlestown, MA 02129
(617) 726-5718
(617) 724-9620 (fax)
sims@helix.mgh.harvard.edu

O

OCULAR DISORDERS

American Council of the Blind
1155 15th Street, NW
Suite 1004
Washington, D.C. 20005
(800) 424-8666
(202) 467-5081
(202) 467-5085 (fax)
http://www.acb.org

American Foundation for the Blind
11 Penn Plaza
Suite 300
New York, NY 10001
(800) AFB-LINE (232-5463)
(212) 502-7600
http://www.afb.org
afbinfo@afb.net

Association for Macular Diseases, Inc.
210 East 64th Street
8th Floor
New York, NY 10021
(212) 605-3719
(212) 605-3795 (fax)
http://www.macula.org
association@retinal-research.org

Carroll Center for the Blind
770 Centre Street
Newton, MA 02458
(800) 852-3131
(617) 969-6200
http://www.carroll.org

Foundation Fighting Blindness, the
11435 Cronhill Drive
Owings Mills, MD 21117-2220
(800) 683-5555
(800) 683-5551
http://www.blindness.org

Glaucoma Research Foundation
251 Post Street
Suite 600
San Francisco, CA 94108
(800) 826-6693
(415) 986-3162
http://www.glaucoma.org

Macular Degeneration Foundation, Inc.
PO Box 531313
Henderson, NV 89053
(888) 633-3937
(702) 450-3396 (fax)
http://www.eyesight.org
eyesight@eyesight.org

Macular Degeneration International
(800) 683-5555
http://www.maculardegeneration.org
mdinfo@blindness.org

National Association for Parents of Children with Visual Impairments
PO Box 317
Watertown, MA 02471
(800) 562-6265
(617) 972-7441
(617) 972-7444 (fax)
http://www.spedex.com/napvi/
napvi@perkins.org

National Association for the Visually Handicapped—New York
22 West 21st Street
6th Floor
New York, NY 10010
(212) 889-3141
(212) 255-2804
(212) 727-2931 (fax)
http://www.navh.org
navh@navh.org

National Association for the Visually Handicapped—San Francisco
3201 Balboa Street
San Francisco, CA 94121
(415) 221-3201
(415) 221-8754 (fax)
http://www.navh.org
staffca@navh.org

National Federation of the Blind
1800 Johnson Street
Baltimore, MD 21230
(410) 659-9314
(410) 685-5653 (fax)
http://www.nfb.org
nfb@nfb.org

OCULO-DENTO-DIGITAL DYSPLASIA

See ECTODERMAL DYSPLASIA

OLIVOCEREBELLAR ATROPHY

Olivocerebellar Atrophy Network Centre for Independent Living
5243 Beach Boulevard
Jacksonville, FL 32207
(904) 399-8484

OPITZ SYNDROME

Opitz G/BB Family Network
PO Box 515
Grand Lake, CO, 80447
(970) 627-8935
(970) 627-8818 (fax)
http://www.gle.egsd.k12.co.us/opitz/index.html
opitznet@mac.com

ORGANIC ACIDEMIA

Organic Acidemia Association
13210 35th Avenue North
Plymouth, MN 55441
(763) 559-1797
(763) 694-0017 (fax)
http://www.oaanews.org
oaanews@aol.com

OSLER-WEBER-RENDU SYNDROME

HHT Foundation International
PO Box 329
Monkton, MD 21111

(800) 448-6389
(410) 357-9931 (fax)
http://www.hht.org
mariannes.clancy@hht.org

OSTEOGENESIS IMPERFECTA

Canadian Osteogenesis Imperfecta Society
c/o Mary Lou Kearney
128 Thornhill Cres
Chatham, Ontario N7L 4M3
(519) 436-0025
(519) 351-4043 (fax)
kearney@kent.net

Osteogenesis Imperfecta Foundation
804 West Diamond Avenue
Suite 210
Gaithersburg, MD 20878
(301) 947-0083
(301) 947-0456 (fax)
http://www.oif.org
bonelink@oif.org

P

PALLISTER-KILLIAN SYNDROME

Pallister-Killian Family Support Group
3700 Wyndale Court
Fort Worth, TX 76109
(817) 927-8854
(817) 927-2073 (fax)

PARKINSON'S DISEASE

Parkinson's Disease Foundation, Inc.
710 West 168th Street
New York, NY 10032
(212) 923-4700
(212) 923-4778 (fax)
http://www.pdf.org
info@pdf.org or relliott@pdf.org

Parkinson Society Canada
4211 Yonge Street
Suite 316
Toronto, Ontario M2P 2A9
(800) 565-3000
(416) 227-9700
(416) 227-9600 (fax)

http://www.parkinson.ca
general.info@parkinson.ca

PATAU SYNDROME
See CHROMOSOME ABNORMALITIES

PENDRED SYNDROME
See HEARING IMPAIRMENT

PITUITARY DWARFISM
See SHORT STATURE

PKU

Association of Neuro-Metabolic Disorders
5223 Brookfield Lane
Sylvania, OH 43560-1809
(419) 885-1809

Association for Neuro-Metabolic Disorders (ANMD)
PO Box 0202/L3220
1500 Women's Medical Center Drive
Ann Arbor, MI 48109-0202
(313) 763-4697

Children's PKU Network
3790 Via De La Valle
Suite 120
Del Mar, CA 92014
(858) 509-0767
(858) 509-0768 (fax)
http://www.pkunetwork.org
pkunetwork@aol.com

National PKU News
c/o Victoria Schuett
6869 Woodlan Avenue, NE
Suite 116
Seattle, WA 98115-5469
(206) 525-8140
(206) 525-5023 (fax)
http://www.pkunews.org
schuett@pkunews.org

POLYCYCSTIC KIDNEY DISEASE
See FAMILIAL POLYPOSIS/POLYCYSTIC KIDNEY DISEASE

PORPHYRIA

American Porphyria Foundation
4900 Woodway, # 780
Houston, TX 77056
(713) 266-9617
(713) 840-9552 (fax)
http://www.porphyriafoundation.com
porphyrus@aol.com

Canadian Porphyria Foundation, Inc.
487 Walker Avenue
Box 1206
Neepawa, MB R0J 1H0
(866) 476-2801
(204) 476-2800 (tel/fax)
http://www.cpf-inc.ca
porphyria@cpf-inc.ca

Erythropoietic Protoporphyria Research and Education Fund
Channing Laboratory
181 Longwood Avenue
Boston, MA 02115
(617) 525-8249
(617) 731-1541 (fax)
http://www.brighamandwomens.org/eppref/
mmmathroth@rics.bwh.harvard.edu

PRADER-WILLI SYNDROME

Ontario Prader-Willi Syndrome Association
1920 Yonge Street, C104
Toronto, Ontario M4S 3E2
(416) 481-8657
(416) 481-6706 (fax)
opwsa@allstream.net

Prader-Willi Foundation, the
223 Main Street
Port Washington, NY 11050
(800) 253-7993
http://www.prader-willi.org

Prader-Willi Syndrome Association
5700 Midnight Pass Road
Suite 6
Sarasota, FL 34242
(800) 926-4797
http://www.pwsausa.org
national@pwsausa

PROGERIA

International Progeria Registry
c/o W.T. Brown, MD PhD
Human Genetics Institure for Research
1050 Forest Hill Road
Staten Island, NY 10314
(718) 494-5333
(718) 494-1026 (fax)
wtbibr@aol.com

PROTEUS SYNDROME

Proteus Syndrome Foundation
4915 Dry Stone Drive
Colorado Springs, CO 80918
(719) 264-8445
http://www.proteus-syndrome.org

PRUNE BELLY SYNDROME

Prune Belly Syndrome Network, Inc.
PO Box 2092
Evansville, IN 47728-0092
http://www.prunebelly.org
lbrokus@prunebelly.org

PSEUDOXANTHOMA ELASTICUM

National Association for Pseudoxanthoma Elasticum
8764 Manchester Road
Suite 200
St. Louis, MO 63144-2724
(314) 962-0100
pxenape@napxe.org

PXE International, Inc.
4301 Connecticut Avenue, NW
Suite 404
Washington, D.C. 20008-2369
(202) 362-9599
(202) 966-8553 (fax)
http://www.pxe.org
info@pxe.org

PSORIASIS

Canadian Psoriasis Foundation
100A-824 Meath Street
Ottawa, Ontario K1Z 6E8
(800) 265-0926

(613) 728-4000
(613) 728-8913 (fax)
cpf-fcp@psoriasis.ca

National Psoriasis Foundation
6600 SW 92nd Avenue
Suite 300
Portland, OR 97223
(503) 244-7404
(503) 245-0626 (fax)
http://www.psoriasis.org
getinfo@psoriasis.org

PYCNODYSOSTOSIS

See SHORT STATURE

R

RESPIRATORY DISORDERS

American Lung Association, the
61 Broadway
6th Floor
New York, NY 10006
(800) LUNGUSA
(212) 315-8700
http://www.lungusa.org

Myotubular Myopathy Resource Group
2602 Quaker Drive
Texas City, TX 77590
(409) 945-8569
http://www.mtmrg.org
info@mtmrg.org.

RESTLESS LEGS SYNDROME

Restless Legs Syndrome Foundation
1904 Banbury Road
Raleigh, NC 27608-4428.
(919) 781-4428
http://www.rls.org

Restless Legs Syndrome Foundation, Inc.
819 Second Street, SW
Rochester, MN 55902-2985
(877) INFO-RLS
(507) 287-6465
(507) 287-6312 (fax)
http://www.rls.org
rlsfoundation@rls.org

RETINITIS PIGMENTOSA

Foundation for Fighting Blindness, the
60 St. Clair Avenue, E
Suite 703
Toronto, Ontario M4T 1N5
(800) 461-3331
(416) 360-4200
(416) 360-0060 (fax)
http://www.ffb.ca
info@ffb.ca

Retinitis Pigmentosa International
PO Box 900
Woodland Hills, CA 91365
(818) 992-0500
(818) 992-3265 (fax)
info@rpinternational.org

RETT SYNDROME

International Rett Syndrome Association
9121 Piscataway Road
Clinton, MD 20735
(800) 818-RETT
(301) 856-3334
(301) 856-3336 (fax)
http://www.rettsyndrome.org
irsa@rettsyndrome.org

Ontario Rett Syndrome Association
PO Box 75014
Bolton, Ontario L7E 1H6
(519) 850-RETT
(519) 850-1272
(905) 857-3016 (fax)
http://www.rett.ca
orsa@rett.ca

ROBINOW SYNDROME

Robinow Syndrome Foundation
PO Box 1072
Anoka, MN 55303
(763) 434-1152
(763) 434-1152 (fax)
http://www.robinow.org
kmkruger@comcast.net

ROMANO-WARD SYNDROME

International Long QT Syndrome Registry
PO Box 653

University of Rochester Medical Center
Rochester, NY 14642-8653
(585) 276-0016
(585) 273-5283 (fax)

**Sudden Arrhythmia Death Syndromes
  Foundation, the**
508 E. South Temple
Suite #20
Salt Lake City, UT 84102
(800) STOP-SAD
(801) 531-0937
(801) 531-0945 (fax)
http://www.sads.org
sads@sads.org

RUBENSTEIN-TAYBI SYNDROME
RTS Canada
111 Twain Drive
Winnipeg, MB R3K 0R2
(204) 227-7879
http://www.rtscanada.org
rtscanada@mts.net

Rubinstein-Taybi Parent Group USA
PO Box 146
Smith Center, KS 66967
(785) 697-2984
(785) 697-2985 (fax)
http://www.rubinstein-taybi.org
lbaxter@ruraltel.net

RUSSELL-SILVER SYNDROME
Russell-Silver Syndrome Network
Division of MAGIC Foundation
6645 W. North Avenue
Oak Park, IL 60302
(800) 3-MAGIC-3
(708) 383-0808
(708) 383-0899 (fax)
http://www.magicfoundation.org
mary@magicfoundation.org

S

SANDHOFF DISEASE
See TAY-SACHS DISEASE

SCLERODERMA
Scleroderma Foundation
12 Kent Way
Suite 101
Byfield, MA 01922-1221
(978) 463-5843
(800) 722-HOPE (4673)
(978) 463-5809 (fax)
http://www.scleroderma.org
sfinfo@scleroderma.org

SCOLIOSIS
National Scoliosis Foundation
5 Cabot Place
Stoughton, MA 02072
(800) NSF-MYBACK (673-6922)
(781) 341-8333 (fax)
http://www.scoliosis.org
nsf@scoliosis.org

SHORT STATURE
Human Growth Foundation
997 Glen Cove Avenue, Suite 5
Glen Head, NY 11545
(800) 451-6434
(516) 671-4055 (fax)
http://www.hgfound.org
hgf1@hgfound.org

Little People of America, Inc.
320 Richey Avenue
Collingswood, NJ 08107
(267) 240-5598
http://www.lpaonline.org
info@lpaonline.org

Little People's Research Fund
616 Old Edmondson Avenue
Catonsville, MD 21228
(800) 232-4423
(708) 494-0055
(708) 494-0062
http://www.lprf.org
lprf@lprf.org

MAGIC Foundation for Children's Growth
6645 W. North Avenue
Oak Park, IL 60302-1376
(800) 3MAGIC3

(708) 383-0808
(708) 383-0899 (fax)
http://www.magicfoundation.org
mary@magicfoundation.org

Parents of Dwarfed Children
11524 Colt Terrace
Silver Spring, MD 20902
(301) 649-3275

SHARE (Source of Help in Airing and Resolving Experiences)
St. Joseph Health Center
300 1st Capitol Drive
St. Charles, MO 63301-2893
(800) 821-6819
(636) 947-6164
(636) 947-7486 (fax)
http://www.nationalshareoffice.com
share@nationalshareoffice.com

Short Stature Foundation
17200 Jamboree Road
Suite J
Irvine, CA 92714-5828
(800) 243-9273
(714) 261-9035 (fax)

SHWACHMAN SYNDROME

Shwachman-Diamond Syndrome Canada
2152 Gatley Road
Mississauga, Ontario L5H 3L9
(877) 462-8907
http://www.shwachman.org
sdscanada@sympatico.ca.

SIBLINGS

Sibling Information Network
249 Glenbrook Road
PO Box U64
Storrs, CT 06269-2064
(860) 486-4985
(860) 486-5037 (fax)

Siblings for Significant Change
United Charities Building
East 22nd Street
New York, NY 10010
(800) 841-8251

(212) 420-0776
(212) 677-0696 (fax)
gerri@ix.netcom.com

Sibling Support Project of the Arc of the United States
6512 23rd Avenue, NW, #213
Seattle, WA 98117
(206) 297-6368
(509) 752-6789 (fax)
http://www.thearc.org/siblingsupport
donmeyer@siblingsupport.org

SICKLE-CELL ANEMIA

American Sickle Cell Anemia Association
Cleveland Clinic
10300 Carnegie Avenue
Cleveland, OH 44106
(216) 229-8600
(216) 229-4500 (fax)
http://www.ascaa.org
irabragg@ascaa.org

Sickle Cell Association of Ontario, the
3199 Bathurst Street
Suite 202
Toronto, Ontario M6A 2B2
(416) 789-2855
(416) 789-1903 (fax)
http://www.sicklecellontario.com
sicklecell@look.ca

Sickle Cell Disease Association of America, Inc.
2626 South Loop West
Suite 245
Houston, TX 77054-2649
(713) 666-0300
(713) 666-0217 (fax)
http://www.sicklecell-texas.org
scatgc@sicklecell-texas.org

Sickle Cell Disease Association of America, Inc.
Eastern North Carolina Chapter
344 Center Street
PO Box 5253
Jacksonville, NC 28540
(910) 346-2510
(910) 346-2614 (fax)

Sickle Cell Foundation of Alberta, the
PO Box 55041
1704 Millwoods Road, SW
New Knottwood, Edmonton, AB T6K 3N0
(780) 450-4943
http://www.sicklecellfoundationofalberta.org
scfoa@shaw.ca

SMITH-LEMLI-OPTIZ SYNDROME

Smith-Lemli-Opitz Advocacy and Exchange
2650 Valley Forge Drive
Boothwyn, PA 19061
(610) 361-9663
http://members.aol.com/slo97/index.html
bhook@erols.com

SOTOS SYNDROME

Sotos Syndrome Support Association
3 Danada Square East
Suite 235
Wheaton, IL 60187-8484
(630) 682-8815
http://www.well.com/user/sssa
sssa@well.com

Sotos Syndrome Support Association of Canada
1944 Dumfries
Montreal, Quebec H3P 2R9
http://www.sssac.com
info@sssac.com

SPINA BIFIDA

Spina Bifida and Hydrocephalus Association of Canada
977-167 Lombard Avenue
Winnipeg, Manitoba R3B 0V3
(800) 565-9488
(204) 925-3650
(204) 925-3654 (fax)
http://www.sbhac.ca
spinab@mts.net

Spina Bifida Association of America
4590 MacArthur Boulevard NW
Suite 250
Washington, D.C. 20007
(202) 944-3285
(202) 944-3295 (fax)

http://www.sbaa.org
agriffen@sbaa.org

SPINAL MUSCULAR ATROPHY

Families of Spinal Muscular Atrophy
PO Box 196
Libertyville, IL 60048-0196
(847) 367-7620
(847) 367-7623 (fax)
http://www.fsma.org
info@fsma.org

Families of Spinal Muscular Atrophy Canada
PO Box 22024
Brandon, Manitoba R7A 6Y9
(800) 866-0016
http://www.curesma.ca
http://www.smacanada.com

Muscular Dystrophy Association
3300 East Sunrise Drive
Tucson, AZ 85718-3208
(520) 529-2000
(520) 529-5300 (fax)
http://www.mdausa.org
mda@mdausa.org

Muscular Dystrophy Canada
2345 Yonge Street
Suite 900
Toronto, Ontario M4P 2E5
(866) MUSCLE-8
(416) 488-7523 (fax)
http://www.muscle.ca
info@muscle.ca

STICKLER SYNDROME

Stickler Involved People
15 Angelina Drive
Augusta, KS 67010
(316) 775-2993
http://www.sticklers.org
sip@sticklers.org

STURGE-WEBER SYNDROME

Sturge-Weber Foundation
PO Box 418
Mt. Freedom, NJ 07970-0418
(973) 895-4445

(973) 895-4846 (fax)
swfball@aol.com

Sturge-Weber Foundation (Canada) Inc.
1960 Prairie Avenue
Port Coquitlam, British Columbia V3B 1V4
(604) 942-9209 (tel/fax)
http://www.sturge-weber.com
sturge-weber@shaw.ca

STUTTERING

See HEARING IMPAIRMENT

SUDDEN INFANT DEATH SYNDROME (SIDS)

Sudden Infant Death Syndrome Alliance, Inc.
1314 Bedford Avenue
Suite 210
Baltimore, MD 21208
(410) 653-8226
(410) 653-8709 (fax)

T

TAY-SACHS DISEASE

Canadian Association for Tay-Sachs and Allied Diseases
569 Laural Drive
Burlington, Ontario L7L 5E1
(905) 634-4101
http://www.catsad.ca
info@catsad.ca

Late Onset Tay-Sachs Foundation
PO Box 5
Flourtown, PA 19031-0005
(215) 836-9425
(215) 836-5438 (fax)
http://www.lotsf.org
mpf@bellatlantic.net

National Tay-Sachs & Allied Diseases Association, Inc.
2001 Beacon Street
Suite 204
Boston, MA 2135
(617) 277-4463
(617) 277-0134 (fax)
http://www.ntsad.org
jayne@ntsad.org

THALASSEMIA

Thalassemia Foundation of Canada
338 Falstaff Avenue
Suite 204
North York, Ontario M6L 3E7
(416) 242-THAL (8425) (tel/fax)
http://www.thalassemia.ca
info@thalassemia.ca

THOMSEN DISEASE

See MUSCULAR DYSTROPHY

THROMBOCYTOPENIA ABSENT RADIUS SYNDROME

Thrombocytopenia Absent Radius Syndrome Association
212 Sherwood Drive
Egg Harbor Turnpike, NJ 08234-7651
(609) 927-0418
(609) 653-8639 (fax)

TOURETTE SYNDROME

Tourette Syndrome Association, Inc.
42-40 Bell Boulevard
Suite 205
Bayside, NY 11361-2820
(718) 224-2999
(718) 279-9596 (fax)
http://tsa-usa.org
ts@tsa-usa.org

Tourette Syndrome Foundation of Canada
194 Jarvis Street, #206
Toronto, Ontario M5B 2B7
(800) 361-3120
(416) 861-8398
(416) 861-2472 (fax)
http://www.tourette.ca/
tsfc@tourette.ca

TREACHER COLLINS SYNDROME

Treacher Collins Foundation
PO Box 683
Norwich, VT 05055-0683
(802) 649-3050
http://www.treachercollinsfnd.org

TUBEROUS SCLEROSIS

Tuberous Sclerosis Alliance
801 Roeder Road
Suite 750
Silver Spring, MD 20910
(800) 225-6872
(301) 562-9890
(301) 562-9870 (fax)
http://www.tsalliance.org/
info@tsalliance.org

Tuberous Sclerosis Canada
45 Bolland Crescent
Ajax, Ontario L1S 3G8
(800) 347-0252 (English)
(866) 558-7278 (Francais)
http://www.tscst.org

TURNER'S SYNDROME

Turner's Syndrome Society of Canada
21 Blackthorn Avenue
Toronto, Ontario M6N 3H4
(800) 465-6744
(416) 781-2086
(416) 781-7245 (fax)
http://www.turnersyndrome.ca
tssincan@web.net

Turner Syndrome Society of the United States
14450 TC Jester
Suite 260
Houston, TX 77014
(800) 365-9944
(832) 249-9988
(832) 249-9987 (fax)
http://www.turner-syndrome-us.org/
tssus@turner-syndrome-us.org

U

UREA CYCLE DEFECTS

National Urea Cycle Disorders Foundation
4841 Hill Street
La Canada, CA 91011
(800) 38NUCDF
(818) 952-2184
http://www.nucdf.org
info@nucdf.org

V

VATER ASSOCIATION

TEF VATER International Support Network
15301 Grey Fox Road
Upper Marlboro, MD 20772
(301) 952-6837
(301) 952-6837 (fax)
http://www.tefvater.org

VITILIGO

National Vitiligo Foundation
700 Olympic Plaza Circle
Suite 404
Tyler, TX 75701
(903) 595-3713
(903) 593-1545 (fax)
http://www.nvfi.org
info@nvfi.org

W

WERNER SYNDROME

See PROGERIA

WHISTLING FACE SYNDROME

Freeman-Sheldon Parent Support Group
509 Northmont Way
Salt Lake City, UT 84103
(801) 364-7060
http://www.fspsg.org
fspsg@mail.burgoyne.com

WILLIAMS SYNDROME

Canadian Association for Williams Syndrome
http://www.caws-can.org

Williams Syndrome Association
570 Kirts Boulevard
Suite 223
Troy, MI 48084-4156
(248) 541-3630
(248) 541-3631 (fax)
http://www.williams-syndrome.org
wsaoffice@aol.com

WILSON'S DISEASE

National Center for the Study of Wilson's Disease
432 West 58th Street
Suite 614
New York, NY 10019
(212) 523-8717
(212) 523-8708 (fax)

Wilson's Disease Association International
1802 Brookside Drive
Wooster, OH 44691
(330) 264-1450
(800) 399-0266
(509) 757-6418 (fax)
http://www.wilsonsdisease.org
info@wilsonsdisease.org

X

XENODERMA PIGMENTOSUM

XP Society
437 Snydertown Road
Craryville, NY 12521
(518) 851-2612
(877) XPS-CURE
http://www.xps.org
xps@xps.org

BIBLIOGRAPHY

Anderson, V. E., W. A. Hauser, J. K. Penny et al. (eds.), *Genetic Basis of the Epilepsies*. New York: Raven Press, 1982.

Atonarakis, S. E., P. G. Waber, S. D. Kittur et al., "Hemophilia A. Detection of Molecular Defects and Carriers by DNA Analysis," *N Engl J Med*, 313(1985): 842.

Applebaum, Eleanor G., and Stephen K. Firestein, *A Genetic Counseling Casebook*. New York: The Free Press (Macmillan, Inc.), 1983.

Arrighi, F. E., E. Stubblefield and P. N. Rao (eds.), *Genes, Chromosomes and Neoplasia*. New York: Raven Press, 1981.

Bailey, J., *Genetics and Evolution, the Molecules of Inheritance*. New York: Oxford University Press, 1995.

Baird, Patricia A., "Genetic Disorders in Children and Young Adults: A Population Study," *American Journal of Human Genetics*, 42(1988): 677–693.

Bank, A., J. G. Mears and F. Ramirez, "Disorders of Human Hemoglobin," *Science*, 207(1980): 486.

Baraitser, M., *Genetics of Neurological Disorders*. New York: Oxford University Press, 1982.

Beighton, Peter, *Inherited Disorders of the Skeleton*, 2nd ed. New York: Churchill Livingstone Publishers, 1988.

———, *The Man Behind the Syndrome*. New York: Springer-Verlag, 1986.

Bergsma, Daniel, *Birth Defects Compendium*, 2nd edition. New York: Alan Liss, 1979.

Blasi, F. (ed.), *Human Genes and Diseases*. New York: J. Wiley, 1986.

Blau, Sheldon, and Dodi Schultz, *The Body Against Itself*. Garden City, N.Y.: Doubleday; 1977.

Blumberg, B., M. Golbus and K. Hanson, "The Psychological Sequelae of Abortion Performed For a Genetic Indication," *Am J Obstet Gynecol*, 122(1975): 799.

Boehm, C. D., S. E. Antonarakis, J. A. Phillips III et al., "Prenatal Diagnosis Using DNA Polymorphisms," *N Engl J Med*, 308(1983): 1054.

Bolsover, S., J. Hyams, S. Jones, E. Shephard, H. White, *From Genes to Cells*. New York: Wiley-Liss, 1997.

Borgaonkar, D. S., *Chromosomal Variation in Man. A Catalog of Chromosomal Variants and Anomalies*. New York: Alan Liss, 1983.

Brock, D. J. H., D. Bedgood, L. Barron et al., "Prospective Prenatal Diagnosis of Cystic Fibrosis," *The Lancet*, 18439 (1985): 1,175.

Carter, C. H. (ed.), *Medical Aspects of Mental Retardation*. Springfield: Charles C. Thomas, 1978.

Cavenee, W. K., A. L. Murphree, M. M. Shull et al., "Prediction of Familial Predisposition to Retinoblastoma," *N Engl J Med*, 314(1986): 1,201.

Children's Defense Fund, *The State of America's Children, Yearbook 1998*. Washington, D.C.: CDF, 1998.

Cohen, Felissa L., *Clinical Genetics in Nursing Practice*. Philadelphia: J. B. Lippincott, 1984.

Conneally, P. M., "Huntington's Disease: Genetics and Epidemiology," *Am J. Hum Genet*, 36(1984): 506.

Conner, M., M. Ferguson-Smith, *Essential Medical Genetics*. Oxford: Blackwell Science, 5th ed., 1997.

Cotlier, E., I. H. Maumenee and E. R. Berman (eds.), *Genetic Eye Disorders: Retinitis Pigmentosa and other Inherited Eye Disorders*. (Birth Defects Original Article Series, vol. 18, no. 6) New York: Alan R. Liss, 1982.

Dalessio, D. J., "Seizure Disorders and Pregnancy," *N Engl J Med*, 3/3(1985): 559.

de Grouchy, J. and C. Turleau, *Clinical Atlas of Human Chromosomes*. New York: John Wiley, 1977.

Der Kaloustian, V. M., and A. K. Kurban, *Genetic Diseases of the Skin*. New York: Springer-Verlag, 1979.

Desnick, R. J., and G. A. Grabowski, "Advances in the Treatment of Inherited Metabolic Diseases," in *Advances in Human Genetics*, vol. 11. New York: Plenum Press, 1981.

Eisenberg, Eileen, and Heidi Eisenberg Murkoff, *What to Expect When You're Expecting*. New York: Workman, 1984.

Emery, A. E. H., and D. L. Rimoin (eds.), *Principles and Practice of Medical Genetics*. New York: Churchill Livingstone, 1983.

Eriksson, A. W., H. Forsius, H. R. Nevanlinna, P. L. Workman and P. K. Norio, *Population Structure and Genetic Disorders*. London: Academic Press, 1980.

Federman, D. D., *Abnormal Sexual Development: A Genetic and Endocrine Approach to Differential Diagnosis*. Philadelphia: W. B. Saunders, 1967.

Feigin, R., and J. Cherry, *Textbook of Pediatric Infectious Diseases*. Philadelphia: W. B. Saunders, 1981.

Finnie, Nanci R., I.C.S.P., *Handling the Young Cerebral Palsied Child at Home*. New York: E. P. Dutton, 1975.

Freiherr, G., "Fetal Surgery: Saving the Unborn," *Research Resources Reporter*, 7(1983): 1.

Friedman, T. F., *Gene Therapy: Fact and Fiction in Biology's New Approaches to Disease.* New York: Cold Spring Harbor, 1983.

Fudenberg, H. H., J. R. L. Pink, A. C. Wang and S. D. Douglas, *Basic Immunogenetics,* 2nd ed. New York: Oxford University Press, 1978.

Galjaard, J., *Genetic Metabolic Disease, Early Diagnosis and Prenatal Analysis.* Amsterdam: Elsevier/North Holland, 1980.

Gardner, K. D., Jr. (ed.), *Cystic Diseases of the Kidney.* New York: John Wiley, 1976.

Garver, Kenneth L., *Genetic Counseling for Clinicians.* Chicago: Year Book Medical Publishers, 1986.

Genetics and Heredity: The Blueprints of Life. New York: Torstar Books, 1985.

German, J. (ed.), *Chromosomes and Cancer.* New York: John Wiley, 1974.

Glasser, Ronald J., *The Body Is the Hero.* New York: Random House, 1976.

Goldberg, M. F. (ed.), *Genetic and Metabolic Eye Diseases.* Boston: Little, Brown, 1974.

Golbus, M. S., "Antenatal Diagnosis of Hemoglobinopathies, Hemophilia and Hemolytic Anemias," *Clin Obstet Gynecol,* 24(1981): 1,055.

Golbus, M. S. and B. D. Hall (eds.), *Diagnostic Approaches to the Malformed Fetus, Abortus, Stillborn and Deceased Newborn.* New York: Alan R. Liss, 1979.

Gomez, M. R. (ed.), *Tuberous Sclerosis.* New York: Raven Press, 1988.

Goodman, Richard M., *Genetic Disorders Among the Jewish People.* Baltimore: Johns Hopkins University Press, 1979.

————, *Planning for a Healthy Baby.* New York: Oxford University Press, 1986.

Goodman, Richard M., and R. J. Gorlin, *Atlas of the Face in Genetic Disorders,* 2nd ed. St. Louis: C.V. Mosby, 1977.

————, *The Malformed Infant and Child.* New York: Oxford University Press, 1983.

Goodman, Richard M., and A. G. Motulsky, *Genetic Diseases Among Ashkenazi Jews.* New York: Raven Press, 1979.

Gorlin, R. J., J. J. Pindborg and M. M. Cohen, *Syndromes of the Head and Neck,* 2nd ed. New York: McGraw-Hill, 1976.

Gottron, H. A., and V. W. Schnyder, *Verebung von Hautkrankheiten,* vol. 7 of "Jadassohn Handbuch." Berlin: Springer-Verlag, 1955.

Graham, John M., *Smith's Recognizable Patterns of Human Deformation,* 2nd ed. Philadelphia: W. B. Saunders, 1988.

Grouse, L. D., "Recognition of Fetal Alcohol Syndrome," *JAMA,* 245(1981): 2,436.

Hagerman, R. J., and P. M. McBogg (eds.), *The Fragile X Syndrome.* Dillon, Colorado: Spectra Publishing, 1983.

Harper, P. S., *Practical Genetic Counseling,* 3rd ed. Boston: Wright, 1988.

Harris, H., *The Principles of Human Biochemical Genetics,* 3rd ed. Amsterdam: Elsevier/North-Holland Biomedical Press, 1980.

Hendin, D., and J. Marks, *The Genetics Connection.* New York: Morrow, 1978.

Hobbins, J. C., P. A. Grannum, R. L. Berkowitz et al., "Ultrasound in the Diagnosis of Congenital Anomalies," *Am J. Obstet Gynecol,* 134(1979): 331.

Holbrook, K. (ed.), "Prenatal Diagnosis of Genetic Skin Disease," *Seminars in Dermatology* 3:3(1984).

Holleb, Arthur I. (ed.), *The American Cancer Society Cancer Book.* New York: Doubleday, 1986.

Holm, V. A., and P. L. Pipes, *Prader-Willi Syndrome.* Baltimore: University Park Press, 1981.

Holmes, L. B., H. W. Moser, C. S. Halldorsson, C. Mack, S. S. Paint and B. Matzilevich, *Mental Retardation: An Atlas of Diseases with Associated Physical Abnormalities.* New York: Macmillan, 1972.

Hook, E. B., and P. K. Cross, *Clinical Genetics: Problems in Diagnosis and Counseling.* New York: Academic Press, 1982.

Horrobin, J. M., and J. E. Rynders, *To Give an Edge: A Guide for New Parents of Down's Syndrome (Mongoloid) Children.* Minneapolis: Colwell Press, 1974.

International Commission for Protection Against Environmental Mutagens and Carcinogens, *Perspectives in Mutation Epidemiology,* 6. New York: Elsevier, 1983.

Ionasescu, V., and H. Zellweger, *Genetics of Neurology.* New York: Raven Press, 1983.

Jackson, L. G., and R. N. Schimke (eds.), *Clinical Genetics, A Source Book for Physicians.* New York: John Wiley, 1979.

Jones, Kenneth Lyons, *Smith's Recognizable Patterns of Human Malformation,* 4th ed. Philadelphia: W. B. Saunders, 1988.

Jones, Peter, M.D., *Living With Hemophilia.* Philadelphia: F. A. Davis, 1974, 1984.

Jorgenson, Yoder and Shapiro, *The Pedigree: A Basic Guide.* Grendel Co., 1980.

Kalter, H., and J. Warkany, "Congenital Malformations, Etiologic Factors and Their Role in Prevention," *N Eng J Med,* 308(1983): 425.

Kelly, T. E., *Clinical Genetics and Genetic Counseling,* 2nd ed. Chicago: Year Book Medical Publishers, 1986.

Kessler, S. (ed.), *Genetic Counseling-Psychological Dimensions.* New York: Academic Press, 1979.

Kevles, Daniel J., *In the Name of Eugenics: Genetics and the Uses of Human Heredity.* New York: Knopf, 1985.

King, R., W. Stansfield, *A Dictionary of Genetics,* New York: Oxford University Press, 5th ed., 1997.

Kirkwood, Evelyn, and Catriona Lewis, *Understanding Medical Immunology.* New York: John Wiley, 1983.

Kolata, G., "Huntington's Disease Gene Located," *Science,* 222(1983): 913.

Knudson, A. G., "Hereditary Cancer, Oncogenes, and Antioncogens," *Cancer Res.* 45(1985): 1,437.

Konigsmark, B. W. and R. J. Gorlin, *Genetic and Metabolic Deafness.* Philadelphia: W. B. Saunders, 1976.

Lammer, E. J., D. T. Chen, R. M. Hoar et al., "Retinoic Acid Embryopathy," *N Engl J Med,* 3/3(1985): 837.

Levitan, Max, *Textbook of Human Genetics.* New York: Oxford University Press, 1977.

Lewontin, Richard C., *Human Diversity.* New York: Scientific American Library, (distributed by) W.H. Freeman, 1982.

Lubs, H. A., and F. De La Cruz (eds.), *Genetic Counseling.* New York: Raven Press, 1977.

Lynch, H. T. (ed.), *Cancer Genetics.* Springfield: C. C. Thomas, 1976.

Lynch, H. T., W. A. Albano, B. S. Danes et al., "Genetic Predisposition to Breast Cancer," *Cancer,* 53(1984): 612.

Macri, J. N., D. A. Baker and R. S. Baim, "Diagnosis of Neural-Tube Defects by Evaluation of Amniotic Fluid," *Clin Obstet Gynecol,* 24(1981): 1089.

Mange, Arthur, and Elaine Mange, *Genetics: Human Aspects.* Philadelphia: W. B. Saunders, 1980.

Marimuthu, K. M., and P. M. Gopinath (eds.), *Conference Recent Trends in Medical Genetics* (held in Madras, India, in 1983). New York: Pergamon, 1986.

Maroteaux, P., *Bone Diseases of Children.* Philadelphia: Lippincott, 1979.

McKusick, V.A., *Heritable Disorders of Connective Tissue,* 8th ed. St. Louis: C.V. Mosby, 1988.

———, *Mendelian Inheritance in Man,* new ed. Baltimore: Johns Hopkins University Press, 1986.

Miles, J. H., and M. M. Kaback, "Prenatal Diagnosis of Hereditary Disorders," *Pediatr Clin No Am,* 25(1978): 593.

Milunsky, A. (ed.), *Genetic Disorders and the Fetus: Diagnosis, Prevention, and Treatment.* New York: Plenum Press, 1986.

———, *Know Your Genes.* Boston: Houghton-Mifflin, 1977.

Milunsky, A., and G. J. Annas (eds.), *Genetics and The Law.* New York: Plenum, 1976.

Mulvihill, J. J., R. W. Miller and J. F. Fraumeni (eds.), *Genetics of Human Cancer.* New York: Raven Press, 1977.

Murphy, E. A., and G. Chase, *Principles of Genetic Counseling.* Baltimore: Johns Hopkins University Press, 1975.

National Center for Education in Maternal and Child Health, *State Treatment Centers for Metabolic Disorders.* Washington, D.C.: NCEMCH, 1986.

———, *Social and Psychological Aspects of Genetic Disorders: A Selected Bibliography.* Washington, D.C.: NCEMCH, 1986.

———, *Starting Early: A Guide to Federal Resources in Maternal and Child Health.* Washington, D.C.: NCEMCH, 1988.

National Center for Health Statistics, *Advance Report of Final Mortality Statistics.* Hyattsville, Maryland: NCHS, 1988.

———, *Advance Report of Final Natality Statistics.* Hyattsville, Maryland: NCHS, n.d.

National Clearinghouse for Human Genetic Diseases, *Prenatal Diagnosis and Genetic Counseling.* Washington, D.C.: NCHGD, n.d.

National Institute of Child Care and Human Development, *Diagnostic Ultrasound Imaging in Pregnancy.* Washington, D.C.: NICCHD, 1984.

———, *Mental Retardation and Developmental Disabilities.* Washington, D.C.: NICCHD, 1986.

National Institute of General Medical Sciences, *The New Human Genetics: How Gene Splicing Helps Researchers Fight Inherited Disease.* Washington, D.C.: NIGMS, 1984.

National Organization for Albinism and Hypopigmentation, *What Is Albinism?* Philadelphia: NOAH, n.d.

National Research Council, *Health Risks of Radon and Other Internally Deposited Alpha-Emitters.* Washington, D.C.: NRC, 1988.

Newmark, M. E., and J. K. Penny, *Genetics of Epilepsy: A Review.* New York: Raven Press, 1980.

Newmark, P., "Testing for Cystic Fibrosis," *Nature,* 318(1985): 309.

Nichols, Eve K., *Human Gene Therapy.* Cambridge: Harvard University Press, 1988.

Nora, James J., and F. Clarke Fraser, *Medical Genetics: Principles and Practice,* 3rd ed. Philadelphia: Lea & Febiger, 1989.

Nyhan, William L., *The Heredity Factor: Genes, Chromosomes, and You.* New York: Lea & Febiger, 1989.

O'Brien, R., and M. Chafetz, *The Encyclopedia of Alcoholism.* New York: Facts On File, 1982.

Paluszny, Maria J., *Autism: A Practical Guide for Parents and Professionals.* Syracuse: Syracuse University Press, 1979.

Porter, I. H., N. H. Hatcher and A. M. Willey (eds.), *Prenatal Genetics: Diagnosis and Treatment* (15th New York State Health Department Birth Defects Symposium, Albany, 1984). Orlando: Academic Press, 1986.

Porter, I. H., and E. B. Hook (eds.), *Human Embryonic and Fetal Death.* New York: Academic Press, 1980.

Powledge, T. M., and J. Fletcher, "Ethics of Prenatal Diagnosis," *N Engl J Med* 300(1979): 168.

President's Commission for the Study of Ethical Problems in Medicine and Behavioral Research, *Screening and Counseling for Genetic Conditions.* Washington, D.C.: U.S. Government Printing Office, 1983.

Pueschel, S. M., *Down Syndrome: Growing and Learning.* Mission, Kansas: Andrews and McNeel, 1978.

Rao, D. C., R. C. Elston, L. H. Fuller et al. (eds.), *Genetic Epidemiology of Coronary Heart Disease: Past, Present, and Future.* New York: Alan R. Liss. 1984.

Reed, S., *Counseling in Medical Genetics.* New York: Alan R. Liss, 1980.

Riccardi, Vincent M., *The Genetic Approach to Human Disease.* New York: Oxford University Press, 1977.

Rimoin, D. L., and R. N. Schimke, *Genetic Disorders of the Endocrine Glands.* St. Louis: C.V. Mosby, 1971.

Rose, N. R., P. E. Bigazzi and N. C. Warner (eds.), *Genetic Control of Autoimmune Disease.* Amsterdam: Elsevier/North Holland, 1978.

Rotter, J. I., "The Modes of Inheritance of Insulin Dependent Diabetes," *Am J Hum Genet,* 34(1981): 835.

Rowley, P. T., "Genetic Screening: Marvel or menace?" *Science,* 225(1984): 138.

Rutter, Michael, and Eric Schopler, *Autism: A Practical Guide For Parents and Professionals.* New York: Plenum, 1976.

Schulman, J. D., and J. L. Simpson (eds.), *Genetic Diseases in Pregnancy: Maternal Effects and Fetal Outcome.* New York: Academic Press, 1981.

Schimke, R. N., *Genetics and Cancer in Man.* Edinburgh: Churchill Livingston, 1978.

Scriver, Charles R., Arthur L. Beaudet, William S. Sly and David Valle (eds.), *The Metabolic Basis of Inherited Disease.* New York: McGraw-Hill, 1989.

——— and L. E. Rosenberg, *Amino Acid Metabolism and Its Disorders.* Philadelphia: W. B. Saunders, 1973.

Shepard, T. H., *Catalog of Teratogenic Agents,* 5th ed. Baltimore: Johns Hopkins University Press, 1986.

Sherlock, P., and S. J. Winawer, "Are There Markers for the Risk of Colorectal Cancer?" *N Engl J Med,* 311(1984): 118.

Simoni, G., B. Brambati, C. Danesino et al., "Efficient Direct Chromosome Analyses and Enzyme Determinations From Chorionic Villi Samples in the First Trimester of Pregnancy," *Am J Hum Genet,* 63(1983): 349.

Simpson, J. L., *Disorders of Sexual Differentiation: Etiology and Clinical Delineation.* New York: Academic Press, 1976.

Smithells, R. W., N. C. Nevin, M. J. Seller et al., "Further Experience of Vitamin Supplementation For the Prevention of Neural-Tube Defect Recurrences," *Lancet,* 8332(1983): 1,027.

Sorsby, A., *Ophthalmic Genetics.* London: Butterworth, 1970.

Spranger, J. W., L. O. Langer Jr. and J. R. Wiedemann, *Bone Dysplasias: An Atlas of Constitutional Disorders of Skeletal Development.* Stuttgart: Gustav Fischer Verlag, 1974.

Stagnos, S., and R. J. Whitley, "Herpesvirus Infections in Pregnancy," *N Engl J Med,* 313(1985): 1270, 1327.

Stanbury, J. B., J. B. Wyngaarden, D. S. Fredrickson, J. L. Goldstein and M.S. Brown, *The Metabolic Basis of Inherited Disease,* 5th ed. New York: McGraw-Hill, 1983.

Stehm, R., and V. Fulginiti, *Immunologic Disorders in Infants and Children,* 2nd ed. Philadelphia: W. B. Saunders, 1980.

Stewart, R. R. and G. H. Prescott (eds.), *Oral Facial Genetics.* St. Louis, Mo.: C. V. Mosby, 1976.

Strachan, T., A. Read, *Human Molecular Genetics.* Oxford: Bios Scientific Publishers, 1996.

Summit, R. L., *Clinical Genetics, A Source Book for Physicians.* New York: John Wiley, 1980.

Taft, L. T., "Mental Retardation Overview," *Pediatr Ann,* 2(1973): 10.

Temtamy, S. A., and V.A. McKusick, *The Genetics of Hand Malformations.* New York: Alan R. Liss, 1978.

Thoene, J., ed., *Physicians' Guide to Rare Diseases.* Montvale, NJ: Dowden Publishing, 2nd ed., 1995.

Thompson, Charlotte E., *Raising a Handicapped Child.* New York: Ballantine, n.d.

Thompson, J. S., and M. W. Thompson, *Genetics in Medicine,* 4th ed. Philadelphia: W. B. Saunders, 1986.

Thompson, Jr., J. N., J. Hellack, G. Braver, D. Durica, *Primer of Genetic Analysis.* Cambridge: Cambridge University Press, 2nd ed., 1997.

Tsuang, M. X. T., and R. Vandermey, *Genes and the Mind; Inheritance of Mental Illness.* New York: Oxford University Press, 1980.

United Nations Scientific Committee on the Effects of Atomic Radiation, *1982 Report to the General Assembly: Ionizing Radiation: Sources and Biological Effects.* New York: United Nations, 1982.

U.S. Department of Health and Human Services, *Congenital Malformations Surveillance.* Atlanta: Centers for Disease Control, 1988.

———, *Leading Major Congenital Malformations Among Minority Groups in the United States, 1981–1986,* Morbidity and Mortality Weekly Report. Atlanta: Centers for Disease Control, 1988.

———, *Premature Mortality Due to Congenital Anomalies— United States,* Morbidity and Mortality Weekly Report. Atlanta: Centers for Disease Control, 1988.

U.S. Department of Health, Education and Welfare, *Antenatal Diagnosis,* NIH Publication No. 79. Washington, D.C.: HEW, 1973, 1979.

Vinken, P. J., and G. W. Bruyn (eds.), *Handbook of Clinical Neurology.* Amsterdam: Elsevier/North Holland, 1970 (vol. 10), 1972 (vols. 13, 14), 1982 (vol. 43).

Vogel, F., and A. G. Motulsky, *Human Genetics: Problems and Approaches,* 2nd ed. Berlin: Springer-Verlag, 1986.

Waardenberg, P. J., A. Franceschetti and D. Klein, *Genetics and Ophthalmology.* Springfield, Ill.: C.C. Thomas, 1961 (vol. 1), 1963 (vol. 2).

Warkany, J., *Congenital Malformations.* Chicago: Year Book Medical Publishers, 1971.

Warkany, J., R. J. Lemire and M. M. Cohen, *Mental Retardation and Congenital Malformations of the Central Nervous System.* Chicago: Year Book Publishers, 1981.

Weaver, David D., *Catalog of Prenatally Diagnosed Conditions.* Baltimore: Johns Hopkins University Press, 1989.

Whaley, Lucille, *Understanding Inherited Disorders.* St. Louis, Mo.: C. B. Mosby, 1974.

Wilson, J. G., and F. C. Fraser (eds.), *Handbook of Teratology,* vols. 1–4, New York: Plenum, 1977.

Wright, E. E., and M. V. Shaw, "Legal Liability in Genetic Screening, Genetic Counseling and Prenatal Diagnosis," *Clinical Obstetrics & Gynecology* (1981).

Wyngaarden, W. B., and L. H. Smith (eds.), *Cecil Textbook of Medicine,* 16th ed. Philadelphia: W. B. Saunders, 1982.

Wynne-Davies, R., *Heritable Disorders in Orthopaedic Practice.* Oxford: Blackwell, 1973.

Yunis, J. J. (ed.), *New Chromosomal Syndromes.* New York: Academic Press, 1979.

INDEX

BIOGRAPHIC SKETCHES

Author and journalist James Wynbrandt has written books on subjects including medical science, history, business, popular music and humor. His articles have appeared in *The New York Times, Management Review, Smithsonian Air & Space, Forbes* and *Aspen magazine* and his reporting and feature writing have been honored by organizations including the Fiscal Policy Council, the International Reading Association and the National Society of Professional Engineers. He lives in New York City.

Mark D. Ludman, M.D., F.R.C.P.C., F.C.C.M.G., is a clinical geneticist with a particular interest in the genetics of cancer and in inherited metabolic diseases. He is presently a Professor and Head of the Division of Medical Genetics in the Department of Pediatrics, as well as a Professor in the Department of Medicine, in the Faculty of Medicine of Dalhousie University in Halifax, Nova Scotia. He is also the Physician Leader of the Maritime Medical Genetics Service, based at the IWK Health Centre there. He is certified as a specialist in both pediatrics and medical genetics in Canada, the United States and Israel.